Strategic Practice Management

Business Considerations for Audiologists and Other Healthcare Professionals

Fourth Edition

Strategic Practice Management

Business Considerations for Audiologists
and Other Healthcare Professionals

Fourth Edition

Robert M. Traynor, EdD, MBA, FNAP
Brian Taylor, AuD

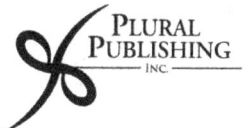

PLURAL
PUBLISHING
INC.

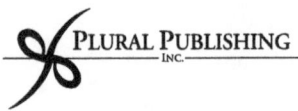

9177 Aero Drive, Suite B
San Diego, CA 92123

email: information@pluralpublishing.com
website: https://www.pluralpublishing.com

Typeset in 10.29/13 ITC Garamond Std by Achorn International
Printed in the United States of America by Integrated Books International

NOTICE TO THE READER
Care has been taken to confirm the accuracy of the indications, procedures, drug dosages, and diagnosis and remediation protocols presented in this book and to ensure that they conform to the practices of the general medical and health services communities. However, the authors, editors, and publisher are not responsible for errors or omissions or for any consequences from application of the information in this book and make no warranty, expressed or implied, with respect to the currency, completeness, or accuracy of the contents of the publication. The diagnostic and remediation protocols and the medications described do not necessarily have specific approval by the Food and Drug Administration for use in the disorders and/or diseases and dosages for which they are recommended. Application of this information in a particular situation remains the professional responsibility of the practitioner. Because standards of practice and usage change, it is the responsibility of the practitioner to keep abreast of revised recommendations, dosages, and procedures.

Library of Congress Cataloging-in-Publication Data

Names: Traynor, Robert M., author. | Taylor, Brian, 1966- author. | Glaser, Robert (Robert G.). Strategic practice management.
Title: Strategic practice management: business considerations for audiologists and other healthcare professionals / Robert M. Traynor, Brian Taylor.
Description: Fourth edition. | San Diego, CA: Plural, [2026] | Preceded by Strategic practice management / Robert G. Glaser, Robert M. Traynor. Third edition. [2019]. | Includes bibliographical references and index.
Identifiers: LCCN 2024040101 (print) | LCCN 2024040102 (ebook) | ISBN 9781635507669 (hardcover) | ISBN 1635507669 (hardcover) | ISBN 9781635504934 (ebook)
Subjects: MESH: Practice Management, Medical—organization & administration | Audiology—organization & administration
Classification: LCC RF291 (print) | LCC RF291 (ebook) | NLM WV 21 | DDC 617.80068—dc23/eng/20240924
LC record available at https://lccn.loc.gov/2024040101
LC ebook record available at https://lccn.loc.gov/2024040102

Contents

A Conversational Foreword

Mueller: First, we'd like to express our appreciation to Drs. Traynor and Taylor for inviting us to be a part of this great effort. We are indeed honored. As seasoned authors and editors ourselves, we fully understand that compiling a textbook of this magnitude is no easy task. Congratulations to you and your contributors for this outstanding fourth edition.

Northern: The contributions of your first three editions to the management of private practices cannot be overstated. Congratulations on this new fourth edition as we are sure it will continue to provide substantive information for those audiologists faced with private practice and clinical management issues.

Mueller: I have to say, I usually skip forewords, and this is my first stab at writing one, but I do remember reading a couple that stood out. One was for Michael Pollack's 1975 *Amplification for the Hearing Impaired,* where Raymond Carhart wrote a 17-page foreword, packed with many pearls that are still relevant today. Another that I recall was by J. D. Harris, again from the 1970s. He cautioned about problems related to the clinical selection of the "best" hearing aid, resulting in some audiologists just throwing up their hands. He summed it up by saying: "If you think that repeated speech testing is a reliable method, you should not only throw up your hands, but also your lunch!"

Northern: We won't even attempt to compete with those two icons. What does make this foreword a little unique for both of us is that a book like this wouldn't even have been written when you and I were getting started in audiology. While there is something here for most everyone practicing audiology, much is geared toward audiologists in private practice and clinical managers. In many cases, private practice in audiology is linked to hearing aid sales.

Mueller: For you younger readers, understand that in the "old days," the Academy of Audiology didn't exist, and neither did state licensure. Hence, the only game in town was to join the American Speech and Hearing Association (ASHA) and obtain the Certificate of Clinical Competence (CCC-A). If an audiologist "sold" a hearing aid in those days, it was considered unethical behavior by the ASHA and resulted in membership expulsion and loss of professional certification. Kenneth O. Johnson, Executive Director of the ASHA, believed that audiology, as a profession, should not profit financially from selling a hearing aid (or any other commercial product) and that the sale of products would certainly compromise and influence our clinical decisions because of the monetary reward. This all changed in 1978, when the ASHA ethical practice rules were changed to permit audiologists to "sell" products, which in turn, encouraged the move of many to enter private practice.

Northern: I recall that Jim Jerger stated at our first American Academy of Audiology Convention in Kiawah Island (1988): "There can be no doubt that the dispensing of hearing aids by audiologists represents one of the most important milestones in our profession. We are all indebted to that handful of courageous individuals who first proposed that audiologists should dispense aids, persevered against formidable opposition, and succeeded in creating what has become an important step forward for the profession."

Mueller: So here we are, almost 50 years after the ban on selling hearing aids was lifted. We are most certainly in a better place. Both for us as professionals and for our patients.

Northern: Drs. Traynor and Taylor indeed have assembled a cadre of experts with broad expertise in practice management that will be useful for readers at every business level. Although this is not a text that one likely reads from cover to cover, it will serve as a solid reference with practical solutions to management problems, and certainly will become the go-to text for AuD courses on this topic.

Mueller: This new edition contains an impressive range of topics covered that provide ample suggestions and guidelines for private practice owners and clinical managers. You will find information on topics such as business planning, policy, procedures, office management, management systems, insurance, accounting, billing and coding in these chapters. You'll also find useful chapters on such innovative topics as audiology assistants, teleaudiology, forensic audiology, and ethics. This fourth edition is packed with tons of new information and new topical areas. And the mega-list of contributors is like a "Who's Who" of practice management.

Northern: From my point of view, practice management is a continuous and ongoing process, much like working on your skiing and golf skills: you can always find ways to improve your *status quo* performance. The successful entrepreneur is constantly seeking a better system for improving efficiency, effectiveness and, of course, profitability.

Mueller: In their opening chapter, Editors Traynor and Taylor discuss why the word "Strategic" is part of their book title. They mention that in the business world, strategic means taking the time to develop a plan, as well as a method of achieving that plan. To analyze, to communicate, to deliberate, to think, to debate, and, perhaps most importantly, to act after doing those tasks. This book is the perfect companion for that journey.

H. Gustav Mueller, PhD
Bismark, North Dakota

Jerry L. Northern, PhD
Spokane, Washington

Acknowledgments

Welcome to *Strategic Practice Management, Fourth Edition.* The text began in 2008 with its first edition. That first edition had only 374 pages, reflecting the knowledge of practice management at the time. Since then, there has been a second edition of 556 pages and a third edition of 768 pages. This fourth edition will meet or exceed 1000 pages of the most up-to-date practice management material written by experts on their specific topics. The text was conceived by Dr. Robert Glaser and myself in the early 2000s as it was obvious that audiologists needed to have a basic orientation to business and effectively build upon that information to be successful. At that time of the third edition, an Academy of Doctors of Audiology survey found that only about 20% of audiology training programs offered their students a course in this area as part of their Doctor of Audiology program. However, with the expansion of audiology private practice, over 40% of AuD programs now offer a business orientation to their students.

As I prepared to write this edition of the text, I learned that my good friend and colleague, Dr. Robert Glaser, former President of the American Academy of Audiology, former professor, VA clinician, 30-year private practitioner at Audiology Associates of Dayton in Dayton, Ohio, and my partner for three previous editions, was unable to participate in this revision. Dr. Glaser's expertise, writing skills, and general collegiality were greatly missed as this volume was created. While Dr. Glaser could not be a co-editor for this fourth edition, he remains a special contributor.

Dr. Brian Taylor and I are extremely grateful to the 20 participants who graciously agreed to improve the profession with this newest edition of one of the most used textbooks for audiology practice management courses in the United States. To Gus Mueller, my longtime friend and colleague, and Jerry Northern, a career-long mentor, my deepest appreciation for writing the Foreword for this edition. Another essential individual to the success of virtually all of the *Strategic Practice Management* editions, but especially this fourth edition, was Krista Buckles Traynor as a contributing editor. We recognize the efforts and special contribution of Krista, who was essential to the completion of this revision with her attention to detail, third-person writing, and offering general suggestions as a former Regulatory Affairs audiologist.

For this fourth edition, my co-editor, Dr. Brian Taylor has been a true partner in its preparation. Dr. Taylor's assistance in offering his experience, expertise, hearing industry, and business orientation to the profession was not only appreciated but added substantially to the discussion of contemporary issues within the area of audiology practice. His daily contact with practitioners kept the essential topics relevant and timely to create an understanding of the current concerns in the ownership and management essential for successful audiology practice.

Robert M. Traynor, EdD, MBA
Fort Collins, Colorado

This book is about time and money: how to allocate your time so you can optimize *both* patient outcomes and revenue in your business. Toward those ends, this book taps into the expertise of some of the best business minds in our profession. I am grateful for the opportunity to work with each of them.

A lot goes into writing a textbook. First, I would like to thank my co-author, Bob, for generously inviting me to partner with him on the fourth edition. A special thank you also goes to Krista Traynor for her editing expertise. I think Bob would agree that this book would not exist without her efforts. Second, I would like to thank each contributor. Each of them brings a wealth of knowledge and skills that are sure to enlighten even the most experienced reader. Finally, I would like to thank my family, especially my wife, Rebecca, for her patience as I completed this project. Writing a book, especially as a "side project," takes time away from doing other things, and I appreciate all her support.

From soup to nuts, everything you need to operate a successful audiology practice can be found between the covers of this book. I hope each reader can take something of value from these pages, apply it to their practices, and enjoy the fruits of their success.

Brian Taylor, AuD
Minneapolis, Minnesota

Contributors

Debra Abel, AuD
Manager, Coding and Contracting
Audigy
Vancouver, Washington
Chapter 17

Amyn M. Amlani, PhD
President
Otolithic, LLC
CEO and Co-Founder
Hearhero, Inc.
Frisco, Texas
Chapter 13

**Dennis A. Colucci, MA, AuD, ABAC,
    FAAA**
Forensic Audiologist
Auditory Disorders and Balance
    Laboratory, Inc.
Dana Point, California
Chapter 22

Alexander Evertz
Hear.com
Miami, Florida
Chapter 4

Nick Fitzgerald
CEO
AUDSEO
Middletown, Florida
Chapter 12

Robert G. Glaser, PhD
Former President and CEO

Audiology and Speech Associates of
    Dayton, Inc.
Dayton, Ohio
Co-Editor Emeritus, Strategic Practice
    Management
Prologue, Chapters 9 and 18

James W. Hall III, PhD
Professor of Audiology
Department of Communication
    Sciences and Disorders
University of Hawaii
Professor of Audiology
Osborne College of Audiology
Salus University
Elkins Park, Pennsylvania
Extraordinary Professor of
    Audiology
University of Pretoria
Pretoria, South Africa
Chapter 21

A. Nichole Kingham, AuD, ABA
Owner/Audiologist
Eastside Audiology
Chief Education Officer
Audiology Academy
Mill Creek, Washington
Chapter 10

Sarah Laughlin, MS
Director, Human Resources
Fuel Medical
Camas, Washington
Chapter 6

Kevin M. Liebe, AuD
President and CEO
Hearing Health and Technology Matters
Cofounder and Producer
This Week in Hearing Podcast
Richland, Washington
Chapter 12

H. Gustav Mueller, PhD
Faculty Appointments
Vanderbilt University
Nashville, Tennessee
Rush University
Chicago, Illinois
University of Northern Colorado
Greeley, Colorado
Foreword

Scott Myatt, MBA, MIM
Founder and CEO
Newman Creek Advisors
Loveland, Colorado
Chapter 25

Jerry L. Northern, PhD
Professor Emeritus (Retired)
Department of Otolaryngology–Head
 Neck Surgery
University of Colorado Medical Center
President, Colorado Hearing
 Foundation
Spokane, Washington
Foreword

Michael D. Page, AuD
Michael Page, LLC
University of Utah
Salt Lake City, Utah
Chapter 23

Brandon T. Pauley, Esq
Member
Brennan Manna and Diamond LLC
Columbus, Ohio
Chapter 2

Stephanie J. Sjoblad, AuD
Professor and Clinical Director
Division of Speech and Hearing
 Sciences
University of North Carolina–
 Chapel Hill
Chapel Hill, North Carolina
Chapter 14

Brian Taylor, AuD
Senior Director, Audiology
Signia Hearing
Minneapolis, Minnesota
Editor Audiology Practices
Academy of Doctors of Audiology
Minneapolis, Minnesota
Adjunct Professor of Audiology
University of Wisconsin
Madison, Wisconsin
Chapters 1, 4, 7, 8, 12, 18, and 19

Thomas J. Tedeschi, AuD
Chief Audiology Officer
Amplifon Americas
Minneapolis, Minnesota
Chapter 16

Krista Buckles Traynor, MA, RAC
Director of Operations
Robert Traynor Audiology, LLC
Fort Collins, Colorado
Contributing Editor

Robert M. Traynor, EdD, MBA, FNAP
President and CEO–Forensic
 Audiologist
Robert Traynor Audiology, LLC
Fort Collins, Colorado
Adjunct Professor of Audiology
University of Arkansas Medical
 Sciences
Little Rock, Arkansas
Adjunct Professor of Audiology
Rush University
Chicago, Illinois

Adjunct Professor Audiology
Salus University
Elkins Park, Pennsylvania
*Chapters 1, 3, 4, 5, 8, 11, 12, 13, and
20*

Brian Urban, AuD
President and Founder
CounselEar, Inc.
Evanston, Illinois
Chapter 15

Michael Valente, PhD
Professor Emeritus
Department of Otolaryngology
Washington University School of
Medicine
St. Louis, Missouri
Chapter 24

Drs. Traynor and Taylor are grateful to those that have preceded us in the profession, encouraging a robust private practice community. In this year of the passing of Dr. James F. Jerger, let us remember his words at the founding of the American Academy of Audiology:

"Let us say, in a clear voice, to those giants of the past upon whose shoulders we now stand, your work was not in vain. We have built upon your solid foundations. The field you conceived is a reality. We, the heirs of your efforts, are proud of the unified profession we have jointly created."

Prologue

Leadership and Successful Practice Management

Robert G. Glaser, PhD

Introduction

Unquestionably, leadership skills permeate all that we do as clinicians. Patients rely on our professional skills as audiologists for the leadership needed to appropriately manage their hearing loss. Leadership skills are equally important in both matching their auditory needs with advanced technologies and managing the critical counseling interface with their family members and significant others in their lives. Leadership is critical to the success of our profession.

There are as many definitions of leadership as there are leaders. In a simple amalgamation, leadership can be defined as a process set into motion by an individual or a team of people to create a meaningful collaboration of focused thinking resulting in action(s) for a common purpose. Agreeing on a definition helps to focus on the topic; however, it is the varied critical elements, the components that create the opportunities for leadership to work its particular magic.

Leadership is complicated, and the process of developing these skills does not evolve overnight. Leaders demonstrate many, distinct characteristics: competence, commitment, positive attitude, emotional strength, vision, focus, discipline, relationship building, responsibility, initiative, people skills; the list goes on. Many of these intermingled factors are intangible, and that is why leaders require so much seasoning to be effective in the venues of their influence.

Clinical Training and Leadership Skills

Talent is never enough (Maxwell, 2007). The fact is that no person reaches their potential unless they are willing to practice their way there. Preparation positions talent and practice, sharpens it. Practice enables development in the clinical domain. Clinicians get better at what they do when they have opportunities to see more patients. That is true, but there must be an important proviso:

Practice creates a better clinician as long as there is a guide, a mentor, a coach straightening the wrinkles and providing feedback on the functional characteristics of their interactions with patients and their families and significant others. Change is never easy but seemingly always essential to success. Guided change is essential to improving clinical skills and, in the long haul, improving patient outcomes. The difficult changes must be done in concert with direction and feedback from another source skilled at evaluation and promotion of better tactical use of whatever talent you bring to the mix. Max DePree, a preeminent leadership expert, recognized that people, in general and no matter the situation, are resistant to change: "We cannot become what we need to be remaining what we are" (DePree, 2004). His directives were clear: To sharpen your talent through guided practice, you need to do more than just be *open* to change; you have to *pursue* change. And that pursuit must be consistent and vigorous and never ending because your competitors are on the same track to improve their talents. Those who sit and wait for change to happen will be covered in dust as those determined to excel on a diet of change and improvement roar pass them in a thunderous stampede.

Selected Characteristics of Leaders

Positive Attitude

"A successful man is one who can lay a firm foundation with the bricks others have thrown at him."

—David Brinkley,
Television Journalist
(Maxwell, 1999, p. 88)

Every profession enjoys a cadre of successful people, whether teaching students, managing a productive research laboratory, or creating opportunities in the many and varied venues where we practice. There will always be those who accelerate the profession by example. Of the individuals who have achieved lasting success in our discipline, there seems to be a singular thread: their positive outlook on life and their profession. Each has overcome difficulties in some fashion, yet each has excelled despite the "bricks others have thrown" in the course of their path to contribution. Maxwell (1999) made two important points about attitude being a matter of personal choice and that attitude unequivocally determines your actions. No matter what happened yesterday, your attitude is your choice today. Attitude becomes the decisive factor for success, because it determines how you act.

Competence

Competence can be defined in a word as "capability" or "expertise." Competence goes beyond words: It is the leader's ability to say it, plan it, and do it in such a way that others know that you know how, and know that they want to follow you (Maxwell, 2007). Leaders are admired for both inherent competence and perceived capabilities. Several key elements must be a part of a leader's armament for success. They are simple elements, easy to accomplish on a consistent basis:

Show Up Every Day

Responsible people show up when they are expected. Highly competent come ready to play every day, no matter how they feel, what kind of circumstances they are facing in their personal or professional life, or how difficult they expect the game to be.

Keep Improving

Highly competent people are constantly engaged in learning, growing, and improving. They do that by asking *why*. After all, the person who knows *how* will always have a job, but the person who knows *why* will always be the boss.

Follow Through With Excellence

Performing at a high level of excellence is a choice, an act of will. As leaders, we expect our people to follow through when we hand them the ball. They expect that and a whole lot more from us as their leaders.

Accomplish More Than Expected

Highly competent people always go the extra mile. For them, good enough is never good enough; they need to do the job and then some, day in and day out.

Inspire Others

Motivating others to perform at high levels is not a skill that develops overnight, nor can it be taught in a classroom. It is a talent commonly learned by watching effective leaders succeed. Excellent leadership has no stops and starts, no clear edges, nothing but smooth transition from concept and plan to effective action completing a well-defined goal.

Engage

Skilled leaders spend their time advancing conversations, not avoiding or ending them. The more you engage others, the better leader you will become both in your clinical efforts and in managing your practice. It is difficult to bring about the type of confidence, trust, and loyalty a leader must possess without being *fully engaged* in person, over the telephone, via email, through social media, or even by sending personal, handwritten notes—likely the most surprising and, therefore, perhaps the most effective example of engagement in this age of rapid, often impersonal informational exchanges.

Communication Skills

"Developing excellent communication skills is absolutely essential to effective leadership. The leader must be able to share knowledge and ideas to transmit a sense of urgency and enthusiasm to others. If a leader can't get a message across clearly and motivate others to act on it, then having a message doesn't even matter."

—Gilbert Amelio,
President and CEO,
National Semiconductor Corp.
(Maxwell, 1999, p. 23)

Your communication skills will make you the kind of leader that people will want to follow—or not. Your message must be clear and well articulated. People will not follow you if they cannot see clearly where you are going and how you intend to get there. Keep your message simple. Before you can convince others to follow, you have to believe in what you are promoting, what it is that is so important to you that it can readily become important to others. The goal of all communication is action. Simply providing information is not enough. Leaders must provide an incentive to listen, an incentive to remember the importance of the tasks ahead and, most importantly, a plan of action and involvement to reach the desired outcome(s). At the root of effectiveness is the ability to communicate meaningful information in a clear and concise manner such that all involved in the processes leading to accomplishing the goals know the path, even when blindfolded.

If you want to become an effective leader, it is best to stop talking and start listening. There is far more to gain by surrendering the floor than by trying to dominate it. As mentioned earlier, there is a seeming rush to communicate what is on one's mind without considering the value of everything that can be gleaned from the minds of others: As my father used to say so effortlessly and consistently—*you can't learn anything with your mouth open.*

Commitment

"Followers expect a leader to face up to tough decisions. When conflict must be resolved, when justice must be defined and carried out, when promises need to be kept, when the organization needs to hear who counts—these are the times when leaders act with ruthless honesty and live up to their covenant with the people they lead."

—DePree (2008)

The obligation inherent in assuming positions of leadership requires personal sacrifice. Consider the many audiologists who have made the commitment to advance their professional acumen by completing their AuD. They have done so not only at financial expense but also in terms of valuable time spent away from family and friends. Consider the incalculable hours as well spent volunteering for professional organizations: Our colleagues sacrifice their time, talent, and personal assets to take on various roles of leadership in our professional organizations. They are involved because they are committed to their profession, what it stands for, what it does for others, and because it is needed to secure our future as important and significant contributors to the health of our nation.

Pursuit

Pursuit is an often-overlooked quality of leadership. Exceptional leaders are never satisfied with traditional practice, static thinking, conventional wisdom, or common performance; they are simply uncomfortable with anything that embraces the status quo. You cannot attain that which you do not pursue.

Myatt (2011a, 2011b) states explicitly, "Leadership is pursuit—pursuit of excellence, of elegance, of truth, of what's next, of what if, of change, of value, of results of relationships, of service, of knowledge and of something bigger than themselves. Smart leaders understand it is not just enough to pursue, but pursuit must be intentional, focused, consistent, aggressive and unyielding. You must pursue the right things, for the right reasons, and at the right times."

Teamwork

"Teamwork makes the dream work."
—Maxwell (2007)

Teamwork divides the effort and multiplies the effect. It is working toward a common goal that joins people in an effort that they might never engage in as an individual. It is an opportunity for growth for all involved, leaders and members of the group as well. Teamwork is not always as easy as getting a few folks together to solve a problem or change a direction. Teams do not usually come together and develop on their own; they require ardent leadership and cooperation within the group. Teamwork, however, is superior to individual effort:

- Teams involve more people, thus affording more resources, ideas, and energy than an individual possesses.
- Teams maximize a leader's potential and minimize weaknesses.
- Teams provide multiple perspectives on how to meet a need or reach a goal, thus devising alternatives for each situation. Individual insight is seldom as broad and deep

as a group's when it takes on a problem.
- Teams share the credit for victories and the blame for losses, fostering genuine humility and authentic community. Individuals take credit and blame alone.
- Teams keep leaders accountable for the goal. Individuals connected to no one can change the goal without accountability.
- Teams can simply do more than an individual.

Ability to Empower

"People under the influence of an empowering person are like paper in the hands of a talented artist."
—Maxwell (2002)

If you are in a leadership role in an organization, your ability to empower others is not an option unless, of course, you plan on running the entire show alone. Empowering others is as critical to the success of the organization as it is critical to the success and effectiveness of the leader. Empowerment has an incredibly high return. When you empower a person to take on a task, lead a team, or research a topic important to organizational advancement, it not only helps the individuals you raise by making them more confident, more at ease in making decisions, and more productive but also frees you to actively promote the growth and health of your organization or practice.

Achievement comes to someone who is able to do great things for themselves. Success comes when they empower followers to do great things *with* them.

Significance comes when they develop leaders to do great things *for* them. But a legacy is created only when a person puts their organization into the position to do things *without* them (DePree, 2004).

A Final Note on the Responsibility for Your Profession

Respect for the future, regard for the present, understanding the past. Leaders must forever move between the present and the future. Our perception of each becomes clear and valid if we understand the past. The future requires our humility in the face of all we cannot control. The present requires attention to all the people to whom we are accountable. The past gives us the opportunity to build on the work of our elders (DePree, 2008).

Although it seems like yesterday, a long time ago as young students, budding practitioners, and teachers and researchers-in-the-making, we accepted the torch of leadership willingly. We recognized early on that there was no substitution for clear communication and effective collaboration within our ranks and across the boundaries of our organizations. We were eager not only to perpetuate our profession but also to improve upon the efforts of those who had come before us. Strong challenges remain today, and each must be met head on and without fear. Our profession requires vigilant stewards willing to accept the torch and make it burn brighter than ever before. Without your

eagerness to accept the responsibility of leadership, our profession will have a restricted future dictated by others seeking to minimize our impact and lessen our rightful place in today's healthcare marketplace. Take the torch and continue the journey. Make us proud.

References

DePree, M. (2004). *Leadership is an art.* Random House.

DePree, M. (2008). *Leadership jazz: The essential elements of a great leader.* Random House.

Drucker, P. (n.d.). BrainyQuote.com. https://www.brainyquote.com/quotes/quotes/p/peterdruck131069.html

Glaser, R. G. (2011). *If not you then who?* Keynote presentation: Ohio Academy of Audiology Fifth Biennial Audiology Conference, Columbus, OH.

Maxwell, J. C. (1999). *The 21 indispensable qualities of a leader.* Thomas Nelson Publications.

Maxwell, J. C. (2002). *Leadership 101: What every leader needs to know.* Thomas Nelson Publications.

Maxwell, J. C. (2007). *Talent is never enough.* Thomas Nelson Publications.

Myatt, M. (2011a). *Forbes.* https://www.forbes.com/sites/mikemyatt/2011/12/19/this-one-leadership-quality-will-make-or-break-you/

Myatt, M. (2011b). *Forbes.* https://www.forbes.com/sites/mikemyatt/2011/12/27/leadership-and-the-power-of-yes/

Traynor, R. M., & Glaser, R. G. (2010). *Positive emergence: Optimization strategies for a difficult economy.* Paper presented at the American Academy of Audiology Annual Meeting, San Diego, CA.

1 Management and Economics Implications for Audiology Practice: The Big Picture

*Brian Taylor, AuD, and
Robert M. Traynor, EdD, MBA*

Introduction

As readers can plainly see from the title of this book, the main topic is *strategic* practice management. Therefore, it should be no surprise that the word *strategic* is doing much of the heavy lifting throughout this book. Before diving into the details of what it means to be *strategic*, it might help to have a working definition of that word. Broadly defined, *strategic* is any subject or issue that directly relates to achieving the long-term goals and interests of a business. To be *strategic* means to take the time to develop a plan, as well as a method of achieving that plan. To analyze, to communicate, to plan, to deliberate, to think, to debate, and, perhaps most importantly, to act after doing those tasks is the working definition of *strategic*.

A well-used adage in the military and in the business world, *hope is not a strategy*, infers that hope will only get you so far. This book is designed to provide the reader with tools that will enable them to never rely on hope

to assess any part of their practice but rather to provide solid knowledge and methods of how to improve it. After all, effective *strategic* managers incorporate continual and incremental improvement by considering the many management and economic implications of how the business of audiology fits into the larger economic landscape. The purpose of this book is to expand the skills necessary to be a better *strategic manager* and, when the time comes, a *better boss*. Since the word *strategic* means to always be analyzing the big picture and planning ahead, this book will examine virtually all of the facets in the management of an audiology practice. The journey to making a living as an audiologist begins in Chapter 1 by clarifying what it means to be both an effective manager and a review of economics.

The Business of Audiology

When entering the profession of audiology, neither the management of a

1

business nor related economic concepts were part of career goals. The focus, of course, was on how and when to provide a myriad of audiological evaluations and interpret those results. Further, energy and focus were devoted to treating hearing and balance difficulties using products and services that suited the best interests of patients. As clinicians move from merely a clinical role to owning and/or managing a clinic, they must realize that the business of audiology is unique. The late Dr. Paul Drucker (1909–2005) was considered one of the world authorities in management, ethics, and business planning. In one of his last publications (2001), he states that business management must always, in every decision and action, put the economic performance of the business first. According to his way of thinking, a business can only justify its existence by the economic results it produces. While this may be true for other businesses, the business of audiology is considerably different in that there are ethical as well as profit considerations that, at times, may be at odds with each other. On one hand, there is a fiduciary responsibility to optimize each patient's hearing and/or balance predicament. On the other, there is a need to make a profit to continue to serve these patients while keeping the audiologist well motivated (Taylor, 2012). This dichotomy sets forth the need for management strategies quite different from many other professions.

In many ways, the business of audiology is an interesting study in contrast. It combines the medical/diagnostic and rehabilitative with the retail and commercial. Each of these traits, all equally important to long-term strategic success, requires vastly different skills sets. For example, the medical/diagnostic and rehabilitative side of the equation requires great attention to detail, impeccable communication skills, and the ability to collect precise information using accurate testing methods—all toward promoting the best interests of each patient. In contrast, the retail and commercial side of the equation requires many of the same skills—to be fastidious and reliable, but in a way that promotes the welfare of people (staff) who work in your business that ultimately contributes to generating revenue and profit while controlling expenses and costs.

Is the Business World Really for Me?

Developing and maintaining an audiology practice can be an exciting and rewarding experience. It can offer numerous advantages such as being the boss and the one to determine salaries, set the schedule, and choose who to hire. But becoming a successful entrepreneur requires thorough planning, creativity, and hard work. So, the first question that must be considered is, "Is running a business really for me?" The answer partially lies in the concepts and skills required to become a successful *entrepreneur*. Entrepreneurs are defined as a person who organizes, manages, and assumes the risks of a business or enterprise. Entrepreneurs who take the risks necessary may be rewarded with profits and growth opportunities.

Haynes (2024) indicates that entrepreneurs play a key role in any economy, using their skills and initiative to anticipate needs and bring new ideas to market. Entrepreneurship is often the result of the actions of a person in search of something new, exploiting their ideas into profitable opportunities by accepting the risk and uncertainty that are inherent to the specific business enterprise. It is also a process of identifying these opportunities within the market and bringing together the necessary resources to pursue these opportunities for long-term gains.

Thus, those audiologists suited for the business world and become entrepreneurs are those who:

- Develop a business model for their audiology practice.
- Acquire the necessary physical and human capital to start a new venture.
- Operationalize their vision for their business venture.
- Are responsible for the success or failure of the business venture.
- Invest their own capital or raise capital from external sources to fund their business.
- Take the blame for failure as well as reap the rewards in case of success.

To be an entrepreneur, the person must have characteristics that will allow them to be successful in areas necessary to facilitate a successful business.

- *Comfortable with taking risk:* Owning a business requires making tough decisions such as what the practice will offer the community, who gets paid first or last, and so forth. Businesses have ups and downs, economies have cycles, and competition has rises and falls. These and other business variables create uncertainty in the future. While some individuals would

rather avoid unstable income and insecurity, others feed on these issues and look to calculated business risks as challenges.

- *Independent:* Business owners need to make a lot of decisions on their own, based upon their instincts, research, and intuition. In everyday business operations, there are often rejection, financial ups and downs, human resource issues, taxes, operational changes, and other hurdles that must be cleared up and the owner is the ultimate decision-maker. If a person enjoys the independence of making their own decisions and trusts their judgment, then it is possible that independent practice might work for them.
- *Persuasive:* Practitioners will need to persuade patients, employees, potential employees, lenders, partners, and others. There are sales skills and political interactions that are necessary to facilitate business and employee harmony. If the new business owner enjoys public speaking, engaging new people, and finding compelling arguments grounded in facts, it is likely that they will be successful in independent practice.
- *Comfortable analyzing financial numbers:* Analysis of data and statistics will often describe the health of the practice by presenting valuable data to managers as to success or failure as well as predict trends and implications that will require business modifications.
- *Able to negotiate:* As a small business owner, there will be a need to negotiate everything from leases to product prices and contract terms to

refunds. Polished negotiation skills will help save money and keep the practice running smoothly.

■ *Creative:* Practice owners need to be able to think of new methods of practice, operation, and concepts of business and offer new services and products before the competition. Solving problems with new ideas and creativity is an essential skill.

■ *Supported by others:* Before starting or managing a practice, it is important to have a strong support system in place. Practitioners will be forced to make many tough, sometimes unpopular, decisions. Families must be on notice that business success can temporarily be the highest priority and that sometimes important family functions may be missed in order to support the business.

Debunking the Truths and Myths

Truths and myths of entrepreneurship, in this case, audiology practice ownership, are a product of working as an employee. Truths are derived from accurate perceptions of bosses and others in charge, while myths are misguided or inaccurate perceptions. Audiologists who put these truths and myths into proper perspective master the essential skills and aptitudes to be entrepreneurs.

Although many individuals have proper perceptions of the truths and myths involved in the motivation for beginning a business, many employees are unaware of the nonclinical work that goes into the management of an audiology clinic. After all, department heads, regional managers, and vice presidents

of operations are just a few of the titles many audiologists assume during their career. In many cases, these titles do not come with any ownership of the actual business, yet as the "managing director," they are required to hire productive individuals, control costs, generate profits, and generally get results. For those reasons, the following misconceptions can be associated with ownership or management of a practice.

Being Your Own Boss

While working as an employee, many audiologists may have believed that it would be better to "work for themselves" or "be their own boss." On the surface, the idea of "being your own boss" in a business seems reasonable. There is no one to tell you what to do, when to do it, how to do it, or if you should do it. Therefore, the idea of "being your own boss" has some face validity to the uninitiated. In reality, "being your own boss" is a myth because a business owner has many bosses, and an audiology practice owner is no exception. This, of course, is especially true if you are managing a department and report on an organizational chart to another person. In that case, you can still assume a "be your own boss" mentality, which means you take ownership of the decision-making process.

In an audiology clinic, there are many bosses, and foremost are the patients, to whom the practitioner is ultimately responsible for providing services and products, as well as follow up the products with warranty service. Practice owners and managers are also responsible to the patients for all other administrative issues, such as keeping malpractice insurance, having a timely return of product deposits, maintaining the competence and certification of not only themselves but also their employees, and virtually everything else that goes with the provisions of high-quality services. The practice's valuable referral sources are another "boss" that requires constant maintenance. Competition for referral sources in the marketplace stresses the importance to turn reports around promptly, keep communications constant, and reinforce the clinic's expertise (Chapter 18). A private practice proverb is, "*If you take good care of your patients and referral sources, they will take good care of you.*"

If the practice has a bank loan, it must be paid no matter if business is good or not, so another "boss" is the banker or the investor in the practice. These bankers or those to whom long-term or short-term loans are owed have a vested interest in the success or failure of the business. Their main goal is to receive a good return on their investment; therefore, their interests may not be the same as the practice goals. While the clinic's goals are to provide the highest quality audiological services and products, these people simply want to be paid and make a profit.

Often the first to observe success or failure of the business is the practice accountant. Since they monitor the books, they are certain to identify what methods and procedures are working within the practice. Therefore, it is a wise practice owner that listens carefully to their recommendations for changes in the provision and pricing of products and services or other business modifications that are essential to the financial stability of the practice, all of which makes the accountant another "boss."

Even the most ethical and conscientious audiology practices can be plagued with legal issues from time to time. Legal issues may involve business structure, leasing space, equipment, employee issues, collections, difficult patients, or payroll taxes. Circumstances may arise, which can create situations where the practitioner must conduct business as indicated by their attorney (Chapter 2).

As discussed later in this text, generally, in patient-centric practice, we work for patients first and foremost, and if we do a good job with our patients, then usually the other bosses will be served as well. Thus, the concept of "being your own boss" is a myth as the audiology practice owner has many bosses, all of whom need to be kept satisfied for a practice to succeed.

Earning a High Salary

A typical reaction, given the costs of services and products, would be that sums of money taken into the practice should generate enough income to increase compensation (Chapters 6 and 14). However, the practice owner's salary is determined by many factors but is mostly dictated by the amount of business conducted or cash flow and control of the fixed and avoidable costs that facilitate the level of the owner's salary. In a new practice, it could very well be that the generation of income will be significant and, accordingly, the salary and benefits will be very high. Realistically, however, a new audiology practice will on average not generate much initial cash flow and, subsequently, not much income for the practitioner until the business is established in the marketplace. Cash flow is limited and as expenses such as rent, utilities, telephone, employees, and payroll taxes need to be paid first, it is not unusual that the owner's salary begins at a lower level than they experienced when working as an employee elsewhere. Another old private practice proverb is, "The owner is always paid last." After some time, it may be possible for the clinic to generate a greater cash flow, meeting all the expenses; then (and only then), salary and benefit increases can be considered for the owner. Entry into private practice does not ensure a higher salary and/or benefits, particularly in the beginning. The survival of the business is foremost and takes priority over how much the practice owner will be compensated. Obtaining a lucrative salary is usually a myth in the beginning and may become a reality as the practice matures.

Setting the Rules of the Practice

Clinicians who have worked for others have often found themselves feeling that they could manage the clinic better than their boss. In their opinion, the clinic should have different hours of operation, better/newer equipment, more or less procedures, less paperwork, better (or different) products, more precise evaluative protocols, higher or lower prices, better credit terms, higher or lower standards, better benefit packages, better policies, and/or various other issues that, in their opinion, should be managed differently. Although these management modifications in policies and procedures seem perfectly reasonable to the employees from their perspective, once they realize the rationales for the positions taken by their employer, they often arrive at the same or similar

decisions they criticized as employees (Chapter 6). Thus, owning a practice and having the ability to change the management technique, policies, and procedures could be either a truth or a myth.

Obtaining Earned Benefits From Manufacturers

Obtaining "benefits" from manufacturers of hearing instruments has become a very controversial issue in the 2020s. These benefits could be earned by selling a specific number of units of a manufacturer's product and thus be rewarded with trips to exotic places, new equipment, low interest loans, special cash accounts, and other benefits without any out-of-pocket expenses. Although these benefits are often considered a normal part of conducting business by manufacturers of most products, audiological recommendations for hearing devices involve a special fiduciary trust relationship. Over the years, ethical practice boards for both national and state audiology organizations have found on numerous occasions that obtaining these benefits is unethical, ruling that these "gifts or benefits" could (and do) influence the clinician's choice of hearing instruments chosen for their patients (Chapter 23). The ethical concern is that a practice manager in need of a few more units to pay for a trip to Europe or this month's payment on the loan might possibly compromise patient care by recommending instruments that count toward the trip when the patient would be better served by another manufacturer's product. Therefore, the American Academy of Audiology, American Speech-Language-Hearing Association, Academy of Doctors of Audiology, and many state licensure boards (Chapter 23) consider the acceptance of accepting these benefits as unethical practice. Owning a practice for the "benefits" offered by manufacturers is most likely a myth, unless owners are willing to risk their profession by compromising their ethical standards.

Taking Time Off

It is good (and necessary) to have time off from work to relax and forget those problem patients, the employees' problems, or the frustrations of paying the month's expenses. However, if the practice is successful, there may not be much time or funds for days off or for personal vacations. In a solo practice, when the clinician is away and only the front office is present, there is no income. Unless the practitioner has additional employees that can keep the doors open and see patients in their absence, time off must be scheduled around the clinic schedule and other low-pressure times, such as holiday periods or when business is usually slow. Even in a practice that has good clerical employees and colleague clinicians, it is difficult to get away for much longer than a week without frustrating situations arising. These difficulties can sometimes be devastating to the practice, so it is best to err on the side of caution and be careful about absences, whether they be elected vacations or necessary emergencies. As in other businesses, audiology practice requires that the owner be available most of the time for business and clinical decisions that are required each day. Often well-meaning employees may make decisions that they feel are in the best

interest of the clinic, but these choices could be inaccurate based upon their lack of knowledge of clinic operations and plans for the future. The business world is unforgiving, and a proprietor or CEO who is absent will be punished severely by the marketplace. Therefore, obtaining more time off is a myth.

Business Management for Nonowners

Much of this textbook is written to address the needs of practice owners, but the reality is that most audiologists will not become owners of their own practice. Not every audiologist has the desire to own their own business. Frankly, under the right conditions, many of the personal and professional rewards associated with ownership can be achieved without actually owning the business (Chapter 7).

Even if a clinician never becomes a practice owner, much of the material in this textbook still applies to the daily work of any manager or director. Experience suggests that when many audiologists get about 5 to 10 years of experience under their belt, they become great candidates to be promoted to a manager or director-level position within a large organization. Once an audiologist assumes a managerial position, even if they continue to see patients in the clinic, their primary focus must shift away from the daily work of patient care to oversight of the daily operation of the business. Tasks such as evaluating financial well-being, marketing, public relations, growing the business, professional development of staff, hiring new staff, and, yes, even firing staff are just a few of the managerial tasks that supplant patient care. It is also essential for the noon practice owner to be familiar with these concepts, and they are covered in the volume.

Manager Versus Leader

Whether a practice owner or someone who carries one of the many titles that indicate management, there are expectations, by virtue of that title, combining the necessary skills of a manager and a leader.

In short, managers must focus on short-term details (e.g., what things need to get done this week or next month for the business to be profitable). On the other hand, leaders are inclined to look more at the big picture, strategically, to evaluate how the future should be shaped through their decisions. In reality, successful practice management requires proficiency in day-to-day management of the elements of a business while simultaneously averting attention away from the "daily grind" of ensuring the *business is equipped to meet the demands of the market 1 or 2 years in the future.*

What Is Management?

Management is defined as the administration of an organization, which may be a for-profit or nonprofit audiology clinic, community hearing center, hospital audiology department, school audiology program, or government-based audiology clinic. Effective management cannot be arbitrary; it must be well planned, consistent, and readily under-

stood by the entire organization. When managing an audiology practice, considerations must be for both the fiduciary and profit responsibilities while developing working management strategies for successful operation within specific markets. Managing is oftentimes a challenging task. Determining the best way to manage an organization has been an issue facing businesses for centuries.

Once these effective management procedures are determined, it is assured that these will need to change over time as the profession of audiology and the market updates according to technology, competitive pressures, government regulations, and patient needs. Over the past couple of centuries, several general theories of effective management have developed. Burrow et al. (2016) have organized basic management theories into specific types: *classical management, administrative management, behavioral management,* and *quality management.*

Classical Management

Classical management was one of the first methods used to apply scientific study to business activities. This method evaluates how work is organized and considers the procedures most effective to complete the job by increasing worker productivity. Clinics that use classical management often use experiments to improve the organization of workspace, procedures, and other factors to increase efficiency. This might involve the use of several types of files or going paperless to become more efficient on the clerical side while changing the protocol for various evaluations and treatment programs to offer more services in less clinical time. Clinics that offer commissions to clerical staff for their phone work or appointment generation may be using a classical type of management.

Administrative Management

Administrative management is involved in establishing the most effective practices for organizing and growing the practice. This method is often used in larger clinics as it sets up multiple levels of management, organizing the practice into specialized departments, such as diagnostic and rehabilitative areas with an administrator responsible for each. Administrative management defines the type of work that must be completed for an effective operation.

- *Authority and Responsibility.* Managers have the authority to assign tasks. They must also give the necessary authority to those assigned to actually complete the tasks.
- *Unity of Command.* Each employee must receive direction from only one manager to avoid conflicts and maintain a clear line of authority.
- *Unity of Purpose.* The goals and direction of an organization must be clear and supported by everyone.
- *Adequate Compensation.* The wages and benefits for every employee should be fair and satisfactory to both the individual and the organization.
- *Esprit de Corps.* Organizations should work to build good interpersonal relationships, a sense of teamwork, and harmony.

Behavioral Management

While some management techniques are directed at efficiency and organization, *behavioral management* is concerned with the effects of changes on employees, specifically focusing on understanding the foundations of employee motivation and behaviors. Sometimes called human relations management, the goal is to cultivate positive relationships with their managers, such that the employees believe they are a valuable part of the organization and are motivated accordingly to do their best work. Practice managers should consistently strive to improve working conditions. Research into behavioral management has repeatedly demonstrated that when employees feel their managers were concerned about them by improving their working conditions, they work harder and with better accuracy in all areas of their responsibilities.

Quality Management

The last half of the 20th century has brought a considerable number of changes in management strategies. As the number of products increased, companies were looking at strategies to improve the speed of production as well as cutting costs. They recognized that effective *quality management* involves using facts and data to make improvements in the process or the products produced. Hearing aid and equipment manufacturers have instituted these quality programs within their operations to make much better products that support our practices. In audiology, quality is increased by advancements in our field and commitment to patient care.

Developing a General Management Strategy

No matter the theory or combination of theories used as a management basis, Burrow et al. (2016) present factors that practice managers must consider when developing a management strategy (Figure 1–1).

The Business

While the type of business might be audiology, there are many varied sizes and types of clinics. Some clinics spe-cialize in hearing instruments, and others offer general audiological services including educational services, aural rehabilitation, and/or cochlear implant follow-up care. Audiologists find themselves in ENT clinics, general hospitals, schools, government clinics, private clinics, and other settings. Each site will have specific advantages and limitations as well as its own management strategy based on the business needs. Financial resources are essential to the provision of quality products and services in any business, especially audiology practices.

The Work

Managers must be prepared to supervise the work of both clerical and pro-

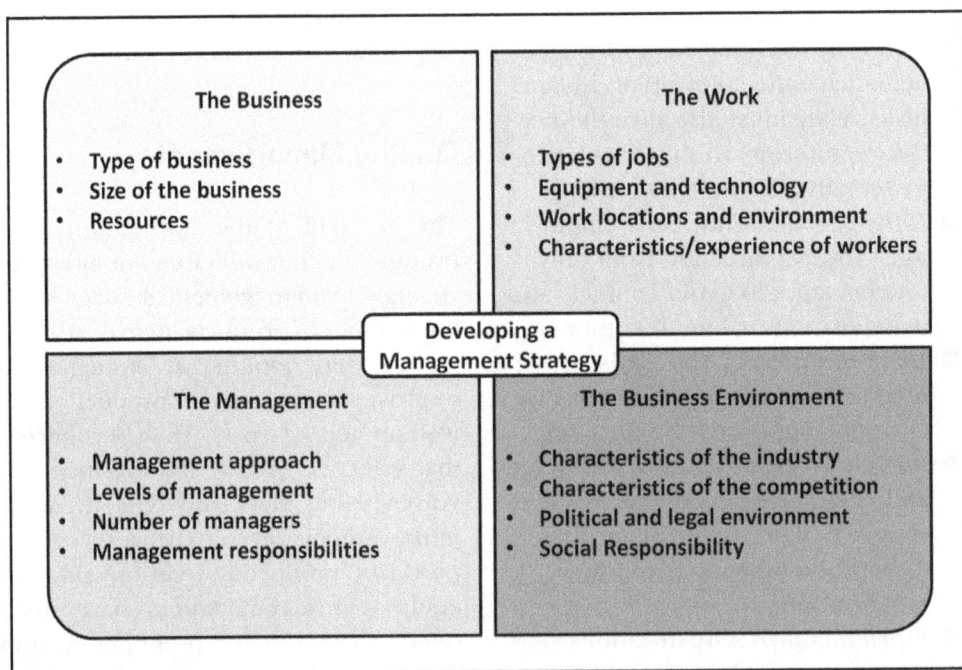

Figure 1–1. Developing a management strategy. *Source:* Adapted from Burrow, J. L., Kleindl, B., & Becraft, M. B. (2016). *Business management* (14th ed.). Cengage Learning.

fessional employees. Diverse types of work require specific types of management. For example, the management of routine clerical tasks, such as answering the phone and organizing files and charts, is quite different from the management of professionals conducting electrocochleography, auditory brainstem response studies, hearing aid fittings, cochlear implant mapping, and operative monitoring. Each of these employee categories includes individuals with varied backgrounds, educational levels, and varied aspirations. Some will be experienced clinicians while others will be new, full-time, part-time, or temporary hires. To provide the best work, employees must be provided with state-of-the-art supplies and equipment that support innovative evaluation with treatment with updates periodically. A small one-location clinic will present very different challenges compared to a multilocation enterprise. In addition to additional employees to manage, larger organizations have greater equipment needs and space maintenance issues and administrative matters, such as vacation, commissions, and benefits, which become more of a concern as the business grows to numerous locations.

The Management

The method of management used depends upon the clinical setting, as well as its size and goals. The previously mentioned management types, *classical*, *administrative*, *behavioral*, and *quality*, or a combination of these, are used by practice managers to maintain the health and viability of the practice. While the responsibilities of manage-

ment will vary according to the number of layers involved, the management type and style are generally determined by the structure and hierarchy necessary for the success of the practice. Drucker (2001) suggested that the basic task of management is marketing and innovation. Thus, management responsibilities will vary not only by the size and type of the clinic but also by the competition within the marketplace.

The Business Environment

The final strategic factor pertains to the characteristics of the business environment. The audiology business climate has changed substantially in the past few years. Increased competition from instrument manufacturers, big box stores, direct-to-consumer and over-the-counter hearing devices, government programs, and insurance companies, as well as cultural changes, have altered the business environment for privately owned clinics. Managers must be prepared with an effective strategy for today's competition while recognizing that future competitive challenges, including political, legal, and regulatory issues, will greatly modify the audiology business landscape.

Management Style

It is management's role to strengthen the bond among employees and assist them in working together as a single unit to ensure satisfaction with job responsibilities. This is best accomplished by understanding employees and striving to fulfill their expectations leading to a stress-free environment in the workplace. Every leader has a unique management style. The following outlines various management styles:

- *Autocratic Style*. Autocrats do not take the ideas and suggestions of their subordinates into consideration. In this management style, the employees are totally dependent upon their bosses and do not have the liberty to make decisions on their own. The employees must adhere to the guidelines and policies formulated by their superiors. While this style offers organization and conformity, it may lead to a lack of motivation among the employees.
- *Paternalistic Style*. Opposite of the autocratic style is the paternalistic style. Here the leaders decide what policies are best that will benefit both the employees and the organization. Paternalistic managers solicit suggestions and feedback from their subordinates before decisions are made, fostering a sense of attachment and loyalty to the organization. Employees stay motivated and enjoy their work rather than treating it as a burden.
- *Democratic Style*. The democratic management style invites feedback from subordinates through open forums discussing the pros and cons of plans and ideas. When the superiors listen to the employees before finalizing plans and operations, it ensures effective and healthy communication between management and employees.
- *Laissez-Faire Style*. In this style, managers are employed just for the sake of it and do not contribute much to the organization. Employ-

ees are not dependent upon the managers; they make decisions and manage their work on their own. Those individuals who have the dream of succeeding in the organization consistently outshine employees who are simply showing up for work.
- *Management by Walking Around Style*. These managers treat themselves as an essential part of the team and take pride in being efficient listeners: They interact with the employees to determine their concerns and take note of their suggestions. The manager is more a mentor and guide than an overseer or boss.

Differences Between Management and Leadership

Most clinicians will be more involved with management than the leadership of their organization. As time and experience builds, they will often become managers exercising the vision of their leaders. After some years, these same clinicians could also become leaders inspiring their colleagues. While leadership and management require each other, the roles are not the same and often confused. To put these business roles into perspective, *Leadership* often represents a person or group of individuals who are responsible for inspiring, guiding, and leading a group of people who are joined for a common cause, while *Management* is defined as a group of people who run an organization. Leadership and management go together as they indirectly require each other for a business to be successful. A leader could also be a manager and vice versa; it all depends on the qualities and the needs of the organization. Bennis (2003) describes the differences between leaders and managers as follows:

■ The manager administers; the leader innovates.
■ The manager is a copy; the leader is an original.
■ The manager maintains; the leader develops.
■ The manager focuses on systems and structure; the leader focuses on people.
■ The manager relies on control; the leader inspires trust.
■ The manager has a short-range view; the leader has a long-range perspective.
■ The manager asks how and when; the leader asks what and why.
■ The manager has their eye always on the bottom line; the leader's eye is on the horizon.
■ The manager imitates; the leader originates.
■ The manager accepts the status quo; the leader challenges it.
■ The manager is the classic good soldier; the leader is their own person.
■ The manager does things right; the leader does the right thing.

As Bennis describes these differences, it is easy to determine that the leader is more for inspiration and ideas that will become policy for managers to execute. Though leadership and management are different, those in these roles commonly work together as both roles are required to accomplish certain goals and objectives.

In today's organizations, a manager is not always only limited to interacting with subordinates and following orders. Many managers inspire, shape, train, and assist in the development of their subordinates. Similarly, many leaders are not just thinking and developing abstract concepts; they may also be managers of the operation, particularly in a small audiology clinical operation. It is believed that leaders and managers must work together or take up additional roles, as they are no longer limited to set definitions. A mixture of both provides the best results in running an organization. (See the Prologue.)

The Economic Divide: Micro- and Macroeconomics

We all like to think that our practices are critically important to current and prospective patients and referral sources and that they are immune from economic circumstances. The reality remains that audiology practices are significantly affected by changes in the economy, and no matter the setting, managers and employees must be aware of the economic environment in which they practice.

Economics is generally split between the analysis of how the overall economy and single markets function. The overall view or "big picture" is called *macroeconomics*. It is concerned with generalized issues such as employment, the current gross domestic product, inflation, and the intricacies of the national debt. In macroeconomics, the big picture is usually a nation and how all its markets interact to generate an overview of national economic conditions. These are referred to as aggregate variables.

Smaller area economics or the "small picture" is called *microeconomics*. Major concerns center on how supply and demand interact within individual markets relative to the provision of local goods and services. In the realm of microeconomics, the object of analysis is a single market or product.

Macroeconomics is part of the 24-hour news cycle and bombards viewers each day with a myriad of incomprehensible terms and economic rationales from around the world. As audiologists, we do not typically attend to these terms, and subsequently, clues to necessary strategic adjustments in our practices become lost in the background noise of the evening news. The calculations and terms that describe the direction and/or health of the economy, known as economic indicators, provide valuable information regarding the strength or weakness of the economy in real time.

Economic Structures

No matter the setting, an audiology practice is simply a business that provides products and services within a specific economic structure. Burrow et al. (2016) set forth three types of economic structures: a market economy, a command economy, and a mixed economy. These economic structures represent a method for governments to decide how to use their resources for what, how, and for whom goods and services will be produced.

Market Economic Systems

A *market economy* is an economic system in which individual buying decisions determine what, how, and for whom goods and services will be produced. For example, the more patients decide to use hearing instruments, the more hearing aids are produced to meet the need. Over the past few years in audiology clinics in the United States, the trend has reversed from recommending mostly in-the-ear (ITE) hearing devices to primarily receiver-in-the-ear (RIC) devices. Consumer purchasing decisions, therefore, have caused hearing device manufacturers to use more of their resources to produce RIC devices than ITE instruments. Thus, in a market economy, individual consumers make their own decisions about what to purchase, and therefore collectively, they inadvertently determine how a manufacturer will use their production resources. In a market economy, such as the free enterprise system found in the United States, individual citizens rather than the government own most of the factors of production, such as land, manufacturing facilities, and other resources. While the United States is an example of a free market system, there are no totally free markets.

Command Economic Systems

Command economies represent an economic system in which a central planning authority, usually under control of the country's government, owns most of the factors of production. This authority determines what, how, and for whom goods and services are produced. Countries that adopt a command economy are often dictatorships or communist regimes where the government rather than consumers decide how the factors of production will be used to meet the needs of the population.

Mixed Economic Systems

No country has a pure market economy or a command economy. Generally, economic systems that use elements of both market and command economic systems fall under the heading of mixed economies. In mixed economies, production decisions for certain goods and services, such as the post office, telephone systems, schools, health care facilities, and public utilities, are government controlled while other goods and services operate within a free market economic system. Virtually all countries in 2024 have some form of a mixed economy, although some have more elements of a command economy. In the United States and Canada, for example, the government plays a smaller role in the economy than it does in the more command-oriented economies such as North Korea and Cuba. Once predominately command economies, countries of the former Soviet Union, Vietnam, and Iran now allow privately owned businesses to operate freely and make their own economic decisions, including what to offer for sale and at what prices.

Market Economies and Economic Cycles

In the United States, our economy is predominately a market economy. Essential to the discussion of how our economy works is an understanding of the *market economy* and *economic cycles*. The United States is thought to be a market economy where prices are set by supply and demand. In a market economy, the amount of a product that is demanded by consumers usually indicates to managers within an industry how much of that product is to be manufactured and distributed to the marketplace.

The assumption is made that market forces, such as supply and demand, are the best determinants of what is right for a nation's well-being. In contrast, the opposite is a *command economy*, where most markets, from hearing aids to toilet paper, are controlled by a committee within the communist party. In command economies, there are often shortages of various products creating huge black markets that meet the product demands of the consumers. As previously presented, the U.S. economy and most other "free" markets are mixed economies and, to some degree, controlled by the government. For example, the U.S. government restricts the sale of alcohol to minors, thus limiting the free market. The same limitation applies to medications that must be prescribed by a licensed physician and dispensed by a licensed pharmacist. These markets, such as the U.S. market and other Western economies, are generally free markets, but there is some government intervention that regulates certain products and services, so they are technically referred to as *hybrid markets*.

Market economies are subject to natural economic cycles, which consist of a pattern of irregular expansion and contraction of the gross domestic product (GDP). GDP refers to the total monetary or market value of all

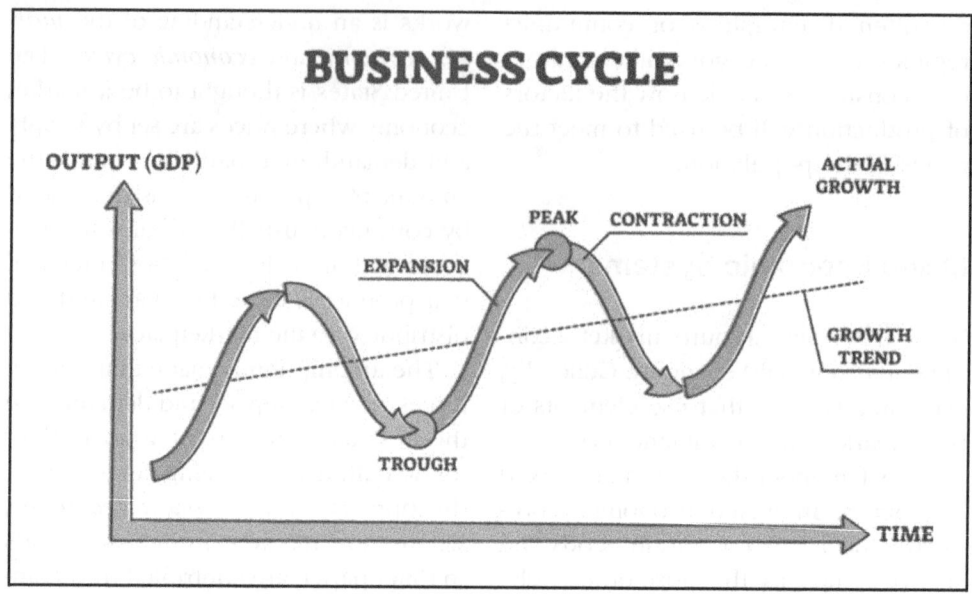

Figure 1–2. Market economic cycles. *Source:* VectorMine/Depositphotos.com.

finished goods and services produced within a country's borders in a specific time period. These business cycles, on average, last about 5 years and pass through four specific stages, *expansion or recovery, peak, contraction or recession*, and *trough*, each of which can vary in length and intensity, with many lasting only a few years. These expansions and contractions in the economy (Figure 1–2) are part of a continuous economic fluctuation that creates periods of prosperity and austerity.

In a recovery economy, businesses flourish, there is high employment, home values increase, and capital is readily available. This increases until the peak or the highest point in the cycle before the economic recession begins.

Recession creates a situation where austerity prevails and business is difficult, people lose jobs, mortgages are foreclosed, and business capital is scarce. A recession period has many different definitions, depending upon the orientation of those offering the definition. Generally, a *recession* occurs when an economic indicator, the GDP, has declined for 6 months or two consecutive quarters, while a *depression* is a serious contraction/recession that lasts longer than 18 months, such as the economic slowdown that occurred in the 1930s and possibly as recently as 2007 to 2013. The *trough* is the lowest point in the economic cycle marking the end of the recession period and the beginning of the recovery period.

Defining Economic Indicators and Their Implications for Audiologists

To fully appreciate some of these terms associated with a market economy and the economic business cycle, it is fundamental to interpret terms known as economic indicators. An economic indicator is a statistic relating to economic activity that allows analysis of economic performance and the predictions of possible future performance. There are many economic indicators, including gross domestic product, the national debt, deficit, interest rates, inflation, deflation, tax increases/decreases, currency value, retail sales, pending home sales, petroleum prices, unemployment, and others available in the news and from various websites. Economic data sometimes depend upon the analysis and point of view or political position. Policymakers, firms, and financial markets all want to know where an economy will likely head in the future. It can be critically important to gauge the current state of the economy and spot indicators of peaks and troughs (turning points) in the business cycle. Further insights can be gained from seeing how it has performed in the past. To assess this, Collin (2021 describes three sets of business cycle indicators used by economists: *leading*, *lagging*, and *coincident indicators.*

■ *Leading indicators* are used to help predict the future course of an economy; generally, the short term is 6 to 12 months ahead or up to 12 to 24 months in the longer term. The turning points of the business cycle are an indicator that tends to move up or move down several months before the economy itself moves. These indicators provide valuable early or advance signals of the likely direction or course of the economy.
■ *Lagging indicators* are those that track changes in the economy but,

typically, do not change direction until a few quarters after the economy moves into or out of a recession.
■ *Coincident indicators* are not so useful for predicting the future course of an economy but do provide valuable insights into the current or prevailing state of an economy.

Leading Economic Indicators

For a leading indicator to be reliable, the relationship between Gross Domestic Product (GDP) (a lagging indicator) and it should be statistically significant and stable over time (i.e., it should consistently lead GDP over time, and movements in this indicator should not be too erratic or volatile). For example, in the United States, treasury note yield, stock market, housing market, retail sales, and manufacturing activity are thought to be leading economic indicators for their reliability in predicting turning points of the U.S. economy.

Treasury Yield

When the U.S. government decides to borrow funds, it issues debt instruments through the U.S. Treasury. While bonds are a generic name for debt securities, treasury bonds, or T-bonds, refer specifically to U.S. government bonds with maturities of 20 to 30 years. U.S. government obligations with maturities above a year and up to 10 years are known as treasury notes. Treasury bills, or T-bills, are U.S. Treasury obligations that mature within a year.

Treasury yields are inversely related to treasury prices. When purchased by an investor, each treasury debt at maturity trades with its own yield (an expression of price). Treasury yield depends upon the effective annual interest rate that the U.S. government pays on one of its debt obligations, expressed as a percentage. Put another way, treasury yields do not simply affect how much the government pays to borrow money and how much investors earn by buying government bonds; they also *influence the interest rates consumers and businesses pay on loans* to buy real estate, vehicles, equipment, and working expenses. Therefore, these treasury yields also show how investors assess the economy's prospects for either a boom or a recession. The higher the yields on long-term U.S. treasuries, the more confidence investors have in the economic outlook because high long-term yields can also be a signal of rising inflation expectations. The U.S. Treasury publishes the yields of all treasury maturities daily on its website.

US Department of the Treasury
Interest Rate Statistics

Stock Market

The stock market has traditionally been viewed as an indicator or "predictor" or leading indicator of the economy. Many believe that large decreases in stock prices are reflective of a future recession, whereas large increases in stock prices suggest future economic growth. The stock market as an indicator of economic activity, however, does not go without controversy. Skeptics point to the strong economic growth that followed the 1987 stock market crash as reason to doubt the stock market's predictive ability.

Theoretical reasons for why stock prices might predict economic activity include the traditional valuation model of stock prices and the "wealth effect." The traditional valuation model of stock prices suggests that stock prices reflect expectations about the future economy and can, therefore, predict the economy. The wealth effect contends that stock prices lead economic activity by causing what happens to the economy.

Illian (2021) summarizes the skeptics in that the stock market eventually catches up to underlying economic conditions, so much so that economic conditions today could be indicative of stock market returns for the next several years. But such a conclusion would contradict the fact that today's stock market prices are any kind of leading indicator; instead, they are a litmus of current feelings about the state of things. So, there are those that believe that the stock market is a leading indicator and those that do not believe that the stock market is an indicator.

Housing Market

Economies and houses are both established on solid foundations, and the relationship between the two means that housing market numbers are part of the daily information diet for investors and traders. Released monthly by

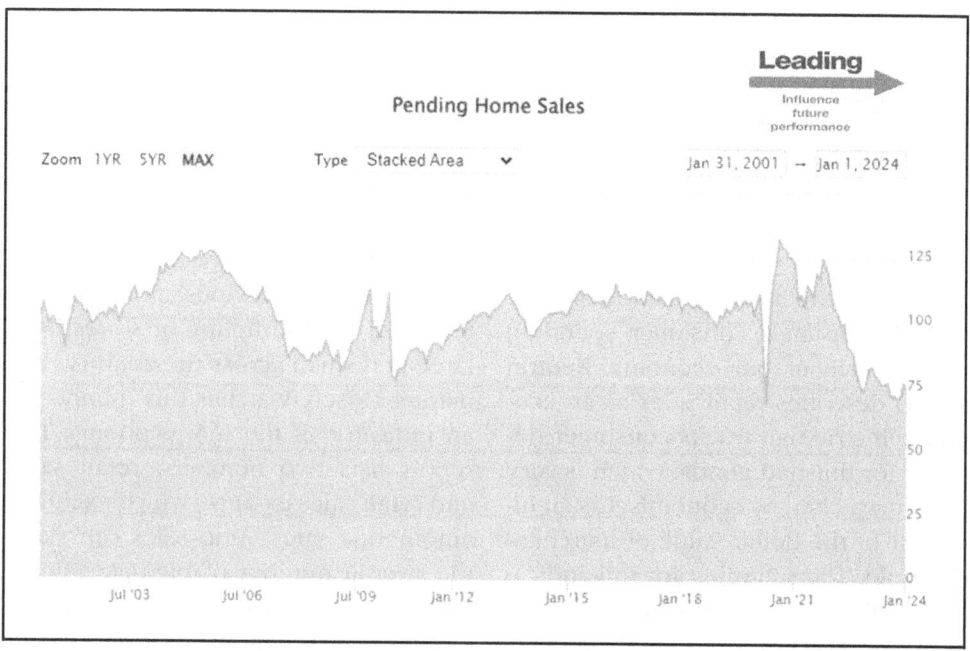

Figure 1–3. Pending home sales index 2002–2024. *Source:* Mortgage News Daily (2024).

the U.S. Census Bureau, housing starts and building permits are among the most widely followed leading indicators. Stronger or weaker-than-expected starts often move equity, bond, and commodity prices, which in turn are indicators as to a recession or a boom economy. People spend big money on not only their homes but also what goes in them, which means that housing data can be a leading indicator of economic activity months in advance.

For example, the housing market was booming until the Federal Reserve began to raise interest rates. Once these new interest rates were in place, the housing market was drastically reduced. There were plenty of houses available at reasonable prices, but the interest rates made payments so high that most people could not afford the house they wanted or where they wanted it. Thus,

it was a major indicator of the recessive economy that inflation had created.

The demand for housing can be an indication of the health of the economy in general. Purchasing a home requires the financial capability to pay the mortgage and maintain the dwelling. As housing demand increases, it can be inferred that people are either making more money or feeling more confident in their ability to make mortgage payments. The *Pending Home Sales Index* was created by the National Association of Realtors (NAR) and tracks homes sales where a contract is signed but the sale has not yet closed (Figure 1–3).

These pending sales are those that are set to close and all contingencies have been waived. This is when the lender, the escrow agent, or attorney will process the loan and title documents to make sure the deal will close on time. The Pending Home Sales Index is a leading indicator of future existing home sales as it typically takes 4 to 6 weeks to close a sale after a contract has been signed.

Retail Sales

Retail sales are an important economic indicator because consumer spending drives much of our economy. Kenton (2024) describes retail sales as an economic metric that tracks consumer demand for finished goods, which is very closely watched by economists as an indicator of the dollar value of merchandise sold. The sampling for this indicator is taken from companies engaged in the business of selling end products to consumers. Comprising 13 types of retailers from food service to retail stores, Kenton presents this figure as a very important data set as it is a key monthly market-moving event that indicates the direction of the economy. It acts as a key economic barometer and whether inflationary pressures exist. Retail sales are measured by durable

and nondurable goods purchased over a defined period. When consumers purchase goods and services, the economy tends to move along rather well.

To monitor these retail sales, the Census Bureau, on or about the 12th of every month, releases the Retail Sales Index, which is a measure of retail sales from the previous month as determined by a sampling of stores both large and small across the country. The market closely watches this number as an indicator of the U.S. economy. The report lists two numbers: retail sales and retail sales ex-auto, which excludes automobile sales. Auto sales can skew the overall number of big-ticket items and are subject to seasonal fluctuations.

Figure 1–4 demonstrates the retail sales index from 2019 to 2024. Kenton (2024) offers a summary of the value of retail sales reports:

- The retail sales data are extremely timely. They are released 2 weeks after the month they cover.
- Retail sales reports get a lot of press. They are an indicator that

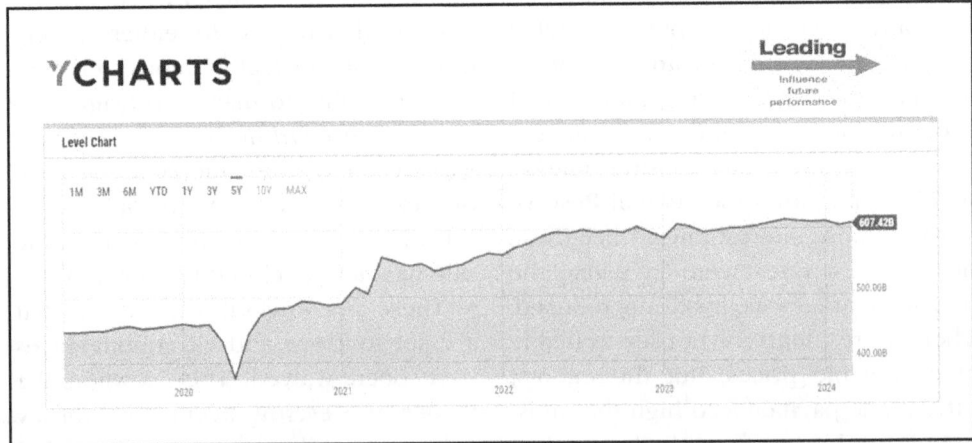

Figure 1–4. U.S. retail sales index 2019–2024. *Source:* Y-Charts (2024).

is easy to understand and relates closely to the average consumer.

■ A revised report comes out later (2 to 3 months on average), amending any errors.

■ Analysts and economists will take out volatile components to show underlying demand patterns. The most volatile components are autos, gas, and food prices.

■ Data are adjusted seasonally, monthly, and for holiday differences.

While the Retail Sales Index can be somewhat volatile and adjustments are often quite large, it is an indication of consumer activity. It does not include services, only products that are manufactured and purchased.

Manufacturing Activity

Manufacturing activities refer to all activities involved in the production, storing, handling, packaging, labeling, and distribution of products to be developed or commercialized. Manufacturing activities may include:

■ Creation and design of the product packaging.

■ Creation and implementation of a commercial inventory and product supply chain distribution strategy.

■ The manufacture of clinical and commercial inventory for the product.

■ The manufacture of a delivery device for the product.

■ The manufacture of the packaging for the product.

■ Quality control and quality assurance of the product.

Obviously, manufacturing activities include a number of activities that re-

quire many operations and employees to conduct those operations. Modifications in manufacturing can be influenced by supply shortage of goods, transportation reduction, chips for vehicles, inflation, high interest rates, consumer slowdown, less fuel supplies, bank defaults, and other economic disruption. Virtually anything that causes issues with the manufacturing process can cause interruptions that lead to economic concerns about a slowdown, which can predict a recession. Conversely, issues that are caused by too much business can also lead to an economic cue that hints that the economy is booming so much that many of these necessary components or other manufacturing concerns are at risk.

Figure 1–5 presents manufacturing activity. Areas below the dashed line represent contraction of the manufacturing activity and areas above the dashed line represent expansion of manufacturing activity. Although manufacturing took a major dip in 2020 due to the COVID-19 pandemic, it recovered in 2021 as a result of a shortage of goods and people purchased items that had not been available during the shortages. After the initial recovery in 2021, manufacturing activity has gone down due to all of those factors mentioned previously above and does not predict a good economy for 2024, as manufacturing has still not recovered into the expansion area. Thus, manufacturing is a good leading indicator of recession or boom economies.

In summary, leading economic indicators represent statistical data showing past or future trends in an economy. They tend to be those that can indicate changes for either boom or recession components of the business

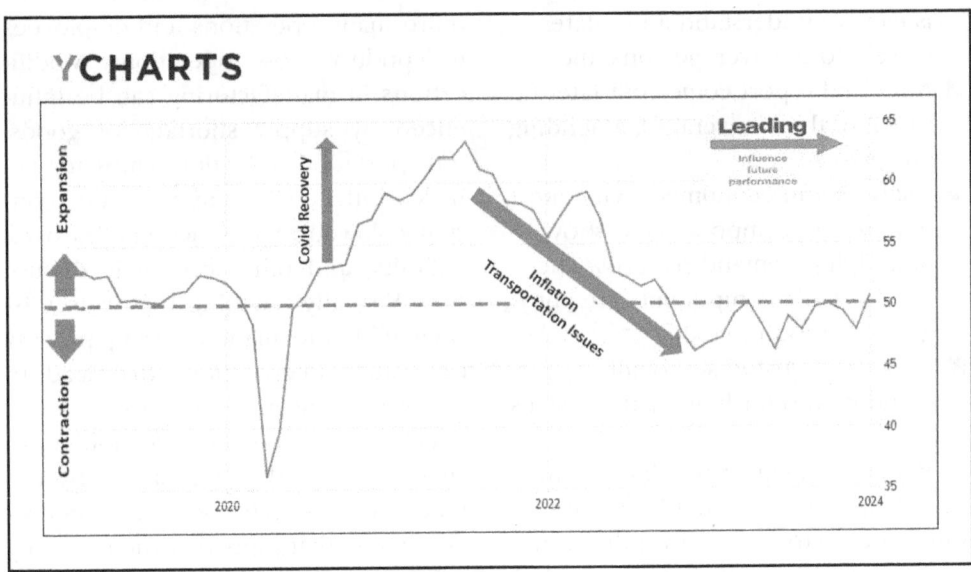

Figure 1–5. Manufacturing activity 2019–2024. *Source:* Y-Charts (2024).

cycle. Audiology practice managers can use these data to predict if it is time for new equipment or locations, new employees, or other major changes in practice patterns. They can also use these to retract various expansions, new procedures, or other projects until the projections are more positive. By reviewing economic data, business investments, purchases, or sales can be considered in view of the current economic cycle.

Lagging Economic Indicators

Lagging indicators can only be known after the event: either a recession or a boom economy. These indicators clarify and confirm an economic pattern that is occurring over time. For example, the unemployment rate is typically one of the most reliable lagging indica-

tors. If the unemployment rate rose last month and the month before, it would indicate that the overall economy has been doing poorly and may well continue to do poorly. The Consumer Price Index (CPI), which measures changes in the inflation rate, is another closely watched lagging indicator. There are few events that cause more economic ripple effects than price increases. Both the overall number and prices in key industries like fuel or medical costs are of interest. Currently, there are lagging costs in food due to a fertilizer shortage as well as feed shortage for livestock.

Gross Domestic Product (GDP)

Fernando (2023) describes the *gross domestic product (GDP)* as the total monetary or market value of all the finished goods and services produced within a country's borders in a specific period. It is a broad measure of overall domestic production that functions as

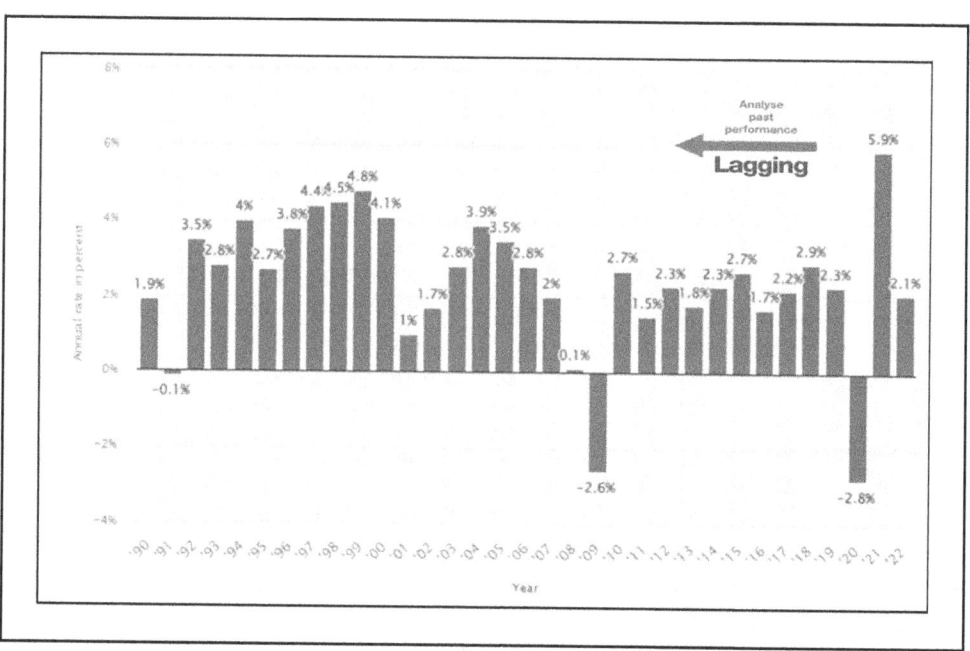

Figure 1–6. Gross domestic product 1990–2022. *Source:* Statistica (2024).

a comprehensive scorecard of a given country's economic health. Although GDP is typically calculated on an annual basis, it is sometimes calculated on a quarterly basis to obtain perspective over a longer period. In the United States, for example, the government releases an annualized GDP estimate for each fiscal quarter and also for the calendar year. GDP is, therefore, a calculation of the total market value of all final goods and services produced in a country each year (Figure 1–6).

The values are usually published quarterly and offer some idea of the performance of the economy during the period. The GDP report is released on the last day of each quarter and reflects the growth in the value of goods and services over the past quarter. Growth in GDP is what is important and the United States. GDP growth has historically averaged about 2.5% to 3%

per year but with substantial deviations. For example, if the GDP calculation is up by 4%, the suggestion is that the economy grew by 4%. Conversely, if the economy is down by 4%, then the economy shrunk by 4% and the value of goods and services became less during the period. During a period termed the "great recession" (2008–2009), GDP had some huge swings ranging from –8% (negative) to 4% (positive) growth presented in Figure 1–6 as 1% in 2008 and –2.6% in 2009. GDP can be figured on the expenditures of companies but is more commonly considered on income since income figures are used for tax reporting. As would be expected during a time when most businesses closed, a huge drop in GDP to –2.8% was seen during the COVID-19 pandemic of 2020–2021 (Figure 1–6).

In the United States and other countries, changes in the GDP affect the stock market either positively or negatively. The market is affected due to the indication of reduced productivity. As the GDP falls, it indicates less demand for goods and services, which affects corporate profits. If the trend continues, companies will lay off or discharge employees, creating unemployment. While GDP is an indication of the performance of the economy, politicians and government agencies often manipulate the data by including some things and leaving out others such that the GDP calculation moves either up or down to suit their needs. For example, particularly in 2008, leaving out the housing market made the figure look much better than if it was figured into the GDP. During the years after the COVID-19 pandemic of 2020–2021, there were many items left out of the GDP to suggest the economy was doing well when it was actually leading to the huge inflation seen in 2021–2022. These manipulations have caused difficulties in reviewing the health of economies, not only in the United States but also around the world.

It is important to differentiate GDP from gross national product (GNP). GDP includes only goods and services produced within the geographic boundaries of the country in question. GNP is the value of all finished goods and services produced by a country's citizens, both domestically and abroad. Thus, the GNP includes goods and services produced by U.S. firms operating in foreign countries.

Interest Rates

The Federal Reserve of the United States is directly responsible for maintaining economic stability. It is the central bank of the United States, created by Congress in 1913 to provide a stable, safe, and flexible financial system. According to the Federal Reserve (2024), their responsibilities fall into four general areas:

- Conducting the nation's monetary policy by influencing money and credit conditions in the economy in pursuit of full employment and stable prices.
- Supervising and regulating banks and other important financial institutions to ensure the safety of the nation's banking and financial system and to protect the credit rights of consumers.
- Maintaining the stability of the financial system and containing systemic risk that may arise from time to time in financial markets.
- Providing financial services to the U.S. government, U.S. financial institutions, and official foreign institutions. Additionally, it plays a major role in operating and overseeing the nation's payment systems.

The most powerful weapon at the disposal of the Federal Reserve is the ability to influence the direction of interest rates. Interest rates are the amounts charged for borrowing money from a bank or other lending institution. The Federal Reserve sets these rates, which are reviewed by the institutions to decide how much to charge customers seeking personal, business, or mortgage loans. The interest rate at which eligible banks may borrow funds directly from a Federal Reserve bank is called the *discount rate*. When discount rates are low, capital is usually easier to acquire, and vice versa,

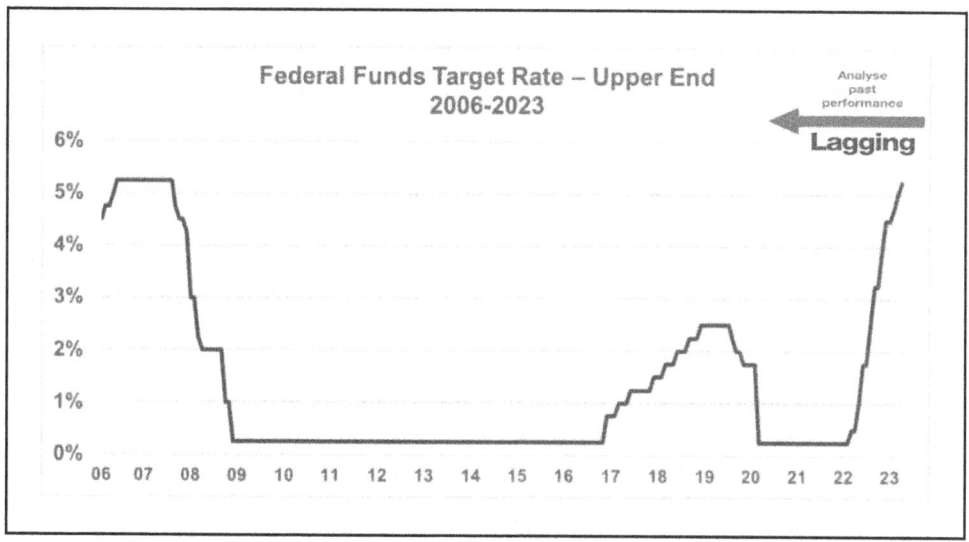

Figure 1–7. Changes in Federal Reserve interest rates 2006–2023. *Source:* U.S. Bank (2023).

when prime rates are higher, capital funds are more difficult to obtain. The interest rate charged to the customer is considered the "retail" interest rate. The difference between the Federal Reserve rate and that charged by the lending institution is bank profit.

Currently, Prime Rate (2024) reports that the Federal Reserve prime rate is 5.25% to 5.50% for funds received by banks through the system (Figure 1–7). So, if a bank needs to purchase funds at 5.50%, they will usually mark up that rate for their very best customers by 3% (some banks charge more and some charge less). This puts the lowest rate for the very best customers at 8.50%, sometimes called the *prime rate*. Business loans are usually higher, particularly for new bank customers and those with less than perfect credit, if they can obtain a loan at all.

So, if the bank charges 8.50% to borrow funds, their profit is still 3.00% on the loan. Typically, when the economy is

in recession and requires stimulation, interest rates are lowered so that funds are more readily available. When the economy is flourishing, it is kept in check by raising interest rates, which controls the flow of capital, which subsequently controls economic growth. Although that seems like a rather simple concept, new and restrictive banking regulations imposed by the government have made the process extremely complex.

Berman (2023) describes the regulations presented in the Wall Street Reform and Consumer Protection Act (also called the Dodd–Frank Bill), which was enacted due to the "great recession" of 2008. Dodd–Frank requires small banks to have more assets to award loans and new underwriting laws involving more documentation, thus adding extra layers of paperwork increasing the length of the loan process. Further, there is no incentive for banks to loan funds to small businesses as there is not much return on investment due to the low interest rates. As a result, during recessionary times, audiologists may find it difficult to obtain funds to purchase practices, finance expansion, and obtain working capital. With these constraints, alternative funding sources have been used by practices such as independent lines of credit and support through hearing instrument manufacturers, buying groups, and others within the industry. While these are ready sources of capital, some ethical issues can complicate their use (Chapter 23). Since funds can be retracted from banks and other traditional lending institutions, and there are ethical issues involved with borrowing from vendors within the profession, other forms of funding have risen to raise capital. While these are usually easily obtainable loans, they carry heavy interest rates and must be reviewed carefully by attorneys to ensure that the lender is legitimate.

Inflation/Deflation

Fernando (2024) defines *inflation* as a rise in prices, which can be translated as the decline of purchasing power over time. The rate at which purchasing power drops can be reflected in the average price increase of a basket of selected goods and services over some time. The rise in prices, which is often expressed as a percentage, simply means that a unit of currency effectively buys less than it did in prior periods. Inflation can be contrasted with *deflation*, which occurs when prices decline and purchasing power increases.

The Federal Reserve causes discount interest rates to rise and fall to reduce the possibility of inflation or deflation. When the economy is in a boom, funds are easier to obtain and interest rates are favorable and, when not controlled, inflation occurs. If the economic stability is out of balance, there can be an increase or decrease in the cost of goods and services, suggesting that the value of money becomes less, *inflation*, or the value of money is greater, *deflation*. The Federal Reserve uses their capability to set the discount rate to control the supply of available funds and the overall (or retail) interest rates. Traditionally, the more funds available at lower interest rates, the more likely inflation will occur. By raising the prime rate, the Federal Reserve makes it more expensive for banks to borrow at the prime rate and thus the "retail" interest rate becomes higher. Subsequently, the higher cost of funds causes money to be scarce and slows the economy down, thus reducing the possibility of inflation.

Inflation is typically measured by the *Consumer Price Index (CPI)*. Fernando (2024) defines the CPI as a measure that examines the weighted average of the price of a basket of consumer goods and services within various economic sectors, such as transportation, food, or medical care. The CPI is calculated by taking price changes for each item in the predetermined basket of goods, averaging them, and then comparing them to the previous period's assessment. Associated with the cost of living, changes in CPI are measured by the higher (inflation) or lower (deflation) cost calculations of these goods and services. The CPI includes roughly 88% of the total population, accounting for wage earners, clerical workers, technical workers, self-employed, short-term workers, unemployed, retirees, and those not in the labor force. Figure 1–8 presents the annual inflation rate over the past 10 years in the United States, reviewing the years 2014 through 2020 when inflation was

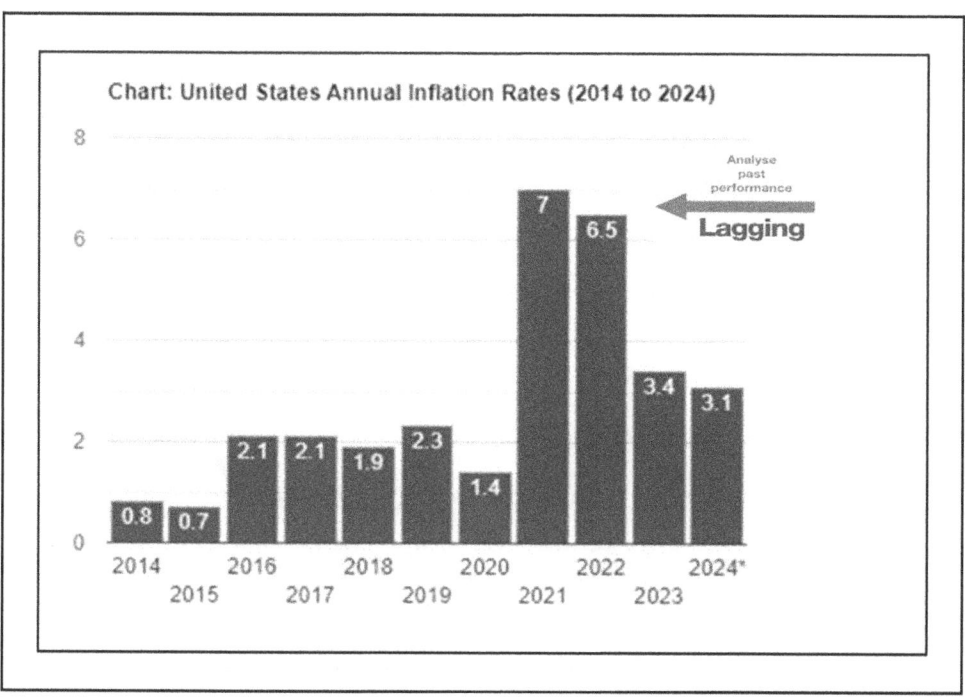

Figure 1–8. Annual inflation rate 2014–2024. *Source:* U.S. Inflation Calculator (2024).

between .8% and 2.3%. Excessive government spending during these years suggested that the *real inflation rate* was 9.1% during this time (U.S. Bureau of Labor Statistics, 2022). Thus, the dollar was worth approximately 10% less in 2022 than it was in 2020.

National Debt

National debt is the total amount of debt that the federal government owes on funds that it has borrowed to keep the country solvent. As Lang (2021) presents in Figure 1–9, this is tremendous: first the COVID-19 spending to keep the country from bankruptcy and then the stimulus packages of the Biden administration, which ramped the nation's debt up to the highest level in history.

At this writing, the U.S. national debt is over $36 trillion and can be easily checked any time for the exact amount at National Debt Clock (2024). This site presents not only the amount the United States owes overall but also how much is owed by each individual citizen, currently hovering over $101,949. Although simply owing money is critical, the public policy problems that created the debt must be adjusted or the country will go bankrupt. Smith (2023) indicates that three major components are essential to controlling additions and reducing the national debt. These major adjustments involve one of three modifications:

■ Print more money.
■ Raise taxes.
■ Reduce government spending.

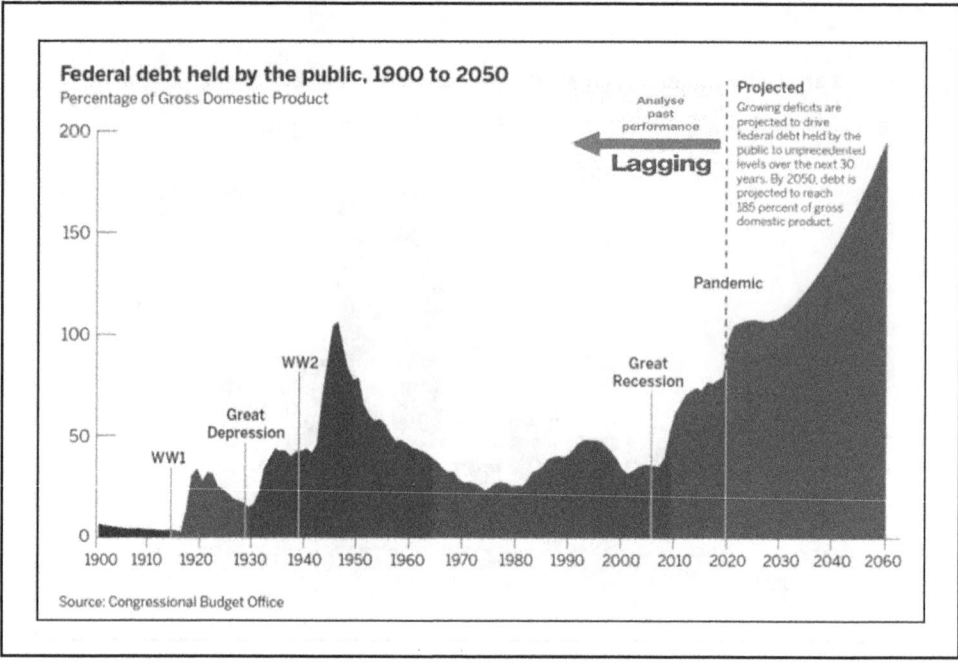

Figure 1–9. National debt 1900–2020, estimated 2020–2060. *Source:* American Banker (2021).

No matter which of these solutions is chosen, none are good for audiology.

Printing Money

The basic issue with the government simply printing more money is inflation and that government bonds that are sold to pay off debt and fund the government would become devalued. People who purchase these bonds (i.e., U.S. Savings Bonds) believe that these government bonds are a safe investment. This notion that the government bonds are a secure investment assumes that inflation is low. If the government prints money to pay off the national debt, it is almost assured that inflation will rise. As inflation increases, people will not want to hold bonds because their value decreases. Subsequently, the government will need to increase the interest rate that they pay those who hold onto the bonds or purchase more. Further, if the government prints too much money and inflation gets out of hand, it will be difficult for entities, such as businesses, to borrow any funds at all. The likelihood of more money being printed to pay the government's obligations is minimal since this process typically leads to rampant inflation, and within a brief period, the currency becomes worthless. Therefore, the options of either a tax increase or reducing government benefits become more realistic methods to solve the problem.

Raising Taxes

Raising revenue seems a logical solution for funding a national debt that is out of control. By increasing taxes, more revenue becomes available to the government to pay down its debt, and in turn, inflation will be reduced, and funds will become more available. Patients, however, are taxed at higher rates, which results in reduced disposable income available for other necessities. Since most audiology patients are in the last one-third of their life, greater taxes reduce their ability to pay for audiological services, purchase hearing instruments, and/or service their current instruments. Practice managers would need to consider cutting expenses, key personnel, and other services, compromising patient care.

Reducing Government Spending

Reduction of government spending limits, entitlement programs such as Medicare, Medicaid, Social Security, and welfare. These government service cutbacks reduce the debt of the government while simultaneously reducing the ability of patients to pay for services. Citizens have paid into these programs most of their lives, and the government has used these funds for other objectives. As such, there may be limited or no funding available when it comes their turn to receive the benefit. By reducing the cost parameters for these programs, the debt can be reduced with funds taken in through taxes rather than borrowing more funds, which increases the national debt. The question then becomes which programs should be cut, how much, and what are the effects of the changes.

While the elimination of these programs is virtually impossible, Medicare and Medicaid reimbursement to all healthcare professionals has suffered significantly, and these cuts have been disastrous to some practices. While these spending cuts are serious issues, a high national debt creates other problems as well, such as reduced value of the dollar, interest rate increases, and inflation.

Deficit Spending

Deficit spending simply refers to the amount that has been borrowed in a specific period. While the government could continue deficit spending and still provide these services, such as Medicare, Social Security, and other government spending projects, currency values are usually the result of a high or low national debt. Currently, if the federal government spends a dollar of their funds and they had to borrow 40 cents of that dollar, then 40 cents of each dollar is the deficit. To present these costs as real numbers, if they spend a trillion dollars, then they must borrow 400 billion of that amount and pay interest on that amount. In most countries, currency reflects their national identity, the value of the specific country's goods and services according to *their* national debt, and the country's political policies. The U.S. dollar has been known as one of the world's most stable and reliable currencies for well over 100 years and is even used in many countries as their currency. As the U.S. national debt has increased, the value of the U.S. dollar has decreased. Mae (2023) states that the dollar has decreased in value by 25% in the past 10 years. Thus, what cost $1.00 in 2013 now costs $1.25, or a car that cost $20,000 in 2013 now costs $5,000 more in 2024 for the same vehicle.

When residing in another country, most people in that country prefer that you pay your bills and other financial obligations in their currency.

It is a system that they understand and use daily as the preferred method of payment. As the national debt has increased over the past 10 years, the value of the U.S. dollar has decreased significantly. For example, in 1999, the dollar was worth $1.80 in Swiss francs (CHF). In May 2017, the same U.S. dollar was only worth $0.97 CHF. This substantial decrease is a direct result of the high national debt brought about by the substantial deficit spending during the past 10 years. In another example, in 1999, the U.S. dollar was on par with the euro (1 U.S. dollar = 1 euro), the currency used by most of the countries in Europe. In May 2017, the same U.S. dollar was worth about €0.89. Audiologists need to be concerned when the dollar is low against European currencies because most amplification products, equipment, and many other products come from these countries.

Unemployment Rate

Unemployment statistics represent an attempt to estimate the number of people who want, but cannot find, work. The data are most often used as measures of labor force utilization and indicators of general economic activity. The use of these measures seems reasonable since unemployment, in principle, means human resources are idled and productive opportunities are foregone. During periods of contraction/recession, an economy usually experiences a relatively high unemployment rate.

Okun's Law

When economists are studying the economy, they tend to focus on two factors: *economic output and jobs.* Because there is a relationship between these two elements of an economy, many economists study the relationship between output (or, more specifically, gross domestic product) and unemployment levels. Arthur Okun, a Yale economics professor who served on President John F. Kennedy's Council of Economic Advisors in the early 1960s, studied the relationship between unemployment and economic production. His study led to *Okun's law*, describing a relationship between GDP and unemployment. Okun's law is an empirically observed relationship between unemployment and losses in a country's production. It predicts that a 1% drop in employment tends to be accompanied by a drop in GDP of around 2%. Likewise, a 1% increase in employment is associated with a 2% GDP increase. Although Okun's law is not derived from any theoretical prediction, observational data indicate that Okun's law often holds true.

Okun's law is not without controversy, and some economists disagree about the exact relationship between employment and productivity. Others such as Fuhrmann (2023) suggest that Okun's law really means the economy must grow at about a 4% rate for 1 year to achieve a 1 percentage point reduction in the rate of unemployment. Kenton (2022) summarizes the use of Okun's law. He feels that it is an observation about the statistical correlation between unemployment levels and overall productivity, and while there have been many times when these variables did not behave as Okun's law predicts, the rule appears to hold true overall.

While there remains considerable theoretical debate as to the causes, consequences, and solutions for unemployment, there is valuable information that can be discerned. If unemployment is rising, it is an indication that the demand for goods and services is down; companies are laying off workers who produce the goods and provide the services, suggesting an impending recession. Conversely, when unemployment is low, the situation suggests there is demand for goods and services, which represents an indication the economy is stable or increasing.

Current Population Survey

The Current Population Survey (CPS), conducted by the U.S. Bureau of Labor Statistics (BLS), is a key source of data on U.S. unemployment. This monthly survey of households provides a comprehensive body of data on the labor force, employment, unemployment, persons not in the labor force, hours of work, earnings, and other demographic and labor force characteristics. The national unemployment rate is derived from this survey and is the number most touted by the media to summarize the state of the economy. The survey presents:

- All people who worked for pay or profit during the survey reference week.
- All people who did at least 15 hours of unpaid work in a family-owned enterprise operated by someone in their household.
- All persons who were temporarily absent from their regular jobs, whether they were paid or not, including those who were on vacation, ill, experiencing child-care problems, dealing with family or personal obligations, on maternity

or paternity leave, involved in an industrial dispute, or prevented from working because of bad weather.

Although unemployment figures can offer some indication as to the ups or downs of the economy, Dollarhide (2023) states that these data do not present the whole picture of unemployment. The CPS method doesn't provide essential details about how American workers are really faring and how race and gender impact unemployment and underemployment. It is essential to examine the many factors not considered by the Current Population Survey, for example, whether an employed person has taken unpaid leave, how many workers are underemployed and not earning enough money to pay their bills, or if a worker has given up on their job search. In her opinion, there are significant issues not presented by these surveys:

- Whether workers have full-time hours. The CPS counts people as employed if they are working at part-time or temporary jobs, regardless of the number of hours worked or whether this employment represents a sufficient or ideal employment situation for that worker.
- Whether workers are "underemployed": Working at a job that requires fewer skills and offers lower pay than the best jobs for which a worker is qualified. These individuals should also be considered involuntary part-time workers.
- Whether a worker has given up looking for a job, even though they need one. These government surveys only count as unemployed those who "do not have a job, have actively looked for work in the

prior four weeks, and are currently available for work." If the worker has a "temporary illness" such as a cold, they are still considered available for work by the survey. Others not considered as part of the labor force in these surveys include prisoners, people confined to nursing homes, members of the Armed Forces on active duty, homemakers, students, and retired persons.

While these data are difficult to use for accurately comparing unemployment across years or periods, comparisons of unemployment from one period to another do not usually reflect the changing population in terms of age, immigration, education levels, and other factors. These are just a few of the problems with relying too heavily on the national unemployment rate as a meaningful indicator of the state of the economy and its workforce. Unfortunately, this often means that the true percentage of people who do not have jobs or do not make enough money to survive is often worse than suggested by the unemployment rates. Unemployment figures can and will be manipulated by the government to reflect a situation that is better than what exists. However, the CPS can be an indication that the economy is either on its way up or down and can offer some suggestions as to how much risk clinicians are willing to take in hiring, expanding, or making other business modifications.

COVID-19 Pandemic Unemployment

The COVID-19 outbreak and the economic downturn it created swelled the ranks of unemployed Americans. Koch-

har (2020) states that unemployment increased by more than 14 million, from 6.2 million in February to 20.5 million in May 2020. As a result, the U.S. unemployment rate shot up from 3.8% in February 2020, among the lowest on record in the post–World War II era, to 13.0% in May 2020. That rate was the era's second highest, trailing only the level reached in April 2020 of 14.4% (Figure 1–10).

The COVID-19 pandemic created huge panic among the workforce that caused many to work from home, create their own businesses, and leave the workforce. During this time, there was great upheaval within the business world to keep employees working so that business could survive. It was extremely difficult to juggle the revenue and keep employees. While this strained businesses, the pandemic led to big changes in employment and operations. Many businesses, including audiology practices, closed while others used ingenuity to stay open and provide services and products under new regulations and operating constraints. For example, audiology clinics had significant changes in how they conducted patient visits, evaluations, and the fitting and servicing of hearing aids. The rise of telehealth interactions and remote fine-tuning of products greatly assisted patient care while accommodating nonexposure to the virus (Traynor, 2020).

Coincident Economic Indicators

Coincident indicators are statistical indicators that usually change simultaneously with general economic conditions

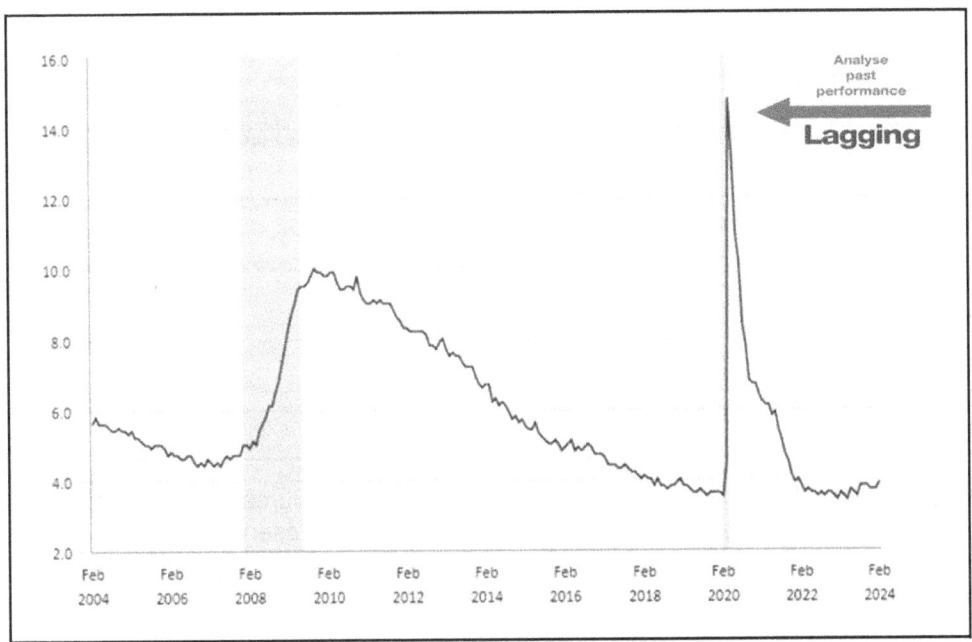

Figure 1–10. Unemployment rate 2004–2022. *Source:* U.S. Bureau of Labor Statistics (2024).

and, as a result, are viewed as reflecting the current state of the economy. While leading indicators look ahead and lagging indicators look behind, coincident indicators reflect the present or very recent past. Personal income is a major coincident indicator of economic health. Higher personal income numbers coincide with a stronger economy. Lower personal income numbers mean the economy is struggling.

Personal Income

Kagan (2023) indicates that personal income refers to all income collectively received by all individuals or households in a country. Personal income includes compensation from a number of sources, including salaries, wages and bonuses received from employment or self-employment, dividends and dis-

tributions received from investments, rental receipts from real estate investments, and profit sharing from businesses. It is tracked as a coincident indicator of the amount of personal income highs and lows, which are directly related to the taxes people pay. The government is interested in this income as it indicates that taxes will be easier to pay if the personal income is high or harder to pay if the personal income is low, all of which is directly related to economic conditions.

Personal income also has a significant effect on consumer consumption because consumer spending drives much of the economy, national statistical organizations, and economists, which is why analysts track personal income on a quarterly or annual basis. In the United States, the Bureau of Economic Analysis (BEA) tracks personal

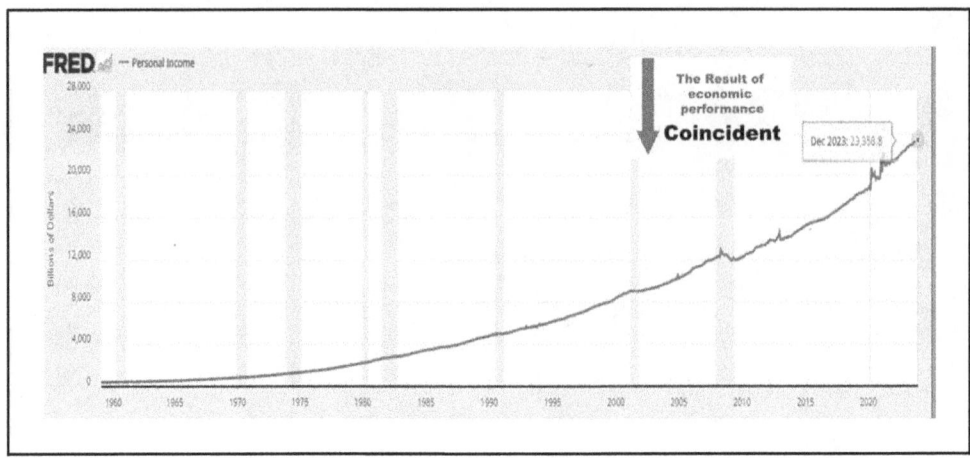

Figure 1–11. Personal income 1959–2023. *Source:* U.S. Bureau of Economic Analysis, Personal Income [PI], retrieved from FRED, Federal Reserve Bank of St. Louis; https://fred.stlouisfed.org/series/PI.

income statistics each month and compares them to numbers from the previous month. The agency also breaks out the numbers into categories, such as personal income earned through employment wages, rental income, farming, and sole proprietorships (Chapter 3), allowing analyses of changing earning trends. Personal income tends to rise during periods of economic expansion and stagnate or decline slightly during recessionary times (Figure 1–11).

Summary

Economics is the primary interest of investors, central bankers, policymakers, and corporate executives. While our first responsibility as audiologists is to our patients, managers and owners would be unwise to not be apprised of and understand the economic conditions in which they live, work, start, or expand practices. Audiology clinic owners should understand economic basics and consider the state of the economy as it affects their clinic operations and profitability.

References

Bennis, W. (2003). *On becoming a leader* (2nd ed.). Perseus Publishing.

Berman, N. (2023). What is the Dodd-Frank Act? Council on Foreign Relations. https://www.cfr.org/backgrounder/what-dodd-frank-act

Board of Governors of the Federal Reserve. (2024). What is the purpose of the Federal Reserve? https://www.federalreserve.gov/faqs/about_12594.htm

Burrow, J. L., Kleindl, B. A., & Becraft, M. B. (2016). *Business management*. South-Western Cengage.

Collin, V. (2021). Leading, lagging and coincident economic indicators. Financial Edge. https://www.fe.training/free-resources/financial-markets/leading-lagging-coincident-economic-indicators/

Dollarhide, M. (2023). What the unemployment rate does not tell us. Investopedia. What the Unemployment Rate Doesn't Tell Us (investopedia.com)

Drucker, P. F. (2001). *The essential Drucker.* Harper.

Federal Reserve. (2024). What is the purpose of the Federal Reserve System? https://www.federalreserve.gov/faqs/about_12594.htm

Fernando, J. (2023). Gross domestic product (GDP): Formula and how to use it. Investopedia. Gross Domestic Product (GDP): Formula and How to Use It (investopedia.com)

Fernando, J. (2024). Consumer Price Index (CPI): What it is and how it's used. Investopedia.com. https://www.investopedia.com/terms/i/inflation.asp

Fred. (2023). Fred economic data: Personal income 1959–2023. Bureau of Economic Analysis, Department of Commerce. https://fred.stlouisfed.org/series/PI

Fuhrmann, R. C. (2023). Okun's Law: Economic growth and unemployment. Investopedia. http://www.investopedia.com/articles/economics/12/okuns-law.asp

Haynes, A. (2024). Entrepreneur: What it means to be one and how to get started. Investopedia. https://www.investopedia.com/terms/e/entrepreneur.asp

Illian, I. (2021). Think the stock market is a leading economic indicator? Think again. Forbes, https://www.forbes.com/sites/forbesfinancecouncil/2021/02/25/think-the-stock-market-is-a-leading-economic-indicator-think-again/?sh=66bb22d83136

Investor Words. (2016). Definition of gross domestic product (GDP). Invstorwords. http://www.investorwords.com/2153/GDP.html

Kagan, J. (2023). Personal income definition and difference from disposable income. Investopedia. https://www.investopedia.com/terms/p/personalincome.asp#:~:text=Personal%20income%20is%20often

%20compared,(GNI)%20and%20personal%20income?

Kenton, W. (2022). Okun's law: Definition, formula, history, and limitations. Investopedia. https://www.investopedia.com/terms/o/okunslaw.asp

Kenton, W. (2024). Retail Sales Index. Investopedia. http://www.investopedia.com/terms/r/retail-sales.asp?lgl=no-infinite

Kochhar, R. (2020). Unemployment rose higher in three months of COVID-19 than it did in two years of the Great Recession. Pew Research Center. How U.S. unemployment during COVID-19 compares with Great Recession | Pew Research Center

Lang, H. (2021). The national debt is big and getting bigger. Does it matter? American Banker. https://www.americanbanker.com/news/the-national-debt-is-big-and-getting-bigger-does-it-matter

Mae, A. (2023). Your dollar buys 25% less than it did 10 years ago: What will it be worth in 10 years? Yahoofinance. https://finance.yahoo.com/news/dollar-buys-25-less-did-210104013.html?guccounter=1&guce_referrer=aHR0cHM6Ly93d3cuZ29vZ2xlLmNvbS8&guce_referrer_sig=AQAAAALJCRffREumc7LiTwdg713lDQEQs6oMSsvWJ_SC8_aE-g2Ht6_oBDkYh-MP7296KJ6b-cL-BG5aFe2G7xsYl3jnvIefj-9ql_pMvrWuTT0vqpxQ2-UQT5k1-onvlAxS-N5eVjhwJVecd9kHpIS3U7LGL104lu_huy3A8L9eANCkHo

Mortgage News Daily. (2024). Pending home sales. https://www.mortgagenewsdaily.com/data/pending-home-sales

National Debt Clock. (2024). The National Debt Clock. https://www.usdebtclock.org/index.html?taxpayer

PMI. (2024). Manufacturing activity. https://ycharts.com/indicators/us_pmi#:~:text=US%20ISM%20Manufacturing%20PMI%20is,manufacturing%20sector%20in%20the%20US

Prime Rate. (2024). Federal Reserve prime rate. Primerate.com. https://www.fedprimerate

.com/#:~:text=United%20States%20
Prime%20Rate&text=target%20range%20
for%20the%20fed,at%205.25%25%20
%2D%205.50%25.

Rodrigo, G. C. (2016). Micro and macro: The economic divide. Finance and Development. http://www.imf.org/external/pubs/ft/fandd/basics/bigsmall.htm

Smith, L. (2023). 5 Ways governments reduce national debt. *Investopedia*. https://www.investopedia.com/articles/economics/11/successful-ways-government-reduces-debt.asp

Statistica. (2024). Gross domestic product 1990-2022. https://www.statista.com/statistics/188165/annual-gdp-growth-of-the-united-states-since-1990/

Stoll, R. (2023). Understanding stock market and economic cycles. Financial Design Studio. https://financialdesignstudio.com/understanding-stock-market-and-economic-cycles/

Taylor, B. (2012). *Consultative selling skills for audiologists*. Plural Publishing.

Traynor, R. M. (2020). Competing in a new era of hearing healthcare Part 4: Differentiating your practice in the COVID era and beyond. *Hearing Review, 27*, 18–22.

U.S. Bank. (2024). Federal funds target rate: Upper end 2006–2023. https://luckbox
magazine.com/topics/3-reasons-the-2023-bull-run-continues/

U.S. Bureau of Labor Statistics. (2022). Consumer prices up 9.1 percent over the year ended June 2022, largest increase in 40 years. https://www.bls.gov/opub/ted/2022/consumer-prices-up-9-1-percent-over-the-year-ended-june-2022-largest-increase-in-40-years.htm

U.S. Bureau of Labor Statistics. (2024). Civilian unemployment rate. https://www.bls.gov/charts/employment-situation/civilian-unemployment-rate.htm

Y-Charts. (2024). U.S. retail sales 2023–2024. https://ycharts.com/indicators/us_retail_sales

2 Legal Considerations in Practice Management

Brandon T. Pauley, Esq

Disclaimer

These materials are prepared for general informational purposes only. It is not intended and should not be used for specific legal advice in a specific factual situation. Questions about the legal issues discussed in these materials should be presented to knowledgeable legal counsel with respect to any given factual situation before deciding on a specific course of action.

Introduction

This chapter is intended to briefly highlight several of the issues facing practicing audiologists. The substance is broad and intended to touch on numerous issues with an emphasis placed on guidance for the aspiring independent practice owner. As with many walks in life, surrounding yourself with knowledgeable and trusted advisors having expertise in certain areas can greatly lessen the stress and uncertainty that naturally comes with being an entrepreneur in the healthcare space. The first section highlights the importance of finding quality advisors, provides an overview of laws applicable to audiology practices, and then delves into various, specific legal issues commonly encountered in audiology.

Securing Professional Advisors

Depending on the selected career (such as becoming an employee rather than starting and operating a business), engaging professional advisors may be necessary to assist with various issues. For example, practice owners are entrepreneurs. Entrepreneurs are forced to wear many hats at any given time, outsourcing to surround themselves with experienced professionals and experts, which can be of great utility. Even as an employee and practice owner, having these established professional relationships can be greatly beneficial. Engaging legal counsel and other appropriate professional advisors to identify and navigate what is relevant to a successful audiology practice and achieving those essential goals and objectives can be critically important. Additionally, those professionals can help provide alternatives to address specific or unique concerns and to recommend solutions.

With a little bit of research and due diligence, professional relationships can be found to assist in the success of the business. The below tips are intended to be a general guide for finding and evaluating professional advisors:

1. *Get Referrals From Trusted Peers and Organizations.* It can be difficult to find a qualified professional interested in the issues of importance to the practice. Referrals from trusted sources are a great way to find these professional relationships. Talk to friends, family, and colleagues who have businesses and see if they have any recommendations. Conduct due diligence by researching potential options.

2. *Conduct Research.* While it is beneficial to have referrals of individual professionals that have been beneficial to others, it is important to conduct the essential research to ensure the professional is a good fit for the business. Read online reviews, check out their website, and reach out for an interview to get a feel for their customer service and professionalism.

3. *Ask About the Professional's Experience With Audiologists and the Hearing Industry.* Especially for legal assistance, relevant knowledge and experience in the audiology industry can be a positive. While broad experience with several businesses, industries, and situations can also be a positive, ask about their experience and expertise with medical practices. An audiology practice will not be too dissimilar from a dental, optometry, podiatry, or chiropractic practice.

4. *Consider Their Pricing Structure.* Pricing is an important factor to consider when choosing any professional, as different professionals will have different fee structures. Work toward obtaining a professional advisor that appreciates the financial position and budget for these services. Although budget is a serious consideration, it is not always better to obtain services from the least expensive professional. Cheapest is not always better and can end up costing more money down the road. The best professionals will cost more, but they may save substantial funds in the long term.

5. *Does the Practice Need a Local Accountant?* Should the accountant be in-house or one who can work remotely? Consider the overall costs. A remote accountant can be from anywhere, including lower cost of living regions where they can charge less. If time zones are not an issue, a nonlocal accountant can be of great assistance. There are significant cost savings by hiring an online accountant as they often present the same quality of services obtained locally.

Discuss advanced technology with them as the software and tools can result in significant savings for the practice. Further, professionals may be able to offer advice on which technology should be used in the practice (Chapter 15). Have a serious discussion about their security management. If the remote accountant cannot discuss the security processes they use, this particular provider could become a weak link, leading to problems.

1. *Ensure There Is a Rapport.* Practice owners work closely with their professional advisors, and it is essential to feel comfortable interacting with them, so consider if this relationship will work over the long term. Practice owners need to feel comfortable calling them and asking them for advice, and if it does not "feel right," then choose another provider. Availability and responsiveness are key components of a quality professional advisor.

2. *Be Open and Honest.* Finally, it's important to be open and honest with professional advisors so that they can provide the best possible services. Share all relevant information about the practice, financial situation, and goals so that they can provide assistance in making decisions in the best interest of the practice and its owner. (One caveat: Not all professional relationships create privilege for such conversations.)

Attorneys

The practice of audiology, especially establishing an independent audiology practice, merges a complex regulatory landscape with the practical issues of entrepreneurism/ownership. For example, an audiologist needs to be keenly aware of business law issues, employment law issues, tax law issues, healthcare law issues, and healthcare regulatory issues, among many other considerations. Awareness of and preparation for these myriad issues will position the audiologist for greater success in practice. When selecting legal counsel, the easiest path is usually to retain someone known personally, or at least known to friends or family. This approach may yield a qualified attorney, but a more systematic search, casting a wider net, enhances the probability of finding the *most appropriate attorney*. Referral services offered by local bar associations and other professionals such as accountants, bankers, and insurance agents are also good resources for identifying qualified candidates to be considered as legal counsel for an audiologist.

Desired qualities for legal counsel, as with any professional advisors, include chemistry and value. The chemistry element of the relationship can be very important and requires affirmative answers to these critically important questions:

- Does the attorney understand the practice owner's specific legal, business, and professional requirements?
- Does the attorney understand the practice owner's approach to problem-solving and their preferences regarding how to address relevant issues that have been identified?
- Does the attorney relate to the practice owner well enough to anticipate questions that have not been asked and to provide access and advice if needed outside of normal business hours?

Significant years of practice dealing with healthcare professionals and associated business issues would constitute relevant experience. A meaningful degree of interaction with other healthcare providers would serve as a basis for industry insight. This can include interaction with other practitioners and institutions and involvement in relevant

---

WHAT ARE QUALITY LEGAL SERVICES?

The "value" component of legal services consists of quality and cost. Quality legal services derive from several pertinent attributes:

- Relevant experience.
- Industry insight.
- Analytical ability.
- Diligence in providing timely advice and appropriate work product.

---

professional organizations, such as the American Health Lawyers Association, and healthcare law committees of local and state bar associations as well as the American Bar Association. Analytical ability and diligence are not characteristics easily ascertained during an introductory meeting or even necessarily by looking at biographical information on an attorney's website. Such characteristics are best determined by speaking with clients the attorney has worked with previously, so references are quite helpful.

The cost of legal services can be significant. Attorneys generally bill hourly at established hourly rates, with certain expenses passed through to their clients. Recently, attorneys are generally more willing to discuss alternative fee arrangements such as fixed prices for specific tasks, so it is worth inquiring about such fee arrangements to make budgeting easier. For example, it is not uncommon or inappropriate to request flat-rate pricing for confined tasks like document preparation or review.

Fees are often a function of geographic area, normally mirroring to some degree the regional cost of living, as well as the size of the law firm. On the coasts or in major cities, fees are usually greater than in the Midwest, smaller towns, and rural areas. Although large firms normally have higher fees than smaller firms, they are also more likely to have attorneys with greater expertise and experience in more focused specialties and greater technical resources within the firm. Reasonable value in legal services, considering the referenced aspects of quality and cost, can be found in any size firm, from solo attorneys to multi-office mega-firms, and should not be presumed according to the size of the firm.

Accountants, Bankers, and Other Advisors

Certain other professional advisors can be very useful in establishing and maintaining an audiology practice. Selection of an accountant, a banker, and an insurance representative should follow a systematic search process similar to that of securing legal counsel.

Accountants

While the primary function may be to assist with the maintenance of books and records and filing taxes, an accountant also helps with cash flow projections and budgeting, as well as with tax and other financial planning and payroll. A skilled accountant that understands the healthcare space can assist managing revenue cycles and compliance with healthcare regulations to craft financial strategies and maximizing revenue.

Banker

A banker can help source money to fund initial operations. A trusted banker can also assist in establishing checking and other relevant business accounts.

A meaningful line of credit or other type of loan will normally require a carefully prepared business plan (Chapter 3) and some type of collateral. If the tangible assets to be owned by the practice do not suffice, a personal guaranty and/or home mortgage may be necessary.

Insurance and Investment Professionals

Insurance agents make recommendations regarding professional malpractice insurance; liability, property, and casualty insurance for the business; and health and life insurance for the owner and any employees. As the practice becomes more profitable, an investment advisor may be helpful to deal with personal investments of the audiologist, as well as investments associated with pension and profit-sharing plans for the owner(s) and other employees (Chapter 6).

Sources of Law and Regulations

It is imperative for practicing audiologists (and all business owners) to recognize and understand laws and legal frameworks that may apply to themselves and the business. As detailed below, U.S. law does not draw from one source alone; instead, it is derived from many (often complex) sources. U.S. law originates from constitutional law, statutory law, treaties, administrative regulations, and common law (which includes case law) at the federal, state, and local levels.

Common Law

The United States follows the common law legal tradition of English law. Judges in the common law system help shape the law through their rulings and interpretations. This body of past decisions is known as case law, which is used by judges to inform their own rulings. In fact, judges rely on precedent (i.e., previous court rulings on similar cases) when determining the ruling in their own cases.

Statutes and Regulations

When a bill becomes a law, it is assigned a law number. Laws are also given legal statutory citation. Laws differ from regulations in that laws are passed by either the U.S. Congress or state legislatures. Regulations, by contrast, are standards and rules adopted by administrative agencies that govern how laws will be enforced. Federal agencies often enjoy broad rulemaking authority when Congress acts to grant them this power. Called "regulations," these agency rules normally carry the force of law, as long as they demonstrate a reasonable interpretation of the relevant statutes. The Administrative Procedure Act (APA) enables the adoption of regulations, which are codified and incorporated into the Code of Federal Regulations (CFR). Federal agencies frequently draft and distribute forms, manuals, policy statements, letters, and rulings. Although these may be considered persuasive authority by the courts, they do not carry the same force as law. It is worth noting that Article VI, Paragraph 2 of the U.S. Constitution is commonly referred to as the Supremacy Clause. It establishes that the federal constitution and federal law generally take precedence over state laws and even state constitutions.

Federal Law

Federal law is created at the national level and applies to the entire nation (all 50 states and the District of Columbia) and U.S. territories. The U.S. federal legal system is made up of codified forms of law, with the U.S. Constitution being the preeminent source of U.S. law. The Constitution establishes the boundaries of federal law, and it must be followed by all citizens, organizations, and entities. The U.S. Constitution forms the basis for federal law; it establishes government power and responsibility, as well as preservation of the basic rights of every citizen.

Federal laws that specifically apply to the practice of healthcare (Chapter 17) and, therefore, impact the practice of audiology directly or indirectly include, without limitation:

- *The Health Insurance Portability and Accountability Act.* Known to its friends and others as "HIPAA" and further amended by the Health Information Technology for Economic and Clinical Health Act (HITECH), sets certain standards relating to confidentiality and protection of patient health information.
- *The Federal Anti-Kickback Statute (AKS).* This act prohibits and makes criminal any offer, payment, solicitation, or receipt of value for influencing referrals to healthcare providers for services or items covered by Medicare or Medicaid.
- *The STARK Laws.* These laws prohibit referrals by physicians in which the referring physician has a direct or indirect financial interest, for certain *designated health services* covered by Medicare or Medicaid.
- *The False Claims Act.* This creates a private right of action—any citizen can bring a claim—for fraudulent billing of the federal government.

In addition, relevant federal legal frameworks and enforcement agencies applicable to audiology services: Food and Drug Administration (regulation of hearing aid devices), Centers for Medicare & Medicaid Services (CMS) and Office of Civil Rights (OCR) (regulation and enforcement of healthcare regulations), and the Federal Trade Commission (regulation of advertising and warranties). See Chapter 17 for more detail regarding these federal laws and their specific application to audiology practices.

State Law

In addition to federal law, each of the 50 states has adopted their own constitutions, state governments, and state courts. Each has its own legislative, executive, and judicial branches. States are empowered to create legislation that is related to matters not preempted by the federal Constitution and federal laws.

Most cases involve state law issues and are litigated in state courts. Relevant state legal frameworks and enforcement agencies applicable to audiology services include:

- Licensing requirements.
- Enforcement of scope of practice.
- No deception or disparagement.
- Unnecessary sales.
- Inducements.
- Incompetence.
- Advertising regulations:
    - Hearing aid sales consumer protection.
    - Disclosures.
    - Rescission.

Local Law

In addition to federal and state law, municipalities, towns or cities, and counties may enact their own laws that do not conflict with state or federal laws. Relevant state legal frameworks and enforcement agencies applicable to audiology services include:

- Zoning—Where can the clinic operate?
- Signage.
- Parking, etc.
- Building standards—is the location properly equipped for healthcare services/equipment?

Employee, Independent Contractor, or Business Owner?

In this section, information is broadly highlighted about employees, the in-

dependent contractor, and/or business owner. Each career path has advantages and disadvantages.

Considerations as an Employee

Choosing a path to become an employee of a healthcare entity or in an academic/teaching capacity is not an uncommon career path and can lead to less (or different) stress and income security. Broadly, an employee agrees to perform work in exchange for a paycheck and perhaps other benefits such as health insurance, vacation, 401(k), and so on. Having clear and understood expectations (for both employee and employer) is critical to ensuring a successful and mutually beneficial relationship.

For an employee, it is still advisable to engage professionals to assist with issues like review of employment agreements, especially if involving noncompetition or other restrictive covenants. Additionally, employees in certain settings enjoy legal protections for family and/or medical leave, so having a trusted resource to advise on rights is always advisable.

The Independent Contractor

Putting an entrepreneurial spirit to work without dealing with the highs and lows of owning a business is the role of an independent contractor. An independent contractor often enjoys the freedom to make their own schedule, pick and choose from potential work engagements, and handle their practice like a personal mini business. As an independent contractor, there would be a need to find independent insurance (health, professional liability, etc.) and arrange for the independent review of business and tax issues. It is easy to blur the lines between whether a worker is an independent contractor or an employee, so ensure there is a firm understanding of these differences prior to accepting a role with an employer.

Owning Your Own Practice and Financing Considerations

Much of the guidance in this chapter is directed to the independent audiologist who is a business (practice) owner. For the purposes of this analysis, these two categories are distinguished by the fact that an independent contractor is in business by themselves engaged by other professionals or practices to perform "for hire" services. While owning a business may involve hiring and maintaining employees of the business, capital (money) is usually required to start up a business. To secure loans from banks or even friends/family, entrepreneurs must be prepared with a business plan demonstrating the use of funds and how those funds will be used in establishing a successful, profitable business (Chapter 3).

While obtaining funds to start a business is difficult and stressful, not all sources of funding are created equal. The borrower must be keenly aware of the conditions of borrowing and legal obligations encountered within the process. A business-to-business loan does not come with the same protections enjoyed in other aspects of consumer life. Rather, a business borrower is expected and deemed to be knowledgeable. Treat the loan paperwork, for startup or ad-

ditional financing in the future, as any other contractual relationship and have it scrutinized by a lawyer. Loans from hearing aid manufacturers are also prevalent in audiology.

Manufacturer Loans

Manufacturer loan agreements have several common sections that create concern from a regulatory and compliance perspective. These include minimum purchase requirements, waivers of interest, and general use of the loan (Chapter 19). Some examples from actual contracts are presented below (specific companies or audiology practices are redacted):

■ *Minimum Purchase Requirements.* "From the Effective Date to [term date] or until all obligations of this Agreement have been met, Customer agrees that no less than the greater of [#]% of its total quarterly hearing aid purchases, will consist of [Products] ordered on accounts affiliated with [Company]. Notwithstanding any other provision in this Agreement, Customer's failure to meet the Minimum Purchase Requirement, in [Company's] discretion, will be a Default entitling [Company] to exercise its remedies."
■ *Purchase Requirements.* "As further consideration for [Company] providing the Loan, while this Agreement is in effect, Business agrees to purchase from [Company] [#] percent of Business's total purchase requirements for hearing instruments, and the Business agrees to purchase from [Company] a total of 1,638 Qualified Hearing Instruments at the average rate of nineteen (19)

units per month (the 'Purchase Requirement')."

■ *Waiver of Interest.* "In the event Customer on average purchases and delivers payment for not less than 80% of their quarterly Net Purchases from [Company] during the Term up to the repayment of the loan and repays the entire principal of the loan, [Company] shall waive all interest accrued as of the repayment date or the last day of the Term hereof."

■ *Use of Loan Principal.* "The Loan Principal will be used to acquire [Business] and to provide working capital for the Customer's business and for any other purpose(s) set forth in a prior written consent of [Company]."

These loan agreement terms are examples of provisions that could create liability per state and federal anti-kickback statutes and ethical codes as described below and in Chapter 23. While similar terms can create similar opportunities for liability, each agreement should be assessed as a whole to understand the complete risk to the individual audiologist.

Choice of Legal Entity and Common Business Structures

Forming a legal entity in which to operate your business can insulate the personal assets of the owner-audiologists from at least the liabilities associated with the practice. This is called the *corporate veil.*

While the corporate veil can function to protect personal assets, it must be understood that it is essential to follow certain formalities to access those benefits. For example, a separate bank account should be utilized for the legal entity (in the name of the legal entity) and maintain books and records for the business. Beware, *personal guaranties* for transactions such as leases, loans, and/or supply agreements with hearing aid manufacturers often require a personal guaranty. A personal guaranty is just that: "Personal" will not fall within the insulation and protection of the corporate veil. It is not uncommon for third parties to require the personal guaranty of an owner of a startup practice for debts incurred until such time that business credit and reputation are established.

Selecting the appropriate business entity is crucial. The business structure affects how much is paid in taxes, the ability to raise money, the paperwork that must be filed, and personal liability. Business structure must be chosen prior to registering with the state. Most businesses will also need to obtain a tax ID number and file for the appropriate licenses and permits.

While it is possible to convert to a different business structure in the future, there may be restrictions based on the business location. This could also result in tax consequences and unintended dissolution, among other complications. Consulting with business counselors, attorneys, and accountants can prove helpful making the appropriate decision as to the specific business structure for practice.

Sole Proprietorship

Business owners are automatically considered sole proprietors if business activities are performed but the business is not organized in any other structure. Failure to formally establish an entity to own a practice would result in sole proprietorship (if a single owner) or a general partnership (if more than one owner). In either such case, all assets of the owner(s) are available to creditors of the practice, subject to applicable bankruptcy laws that vary from state to state but may permit certain categories or amounts of assets to be protected from bankruptcy creditors.

Sole proprietorships do not produce a separate business entity. This means business assets and liabilities are not separate from personal assets and liabilities. The business owner can be held personally liable for the debts and obligations of the business. Sole proprietors may still obtain a trade name, but it may be more difficult to raise money as stock cannot be sold, and banks are hesitant to lend to sole proprietors. However, although there are some drawbacks, sole proprietorships can be a good choice for low-risk businesses and owners who want to test their business idea before forming a more formal business.

Partnerships

Partnerships are the simplest structure for two or more people to own a business together. There are two common kinds of partnerships:

- Limited partnerships (LP).
- Limited liability partnerships (LLP).

Limited partnerships have only one general partner with unlimited liability, and all other partners have limited liability. The partners with limited liability also tend to have limited control over the company, which is documented in a partnership agreement. Profits are passed through to personal tax returns, and the general partner, the partner without limited liability, must also pay self-employment taxes.

Limited liability partnerships are similar to limited partnerships but give limited liability to every owner. LLPs protect each partner from debts against the partnership; thus, they will not be responsible for the actions of other partners.

Partnerships can be a good choice for businesses with multiple owners, professional groups (like attorneys), and groups who want to test their business idea before forming a more formal business.

Limited Liability Company (LLC)

A limited liability company takes advantage of the benefits of both the corporation and partnership business structures. LLCs protect the owner from personal liability in most instances, such as personal assets like vehicles, houses, and savings accounts. These assets will not be at risk in case the LLC faces bankruptcy or lawsuits. Profits and losses can get passed through to your personal income without facing corporate taxes. However, members of an LLC are considered self-employed and must pay self-employment tax contributions toward Medicare and Social Security.

LLCs can be a good choice for medium- or higher-risk businesses, owners with significant personal assets they want protected, and owners who want to pay a lower tax rate than they would with a corporation. If the LLC structure is chosen, an LLC operating agreement may provide that allocations and distributions are to be made other than pro-rata with equity/capital ownership. Additionally, there is no limit on the number of or nature of owners in a LLC, whereas an S Corporation may be owned by no more than 100 owners, including individuals or qualified trusts.

Corporations

Generally, corporations are either a C Corporation or an S Corporation. These corporations are a legal entity that is separate from their owners. By default, a corporation will be considered a C Corporation unless an S Corporation election is affirmatively made by the owner(s).

Corporations can make a profit, be taxed, and be held legally liable. Corporations require more extensive recordkeeping, operational processes, and reporting. Unlike sole proprietors, partnerships, and LLCs where profits may be passed through to its owners, corporations often pay income tax on their profits. In some cases, corporate profits are taxed twice:

■ First, when the company makes a profit.
■ Second, when dividends are paid to shareholders on their personal tax returns.

Corporations have a completely independent life separate from their shareholders. If a shareholder leaves the company or sells their shares, the corporation can continue doing business relatively undisturbed. Corporations have an advantage when it comes to raising capital because they can raise funds through the sale of stock, which can also be a benefit in attracting employees. Corporations can be a good choice for medium- or higher-risk businesses, as

well as those that need to raise money, and/or be positioned for private equity acquisition.

An S Corporation, sometimes called an *S Corp*, is a special type of corporation that is designed to avoid the double taxation drawback of a regular *C Corp*. An S Corp allows profits, and some losses, to be passed through directly to owners' personal income without ever being subject to corporate tax rates.

Not all states tax S Corps equally, but most recognize them the same way the federal government does and tax the shareholders accordingly. Some states tax S Corps on profits above a specified limit, and other states do not recognize the S Corp election at all, simply treating the business as a C Corp. S Corps must file with the IRS to obtain the S Corp status, which is a different process from registering with their state. If a shareholder leaves the company or sells their shares, the S Corp can continue doing business relatively undisturbed. S Corps can be a good choice for a business that meets the criteria to file an S Corp election.

Accountants and tax attorneys, who should be consulted prior to or during the entity formation process, often have preferences regarding the selection of the form of an entity, a threshold question being whether a "flow-through" of tax attributes is desired. "Flow-through" entities include LLCs (unless they elect otherwise), as well as any corporation (including professional corporations) electing to file with the Internal Revenue Service as an "S Corporation." The flow-through entity is not separately taxed for federal income tax purposes, and all revenues and expenses of the entity are attributed to the owners in proportion to their respective ownership interests (or as they may otherwise agree in certain circumstances). Accountants for the entity will prepare a Schedule K-1 annually for each owner, which provides the information needed for such owner's personal income tax return. Conversely, a corporation not properly electing "S Corporation" status (known for these purposes as a "C Corporation") would be separately taxed for federal income tax purposes. Income of a C Corporation is not attributed to owners unless they actually receive funds as compensation (which would be deductible to the entity but only to the extent the amounts are "reasonable") or dividends (which would not be deductible to the entity), and expenses would not "flow through" to the owners and be deductible on their personal federal income tax returns. An S Corp can also be understood as a tax status. It is also possible for an LLC to be taxed as a C Corp or S Corp.

Why Incorporate?

As a medical professional, it is possible to encounter various claims alleging some sort of liability for personally and/ or for the practice. As mentioned above, the "corporate veil" is a concept that insulates the practice owner and their individual assets against claims against the business. Two common claims relate to contract and tort claims.

Litigation and Dispute Resolution

Risk management for an audiology practice, like most businesses, is addressed primarily by complying with applicable professional standards of care and by procuring appropriate insurance. Malpractice is an obvious risk, but insurance to cover nonprofessional liabilities of the practice, as well as property or casualty losses, life, health, and disability of owners and/or employees, must also be considered. The most important action business owners can take is to implement a process and procedure for reviewing treatment, outcomes, and modifying the practice accordingly.

Sometimes events lead to disputes with third parties that cannot be resolved informally by an insurer or otherwise, in which case selection of the method of, and venue for, dispute resolution can be very important. Contractual arrangements described above can be structured to require mediation and/or arbitration as alternatives to litigation in a judicial setting. Even in situations where the dispute is not governed by mandatory alternative dispute resolution, the parties can agree at the time of the dispute to utilize such alternative methods.

Mediation is nonbinding, but mediators are quite often former judges who can help the parties see the weaknesses of the parties' respective arguments, as well as likely results of a prolonged and costly formal litigation process. This process often yields a compromise that is mutually advantageous (compared to proceeding with litigation, such as a trial) and mutually acceptable.

Arbitration can be binding, with the decisions enforceable in court. While arbitration has historically been promoted as less expensive than formal litigation, that is often not the case, since their standards for conducting arbitration, the rules of evidence, discovery, and other matters (that are well defined in the judicial process) can take significant time and energy to negotiate during the arbitration process. Arbitration does have the benefit of being a confidential process, which is usually desired by healthcare professionals. Lawsuits are generally available for public access and publicity in the media if deemed newsworthy by media outlets.

The location or venue for any dispute to be heard, whether judicial, arbitration, or mediation, can be preagreed if the parties to the dispute have an underlying written contractual arrangement. This may be of limited relevance to audiology practices because patients customarily reside in the same jurisdiction as their audiologist and insurance payers usually are unwilling to negotiate to modify their standard contractual terms, which include having the venue and area of judicial proceedings in the location of their principal office.

Contract Claims

A breach of contract is not doing that which has been agreed upon. Breach of contract happens when one party to a valid contract fails to fulfill their side of the agreement. If a party does not do what the contract says they must do, the other party can seek remedy for any damages sustained. A breach of contract claim is generally dependent on the following elements:

1. The existence of a contract.
2. Performance by the plaintiff or some justification for nonperformance.
3. Failure to perform the contract by the defendant.
4. Resulting in damage to the plaintiff.

First, there must be the existence of a contract—whether an oral contract or a written contract. Second, the plaintiff must show that they performed the duties under the contract. If both parties claim a breach of the contract, then there may be no relief unless one party's breach was more severe than the other's. Third, the plaintiff must show the provision or term of the contract that the defendant breached and how the contract was breached. Finally, if the plaintiff shows all three of these things, they must show that they have been damaged in some way and the amount of this damage. To avoid a breach of contract lawsuit, business owners should check any contract they sign to ensure the language of the contract is clear and precise. The individual and other parties signing the contract should understand the expectations outlined in the contract and that those expectations are attainable. Lastly, to be binding, a contract needs to be legal. If not sure, work with a lawyer specializing in contract law before anyone commits to signing the contract. Avoid breach of contract lawsuits by carefully selecting the people or companies that are contracted for products and services. Perform due diligence prior to entering these binding agreements.

Tort Claims/Professional Liability Claims

"Tort" claims resulting from business operations, such as someone slipping and falling at the office, would also be a type of liability from which owners of a corporation or limited liability company would be protected personally. A

tort claim is generally dependent on the following elements:

1. The accused had a duty to act in a way that did not cause you to become injured.
2. The accused committed a breach of that duty.
3. An injury occurred to you.
4. The breach of duty was the proximate cause of your injury.

Claims relating to professional services would normally be pursued against the individual audiologist, as well as against the practice, so a limited liability form of entity will likely not provide a barrier for such claims putting personal assets at risk. While professional liability insurance is required, there must be an allegation that either the audiologist and/or the practice made an error or omission in the course of rendering professional services that resulted in harm to a third party.

The Function of the "Corporate Veil"

As discussed previously, the corporate veil protection is a presumption, which can be overcome by showing that the business was really being operated as an alter ego of the owner(s), without its separate existence being respected by the owner(s). The "piercing the veil" concept of holding the owner(s) liable for liabilities of a corporation or LLC most frequently arises when money received or paid by the practice is not properly tracked, documented, or properly accounted for or when contracts are signed in the name of the owner(s) rather than in the business name. Maintaining corporate books and records, as well as separate business bank accounts, and observing traditional formalities for business activity will help ensure the corporate veil is effective.

Compensation and Benefits

Since each owner in a multiple-owner scenario is usually concerned about the productivity of the other owners, compensation structures often involve a base salary or draw, with a supplemental compensation formula to reflect the relative productivity of each owner. Occasionally, a healthcare practice will simply allocate compensation on a pro-rata basis each year; this works only when each owner takes their responsibilities to the others seriously and peer pressure keeps the owners at comparable and positive rates of productivity. However, unless the chemistry among owners makes such an approach possible, agreeing to some productivity and quantifiable measurement standards will be needed to serve as the basis to make at least annual compensation adjustments.

A variety of employee benefit plans, many using pretax dollars, can enhance the compensation arrangements and financial security for owners as well as nonowner employees (Chapters 6, 8). Defined contribution retirement plans, such as 401(k) and profit-sharing plans, are common for employers of all sizes while Simplified Employee Pension Plans (or SEPs) and SIMPLE-IRA plans may be particularly attractive to employers with few employees. SIMPLE-IRAs and 401(k) plans permit employees to contribute up to a certain amount of pretax dollars to their account in the plan. Subject to legal restrictions, these plans as well as profit-sharing plans and SEPs permit employers to match or otherwise contribute to their employees' retirement accounts. Noncontributory defined benefit plans are less common for closely held companies than defined contribution plans, but that is a potential benefit plan as well. While substantial healthcare reform changes are currently being debated, health insurance is currently a typical benefit, with some portion contributory by all employees—the magnitude of employer subsidy to be determined by the owner(s). Flexible benefit plans (sometimes known as "cafeteria" or "Section 125" plans) permit pretax contributions by employees to pay group insurance premiums and otherwise noncovered health costs, including deductibles, copays, and child-care expenses. Other employee benefits to be considered include dental insurance, disability insurance, and life insurance. Benefit plans must be carefully designed to avoid violating government-imposed nondiscrimination tests that are intended to protect lower-paid employees. Consultation with benefits specialists, whether attorneys or accountants, is imperative for a practice entity to navigate these hurdles.

Whether subsidized by the employer as an employee benefit or not, estate planning is important for all the usual reasons of making sure desired allocations are provided for and taxes are minimized. It is important to periodically revisit the estate planning process as financial resources, survivor needs, and intended beneficiaries evolve. A qualified estate planning attorney (optimally affiliated with the attorney retained for organizational purposes so planning for business succession can be coordinated with estate planning) can ensure wills

and associated documents meet desired goals in consideration of applicable federal and state estate taxes, trusts for life insurance, dependents or others, and living will and other healthcare planning documents, which are generally governed by state law.

Relationships With Patients

The patient relationship is a professional one, as well as contractual. All audiologists should understand the boundaries set out for them by their state's Board of Audiology regarding the applicable Code of Ethics or other similar rules governing the patient relationship. Each state has its own distinct governing body, and any practitioner should seek their state's applicable board to locate and consider materials and guidance related to the standard of practice expected in each state. Each state has specific rules and regulations that govern audiologists and establishes the applicable Code of Ethics for audiologists. Audiologists must be very familiar with these types of rules, so as not to overstep or violate a rule that could put their license to practice at risk.

Providing new patients with contractual terms upon initiation of the relationship, usually as part of the application/information forms, is important. This is particularly true in the context of establishing primary payment responsibility. Applicability of insurance coverage is often not clearly discernable until after services are provided and claims are submitted, because of employment status and satisfaction of premium payment obligations. Within certain parameters, insurance companies may deny coverage to patients when employment of the primary covered person with the subscribing employer has terminated or when that employer has failed to pay premiums. At the time of service, the audiologist may not know these facts, which can substantially impact payment for services rendered or instruments dispensed.

Other Contractual Relationships

Contracts of all types are vitally important to a business. Contracts govern relationships with patients, suppliers, vendors, and all other third parties. A properly drafted contract will clearly identify what is expected of each party and the agreed terms by which to do business. If a party breaches their obligations as set forth in the contract, the business can suffer considerable disruption and significant liability.

Insurers/Payors

Unless the practice intends to operate on a cash payment basis only, which would be challenging for patients (who will generally expect to use their insurance coverage), an important aspect of any healthcare practice these days is relationships with insurance companies and other payors. The major national health insurance companies will provide their standard provider agreements. The goal of reviewing such agreements is usually not negotiation since respective bargaining power of the parties is customarily quite disparate. However, pay close attention to reimbursement rates and any requirements to provide complimentary services. For such provisions, many

states have specific laws and regulations regarding these types of contracts and the provisions that must be contained therein. Resources are available on the applicable state's department of insurance website.

Ear, Nose, and Throat Physicians (ENT)

As an independent contractor or business owner, it may be necessary to actively manage your contractual relationships with the ENTs for whom services are provided. While a chosen attorney will assist in preparing or reviewing a contract that adequately protects the business, it may be necessary to promote the practice to ensure the relationships with the ENTs remain strong. To do this, it is essential to maintain consistent and open communication with these ENT colleagues. Both parties to the relationship will benefit.

Regulatory Compliance

The practice of audiology is subject to state licensure or registration. Since criteria vary from state to state, it is very important to become familiar with the requirements of the state(s) in which a license is desired and to ensure that such requirements are met before making application for a license. A careful review of the state law and administrative rules should provide the required information; all such information should be available on the applicable state board website. If not, contact the executive director at the licensing board for specific clarifications.

In addition to state licensure, the practice of audiology is subject to various federal, state, and local laws and associated rules, some unique to the healthcare industry and others applicable to general businesses. This fundamental information is presented elsewhere within this text, with some detail in Chapter 17.

General HIPAA Issues

To improve the efficiency and effectiveness of the healthcare system, the Health Insurance Portability and Accountability Act of 1996 (HIPAA), Public Law 104-191, required the Department of Health and Human Services (HHS) to adopt national standards for electronic healthcare transactions and code sets, unique health identifiers, and security. At the same time, Congress recognized that advances in electronic technology could erode the privacy of health information. Consequently, Congress incorporated into HIPAA provisions that mandated the adoption of federal privacy protections for individually identifiable health information. Several sections of HIPAA are pertinent to audiologists: Transaction and Code Sets, Privacy Rule, and Security Rule. Importantly, HIPAA remains subject to review and update. A 2009 update included many new and significant HIPAA privacy and security requirements on covered entities, business associates, and other entities. These changes all fall under HITECH.

In 2024, the HIPAA Privacy Rule was updated to strengthen protections for reproductive health information. This highlights the importance to stay up to date.

Privacy Rule, Security Rule, and Business Associates

A key portion of HIPAA, the Standards for Privacy of Individually Identifiable Health Information of HIPAA, sets forth the standards for the protection of certain health information. This portion of HIPAA addresses the use and disclosure of individuals' health information ("protected health information" or PHI) by organizations subject to the HIPAA, which are known as "covered entities." If a covered entity uses the services of another entity to, for example, perform a function or activity involving the use or disclosure of PHI, the other entity will be considered a "business associate" under HIPAA. Originally, under the HIPAA regulations, a business associate was not directly regulated by HIPAA or subject to HIPAA's civil and criminal penalties (but the business associate could have been contractually liable via a business associate agreement). Under HITECH, the HIPAA requirements apply directly to business associates in the same way that they currently apply to covered entities. In other words, a business associate of a covered entity would be subject to the same penalties as a covered entity, even though it is not a health plan, healthcare provider, or healthcare clearinghouse.

Disclosure Exceptions for Treatment, Payment, and Healthcare Operations

The primary exception to the HIPAA privacy rules relates to routine disclosures of a patient's PHI for the purposes of treatment, payment, or healthcare operations (often referred to as TPO). The general rule covering these disclosures is that a covered entity must issue a general privacy notice explaining what types of disclosures they make for routine purposes. An example of an application that pertains to audiology would be a clinical audiologist and an educational audiologist exchanging information on a mutual patient. For all other disclosures of a patient's PHI, a specific exception must apply, or an authorization must be signed by the patient. To be a valid authorization, it must, among other things, specify the patient's name, address, date of birth, the name of the requesting facility, what information/test results are requested, the expiration date of the authorization request, and the name/address of the recipient. The patient's right to revoke the authorization and notification if the PHI may be re-disclosed by the recipient need to be addressed in the authorization as well.

Permission to Evaluate and Treat

Inevitably, providers encounter patients who do not seek audiologic treatment under their own volition but by a well-meaning relative or friend. The patient has the ultimate right of determining treatment. When that patient is incapacitated and unable to make their own decisions, clinicians may rely upon a person who has been designated as the patient's attorney-in-fact under a power of attorney (POA) to make decisions on behalf of the patient. It is suggested that clinics include a place for the patient or their attorney-in-fact signature on the practice registration form, indicating the patient or attorney-in-fact is granting the clinic and their providers permission to provide the necessary audiologic diagnosis and treatment options. For those

18 years or younger, a note granting permission to evaluate and treat is required from the parent or guardian to provide audiologic services in that parent or guardian's absence.

Privacy Officer

Every office providing healthcare in compliance with HIPAA has specified on their Notice of Privacy Practices (NPP) the name of their privacy officer. The privacy officer is to be used if a patient has a complaint that can then be addressed in-house. Should a patient wish to exercise their right to review their chart and request a change or otherwise amend their records, they will do so in accord with the designated privacy officer. The change or amendment to the record will be accepted or rejected by the privacy officer, who will document the full transaction in the record. The patient may file a complaint if they disagree with the ruling of the privacy officer.

Enforcement and Penalties

Both civil and criminal penalties are possible for violations of HIPAA. Specifically, the Secretary of Health and Human Services (Office for Civil Rights) may impose civil fines up to a maximum of $25,000 per calendar year and the Department of Justice could assert criminal penalties ranging from a $50,000 fine and 1 year in prison to a $250,000 fine and 10 years in prison. Notwithstanding those potential penalties, HIPAA does currently provide exceptions for lack of knowledge or where the violation was cured within 30 days.

In addition to the federal agencies that may bring actions, HITECH gives authority to state attorneys general to bring civil actions against covered entities for violations of HIPAA and to obtain damages on behalf of the residents of their state. Notwithstanding, if the secretary of Health and Human Services has instituted an action against a person with respect to specific violations of HIPAA, no state attorney general may bring an action. Damages for an attorney general action can amount to $100 per violation, with a maximum of $25,000 for violations of an identical requirement during a calendar year and include attorney's fees for the state.

No Surprises Act

The No Surprises Act is a federal consumer protection law that helps control the practice known as "surprise billing" for medical care. The act was signed into law on December 27, 2020, as part of the Consolidated Appropriations Act of 2021. Most sections of the legislation became effective on January 1, 2022.

- *Part I of the No Surprises Act.* Part I establishes new protections from surprise billing and excessive cost-sharing for consumers for emergency services and certain nonemergency inpatient services.
- *Part II of the No Surprises Act.* Requires healthcare providers and facilities to provide a good-faith estimate of charges to uninsured or self-pay individuals. It also details the federal arbitration process/ independent dispute resolution process that providers, facilities or providers of air ambulance services, and health plans or issuers will use

to determine final payment beyond allowable patient cost-sharing for certain out-of-network healthcare services in situations where the No Surprises Act prohibits surprise billing.

When a person with health insurance coverage obtains care from an out-of-network (OON) provider, their health plan usually does not cover the entire OON cost, leaving the person with higher costs than if they had been seen by an in-network provider. In many cases, the OON provider may bill the individual for the difference between the billed charge and the amount paid by their plan or insurance, unless prohibited by state law.

A "balance bill" may come as a surprise for many people. This can happen when a person with health insurance unknowingly gets medical care from a provider or facility outside their health plan's network. Surprise billing happens in both emergency and nonemergency care.

Fraud and Abuse Laws

Federal fraud and abuse laws will apply to any provider of Medicare, Medicaid, or other federal healthcare reimbursable services. There may be some audiology practices that will not be serving any Medicare/Medicaid patients, so these laws may not apply to those entities. However, most state laws mirror the federal fraud and abuse laws, and certain third-party payors include language akin to the federal laws. The key fraud and abuse laws include the Anti-Kickback Statute, the Civil Monetary Penalties Law, and the Stark Law.

The Anti-Kickback Statute (AKS)

The Federal Anti-Kickback Statute (42 U.S.C. §1320a-7b) was enacted to prohibit transactions that are intentionally designed to exploit federal healthcare programs. The AKS is an intent-based law that can result in criminal liability. AKS prohibits knowingly and willfully offering, paying, soliciting, or receiving remuneration to induce or reward referrals for items or services covered by a federal healthcare program.

Specifically, §1320a-7b(b)(2) defines an illegal remuneration as "whoever knowingly and willfully offers or pays any remuneration (including any kickback, bribe, or rebate) directly or indirectly, overtly or covertly, in cash or in kind to any person to induce such person—(A) to refer an individual to a person for the furnishing or arranging for the furnishing of any item or service for which payment may be made in whole or in part under a Federal health care program, or (B) to purchase, lease, order, or arrange for or recommend purchasing, leasing, or ordering any good, facility, service, or item for which payment may be made in whole or in part under a Federal health care program, shall be guilty of a felony and upon conviction thereof, shall be fined not more than $100,000 or imprisoned for not more than 10 years, or both."

The statute applies to both the giver of the remuneration and the giver of the referral if the referral is for services reimbursable by a federal healthcare program, including Medicare or Medicaid. If even *one purpose* of an arrangement is to induce or reward referrals, then the AKS has been violated. The bar for violations is low and easy for the government to meet in an enforcement context.

The Department of Health and Human Services has promulgated *safe harbor* regulations that define practices that are not subject to the AKS because such practices would be unlikely to result in fraud or abuse. The safe harbors set forth specific conditions that, when met, ensure entities involved of not being prosecuted or sanctioned for the arrangement qualifying for the safe harbor.

Beware: Safe harbor protection is afforded only to those arrangements that precisely meet all of the conditions set forth in the safe harbor. If all conditions of a safe harbor are not met, the activity or arrangement is not automatically illegal. Rather, the particular safe harbor does not apply and the intent of the parties may be examined to determine applicability of the statute. In audiology, hearing aids purchased in exchange for a gift or some other incentive may be tainted under the federal AKS (Chapters 17, 23).

An audiologist could be at risk for prosecution under the False Claims Act for violating the AKS if they purchase the hearing aids required for the incentive, participate in the incentive (accept the benefit, underwritten by the manufacturer or distributor in exchange for the hearing aid purchase), and then dispense one of those hearing aids to a patient who was reimbursed, in whole or in part, by Medicare or Medicaid.

The False Claims Act

Under the False Claims Act (18 U.S.C. §287), it is a criminal offense to submit false claims to the federal government. A separate law (31 U.S.C. §3729 *et seq.*), also known as the False Claims Act, provides a civil cause of action against anyone making a false claim to the federal government. Violations include the following types of actions:

■ Submitting claims for services that were not rendered.
■ Submitting claims for services that are not medically necessary.
■ Not billing with the appropriate provider number.
■ Billing for services known to be noncovered.
■ Falsifying a patient's diagnosis.
■ "Upcoding" or billing for a service at a higher rate.
■ "Unbundling" bundled codes.

In addition to criminal and civil penalties, violations may result in the revocation of privileges to provide services to a private insurer and revocation of state license(s). The key point to take away from this section is to accurately bill for only services that are necessary in the quest to determine the diagnosis. The Office of the Inspector General, in its pursuit of fraud and abuse, is on the lookout for false claims, especially claims submitted for services not rendered (Chapters 17, 23).

The Stark Law

Section 1877 of the Social Security Act, also known as the Physician Self-Referral law or "STARK," (1) prohibits a physician from making referrals for certain "designated health services" (DHS) payable by Medicare to an entity with which they (or an immediate family member) have a financial relationship (ownership or compensation), unless an exception applies, and (2) prohibits a physician from filing claims with Medicare (or billing another individual,

entity, or third party payer) for those referred services.

Since the inception of STARK, the Department has provided rules and guidance applicable to STARK. To date, there have been three phases, each of which provides some level of guidance as to how STARK applies to particular situations. Within these phases, there are a number of specific exceptions to STARK, but in order for an exception to apply, all of the applicable elements must be met. The Stark Law could be implicated for audiology services because certain audiology services may be considered designated health services. However, although audiologists are doctors of audiology, they are not considered physicians under federal law.

Since referrals and a financial relationship are the triggers for a violation of STARK, the definitions of these terms are integral to this analysis. Section 1877(h)(5)(c) defines "referral" as a request by a physician for an item or service for which payment may be made under Medicare Part B, including a request for a consultation and any DHS ordered or performed by the consulting physicians or under the supervision of the consulting physician, and the request or establishment of a plan of care by a physician that includes the furnishing of DHS. Section 1877(h)(1)(A) defines "compensation arrangement" generally as any arrangement involving any remuneration between a physician (or an immediate family member of such physician) and an entity. Section 1877(h)(1)(B) states that "remuneration" includes any remuneration, directly or indirectly, overtly or covertly, in cash or in kind.

STARK is a civil, not a criminal, law. Violations may result in denial of reimbursement, mandatory refunds of federal payments, civil money penalties, and/or exclusion from federal and state healthcare programs. To violate STARK, there must be a referral by a physician (or their immediate family member) to an entity in which the physician (or their immediate family member) has a financial interest for the furnishing of DHS. In this context, audiologists are not considered "physicians," so STARK generally does not apply to referrals by audiologists to other providers. The only audiology services that fall within the definition of DHS are audiology services furnished as hospital inpatient or outpatient services. However, as the entity furnishing DHS is the entity that receives payment from the Centers for Medicaid & Medicare Services (CMS), and as CMS reimburses the hospital for inpatient and outpatient services, it is the hospital (not the audiologist) that must comply with STARK (Chapter 17).

State Fraud and Abuse Laws

Many states have codified their own versions of fraud and abuse laws. For example, the Ohio Administrative Code gives the Ohio Speech and Hearing Professionals Board the power to reprimand, place on probation, deny, suspend, revoke, or refuse to issue or renew the license of an applicant or a licensee that "[obtains] a fee through fraud, deception, or misrepresentation or accepting commissions or rebates or other forms of remuneration for referring persons to others" (OAC 4753-3-08(E)(3). Additionally, Pennsylvania only provides for two narrow exceptions for the bona fide lease of office space and properly disclosed discount exception. It is vitally important that the state law is un-

derstood in the state where the practice resides.

Licensure

Audiologists are regulated by state licensure or registration in all 50 states. These laws and administrative rules set forth minimum qualifications, competencies, and continuing education requirements to practice audiology. It is incumbent on every licensed or registered healthcare practitioner to understand their respective laws and rules, which can be found on the website for the applicable state board.

A registered or licensed healthcare practitioner is burdened with reading, understanding, and accepting all tenets of the laws and rules governing the professional involvement in the care of patients. Should a licensee or registrant violate the laws or rules, the consequences may include restriction or loss of the license to practice. This also applies to those who come under direct supervision within the practice. Licenses and registration certificates carry the weight of law and the billing for services performed without a license is fraud, subject to criminal penalties.

Certification

State laws require healthcare practitioners to be licensed to practice their specialty within the broad range of opportunities that comprise the delivery of healthcare in their respective states. Certification is voluntary. By submitting to a process of certification, usually offered in accord with a professional organization, the applicant indicates their specific credentials and preparation to meet the requirements for the certificate. Certification is an affirmation awarded to an individual by a body of peers. It recognizes specific accomplishments and may define an area of specialty preparation or advanced study.

Miscellaneous Business Law Issues

The Ethical Practice Guidelines on Financial Incentives for Hearing Instruments position statement, adopted by the American Academy of Audiology and the Academy of Doctors of Audiology in 2003, defines, for the members of these organizations, the ethics and legality of the acceptance of trips, cash, and other gifts in exchange for recommending items that may be paid for by a federal healthcare program. Abiding by these guidelines protects the audiologist from inadvertent violations of the AKS. It is recommended that all audiologists read these guidelines as well as adopt them in their clinical practices (Chapter 23).

Payer Relationships

The audiology industry has seen the growth of third-party involvement in the hearing healthcare reimbursement process. Programs are being offered by traditional commercial payers and their subsidiaries, Medicare and Medicaid contractors, government entities, worker's compensation programs, and third-party administrators. As a result, audiologists and audiology practices are being presented with numerous opportunities to be involved as providers of care in these programs. It is important for the audiologist or audiology practice to consider each opportunity carefully when determining whether signing a third-party contract will be a good decision for the practice.

Some considerations: Can the practice afford to provide the level of care, at the agreed-upon rates, required by the plan? Is the plan offering a funded or unfunded (discount) benefit? How many current patients are now being represented by this payer? How many dollars do those patients represent? Can the practice afford to potentially lose the patients and their dollars? How does the reimbursement from the payer compare to what the practice used to receive from the insurer and the patient? Do any of the payer program terms conflict with the terms of other managed care arrangements? Does the payer give the provider access to a payer and their patients that the practice was unable to contract with on your own? (See Chapter 16.)

Employment Law

Relationships with employees raise a number of legal issues. Employment law is governed by a menagerie of federal, state, and local laws, as well as contractual arrangements. An employee handbook is always a good idea, even if there are few employees, to establish a baseline of expectations for performance and conduct. Otherwise, it is always risky to rely on unstated, potentially ambiguous, and/or misunderstood aspects of the employment relationship.

When permitted by state law, confirmation on the employment application or in an employee handbook that an employee is an "at will" employee can be key to the right of the employer to terminate employment for any or no reason. Please be aware that termination can never be for an illegal reason and without proper justification, such as discriminating based on age, race, sex, or another protected class of individuals.

Furthermore, an arrangement not reflected by an employee manual or other written document permits an employee to assert that the parties understood there would be no termination by the employer without "cause." Addressing adverse employment claims/litigation are inconvenient and costly to an employer. A matter devolving into a contentious "she said, he said" will expend significant time and energy proving a valid "for cause" reason for termination. When the employment is "at will" in writing, it will be much easier to rid the practice of an otherwise incompatible or unproductive employee. While formal employment agreements for key employees may be an unnecessary cost, an operational practice with more than one professional may be well served by written agreements with the professionals and perhaps other key employees to specifically cover duties, base salary, bonuses, benefits, and termination transition issues, among other things.

Other topics covered by employer-employee documentation normally include confirmation and acknowledgment of the ownership of patient records, as well as financial, personnel, and other proprietary business information of the employer. The terms usually confirm the employee's agreement that such information is confidential and proprietary and not to be used other than in the normal course of the employer's business and is not to be removed from the employer's premises. Required compliance by the employee with identified standards of care is often set forth in such documentation as well (Chapters 6, 9).

Cybersecurity and Data Privacy

Small, independent healthcare organizations tend to have limited resources for managing their cybersecurity practices, but they are no less subject to HIPAA and state law obligations for data privacy and cybersecurity. Healthcare businesses are often targeted by criminal hacker for cyberattacks and those attacks can be very disruptive and costly. In addition to outside threat actors, many data incidents occur from within the organization due to lax policies and procedures and/or careless personnel. For example, if a small provider practice loses a laptop with unencrypted personal health information (PHI), a reportable breach could result. Such a breach could have consequences for the patients and the practice's reputation. Implementing policies and procedures for employees and basic technical tools like antivirus and firewalls for the network is important for limiting vulnerability to such incidents (Chapter 15).

Real Property—Leasing and/or Ownership

In most practices, a physical location for an office will be necessary. While purchasing an existing building or constructing a facility on purchased property are alternatives, a conventional startup practice will simply lease space.

Legal counsel with real estate experience will be useful for identifying usual terms and conditions for the lease within the specific geographic area. Material terms to be considered include rent (and provisions for, and any limitations on, increases and expense pass-throughs); respective maintenance obligations of the landlord and tenant, including exterior and common areas; rights of each party to terminate or modify the lease; provisions on subleasing or assigning the lease; any limitations on use of the facility (even if the practice is permitted, currently inapplicable prohibitions may be a problem for potential future assignees or subtenants); and allocation of risk associated with the facility, as may be reflected by indemnification and/or insur-

ance provisions. It is important to inform the practice's legal counsel if the landlord is also a referral source; this information will assist the attorney to properly identify all relevant regulatory issues such as AKS implications.

Events such as a fire, a major water leak or flood, or a power outage or surge can interfere with a tenant's ability to use the leased space and operate the facility. Leases characterized by a landlord as "standard form" often give only the landlord (1) a right to terminate a lease in the event of a casualty, (2) a period of time to decide whether or not to restore damaged premises, and (3) a further period of time to affect the restoration (6 to 9 months is common). In addition, the landlord's lender, usually the payee of landlord's insurance proceeds in the event of a casualty, may decline to make such proceeds available for restoration. A tenant with some degree of bargaining power may be able to procure a commitment from the landlord's lender, by means of subordination, nondisturbance, and attornment agreement described below, that insurance proceeds will be made available for restoration if certain conditions confirming the lender's security are met. In any event, a tenant should consider what (if any) portions of the leased space are essential to operation of the practice and options for alternative temporary space if the need arises.

The subordination, nondisturbance, and attornment agreement mentioned above provides that even if the landlord defaults on its financing arrangements with the lender, including a mortgage on the leased premises, the tenant may continue to occupy the premises if the tenant continues to comply with its obligations, including payment of rent, under the lease. Without such an agreement, such a lender may evict a tenant of a defaulting landlord in certain circumstances. Most tenants do not ask for such an agreement, but in cases where substantial improvements are being made to the premises or other suitable space is difficult to find, it is worth requesting.

If a need for additional space is reasonably anticipated in the foreseeable future to accommodate expected growth in the practice, it is not unusual to ask for an option or at least a right of first refusal in the lease on identified space adjacent to the currently leased space. Additionally, the lease can be written to include the right of first refusal regarding the sale of the building, so as to give the practice the opportunity to purchase the building before a third party does.

If improvements to the leased space are required before occupancy, the landlord and tenant must agree upon what improvements will be made, who will secure the contractors to make the improvements, and who will finance the improvements. The landlord may agree to give the tenant an allowance or to finance the cost over the lease term with the tenant making periodic payments to the landlord. If the tenant is responsible for construction of the improvements, the tenant will need to obtain all necessary governmental approvals (e.g., building permit) and confirm that the improvements will comply with applicable legal requirements (e.g., zoning, Americans with Disabilities Act). These issues can be dealt with in the lease itself or in an incorporated and mutually signed side letter.

One should seek to negotiate more favorable terms and conditions to some degree. Commonly negotiated terms include the rent rate and duration of a lease. Note that even if a lease does not contain obviously problematic restrictions on use of the premises, local zoning laws may have such restrictions, so a look at the local zoning map and related definitions and regulations may be prudent but usually reserved to cases where the property is being purchased.

Acquisition and/or Sale of Business

Audiologists, like attorneys, physicians, and other professionals, often retire only with reluctance. It is perhaps the love of the practice and/or perhaps the lack of desirable alternative activities. Nevertheless, planning for retirement may be most effectively accomplished years in advance by anticipating postretirement financial needs in the context of investments (personal and deferred plans) and liquidity of ownership interest in the audiology practice. The liquidity of the ownership interest in the practice is also relevant if practicing with the practice group turns out to be unsatisfactory and a change in practice environment is desirable.

If buying or selling a business, the following factors are generally considered in selecting whether you should do a stock purchase (or membership interest purchase in the case of an LLC) or an asset purchase:

- The degree of liability being assumed by the buyer.
- Whether the purchase should transfer the entirety of target's assets or only some assets.
- Whether the purchase price will be paid upfront or via a (secured or unsecured) promissory note and tax implications.

First, conduct meaningful due diligence: Learn about their financials (preferably audited financials), learn about their business relationships and contracts, learn about their employees, review their corporate maintenance and recordkeeping, identify and discuss any outstanding liabilities or debts, and make sure to get a robust sense of revenue trajectories and the condition of any physical assets. Consider a business appraisal if unsure about the value of the business.

The key terms will likely revolve around whether the purchase price will be paid upfront, whether a portion will be paid upfront with the remainder subject to a promissory note, or whether the entire transaction will be paid via promissory note (this is not recommended).

Liabilities of the target practice are also of significant concern. If the transition involves a sale of assets, a buyer and seller might negotiate the assumption of limited, known liabilities, but usually will not assume any and all liabilities. Liabilities not assumed by a buyer of assets will remain with the seller and generally must be paid off by the proceeds from sale. If the practice is conducted within an entity with limited liability, the entity generally may be dissolved and remaining assets distributed to the owner(s), as long as sufficient assets are retained by the entity to cover all known liabilities (Chapter 25).

Buy/Sell Arrangements With Co-Owners and Retirement Scenarios

In circumstances where a practice has co-owners, it is not uncommon to have buy-sell arrangements in a shareholder agreement or operating agreement. These provisions usually contemplate retirement or other exit scenarios from the practice along with limitations as to how such ownership can be divested. Further, it is common to agree on a valuation method and payment terms for the price.

In a solo practice without a co-owner, similar transition upon retirement arrangements can be made with a nonowner employee audiologist or the owners of another practice. In a sale to an unrelated party, be prepared for a due diligence process, during which the prospective buyer thoroughly reviews and assesses the legal and business records of the practice; if they are in order, the process will cause significantly less angst.

To cover situations where the goal is not retirement but rather voluntary or involuntary withdrawal from an incongruous practice group, the same sort of buy-sell arrangement, or an employment agreement if one exists, can be used to address comparable issues associated with the departure. Customarily, this mechanism involves a sale of the equity interest directly or indirectly to the remaining owners (often via redemption by the practice entity) on a valuation basis that takes into account three major areas of interest:

■ Existing cash and cash equivalents of the practice.
■ Receivables associated with the departing professional.
■ Existing debt of the practice incurred to facilitate generation of such receivables.

If the departing audiologist is a recent graduate leaving a group practice after a relatively brief period of time, the event can be more simply structured as a "walk-away" with no payment for the proportion of receivables and no offset for existing pro-rata debt.

In any retirement transition, issues to be considered include accounts receivable attributable to the efforts of the retiring owner. Patient transition is a major issue since consideration needs to be given for the continuity of the patient's care, how best to retain the patient in the practice, and how the patients will be advised of the transition. Patients will ultimately have the option to remain with the practice or seek alternative care.

Tax effects of any such transition must also be considered. General rules include that sale of a capital asset, such as shares of corporation or interest in a LLC, yields capital gains, while the sale of an entity's assets yields tax consequences based upon the nature of the assets sold. Note that assets sold by a "C Corporation" will be taxed at the corporate level and that any subsequent distribution to shareholders may be non-deductible to the corporation and taxable as ordinary income to the shareholders. Finally, payments to former owners may not be deductible to the entity, depending upon the structure and terms of the buy-out. This can leave the continuing owners with the burden of funding the buy-out with after-tax dollars.

The term *"tail" malpractice insurance* covers claims made after expiration of "claims made" insurance coverage but relates to events occurring during the coverage period. Alternatively, *"occurrence" coverage* by definition covers events occurring during the coverage period, regardless of when the resulting claims are ultimately made. Since most currently sold malpractice policies are *"claims made"* rather than *"occurrence" based*, tail insurance is usually an important (albeit potentially costly) safeguard and should be considered whether simply leaving an existing practice or retiring from practice. It is important to make sure the insurance agent explains the alternatives and implications of tail coverage as you purchase or modify insurance coverage prospectively.

Record retention is another retirement consideration. This is less of a concern if the practice and associated obligations are assumed by co-owners or by a buyer of the practice. However, if practice-related obligations are not assumed by others at the time of retirement, and patients are simply referred to alternative providers, existing records should be retained as may then be required by previous contracts with payors, applicable law, and relevant professional standards (Chapter 25).

Suggested Reading

For further information on the foregoing topics, we recommend the following online resources:

Professional Associations:

■ Academy of Doctors of Audiology (https://www.audiologist.org)
■ American Academy of Audiology (http://www.audiology.org/)

Government Resources

■ CMS—Medicare Fraud and Abuse (https://www.cms.gov/Outreach

-and-Education/Medicare-Learning
-Network)

■ HHS Information Privacy (https://
www.hhs.gov/ocr/privacy/)

■ HIPAA (https://www.hhs.gov/hipaa
/index.html)

■ HITECH Act Summary (http://www
.hipaasurvivalguide.com/hitech-act
-summary.php)

■ HIPAA and Telehealth (https://
www.hhs.gov/hipaa/for-profession
als/special-topics/telehealth/index
.html)

■ Bureau of Labor Statistics—Audiologists (https://www.bls.gov/Oes
/current/oes291181.htm)

Strategic Business Planning

Robert M. Traynor, EdD, MBA

Introduction

Independent audiology practice is a rapidly expanding sector of the profession. The audiologists choosing this path are truly fostering the successful transition of audiology into an entrepreneurial business-oriented doctoring profession. While there are still some issues such as insurance and government regulations that limit practice to some extent, audiology is now taking its place alongside other doctoring professions such as optometry, dentistry, and chiropractic. While quite different from these other professions, audiology has become a stand-alone professional business enterprise poised to treat the huge Baby Boomer hearing-impaired population.

As in the past, there are simply not enough audiologists to serve the hearing-impaired population. The advertising that was generated by the discussion of over-the-counter (OTC) hearing aids from 2015 until October 2022, when the Food and Drug Administration established a regulatory category for these devices to increase the public's access to hearing aids, has added to the demand for audiologists and their clinical and rehabilitative skills. With the current backlog of audiologists, it would be easy to have an "if you build it they will come"

attitude since there is likely enough patients available to build business and support professional ambitions until 2050 (Figure 3–1).

Windmill and Freeman (2017, 2019) state that while a laissez-faire business attitude worked rather well in the past, the changing competitive environment now requires more planning to begin a startup audiology business or to expand and/or modify an existing one. There are many changes that have occurred over the years leading to the necessity for business planning in audiology. Some of these sources include:

- The modification of government regulations relative to the provision of hearing and balance services.
- The difference in the attitude toward the treatment of hearing loss of Baby Boomers and their Gen X children compared to previous generations. The need to stay social and interactive, along with the changes in technology, causes these groups to look at hearing loss as a more treatable disorder as in the past.
- Retail and Internet over-the-counter hearing aid sales.
- Direct-to-consumer hearing aid sales.
- Competition from the big box stores such as Sam's Club and Costco.

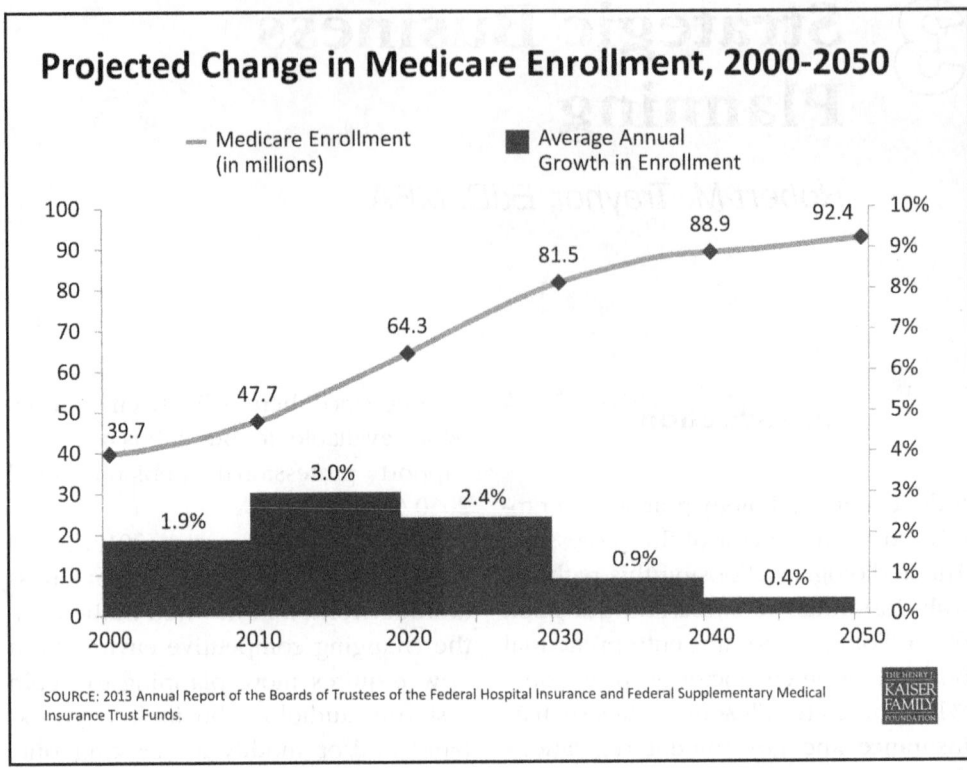

Figure 3–1. Projected market for audiology services 2000–2050. *Source:* 2013 Annual Report of the Boards of Trustees of the Federal Hospital Insurance and Federal Supplementary Medica; Insurance Trust Funds, The Henry J. Kaiser Family Foundation.

- Competition from hearing aid manufacturers' "outlet" stores, such as Connect Hearing and Hearing Life.
- Increasing competition from audiologists entering into private practice.
- Increasing competition from government clinics, such as the Veterans Administration.
- Increasing competition from insurance companies.
- Patients using Medicare Advantage hearing aid benefit programs.

The profession of audiology is now, more than ever, recognized by the general public and individuals seeking resolution of their hearing difficulties, but the profession is generally less familiar to bankers and other prospective lenders. Financial institutions, such as bankers and venture capitalists, loan money to unfamiliar businesses every day, so they apply a specific set of rules when evaluating each of these investment opportunities. One of the "rules of the road" is the review of a business plan. Even in the best of times, the prevailing attitude among lenders is that of skepticism. In order to raise capital for an existing or new audiology practice, the practitioner must present an extremely convincing business plan (Berry, 2023). Practitioners seeking funds must develop a plan that clearly establishes their fundamental business strategy for the generation of revenue. The challenge is to construct a conservative, straightforward, concise, yet detailed business plan that will demonstrate the lucrativeness of the investment opportunity to the lender. A well-thought-out business plan has become an essential component of the business rules of engagement and the basic link between prospective lenders and the entrepreneurial audiology practitioner. Indeed, Benjamin Franklin's famous saying "Businesses that fail to plan. . . . Plan to fail" is now truer than ever.

When initiated, a business plan is simply an idea, often discussed with a friend, family, or colleague, and starts with a conceptual framework or pre-planning exercise. This preplanning builds a general concept of the practice by reviewing the business climate, the products and services to be provided, the populations to be served within a specific venue and market area, projected costs, and an estimate of the projected income. Once the preplanning concepts are solidified, a detailed formal business plan is developed from the preplanning exercise that will determine the operational and economic realities of the practice concept. The formal plan must be exhaustive in its clarity of concept and present an accurate, yet conservative, depiction of the 3-year startup phase and beyond.

Although business plans are generally assumed to be necessary for obtaining funds for a private practice, they are also compulsory for other settings that may be referred to by another name, such as a "New Program Proposal" or "Departmental Prospectus." These alternative plans may be labeled with other titles specific to the business concept under consideration but are nonetheless a business plan. In an educational setting, a New Program Proposal may be used to present the clinical and financial benefits of offering a new service to students. In a hospital setting, a Departmental Prospectus might be used to conceptually present a new service, the costs of providing that service, and the financial benefits to the department and ultimately the organization. Regardless, business plans are utilized to establish and set forth the operational and fiscal requirements necessary to maintain the new or expanded enterprise and, most importantly, financial benefit.

The purpose of this chapter is to present a rationale for developing a business plan for startup and existing audiology practices. It offers a solid structure to follow, tips for success, and checklists to ensure that all the planning has been accomplished. While there are a myriad of computer programs available to facilitate business planning, it is highly recommended that those preparing a business plan consider the use of websites such as LivePlan that offer essential expertise, videos, and other tools at a reasonable cost and are MAC or PC computer compatible (LivePlan, 2024). These relatively inexpensive yet very sophisticated websites bring the

expertise of seasoned business professionals to the table as they lead the preparer from the most basic business planning concept to its completion.

What Is a Strategy?

Organizations that succeed and organizations that fail have one link, strategy. What goes into a strategy? Cohen (2010) discusses Drucker's concept of strategic development as "the continuous process of making entrepreneurial (risk taking) decisions systematically in the present with the greatest knowledge of their futurity while organizing systematically the efforts needed to carry out these decisions through organized systematic feedback."

Drucker presents that strategizing or strategic development is a continuous process that involves risk-taking decisions. These decisions must be made in the present for things that will happen in the future, and of course, the only thing we know about the future is that it will be different from the present. Thus, when making decisions as to how to approach the situations created by a new business, Drucker feels that an organized and detailed plan (i.e., a business plan) must be generated to ensure that all future variables are covered, at least to the extent that they can be predicted. Finally, he felt that all planning and strategizing was a moot point without systematic feedback to make modifications if the future did not actually turn out as predicted. The directors of a clinic, a private practice owner, or others in charge of the clinic are the leaders, and the leaders are re-

sponsible for pointing out the general direction for the implementation of the strategy.

What then is a strategy? Cohen (2010) describes it as more than a combination of objectives, resources, and well-thought-out approaches to where the plan hopes to go, but rather it is a roadmap that guides the organization forward to the future.

Arrival at a strategy involves asking some questions (Cohen, 2010):

1. What opportunities does the practice want to pursue and what risks is it willing to take?
2. What is the scope and structure of the business concept, including the right balance among such aspects as specialization, diversification, and integration?
3. What is the acceptable trade-off of time and money and in-house execution as opposed to merger, acquisition, joint venture, or other external means to reach the desired objectives?
4. What organizational structure is appropriate to economic realities, opportunities, and performance expectations?

Why Plan?

It is impossible to predict the precise economic and competitive future for an audiology practice, but planning the business allows the potential owner to strategize, as much as is possible, what future issues may contribute to the success or failure of the business. Since businesses are influenced by many outside factors and evolve over time, a busi-

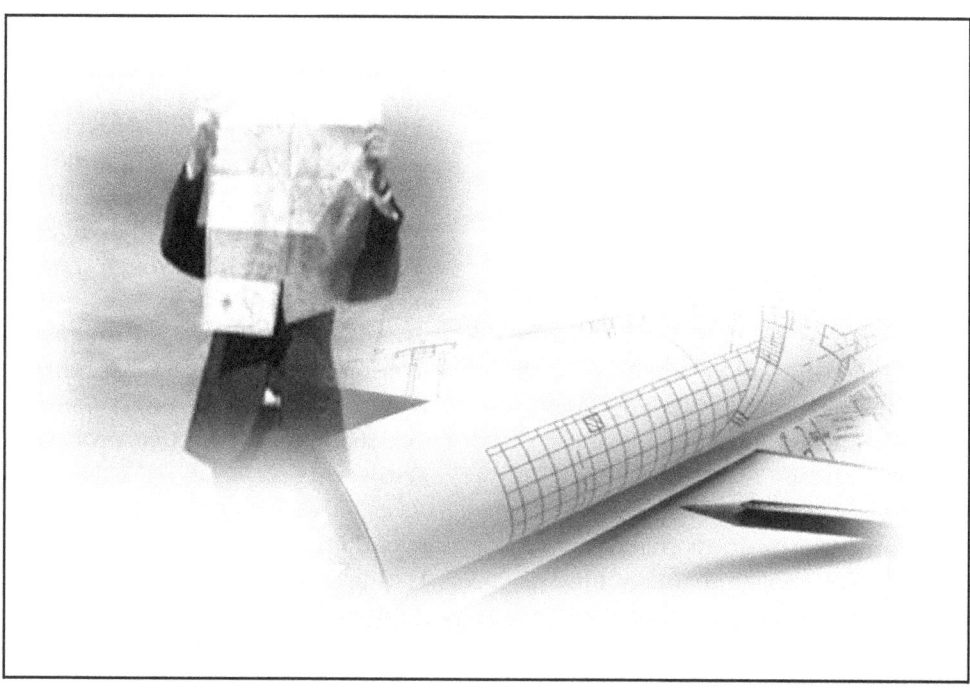

Figure 3–2. A business plan is blueprint or a roadmap for success.

ness plan should be a *work in progress.* Even if a practice is successful, a current business plan should be maintained to ensure fresh knowledge of the elements affecting continued success. Many factors critical to business success depend upon the planning process, such as obtaining outside funding, credit from suppliers, management of the operation's finances, and promotion and marketing.

Some prospective business owners assume that if they are not going to seek financial support from lenders or investors to fund their practice, it is not necessary to prepare a business plan. Not true, *every* business should have a plan, sometimes called a blueprint of the project, or as Cohen (2010) calls it, a *roadmap,* no matter if it funded by third parties or with personal funds (Figure 3–2).

Berry (2023) indicates that prospective business owners, in our case practice managers, should know the obvious reasons for planning, but several other issues must be considered when establishing or expanding a business. The following considerations are 14 answers to the question, "Why Plan?":

1. *Grow a startup or existing practice 30% faster.* Establish strategy and allocate resources according to strategic priority. Review the benefits of the expansion, the costs involved, competition in the expansion area, and the prospective revenues required.

2. *Planning is a necessary part of the fundraising process.* Lenders want to see a plan as to how *their* funding will be spent and review how long it will take for the practice to

make a profit. They will expect the business plan to cover their main points of interest, which usually vary from reviewer to reviewer and institution to institution.

3. *Having a business plan minimizes the risk.* Whether it is a startup or not, investors need to see a business plan before they decide whether to invest. Practice owners and their investors sign up for risk or the uncertainty that goes along with starting a business. Even if the lender is "Rich Uncle Harry," they always know risk is involved in any new business or expansion. They also realize that creating and reviewing a business plan regularly is the accepted method for uncovering weak spots, flaws, gaps, and inaccurate assumptions, which allow for redirection of the practice when profits are not generated as expected.

4. *Craft a roadmap to achieve important practice milestones.* A business plan is like a roadmap (or a "google map") for practice. It assists in setting, tracking, and reaching business milestones or goals. For a business plan to function as a guide, it should outline the company's short- and long-term goals to ensure progress (or lack thereof) and allow the owners to make the necessary adjustments to stay on a successful, profitable track, avoiding the costly detours. In fact, one of the top reasons why new businesses fail is due to *bad business planning*. Combine this with *inflexibility*, and it is surely a recipe for a business disaster. Planning is not just for startups; established practices benefit greatly from revisiting their business plan. This process keeps them on track, even when the overall business cycles, insurance programs, competition, government regulations, and other factors cause the market changes.

5. *A plan helps decide if the practice idea can become a revenue-generating business.* To turn an idea into reality, there must be an honest and accurate assessment of its feasibility. Part of that process is to verify:

- Is there a market for the audiology practice at the proposed location?
- Who is the target audience for these audiological products and services?
- Why will customers (patients) come to *this* practice and not go where they have received these products and services in the past?
- How will this practice gain an edge over the current competition?
- Can this practice be ethically run profitably?

A business plan forces owners to take a step back and look at the practice objectively, which makes it far easier to make tough decisions down the road. Additionally, a business plan helps identify risks and opportunities early on, providing the necessary time to design strategies to address these issues. Finally, a business plan assists owners as they work through the nuts and bolts of how the practice will succeed financially and, most importantly, if it can become a sustainable business venture over time.

6. *Big spending decisions can be made with confidence.* As the practice grows, there are essential major decisions, such as when to hire new employees, when to expand to a new location, the feasibility of adding new procedures within the practice, or affording a major equipment purchase and other expenditures. If the owners are regularly reviewing the forecasts mapped out in the business plan, these decisions will be made with better information to avoid costly choices.

7. *Practice cash-flow challenges are faced earlier with a good business plan.* The other side of those major spending decisions is understanding and monitoring the practice cash flow. The *cash-flow statement* is one of the three key financial statements that are integral to a business plan. The other two important statements are the *balance sheet* and *income statement (P&L)* (see Chapters 7, 11). Reviewing the cash-flow statement regularly as part of the routine business plan review will present potential cash-flow challenges earlier so action can be taken to avoid a cash crisis, resulting in an inability to pay the bills.

8. *Allow the practice brand to be positioned against competition.* Competitors are one of the factors that need careful consideration when starting a new audiology practice or any business (see Chapters 4, 5). Obtaining competitive intelligence requires much research and is an integral component of writing a meaningful business plan. Obtaining competitive intelligence

requires business planners to ask questions such as:

- What is the competition doing well? What are they doing poorly?
- What can be done to set this new or expanded practice apart from the existing competitors?
- What can be learned from the experiences of the competitors?
- How can this practice stand out from the competitors in the marketplace?
- In which key business areas can the new or expanded practice outcompete the competition?
- Who is the target market for the new or expanded practice?

Finding answers to these questions helps solidify a strategic market position and identify methods to differentiate the practice from the competition. It also proves to potential investors that competitive research has been conducted and the owners understand how to compete within the existing marketplace.

9. *Determine financial needs and revenue models.* A vital component of starting any business is understanding the expenses and how the practice will generate enough revenue to cover those expenses. Creating a detailed business plan assists in reviewing these expenses compared to the revenue while defining other ongoing financial considerations. Without a business model, it is difficult to know whether this practice idea in a particular location will generate revenue. By detailing a plan to make money, you can

effectively assess the viability and scalability of the business can be assessed. These issues should be completely understood early to avoid unnecessary risks to begin a practice confident that it will be set up correctly for success.

10. *Assist in thinking through the proposed practice marketing strategy.* A business plan is a great way to document the marketing plan for the practice. This ensures that all marketing activities are aligned with the practice's overall business performance goals. The practice will not be successful without a steady flow of patients and a strategy for acquiring those patients. The business plan should include information about the target market, the marketing strategy, and, moreover, the marketing budget. Details should include a plan to attract and retain patients, acquire new referral sources, and effectively use digital and other marketing techniques (see Chapter 12). A documented marketing plan automates business operations, keeps the practice on track, and ensures efficiency in the use of marketing funds.

11. *Clarify the vision for the practice and ensure everyone is on the same page.* To create a successful practice, a clear vision and plan are essential. This is all detailed with the mission statement defining the purpose of the practice and the personnel plan outlining the roles and responsibilities of current and future employees. Together, they establish the long-term vision for the practice and who and what will be necessary

to succeed. Additionally, the business plan is a great tool for getting the team synchronized. Through consistent plan reviews, it is also easy get everyone on the same page and direct your workforce toward tasks that truly move the needle toward success.

12. *Future proofing of the practice.* A business plan helps evaluate the current situation and make realistic projections for the future. This is an essential step in growing the practice, and it is often overlooked. With a business plan in place, it is easier to identify opportunities and make informed decisions based on data. Therefore, it requires outlining the goals, strategies, and tactics to focus the organization on important emerging matters. By regularly revisiting the business plan, especially during varying business cycles, market competition, or government regulation changes, the owners are better equipped to handle business challenges and pivot to other strategies faster. The management will also be in a better position to seize opportunities and follow new best practices as they arise.

13. *A business plan allows the tracking of progress and measures success.* An often-overlooked purpose of a business plan is as a tool to define success metrics that determine if business milestones or goals are met. A key part of writing a business plan involves a viable financial plan. This includes financial statements such as profit and loss, cash flow, balance sheet, and sales forecast (see Chapter 11). By housing these financial

metrics within the business plan, there is an easy way to relate the practice strategy to actual performance. Managers can track progress, measure results, and follow up on how the practice is progressing. Without a business plan, metrics, and milestones or goals, it is almost impossible to gauge whether the business is on track or not. Additionally, by evaluating the practice's successes and failures, owners can learn what works and what does not for incorporating strategic adjustments in the business plan. In short, a business plan offers a framework for measuring success to determine if the metrics indicate that milestones have been met. It also assists in building a "lessons learned" knowledge database to avoid costly mistakes in the future.

14. *The business plan is an asset if selling the practice is a future goal.* Down the road, owners might decide to sell the practice or position the clinic for acquisition. Having a solid business plan will assist the managers in making the case for a higher valuation. The practice is likely to be worth more to a buyer if it is easy for them to understand the business model, target market, and the overall potential for growth.

A business plan forces objective thinking and an opportunity to stand back and review the business as an outsider, critically considering the positives and negatives. At the end of the planning process, there is usually a more realistic perspective *of the effort* this practice will require and if it is a venture that will be worth the time, energy, and funds to be invested when compared with the generated profit. To audiologists, often not familiar with business, the task of business planning is formidable and intimidating, but it can foster new business strategies and concepts not previously considered. Written business objectives enable continuous focus on the practice so that the vision is not lost once the practice is up and running. A theme that is throughout this chapter is that it is no longer necessary to get a book and learn business planning. It is not even necessary to find a software program to learn and complete a business plan as there are extremely good websites, such as Liveplan.com, that take the novice from beginning to end in the business planning process. When there is a roadblock in the development of the plan, videos are often available to explain the concept, such as competition, marketing, and the even the greatly detested financials.

Preplanning for an Audiology Practice

Before a formal business plan is generated for an audiology practice, a strategic preplanning exercise should be conducted. This preplanning allows the practitioner to consider resources and the general economic climate as they design the type of audiology practice that will be viable within the community. The practitioner should be able to conceptualize the answers to four critical questions:

- What service or product does this business provide and what need does it fulfill?

- Who are the potential consumers for these products or services and why will they buy from this practice?
- How will these consumers be reached?
- Where will the financial resources to start up, run, and maintain the practice or the expansion come from?

An organizational concept that greatly assists in preplanning is offered by Harrison and St. John (2004) and has been updated by Traynor (2008, 2013, 2019) as a model for an audiology practice. The model, presented in Figure 3–3, describes a simple exercise that, in this example, has been applied to a new audiology practice.

The model presents preplanning as a process where the prospective practice owner analyzes and learns from external and internal environments to formulate goals. It is essential to establish a direction for the practice by creating strategies that are intended to assist in the achievement of those formulated goals and then safely execute those strategies.

Internal and External Analysis

The preplanning process begins with an analysis of the internal resources available. This can include personnel, office policies, equipment, physical location, space, and capital. Reviewing these internally controllable resources allows for the development of a *realistic* conceptual plan that transfers easily into the formal business plan. Similarly, external limitations require analysis, including the economic climate, competition, suppliers, referral sources, and insurance companies that influence the preliminary plan but are out of the control of the prospective practitioner. While there is usually no control over these factors, it is essential to the overall success of the business to formulate solid strategies to face these critical issues.

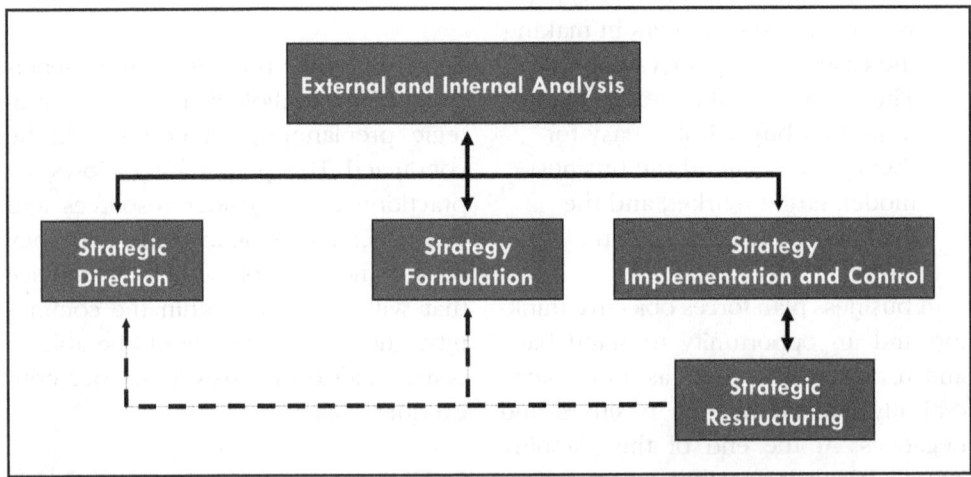

Figure 3–3. Strategic preplanning (Harrison & St. John, 2004; Traynor, 2008, 2013, 2019).

Strategic Direction

Another component of the preplanning exercise is the practice's direction. This exercise analyzes the type of a practice offered to the marketplace and involves asking the basic question, "What type of an audiology practice do I want?" Part of that discussion should also be other questions including, "Should the practice specialize in general audiology, hearing instrumentation, the pediatric population, adults, or both?" "Should the new clinic offer balance services, ABR, middle ear and/or cochlear implant device follow-up, and fine tuning?" "Should the practice offer operative monitoring?" In general, what brand of audiology should be offered to fill the void or improve the available services in the marketplace? Cohen (2010) indicates that Drucker called this exercise "looking out the window." Drucker suggests that this involves finding and assessing the target market, considering cultural, ethnic religious, racial, and social variables. Other issues considered would be demographics, buying group participation, competitors, referral sources, technology, economics, politics, and legal issues.

Strategic Formulation

Once the overall strategic direction of the practice is outlined, it is necessary to consider the methods of interfacing with the market, referred to as *strategic formulation*. Preplanning decisions necessary at this point involve whether marketing techniques such as print media, television, radio, and digital media (social media, websites, etc.) will be incorporated. Physician market-

ing should be considered a must to establish a firm referral base—to get the "word" out that there is a new practice in town offering something unique and different is imperative (Chapter 12). The prospective practitioner will also need to develop a pricing strategy that is appropriate but also aggressive for the locality to position the brand within the marketplace (Chapters 13 and 14). Decisions pertaining to patient centrism, risk management, and ethics must also be part of the refinement. All of these factors correspondingly apply to an expansion practice where the emphasis most likely would be offering new procedures, additional staff, extended clinic hours, a renovated office space, and/or additional clinic locations.

Strategy Implementation Control

Planning the implementation of the strategy involves a final review of what will be necessary to offer the practice into the marketplace. Final decisions regarding personnel and their qualifications, services and treatment programs, equipment and space, and financing must be made. Although there may be one implementation strategy that appears to be useful during the preplanning stage, others may present themselves during the exercise and following the initiation of the formal business plan, as described in the following section.

Strategic Restructuring

As the market and practice patterns change, it may be necessary to revisit the preplanning process to restructure or fine-tune the concept before the development of the formal business plan or a formal update of an existing business plan. Prior to consideration of a formal business plan, a preliminary strategic preplan must be formulated and sometimes even reformulated to fine-tune the unique, well-developed arguments for the proposed success of the practice or project.

Preliminary Considerations in Developing the Formal Business Plan

Berry (2023) indicates that a business plan is any plan that works for a business to look ahead, allocate resources, focus on key points, and prepare for problems and opportunities. A normal or customary business plan includes a standard set of elements, but formats and outlines vary somewhat according to the type of business that is to be planned and, sometimes, according to the software used to prepare it. Generally, a formal business plan will include components such as descriptions of the company, product or service, market, forecasts, management team, and financial analysis.

The formal business plan is a succinct document that addresses how to build and maintain a practice or develop a business project by postulating the specific components of the longitudinal business strategy developed in the preplanning exercise. Specifically, the plan describes to *stakeholders* (those concerned with the long-term success of the venture) how the practice will function within the marketplace. These formal plans also present what is being sold, by whom, the specific background and qualifications of those involved in the company, prospective customers, where they can be found, what is needed to build the business, and how the practice plans to promote and determine the viability of the venture within a designated market. Not only is formal business planning a clarification of the practitioner's goals, but it establishes a plan of action for reaching those goals by taking the preplanning general concepts from the "cocktail napkin" and turning them into specific well-planned ideas.

Since the practice or project business plan is so important, there are components that must be avoided. Offered in Traynor (2008, 2013, 2019) are some dos and don'ts relative to business planning.

Formal Business Plan Dos

■ A mission statement must be crafted to reflect the purpose and long-term vision and goals of the practice.
■ As part of the strategy, formulate concrete goals, responsibilities, and deadlines to guide the practice from startup through 3 to 5 years.
■ Milestones must be established and, once achieved, describe other actions that can develop such as obtaining more or updated equipment or hiring another audiologist contingent on attaining specific revenue milestones.
■ Assign action to achieve goals and milestones to a specific individual in the practice for implementation and monitoring progress.
■ The competition must be exhaustively researched and accurately characterized.

■ Describe why this business is unique and differentiate it from the other practices in the area.

■ As part of the implementation of a business plan, schedule times for evaluation and assessment of the plan—at least quarterly in the first 3 years, semiannually thereafter.

■ Good business plans provide a practical *roadmap* with clear metrics for achieving goals and objectives relative to the mission of the practice.

Formal Business Plan Don'ts

■ Use a business plan to show how much is known about the business.

■ Have an executive summary more than 1 page.

■ Exceed 25 pages; lenders will avoid reading a plan that takes up too much of their time.

■ Overhype the opportunities; keep enthusiasm visible in the document but avoid the temptation of overselling the product.

■ Set forth unattainable goals; be realistic relative to the demographics and the patients and referral sources to be served.

■ Underestimate the need for the services to be provided.

■ Underestimate or lose sight of the competition.

■ Develop unrealistic or unattainable financial projections; be conservative in estimates and projections.

■ Underestimate the effects of reducing margins on hearing instruments and the necessary strategy to counteract the trend.

■ Assume that hearing instrument manufacturers would rather deal with the clinic rather than directly with the consumer of their products.

Formal Business Planning: The Advantages and Utility of a Business Plan

Since the 1970s, audiologists with entrepreneurial spirit have understood that the business plan was, and remains, a highly stylized document involving a logical progression of information in a commonly accepted format. The content requirements may have changed somewhat over the years, largely as a function of changing technologies and advancing clinical protocols; however, these changes have resulted in additional opportunities to generate revenue. Furthermore, there is improved accessibility to informational statistics important for defining the patient base, potential sources of patient referral, insurance information, and general demographic data, including increasingly critical information about products and services provided by competitive practices.

In business plans today, lenders expect an exhaustive market analysis. They will expect to know what the marketing and promotional plans will be at startup and over at least a 3-year period. Funders will want to understand the milestones for the practice over that 3-year period and, if they are providing serialized financial support, how those milestones will be achieved and validated before each note is reissued and more funds are transferred to the practice. Another critical component of the plan is a complete forensic on the competition and how this specific venture exceeds the competition. Discussion of how this practice will provide that information to referral sources and potential patients so that they will choose this practice for their hearing and balance needs must be included. Staffing projections and equipment costs, including clinical and business equipment, office furnishings, informational technologies to be instituted at startup, website development, and planning for a consistent Internet and social media presence, will need to be addressed in the plan. Anything less will constitute a lack of due diligence in the eyes of potential lenders.

In short, the comprehensive business plan develops all the components of a successful practice based on the vision of the person seeking financial support. The audiologist seeking funding must be able to answer a single question about the business plan. The question: "If you were a venture capitalist or a banker with money to invest, would you invest in this practice?" To put it another way, did the business plan develop an opportunity for a lender to become a partner in the venture with limited risk based upon the due diligence set forth in the business plan? If the business plan contains the appropriate balance of information, realistic projections, well-developed demographics, and information about services available within the market, the answer to the question will be simple.

Business plans are a management and financial blueprint of the practice that clearly identifies and defines the goals while precisely outlining the methods of achieving those goals. The business plan is also a document that may be critical to the startup of the practice, but it is also critical to the ongoing good health

of an existing practice. This is a misconception. Some believe the business plan is no longer of use after startup funding has been obtained. Rather, it should be considered a living and growing document to be renewed and updated from time to time as the practice grows and flourishes. The business plan should be in close-to-current form at all times so that when the need for expansion capital arises, the plan will be ready to submit with minimal revision. It should be kept handy and reviewed occasionally as a reminder of where the venture began, how it is evolving, and whether or not the practice is on its planned schedule.

Business Plans Change With Market Changes

The business plan at 3 years' post startup will likely be considerably different from the original. As roadmaps, google maps, and blueprints change with the addition of new highways or structural modifications, so do the business plan. As the venture flourishes, hits bumps in the road, encounters market changes, experiences boom and recession business cycles, and faces new competition and government regulations, the practice owner may need to consider an office relocation or addition of a second or third location.

Particularly true in the 2024 healthcare environment, change is an inevitable part of conducting audiology business and must be embraced in the business plan with flexibility. In a matter of a few years, an office location once considered the best spot in the target demographic can change abruptly for several reasons:

- A hospital can internalize a large family practice group, immediately dictating their referral patterns to providers participating in the hospital's network or provider panel.
- Older patients move to assisted living facilities or move in with their children outside a reasonable drive time to the practice.
- Competitive practices move into the area and begin to dilute a once exclusive referral base.

Other market changes are driven by factors well outside the realm of healthcare. For example, if the practice is dependent on a large, single employer and the plant closes or moves to another state, the impact on the entire community and the healthcare market will be felt across the board, and perhaps, especially so in the audiology practice. In the case of an impending plant closing, the business plan should be revisited to consider adjustments in marketing to those workers and retirees who will remain in the area following the closing or issuing of information about the need to take advantage of their hearing care benefits while their insurance benefits remain in full force. Adapting to changing market parameters is vital to the long-term survival of many practices today, not just audiology, but in primary care and other medical specialties as well.

Formal Business Plan Format for an Audiology Practice

While business plans conform to generally accepted guidelines of form and content, the specific format may vary depending on the nature of the business and the business planning software or website used to construct the plan. No matter the programs used, healthcare business plans require specificity of the patient population to be served, the referral sources as pathways to the market, equipment and personnel necessary to provide the services, and in-depth analyses across each market segment of care. A business plan specifically adapted for audiology practices is proposed below:

- Executive Summary
- Vision & Mission Statement
- Practice Overview
- Market Assessment
- Competition Analysis
- Personnel/Human Resources
- Operational Plan
- Financial Components

Executive Summary

The *executive summary* is the single most important segment of any business plan. It is the section that is read first and creates the first impression. If it is well crafted, it may become the basis for the decision to fund or not to fund an audiology business venture or to continue review of the plan. The executive summary must not exceed two pages; preferably, it should be completed on one page. It needs to be precisely written and should generate a wide enough snapshot of the practice to provide the reader with the most important business facts and concepts that are or will become the practice. Schooley (2023) states that an executive summary is a business plan overview that succinctly highlights its most essential elements. It provides the reader with an overview of the business plan. The executive summary can be thought of as an introduction to the business. It is suggested that the best format for constructing the executive summary is to put the issue, or the problem, and the purpose into the first paragraph to formulate interest in the reader. The scope and limitations as well as the alternatives or procedures will go in the next paragraphs, while the significant considerations, analysis, and decisions will comprise the final paragraphs. Care must be taken to only include the significant points, as extra information in these areas is not appropriate and should be reserved for deeper discussions in the following sections of the business plan. Since each segment of the executive summary should contain key facts and information gleaned from the other portions of the business plan, experts agree that *the executive summary should be written last*. Each paragraph should mirror each section of the business plan.

Schooley (2023) offers five specific general suggestions for writing the executive summary of a business plan:

1. *Write the business plan first.* The executive summary is ALWAYS written last. It will briefly cover the most essential topics the business plan covers. For this reason, the entire plan should be written first, and then the creation of the executive summary. The executive summary should *only cover facts and details included in the business plan.*

2. *Write an engaging introduction.* What constitutes "engaging" depends on your audience. The introduction must be relevant to the practice and, importantly, capture your audience's attention. Therefore, it is essential that the executive summary be tailored to the audience for which the plan is intended, such as bankers, venture capitalists, "rich Uncle Harry," or a prospective buyer of the practice (Chapter 25). It is also crucial to identify the business plan's objective and what the reader can expect to find in the document.

3. *Write the executive summary.* Go through the business plan and identify critical points to include in the executive summary. Touch on each business plan key point concisely but comprehensively. Mention the marketing plan, target audience, company description, management team, and more. Readers should be able to understand the business plan *without reading the rest of the document*. Ideally, the summary will be engaging enough to convince them to finish the document, but they should be able to understand the basic plan from the summary.

4. *Edit and organize your document.* Organize the executive summary to flow with the business plan's contents, placing the most critical components at the beginning. A bulleted list is helpful for drawing attention to your main points. Double-check the document for accuracy and clarity. Remove buzzwords, repetitive information, acronyms, qualifying words, jargon, passive language, and unsupported claims. Verify that the executive summary can act as a standalone document if needed.

5. *Seek outside assistance.* Since most entrepreneurs are not writing experts, have a professional writer or editor look over the document to ensure it flows smoothly and covers all critical points. In addition to the web-based business planning program, there are many suggestions online for precise detail in writing the executive summary.

Vision & Mission Statement

Morelock (2024) presents that vision and mission statements are just as vital as a map. She states, "To succeed, you need to understand where you are going and how you will get there. And, if your employees don't know the difference between the two, you'll end up 1,000 miles off track."

The *vison and mission statement* should be considered the starting point of the business plan.

The difference between a mission statement and a vision statement is that a mission statement focuses on a company's present state while a vision statement focuses on a practice's future. These statements are essential to the business plan for several reasons. First, the statements can assist in focusing on what is essential to success. Stakeholders may know the goals and objectives for the potential practice or project, but often when dealing with the day-to-day frustrations that plague all businesses, especially healthcare practices, even the most motivated can become discouraged. The vision and mission statements remind the stakeholders of what is important and keeps them focused and bound together for a common purpose. Second, these vision and mission statements offer other individuals, such as lenders, employees, and even patients, a snapshot of what the new practice or project hopes to accomplish. Not only do these statements serve as a constant reminder of what is essential to the practice or project, but the statements foster an atmosphere where employees and stakeholders see the organization as "theirs."

It is only common sense that people will generally believe in something more completely if they had a hand in developing it. Presenting a clear and compelling *vision statement* can:

- Define the optimal desired future state—the mental picture—of what the organization wants to achieve over time.
- Provide guidance and inspiration as to what the organization is focused on and achieving in 5, 10, or more years.
- Provide a basis for developing the other sections of the business plan.

A concise *mission statement* can:

- Serve as an internal guidance statement for practice employees.
- Inform those who come to the practice about the clinic's philosophy and commitment to excellence in all aspects of the services provided.
- Convert the broad dreams of the vision into more specific, practical, action-oriented behaviors.
- Explain goals to stakeholders in a clear and concise manner.
- Enhance the practices' image as being competent and professional, thus reassuring patients and funding sources that their investment was a smart choice.

These statements are fundamental to the business planning process. The vision is a loftier theoretical, often esoteric, goal statement that is written succinctly in an inspirational manner that makes it easy for all employees to repeat it at any given time. Some examples of these might be:

- *Our Vision is a World without Hearing Loss.*
- *Imagine a World where Noise did not Create Hearing Loss.*
- *Our Vision is a Whole World Completely in Balance.*

Mission statements are more practical defining the state or purpose of the practice. The mission statement is a derivative of the vision statement. Typically, these are high-level statements and are usually written in the form of a sentence or two, and they pertain to a shorter time frame, usually 1 to 3 years. It is a statement that means something to all employees and stakeholders and should be easily repeated by all involved. Mission statements address:

- *WHAT* it does.
- *WHO* it does it for.
- *HOW* it does what it does.

A sample mission statement would be: *Audiology Associates will work honestly and diligently every day to exceed the expectations of our patients and referral sources by providing the best hearing and balance care in our community.*

Some companies list both their vision and mission statements on their websites. It is good practice to post them in the clinic so that all are aware of both the vision and the mission of the practice. While some companies tend to blend these statements, in practice,

the mission statement becomes a proclamation of the general nature and direction of the business and reflects the quality policy. It is an assertion integral to the concepts presented with the business plan and sets the tone for the overall project.

Practice Overview

The opening section of the *practice overview* should describe the profession of audiology and its important contributions to contemporary hearing and balance care. This should be no more than a couple of pages. For startup companies, this section will be brief, so it is necessary to focus on why the practice should be started and the reason for existence.

For an expanding practice, this section should contain the developmental stages to date and a brief summation of the history of the practice, its evaluations and products, the overall market that it serves, the management, accomplishments, and challenges the practice has endured. It is a good idea to include why the practice was started, what products were initially offered, and how the company has progressed to its current position. An overview of the business side of the practice might also include a summary of financial statements such as revenues, gross operating profit, and net income for the last 5 years to support growth statements. The business discussion should include any major changes in the balance sheet (Chapter 11) and a discussion of major assets that have been acquired over time. Further, office locations, Internet presence (website, Facebook, X (formerly Twitter), LinkedIn, and other social media, etc.) (Chapter 12), legal business structure (sole proprietorship, LLC, etc.) (Chapter 2), and a list of principals participating in the practice are part of this discussion.

In practice overviews, there is usually an expansive narrative describing the problem that the patients want solved, in this case a hearing, tinnitus, or balance issue. Diagnostic and treatment procedures, hearing instrument assessment and assistive device selection, and fitting and follow-up care should be presented so that the reader readily understands the operational core of the practice and clinical opportunities available to patients, as well as referring practitioners.

It is also helpful to the reviewer if a patient takes the path from referral source to the audiology clinic and through the examination, interpretation, and counseling process. Pathway descriptions will vary depending on the patient's needs and the procedures offered by the clinic. This description will illustrate the many interactions between the patient and clerical and clinical staff members, specialized environments, and the equipment used in the clinical process.

The practice overview should characterize treatment trends in audiology and relate them to the needs of patients in the market area, such as prescription hearing aids, over-the-counter devices, and assessment trends, such as extended high-frequency and speech-in-noise assessments. It must establish the practice's competitive edge whether based on personnel with advanced degrees and licenses, specific assessment, or therapeutic protocols not offered by others in the market (e.g., tinnitus assessment and treatment, preventative noise control, central auditory testing and treatment, vestibular assessment and treatment, operative monitoring, group aural rehabilitation), or a unique

marketing approach to primary care physicians, dentists, chiropractors, nurse practitioners, and other professionals that have not been considered. The reader of this section should have a clear picture and an appreciation for what differentiates this practice or project from the competition.

Market Assessment/Analysis

The *market assessment/analysis* is essential to all business plans and one of the most important reasons to devise a business plan. The market analysis is a thorough qualitative and quantitative assessment of the current market. It provides an understanding of the volume and value of the market, potential customer segments and their buying patterns, the position of the competition, and the overall economic environment, including barriers to entry and industry regulations. While a detailed market analysis is expected within a business plan, it is actually a process that should be ongoing so that the managers are apprised of the changes in the marketplace as they happen rather than being surprised.

An in-depth knowledge of the market is essential to a successful business plan. It verifies that the managers understand their market and those within it so that they can successfully target them for the business venture. Parsons (2024) indicates that a market assessment/analysis can seem like a daunting task, but it can be broken up into four simple elements:

1. *Industry overview.* This component within business plans describes the current state of the hearing industry, the future

perspective of the profession, and private practice in general.

2. *Target market.* The target market is future patients that the practice will serve. This component asks, "Who are the actual customers?" The plan should present how many there are in the location of the practice and their needs, especially those needs not being met by the current businesses in the area. The population should be described by a market segmentation review that includes demographics, geographics, psychographics, and behavioral graphics of the target population.

3. *Competition.* Each of the competitors and their positioning, strengths, and weaknesses need to be presented in detail with a description of how the startup or expansion projects compete with them.

4. *Pricing and forecast.* Pricing, either itemized, bundled, or a combination of these concepts, will assist in determining how to position the practice within the market and speak to some degree regarding competitive concerns. Forecasting will show what portion of the market the practice hopes to obtain, which will allow for estimates of revenue.

Industry Overview

In this step, describe the hearing industry and discuss its direction for the future. The business plan should present key industry metrics such as size, trends, and projected growth. While part of the overall process is similar to the market assessment/analysis section of the plan, analyzing the industry is different from market assessment/analysis. The focus of this section is the whole industry, all businesses including the new practice or expansion to be created. It is not a discussion of the patients/customers but an overview of the industry as a whole. Although the focus is on audiology, it must also include businesses that *look like audiology clinics* to consumers but are *simple sales operations*, such as big-box stores, manufacturer sales outlets, traditional hearing aid dispensers, Internet/brick/mortar over-the-counter operations, and direct-to-consumer product sales. Specifically, the industry overview verifies to the investors that the applicants understand the larger competitive landscape of the profession. More importantly, it assists the managers of the startup or expansion project to understand if there is to be more demand for audiology products and services in the future, as well as the competitive environment. A valuable source for this information is websites, ads, and market communication by various national competitors, audiology journals, podcasts, LinkedIn, and other media sites as well as the online U.S. census and Medicare data. While there are some free sources for this information, such as MarkeTrak (Carr & Kihm, 2022), some very expensive marketing studies, such as Ariston (2024) and others, can be purchased to add if very detailed data become necessary.

Some variables that could be considered are the current population, overall estimated growth or decline of the target market, expected growth in the workforce versus estimated numbers of retirees, predicted changes in local industries such as a trend for closures of factories or businesses, or increase in technological firms or medical device/drug companies. Citations from Windmill and Freeman (2017, 2019) are important here as they have documented the numbers of patients requiring hearing care until 2050. Other segment factors could include the number of daily commuters and travelers passing through the chosen service area in need of services.

Recently, there have been some revolutionary legislative proposals to bring audiologists to the practitioner level (Chapter 17). If this happens, it will be necessary to explain this status and the difference between audiology practice with and without this status. The addition of practitioner status will enhance the approval prospects and, when it becomes reality, should be reflected in all audiology business plans (Medicare Audiology Access and Improvement Act, 2024; ADA, 2024).

Market growth should generally be viewed as a percentage change in purchase patterns. Market forecasts start with the total number of possible purchasers in each market segment and the percentage change projected over the next 3 to 5 years. There are great projections offered both in print and online about once per year in both *Hearing Review* and *Hearing Journal* as well as other publications. Government websites are also an excellent source of population estimates of cities, counties, states, regions, and even the overall United States. In some instances, however, not all of the required information for business planning is readily available or public. To provide detailed market estimates in these situations, it may be necessary to dig deeply into the literature and Internet files or purchase very expensive

information from private marketing groups to provide the detail required for conservative forecasts necessary to impress some lenders.

As for market growth, Souza (2014) and Windmill and Freeman (2017, 2019) both predict that over the next 30 years, the percentage of the U.S. population over 65 years of age is expected to double and those over 85 years is expected to triple. Older adults are not only living longer but also working longer and staying socially active later in life. In their efforts to be contributors and stay active, the rate at which these adults seek help is likely to drastically increase, driven by their communication needs and improved access to healthcare. Thus, the market is only going to get substantially larger over the next 30 years.

Use of these contemporary online data within an industry overview will demonstrate to investors and funders that there is not only an increasing market for audiology products and services but that the stakeholders are incorporating the latest, most accurate data into their business forecasts.

Target Market

Defining the target market is the most important section of your analysis. While this chapter focuses on the business planning process, Chapter 12 focuses on the details of marketing an audiology practice and may be of benefit as the business plan is developed. This component of the market assessment/analysis is the area where the ideal patient/customer for the practice is discussed. To discuss the diversity of patients seen in an audiology clinic, it may be necessary to conduct a market segmentation (Chapter 12). This is where similar types of patients/customers are grouped into segments and the attributes of each of the segments are described with their contribution to the overall practice. Begin broadly and refine the research by following the elements of the population proposed as patients/customers. These elements include:

■ *Market size.* Unlike industry size, usually measured in dollars, the market size for an individual practice refers to how many potential patients/customers there are within the market area for products or services of the practice.

■ *Demographics.* Describe the typical patient/customer's age, gender, education, income, and more. This is a description of the perfect patient/customer for the practice.

■ *Location.* This area describes the location of these patients/customers. Maps of a specific region, state, city, county, and so on are a useful addition and desirable. This discussion should include a presentation of the cultural characteristics of the area, small town, large town, or city, as well as the sports, recreational activities, and specifics that make the location of interest for a practice. For example, a business plan for a practice in a vacation retreat is quite different from a practice in a small town or large city.

■ *Psychographics.* In this area of the plan, a presentation of inside the mindset of the area's patients/customers is presented. Describe their needs and how they will possibly react to the idea for this type of practice in their community. What

do these people like or dislike, how do they live, and what is their personal style? This component can assist in describing the necessity and the rationale for the practice as it meets the existing competition.

■ *Behaviors.* This is essentially an extension of some of the psychographic information. Explain how patients/customers shop for and purchase hearing care products and services.

■ *Trends.* As in all businesses, customer behavior is always changing. If there are trends, such as over-the-counter (OTC) or direct-to-consumer (DTC) products, third-party insurance programs, itemizing of costs, and other trends in the target market, they should be detailed in this section.

Competition

Distinguishing a new practice from the crowd of competitors is not merely important; *it is the key to both the short- and long-term success of the practice.* Potential investors expect a comprehensive assessment of the competition in the defined market area. In addition to the current landscape of competitors and the marketing program, investors will also want to know about the possible changes that may be coming to the marketplace that could affect the success of the proposed practice over time. Thus, the market assessment/analysis is not complete without a detailed description and introspection of the competition within the market.

Beyond knowing who the other competitive practices/businesses are in the area, a good market analysis involves obtaining competitive intelligence. Presented more completely in Chapter 4, competitive intelligence is the action of defining, gathering, analyzing, and distributing intelligence about products, patients, competitors, and any aspect of the environment needed to support those in the practice design that implements strategic decisions. Competitive intelligence essentially allows the practitioner to understand and learn what is happening in the local marketplace world. Competitive intelligence will point out competitors' weaknesses that can be exploited for advantage opportunities.

All hearing care professionals survive on referrals from the medical, chiropractic, dental, nursing, and other communities, so part of the intelligence gathering should also be a discussion with community professionals regarding their satisfaction with the current services available, so a plan to obtain referrals from these professionals can be created. With this knowledge, the new practice or expansion can differentiate itself by offering products and services that fill gaps competitors have not addressed. The use of competitive intelligence in the business plan demonstrates that the stakeholders are aware of the current methods and procedures for obtaining information about those that are competing or will compete with the practice.

When analyzing the competition, consider the following areas:

■ *Direct competition.* There is increasing direct competition from audiology practices providing the same products and diagnostic/rehabilitative services as more audiology practitioners enter the market with their own independent clinics. Moreover, competition is now for-

midable from otolaryngology practices, big-box stores (Costco, Sam's Club/Walmart, etc.), government audiology clinics (Veterans Administration), insurance companies, hearing aid manufacturer–owned stores and clinics, Internet hearing aid sales, direct-to-consumer sales, and hearing aid dispensers. These are all companies offering very similar products and services that look to patients/customers to be the *same as the practice or expansion being considered.* Potential patients/customers are likely current patients within these other businesses, so the business plan needs to address how the new practice will differentiate from these competitors.

To best typify the competition in the market within a business plan, specific competitors must be listed with an estimate of their market share and a consideration of their advertising in various media, including their website, search engines, Facebook page, and so on. Further, each of the competitors should be characterized by their clinical offerings, the qualifications of the providers in the practice, and a candid, unbiased assessment of their strengths and weaknesses. Qualifications and other information can be gleaned from licensure boards, advertising, former patients, and current vendors who have had interactions with them.

Offering an assessment and treatment protocol for tinnitus, central auditory disorders, or disequilibrium can offer a new or expanded practice an important edge in a market where other providers do not offer the service or fail to advise the healthcare community about its availability and efficacy. Patients with tinnitus, central auditory, and disequilibrium are vexing problems for primary care practitioners. If they have an audiologist in the community who has made known to them that their practice welcomes patients with the complaints of tinnitus or dizziness, the referrals will begin and continue if the services and treatment exhaust the patient's need for clinical attention, valid diagnostic and therapeutic intervention, or referral for further treatment. Primary care physicians not only appreciate that their patients undergo extensive evaluation, competent counseling, and explanation of their difficulty but also that their patients have some chance of remediation.

■ *Indirect competitors.* Consider indirect competition as alternative solutions to the problems solved by the practice or expansion being proposed. This is particularly important for companies that are inventing brand-new products or services. For example, the offering of Epley maneuvers could be an alternative treatment for positional vestibular disorders against physical therapy (PT) clinics in the area, or virtual reality goggles for vestibular assessment and/or rehabilitation might be another innovative system to offer to the area competing with PT clinics.

Additionally, the credentials of an audiologist are quite different from those of a hearing aid dispenser, or maybe your practice or practice expansion offers assessments such as distortion product otoacoustic emissions and extended high-frequency audiometry or speech-in-noise testing not available anywhere else in the area. All of these differences should be pointed out in the business plan to present to the reader of the plan the rationale as to why patients/customers will go to this clinic and not the competition.

■ *Emphasize how this practice is different and why these patients/customers would come to this practice instead of the competition.* The new startup or the practice expansion does not want to be the same as the competition. Ensure to include a discussion within the business plan as to how this practice or expansion, with its focus toward audiological products and services, is different from the competition. The difference could be credentials, location, expertise, itemized pricing (Chapter 13), or other differences that will attract patients/customers from the competition.

■ *Barriers to entry into the market.* As part of the Porter's Five Forces discussion in Chapter 5, barriers to entry are discussed in detail. In the business plan, however, it is necessary to describe how others will not be able to compete with this practice or expansion's market orientation and methods. Describe the protections that prevent new companies from competing, for example, possibly location, equipment, expertise, practice orientation, or other special features that make this company unique from all others and difficult to duplicate.

■ *Pricing and forecast.* The final step in a market assessment/analysis is to figure out the pricing of products and services (Chapters 13 and 14) and create a sales forecast. In pricing products or services, first ensure that the price is more than the costs to deliver the products and/or services. This includes all fixed, variable, avoided, and sunk costs that are essential to running the business.

Further, consider the message that pricing sends to consumers. Consumers equate high prices to quality. If using a high pricing or "market skimming" scheme, the marketing signals a high-quality product or service. External and internal visual effects, logo, and patient experience should exclaim high-quality during the entire process.

On the other end of the spectrum, if competing as a low-priced alternative to other products or practices, other messaging needs to present the same unified message and not promise more than can be delivered for the low price.

■ *Forecasting for initial sales volume.* Once pricing options have been chosen, consider how many products or services will be sold. Often, new businesses or expansions do not begin rapidly; they need time to "ramp up" to a productive level. Start small, maybe even at a loss initially, but with the correct strategy and marketing, the practice will evolve and business will get better, revenues will increase, and the business will finally "take off." Since there are no readily available benchmarks for practices in various locations within the industry, most of these forecasts are conducted with estimates for numbers of patients, product, and service sales monthly, as well as yearly.

These estimates should be conservative. While these estimate performance characteristics are totally speculative, those that read business plans are aware of this concern. The financiers will look for a conservative estimate of the numbers of patients, sales, revenues, and insurance reimbursements compared to expenses, especially in the first few months and the first year. If a loss is predicted for the first year, the plan needs to outline how this loss will be mitigated. Will it be from personal funds or loan funds, and so forth? They will also want to see that business gets better later in the first year and in subsequent years. Revenues should not be overestimated as this will be viewed by the lenders as unrealistic, suggesting the managers do not know their business. For some projects with current revenue, web-based programs, such as LivePlan.com can automatically gather existing data to assist in the comparison of the business plan forecast to the accounting data.

Another productive method in researching competition is to discuss the competition with prospective consumers and ask them what is missing from the provision of audiological products and services within the market. Not only consumers but stakeholders, such as referral sources, suppliers, and others, are also good for competitive intelligence. Of course, spending some time on "Google" for intelligence-gathering activities (Chapter 5) to figure out what else is in the current and predicted market is also valuable.

Personnel/Human Resources

Although job descriptions should not be included in their entirety in this section, the reader must understand the need for each position, the qualifications required, and the work product expectations of each position. Regardless of the number of positions filled at the outset of the practice, every position filled or anticipated should be described. Metrics or milestones should be established in concert with timelines to hire additional personnel. For example, the addition of an audiologist may be considered when specific patient bookings exceed a 2-week waiting list (the metric) on a consistent basis or when fiscal reserves reach a specified point with monthly or quarterly revenues reaching specific levels (another metric). First and foremost, the perceived need should be weighed against financial facts. The practice should generate enough opportunity for billable time to support another audiologist, audiology assistant (Chapter 10), or additional front office personnel to meet increasing billing and insurance claim submissions. These issues represent positive indicators of human resource growth.

Four traditional steps should be considered in the human resource component of the business plan.

■ Prepare a human resource forecast based on how many employees are necessary over time.
■ Develop a human resource inventory of initial hires.
■ Develop a job analysis of employee responsibilities.
■ Prepare a comprehensive plan of how to integrate new employees into the practice.

First, anticipate how many employees will be required in the future. For existing practices, this number will be more accurate as there is a historical perspective of past growth. For new practices, the forecast will be based upon knowledge of the practice of the profession and of market fluctuations. *Second* is the development of a human resource inventory, or how many employees are required to execute the project or a startup practice. Initially, this is rather easy as it is often only one person, the practitioner. As the practice grows, however, it is necessary to consider the necessity of new employees, such as a receptionist or another audiologist and how they will be assimilated into the practice, as well as which milestones should be achieved before hiring them. *Third* is the consideration of what each of these individuals will be required to do. These job responsibilities may change over time as the practice or project grows. A comprehensive plan for human resources, *Step 4*, may be the most time-consuming, but it is the most critical component of the human resource section, offering a plan to successfully integrate or "on board" new employees into the practice. It should include budgeting for future wages and training techniques to bring current employees up to and maintain the required skill levels. For employees who are yet to be hired, prioritization as to which types of employees should be hired first, next, and last must be considered. These steps should be integral to the business plan and reviewed periodically to update the human resource requirements as the practice's needs change.

Operational Plan

This section is usually the most difficult to write. It describes how the practice will perform in the market, what services it will provide, immediate and long-term equipment needs, whether clinical or office equipment will be leased or purchased, and front office operations. It emphasizes the physical necessities for the operation of the practice, such as physical location, facilities, and equipment, as well as inventory requirements and suppliers. It also should describe the flow of a typical patient through the clinic from the first phone call to their exit. It is advantageous to divide this section into two categories: Development and Production.

Development

Development begins by presenting what has been done so far for the startup company or the expansion project and what still needs to be done to become operational. Elements of the developmental plan are as follows:

- *Clinical production.* Include a discussion of the advantages and limitations of the various evaluations offered and the risks involved in the provision of these services and products.
- *Audiology Association memberships & credentials.* It is beneficial to present a biographical sketch of the licensing and certification requirements of the practitioners, in addition to organization affiliations. This demonstrates capability to manage the clinic and an awareness of the local, regional, or national standards and regulations necessary to practice the profession.
- *Suppliers.* List all potential suppliers and the reason for choosing them. Typical reasons might be technology, reliability, prices, terms, and

conditions. It is also beneficial to describe alternative arrangements if these suppliers do not deliver expected results (Chapter 19).
- *Quality control.* How will the practitioner control the quality of the services and products provided? While this may be easy in the beginning, as the practice grows to other locations and others are providing the services, a process is necessary to ensure that high-quality products, evaluations, and rehabilitative treatment are provided to each and every patient.

Production Process

The *production process section* expands on the development section and presents the details of day-to-day operations. The goal of this section is to demonstrate an understanding of the clinical processes and skills necessary for the business' operation:

- *General.* Conduct an outline of the practice's day-to-day operations, including the days and hours of operation.
- *Clinical workflow.* A high-level, step-by-step description of how the clinic operates. State what happens from the time a patient calls for an appointment to the time they leave the office satisfied with their evaluation or products. This would include some of the evaluation process such as amplification requirements, levels of technology, discussion of other hearing issues, and/or rehabilitative procedures.
- *The clinic.* Space requirements and location are discussed in this section. Include drawings of the

building, space allocations, and tenant modifications if applicable. Drawings and sketches are typically suppled in the appendix. Discuss how the space is efficiently utilized and how the location of the practice provides easy access and ample parking.

■ *Equipment.* Provide a detailed description of all the equipment and its function. It is also essential to include worth and cost and explain any financing arrangements, such as leased or purchased.

■ *Assets.* If the space is owned, the practitioner should make a list of all assets such as land, building, inventory, furniture, equipment, and vehicles. If necessary, include legal descriptions in the appendix. Integrated software that tracks patient data and any patient-interface aspects should be described, in addition to billing and financial management software. The lender or investor will be especially interested in the practitioner's contribution to the startup costs of the project.

■ *Special requirements.* If the practice has any special requirements, such as water or power needs, ventilation, drainage, floor reinforcement, and handicap parking, these details are part of the operation plan, especially if it involves extra funds.

■ *Supplies & services.* Outline all venders of supplies and calibration services and describe the qualification procedures. Explain what terms have been negotiated with suppliers and the plans for controlling costs in the new practice.

■ *Production.* Describe the time allocated for each unit of service (i.e., specify the time allotment to conduct a hearing or balance evaluation, hearing aid consultation, or fitting compared to the cost per clinical unit hour). A brief description of the diagnostic utility and clinical necessity of each service by CPT code should be included to orient the reader to the breadth and importance of the care to be provided. Special procedures linked to specific equipment should be described relative to their anticipated use. Hearing instrument fitting and follow-up care should be explained with conservative projected numbers of instruments to be fit over the course of the first 3 to 5 years. If the practice begins with limited services, indicate the services to be added later and discuss the timeline and/or a decision metric or milestone that will permit service expansion.

■ *Inventory.* Although most audiology clinics do not have much inventory, if applicable, discuss how the inventory will be controlled.

■ *Feasibility.* Describe any product, price, prototype, or other testing that may become part of the practice protocols.

■ *Cost.* Present product-cost estimates relative to revenue. This section could also include a discussion of insurance discounts and buying group relationships and how they will impact the revenue of the practice.

The headings above may be used as subheadings with details in paragraph format. If a topic does not apply to a specific practice, omit it. Brief and concise must be the watchword of this section. It is best to include all those involved in the practice, including the practice attorney and accountant, to read, review, and comment on how the business is defined.

Financials

The financial section of a business plan is one of the most essential elements of the plan, and it seems to create the most difficulty for audiologists. Wasserman (2024) indicates that a business plan is all conceptual until the numbers and terms are presented. While the marketing plan and strategies are interesting to read, they mean nothing if there is no financial justification of the practice with positive figures on the bottom line. Thus, this portion of the plan determines if the proposal is viable.

The purpose of the financial section is twofold. First, it is mandatory if seeking funding from venture capitalists, investors, or even smart family members. Investors want to see numbers that present rapid growth and/or an exit strategy, during which they can make a profit. Any bank or lender will need to see these numbers to ensure that the loan can be repaid. Second, and most important, it is for the benefit of the owner, in predicting future financial success.

This section requires realistic and objective projections based on as much factual information as possible. Care must be taken to not overstate or inflate revenue projections, numbers of services to be provided, or numbers of instruments to be dispensed. Revenue projections should be based on anticipated referrals and self-referred patients over a specified time period. Incremental numbers of new patients

should be discussed as a function of proposed marketing efforts. A credible financial section for a business plan must be realistic. The financial forecast is not necessarily compiled in sequence, and it is most likely not going to be presented in the sequence that it is compiled. Berry (2008) presented that it is typical to start in one place and jump back and forth. For example, the cash-flow plan might mean going back to change estimates for sales and expenses. Berry further indicates that the financial section consists of six steps, and it is often necessary to revisit previous steps to arrive at the final financial data ultimately presented in the business plan. These steps are as follows:

- *Start with a sales forecast.* Set up a spreadsheet projecting sales over the course of 3 years. Differentiate separate sections for each line of sales, such as evaluations or hearing devices and other products, and columns for every month for the first year and on a monthly or quarterly basis for the second and third years. Berry suggests creating a spreadsheet with blocks for unit sales, a second block for pricing, a third block that multiplies units times price to calculate sales, a fourth block that has unit costs, and a fifth that multiplies units times unit cost to calculate cost of sales (also called COGS or direct costs). This allows for the calculation of gross margin. Gross margin is sales less the cost of sales and is a useful number for demonstrating the viability of a practice.
- *Create an expense budget.* It is fundamental to understand the

costs involved to make the sales forecasted. Differentiations must be made between fixed costs (i.e., rent and payroll) and variable costs (i.e., expendable materials: probe tips, electrodes, earmold impression material). This provides an idea of the costs relative to the gross margin, and lower fixed costs mean less risk. Also included in the budget must be an estimate of interest and taxes. Berry (2008) suggests multiplication of the estimated profits times a "best-guess" tax percentage rate to estimate taxes and multiplication of the estimated debt balance times an estimated interest rate for the estimation of interest.

■ *Develop a cash-flow statement.* This statement presents the physical dollars moving in and out of the business. This is based partly on sales forecasts, balance sheet items, and other assumptions. In an existing practice, there are historical documents, such as profit and loss statements and balance sheets from years past upon which to base these forecasts. If starting a new practice and historical financial statements are not available, the practitioner should start by projecting a cash-flow statement broken down into 12 months. Cash-flow projection uses a realistic ratio of invoices paid in cash, out 30 days, 60 days, 90 days, and so on. Surprises such as only collecting 80% of invoices in the first 30 days when the business was counting on 100% to pay expenses can be devastating, especially at the beginning of a new practice, and insurance companies are noted for paying slowly. Some business planning software programs, such as LivePlan.com, offer formulas that are built into the projections to assist in making these forecasts.

■ *Detail income projections.* This is the pro forma profit and loss statement, detailing forecasts for the practice or project for the upcoming 3 years. This statement uses the numbers from the sales forecast, expense projections, and cash-flow statement. Recall that sales, less cost of sales, is gross margin, and gross margin, less expenses, interest, and taxes, is net profit (Chapter 11).

■ *Deal with assets and liabilities.* Assets and liabilities that are not included in the profit and loss statement must be addressed for projection of the net worth of the business at the end of the year. Compiling the balance sheet begins with assets and an estimate of cash on hand month by month, accounts receivable, any possible inventory, and substantial assets such as land, buildings, and equipment. As for liabilities, or debt (the right side of the balance sheet), current bills that are not yet paid (accounts payable) are entered in addition to the debt that is owed for long-term outstanding loans. This and the contributions that have been made to the practice at this point will make up the rest of the balance sheet.

■ *Breakeven analysis.* The breakeven point is when practice or project expenses match sales or service volume. The 3-year income projection will enable the practitioner to undertake this analysis. If the practice is viable, after a certain period of time, the overall revenue will exceed the overall expenses, including interest. The breakeven point is important for investors who want to know if they have financed a fast-growing practice with an exit strategy. Breakeven points should be defined based on numbers of referrals, procedures completed, and instruments dispensed over a specific timeline.

As the financial section is prepared, common sense should prevail: If it is unlikely there will be referrals to support an auditory evoked potential or a videonystagmography system in the beginning of the practice, there is no need to allocate funding for its purchase until such time that anticipated referrals can support its use.

Cloud-Based Business Planning

Over the years, many methods of teaching and learning business planning have been used with variable success. Initially, business planning books and other printed materials presented theoretical material to create a business plan but with intermittent success. Later, computer programs were generated from a number of sources that offered a substantial improvement but lacked the capability for all computers to use the same operating systems. While these programs offered a more complete method of incorporating the theoretical concepts of business planning into a practical document for those that were not business savvy, they were also expensive. Recently, cloud-based business planning programs have become available to present the process from beginning to end with videos for each stage.

While others will likely surface over time, one such program is www.live plan.com. LivePlan, offered by Palo Alto Software, was the first of its kind to present a professional business planning process to those that have no background in the planning process. While it offers professional plans for about 500 types of businesses, currently there is not a sample for an audiology practice. The principles are, however, very easily applied to developing a business plan for a new practice or expansion of an existing practice or other types of enterprise, such as a new program for a hospital or school district. With the use of LivePlan, the practitioner does not need to know anything about professional business planning because it guides and eases students into the planning process, as well as aids in developing a pitch for the practice, forecasting the market, and outlining the competition and financials through quality video and easy text instruction. Additionally, for a minimal cost, it generates graphs and tables necessary to complete a professional business plan worthy of presenting to bankers and investors.

Summary

Lenders reviewing the business plan of startup practices want to be convinced that the proposed venture will reach the financial projections detailed in the plan. In short, they want to be convinced that their participation as a financial partner will result in a successful practice or project. If the plan is done well, it will provide readers with a measure of confidence and an incentive to lend the monies needed to fund the venture. The document should be straightforward and as short as possible, as well as offer realistic financial data supported by comprehensive due diligence about the opportunities for success in the market.

As a vital and living document, the business plan should be revisited periodically and updated accordingly. If the plans for the practice change, the business plan should reflect that change. One should consider sending a revised business plan to the lenders, attorney, and accountant to keep them informed and confident that the business portion of the practice is being managed diligently with the same level of completeness that the clinic manages its patients.

References

ADA. (2024). Medicare Audiology Access and Improvement Act of 2024. Academy of Doctors of Audiology. https://audiologist .org/resources/advocacy/maaia

Ariston. (2024). Hearing aids market—global outlook & forecast 2024-2029, 4th edition. Ariston Advisory and Intelligence. https:// www.arizton.com/market-reports/ hearing-aids-market-analysis-2024

Berry, T. (2008). The plan as you go business plan. Entrepreneur Media. Palo Alto Software. https://www.amazon.com/Plan -As-You-Go-Business-Plan-Tim-Berry/ dp/1599181908/ref=sr_1_2?s=books &ie=UTF8&qid=1483012829&sr=1-2

Berry, T. (2023). 14 Reasons Why you need a business plan. https://www.bplans.com /business-planning/basics/why-you-need/

Carr, K., & Kihm, J. (2022). MarkeTrak— tracking the pulse of the hearing aid market. *Seminars in Hearing*, *43*(4), 277–288.

Cohen, W. (2010). *Drucker on leadership*. Jossey-Bass/Wiley.

Harrison, J., & St. John, C. (2004). *Foundations in strategic management* (3rd ed.). Thompson-Southwestern.

LivePlan. (2024). LivePlan website. www .liveplan.com

Morelock, A. (2024). Vision vs. mission statements: Why it's important to know the difference? *Insight Global*. https://in sightglobal.com/blog/vision-vs-mission -statements/

Parsons, N. (2024). How to conduct a market analysis in 4 steps—2024 guide. LivePlan. com. https://www.liveplan.com/blog/mar ket-analysis-in-4-steps/

Schooley, S. (2023). 5 Steps for writing an executive summary. *Business News Daily*. https://www.businessnewsdaily.com /15814-write-an-executive-summary.html

Souza, P. (2014). Hearing loss and aging: Implications for audiologists. National Institute on Deafness and Other Communication Disorders (R01 DC60014 and R01 DC12289). http://www.asha.org/Ar ticles/Hearing-Loss-and-Aging-Implica tions-for-Audiologists/

St. Clergy, K. (2016). Helping practices grow with patient education. MedPB, Medical Practice Builders. http://www.medpb.com /about-us/educated-patients-kevin-st -clergy/

Traynor, R. M. (2008). Strategic business planning. In R. Glaser & R. Traynor (Eds.), *Strategic practice management* (2nd ed.). Plural Publishing.

Traynor, R. M. (2013). Strategic business planning. In R. Glaser & R. Traynor (Eds.), *Strategic practice management* (2nd ed.). Plural Publishing.

Traynor, R. M. (2019). Strategic business planning. In R. Glaser & R. Traynor (Eds.), *Strategic practice management* (3rd ed.). Plural Publishing.

Wasserman, E. (2024). How to write the financial section of a business plan. Studocu. https://www.studocu.com/en-au/docu ment/swinburne-university-of-technology

/advanced-innovative-business-practice
/bus30024-assignment-1-business-im
pact-sdgs/25608573?origin=viewer
-recommendation-2

Windmill, I., & Freeman, B. (2017, April). *Projected change in Medicare enrollment 2000-2050.* Paper presented at the 2017 American Academy of Audiology.

Windmill, I., & Freeman, B. (2019). Medicare, hearing care, and audiology: Data-driven perspectives. *Audiology Today, 31*(2), 18–26.

4 Competition: Strategies for Differentiating the Audiology Practice

Brian Taylor, AuD, Alexander Evertz, and Robert M. Traynor, EdD, MBA

Introduction

To fully understand and appreciate the benefits of competition, it helps to illustrate how audiology might be practiced in a planned economy such as Cuba. As many know, Cuba has been a communist country with a centrally planned economy for more than 60 years. Cuba is a place where all citizens obtain free healthcare, but it comes with some compromises. Although all citizens are entitled to free healthcare, including hearing care, unelected municipal authorities decide how the funds set aside for healthcare will be divided across the entire population. These same authorities also prioritize the types of services that citizens can obtain based on the severity of their condition. Since hearing loss is seldom a life-threatening condition, it receives low-priority status within their planned system. Consequently, "free" hearing care for adults is rather spartan, with no choice of hearing aid technology levels or form factors and minimal, cookie-cutter follow-up care. Additionally, since all the healthcare workers, in-

cluding audiologists, are employed by the government (private healthcare businesses are forbidden), there are no opportunities for entrepreneurs to provide competition to the existing service model, businesses that may provide better care, faster service, and more innovative devices. In short, because of a lack of competition, people with hearing loss are woefully underserved, with sparse choices and barebone services.

This chapter is devoted to the benefits and challenges of competitive free markets. As the chapter outlines, both persons with hearing loss and clinicians benefit from a competitive free market system with oversight from regulatory bodies. Competition is the lifeblood of a thriving market-based economic system. It provides customers with abundant choices and workers and entrepreneurs with greater opportunities. Moreover, healthy market competition is fundamental to a well-functioning U.S. economy. Basic economic theory demonstrates that when businesses must compete for customers, it usually leads to lower prices, higher-quality goods and services, greater variety of choices, and more innovation. Competition is good not only for customers, but it is also beneficial to employees, including audiologists. When firms compete to attract employees, they must increase compensation and improve working conditions. Just about everyone wins in a well-regulated, free-market system.

When there is insufficient competition, dominant businesses can use their market power to charge higher prices, offer decreased quality, and block potential competitors from entering the market—meaning entrepreneurs and small businesses cannot participate on a level playing field and new ideas cannot become new goods and services. Former Supreme Court Justice Louis Brandeis (1856–1941) coined a term, "The Curse of Bigness," to describe how concentrated power, when in the hands of just a few powerful people or businesses, is a menace to both customers and employees. Some economic experts believe that the market for hearing aid suffer from this "Curse of Bigness" (Brandeis, 1934). As a Fellow at the Open Markets Institute Stoller (2021) states, "The five leading hearing aid manufacturers control more than 90% of the market." One objective of this chapter is to look more carefully at this Curse of Bigness and discuss the attributes of competition.

The positive and negative attributes of the hearing aid industry as it currently looks in 2024 with its corporate roll-ups and continued vertical integration will be presented in this chapter. However, the beginning of the journey to understanding competition must begin by a discussion of the key aspects of a free-market economy and how entrepreneurs can leverage their competitive advantages to create value for customers.

The Discipline of Market Leaders: Making Hard Choices

The assumption behind a free-market economy is that supply and demand are the best determinants for an economy's growth and health. Supply and demand influence three fundamental aspects of an economy:

1. What goods and services should be produced.
2. How many goods and services should be produced.
3. At what price the goods and services should be sold.

These factors also influence other economic decisions, such as how many workers companies should employ and what these workers ought to be paid.

In contrast, command economies like the Cuban healthcare system utilize central planning, relying on a dominant authority to make all economic decisions. In a planned economic system, a group of bureaucrats decides all three of those fundamental aspects of the economy. In a truly free market (zero government intervention), all resources are owned by individuals. The decisions about how to allocate their resources are made by those individuals rather than by central governing bodies. This economic theory, known as laissez-faire, asserts that governments should have no hand in business. In this theory, their interventions often lead to market inefficiencies.

In reality, the government always has some involvement in regulating free-market economies, so there are no recognized economies that are 100% free. However, government is limited in how it regulates transactions within a market economy. Most of the rules it enacts are to protect consumers, the environment, market participants, and national security. Additionally, the amount of government oversight and regulation on the economy of a certain sector of the economy tends to change depending on popular opinion and political administrations.

The advantages of a market economy include increased efficiency, productivity, and innovation. Unlike other types of economies, a market economy increases business efficiency and competition. Governments, in their limited roles, work to promote this by creating and enforcing legislation that places limits on activities that detract from a competitive environment. They also support business efficiency but regulate how businesses treat consumers and workers to maximize efficiency. In the hearing aid industry, two federal agencies, the Food and Drug Administration (FDA) and the Federal Trade Commission (FTC), provide oversight of hearing aid manufacturing processes, product claims, and marketing claims. On the other hand, states, through their licensing guidelines, regulate the clinical audiologist's ability to practice.

Efficiency is usually measured in terms of costs and profits. High efficiency is typically viewed as low costs and high profits, whereas low efficiency is viewed as high cost and low profits. Competition plays a role in efficiency because it forces businesses to do whatever is necessary to lower costs, control more of the market, and achieve higher sales to increase profits, as long as it is legal. Increased productivity is also associated with a market economy. In any econ-omy, people need money to purchase goods and services. In a market economy, this need leads to increased motivation because workers want to earn more money to supply their needs and to live comfortably.

People motivated to work increase productivity and output for the economy. In a command economy, where a central authority or government sets wages, levels of production, prices, and investments, there is less worker motivation because no matter how much harder they work, they will not see additional monetary benefit.

A third component of a market economy is innovation. Firms and individuals are encouraged to innovate to gain a competitive advantage and increase their market share. With money as a primary motivating factor, companies look to create new products and technologies to generate more revenue, higher incomes, and more profit. Innovation also leads to a greater variety of goods and services, which provides a broader selection for consumers.

Market Leadership: How Should This Company Be Known in the Market?

Since businesses in a market economy are owned by individuals, it is imperative for these individuals to have a strategy or plan that enables their business to be profitable. One approach to differentiating a business from competitors was provided by Treacy and Wiersma (1995), suggesting that the most financially successful companies focused on customer satisfaction rather than shareholder profits.

Perhaps their most important insight with respect to competition was that all successful businesses focus on these three dimensions of value but choose just one of them where they can truly excel.

1. *Customer Intimacy*—knowing as much as possible about the people who need the product and services and delivering an engaging customer experience.
2. *Product Leadership*—bringing to market the most innovative products and services that deliver superior outcomes to customers.
3. *Operational Excellence*—running the most cost-efficient business that yields low prices for consumers.

Notice that all three of these dimensions offer something of remarkable value to the customer. The authors pose that any successful business needs to maintain at least "acceptable" levels of performance in each of the three dimensions, but each business must choose one of them to become a market leader in its field. Their model suggests that if the business truly wants to excel in one of the three disciplines, you will have to make sacrifices in the other two. How does the discipline of market leaders apply to managing an audiology practice? Choose one of these three dimensions and become recognized in the community for it. The lesson for aspiring owners and managers of audiology practices is this: No one has an infinite number of resources; therefore, they cannot be all things to all people. They must carefully evaluate their competition and understand what they do well while simultaneously assessing their practice's own strengths and weaknesses. After careful analysis, choose one of the three dimensions of value in which the practice can become the market leader. Once this hard choice has been made, allocate resources to make it happen.

Development and Implementation of a Competitive Strategy

Competition in the market is unfamiliar territory for audiologists that creates some fundamental challenges. Practitioners have spent most of their time developing theoretical and experiential clinical skills to treat their patients. Unfortunately, in the current hearing care market, a doctoral degree, good clinical skills, and expertise in the treatment of patients are not enough to achieve success as an independent private practitioner. Often audiologists come into their practice with lofty goals, without much thought and/or expertise as to how to achieve them. Competing involves creating value for patients while leveraging clinical, physical, business, and financial resources. This chapter reviews many of the specific aspects of competition in the hearing healthcare profession with an emphasis on how the various large industry corporations affect the development and execution of a coherent clinical strategy. Chapter 5 takes a broader view of competition and how to conduct a strategic analysis of an audiology practice.

Understanding the Competition and Creating a Market Niche: Factors to Consider

Perhaps the most essential element of devising any strategic imperative in an audiology practice is understanding the customer. Peter Drucker, a foremost 20th-century business scholar, stated that the purpose of any business is to create a customer (Drucker, 1954). In the case of any audiology business, that process begins with studying the market for hearing and balance and addressing the question: Who is the customer?

Current statistics about the worldwide prevalence of hearing loss provide a beginning for this discussion. The World Health Organization (WHO) published a World Report on Hearing in 2021, which stated that hearing loss of all levels currently affects more than 1.5 billion people worldwide. The WHO also reported that 430 million people live with disabling hearing loss, moderate or worse in the better ear. Those figures indicate that over 80% of ear and hearing care needs around the world remain unmet. Additionally, the WHO reported that unaddressed hearing loss poses an annual cost of $980 billion each year globally (WHO, 2021).

In the United States, consider the number of prospective patients in each age category. Current statistics by the National Institute on Deafness and Other Communication Disorders (NIDCD, 2021) indicate the following:

- 2% of adults aged 45 to 54 have disabling hearing loss.
- 8.5% of adults aged 55 to 64 have disabling hearing loss.
- 25% of those aged 65 to 74 have disabling hearing loss.
- 50% of those 75 and older have disabling hearing loss.

Now digest the above data into the number of potential individuals in the market for hearing care, assuming that the total U.S. hearing impaired population is about 10% of the overall population or about 32 million individuals. Calculations would suggest the following potential market for hearing care services and products as approximately:

- 900,000 people aged 45 to 54.
- 3,000,000 people aged 55 to 64.
- 5,500,000 people aged 65 to 74.
- 9,300,000 people aged 75 and older.

While these numbers present a total U.S. market of about 102 million individuals that have some form of hearing loss, it does not account for the fact that since January 2006, each day, about 10,000 individuals turn 65 years of age, netting about 250,000 new individuals per year potentially requiring hearing care. Demographic statistics suggest that this yearly increase in potential patients will continue until 2030. When binaural fittings are considered, huge numbers of hearing aid units will be required to accommodate the increasing population, making the hearing industry a potential target for big business. International markets have similar increasing numbers, particularly Europe and Australia, as well as many developing nations.

In support of these data, Grand View Research (2023) has found that the global market size for hearing devices

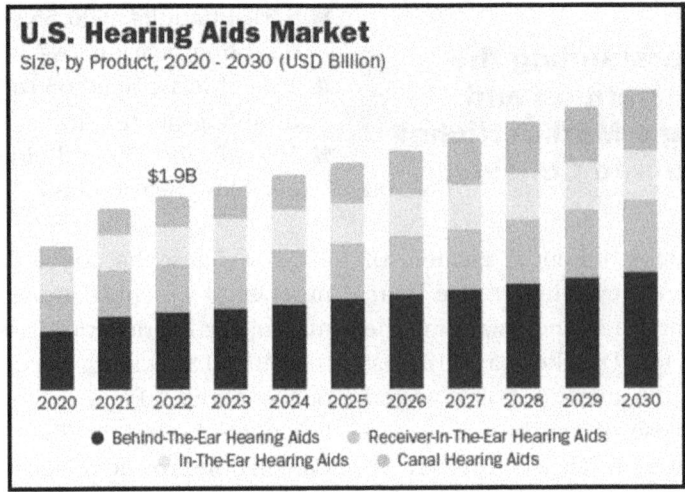

Figure 4–1. Predicted hearing aid market 2024–2030. *Source*: Grand View Research (2023).

was estimated at USD 7.96 billion in 2023 and is projected to grow at an annual growth rate of 6.78% from 2024 to 2030 (Figure 4–1). The market growth (or market penetration) can be attributed to the increasing adoption of hearing aids devices, growing awareness regarding technologically advanced devices for auditory impairment, and the increasing prevalence of hearing loss due to the growing geriatric population.

Hearing Aid Market Penetration

Defined by Kenton et al. (2024), market penetration is the number of sales or adoption of product or service compared to the total theoretical market for that product or service.

For the past 40 years or so, penetration of the hearing aid market has been an issue. Staab (2014) reported that market penetration (also known as hearing aid uptake) had been relatively flat in

the hearing industry for the past 40 years. This supports the Schroeder (2009) data indicating that market penetration in 2008 was 24.6%, suggesting that about 75% of those requiring hearing care were not receiving it. Taylor (2016) offered insight into the details of patient uptake of hearing aids according to the severity of hearing loss, presented in Figure 4–2 as:

- Profound hearing losses make up about 1.6 million people: 70% or 1.1 million use hearing instruments, and 30% or 500,000 do not use hearing devices.
- Severe hearing losses make up about 6.4 million people and about 50% or 3.2 million use hearing devices, but 3.2 million do not use hearing devices.
- Mild to moderate hearing losses make up 24 million people and only 10% or 2.4 million use hearing devices, and 90% or 21.6 million do not use hearing devices.

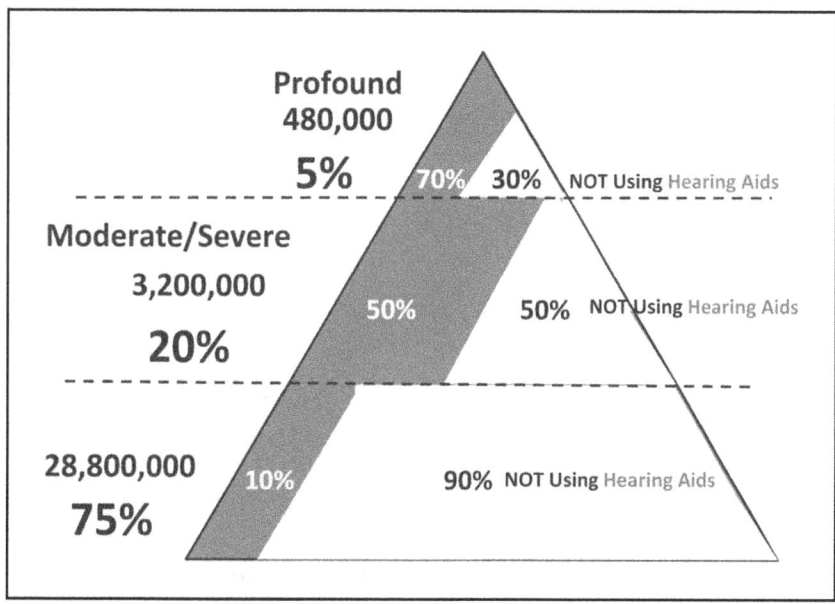

Figure 4–2. Hearing loss prevalence as a function of degree of hearing loss and predicted uptake rates of hearing aids for each. *Source*: Taylor (2016).

From the numbers illustrated here, there was a potential market of approximately 28 million individuals who do not use hearing aids in the United States, indicating a potential overall U.S. market for hearing aids at 55.4 million devices. Regardless of the specific reported uptake rate (statistics on this rate vary because of differences in how hearing loss is defined), it has been well known there is a huge unmet need for hearing-related services, as somewhere between 70% and 90% of those who could benefit for hearing aids and related services *have not acquired them.* Humes (2023) still reports that 85% of those with self-reported hearing difficulties do not wear hearing aids.

Audiology clinics in 2024 are very busy, and the market is on the rise despite a poor economy. The news reports and "hype" that has surrounded the hearing industry since the original PCAST (2015) discussion of hearing aids, legislation, and 2022 final implementation of the OTC Act (2017) have injected the market with substantial visibility. Part of this legislation eliminated the mandatory physicians' recommendation that has been required for acquisition of hearing aids, making the acquisition process less frustrating. Cultural changes in the United States are contributing to the increase of hearing aid use in that stigma, though still an issue, is significantly reduced with the aging of the U.S. population and market penetration.

In his discussion of market penetrations, Edwards (2020) proposed that the untapped market for hearing care services is much more expensive than previously believed. To explain the theory of the two variables (degree of hearing loss and hearing difficulties), a four-quadrant

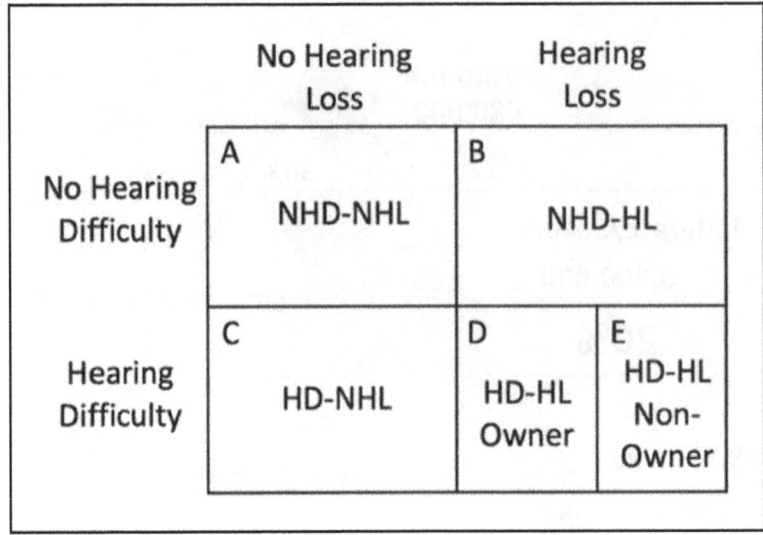

Figure 4–3. The population segmented by hearing loss and self-reported hearing difficulty. HD = hearing difficulty; HL = hearing loss on audiogram; NHL = no hearing loss. *Source*: Edwards (2020).

matrix is used as a method to fully capture the unmet need for hearing devices and professional services (Figure 4–3).

Edwards (2020) argues that it is only the individuals who fall into the lower-right Quadrant D/E who have sought care from an audiologist. Note that Quadrant D/E is divided into two groups: sub-Quadrant D represents those who have acquired hearing aids, and sub-Quadrant E represents those who did not. This entire quadrant (D/E) comprises about 5% to 6% of the entire U.S. adult population. About half of those in the D/E quadrant have sought care from an audiologist and been informed during the appointment that they would benefit from hearing aids but rejected that recommendation.

Next, focus on the bottom-left quadrant, labeled C in Figure 4–3. These are individuals who have normal audiograms (pure-tone average better than 25 dB HL), but they self-report difficulty with their hearing in acoustically challenging situations. According to Edwards's analysis, approximately 12 to 15 million American adults fit into Quadrant C. Although this group struggles with communication in specific listening situations and often seeks help from audiologists, historically, they have not been considered candidates for hearing aids. Individuals in Quadrant C, however, might be excellent candidates for hearing aid substitutes such as hearables and other amplifiers sold over the counter.

Now, focus on the top-right quadrant, labeled B. These are individuals who are hearing aid candidates according to their audiogram but have not sought the care or guidance of an audiologist because they do not report or perceive any discernable hearing difficulty. Rather than acquiring hearing aids, those in the Quadrant B might value an initial interaction with an audiologist to facilitate a better understanding of how hearing loss is impacting their health and wellness before actually pursuing the use of hearing aids. It is also possible that individuals in Quadrant B, because they might be in denial about hearing loss, would prefer to not call attention to their condition and prefer to dabble with over-the-counter hearing aids from the comforts of home.

Finally, consider that Quadrant A in the top left of Figure 4–3 comprises individuals with normal audiograms and no self-reported hearing difficulties. Although the overwhelming majority of people in the community fall into Quadrant A, there are still opportunities to educate this group about the use of hearing protection and the importance of periodic hearing screenings.

Each of the four quadrants illustrated in Figure 4–3 values something different and unique for audiologists. By thinking about persons with measured hearing loss on the audiogram and self-reported hearing difficulties as separate, yet overlapping categories of potential consumers, Edwards has expanded understanding of different segments of the market and how each individual's *perception of value differs*, depending upon the quadrant into which they fall. Since individuals within each quadrant value something different in this four-quadrant approach to understanding the market for hearing care, it becomes an effective beginning for the development of a sound business strategy. After careful analysis, using this four-quadrant approach, the audiology practice owner may decide to attract any one of these four different market segments to their practice.

Given the unmet need presented in Figure 4–1 and the unaddressed value propositions of various market segments offered by Edwards in Figure 4–3, it should be no surprise that there are potentially several new startup businesses looking to enter the hearing care space. After all, a key tenet of free-market capitalism is to create a business that serves an untapped segment of the market. Today, these startups comprise over-the-counter and direct-to-consumer hearing aid companies, as well as other firms that attempt to offer something of value (e.g., app-based auditory training) to the underserved segments outlined in Figure 4–2. On the other hand, existing mainstays (e.g., hearing aid manufacturers, large retail hearing aid chains) are likely to see opportunities to capture more business by tapping into underserved segments of the market or by operating more efficiently. In times when an industry has expanded, the use of two strategies, consolidation and vertical integration, will facilitate efficiency (profitability), allowing existing companies within that industry to thrive.

Thus, at this writing, the outlook for the end of the "flat" market is promising, with traffic in practices now increasing according to the Grand View Research 2024–2030 predictions presented in Figure 4–1.

Industry Consolidation: Horizontal and Vertical Integration

One of the peculiarities of the profession of audiology is that an essential business partner of the independent clinical audiologist, hearing aid manufacturers, is oftentimes also a competitor. This section of the chapter explains why hearing aid manufacturers, which have a vested interest in maintaining effective

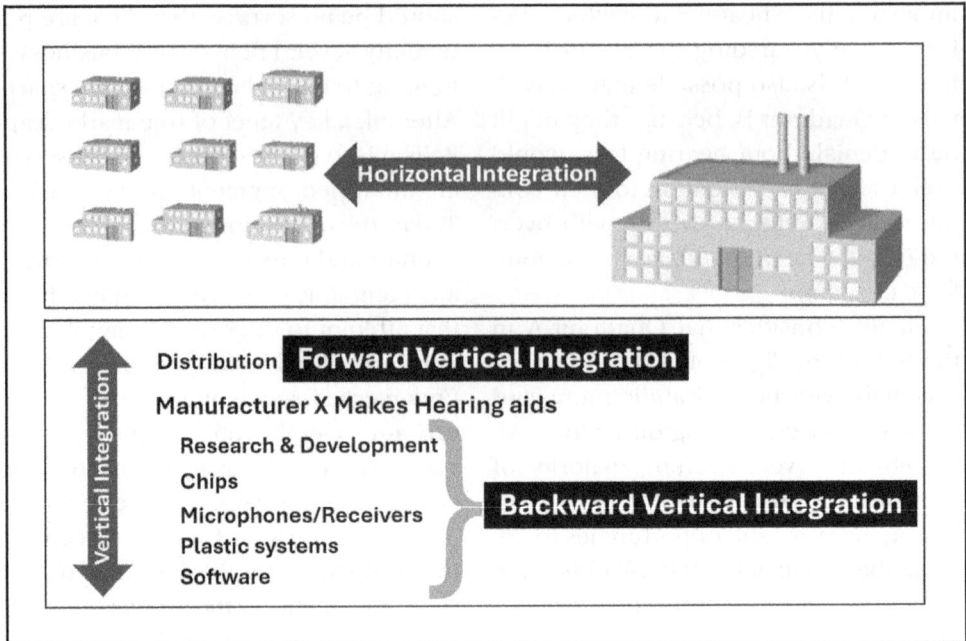

Figure 4–4. Horizontal and vertical integration.

relationships with clinical audiologists who dispense their products, are also competitors. The story of this rather odd relationship between manufacturers, audiologists, and dispensers of hearing aids revolves around the concepts of consolidation.

The huge increase in the hearing-impaired population had been predicted for many years, but during the time when the market was flat in the early 2000s, there were some winners and some losers that made consolidation within the hearing care industry inevitable. As the profits of large hearing aid manufacturers began to shrink, the natural industrial consolidation process becomes the place for these companies to secure new profits from acquisitions and mergers. While a frustration to established markets and traditional methods of doing business, consolidation is a natural result of an age-old industrial business cycle.

Whiting (2024) describes *industry consolidation* as a process whereby companies purchase or obtain controlling interest in other companies within the same industry, resulting in the reduction of the number of competitors within that industry. The main goal for these corporate consolidators is to grab market share, cut costs, boost productivity, gain patents and technology, and improve investment returns through scale economies. By the simple process of becoming larger, the purchasing company can become more efficient in the production and distribution of its products. Industry consolidation may be categorized into either *horizontal or vertical integration* (Figure 4–4):

■ *Horizontal integration* combines similar firms and products within a particular market segment, and the purchasing company becomes larger, often resulting in a greater market share.

■ *Vertical integration* consolidates companies so that each member of the supply chain produces a different product or service and combines to satisfy the common needs of the corporation.

Forward integration is a vertical integration business strategy whereby business activities are expanded to include control of the direct distribution of a company's products direct to the consumer. A good example of forward integration is the sale of hearing instruments directly to the consumer by manufacturers and bypassing the audiologist or other "resellers." Forward integration is an operational strategy implemented by a company that wants to increase control over its distribution channels so it can increase its market power. For a forward integration strategy to be successful, a company needs to gain ownership over practices that were once customers, such as the purchase of independent audiology clinics or a hearing aid dispensing practice. The UN Trade and Development (2014) reports that the U.S. Federal Trade Commission (FTC) supports industrial consolidation as benefiting competition and consumers by allowing firms to operate more efficiently. Others in the same report note that mergers and consolidation can lead to monopolistic positions, which may lead to higher prices, decreased innovation, and/or a drop in the quality or availability of goods or services.

Myers (2014) indicates that industry consolidation is almost inevitable. Over time, most industries, no matter their products or purpose, will consolidate into the largest three to five dominant companies while the rest of the smaller players will be rendered almost irrelevant as they retreat into specialty niches. Consider homebuilders, airlines, autos, computer software, or virtually any mature industry and they all began with thousands of players. As the industries grew, over a decade or several decades, these smaller companies predictably consolidated into larger and larger companies.

This natural industrial consolidation, both horizontal and vertical, has been going on for the past 25 years in audiology and the hearing industry. While this process is considered a normal part of a maturing industry, the transformation of the hearing care industry is not unlike that of the 20th-century automobile industry consolidation.

Automobile Industry Example

A good example of this natural industrial consolidation process is the auto industry. Consider that in the early part of the 20th century, there were literally hundreds of small automobile companies in the United States. Between 1896 and 1930, there were over 1,800 automobile companies created. For a few years, they all flourished as companies struggled to manufacture enough cars to meet consumer demand. Initially, the need for vehicles was so great that consumers did not care too much about brand, only that it was available, affordable, and reliable transportation. After a few years, the excessive demand for vehicles diminished, and by the late 1920s, these small automobile companies struggled against each other as well as the larger, more efficient competitors for essential manufacturing materials and market share. Many of these smaller, less efficient companies eventually went out of business or were purchased by larger, better-managed automobile companies. In an effort to compete with these larger companies, the surviving smaller manufacturers banded together into buying groups to purchase their manufacturing materials in bulk and, in return, they were given very favorable prices. Although those that banded together had to deal with buying group politics and other issues, the nonbuying group participants paid a higher price for component parts, metals, and rubber as well as other essential materials and, subsequently, had less funds for marketing and other operating expenses.

There were many innovators in the automobile industry, but a major contributor to the industrial consolidation process was General Motors under the leadership of Alfred P. Sloan Jr. In the 1920s and 1930s, Sloan and his staff invented the concept of *planned obsolescence* by putting a new emphasis on styling, exemplified by the annual largely cosmetic model changes and a planned 3-year major restyling that coincided with the life of the factories' production tools. The goal was to make consumers dissatisfied enough to trade in and, presumably, up to a more expensive new model long before the useful life of their present cars had ended. Sloan's stated philosophy was "the primary object of the corporation was to make money, not just to make motorcars" (Foner & Garraty, 1991). By the 1950s, industrial consolidation and other innovative corporate philosophies had dwindled the competition down to three major competitors in the auto industry, General Motors, Ford, and Chrysler. Later, having horizontally consolidated as much as possible, ver-

tical consolidation began and flourished as the automobile manufacturers began their purchase of parts from companies that used to make the engines and other components of the vehicles. Forward integration process also began by purchasing dealerships to offer their products directly to the consumers without sharing the profit with a dealership owner. This process was so successful that eventually, the manufacturers owned the dealerships, where they could manufacture the products with components from companies that they owned and sell the finished vehicle directly to the consumer without the "middleman" taking a share of the profits. This put the big three auto manufacturers in full control of both the manufacture and the distribution of their products, greatly increasing profits.

Consolidation Within the Hearing Industry

The consolidation process began in the late 1990s as companies began their horizontal process of purchasing competitive companies. They are interested in these other companies to increase their business by the acquisition of patents, new technologies, better discounts for manufacturing materials, more efficient manufacturing processes, better product distribution systems, and updating their sales and research and development employees. Vertical integration over the past 25 years has ebbed and flowed in our profession. While the beginning of the vertical process was backward integration, acquiring companies that had special patents for memories and programming made microphones and receivers, chips, plastics, technologies, software de-

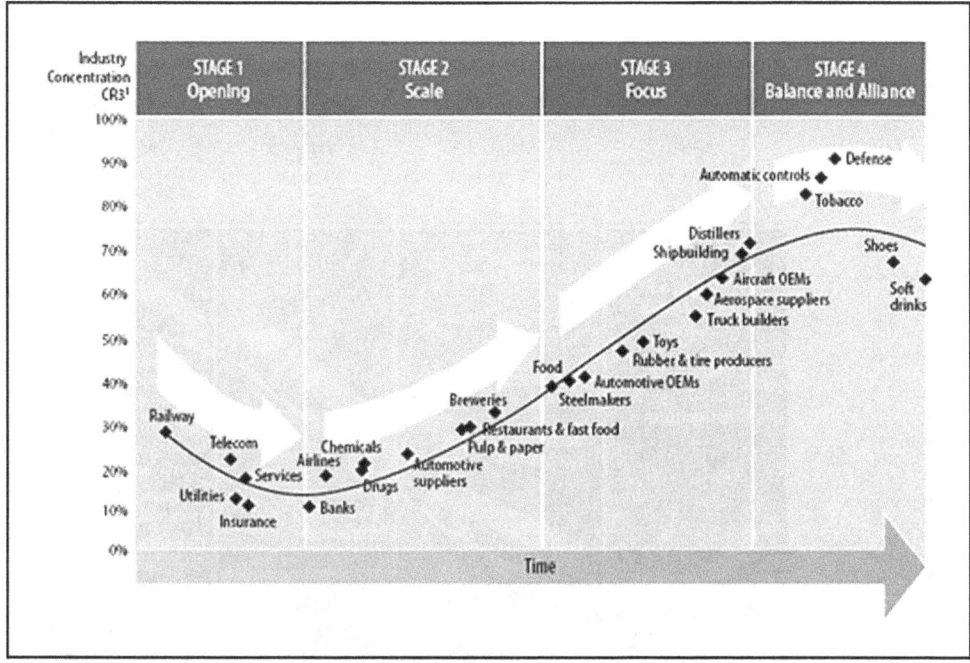

Figure 4–5. Four stages of industrial consolidation. *Source*: Deans et al. (2002).

velopers, and those researchers and engineers that created some of the most innovative technologies. For these acquisitions, it was easier and less expensive to acquire the new companies rather than reinvent these concepts and processes.

Later, as many of the original private practice owners retired, their businesses were acquired by these larger industrial entities and rolled up into a large chain of corporate-owned clinics as part of their forward integration process. When this occurred, hearing aid manufacturers became direct competitors with many of their independent customers who buy hearing aid products from them. As a result, like the automobile industry of a hundred years ago, audiologists and dispensers began moving to buying groups to purchase products and supportive services to reduce their product costs to remain competitive.

Industrial Consolidation of the Hearing Aid Industry

Although this horizontal and vertical consolidation seems to have taken place in a rather short time, it is an inevitable process of the normal growth and development of an industry. Deans et al. (2002) present that once the industrial consolidation process begins, there are four stages of progression, presented in Figure 4–5.

- Stage 1—Opening. Building products that do a good job for the end user.
- Stage 2—Scale. Companies building reputations. Major players purchase weaker ones and empires begin to form (horizontal integration).
- Stage 3—Focus. Successful companies begin purchases of allied companies (horizontal integration).

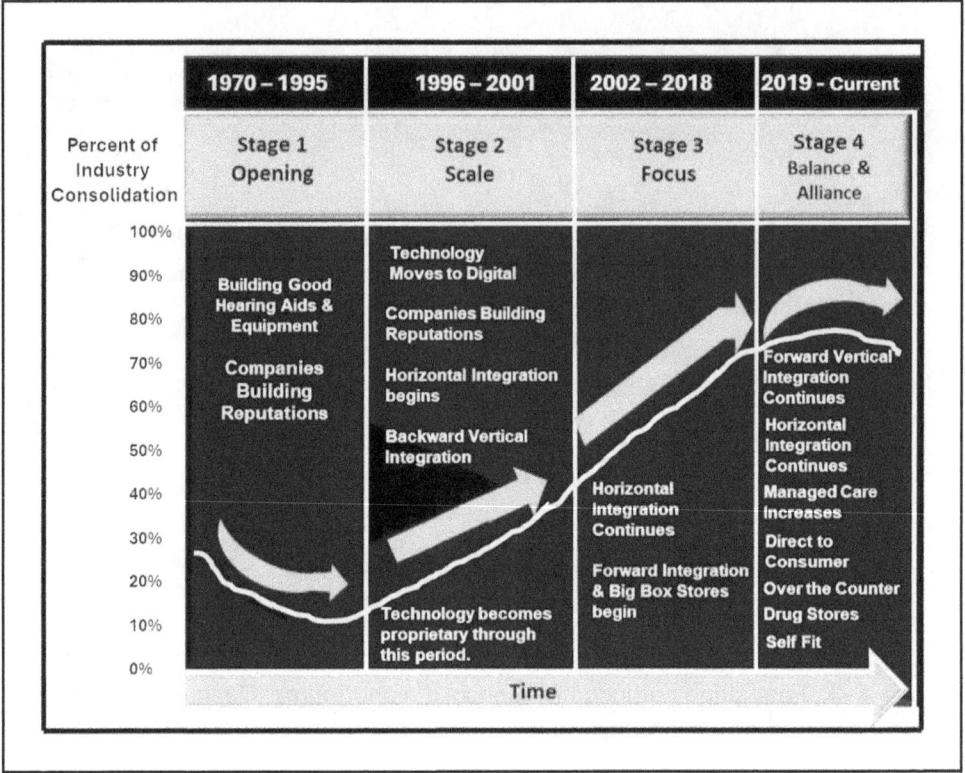

Figure 4–6. Four stages of hearing aid industrial consolidation. *Source*: Adapted from Deans et al. (2002).

Vertical and forward integration begins.

■ Stage 4—Balance and alliance.

The application of the model offered by Deans et al. (2002) offers a method by which the hearing aid industry consolidation can be explored.

Reviewing the various stages of industrial consolidation, the following might be a reasonable model to discuss the process as it has occurred in the hearing industry (Figure 4–6).

Stage 1: Opening

The *opening stage* of the consolidation process begins while still working with conventional analog circuitry in the 1970s. While manufacturers were formidable competitors in the marketplace, their altruistic motives were paramount in their attempt to provide the most technologic, reliable, and beneficial products for the hearing impaired. Some hearing care manufacturers were building reputations for better products over others, and due to competitive issues, horizontal consolidation begins as more efficient companies purchase technologically outdated competitors. During this period, consolidations were primarily conducted to obtain patent rights as well as for hardware, software, and programming innovations. Further, it was also to acquire famous brand names that had not kept up with sales and marketing of their products or that were financially troubled.

Stage 2: Scale

The *Stage 2 or scale* period begins as digitally controlled; analog circuits were available to the marketplace in the late 1980s. As the market moved to digital products in the mid-1990s, some hearing care manufacturers were building reputations for better products over others, and due to competitive issues, horizontal consolidation begins as more efficient companies purchase technologically outdated competitors. During this period, consolidations were primarily conducted to obtain patent rights as well as for hardware, software, and programming innovations, but as the horizontal consolidation continues and backward vertical integration begins, it will be to basically steal any technology, process, or specialized employees that will assist the company in becoming one of the major manufacturers in the industry. Part of this process was to acquire famous brand names that had not kept up with sales and marketing of their products or that were financially troubled and to use that company's reputation to build their business. This was summarized by Kirkwood (2011), who stated that "as in virtually every industry, hearing care has seen a trend of larger hearing aid manufacturers buying up smaller ones." Kirkwood noticed that there was one especially hectic period of consolidation from 1999 to 2001, highlighted by:

- Beltone purchased the hearing aid division of Philips Electronics.
- Starkey Laboratories purchased Micro-Tech.
- Siemens Hearing acquired Electone.

- GN Store Nord A/S purchased ReSound and Beltone.
- Unitron Industries acquired Argosy and Lori Medical.
- Phonak AG (now Sonova Holding) purchased Unitron.

Stage 3: Focus

Stage 3 or the focus phase began somewhere around the year 2002. At this point, hearing care corporate executives were no longer altruistic about the hearing impaired but had adopted the "Alfred Sloan philosophy" that "the primary object of the corporation was to make money, not just to make hearing aids."

Through the first two decades of the 21st century, consolidation within the hearing aid manufacturing sector of the hearing care industry waned; after all, there were far fewer small independent hearing aid manufacturers left to acquire. It was during this time, 2002 to 2018, however, when other sectors of the industry, including large retail dispensing chains, buying groups, and equipment distributors, emerged as targets of further consolidation. Stage 3 or the focus period also began the movement of hearing instruments into big box stores, such as Costco, Walmart, HearUSA, Connect Hearing, and other large sales operations that now account for a significant share of the current hearing care market.

New Internet companies came on the scene with some of the initial direct marketing to consumers as the FDA began relaxing their requirements for a physician's examination prior to being fit with hearing aids due to the over-the-counter hearing aid legislation of 2017 (OTC Act, 2017). These Internet companies were anything from low-priced, direct-to-consumer hearing aid sales operations with no support to customers or others that offered customer interaction with virtual dispensers across the country available to provide fitting and follow-up support as part of their purchase. The focus period also heralded the beginning of forward integration by some of the Big Five, which served to increase corporate profits in the face of a stalled market for amplification, equipment, and other hearing care products. As in the auto industry, the corporate retail acquisitions were dispensing practices where owners were retiring or in financial difficulties. Building upon their early success, forward integration spread to all the Big Five hearing care manufacturers.

Private practices were being bought in huge numbers by manufacturers to form major retail outlets for their products, such as Hearing Life, Connect Hearing, and others. By the end of 2018, there were six major manufacturers of hearing aids left in the group of major players that not only owned component manufacturers but were competing fiercely with their customers in the private practice sector. Companies that had survived the consolidation process were known as the "the Big Six": Starkey, GN Resound, William Demant, Sonova, Widex, and Signia.

Stage 4: Balance and Alliance

Stage 4 or the balance and alliance phase seems to have begun about 2019 and continues into the mid-2020s. This phase of consolidation begins with the merger of Signia and Widex in 2019 into WS Audiology. This most recent flurry of acquisitions has now left a group of five incumbent companies, now referred to as "The Big Five," currently dominating the business of hearing care worldwide. The companies that form the "Big Five" are Sonova, William Demant, GN Store Nord, WS Audiology, and Starkey. The Big Five group also began to purchase buying groups that had been established by independent hearing care professionals to keep their costs within reason, allowing these companies insight into the independent practice and control over some components of the market where there had been little influence in the past. Initially, this process was very controversial due to state legal and licensing issues. The Internet was also found to be an innovative new distribution channel, attracting new customers in an otherwise stagnant market. Companies such as hear.com, a direct-to-consumer hearing aid retailer, was acquired by WS Audiology.

By the entry into Stage 4, the hearing industry has been significantly consolidated and most are working with big-box stores, some using their name brand (such as ReSound from GN Store Nordic, Phonak from Sonova) and others using one of the brands that they purchased in the consolidation phase (such as Bernafon and Sonic Innovations from William Demant). In many states, many now own or have major financial interests in buying groups, such as CQ Partners (William Demant) and Audigy (GN Store Nordic). There is now a myriad of Internet companies, such as Hearing Planet (owned by Sonova) and hear.com (owned by WS Audiology), which use many innovative distribution techniques, including direct-to-consumer virtual care. The forward integration process has developed into a lucrative corporate profit center that openly competes with their own business divisions, such as Connect Hearing (Sonova), Hearing Life (Demant), and All-American Hearing (Starkey).

To complicate matters even more, small retail chains are often owned by one of the large corporate entities but are disguised to look like independent practices. These small regional chains have been purchased outright by the manufacturers but allowed to keep their original name, operating procedures, and the old employees but operate as a corporate retail store, further disguising corporate retail activities. Additionally, many of these large corporations have a vested interest in small independent practices. By acting as a bank, the so-called "Big Five" hearing aid manufacturers provide loans to small independent practices. These loans are used by the independent practice to expand their operation in exchange for unit commitments to the manufacturer providing the loan. Although the manufacturers do not own these practices, they are essentially locking in business with independent practices in a way that is similar to how they secure market share through owned retail locations.

With the advent of over-the-counter hearing aid regulations in October 2022, large corporations now have a vested financial interest in this new segment of the market. Many of the Big Five manufacturers not only own hearing aid brands but also have a financial stake in OTC devices (Sony/WS Audiology, Sonova/Sennheiser, GN Resound/Jabra), diagnostic equipment (Demant), and managed care.

Industry Consolidation in 2024

Initially, these large hearing care companies were simply manufacturers of hearing aids. As the industry consolidated over the past 30 years, however, these hearing aid companies began buying other smaller hearing aid companies to expand their brand portfolio as well as related entities such as equipment manufacturers, retail clinics, and buying groups. These were businesses that could move a particular hearing aid brand to the forefront for sales as technology was a major driver of the hearing aid business during the consolidation period. Additionally, by adding specific brands of hearing instruments to a manufacturer's portfolio, they could immediately enter and become competitive in an otherwise formidable domestic or international market.

Figure 4–7 illustrates all the consolidation and forward integration that has occurred through June 2024. Note there are eight major corporations illustrated in Figure 4–7. To qualify as one of these corporations shown in the figure, the firm must own more than one type of business inside the industry. (The smaller companies that own a single entity or brand are listed at the bottom of Figure 4–7.)

Beginning at the top right of Figure 4–7, review each of these eight large corporations in a clockwise manner. For each of these eight corporations, the brands or divisions that they own or for which they have a large financial stake are illustrated. Although there are eight corporations depicted, five of them, Demant, GN, Sonova, Starkey, and WS Audiology, are traditional hearing aid manufacturers commonly known as the "Big Five."

Demant

The Demant Group was founded in 1904 by Hans Demant, under the name Oticon. It is a holding company that is

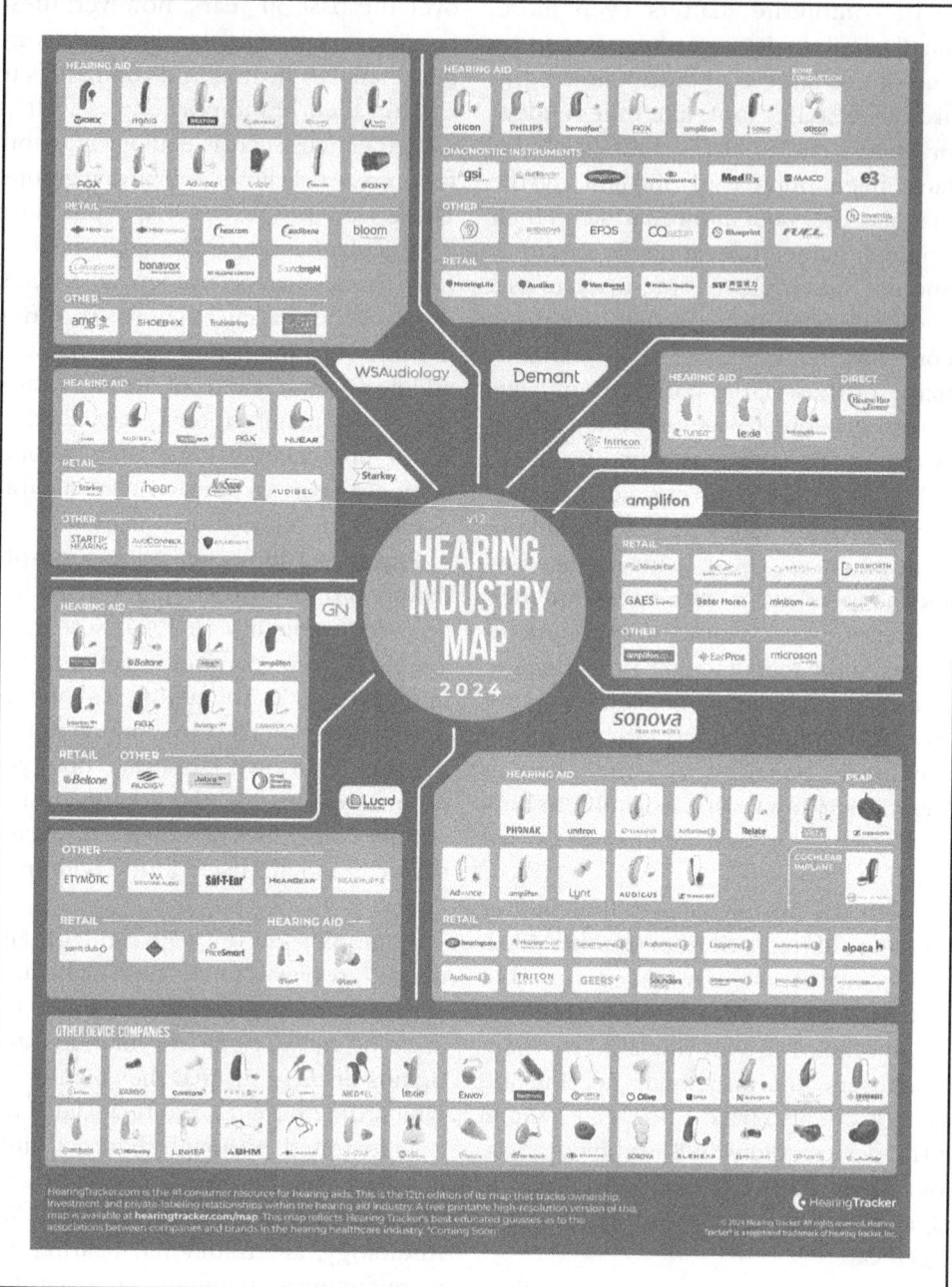

Figure 4–7. Hearing Industry Map 2024. *Source*: Reprinted with permission from Aram Bailey, Hearing Tracker (2024).

traded on the Danish stock exchange. The company focuses on three separate business units: hearing aids, retail hearing aid centers, and equipment. Many of their largest brands are shown in Figure 4–7.

Itricon

Located in Arden Hills, Minnesota, Intricon supplies electronic components to other major brands that they use to build hearing aids. Some of their major brand suppliers are listed in the Intricon section of Figure 4–7.

Amplifon

Amplifon was founded in 1950 by Algernon Charles Holland, a former official of the British special forces. Based in Milan, Italy, Amplifon is the world's largest hearing aid retailer. Traded on the Italian stock exchange, Amplifon has an 11% global market share and is present in 29 countries. The company operates through a network of about 5,150 direct points of sale, 4,000 shop-in-shops and corners, and 1,800 stores affiliated with the network, employing 16,000 employees overall. Miracle Ear is their best-known American brand.

Sonova

Sonova Holding AG (Phonak Holding AG before August 2007) is a Swiss holding company. Founded in 1947 by Ernst Rihs, he renamed the company Phonak in 1977. Sonova consists of more than 30 constituent companies, many of which

are shown in their section of Figure 4–7. Additionally, Sonova has a strategic partnership with Sennheiser OTC hearing aids.

Lucid Hearing

A relatively new "kid "on the block, Lucid Hearing, founded in 2009, grew out of the small independent hearing aid company, Liberty Hearing Aids. Currently, Lucid Hearing does most of their business in the OTC market. Some well-known legacy companies, including Etymotic Research and Westone, currently fall under the Lucid Hearing umbrella. They also have a strong presence in Sam's Club as their major distribution outlet.

GN Group

Resound was founded at AT&T Bell Labs in the 1970s. In the 2000s, Resound was acquired by GN Store Nord A/S, a Danish company. It is publicly traded on the Danish stock exchange. Today, the GN Group consists of GN Store Nord A/S, GN Hearing A/S, and GN Audio A/S. In 2000, the GN Group acquired Beltone, one of the largest retail hearing aid chains in the world.

Starkey

Founded by Bill Austin in 1967, Starkey is a privately owned American hearing aid manufacturer based out of Eden Prairie, Minnesota. In addition to several private label hearing aid brands, Starkey owns several retail locations managed by their subsidiary, Audibel.

WS Audiology

WS Audiology was created with the merger of Signia and Widex. WS Audiology is a privately owned manufacturer of hearing aids with headquarters in Denmark and Singapore with roots going back to 1878 and Siemens AG. Siemens, now Signia, has a long-time partnership with the Miracle Ear brand, owned by Amplifon, to manufacture and private label their hearing aids. In addition to their two major hearing aids brands, Signia and Widex, WS Audiology owns a managed care company (Tru-Hearing), a direct-to-consumer retail company (hear .com), and several retail chains, including HearUSA. Additionally, WS Audiology has a strategic partnership with Sony OTC hearing aids.

A key characteristic of consolidation and forward integration is that the most profitable companies in an industry, because they have ample amounts of cash, acquire smaller companies that can effectively distribute more of their product. In the hearing aid industry, the most profitable entities have been the manufacturers who have acquired (or rolled up) smaller retail locations and merged them into large retail chains. Additionally, hearing aid manufacturers have acquired buying groups, managed care companies, and an assortment of other firms that are part of the larger hearing care industry. The following examines some of these integrated businesses in more detail.

Retail Chains and Big-Box Stores

To fully appreciate forward/vertical integration in the hearing aid industry, it might help to start with an example from another sector of the economy most of us are familiar with. Imagine you own a large brewery. One of your central challenges would be finding liquor stores that are willing to sell your beer. Of course, many other breweries have really great tasting beer like yours. It is a crowded market with so many outstanding brews. Competition is fierce, as each liquor store has only so much shelf space in which to display and sell beer. Now, as the owner of a brewery who is faced with this fierce competition to have your beer placed on store shelves, it would be tempting to lower your prices. By lowering your price, you might find more stores willing to get a "good deal" and stock your beer over others. The problem, however, is that by lowering your prices, you risk losing money making your beer. Losing money is the path to going out of business. Rather than lowering your prices, you must look for other ways to win space on the shelf. Maybe it is with a catchy name of your latest ale or a colorful logo. Maybe it's a novel new pale ale that no one else can make. The problem is everyone is making really good beer, devising similar marketing strategies, and pricing their beer competitively. This competitive dilemma is easily solved with the brewer who has the deepest pockets and can buy the liquor stores that sells their beer.

This example is similar to how the hearing aid industry works: Manufacturers own retail hearing aid dispensing chains. That is, through the purchase of retail locations, they own a large share of the distribution of their product. Manufacturers buy stores or clinics that dispense hearing aids, and because they now own those stores and clinics, they can dictate the brand of hearing aids dispensed. This is known as vertical integration, and it has been occurring in the hearing aid industry for more than 25 years. As Figure 4–7 shows, every major hearing aid manufacturer owns or has a large financial stake in retail locations. Manufacturer-owned retail chains have one large competitive advantage: They can sell their products in their stores at a lower cost than that of an independent audiologist. However, these retail chains have a couple of potentially huge downsides: They limit consumer choices (imagine going to your liquor store and seeing only one brand of beer available). Independent audiologists can exploit this downside by simply offering a wider range of product choices.

Another large corporate entity like manufacturer-owned chains are big-box stores. Big-box stores such as Costco, which is the largest retailer of hearing aids, stand out from the competition because of their buying power and economies of scale. Because big-box chains like Costco sells hundreds of hearing aids each day in their thousands of hearing aid centers around the United States, they command tremendous buying power. This means they can ask manufacturers for extremely low wholesale prices in exchange for having hundreds of hearing aids sold in a turnkey manner. This turnkey operation means that each of the thousands of Costcos around the country is fitting and dispensing hearing aids in the same way. This makes it less expensive for hearing aid manufacturers to train and update Costco-employed clinicians. All these reasons make doing business with Costco and other big-box retailers very appealing if you are a hearing aid manufacturer.

Costco's secret sauce is the combination of low prices for high-quality name-brand prescription hearing aids and consistently good service in its hearing aid

centers. Costco stays ahead of the pack by performing real ear measures on every hearing aid fitted and by offering competitive return policies and product warranties. Costco uses its buying power and distribution clout to offer lower prices for hearing aids than most national chains and private hearing aid practices. It also has substantial advantages when it comes to not having to shoulder the same marketing and overhead costs as private practices or clinics—enabling Costco to discount hearing aids steeply. For example, Costco employs a shop-in-shop model, which minimizes overheads like rent versus traditional brick-and-mortar clinics. Given their buying power and economies of scale, Costco has a huge competitive advantage on price. This means that audiologists in private practice and small clinics must be agile and clever in how they differentiate themselves in the marketplace.

Differentiating a practice within a marketplace competing with Costco involves some analysis using many of the principles outlined in Chapter 5. To conduct a thorough strength, weakness, opportunities, and threats (SWOT) and three-circle analysis, developing a comprehensive competitive strategy is critical. As a general rule, there are opportunities to position an independent practice nicely against big-box retailers because with their lower prices come some important trade-offs for customers:

■ A regular Costco Wholesale warehouse club membership, starting at $60 per year, is required to buy and get service from its hearing aid centers.

■ Costco does not always carry the latest and greatest versions of name-brand hearing aids because manufacturers usually provide them first to private audiology practices.

■ While Costco generally gets decent grades for dependable service, it is less likely the hearing aids will be fitted by a doctor of audiology and more likely by a state-licensed hearing aid dispenser with substantially fewer years of schooling.

■ Costco dispensers generally do not have as much time for patients or "skin in the game" as might a typical owner or partner in a private practice.

■ Costco's dispensing model is geared more toward higher volume than comprehensive hearing care. People with more complex/severe hearing losses will benefit from the specialized diagnostics and individualized attention (i.e., numerous follow-up visits, assistive technologies, aural rehab, tinnitus treatments, etc.) offered by audiology practices.

■ Costco hearing aid centers tend to be barebones and have a look and feel more akin to a car tire center than a healthcare center.

By focusing on providing a memorable patient experience, comprehensive care, and other elements of "high-touch" service, independent-minded audiologists can compete and thrive against big-box competition.

Managed Care

One of the biggest changes in the U.S. hearing aid market over the past 10 years has been the rise of managed care. According to experts, in 2024, managed care accounted for 21% of wholesale distribution in the U.S. market, up from around 8% in 2017. Typically, in managed care, the insurers, or more often third-party administrators (TPAs) on behalf of the insurers, negotiate wholesale prices of devices directly with hearing aid manufacturers. The insurers/TPAs then rely on a network of retail stores or independent clinics, who participate in their program. Managed care companies direct their policyholders to audiologists, who are part of these managed care/TPA networks. Clinicians, in turn, receive a fixed fitting fee in exchange for providing audiologist service to the policyholders. Managed care and TPA businesses make money through the difference in the fees received by the insurance plan and customer (copay) versus the wholesale cost of the device, the fitting fee, and administrative costs (Chapter 16).

Given that many manufacturers illustrated in Figure 4–7 own large segments of the managed care hearing aid business, this serves as a great example of *forward integration*. WSA Audiology is the biggest player in managed care given they own TruHearing, the largest TPA. It is likely that most units sold through TruHearing are WSA products in the same way that most hearing aids sold through manufacturer-owned stores are that manufacturer's products. Sonova is the next largest player in the managed care arena. Sonova also manufacturers the hearing aid for Epic's own brand hearing aids, Relate. It is assumed that they have about a 30% share in managed care. GN has talked about a fair share in managed care outside of some players such as TruHearing. Therefore, the estimate is that they currently have a 10% to 15% share in the overall managed care market. Demant likely under-indexes in managed care, and we estimate a man-

TPA	Ownership	Lives covered	Insurance plan partnerships	Retail partners	Service included	Brands offered
TruHearing	WSA	160mn+	100+	7,250+	1y unlimited follow-ups	Phonak, Oticon, ReSound, Signia, Widex, Starkey
Epic Hearing Healthcare	UnitedHealth	Not disclosed	Not disclosed	7,000	Initial visit + 3 follow-ups	Phonak, Oticon, ReSound, Signia, Widex, Starkey, Beltone, Rexton, Unitron
NationsBenefits	Independent	Not disclosed	Not disclosed	8,000+	Initial visit + 3 follow-ups	Phonak, Oticon, ReSound, Signia, Widex, Starkey, Beltone, Unitron
Hearing Care Solutions	Independent	Not disclosed	Not disclosed	4,500+	1y unlimited follow-ups	Phonak, Oticon, ReSound, Signia, Widex, Starkey, Beltone, Rexton, Unitron
Amplifon Hearing Healthcare	Amplifon	50mn	80+	6,000+	1y unlimited follow-ups	All 5 major manufacturers

Figure 4–8. The major third-party administrators (TPAs) and their attributes.

aged care unit share around 15% versus their overall market share of around 20%. Figure 4–8 outlines many of the key players and their attributes in the managed care hearing aid market.

This issue brings the question, "How do managed care companies and their third-party administrators who broker business relationships with audiologists compete?" The simple answer is related to reimbursement. Recall that reimbursement is the amount of money managed care companies agree to pay the audiologist for specific procedures and products they provide at negotiated rates. Managed care contracts tend to keep prices down for their members; therefore, a person with hearing loss can often save hundreds of dollars of out-of-pocket costs when they buy hearing aids through a managed care program rather than in the "private pay" market. In turn, to keep costs low for members, managed care contracts also keep the reimbursement rates low for audiologists who participate in their programs. For audiologists who run an efficient business by keeping their own operating expenses in line, managed care reimbursement rates, even though they are lower than the private pay market, can be profitable. One reason for this is related to volume: If there is a large membership base of a certain managed care company in the practice's geographic area, this can lead to an influx of business that flows into the practice without any marketing expense. In contrast, audiologists who opt out of certain managed care contracts because the reimbursement is too low will find themselves competing directly with these managed care companies in which they are not members.

If practitioners become concerned with the low reimbursement rates and frustrations with managed care programs, review Chapter 16, which outlines methods and procedures for working within these programs at a profit.

Buying Groups

Another entity in Figure 4–7 is buying groups. Buying groups rely on buying power to provide their members with lower-cost hearing aids. Additionally, most buying groups offer business support in the form of turnkey marketing collateral, operational analytics, and human resources. From a competitive perspective, buying groups, through their ability to provide members with lower wholesale prices, are a competitive advantage for their membership. Unless a buying group offers exclusivity (e.g., territory is protected and limited to one member per city), they are not a competitive obstacle. Since it is easy to join a buying group and enjoy better wholesale pricing as a perk to membership, buying groups usually benefit independent practices.

Direct-to-Consumer and Internet-Based Businesses

If born after 1950, chances are good that you have spent some time playing with Mr. Potato Head. For many, Mr. (and Mrs.) Potato Head is an American icon, fondly known to consist of a plastic model of a potato to which a variety of other plastic parts can attach, typically ears, eyes, shoes, hat, nose, pants, and mouth. Any child playing with Mr. Potato Head can mix and match these items as they wish. Oddly enough, with the rise in a variety of direct-to-consumer hearing devices and remote telecare options, consumers, much like a play date with Mr. Potato Head, can mix and match the various components of hearing healthcare. These consumer options are another source of both competition and opportunity for the independent-minded audiologist. Because they provide consumers with alternative, direct-to-consumer, and other Internet-based business models that sell over-the-counter hearing aids, they are considered a substitute for prescription hearing aids and the traditional brick-and-mortar clinic.

Recently, Brice et al. (2023) created a framework that helps to better understand how persons with hearing difficulties can combine or blend the various elements of their own journey toward better hearing. This framework, illustrated in Figure 4–9, suggests there are four elements of hearing care: Technology (hearing devices), Service (assistance, counseling), Channel (the way in which technology and service are delivered), and Reimbursement (the transaction process). All four of these elements exist independently of each other. Persons with hearing difficulty can pick, choose, and even change on a whim how they want to engage with each of these elements. Additionally, each element exists on a continuum, as Figure 4–9 depicts, with clinic-driven care on one side and consumer-led, self-directed care on the other.

This framework allows us to see how technology, service, and channels can be mixed and matched, depending on the needs or wishes of the person with

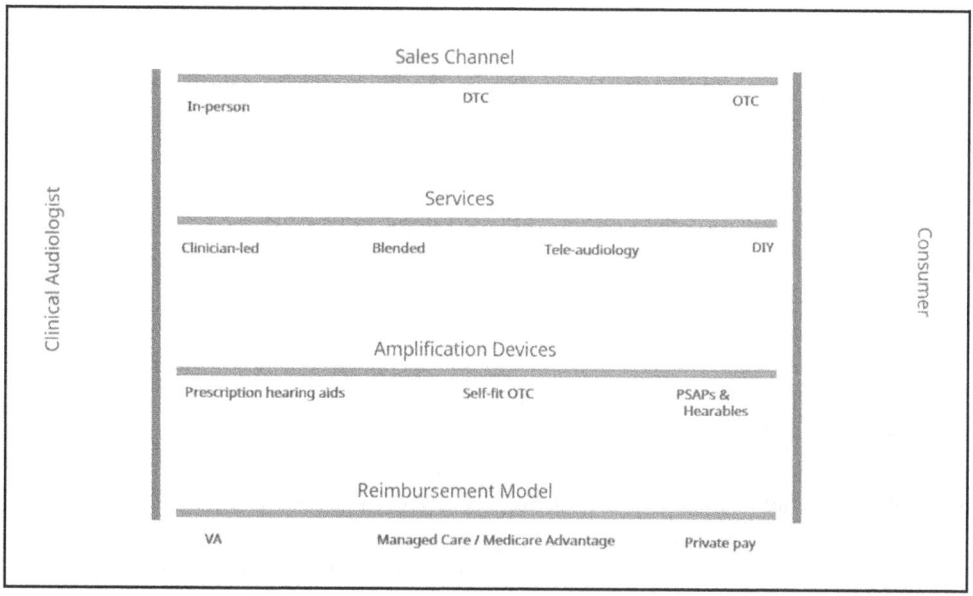

Figure 4–9. Types of retail operations owned by manufacturers.

hearing difficulty. For example, someone could begin their journey with the purchase of hearables online and eventually find their way into a clinic for an assortment of professional, counseling-related services—delivered in person. The decoupling of device sales from service, as well as where people can acquire these services (in a clinic, online), presents new forms of competition, but they also provide opportunities for those audiologists who want to offer stand-alone services or dispense OTC hearing aids through a website.

Hearing Instrument Specialists

Another source of competition is hearing aid dispensers. Hearing aid dispensers, also known as hearing instrument specialists, are often employed by retail chains, medical centers, and smaller independent practices to fit hearing aids.

Like audiologists, dispensers can also own their own practices. Hearing instrument specialists have their own professional organization (International Hearing Society) and their own ethical code and credentialing process. To the consumer, the differences between audiologists and hearing aid specialists are quite subtle, so it is easy for them to get confused about which expert they are seeing. However, there are some key differences in what these two professions can offer. Basically, a hearing aid specialist can test hearing and fit hearing aids. In contrast, an audiologist can assess and diagnose a wider range of hearing and balance problems. Both professions are licensed by all 50 states.

Because hearing aid dispensers, who receive less academic training than audiologists, can dispense hearing aids just like audiologists, they are considered a competitor in the market. Bray and Amlani (2022) project that in 2025, there will be approximately 15,000 audiologists and 12,500 hearing aid dispensers practicing in the United States. However, given the high costs of tuition to obtain a doctorate in audiology compared to the lower cost, more apprenticeship-based training of hearing aid dispensers, the number of audiologists is projected to shrink, and the number of dispensers will increase over the next decade. Nationally, the ongoing shortage in the audiology workforce is being offset by rapid growth in the hearing instrument specialist workforce. As of 2023, Bray and Amlani project there will be about 16,000 audiologists and an equal number of dispensers as the number of dispensers continues to increase, while the number of audiologists will remain the same. By 2039, they project there will be about 3,000 more dispensers than audiologists. Given a shrinking number of audiologists in the face of an aging population in need of hearing care services, Bray and Amlani's projections suggest the competition between audiologists and hearing instrument specialists will evolve. Given the scope of practice differences between the professions, it is possible that a growing number of entrepreneurial audiologists will oversee the testing and fitting of hearing aids by dispensers. Regardless of the differences between the two professions, there are opportunities for them to work together to deliver high-quality care to the market. Like hearing aid manufacturers, hearing instrument specialists can be viewed as both competitors and partners. All parties have a vested interest in growing the market for hearing devices and related services, but in many places, they compete for business.

Now that the various entities that compete directly with audiologists in the marketplace have been reviewed, attention can be turned to *how to stand apart* from whoever the competition might be in the geographic or virtual footprint that is serviced. The following section discusses how knowledge of the competition, combined with carefully planned strategic actions, can be used to differentiate a practice in the eyes of consumers.

The Kernels of Strategy

Strategy is problem-solving. It is how you overcome the obstacles that stand between where you are and what you want to achieve. What has been discussed so far—*competition*—is simple yet critically important to overcoming obstacles. All the time and energy used to better understand the competition is wasted if it is not applied to trying to create value for customers or solve a problem that stands in the way of operating a profitable business.

Strategy is designing a way to deal with a challenge. A good strategy, therefore, must identify the *challenge* to be overcome and design a way to overcome it. To do that, according to Rumelt (2011), the kernel of a good strategy contains three elements: a *diagnosis*, a *guiding policy*, and *coherent action*.

- A *diagnosis*. Defines the challenge or scope of the problem being faced. What is preventing the person from reaching their goals? A good diagnosis simplifies the often-overwhelming complexity of reality down to a simpler story by identifying certain aspects of the situation as critical.
- A *guiding policy*. An overarching approach chosen to cope with or overcome the obstacles identified in the diagnosis. Like the guardrails

on a highway, the guiding policy directs and constrains action in certain directions without defining exactly what shall be done.

■ *Set of coherent actions.* These dictate how the guiding policy will be implemented. The actions should be coherent, meaning the use of resources, policies, and maneuvers that are undertaken should be coordinated and support each other (not fight each other or be independent from one another).

The application of these kernels of strategy builds an audiology practice that stands out from retail chains and big-box retailers—a strategy that allows the audiologist to remain independent, profitable, and practicing to their highest scope. The rest of this chapter is devoted to a case study that demonstrates how to develop a set of coherent actions, using knowledge of the competition that enables an audiology practice to stand apart in the eyes of the consumer from others.

A Case Study in Competition and Strategy

■ *Details:* A hypothetical practice, Smith Family Hearing, is located in a relatively affluent metro area in which there are more than a dozen other hearing care clinics and retail stores within an hour's drive of their location. Smith Family Hearing is looking for ways to become more profitable and differentiate themselves from the dozens of other locations.

■ *Diagnosis:* The market is overcrowded with practices that dispense hearing aids in a cookie-cutter fashion. Each practice primarily advertises low-cost hearing aids through direct mail and television advertising. This strategy has commenced a race to the bottom in which all key players compete on price and all clinical providers are undifferentiated. Faced with plummeting costs, due in no small part to managed care contracts, Smith Family Hearing sees an opportunity to compete on service and experience, rather than price. Diagnosis answers the question, "What is going on?"

■ *Guiding policy:* Smith Family Hearing will rely on the maxims set forth in the book, *The Discipline of Market Leaders*, discussed earlier in this chapter (Treacy & Wiersma, 1995). By concentrating on customer intimacy and operational excellence, they can narrow their focus on achieving a specific number of goals that align with their guiding policy. Guiding policy answers the questions, "What are we trying to do?" and "Why are we trying to do it?"

■ *Coherent actions:* A series of coordinated tasks and processes that are executed by staff and other key stakeholders of Smith Family Hearing. The following are some coherent actions they created that are aligned with their guiding policy. Coherent actions answer the question, "How are we going to do it?"

Guiding Policy: Customer Intimacy and Operational Excellence

The current status of the marketplace for hearing care services (low uptake rates, rising popularity of managed care, the availability of direct-to-consumer alternatives) means that competition is steeper than ever. Since competition is fierce, it is imperative that audiologists have a keen idea of how to differentiate their practice in order to stand out from the pack. The end of this chapter provides some practical guidance on how to create strategies that are designed to differentiate an audiology practice from the competition in the second and third decades of the 21st century. Given new competition pressures from direct-to-consumer retailers and over-the-counter hearing aids (many of which are owned by hearing aid manufacturers), the rising popularity of managed care, the increasing number of hearing instrument specialists, and the use of social media to capture attention of the marketplace, it is absolutely essential for audiologists to carefully consider their own business strategy.

Recall at the beginning of this chapter, a concept was introduced, the discipline of market leaders indicating that market leadership is obtained in one of three places: customer intimacy, product innovation, or operational excellence. Given the relatively level playing field associated with product innovation in the audiology field—there is no clear brand that shines above the others with respect to innovation—therefore, a viable competitive strategy requires a maniacal focus on either customer intimacy or operational excellence.

First to consider is *operational excellence*. It should go without saying that a big part of running an efficient business is managing costs and maximizing revenue. From a practical standpoint, there are three major areas where costs can be carefully managed and where revenue flow is optimized:

1. *Office traffic.* The number of patients visiting the practice.
2. *Revenue generation.* The number of revenue-generating procedures or devices sold—testing revenue and hearing aids sales.
3. *"Time over target."* The per hour revenue generated from these activities. Since office traffic, which is often a function of advertising and marketing, is the source or headwaters of productivity, the following "gameplan" is offered for how operational excellence for marketing can be executed in a modern audiology practice.

Coherent Policy 1: Digital Marketing in Audiology

Today, people of all ages, from the young to the elderly, are actively engaging online. In 2024, 96% of individuals aged 50 to 64 and 88% of those 65 and older are active online within the United States, demonstrating a significant online presence among older generations (Chapter 20). This trend underscores the importance of digital marketing for all businesses with an elderly target group, including audiology practice. Its role extends beyond merely attracting more patients to foster growth; it also plays a critical part in raising awareness. In an industry where many potential customers have yet to act, digital marketing addresses the crucial challenge of ensuring that individuals experiencing hearing loss are aware of and have easy access to the benefits of hearing aids.

Understanding the consumer's state of mind is pivotal to effective marketing. Today's consumers are not just looking for products; they are seeking solutions that seamlessly integrate into their lifestyles and address their specific concerns. In the context of audiology practice, this means recognizing the unique needs, emotions, and hesitations of potential hearing aid wearers (Chapter 12).

The current population of potential hearing aid customers can be generally characterized as:

- **Connected:** 50% of individuals over 50 spend more than 15 hours online per week. This group is active on online shopping platforms and social media, even more so than millennials.
- **Affluent:** They possess the financial means and willingness to invest in quality products. This demographic is projected to remain the most affluent generation until at least 2030.
- **Busy:** They lead busy lives and have limited time for lengthy processes.
- **Younger:** They are younger than previous generations of hearing aid users, typically between 50 and 70 years old, indicating a shift in the customer base.
- **Demanding:** Consumers expect the highest quality in both service and product and are not hesitant to compare options and voice their opinions.
- **Active:** They are often still professionally engaged, travel frequently, and participate in a variety of hobbies and social activities.

tomers' state of mind from being unaware of their hearing loss to the decision to seek assistance. The stage of awareness influences how potential customers can be engaged through various marketing strategies, divided broadly into "push" and "pull" tactics.

In push marketing, the strategy is proactive and targets potential customers that may not yet be actively seeking hearing aids. The objective here is to spark interest and create awareness about hearing solutions. By informing them about the latest advancements and benefits of hearing care, aim to cultivate a desire for hearing aids before the need becomes apparent. Effective channels for push marketing include Display, Google Display Network (GDN), Acquisition Email, and social media.

Conversely, pull marketing targets individuals that acknowledge their hearing loss and are actively seeking solutions. These customers are in the decision-making phase, ready to interact with content that will lead them to a purchase. Pull marketing ensures these potential customers find compelling reasons to choose an audiology practice over competitors. Key channels for pull marketing include Search Engine Optimization (SEO), Customer Relationship Management (CRM), Search Engine Advertising (SEA), and Direct Marketing. Figure 4–10 summarizes the push and pull of marketing (see Chapter 12).

Different Online Marketing Channels Reach Different Customer Groups

Marketing that is customer-centric goes beyond traditional selling points; it requires a deep understanding of the cus-

Tackle the Fears, Prejudices, and Misconceptions Head-on

Stigma surrounding hearing aids consistently prevents people from addressing their hearing loss. Many hesitate or completely avoid seeking help due to

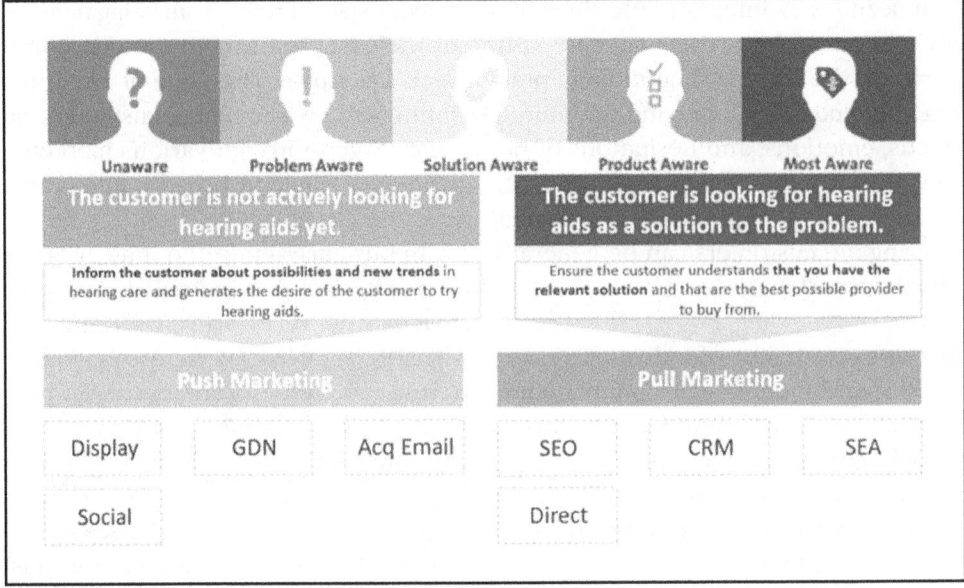

Figure 4–10. Push-and-pull marketing.

deep-seated prejudices associated with hearing aids. Instead of ignoring these misconceptions, it is crucial to tackle them head-on. The objective is to transform these biases into positive messages that capture customer interest, sparking moments of realization and surprise. These positive messages are consistently reinforced at every stage of the customer's journey, from the initial advertisement through all subsequent appointments, ensuring a shift in perception.

Common Fears and Misconceptions

The most common prejudices against hearing aids arise from misconceptions about their appearance, functionality, and the associated stigma of hearing loss. These misconceptions largely stem from older models, which differ significantly from today's advanced devices.

Below are some of the most prevalent misconceptions:

- "Hearing aids are big and bulky."
- "Hearing aids are only for old people."
- "Hearing aids help only against severe hearing loss."
- "Hearing aids are not worth the investment."

Reframing Misconceptions Into Positive Marketing

The following are a few examples of how to counteract the common misconceptions with effective marketing campaigns and positive reinforcement during appointments.

To combat the idea that "hearing aids are big and bulky," marketing efforts should showcase sleek, invisible, in-the-ear models or small receiver-in the-ear

(RIC) devices through compelling imagery. This helps to shift perceptions toward the discreet and advanced design of modern devices.

Addressing the belief that "hearing aids are only for old people," marketing should highlight younger users and showcase modern features like Bluetooth connectivity. This can make the devices more relatable to a broader demographic.

To challenge the notion that "hearing aids are not worth the investment," offering a free trial can be an effective way to demonstrate the immediate improvement in quality of life that these devices provide. In addition, it offers the customer the chance to experience the value of hearing care themselves.

Positive marketing is crucial, but it's equally important to reinforce these messages across all subsequent touchpoints. This includes not just appointments but also emails, SMS messages, and printed materials provided to the customer during the initial weeks of trying out new hearing aids.

Be Action-Oriented and Provide High-Quality Information

A landing page is the designated entry point for a website, specifically designed to receive and convert traffic from marketing campaigns. Best practices recommend creating separate landing pages for different marketing channels or even specific campaigns. This strategic segmentation ensures that each landing page delivers messages tailored to resonate with the advertisement and channel from which the customer originated.

Furthermore, maintaining separate landing pages facilitates A/B testing—allowing marketers to experiment with various ad formats, headlines, and calls to action (CTAs). This structured separation helps marketers analyze which versions generate the most engagement and assess the success of individual campaigns.

A well-constructed landing page offers engaging, insightful content that not only informs but also motivates the visitor to take action, effectively transitioning them from casual browsers to potential customers (Figure 4–11).

1. **Headline:** The headline is the first element that visitors encounter, so it must immediately capture their attention and align seamlessly with the ad copy that brought them to the page. This synchronization ensures that there is no disconnect between the visitor's expectations and the page's content, providing a smooth transition.

2. **Call to Action:** The call to action should be distinctly clear and concise, ensuring that signing up feels like a logical step for the visitor. It must be prominently displayed on the page, utilizing strategic colors or placement to catch the eye immediately. Additionally, the process should involve minimal effort, presenting a low barrier to entry. For example, opting for a simple form fill-out rather than a phone call can significantly reduce hesitation.

3. **Image:** The chosen image must feature the hearing aid, illustrating the product that customers are considering. It should grab the visitor's attention and be strategically positioned to direct the viewer's gaze toward the CTA.

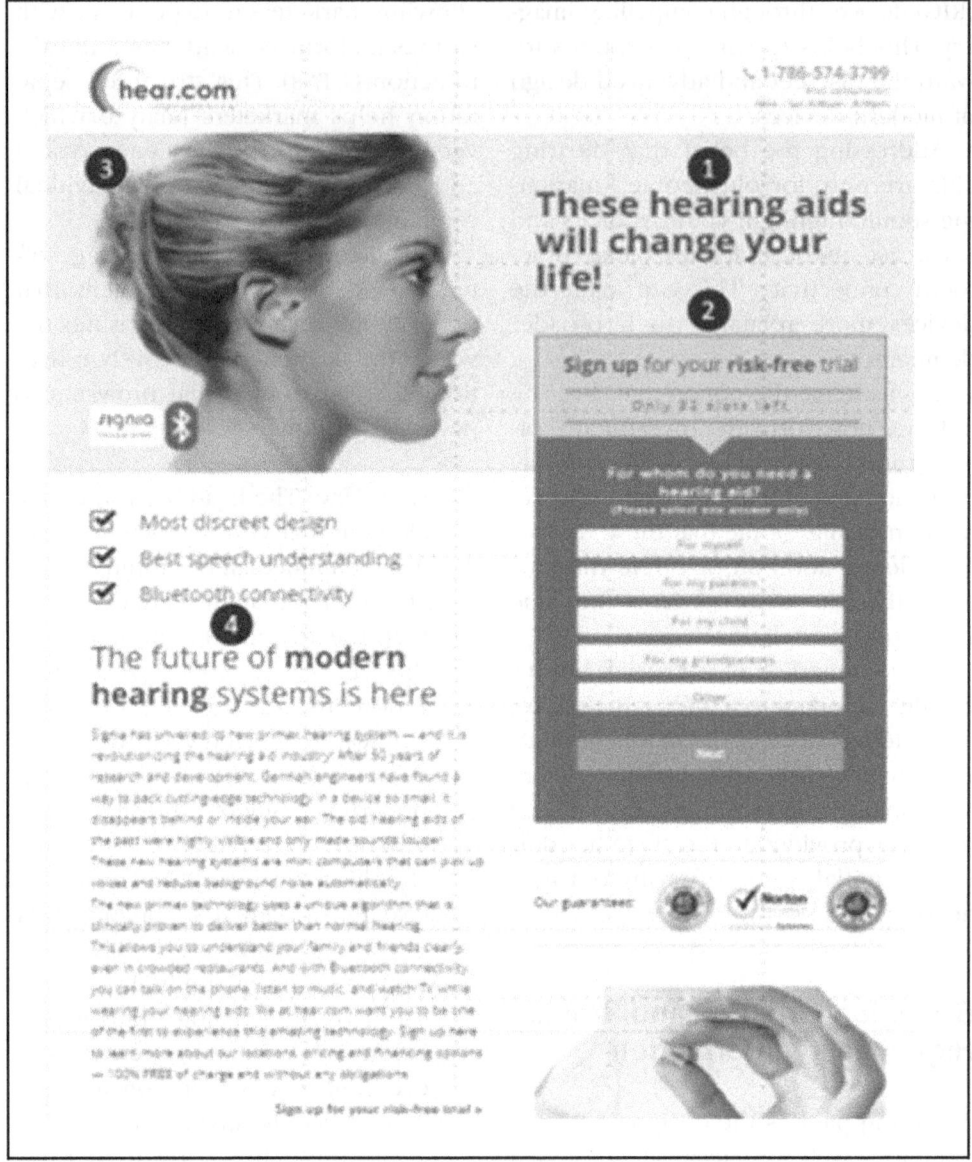

Figure 4–11. Action-oriented—information copy. *Source*: Hear.com.

This placement optimizes the visual flow, smoothly guiding visitors toward the desired action and reinforcing a direct link between the product's benefits and the call to action.

4. Copy: The copy of the landing page should be short yet informative, providing essential information about the product and clarifying the reasons for the visitor to take the next step. This text should explain what the product is, its key benefits, and how it can solve the visitor's particular needs or problems.

Momentum Is Key

In today's rapid information exchange (e.g., 30-second TikTok videos) and quick service environment (e.g., Amazon deliveries arriving at our doorstep within a day, sometimes hours), maintaining customer interest after their initial engagement is more important than ever. Once a customer has responded to digital marketing efforts, timely follow-up actions are essential. This is comparable to managing a queue in a retail store; if the wait is too long, customers lose interest and may decide to take their business elsewhere.

It is important to recognize that even if a consumer understands why a hearing aid is beneficial, this does not necessarily mean they are ready to make a purchase. They may still harbor reservations, often operating under a "not yet" mindset, constantly looking for reasons to delay action. Even in the late stages of the journey, they are still looking for a way out.

Momentum is particularly important for customers who come through online advertising. These individuals are often not as committed as those who might walk into your clinic in person. Reflecting on the customer awareness scale discussed in the previous chapter, online customers typically fall into the earlier stages of awareness. They require more guidance and encouragement to move through the decision-making funnel compared to walk-in customers who have already taken more proactive steps toward purchasing.

Do Not Underestimate the Power of the Phone

Following up quickly after a customer has shown interest is essential. While emails and SMS are efficient ways to reach out, they lack the personal touch that can make a significant difference in customer engagement. This is where the power of the phone comes into play.

A phone call adds a human element to the interaction, which can profoundly impact the customer's experience. It allows for a real-time, two-way dialogue that not only confirms details or schedules appointments but also delves deeper into the customer's needs and the reasons behind their interest.

This human touch point is crucial; it introduces a personal dimension that automated messages simply cannot replicate. The voice of a friendly, knowledgeable expert on the other end of the line can elevate initial curiosity to serious consideration. While not necessarily prompting an immediate purchase of hearing aids, this interaction can encourage a commitment to visit the clinic for further discussion.

Stay close, follow up regularly, and focus on solving the very hearing problem that made them reach out. Digital marketing does more than just attract new patients to the practice; it is a crucial tool for nurturing long-term relationships that boost customer satisfaction and promote business growth. It is essential to maintain ongoing communication with customers, whether they have previously purchased hearing aids or disengaged during the process previously. Each interaction should be viewed as an opportunity to deepen the relationship.

In this context, it is vital to leverage technology to its fullest potential. Utilizing a Customer Relationship Management (CRM) system can play a pivotal role here. The CRM is not just a tool for organizing customer information; it is a powerful marketing channel that helps personalize communication, track customer engagement, and anticipate needs based on past interactions.

A well-managed CRM system is arguably the most powerful marketing channel available. Over time, a robust CRM strategy can generate 40% to 50% business, making it not only the most impactful but also the most cost-effective channel. Given its significant potential for business growth and customer retention, the CRM system deserves special focus.

Measure Everything, Every Step of the Journey

Tracking and analyzing every facet of online marketing efforts is critical to understanding the effectiveness of each dollar spent. By meticulously measuring various metrics, businesses can pinpoint which campaigns are successful and which should be discontinued.

To effectively manage the digital strategy, focus on several key performance indicators (KPIs), including quantitative metrics, conversion rates, and customer satisfaction. Quantitative metrics provide insights into the growth and scale of online business, offering a comprehensive view of your overall progress. Conversion rates are essential for assessing the efficacy of marketing tactics, pinpointing the stages at which potential customers may be dropping out, and identifying opportunities for optimization. Lastly, measuring customer satisfaction is critical for evaluating the quality of the experience,

which is pivotal for customer retention and enhancing the brand's reputation.

Tracking Key Performance Indicators Along the Customer Journey

The customer journey typically begins with ad views and website visits, metrics tracked using tools like Google Analytics. Ad views count the number of times the ads are displayed, offering insights into the reach of the campaign. Tracking the number of unique website visitors helps assess how effectively these ads and organic search efforts are attracting traffic.

As the journey progresses, linking generated leads, booked appointments, and sales directly to the marketing campaigns is crucial. This connection is key to understanding the effectiveness of different channels and campaigns. Although aggressive marketing might initially drive traffic, it can also lead to higher dropout rates later on. Therefore, it is important to track net sales, excluding any customers returning their hearing aids.

As the marketing is expanded, it is crucial to monitor conversion rates at each stage of the customer journey. Tracking these rates helps pinpoint where potential customers are dropping out and highlights opportunities for improvement. For example, the click-through rate (CTR) measures the percentage of viewers who click on the ads, indicating how compelling the ads are. It is also important to track conversions from visitor to lead, lead to appointment, and appointment to sale. Low conversion rates at any stage of the customer journey may indicate that a specific touchpoint is not optimized, does not fully meet customer expectations, or that earlier stages may not align perfectly. For example, if a hearing test is advertised but primarily promotes hearing aids, this mismatch could confuse potential customers, leading to drop-offs. Therefore, it is crucial to ensure a coherent narrative that links each touchpoint, smoothly guiding customers through the journey.

The financial efficiency of marketing campaigns is evaluated by tracking specific cost metrics such as Cost Per Click (CPC), Cost Per Lead (CPL), and Cost Per Sale (CPS). The CPS metric is particularly relevant, as it indicates how much investment is required in online marketing to generate one sale, thus providing a clear measure of the marketing activity's profitability.

Introducing Net Promoter Score

Net Promoter Score (NPS) is a standardized metric used across various industries to measure customer satisfaction and loyalty. It is based on a single question: "On a scale of 0–10, how likely are you to recommend our company/product/service to a friend or colleague?" The simplicity of this question allows organizations to quickly gauge their customers' overall perception and satisfaction with the service they are receiving.

NPS categorizes respondents into three groups based on their ratings:

- Promoters (score 9–10): Loyal enthusiasts who will keep buying and refer others, fueling growth.
- Passives (score 7–8): Satisfied but unenthusiastic customers who are vulnerable to competitive offerings.

- Detractors (score 0–6): Unhappy customers who can damage the brand and impede growth through negative word of mouth.

To calculate the NPS, subtract the percentage of detractors from the percentage of promoters. The result is a score ranging from –100 (if every customer is a detractor) to 100 (if every customer is a promoter).

$$NPS = (\% \text{ of Promoters}) - (\% \text{ of Detractors})$$

As a benchmark, the Marketrak 2022 survey indicates that the average Net Promoter Score (NPS) in the U.S. hearing care market for buying customers is 25. In online marketing, building trust is crucial to convincing potential customers to enter their personal details on the website. They often consult review platforms such as Google, Trustpilot, and the Better Business Bureau to gauge the credibility and reliability of a company. Therefore, maintaining high customer satisfaction is crucial. The NPS serves as an effective tool for tracking customer satisfaction, helping identify how well the business meets customer expectations and where improvements can be made to enhance the overall customer experience.

Coherent Policy 2: Building Your Brand Around Customer Experience

Next, is a discussion of what is perhaps the only way to differentiate audiology practice in today's highly competitive business environment: the brand. In this case study, Smith Family Hearing, after a careful analysis of the competition and a diagnosis of the problem, decided to build their brand around patient experience. In this example, their brand is a promise to patients of a remarkable, transformative experience. Whether recognized or not, the practitioner, as an individual, is a brand. Prior to marketing's influence on a practice, most audiologists termed this as their reputation. Today, reputation is still a critical component of the value of a brand (i.e., *brand equity*). The key difference now is that many other elements influence a patient's perception of value (i.e., *brand value*). Once upon a time, bedside manner and clinical skills were the key determinants. In the modern era, you must go far beyond bedside manner to effectively manage and build your brand as an audiologist.

Individuals have been brands forever, and today's ability to communicate seamlessly with a target audience has allowed people to build their brands in ways that were unthinkable just 10 or 20 years ago. Taylor Swift is an excellent example of someone who has leveraged her performance talent through social media to capture millions of friends and followers across YouTube, Facebook, X, and Instagram. Ask any "Swifty" what she means to them.

Many audiologists have been led to believe that advertising equals marketing. Advertising is simply one form of marketing. This distinction is fundamental to the approach to branding, which includes not just promotional activities but everything performed within and outside of the practice. Business cards, office layout, virtual layout (more commonly known as the website), staff's behavior, and community involvement are all integral components of brand and should be intentionally thought out.

For example, do not call the area where patients gather after they arrive a *waiting room*; the phrase itself (and associated activities) likely detracts from brand equity, because nobody wants to wait in an era when they can instantly perform Google searches with the smartphone in the palm of their hand. A related tip: change the name and the function of what happens between the patient's arrival and being taken back to the assessment room for a case history. Respecting people's time is a solid strategy by which to build patients' perception of value.

Too often, an audiologist and the practice try to be too many things to too many people. The problem is that, trying to appeal to everyone, actually appeals to no one (Chapter 5). It is a common mistake that comes from a fear of being too narrow in focus and/or a fear of being seen as exclusionary or elitist. This chapter has attempted to show that only after understanding what competitors do well can the process of differentiation begin. Much of the differentiation, then, starts with branding the practice.

Coherent Policy 3: Implementation of Best-Practice Standards

Practice standards have existed in most professions for many decades, if not longer. It is important for a profession to define standard methodologies for services commonly provided. Family hearing centers recognize that when providers perform tasks differently, it leads to chaos in a healthcare system: Other healthcare providers have difficulty coordinating care, teamwork becomes difficult for support staff, and patients notice inconsistencies in outcomes.

Clinical standards reduce risk for providers by minimizing adverse events. They promote faith in a profession because patients and other providers know what to expect. They support education and help to codify routine tasks for payers and regulators. They do not restrict practice because it is recognized that all patients are different, and providers must utilize an array of tools to meet their needs. For this reason, there are clinical guidelines. Clinical guidelines provide a framework for patient care that allows for individual differences and multiple pathways to achieve positive outcomes. For these reasons, family hearing care centers make the decision to follow all clinical standards published by the Audiology Standards Organization. Each standard is freely available to download on the APSO website at https://www.audiologystandards.org, as is the standards creation process. All patient-facing staff will be instructed on the standards and provided an opportunity to incorporate these standards into their daily work.

Coherent Policy 4: Implement Block Scheduling

Block scheduling is a method of creating a work schedule in which the workday is divided into blocks of time and each block is assigned a specific type or subtype of activity (i.e., hearing aid evaluation, private pay hearing aid evaluations, hearing aid fitting, check & clean, outbound calling, etc.). The level of detail for each block category can be tailored to an individual practice, but the overarching goal of block scheduling is still the same: to ensure the necessary time to complete a given business activity is set aside as well as ensure the task is completed in time to meet business objectives. For example, a practice has drastically increased the number of patients it has seen this year over last year, but they ended up making less money. A likely culprit is the practice is treating more patients utilizing third party–administrated benefits or insurance with a low reimbursement rate. Block scheduling would be a potential solution if used to ensure that the practice sees the necessary number of private pay patients required to hit revenue targets.

The block scheduling process helps a practice attain business goals by being more efficient with how time is spent—time is set aside for appointments that tend to generate ample revenue. Additionally, this process of establishing block schedules breaks down the important annual financial goals into the daily necessary steps or subgoals. Because the annual revenue goal has been broken down into daily subgoals, managers will quickly be alerted to any deviation to the plan the same day that the deviation occurred. With the alerts being executed in real time, management can quickly take corrective actions to get the business back on track to meet goals.

Another helpful practice that uses similar mechanics to block scheduling is called reverse block scheduling. This process helps limit specific activities that, when in overabundance, can hinder or prevent a practice from meetings its financial goals. An example is treating patients using third-party or fitting fee payment options versus private pay.

Whereas all patients are important, a practice must balance financial solvency with community commitment to keep serving any patients. That is, if a business becomes insolvent and goes out of business, it cannot serve any patients at all. The bitter reality in most practices is that third-party insurance contracts, although they are often an essential component of business, are substantially less lucrative than private pay opportunities. Thus, block schedule ensures there is sufficient time on the schedule for private pay opportunities.

Summary

As this chapter attempts to illustrate, understanding the competition is critically important to differentiation of a practice and the creation and execution of a coherent strategy. Although it is critically important to have keen knowledge of the competition and the business dynamics that shape it, competition is just one component of having a strategy. In short, a strategy is nothing more than a plan. This chapter provides insights on how an analysis of competition fuels the development of a strategy that answers the *what*, *why*, and *how* of a business.

A coherent strategy based on a careful analysis of the market is needed if one wants to stand out from the pack. Further, the core of any strategy is a three-part process. One, discover the critical factors of the problem or challenge. This starts by understanding the competition and conducting a SWOT analysis. Two, coordinate the resources, including personnel, financial, marketing/branding, or operations that will be used to over-come the challenge or solve the problem. Three, execute a clear course of action that addresses the problem or challenge. Whatever the course of action, be sure that it is continually monitored and amended as needed in order to ensure all goals are achieved. By combining the information and insights from this chapter, along with those in Chapter 5 and Chapter 12, you will be able to analyze any market and then create and implement your own strategic plan.

As much as competition can be a source of stress and anxiety when audiologists are faced with making tough decisions inside a practice, competition in a free-market system provides a tremendous opportunity for consumers in the form of more choices and lower prices. Competition also brings out the best in audiologists, who must "raise their game" and look for ways to bring value to untapped markets, as well as innovative services to those who need them. It all starts with a sound strategy.

References

Bray, V., & Amlani, A. (2022). A new analysis of the audiology workforce, benchmarked to other healthcare professions. *Audiology Practices*, *14*(4), 42–51.

Brice, S., Saunders, E., & Edwards, B. (2023). Scoping review for a global hearing care framework: Matching theory with practice. *Seminars in Hearing*, *44*(3), 213–231.

Brandeis, L. (1934). *The curse of bigness*. Viking Press. https://orionmagazine.org/article/the-curse-of-bigness/

Deans, G., Kroeger, F., & Zeisal, S. (2002, December). The consolidation curve. *Harvard Review*. https://hbr.org/2002/12/the-consolidation-curve

Drucker, P. (1954). *The practice of management.* Harper & Brothers.

Edwards B. (2020). Emerging technologies, market segments, and MarkeTrak 10 insights in hearing health technology. *Seminars in Hearing, 41*(1), 37–54.

Foner, E., & Garraty, J. (1991). Readers Companion to American History: Automobiles. Houghton Mifflin Harcourt Publishing Company. *History.com.* http://www.history.com/topics/automobiles

Grand View Research. (2023). Hearing aid market analysis—2024–2030. Grandview Market Analysis. https://www.grandview research.com/industry-analysis/hearing-aids-market

Humes, L. E. (2023). U.S. population data on self-reported trouble hearing and hearing-aid use in adults: National Health Interview Survey, 2007–2018. *Trends in Hearing, 27,* 23312165231160967.

Kenton, W., Kelly, R., & Overcast, K. (2024). Market penetration: What it is and strategies to increase it. *Investopedia.* https://www.investopedia.com/terms/m/market-penetration.asp

Kirkwood, D. (2011). Though the "Big Six" hearing aid makers are intact, consolidation isn't over in the hearing industry. Hearing Health and Technology Matters, Phoenix, AZ, September 27, 2011.

Myers, W. (2014). How to win in the midst of an industry consolidation? Crown Business. https://crownbiz.com/how-to-win-in-the-midst-of-an-industry-consolidation/

National Institute on Deafness and Other Communication Disorders. (2023). Quick statistics about hearing. https://www.nidc .nih.gov/health/statistics/quick-statistics-hearing

OTC Act. (2017). S.670—Over-the-Counter Hearing Aid Act of 2017. United States Congress, Washington, DC. https://www .congress.gov/bill/115th-congress/senate-bill/670

PCAST. (2015). PCAST recommends changes to promote innovation in hearing technologies. https://obamawhitehouse.archives .gov/blog/2015/10/26/%E2%80%8Bp cast-recommends-changes-promote-inno vation-hearing-technologies

Rumelt, R. (2011). *Good strategy bad strategy: The difference and why it matters.* Crown.

Schroeder, A. (2009, November). *To hear or not to hear: Barriers to better hearing.* Paper presented at the Convention of the American Speech Language Hearing Association, New Orleans, LA.

Staab, W. (2014). Hearing aid market penetration. Hearing Health and Technology Matters, LLC. https://hearinghealthmatters .org/waynesworld/2014/hearing-aid-market-penetration/

Stoller, M. (2021). Silencing the competition: Inside the fight against the hearing aid cartel. https://www.thebignewsletter.com /p/silencing-the-competition-inside

Taylor, B. (2016). Hypersound hearing solutions. Webinar. https://www.google.com /search?q=Hypersound+hearing+solutions .+Webinar.&oq=Hypersound+hearing+so lutions.+Webinar.&gs_lcrp=EgZjaHJvbWUy BggAEEUYOTIHCAEQIRigATIHCAIQIRig ATIHCAMQIRigATIHCAQQIRigAdIBCDE 1MDZqMGo3qAIIsAIB&sourceid=chrome &ie=UTF-8#fpstate=ive&vld=cid:4a1d43ed ,vid:9e6FrETnWrA,st:0

Treacy, M., & Wiersma, F. (1995). *The discipline of market leaders.* Addison-Wesley.

UN Trade & Development. (2014). Intergovernmental Group of Experts on Competition Law and Policy, Roundtable on: The Benefit of Competition Policy for Consumers Contribution by USA. Fourteenth Session Geneva, 8–10 July 2014.

Whiting, A. (2024). Industry consolidation: Why and when does it happen? Dealroom. https://dealroom.net/blog/industry -consolidation

WHO. (2021). *World report on hearing loss.* World Health Organization.

5 Analysis of the Audiology Practice

Robert M. Traynor, EdD, MBA

Introduction

In the 1970s, audiologists became aware that hearing devices and services should be provided in a practice setting where the devices could be dispensed as part of an overall aural rehabilitation program. At that time, the competition consisted mainly of hearing aid salespeople or academics that recommended hearing devices from a university audiology clinic. With the advent of the Doctor of Audiology degree in the mid-1990s, the number of audiology practices began to increase, and audiologists realized the financial benefits of owning their own business. Over the next 20 years, these audiology practices thrived, and patients benefited from increased access to high-level, professional hearing care. As the field of audiology was developing, consolidation of the manufacturers within the hearing industry was proceeding behind the scenes without much notice, until forward integration (manufacturers starting their own clinics) and the advent of the big-box store began (Chapter 4).

Recently, the landscape of the hearing industry has seen some drastic changes. Competition for hearing care products and services now bombards audiology practices from many differ-ent directions due to several factors that contributed to elevate the profile of hearing loss as a significant public health issue during the period from 2015 to 2022. This heightened awareness was attributed to:

1. *Technological advancements:* The introduction of new and improved hearing aid technologies attracted media coverage. Innovations in medical devices, such as more advanced and discreet hearing aids, played a significant role in bringing hearing loss into the spotlight (Skibinsky, 2020).

2. *Public health campaigns:* Organizations like the World Health Organization (WHO) conducted campaigns to raise awareness about hearing loss. For example, WHO estimated that over 466 million people worldwide had disabling hearing loss as of 2020, with this number expected to double by 2050. Such statistics often garnered media attention and highlighted the growing public health challenge (Skibinsky, 2020).

3. *Celebrity advocacy:* High-profile individuals and celebrities speaking out about their experiences with hearing loss helped to destigmatize the condition and bring it

into mainstream conversations. Media outlets often covered these personal stories, which increased public interest and awareness.

4. *Legislation and policy changes:* In some regions, changes in legislation, such as the Over-the-Counter Hearing Aid Act in the United States, which was passed in 2017 and implemented in 2022, led to increased media coverage. This act allowed hearing aids to be sold over the counter, making them more accessible and affordable, which was widely covered by the media (Caporuscio & Lawrenz, 2022).

5. *COVID-19 pandemic:* The pandemic also contributed to the focus on hearing health, as people experienced complications related to COVID-19, including hearing loss and tinnitus. This connection was reported in various media outlets, bringing more attention to the issue. This increased visibility has been crucial in raising awareness, reducing stigma, and encouraging people to seek treatment for hearing impairments and has resulted in audiology clinics being extremely busy with patient backlogs during 2023 and 2024.

As noted above, the one major change in the audiology market came in late 2022 when the Over-the-Counter Hearing Aid Act of 2017 became effective in the United States. This legislation drastically changed the landscape of an already competitive hearing aid market forever. This legislation created a whole new category of products while dropping the physician's prescription requirement for those over age 18 years of age. This legislation, among other legal modifications, mandated two general categories of amplification:

■ Over-the-counter (OTC) hearing aids for those with mild to moderate hearing losses.
■ Prescription hearing aids for those that have more severe hearing losses.

While the over-the-counter category is open to virtually anyone and any type of product meeting the legal specifications for mild to moderate hearing loss, prescription products are designed for those with more severe losses. Since severe and greater hearing losses require more expertise in their fitting and aural rehabilitative invention in their use, they may only be provided by licensed professionals. Although audiology clinics should provide all types of hearing products from both categories, it becomes even more important to understand how a particular practice compares to other practices in the market. The techniques presented in this chapter may be used for practice comparisons and/or the development of a detailed strategic competitive strategy in either category within a local, national, or international market.

Benefits of Competition

While it does not seem logical, competition can be beneficial to an audiology practice and the profession in general. As an introduction to this topic, a short discussion of the history of competition in the field of audiology is in order.

To fulfill the needs of the ever-growing population of hearing-impaired individuals, the market now consists of not only local audiologists but also traditional hearing aid salespeople, big-box stores, and manufacturers' clinics. Additionally, there are recent avenues for patients to address their hearing difficulties such as direct to consumer, the Internet, pharmacies, and even some grocery stores. A big change in the competitive market is that competitors are not just local but national and even international, complicating the landscape.

Although competition is often viewed as negative, a lot can be learned by acknowledging what can be gained from recognizing the potential benefits. Three important factors to consider are:

- Competition *teaches* practice owners about their business.
- Competition *fosters an understanding of the core market*, such as who the patients are, what their needs are, and how those needs are going to be met, no matter if they reside in the OTC or prescription camp.
- Competition *challenges* practitioners to learn new innovative products, procedures, and treatments that will facilitate better hearing and balance care.

What Competition Teaches About Business

Competition teaches business owners how to review their market offerings in terms of quality, pricing, and support. While all businesses need to be concerned about competition, an introspective review of a business is always a good idea. It allows for the critical review of the how business is conducted, the status of equipment, employees, hardware products and services offered, possible new offerings, manufacturer changes, or other necessary modifica-

tions to the business to keep the brand in front of the market.

Understanding the Core Market

To grasp what the *core of a market* is, the practice's "main" or "essential" activity must be determined. It is essential to evaluate what is performed, on whom, and how it is performed. This knowledge generates a market-sensing process that consists of gathering marketing intelligence and then acting on that information. In audiology practice, competition forces clinicians to review the complexion of their patients and how the practice will fulfill their wants, needs, and demands (Chapter 12). These reviews involve identifying the causes of revenue ups and downs since the last review. It is important to consider changes in patient population, such as generation, aging, technical savvy, and other issues within the patient population. Are there differences in how the practice should approach patients in the current market compared to previous years? What changes are being implemented by competitors that need to be incorporated within the practice? Practices should strive to be the innovators within their market, and this is achieved by constant product and service review.

Competitive Innovative Challenges

Another benefit of competition is the challenge that it presents to practices and practitioners to be at the "top of their game." This encourages continuing education in the discipline and continued upgrading of equipment within the practice. Armed with core market knowledge, the practitioner can investigate innovative new offerings using both traditional techniques and artificial intelligence (AI) methods to organize and conduct business differently. This might involve redefining the target market, prospecting for new patients, and experimenting with new product and service delivery models that might enhance the practice.

Competition teaches practitioners to manage their clinics more efficiently by pressuring the practice owner to evaluate whether routine procedures such as ordering and product delivery are conducted in a timely manner, if waiting room time needs to be reduced, and whether payment terms are convenient, among other issues. The need to compete in a demanding, fluctuating marketplace spurs innovation for procedures, products, pricing, and marketing strategy. Competition can be the incentive that causes a practice to flourish and become a market leader.

Implementing many of these efforts often involves funding for attendance at both virtual and face-to-face training sessions to add to or renew professional skills and certifications. Continuing education is essential to stay competitive, and according to Weave (2024), it also offers the following benefits to those that practice the profession as well as to patients:

- Enhances clinical skills and knowledge.
- Ensures compliance with industry standards.
- Maintains competence in a chosen specialty.
- Allows access to the latest research.
- Results in continuing education units (CEUs) to meet licensure requirements.

- Continues to remain competitive in the field.
- Improves patient outcomes through updated practices.
- Allows networking and collaboration with industry professionals.

Beginning the Practice Analysis

Before a competitive strategy can be constructed, it is fundamental to know where the new practice or existing practice stands in the marketplace. Methods for the analysis of a practice's position within a specific market have been offered by Traynor (2019). Based upon sound competitive intelligence and the use of the SWOT (strengths, weaknesses, opportunities, and threats) analysis (Traynor, 2019), Porter's Five Forces (Porter, 1980/1998, 2008; Traynor, 2019), and the three-circle technique (Traynor, 2019, Urbany & Davis, 2010), a practice's competitive position may be determined. Once the market position and strengths and weaknesses of the practice are known, practice managers are then challenged to take the necessary business steps to implement the strategy to compete within that market. For either a new or existing practice to survive in this highly competitive entrepreneurial environment, now consisting of two separate categories (OTC vs. prescription), there must be a business strategy set into place based upon a substantial market study.

Each market or community has unique cultural and business cosmetics. The development of an effective competitive strategy first requires a comprehensive review of the global cosmetics of the hearing care community with a focus on the specific market in question. What kinds of practices are competing with one another: audiologists, traditional dispensers, franchises, big-box stores, manufacturers' corporate sales operations, the Internet, direct to consumer, or others? Knowledge of the special differences among these businesses and the practice that the entrepreneur initiates or hopes to expand is paramount in the construction of a competitive strategy.

ified substantially since the last edition of this text. As presented in Figure 5–1, the analysis of a practice involves several considerations and procedures to arrive at an accurate assessment. This assessment allows management to digest the information into strategies to interact with the market for the continued success of the practice.

A dissection of this model into practice applications for analysis of a practice is essential.

A Model for Competing in the Hearing Healthcare Market

A model for the analysis of a practice has been developed over several years (Traynor, 2013, 2019) and has been mod-

General Competitive Considerations

Initially, it is essential to first review and capitalize on some of those underlying gut feelings about a competitive community prior to conducting the more specific analysis of the practice

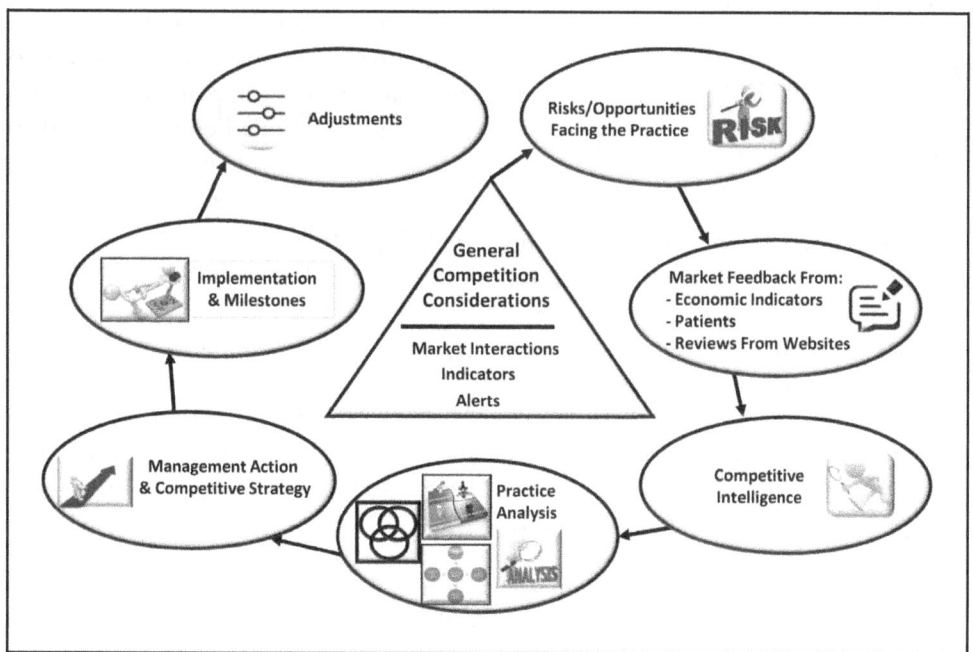

Figure 5–1. Model for competing in the hearing healthcare market.

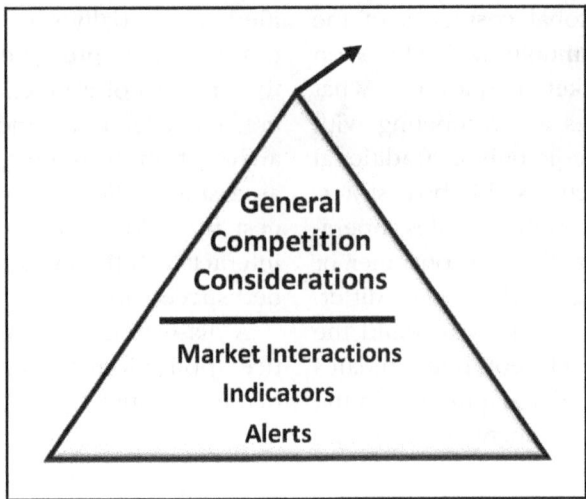

Figure 5–2. General competitive considerations.

(Figure 5–2). These general feelings are a component of competitive intelligence (CI) discussed later, but typically these cursory messages fall into three categories:

- Market interaction
- Indicators
- Alerts

Market Interaction

Market interaction is the word on the street that a practitioner hears from the market. This is simply just general information that is often obtained from patients and others around the community about the competition. Who is sending direct mail, what does it say, and what types of offers are patients receiving from others in the community? Which insurance companies tend to be in the area and what are their programs? This initial market interaction is simply a surface view of the actions of others and their reputation.

Indicators

These are considerations after digesting the cursory information about the market interactions. The indicators cause practitioners to ask themselves: What could we or should we do about the marketing being conducted within the community and beyond? How should the practice, if at all, react to the advertising or statements being presented to prospective patients in their mailbox, word of mouth, online, and elsewhere? With these indications, how does a clinic approach the problem if there is one?

Alerts

There are often alerts or challenges that must be met, such as a competitor's open house that was successful. What are they doing that this practice is NOT doing? In the market, there could be a new product or procedure that is attracting new patients to a competitor. This alert would likely trigger the full practice analysis.

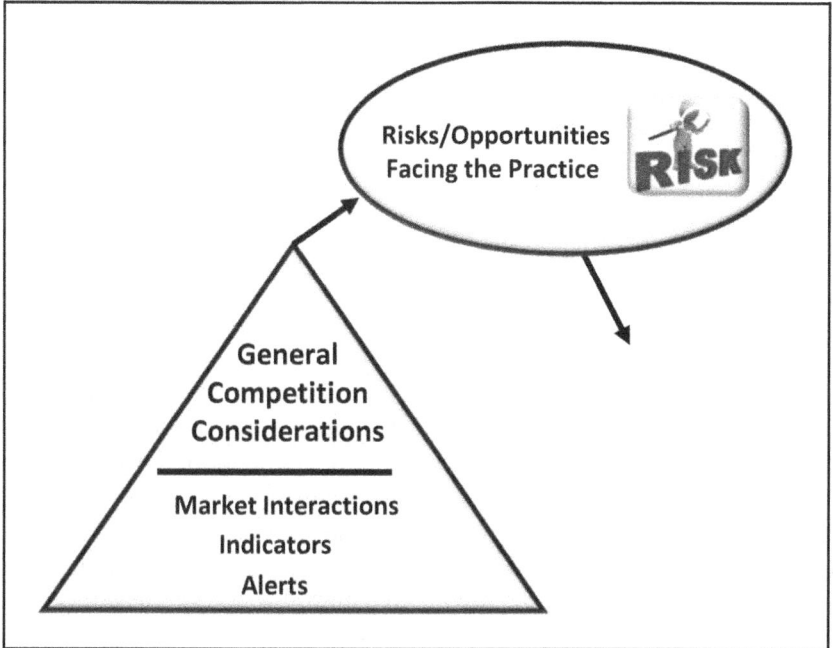

Figure 5–3. Risk/opportunity considerations.

Specific Considerations for Competing in the Hearing Healthcare Market

Throughout the discussion of a practice's competitiveness refer to Figure 5–3. This model offers a structured method for considering risks, detailed feedback from the market, competitive intelligence, analysis of the practice, management action and competitive strategy, implementation of the new strategy and checking the milestones for success or failure, and adjustments.

Risks in Audiology Practice

As a starting point, it is first necessary to consider the business risks involved in audiology private practice. Risk, in

this context, may be defined as the possibility that a company will have lower than anticipated profits or that it will experience a loss rather than a profit. A review of risks involved in audiology practice include economic cycles, social demographic changes, legislative changes, new technology, and changes in competitive behavior. Risks often become opportunities for startup practices and expansions, depending on the variables encountered.

Risks of Economic Cycles

As mentioned in Chapter 1, economies all have recessions and boom periods. Beginning a practice in a boom period has less risk than entering a startup business in a recession. Recessions mean that funds for the purchase of the practice or for expansion are usually more difficult to find and the "would-be" patients will not have as much discretionary income to afford the products and services of an audiologist unless they have special insurance or savings (Chapter 1). This may or may not be a risk as it is dependent upon the prevailing economic conditions when the practice is purchased, sold, or expanded.

Risks of Social Demographic Changes

According to Windmill and Freeman (2013), Medicare enrollment will continue to rise until at least 2050 (Figure 5–4).

First, the Baby Boomers and then their children (Generations X and Y) will be seeking audiological services as they age, in addition to those that have problems where assessment and treatment are required for hearing and balance disorders. Additionally, only about 10% of mild to moderate hearing-impaired individuals who could use hearing devices effectively are using them. While there is a significant group that will consider the OTC products, many will decide that the purchase of OTC products is best conducted from an audiologist. Further, there is still a huge population that could use hearing aids for their moderate or worse hearing loss as only about 50% of this population

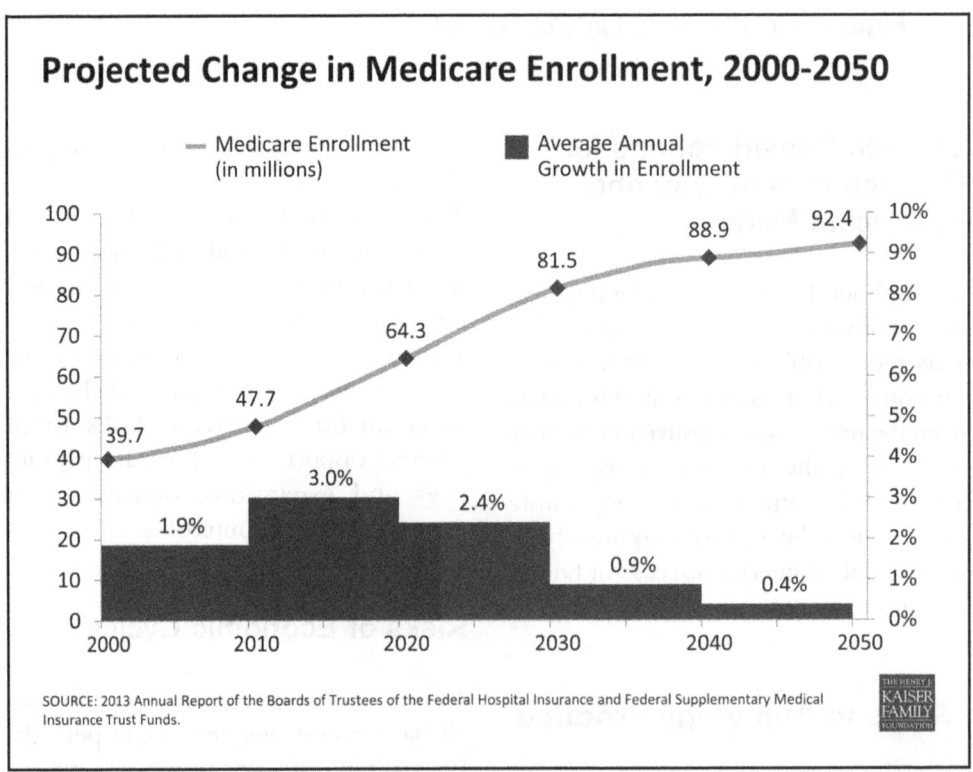

Figure 5–4. Projected Medicare enrollment 2000–2050. *Source:* 2013 Annual Report of the Boards of Trustees of the Federal Hospital Insurance and Federal Supplementary Medica; Insurance Trust Funds, The Henry J. Kaiser Family Foundation.

currently use amplification. Therefore, these factors have been considered to be more of an opportunity than a risk for quite some time.

Risks of Political Climate and Legislative Activity

Government regulations can cause drastic changes in the climate relative to healthcare. The latest example is the Over-the-Counter Hearing Aid Act of 2017. While most clinics have not been affected by this legislation, there may be other legislation that may bring audiology to the forefront. This would be the Medicare Audiology Access Improvement Act (S. 2377) of 2023, which, at this writing, is still a possibility for passage in the 118 Congress (Chapter 17). This bill would bring audiology to the provider level and open up Medicare and other insurances to the audiology scope of practice. It is expected to pass in either this congress or the next one. Although the political climate in 2024 is quite volatile, it is expected to pass soon. Once this legislation passes, it will be a substantial enhancement of the audiology scope of practice that can be reimbursed by Medicare and other insurances. Further, it will bring the profession to the same level as optometry, dentistry, chiropractic, nurse practitioners, and other allied health professions. Thus, the outlook in the near term for legislative governmental interference in the profession is far less risk and more opportunity.

Risk of Technology

Technology may be a risk or an opportunity. Some hearing aid manufacturers have already used artificial intelligence (AI) in their products in 2024. More generations of products will certainly use more AI as part of their processing and other functions. Additionally, cochlear implants will likely be used more often in situations that are currently being served by hearing aids. This could possibly reduce the number of hearing aids sold by audiology practices. While this is a future risk possibility, it is also an opportunity as patients of these products will need assessments, aural rehabilitation, and programming designed for them. Technology has, over the past 40 years, offered opportunities for audiology practices with advancements in equipment as well as testing procedures. Thus, technology might be a risk for practices, but being in touch with the core innovations in professional practice can facilitate a significant business opportunity.

Risk of Competitive Behavior Modifications

With changes in all areas of practice, there will be modifications in how audiology practices compete with each other, as well as against all of the other competitors in the marketplace. It is a challenge for practice owners to modify their clinical offerings to the market that match the changes that will come to the profession over the time that they own their practice. Thus, a change in practice patterns is inevitable, but for those practice owners who stay in touch with their core market, these necessary changes in offerings will result in significant opportunities for success.

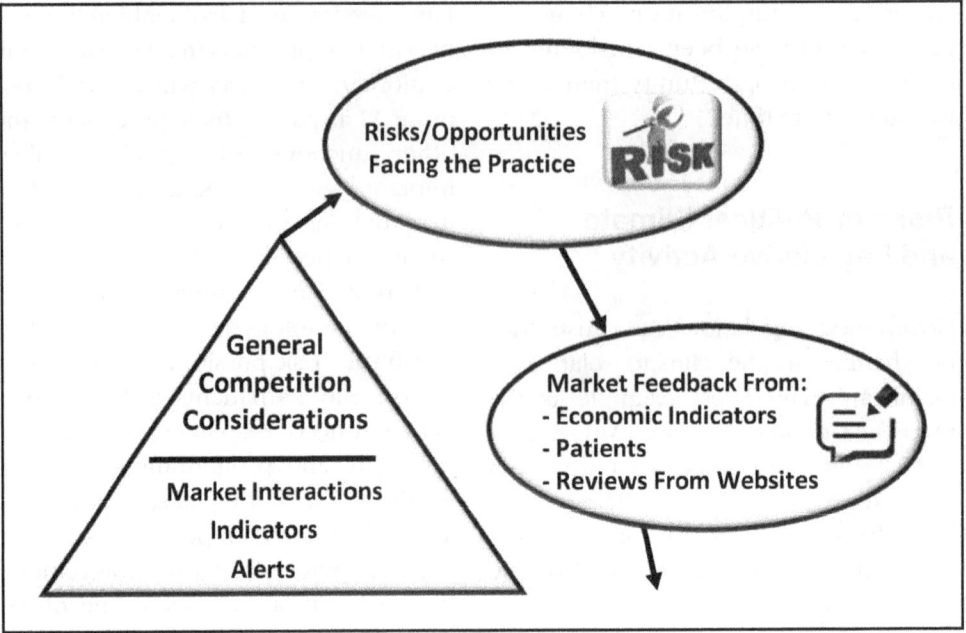

Figure 5–5. Market feedback.

Market Feedback

This consists of information supplied by patients, referral sources, families, and others regarding the current marketing efforts, treatment, products, and support. Clinicians need to listen to their patients and their interactions with other businesses within the community. This includes reviewing competitive marketing, direct mail, and other advertising that is available (Figure 5–5). Does the practice offer services to a broad range of patient types, and are products or services of high quality? The one question drastically important is: Will you consider this clinic again for hearing aids or other services offered by this provider?

Likely the latter is the most important as when patients are unsatisfied and do not indicate their dissatisfaction, they just go elsewhere. Morrow (2024) presents that although silent customers do not complain to management, they most certainly will share their experiences with their friends, neighbors, and co-workers. A customer who is dissatisfied will tell between 9 and 15 people about their experience, with over 1 in 10 telling 20 people about their bad experience. The impact of negative word of mouth can be more devastating than ever as online and social tools that amplify word of mouth are increasingly more powerful. Seventy-six percent of consumers are using online reviews before determining which business to use. Thus, a negative review could be devastating in today's viral world of social media (Chapter 12).

Competitive Intelligence

Once the risks are considered, it is time to conduct competitive intelligence, pre-

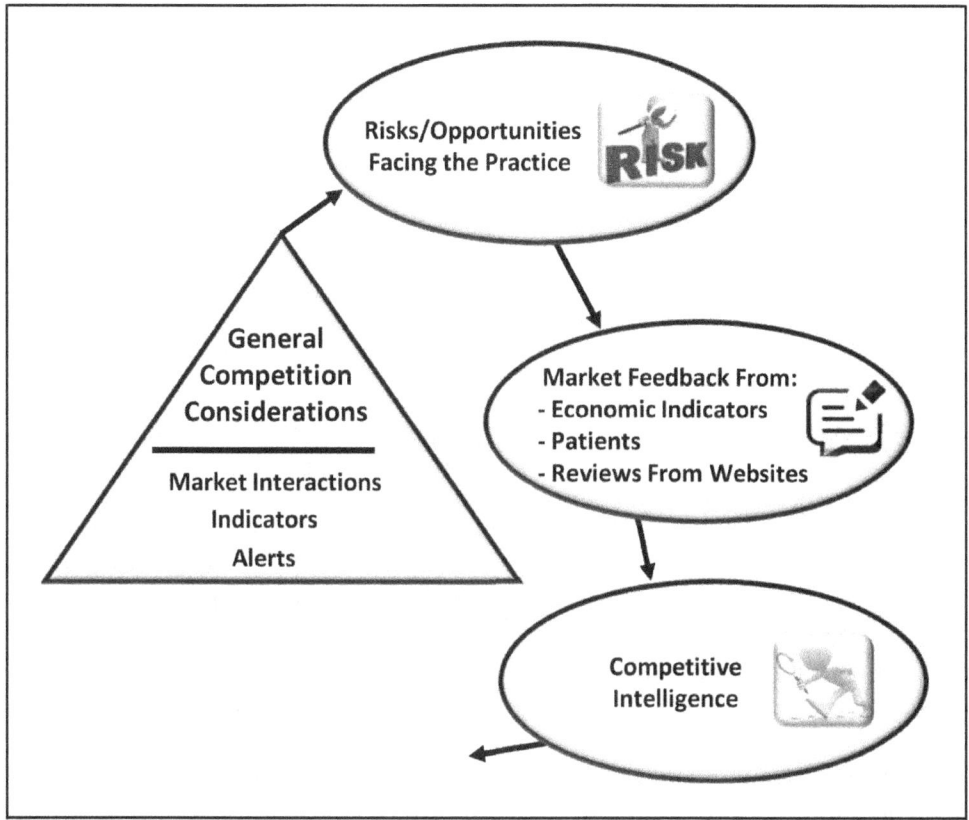

Figure 5–6. Competitive intelligence.

sented in Figure 5–6. This component of the analysis is an in-depth look at the competitive forces within the market and how they are competing against the practice. Obtaining this information is fundamental to the analysis as it sets up a defense against major competitors and/or the whole market.

Napoleon Bonaparte once said, "War is ninety percent information." Competition in the marketplace is a bit like a war between the practice and its competitors. This competitive war, like most wars, is for survival. In this case, it is to survive as an independent private practice. It is necessary to obtain and use these data, much like intelligence officers use information in wartime to win business battles and ultimately the

war against the competition. Therefore, the next step in the model is gathering competitive intelligence. The term *competitive intelligence* was coined by Gilad (2004), an ex-Israeli intelligence officer turned Harvard MBA businessman in the 1990s, who used warlike methods to gain information on the competition. The term *competitive intelligence* engenders images of fictional secret agents using an impressive array of sophisticated gadgetry to eavesdrop on their competitors. While it is a bit like business espionage, the process is ethical, legitimate, essential, and 95% available using public documents.

In audiology and hearing care, the continuous monitoring of the hearing industry is necessary to identify current and future competition. As in war, this information is used to develop tactical methods of engagement, actively seeking information from competitors so the practice can respond appropriately to their offensive marketplace moves. The challenge is to build a network by utilizing a formalized process for gathering information. Tyson (2010) indicates that competitive intelligence transforms random bits and pieces of data into strategic knowledge. In business, the process gathers information about:

■ The current competitive position and the probable future plans of competitors.
■ The driving forces within the marketplace.
■ Specific competitive products and technology.
■ The economic, political, and demographic influences that have an impact on the market.

Tyson further describes competitive intelligence as gaining an understanding of the strategies and mindsets of key competitors by developing a sense for their probable reaction to market developments or a marketing initiative generated within a specific practice. Gaining this knowledge involves continuous monitoring of competitors, consumers, suppliers, and other market forces, such as new product categories, so that the practice is never surprised by the action or reaction of the competition. Competitive intelligence involves more than just studying the competitors; it is the process of studying anything that helps make the practice more competitive.

Competitive intelligence has been thought of as a technique for big business to compete against other large corporations, but it can be extremely useful to a small practice in today's highly competitive hearing care market. Fleisher and Bensoussan (2015) defined *competitive intelligence* as a process by which actionable information is gathered about competitors and the competitive environment. According to these authors, within profit-seeking enterprises, there are four main categories of competitive intelligence. Presented in Table 5–1, these four areas are broken down into specific areas of study.

Levels of Competition

Figuring out the competition used to be far easier. The commercial hearing aid dealers were more sales oriented and the audiologists were more rehabilitative oriented. While that is still true to some extent, figuring out the motivation of both of these groups as well as others involves the application of analytical art and science. The following applies Fleisher and Bensoussan's categories to the hearing industry (Table 5–1). Hearing care involves competition at many levels:

■ *Specific product level.* Virtually all competitors in the market, such as independent audiologists, big-box stores, manufacturers' outlet stores, hearing aid dispensers, direct to consumer, and Internet sales, often appear to be the same to consumers (Chapter 12). While they realize there are many different brands of products, they are not generally aware of the inherent differences among them or the differences

Table 5–1. Categories of Business and Competitive Analysis

Scope of Analysis	Specific Targets
Levels of competition	• Specific product level • Needs-based/generic level • Share of wallet/mind/attention
Environment	• Competitive • Consumer/patient • Economic • Political, legal, regulatory • Social • Scientific
Technology	• Innovative products and methods
Decision levels and implementation	• Strategic decisions • Tactical decisions • Micro decisions

among the various types of businesses and clinical practices that provide them. Consumers are also typically unaware of the credentials and experience of some providers versus others. Competition on the product level requires knowledge of products, services, expertise, location, prices, policies, education, and other competitive factors, but again, particularly to first-time customers, all the products and places to obtain them all look the same. In this area, it is particularly necessary to differentiate prescription products and services from the competitors and concentrate on amplifying those differences to consumers.

■ *Needs-based/generic level.* This is a level of competition that seeks to satisfy the same functional group but considers any type of product or service that might be chosen instead of prescription hearing aids, especially OTC devices. Intelligence

as to the benefits and limitations of these competitive OTC treatments is essential to success as they have definite limitations, and those that use these products will at some time be ready to move to prescription products. Intimate knowledge of these products and the support offered by those competitors offering them is fundamental for the development of competitive strategies as well as the incorporation of them into the practice.

■ *Share of wallet/mind/attention.* The broadest level of competition is any other type of product that might cost the same but is a substitute for hearing care, such as OTC products. For example, once the arguments for treatment have been presented, the consumer might choose to use the funds to go on a cruise with OTC instruments rather than seek prescription hearing care. Personal decisions are tough competition, and sometimes success against competitive products and services may only be obtained when the hearing problem begins to affect the consumer's everyday lifestyle.

Environment

Within the market environment, factors stand out for any competitive situation. Knowledge of the actions and reactions of competitors to environmental issues can create a competitive edge for the practice. Environmental factors involve the following areas:

■ *Competitive.* An assessment of the current and prospective competitors and the specific methods by which they compete should be conducted.
■ *Consumer.* The practice's current and potential patients, as well as a perspective of the competitor's patients regarding their similarities and differences, should be reviewed.
■ *Economic.* The leading, lagging, and coincident economic indicators such as gross national product, inflation, financial markets, interest rates, price regulations, fiscal and monetary policy, and currency exchange rates need consideration as these indicate the health of the economic conditions where the competition exists.
■ *Political, legal, and regulatory.* There are changes that can happen "in the rules of the game." Institutions, governments, pressure groups, and stakeholders influence how business is conducted. These changes, for example, are now used to allow sales of OTC hearing aids in drug stores, direct to consumers,

the Internet, and elsewhere as the result of the recent legislation and the rescinding of the medical clearance regulation.
■ *Social.* Changing demographics, wealth distribution, attitudes, and cultural and social characteristics can alter buying habits. For example, recognizing the differences in the Baby Boomer population versus the previous and/or next generation of hearing-impaired patients should be taken into consideration when developing a competitive treatment plan.
■ *Scientific.* Emerging and changing technologies, such as the possible transition from traditional amplification to implantable products, new electronics, such as Auracast, must be considered in gaining a place within the competitive market.

This information can be obtained by publications, advertisements, presentations, chat forums, word-of-mouth discussions, trade journals, manufacturer meetings, and training sessions.

Technology

The technology area of competitive intelligence is principally concerned with new or emerging technological capacity by the evolution of science, scientific activity, or artificial intelligence such as basic and applied research that leads to alternative approaches to hearing rehabilitation and other procedures. Some clinics and franchises as well as manufacturer sales operations will attempt to imply that these methods are proprietary, but good competitive intelligence will alert the practitioner when this is happening and even anticipate its existence. Innovative fitting methods and hearing technologies are made known to most practices when presented to the marketplace, such as at conventions and invited seminars. The key is knowing when these techniques, products, and other procedures are available.

Decision Levels and Implementation

Management decisions are integral to the success of a practice and will likely affect its differentiation in the marketplace. Based upon the intelligence available, there are decisions that must be made at various levels.

- *Strategic decisions.* Strategic decisions are usually made by the owner of the clinic, usually with input from staff based upon their knowledge from many areas, including insurance claims, hearing aid programs, and lease versus purchase. Strategic considerations involve all these areas but ultimately depend on the budget available. These decisions set the policies of how the practice will approach the competition.
- *Tactical decisions.* In small practices, these decisions are made by the owner, assisted by staff, and implemented within the overall strategic policy for marketing, accounting, product branding, and service offerings.
- *Micro decisions.* These are the day-to-day decisions made by staff based upon routine encounters with patients. These encounters often generate valuable feedback to the practice principles about the competition, the practices' policies,

and operational issues that can be beneficial in decisions to maintain or modify practice procedures, products, and services.

The Goals and Type of Competition

While the foregoing relates to the theory of competitive intelligence, a method to categorize this necessary information is presented in Figure 5–7. In the sample, there is a practical identification of the type of competition, including their goals and objectives, their strategies and tactics, strengths and weaknesses, and their reactivity and hostility.

Who Is the Competition?

Initially, the concern is identifying the kind of competition in the marketplace. Competition may come in many forms, and most of these forms are not the same, some not even similar. At this stage in competitive intelligence, it is necessary to find out as much as possible about the type of competition that is being encountered.

What Are the Goals of the Competitors?

The goals of the competition are, of course, to make a profit and stay in business by competing with the owner's clinic. If they are an audiologist that has become aggressive in the market, they may be after the clinic's referral sources. If the competition is a sales operation, either a manufacturer or a retail outlet for OTC products, they are simply out in the consumer market to obtain customers, often on a "one-shot"

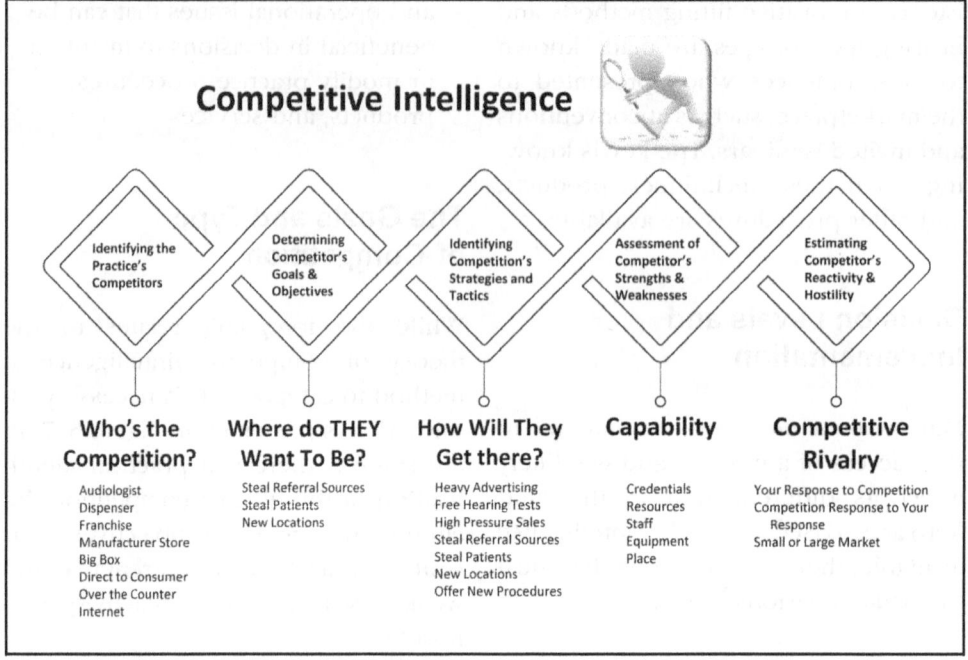

Figure 5–7. Specific competitive intelligence areas.

journey toward more sales. Other times, it can be other traditional hearing aid sales or other audiologists simply attempting to steal patients away for the practice or to their new location. Gather as much information as possible about these operations to determine their weaknesses and use that information along with other data to exploit them. All possible retaliations, both subtle and obvious, can be used to reduce and hamper them from meeting their goals against the owner's practice.

What Is the Strategy of the Competition?

Competitors have various strategies that must be investigated. Are they heavy advertisers, high-pressure sales, or visiting physicians aimed at stealing referral sources? Are they possibly offering products, procedures, or services that are

now allowing their differentiation to be an obvious departure from the offerings within the owner's clinic? The task is to identify the activities being used by a particular competitor to target a clinic and how a practice's marketing projects can be utilized to negate their efforts. Thus, the owner's practice must gather as much information as possible to successfully combat the attacks against the business.

The Competition's Capability to Meet Their Goals

The concern in this area is the capability of the competition to reach their goal of success at the price of the owner's practice. Do they have the credentials, funds, staff, location, and tenacity to compete against the clinic? Usually big-box stores, major retailers, and manufacturers have the funds but not some of the specific knowledge needed to compete against an audiology clinic.

Competitive Rivalry

After the gathering of competitive intelligence, how will the competition react to the retaliation of the owner's clinic to the aggressive marketing being conducted against the practice? While audiologists are governed by certain ethical standards for advertising and competition, it is essential that owners consider what the competitors will do if they market in certain directions. These are careful decisions that must be made with the appropriate data.

Where Do I Find This Competitive Intelligence?

The hardest part for most practice managers is finding the information neces-

sary to gain the real answers to some of the questions about competitors. Competitive intelligence is mostly available from accessible sources (Figure 5–8). General competitive information comes from sources such as trade journals and trade organizations discussing the latest technology and industry trends. Traynor (2019) categorizes the review of competitive intelligence into three areas:

Internal Environment of Competitor Clinics

Information that offers an advantage to the practice is a review of all that can be found about the competition. Does the competition have personnel who have difficult personalities, low-level technologies and skills in the field, or less expertise? Are their clinical procedures cumbersome or not well organized or best practice? Does

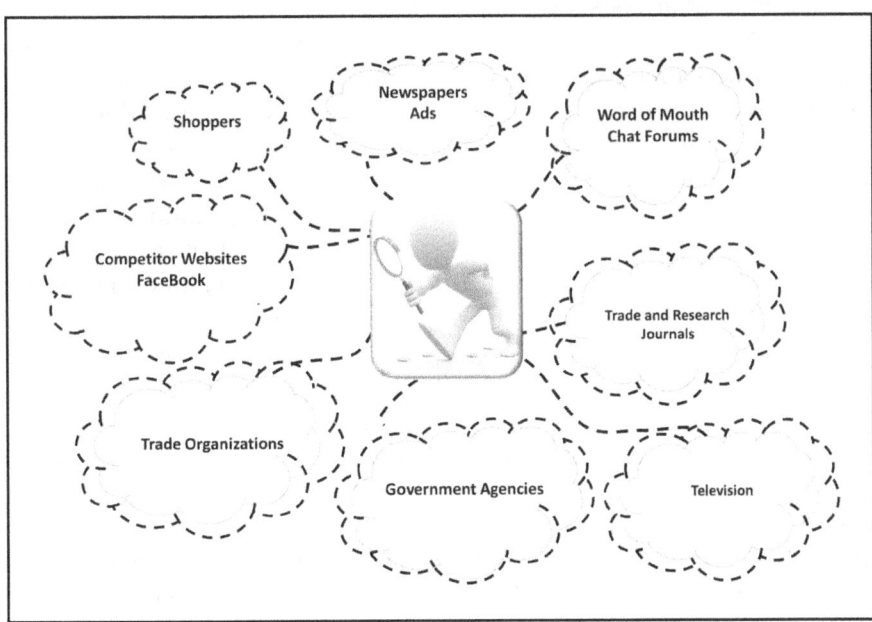

Figure 5–8. Sources of competitive intelligence.

the competition have a shabby or outdated facility where they practice? Does the competition appear to have financial problems?

Knowledge in all of these areas is advantageous to finding methods and areas to attack the competitors.

The Microenvironment of Competitive Clinics

This competitive intelligence information involves the patients and their experiences with competitors. Patients may be unsatisfied, satisfied, or elated with the clinical services and supportive operations they find within the competitive clinics. Patient reports as to how they are served by these competitors offer valuable information that can be explored. How does the clinic do a better job than the competition with patients that are either unsatisfied or satisfied offer an opportunity? If patients are elated, what does the competition do better?

In most markets, there is severe competition for referral sources. Investigate the perception of the competitive clinics and use this information to take advantage of the opportunity to make the referral source look knowledgeable and caring by providing better clinical services and support than the competitors.

Some suppliers are better than others. Sometimes it is the products, prices, or support offered that can make a major difference in the perception of patients. Explore the competitive products and find out their advantages and disadvantages relative to those offer by the clinic. A better product for a similar price can be a significant competitive advantage.

It is beneficial to understand how the competition relates to the other competitors within the marketplace. This rivalry is often fierce and can be problematic for the competition in the market. Reservation responses to ads can sometimes be an opportunity attract new patients into the clinic.

Macroenvironment Clues to the Competitors

These are the "big picture" issues such as politics, the economy, social-cultural concerns, and changes in technology. In many cases, these issues are at the forefront of the news. Changes in the political climate may be that audiology is granted practitioner status, and maybe the economy gets better or worse. Sociocultural factors can be monitored with social media and other mediums providing information about these needs within the market. Further, technological changes can be monitored in the news, review sites, the literature, and reports from consumers.

For specific information in various areas, a review of competitive newspaper and online ads, online hearing aid and hearing healthcare chat rooms, competitive websites, and Facebook pages offers a wealth of information. If information is unavailable from these traditional sources, the use of a "faux" shopper can be of great assistance in gaining information relative to treatment techniques, prices, and other valuable insight into the competition. The more information available to the practice manager as they make their analysis of their practice compared to competitors, the more sound the competitive strategy.

Practice Analysis Methods

Based upon the competitive intelligence gathered from each competitor, the existing practice or proposed new practice should be analyzed in detail so that there is evidence it will stand up to competitors. While there are many methods for reviewing general hearing care market competition, the SWOT analysis, Porter's Five Forces, and the three-circle analysis offer great assistance (Figure 5–9).

The SWOT Analysis

A common method of studying the market is a classic technique used in most businesses that reviews the *strengths (S), weaknesses (W), opportunities (O), and threats (T) (SWOT)*. SWOT analysis is a renowned tool for the audit and analysis of the overall strategic position of a business. Probably created in boardrooms in the 1950s or 1960s, this method was used to identify the strategies that create a firm business model so that an organization's resources and capabilities align with the market in which it operates.

SWOT is the foundation for evaluating the internal potential and limitations as well as the probable opportunities and threats from the external environment. SWOT is a strong but subjective tool that attempts to synchronize the practice with the marketplace by building practice strengths, reversing weaknesses, maximizing the clinic's response to opportunities, and overcoming the threats to the practice by identifying core competencies and setting objectives.

SWOT analysis helps in strategic planning in the following manner:

- Provides a source of information for strategic planning.
- Builds on the practice's strengths.
- Attempts to reverse the practice's weaknesses.

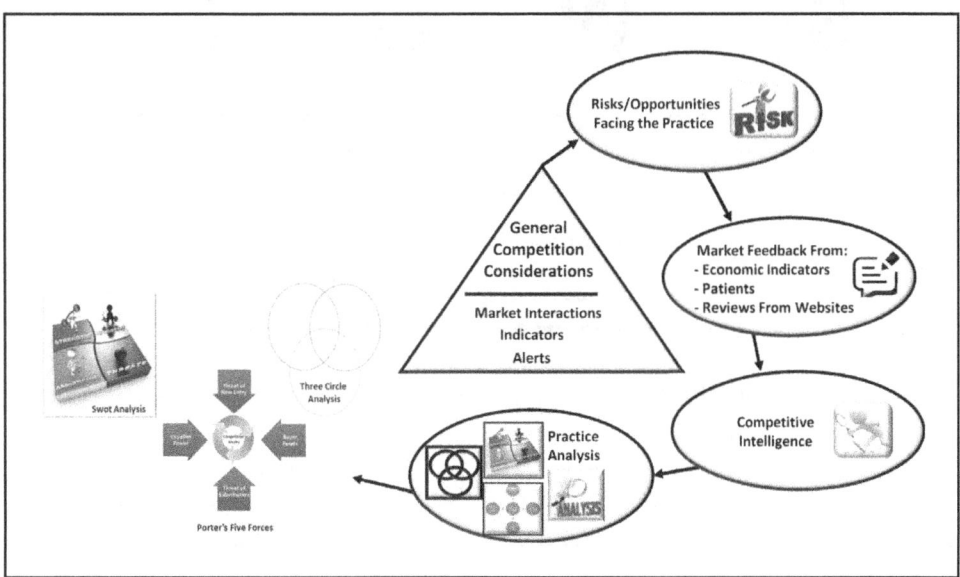

Figure 5–9. Analysis of the practice.

■ Maximizes the practice's response to opportunities within the market.
■ Overcomes the threats to the practice's success.
■ Identifies core competencies of the practice.
■ Assists in setting the objectives for strategic planning.

Although a SWOT analysis is useful in the study of a market and the practice's place within it, the method does have some limitations:

■ Does not specify how the clinic can identify these strengths, weaknesses, opportunities, or threats.
■ May present an oversimplified, subjective view of the situation that puts too much or too little emphasis on the competition.
■ Even if the SWOT is done correctly and with much diligence, many strengths and weaknesses are difficult to measure objectively.

Limitations notwithstanding, the assessment of a practice's strengths, weaknesses, market opportunities, and threats through a SWOT analysis is a relatively simple process that can offer powerful insight into the potential and critical issues affecting a business. Presented in Figure 5–10, the SWOT analysis begins by conducting a general inventory of internal strengths and weaknesses in the practice. After a careful review, the external opportunities and threats are considered within the constraints of the overall market. As the SWOT analysis begins, it is best to not elaborate on the topics, so bullet points are used to capture the major relevant factors in each of the four areas. Figure 5–11 presents a sample SWOT analysis of an audiology practice.

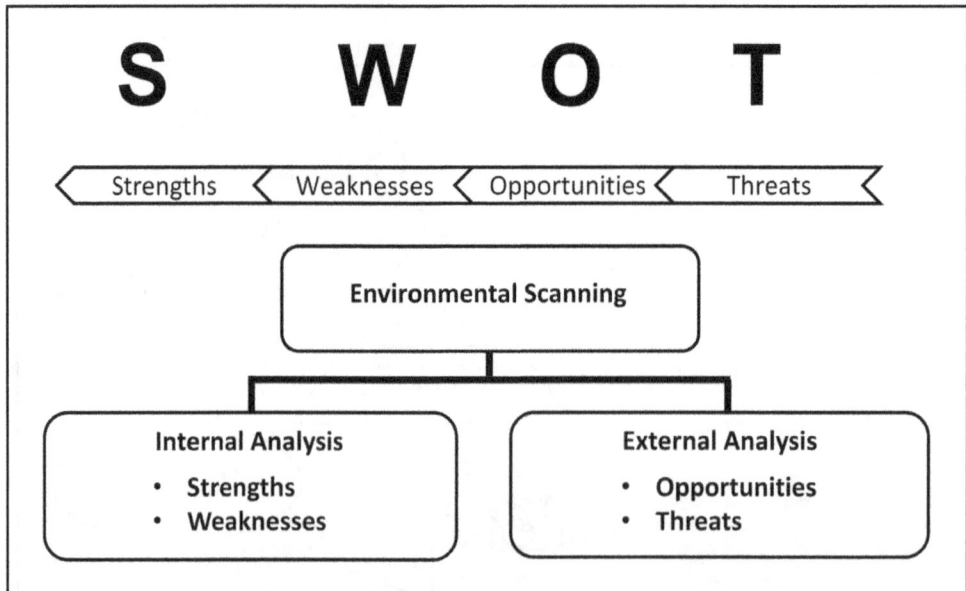

Figure 5–10. General components of a SWOT analysis.

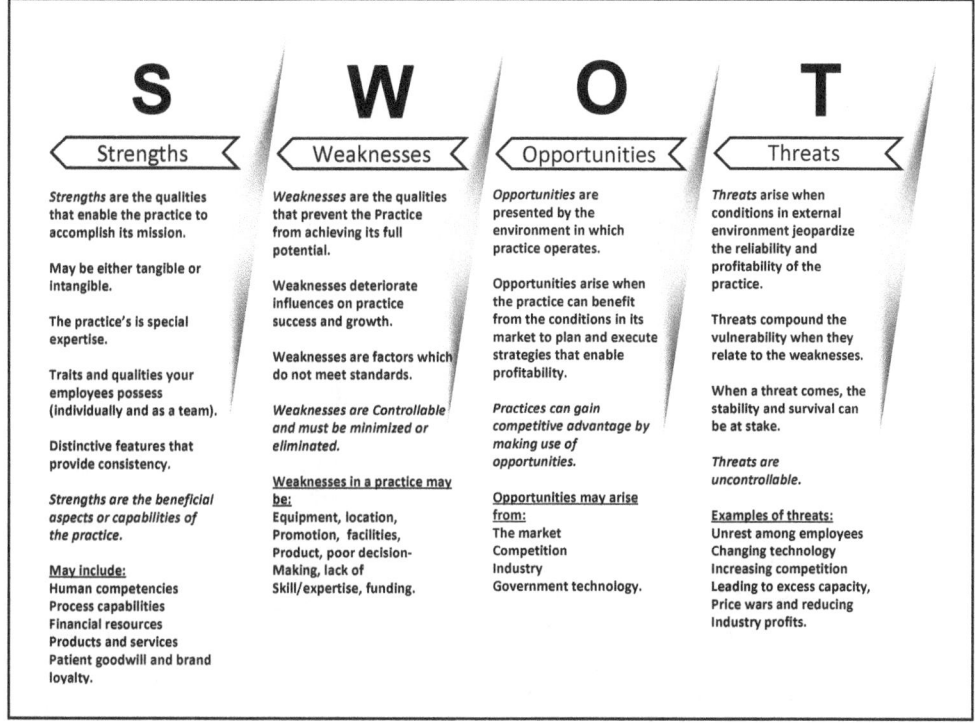

Figure 5–11. Specific components of a SWOT analysis.

Strengths

Strengths are the qualities that enable the practice to accomplish its mission serving the hearing impaired. This is the basis upon which continued success can be conducted, continued, and sustained. Strengths are the beneficial aspects or capabilities of the practice that include human competencies, process capabilities, financial resources, products and services, customer goodwill, and brand loyalty. Examples of organizational strengths of a practice might include but are not limited to vast financial resources, broad evaluation capability and product line, no debt, and committed employees and education level.

Weaknesses

Weaknesses prevent practices from achieving full potential by not meeting the standards the business plan has outlined. Weaknesses in a specific practice may be a minimal array of products, depreciating and out-of-date equipment, insufficient knowledge of specific areas of expertise, narrow product range, and poor decision-making. Weaknesses, however, are controllable and can be minimized or eliminated. Managers must recognize the drawbacks early on and act quickly to find a means to overcome, for example, problems such as overwhelming debt, high employee turnover, or antiquated equipment.

Opportunities

Opportunities that will result in a profitable practice are often presented by the conditions in the environment where the practice operates. Practices can gain competitive advantage by making use of opportunities. The practitioner must be prepared to execute strategies whenever opportunities surface from sources such as the market, competition, industry/government, and technology.

Threats

Threats arise when conditions in the environment jeopardize the reliability and profitability of the practice's business. Threats are compounded by vulnerability when they relate to un-covered weaknesses. Unfortunately, threats are uncontrollable, and the stability and survival of the practice can be at stake. Examples of threats can be ever-changing technology, increasing competition leading to excess market capacity, price wars, and a reduction in industry profits.

Items of Control: Strengths and Weaknesses Assessment

Strengths and weaknesses involve an internal qualitative analysis. When identified, these considerations will assist in determining whether a practice can manage the opportunities and threats (Figure 5–12). As indicated earlier, strengths can be anything that will increase market share or financial per-

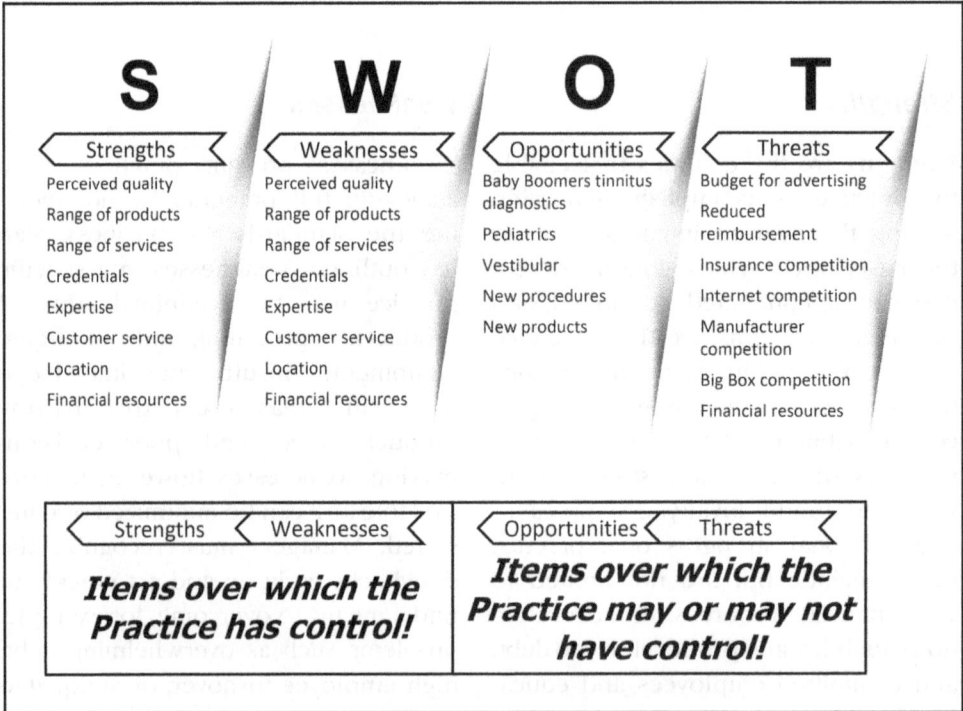

Figure 5–12. Items of control in the SWOT analysis.

formance, while weaknesses are problems that will hurt potential market share or the financials. These issues are usually familiar to the practitioner; however, closeness to the issues sometimes clouds judgment. Often, the practitioner has difficulty recognizing some of the obvious marketing problems, which is one of the inherent limitations of the SWOT analysis. Caution must be exercised that this closeness to the issues does not impact upon the analysis clouding the real picture of practice strengths and weaknesses. Analysis of these internal factors is essential and should center on:

■ The practice's operational leadership effectiveness in the community.
■ The financial strength of the practice to combat the threats and take advantage of the opportunities available.
■ The practice's physical capabilities for the location such as facility space, personnel, and equipment.
■ The responsiveness and motivation of the workforce in the practice.

Items of Control: Opportunities and Threat Assessment

The analysis of opportunities includes a review of problem-solving, product use cycles, creative methods of providing services and products, and ideal scenarios. Since opportunities are external to the practice analysis, a review of the practice's opportunities should center on market-oriented factors such as:

■ Practice market share.
■ The practice's ability to meet the needs and trends of the market.

■ The value the practice brings to the target market.
■ Quality of the practice's products.
■ Quality of the practice's customer service and support.
■ Quality/effectiveness of past promotions and other marketing efforts.
■ Pricing as compared to others for the value obtained.
■ The practice's geographic advantage.

While conducting the SWOT analysis, the following should be considered when reviewing threats:

■ The practice philosophy or mission.
■ Product (both goods and services) features, benefits, and quality.
■ The competitive advantage of the practice.
■ How the services are conducted and products dispensed in addition to patient and referral source satisfaction.
■ Practice pricing structures.
■ Target market awareness of the practice and services.
■ Target market's attitudes toward audiology, hearing aids, and new referral sources.
■ Target market's brand loyalty or lack thereof to the practice.
■ The competition's activities regarding new product launches, price changes, or new companies.

Reviewing these areas offers the audiology practice manager a good start in evaluating practice procedures, their place in the market, and the possible threats to be encountered. These are concerns that may or may not arise but can be a major problem if not considered as part of the analysis. Since the owner dictates the management of the practice and usually conducts the SWOT analysis, is important to use the SWOT analysis as a *guide* toward better management but NOT as a *management prescription* for success. Successful businesses build on their strengths, correct their weaknesses, and protect against internal and external threats.

Porter's Five Forces

Another classic method of *studying the market* was developed by Porter (1980/ 1998, 2008), a Harvard business professor. Porter's Five Forces (Figure 5–13) is a powerful tool that is used to review the overall market as well as assess the *competitive risk* by business professionals in virtually every industry. Within Porter's Five Forces, an industry is defined as a group of firms that produce products that are close substitutes for each other, such as audiology clinics versus hearing aid dispensaries within a specific area. These industries are not a closed system because competitors exit/enter the market continuously. The suppliers and buyers exert significant influence

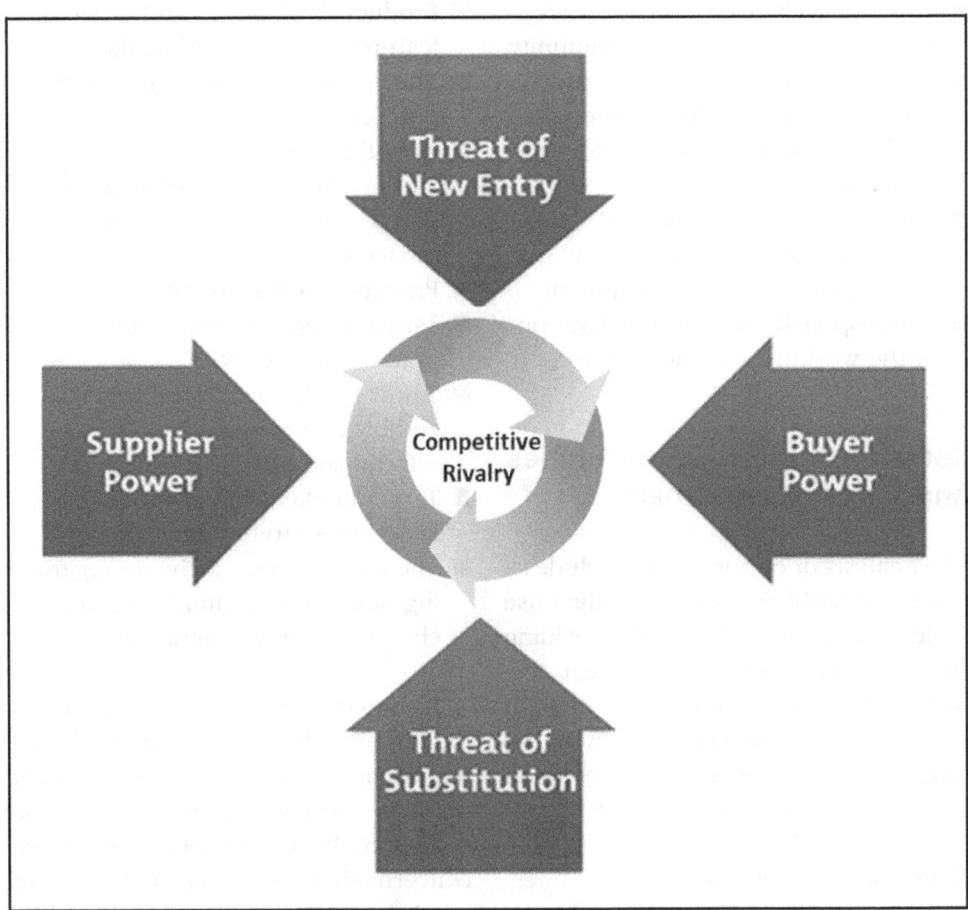

Figure 5–13. Porter's Five Forces.

on profitability and overall success, and they offer an outlook for future success or failure. Porter's model is simple and allows for the study of the market and an assessment of how a brand competes within an industry or, in this case, a specific audiology marketplace.

To accurately study a market and assess its competitive nature, it is necessary to understand where the power lies among competitors within a market. Porter stresses that understanding the structure of the market is fundamental to the formulation of an overall competitive strategy. Changes in a market structure are usually slow and evolve over time but nevertheless can result in social or cultural changes to the method and procedures of how business is conducted. These are usually due to political, labor, or economic issues but can also be the result of natural industrial consolidation and/or forward integration. Porter's classic model reflects strategy through an un-derstanding that the opportunities and threats can and will change over time.

In his model, Porter identifies five specific competitive forces that shape virtually every market no matter how large or small, and these forces determine the intensity of competition and, hence, the profitability and attractiveness of a specific business opportunity. Porter's model assumes these five forces determine the competitive power within a specific business, and by applying these driving forces, a manager or practitioner can derive a plan that will influence or exploit characteristics and situations within their industry. An overview of Porter's model is presented in the box and presents the relationships of the five forces:

- Threat of new entrants.
- Bargaining power of buyers.
- Bargaining power of suppliers.
- Threat of substitutes.
- The rivalry within the industry.

DECISIONS ON HOW TO COMPETE

The practice manager's decision-making process also reviews some of the classic lessons of how to compete. Urbany and Davis (2010) present six lessons that are essential thoughts and discussions when managers are developing their competitive strategy. These basic lessons include the following:

Lesson 1: *All product options can be broken down into features and benefits. Consumers purchase benefits, not features.* For example, consumers do not purchase a feedback manager; they purchase no squealing. They do not purchase directional microphones; they purchase less background noise.

continued on next page

continued from previous page

Lesson 2: *Certain features must be available for the practice to even be in consideration.* For example, the product must be digital, and it must help the consumer to hear better.

Lesson 3: *Other attributes and benefits provide differentiation.* While hearing devices must have certain attributes, others make them stand out among the competition. The idea that hearing aids can connect directly to iPhones, television, or microphones or be rechargeable differentiates not only a manufacturer's product within the marketplace but also the practice that the first into their market with these innovative products can differentiate themselves from competitors.

Lesson 4: *The once differentiating features will eventually become common to all products.* Competition evolves around the ebb and flow of new features such as feedback management, automatic volume controls, programmability, multiple memories, connectivity, and others that once were innovative are now expected. Features that provide expected benefits are essential to even be in consideration for purchase.

Lesson 5: *It is fundamental to put the meaning into the benefits created by the features!*

- *Functional:* Does the product or service provide some basic service or value that the patient values? . . . Hearing?
- *Place:* Is there value for the consumer in the convenience and accessibility of location for acquiring this brand? Instant delivery, easy access for follow-up?
- *Financial:* Are there financial benefits to the consumer? Value for money?
- *Information:* Does the consumer feel "informed" in the purchase of the product or service? Does this provider have enough expertise to take care of my situation?
- *Time:* Did the consumer perceive value in the time taken with them or in the speed and general timesaving by coming to this practice? Waiting time in waiting room? Waiting time for product? Did the clinician get right the first time?
- *Relationship:* Does the consumer feel connected to this clinic, the product brand, specific clinician, and/or employees?

continued on next page

continued from previous page

■ *Experiential:* Does the consumer get particular enjoyment or satisfaction from the visits to the clinic? Expertise, good experience with reception, clinical interactions, etc.

■ *Symbolic:* Is the patient proud of this specific brand, the clinic, or being seen by this particular provider?

■ *Psychosocial:* Does the patient relate to other people through consuming this product or service. To they hear, receive love, communication, and other benefits.

Lesson 6: *Features are only important if they produce hearing, enjoyment of life, quality of life, better lifestyle, ease of use, and/or the perception of being less old.*

Threat of New Entrants

Porter's first concern is *New Entrants* into the industry (Figure 5–14). New entrants into an industry add capacity and more places for patients to go for care, thus thinning out the patient population that would possibly consider an existing practice within the industry. In this case, if the capacity added to the marketplace is greater than the growth in demand by the hearing impaired for services and/or products, this added capacity within the marketplace reduces the profitability of the whole market. Essentially, the easier it is for new companies to enter the market, the greater the chance for more competition. New entrants can emerge at any time, changing a market's character for market share, price, and customer loyalty, thus disrupting other critical balances within the business environment. There is always a latent pressure for reaction and adjustment among the existing businesses (that Porter calls incumbents) within the

market. The threat of new entries into the market will depend on the extent to which there are *barriers to entry*. A new entrant needs to understand that the objective of competitive strategy for incumbent practices is to have strong and durable barriers to entry of others into the market, which they will utilize when threatened.

Significant barriers to entry in most industries include:

■ *If significant capital is required to start a company, an obstacle may need to be overcome.* Some industries require huge amounts of capital to begin operations and follow up with marketing efforts to facilitate entry. Especially in times when capital is scarce and significant amounts are required, funding can be a major barrier. In the hearing industry, establishing a clinic takes minimal capital and manufacturers are willing to loan funds to practitioners to sell their products; thus, the threat of new competition is always a possibility.

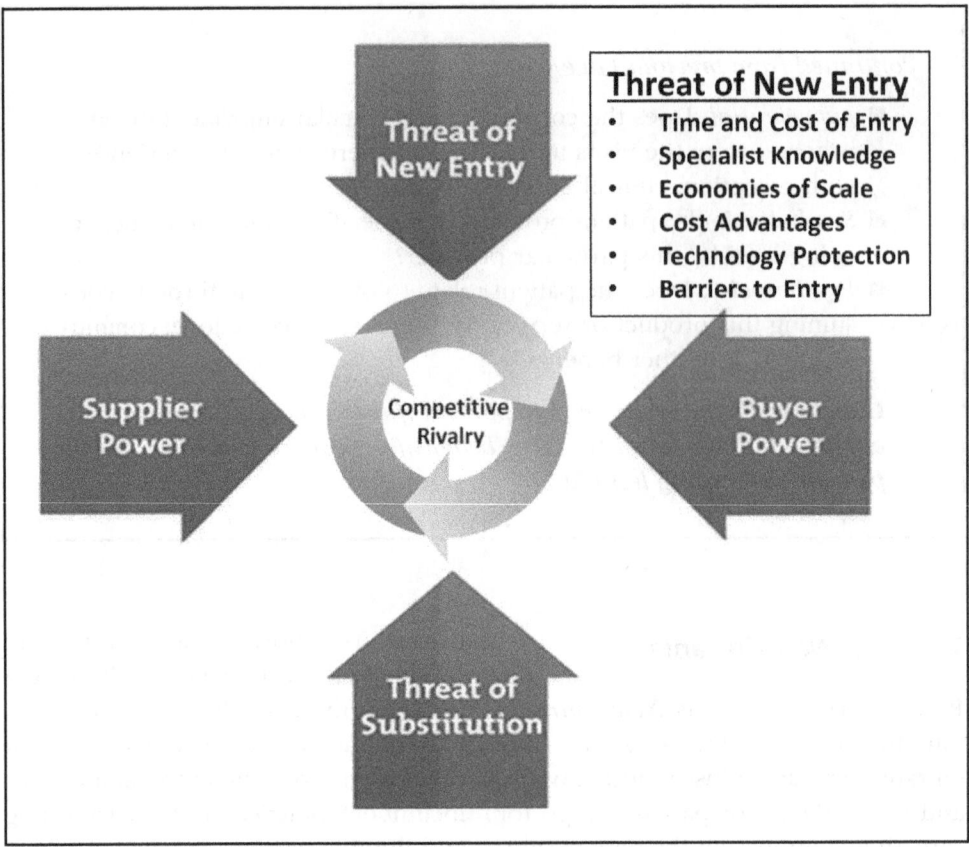

Figure 5–14. The threat of new entry. Components of Porter's Five Forces (Porter, 1980/1998, 2008). *Source:* Adapted from Mind Tools (2024).

■ *If obtaining enough product volume (economies of scale, i.e., patients), is an issue, success is impeded.* Practices that have been in the marketplace have developed essential business skills to stay profitable. If new businesses are not capable of attracting enough consumers, volume will suffer and subsequently profitability. Similarly, if the cost of doing business is more than other existing clinics within the market, the costs presented to each new consumer will be priced too high and the business will suffer.

■ *If access to resources, such as trained professionals, products, and expertise is limited, risk increases.* Often access to valuable resources can be controlled by competition. These may be product brands or experienced clinical staff. If the new market entrant is not able to access some of these essential components, they will be seen as substandard and, without significant compromise in price, sales will lag behind other clinics in the market, thus increasing the risk of success by the entrant.

- *If access to distribution channels is controlled, access to sources is limited.* New entrants into the market need access to the traditional distribution channels, such as referral sources and insurance contracts, or they must discover new ones to be successful. If the distribution channels are controlled by another clinic within the market, entrance can be difficult and consequently a barrier.
- *If the consumers believe that switching to another clinic would not be cost-effective.* Some consumers are brand loyal and prefer not to switch to a new entrant within the market. Additionally, if the costs to the consumer in terms of relationship, expertise, price, environment, ease of access, trust, and other issues are too high, the new clinic will not be adopted by the market.
- *If there is government intervention within the industry, new entry may be prohibitive.* Governments often rule over who may sell certain products. For example, there are drastic government plans to overhaul regulations regarding over-the-counter hearing aids and personal sound amplification products (PSAPS) that may influence the methods by which hearing aids are acquired by the public. Changes in government regulations can have significant effects on the business of audiology, resulting in the need for modifications in practice patterns and even the viability of independent audiology practice. Additionally, there are Medicare and Medicaid rules relative to service and product provisions that can be prohibitive to a new entrant.

Bargaining Power of Buyers

The *bargaining power of buyers* determines how customers can impose pressure on product or service margins and volumes (Figure 5–15). In most cases, a buyer of a product will shop around for the best deal, causing downward pressure on prices. A buyer's bargaining power is likely to be high in the following situations:

- *If switching to another practice means lower costs.* When buyers (patients) can easily switch to another practice with relatively low cost and frustration, they are empowered to purchase from the lower-cost provider. Some age groups, such as Baby Boomers, are not brand loyal in their business relationships and can be easily lured by a better deal elsewhere (Thornhill & Martin, 2007), even if it means less product and service. With today's commoditization trends, it is even more important to listen to the wants and needs of the patient so that they will not consider the competition.
- *If buyers purchase in large volume.* In the community hearing marketplace, buyers can be large key customers, such as insurance companies or referral sources that want the best for their patients. Insurance companies will seek the best deal possible to ensure the best possible treatment for their customers by requiring a credentialing process discount. The more competition, the more advantageous it is to accommodate these inconveniences and discounts. Insurance companies

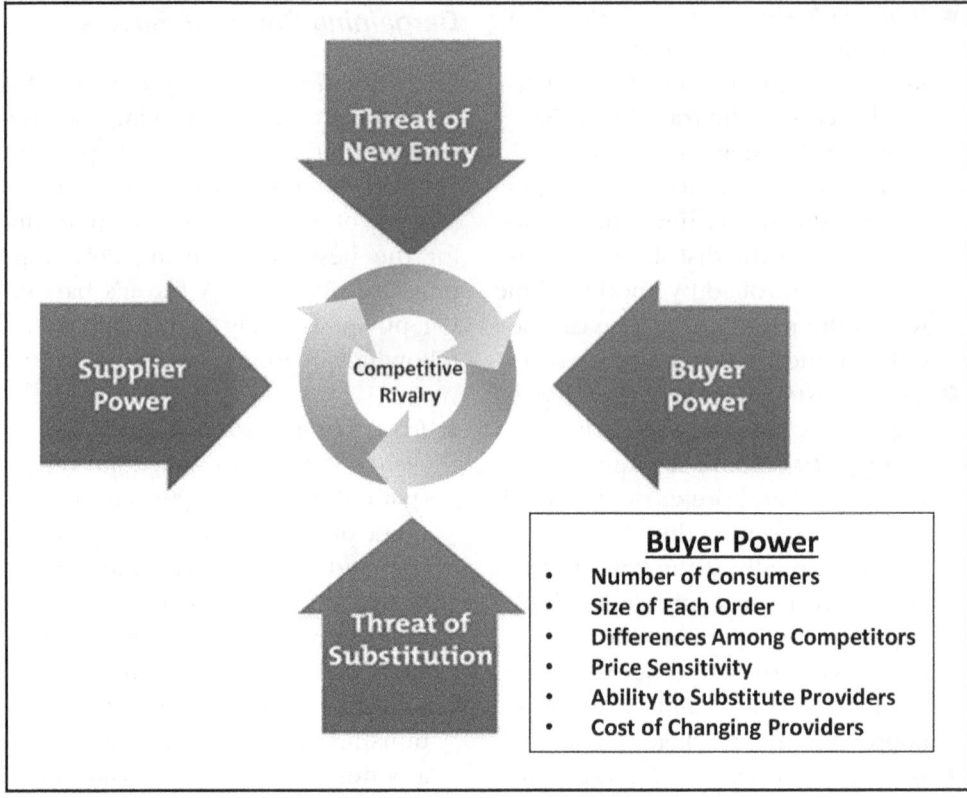

Figure 5–15. Buyer power. Components of Porter's Five Forces (Porter, 1980/1998, 2008). *Source:* Adapted from Mind Tools (2024).

wield many patients and can bring business to the clinic when it is scarce. Referral sources are a continuing source of patients; thus, it is always in the clinic's best interest to demonstrate that the practice is worthy of their referrals by generating timely reports, providing impeccable follow-up care, and having fair and reasonable pricing.

■ *If the industry comprises many small operators.* A greater number of competitive clinics (suppliers) ensure more price competition. Therefore, the pressure is higher to keep costs down and incentives high, such as longer warranties and more service.

■ *If the supplying clinics operate with high fixed costs.* Some clinics have high operating costs and cannot make modifications to their purchase terms without compromising their cash flow and thus their possible business success. These clinics will have more difficulty meeting the price and incentive pressures in a high buyer power environment.

■ *If the product (audiology, hearing aids, accessories, etc.) is undifferentiated and can be easily replaced by substitutes.* Products or services that are essentially the same can be purchased from any clinic (supplier) for the lowest possible price.

Differentiation is the key to success. Clinics must provide faster service and more sophisticated technology than their competitors, exceed in their level of expertise, have state-of-the-art equipment, offer a convenient location with ample parking, and have handicapped accessible ramps. These differentiations will attract consumers to another clinic when buyer power is high.

■ *If switching to an alternative product is relatively simple and price is not the issue.* As suggested earlier, it is a minor issue to switch audiologists; therefore, the products must exceed the buyer's expectations, or they will be motivated to go somewhere else.

■ *If buyers are price sensitive.* While some communities are affluent, others are not and extremely price sensitive. Although some consumers would like to have the highest technology, they simply cannot afford it; therefore, it is essential to have some low-cost options for those that do not have the resources.

Essentially, the concern with *Buyer Power* is the ease with which buyers can drive prices down. The degree that the consumer (patients) has power to control costs is diametrically determined by the number of clinics in the marketplace, the number of buyers, and frequency of purchase. Additionally, if the "buyer" is the referral source and/or insurance company, they have greater power to dictate agreement terms.

Bargaining Power of Suppliers

A new or existing business must appreciate the *bargaining power of suppliers* to compete in today's economy and establish a foothold for future positioning (Figure 5–16).

The term "suppliers" comprises all the competitive clinics, dispensers, and other facilities that appear to consumers to provide the same goods or services. Supplier bargaining power is likely to be high when:

■ *The market is dominated by only a few suppliers.* In a market where there are few clinics, there is less chance for negotiation since there are ample consumers requiring services and products.

■ *There are no substitutes for certain products.* It is well known that audiologists can fit 85% of their patients with one brand of product. For some patients, however, there are no substitutes for the products that are needed or desired. Phonak's Lyric is a good example because if the consumer wants this device, they must go to a clinic to obtain it. While the FDA has approved patients to self-fit Lyric instruments, consumers must be seen in specific clinics to obtain these devices. The same may be true if a rechargeable device or other new/novel featured device is preferred. For these and other evaluations or instruments, the clinic dictates price, availability, and terms of use because there are no alternatives.

■ *The supplier's customers are fragmented, so their bargaining power is low.* The example here is of a consumer that has an insurance benefit. If there are not many patients with the same insurance benefit, it is not profitable for the clinic to participate in the provision

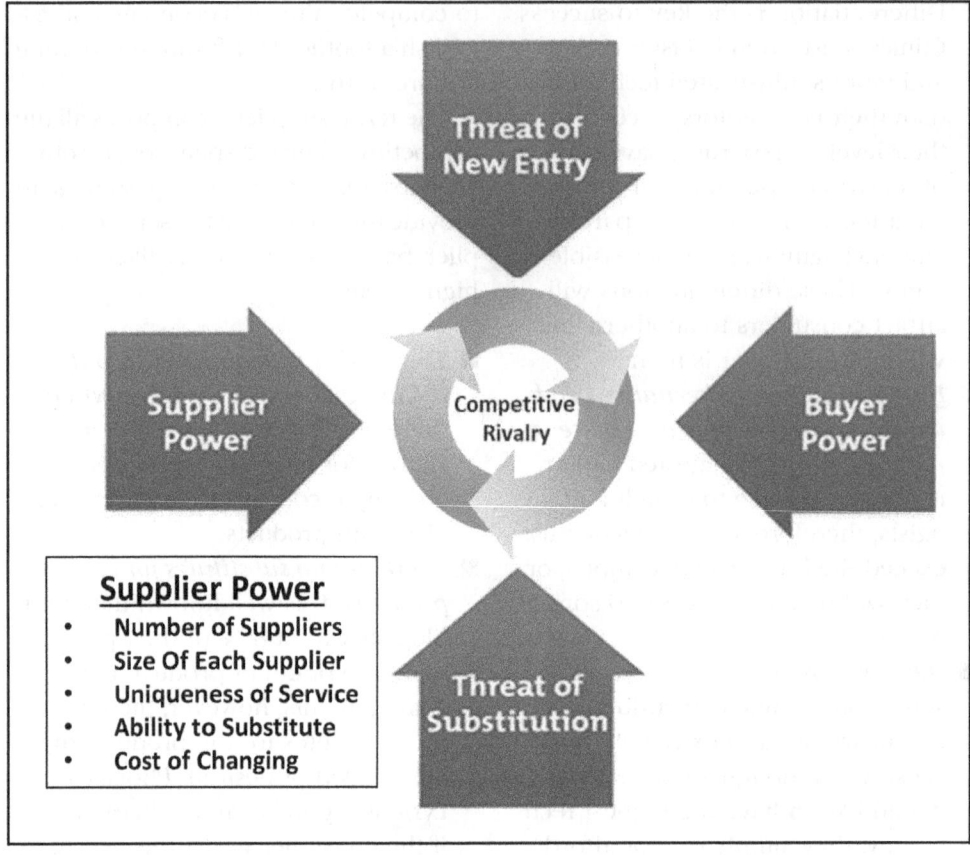

Figure 5–16. Supplier power. Components of Porter's Five Forces (Porter, 1980/1998, 2008). *Source:* Adapted from Mind Tools (2024).

for that insurance company (Chapter 16). These insurance companies often want discounts and increased services over and above what is profitable for the clinic. Since there are no other choices for the consumer, the clinic has the power to not accept the insurance benefit and offer the services and/or products at the going rate.

■ *Switching costs from one supplier to another are high.* Switching costs are not usually high and are generally in the buyer's favor for audiology services, but the exception is

when there is only one supplier of a specific evaluation or device. Especially in rural areas where there is only one supplier and others are miles away, there is high supplier power because with switching comes the inconvenience of driving many extra miles to obtain treatment.

Basically, *Supplier Power* is how easy it is for clinics to drive up prices. Independent clinics are compelled to raise prices if there is no competition in the market, a unique product or service is offered, there is control over the buyers within the market (e.g., denying insurance), and the cost of switching from one clinic to another is high.

Threat of Substitutes

The *Threat of Substitutes* exists if there are alternative evaluations or products available for the same purpose with lower prices that have better performance parameters than incumbent products (Figure 5–17). These new evaluations or products could potentially attract a significant proportion of market volume and, hence, reduce the potential sales volume for existing companies.

A recent example is the advent of OTC hearing aids. Prior to the introduction of OTC products, mild to moderate prescription fittings were very common. Since prices for OTC devices are more affordable than prescription devices and may provide ample benefit to patients with these mild hearing losses, theoretically, this was thought to cause a reduction in the number of sales for mild to moderate prescription devices. In the early OTC markets, the product performance has been substandard.

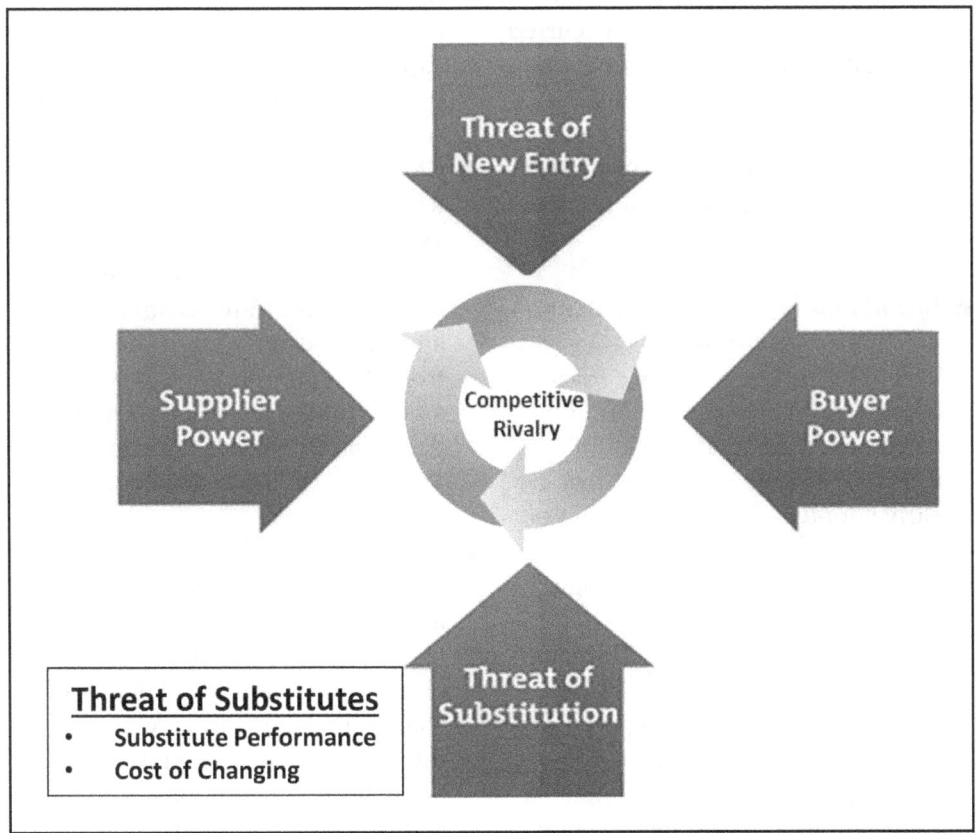

Figure 5–17. The threat of substitutes. Components of Porter's Five Forces (Porter, 1980/1998, 2008). *Source:* Adapted from Mind Tools (2024).

Combined with a substantial amount of advertising prior to the introduction of OTC products, this has increased the market for prescription devices. It is possible, however, that if OTC products improve, consumers will see them as a direct competitor to prescription devices.

Another example of substitutes in audiology occurred in the 1980s and 1990s when auditory brainstem response (ABR) was used to evaluate patients for suspected acoustic tumors. By the late 1990s, the use of ABR gave way to the use of magnetic resonance imaging (MRI). The MRI was a better choice for the physician as they could directly view the presence of a vestibular schwannoma tumor. This also occurred when analog hearing aids progressed to programmable, then to digital. Comparable to the threat of new entrants, according to Porter (1980/1998, 2008), the threat of substitutes is determined by factors such as:

■ *Brand loyalty of customers.* Many patients are brand loyal as they have their personal reasons for using a particular clinic or audiologist for their treatment. While there is a fraction of buyers that are early adopters, looking for a better product each day, most will take the advice of their trusted audiologist regarding what to use and when to purchase. Substitutes for traditional amplification are on the horizon and clinics need to be prepared for this change as they have for preceding products. Cochlear implants are a well-established intervention for profound sensorineural hearing loss, but they are increasingly being used for single-sided deaf-

ness in Europe. Auditory brainstem implants are an alternative when a cochlear implant is contraindicated. Medical devices such as middle ear and bone conduction implants are becoming more and more popular, and other devices are being investigated such as cochlear direct drive devices that require implantation of a micro-actuator through a cochleostomy. Clinicians must be prepared to manage these patients because these devices are being shown to provide good audiological outcomes, especially when surgery is simple, straightforward, and constantly evolving. The brand loyalty of the consumers to a particular clinic may depend on the clinic's capability to deliver services for these innovations that may become substitutes over time.

■ *Close consumer relationships.* Clinics need to keep consumers happy as this will determine how easily they will switch to substitute products when they are recommended and become available. The benefit from their current devices will be a determining factor in a patient's decision to consider the supplier's advice to use these new and innovative products.

■ *Switching costs for consumers and clinics.* The costs of switching to an implantable product are probably high for the patient and depending on the innovation may initially price itself out of the market. Costs for the clinics would also most likely be high due to additional training and expertise for follow-up support. Costs notwithstanding, there is a threat from new products on the horizon, and it will be necessary to know and deal with these new products/evaluations or the clinic will not survive.

- *The relative price for performance of substitutes.* Clinicians must be able to decide if a high-end product is appropriate for a patient or whether an implantable device is desirable over a traditional hearing instrument. Value for money is always a concern when recommending a new type of product. The clinician should weigh the benefits and risks when determining whether to provide the new products and/or services and whether a referral to the otologist is in the patient's best interest.

- *Current trends.* There are some trends that must be followed if the clinic is to be in the market and others that are simply fads. It is up to the clinic and their staff to decide which of these innovations truly creates a lasting difference and which is simply innovative but of no real benefit.

The *Threat of Substitution* is dynamic and ever-changing. There are new inventions every day that may significantly threaten a standard of the industry and even replace them. The traditional digital hearing instrument may soon be ancient history. Since there is a continuous threat of substitutions for most of what audiologists do and recommend each day, it is essential that fervent monitoring of these changes be conducted on a regular basis.

Competitive Rivalry

Competitive Rivalry or Rivalry Among the Incumbents refers to the intensity of competition among existing players (incumbents) within the market (Figure 5–18).

Rivalry is fueled by the number and diversity of competitors, the growth of the market, those with high advertising budgets, high fixed costs, and a general overcapacity within the market for services and products. A highly competitive business climate, often the result of high buyer power, presents severe pressure on prices, margins, and therefore profitability for every clinic in the market. Rivalry among existing market competitors is likely to be high when:

- *There are many incumbents about the same size.* Rivalry tends to be high when there are many clinics offering products perceived the same by consumers. One receiver-in-the-canal, in-the-ear, in-the-canal, completely-in-the-canal, invisible-in-the-canal (RIC/ITE/ITC/CIC/IIC) looks about the same as another, and the more clinics there are in the market, the easier it is for patients to believe that there is no difference among them, and one facility is as good as another to obtain these devices.

- *The incumbent companies have similar strategies.* Competition is high from most of these companies as they have similar strategies. Many clinics use a referral strategy and chase each other's referral sources. Others have huge marketing budgets and rely on attracting new consumers through full-page ads each week in the print media or television. Basically, they are using a differentiation strategy by attempting to present their product as different from others. Competition for

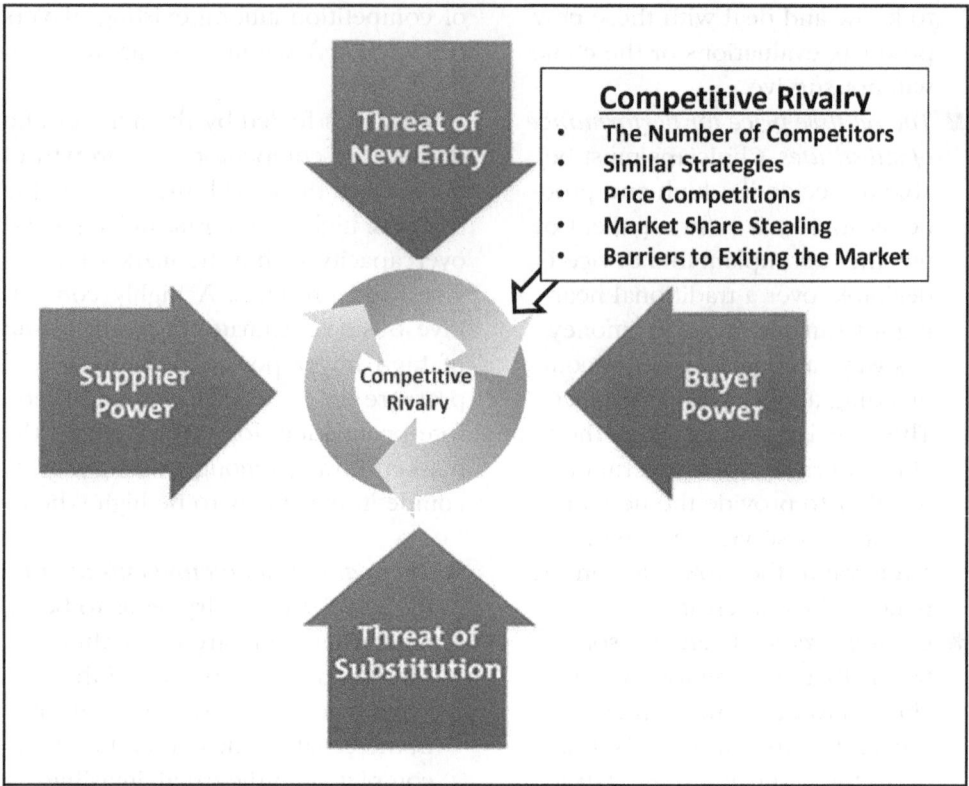

Figure 5–18. Competitive rivalry. Components of Porter's Five Forces (Porter, 1980/ 1998, 2008). *Source:* Adapted from Mind Tools (2024).

differentiation among amplification, assessment, and other audiological products is fierce and essential for survival.

■ *There is not much differentiation among incumbents and/or their products, and thus the price competition is intense.* There is fierce competition for differentiation of products but, simultaneously, there is the continuous commoditization of amplification that attempts to un-differentiate products. For practices where differentiation is minimal, there is intense price competition, while for those practices that are successfully differentiated, price is not a major issue.

■ *Low market growth rates indicate that the growth of a particular company is possible only at the expense of a competitor.* For quite some time, the market for amplification has been stagnant. This stagnant market suggests that the growth of a company that supplies evaluations and amplification products will only grow at the expense of another incumbent. Since there is considerable market share stealing going on among the major incumbents, intense rivalry exists in the hearing marketplace.

■ *Barriers for exit are highly expensive.* In addition to the high cost of obtaining qualifications to practice, such as an AuD, there are the costs that went into the practice, often funded by a manufacturer. These are loans that will require repayment and serve as a barrier to exiting the market until the clinic cannot support itself.

Once there is an overall analysis of the strengths, weaknesses, opportunities, and threats using a SWOT and an overall look at the market climate with Porter's Five Forces, it becomes necessary to perform an analysis of each competitor, which can be conducted with the three-circle analysis (Urbany & Davis, 2010).

Three-Circle Analysis

The *Three-Circle Analysis* incorporates Venn diagrams to compare each competitor with the largest market share to the practice, so that there is detail of the competitive needs for the practice. The premise is that a business that develops the best understanding of the value sought by consumers has a competitive advantage. The authors recognize that in today's highly competitive hearing care environment, markets are volatile and uncertain with shifting consumer desires and demands.

The Urbany and Davis three-circle model facilitates a rapid grasp of the practices' competitive situation and focuses its attention on the most critical strategic concepts in winning the competitive battle. The model systematically considers four key drivers. First, the model defines, builds, and defends the unique value advantage or value disadvantage that is created by the practice.

Second, it reviews, reveals, corrects, and eliminates value that is required by the market but failing within the practice. Third, it potentially neutralizes any unique market value that is created by the competition and, finally, explores and exploits the possible growth opportunities through an understanding of the unmet needs within the market. The three-circle analysis begins with the consideration of three important factors:

- The practice offerings.
- Patient needs and/or expectations from the practice.
- The competitor offerings.

In the example in Figure 5–19, the bottom circle for competition is represented by Costco as a formidable competitor compared to the practice (Audiology Associates, Inc) in the left circle and, finally, patient needs represented by the right circle.

The next step in the analysis is to begin entering detailed information, keeping in mind the interrelationship of each player within the model, Costco, the practice, and the patient:

1. Hearing care professionals know the needs of their patients. Those needs should be listed remembering that these are the same needs for any practice being analyzed. To be correct, for consumer issues that remain unclear, patients should be asked what is important to them.
2. Competitive intelligence needs to be obtained on the competitor and entered into the model.
3. The main features of the products and services of the practice are then added for comparison to the competitor.

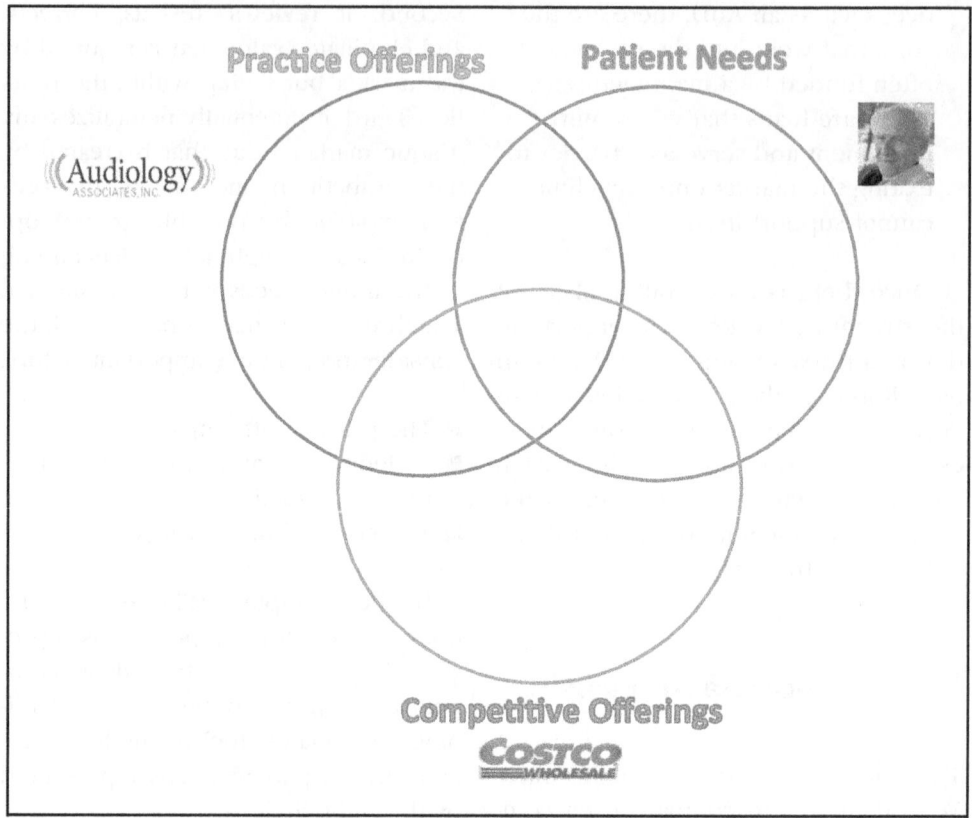

Figure 5–19. The three competitive circle analysis (Urbany & Davis, 2010).

Figure 5–20 begins with each area within the circles assigned a letter A to G.

Area letters represent the following issues about the practice, patient, and competitor:

- *Area A—The practice's points of difference from the competitor.*
- *Area B—The points of parity between the practice and the competitor.*
- *Area C—The points of difference between the practice and the competitor.*
- *Area D—Patient unappreciated differences for both the practice and the competitor.*

- *Area E—Patient unappreciated differences for the practice.*
- *Area F—Patient unappreciated differences for the competitor.*
- *Area G—Unmet patient needs by both the practice and the competitor.*

Figure 5–21 completes the areas relative to patient needs from Audiology Associates compared to Costco.

- *Area A* outlines the specific values that the practice brings to the market and separates it from the competitor. These issues may in-

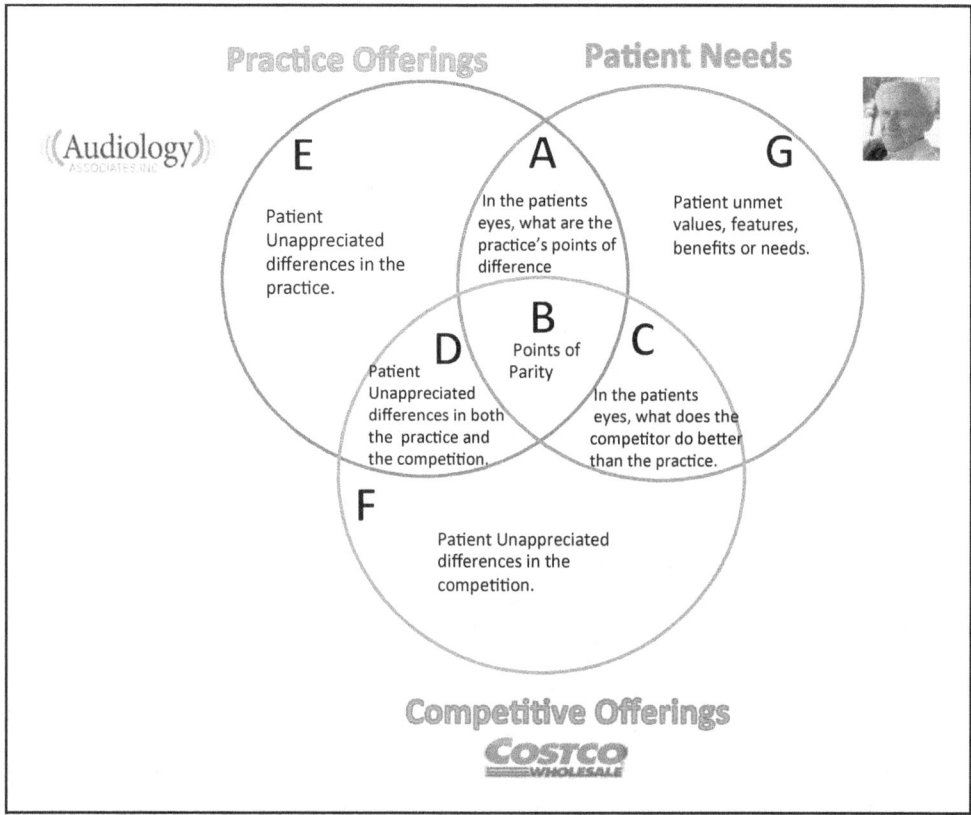

Figure 5–20. The areas within the circles (Urbany & Davis, 2010).

clude education, experience, product knowledge, hearing knowledge, detailed hearing evaluation, cerumen removal, clinical environment, equipment, privacy, relationships, and longevity.

■ *Area B* lists all the areas of parity, or where the competitor and the practice are similar, such as premium technology, warranties, free loss and damage, hearing testing, free demonstrations, free cleaning, and probe microphone verification.

■ *Area C* points out the differences between the competitor and the

practice. In the case of Costco, their major point difference is that of price, and secondary issues would be the 2-year return policy and their national brand. The challenge for the practitioner is to accurately perceive the competitive differences from the patient's perspective. For example, the practice may be quite different from the competition, but those differences are not really seen as different by the patients. There can also be the situation that the practice is different from the competitor in ways that matter to patients, but there are no

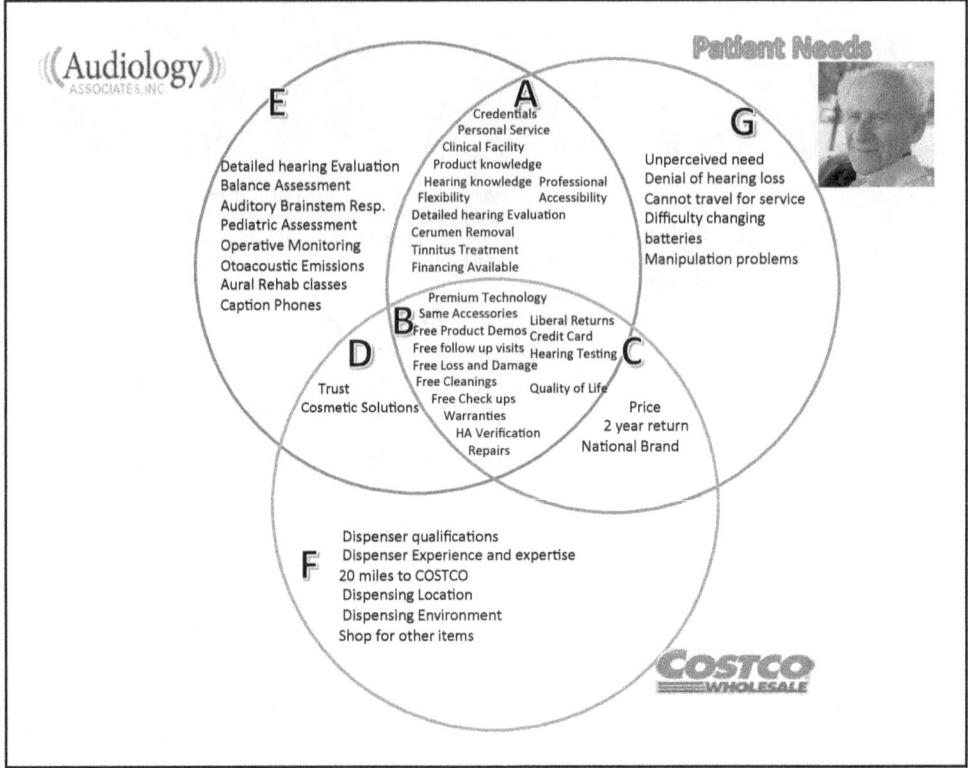

Figure 5–21. Three-circle comparison: audiology associates to Costco (Urbany & Davis, 2010).

resources or capacities to build or sustain those important differences.

- *Area D* describes those benefits that are unappreciated by the consumer such as trust, service, and cosmetic solutions.
- *Areas E and F* are areas of consumer unappreciated differences for the practice and the competitor, respectively. These are issues that are not well known or appear to be the same offering by the practice and the competitor that are not the same.
- *Area G* reflects the benefits that will likely not be achieved by either the

competitor or the practice, such as normal hearing.

The example in Figure 5–21 reflects a typical three-circle analysis with comparison to Costco, but the practice should exercise a three-circle analysis against each of the major competitors within the market area.

Management Action & Competitive Strategy

The objective of a strategy should be to modify competitive forces in a way that improves the position of the practice based upon the data that have been gathered (Figure 5–22). Strategic development is based upon the practice manager's assimilation of market indicators, feedback and alerts gleaned from the generic knowledge of the market, the risks, competitive intelligence as well as conducted analytics of the SWOT, Porter's Five Forces, and possibly a three-circle analysis against the biggest competitor.

Competitive advantage refers to any characteristic that allows a company to outperform its rivals. This may be achieved through several means, such as offering lower prices, providing superior quality or innovative new products, or delivering exceptional customer service. The ultimate goal is to create a unique and sustainable position in the market that competitors cannot easily replicate. Porter (1980/1998, 2008) suggested there were three potentially successful generic approaches to outperforming other businesses within an industry such as audiology (Figure 5–23):

■ Stuck in the middle
■ Focus
■ Overall cost leadership
■ Differentiation

It will take one of these generic strategies to build value for the consumers who visit the practice. Although these strategies can be implemented at the same time, they rarely are executed together. Everyone associated with the practice must be on board with the strategy as successful implementation requires total commitment from the clinical operations team, including the professionals, clerical employees, and supportive family members.

Stuck in the Middle

Probably the worst place to be, strategically, is "stuck in the middle" with no direction. Any business, including audiology practices, must orient to a generic strategy, have cost leadership, focus on a target market, or achieve differentiation (a uniqueness) to be successful. Attempting to be all things to all types of patients is a strategy for failure. As strategies go, any business, including audiology practices, should choose one and move in that direction because the worst place to be is "stuck in the middle" with no direction. Audiology practices that are "stuck in the middle" must make a fundamental, strategic decision to move forward with a decision to focus on a specific area or areas of practice, become an overall cost leader, or differentiate their practice or become irrelevant in the market.

Focus Strategy

Porter's definition of a "Focus Strategy" is the ability to deliver the same benefits as competitors but to a specific market that is underserved, such as a particular patient group, segment of a product line, or geographic area. Although the other two generic strategies are aimed at the total community market, this strategy focuses on a *specific target*. In audiology practice, the business is fine-tuned for a specific audience and to the benefit of a specific group or groups of patients. Focusing involves specializing

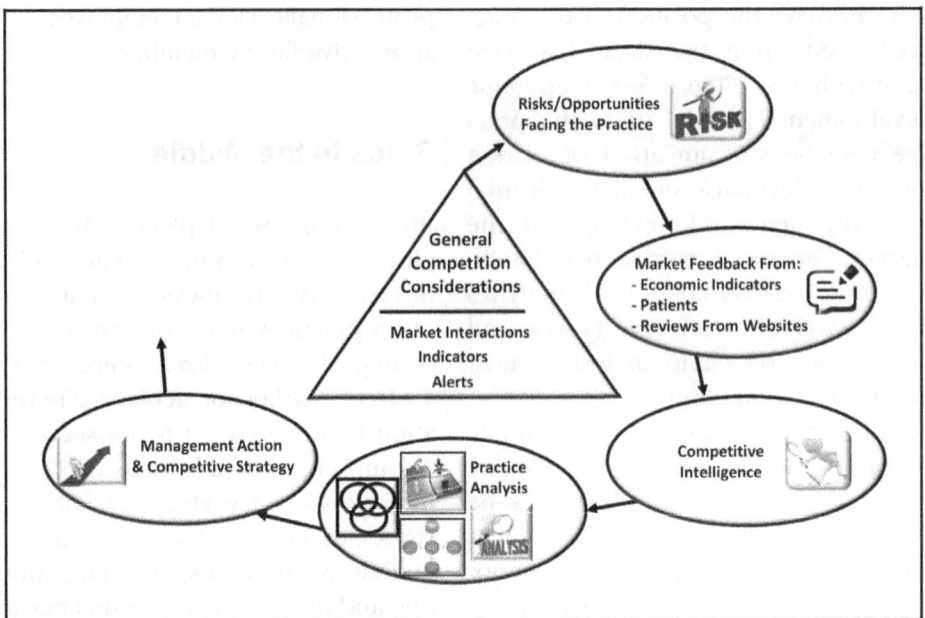

Figure 5–22. Porter's Generic Competitive Strategies.

in a specific area of practice such as the treatment of pediatrics, balance, tinnitus, industrial and recreational noise control, nursing homes, rural populations, mobile vans, and other niche markets that can be exploited. Often practices can obtain a "first mover advantage," allowing the establishment of strong brand recognition, product/service loyalty, and special expertise before other entrants. These may be products that are not available to other audiology clinics or those that have not been seen in the community in the past. In audiology past examples were the Lyric products, which took some time to become available in most markets. Later it was the availability of Bluetooth connections for telephones and televisions. In the future, it will be Audiocast connections as they become available to all hearing instrument products. There are several advantages in being the first practice to

execute a focus on a specific area of the profession:

- The practice that establishes a best practice standard for a focus or niche specialty will be a step ahead of the local competitors.
- Achieving a strong impression with patients and their families with demonstration in specialized expertise, innovation, and available benefits will lead to brand recognition and extreme patient loyalty.
- Specialization will lead patients to switch from other area practices to obtain the product or procedure that is now a unique offering.

Focusing involves obtaining specialization in one or more areas of expertise that can require further study or credentials. While extra training or certification may be required, focusing will often in-

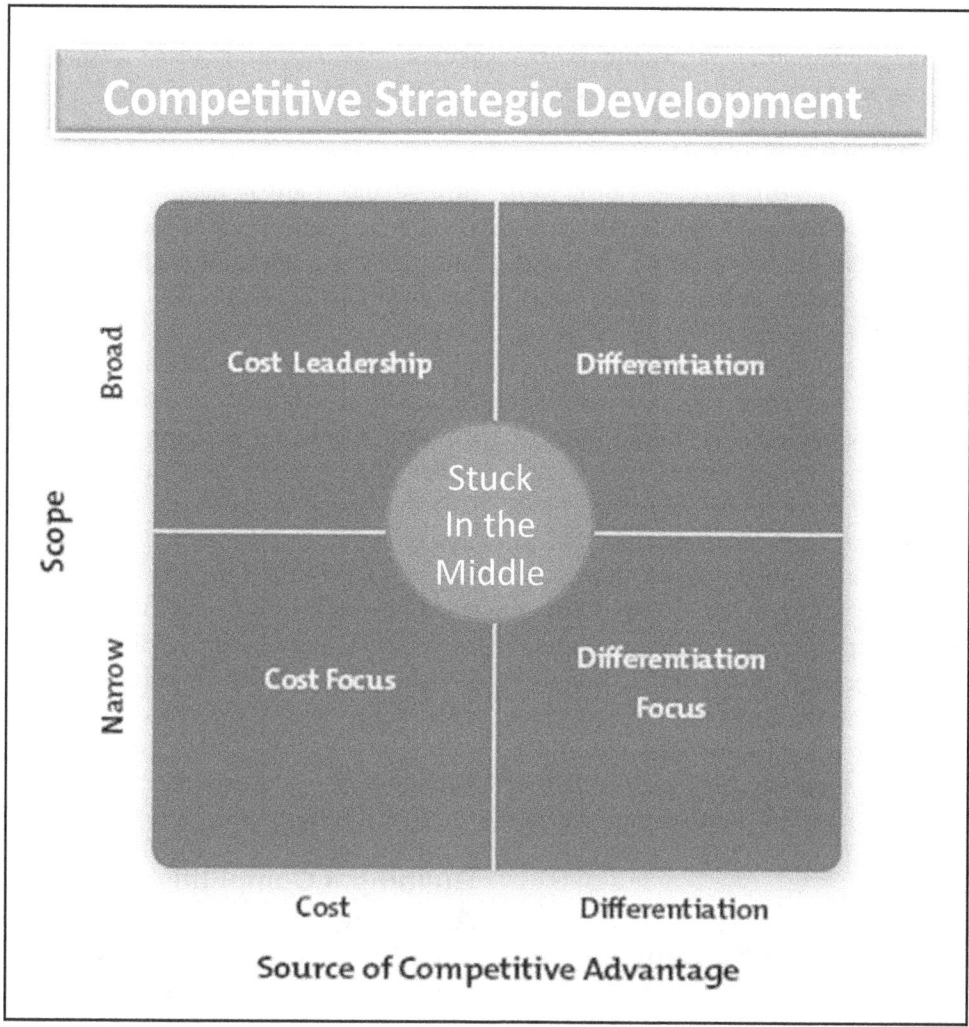

Figure 5–23. Practice resources.

Cost Leadership Strategy

To be the cost leader, there must be a great deal of managerial attention to product cost control. Providing the same quality products, services, and other supportive functions at a lower cost relative to the competitors becomes the theme running through the entire business (Porter, 1980/1998). Baldwin (2024) indicates that a low-cost strategy is centered on the capability of the company to produce and deliver a product or products of competitive quality at lower costs.

Market research suggests that generally, consumers are price sensitive, and if a product can be delivered for equal benefit for less cost than the competition,

crease the number of referral sources due to the unexpected special treatment, service, or product for their patients.

more sales will be generated. One of the advantages of low pricing is that it often leads to a more consistent or predictable demand because suppliers and/or retailers can more effectively control and forecast production, as well as predict inventory needs and shipping costs, thus stabilizing demand. Hurwich (2011) cautions that, while this strategy works in some markets, it does not make sense where demand is so high that price increases are warranted or when demand declines to the point that price discounts are needed to reduce inventories. In the hearing industry, it is obvious that Costco, Walmart, and other big-box stores are leaders in the cost leadership strategy. Depending upon the market, products offered through these outlets are usually about one-third less in cost than through a typical audiology clinic. Experience suggests that practices that attempt to be the cost leaders do not survive.

Differentiation Strategy

Likely the most important of Porter's generic strategies for a healthcare practice is differentiation of the product and/or service offerings that will be perceived as a distinctive experience, with unexpected quality and performance, and service that is truly unique from the competition, adding a special value (Traynor, 2019). In a product differentiation strategy, the practice still considers cost control, but costs are neither the focus nor the primary target. Differentiation provides insulation against the competition by generating brand loyalty to the practice or the practitioner that results in a lower sen-

sitivity to price. This is usually coupled with a lower market share as it requires a perception of exclusivity but yields higher margins with which to deal with suppliers. Thus, the patient's perception is that there is no other place to obtain the product or service with the same differentiation; thus, they are less sensitive to the overall costs of the final product.

Most product manufacturers are differentiation strategy companies. It is obvious when scrutinizing marketing materials, presentations, and journals that the major effort in the hearing industry is that of differentiation. While a differentiation strategy may be coupled with a lower market share, the requirement is a perception of exclusivity, which will generally yield higher margins. If successful, it allows charging a premium price for higher-quality products, services, and expertise.

Building a Competitive Advantage

Competitive actions taken by practice managers involve complex decisions and must include deliberation of the following:

- Overall practice resources available.
- Distinctive competencies of the practice.
- Specific capabilities of the practice with the available resources.

Practice resources include four generic areas that are fundamental to building a competitive advantage and essential to the health of any business. Without strength in these four fundamental resource areas, a practice will

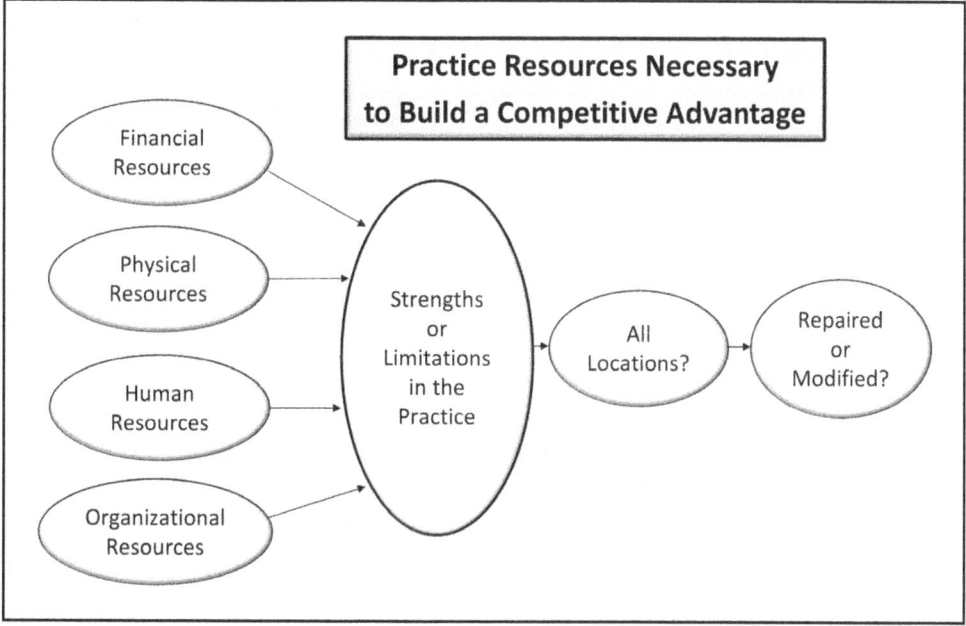

Figure 5–24. Model for competing in the hearing healthcare market.

have difficulty maintaining any type of competitive advantage, regardless of the strategic decisions offered by management (Figure 5–24).

Practice resources comprise:

■ *Financial resources*. This includes steady cash flow, a strong balance sheet, superior past performance, and the capability to inject cash when necessary to facilitate various projects, such as a campaign against the competitors.

■ *Physical resources*. This relates to the physical premises of the practice, including the atmosphere, location, parking, equipment, and other physical parameters of the practice.

■ *Human resources*. Human resources include business management capabilities of the owner and a well-trained and motivated staff with certified doctoral-level professionals

to ensure the best possible experience for patients.

■ *Organizational resources*. A practice that has been established for a long time will have a reputation or a well-known "brand" in the community. The clinic would be trusted and be known for its clinical competence, products, excellent customer service, flexibility, and other specifics of operation that make them stand out among the competitors.

Various markets and personnel can create very different competitive situations; therefore, all locations need to be evaluated for their resource capabilities. Limitations in the resource areas must be modified or corrected for a practice to be successful in building a competitive advantage.

Another area of concern involves the distinctive competencies that allow

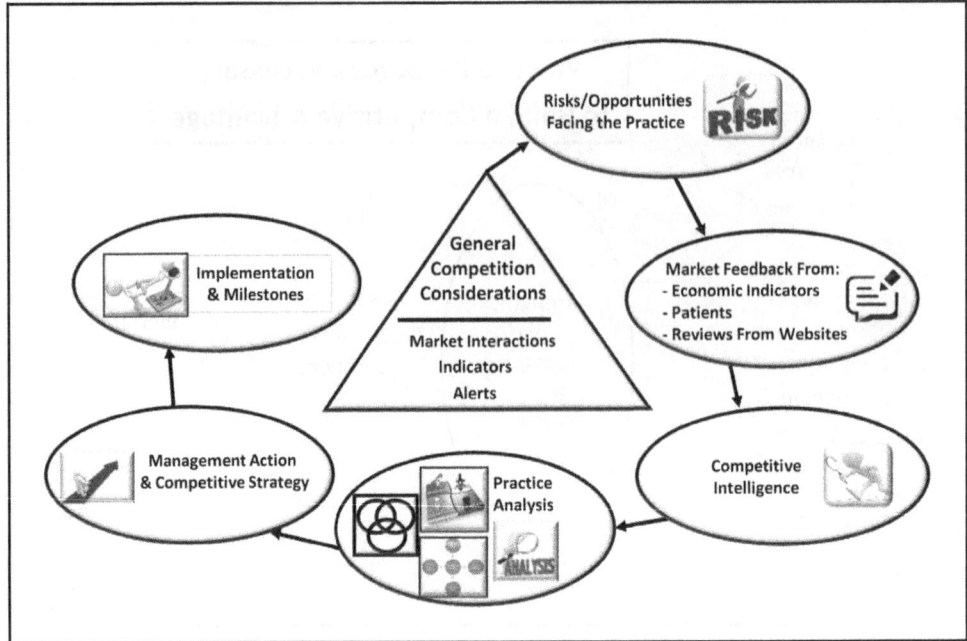

Figure 5–25. Implementation and monitoring of milestones.

the practice to consistently perform at a higher level than its competitive counterparts. These areas could include technology, marketing activities, or management capabilities.

Implementation and Milestones

Based upon all of the data, information, and general feelings for the market, the strategy is then implemented. Milestones such as the number of patients seen in the clinic, the number of products dispensed, or services conducted must be monitored to facilitate knowledge that the new strategy against the competitive forces within the market is successful. If the chosen strategy is not successful by monitoring the milestones, then either an alternative strategy is chosen, or the analysis begins all over again (Figure 5–25).

Adjustments

The process of practice analysis should be conducted about every 6 months and even sooner if the practice owner feels an analysis is necessary to be competitive within their market. Additionally, the best assessment can have flaws and require modification or minor changes. The reasons for a flawed new competitive strategy are many, considering all of the risks discussed earlier in this chapter, as any of those risks could contribute to a need to revisit the analysis. If further analysis is necessary, it is recommended that the owner follow the steps

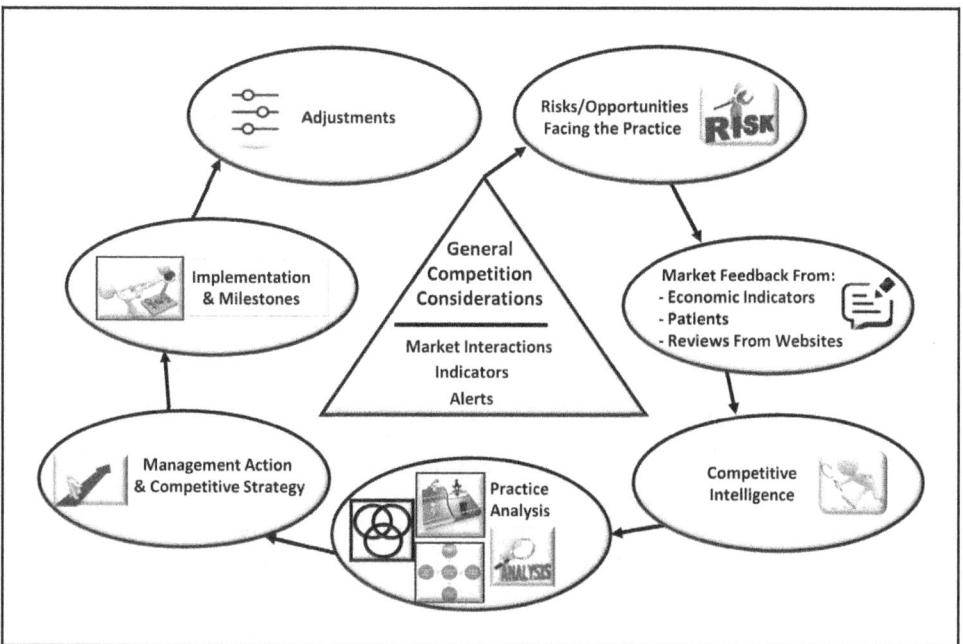

Figure 5–26. Adjustments according to milestone indications.

outlined in this chapter to determine the new competitive concerns and modify the current strategy (Figure 5–26).

strategy can be created to combat the threats to an owner's practice.

Summary

This chapter has described the components of a detailed practice analysis using a model that calls for consideration of general market thoughts, competitive risks, and obtaining competitive intelligence. The process further considers the use of the SWOT analysis, Porter's Five Forces, and three-circle analysis to review what the competitors are doing and how they have impacted the owner's practice. Once these data are known and reviewed by management, then a solid competitive

References

Baldwin, M. C. (2024). Strategy: Low cost or differentiation. *Simplified strategic planning blog*. http://www.cssp.com/strategic planning/blog/strategy-low-cost-or-dif ferentiation/

Caporuscio, J., & Lawrenz, L. (2022). Blue Monday. *South Florida Reporter*. https:// southfloridareporter.com/what-to-know -about-the-monday-blues/

Carbone, L. (2004). *Clued in: How to keep customers coming back again and again.* Pearson Education, Inc.

Carbone, L. (2016, October). *Creating an experience.* Workshop for Positioning your Practice for Success, Unitron, New Orleans, LA.

Fleisher, C., & Bensoussan, B. (2015). *Business and competitive analysis: Effective application of new and classic methods* (2nd ed.). Pearson Education.

Gilad, B. (2004). *Early warning.* American Management Association. https://en.wikipedia.org/wiki/American_Management_Association

Hurwich, M. (2011). Everyday low pricing. Strategic Pricing Management Group. http://spmgblog.blogspot.com/2011/04/every-day-low-pricing-pros-and-cons.html

Kernez, R. (2024). Competitive advantage: The key to business success. Forbes communication council. https://www.forbes.com/sites/forbescommunicationscouncil/2024/02/07/competitive-advantage-the-key-to-business-success/?sh=149d573538d2

Mind Tools. (2024). *Porters five forces: Assessing the balance of power in a business situation.* https://www.mindtools.com/pages/article/newTMC_08.htm

Morrow, L. (2024). *What's more dangerous than a dissatisfied customer? A silent one.* Market Connections. https://www.marketconnectionsinc.com/dangerous-silent-cusomer/

Porter, M. (1998). *Competitive strategy.* Free Press. (Original work published 1980)

Porter, M. (2008). *On competition.* Harvard Business Press.

Skibinsky. (2020). Medical device marketing strategies that work best. LLDGT. https://alldgt.com/medical-device-marketing/

Thornhill, M., & Martin J. (2007). *Boomer consumer.* LOINX Corporation.

Traynor, R. (2013). Chapter 1: The economic realities and competitive landscape of audiology private practice. In R. Glaser & R. Traynor (Eds.), *Strategic practice management* (2nd ed.). Plural Publishing.

Traynor, R. (2019). Chapter 3: Competition in audiology practice. In R. Glaser & R. Traynor (Eds.), *Strategic practice management* (3rd ed.). Plural Publishing.

Tyson, K. (2010). *The complete guide to competitive intelligence* (5th ed.). Leading Edge Publications.

Urbany, J., & Davis, J. (2010). Grow by focusing on what matters. In M. Carpenter (Ed.), *Strategic management collection.* Business Expert Press.

U.S. Congress. (2017). S.670—Over-the-Counter Hearing Aid Act of 2017: 115th Congress (2018), Became law October 2022. https://www.congress.gov/bill/115th-congress/senate-bill/670

Weave. (2024). The landscape of audiology continuing education. https://www.getweave.com/audiology-continuing-education/

Windmill, I., & Freeman, B. (2013). Demand for audiology services: 30-yr projections and impact on academic programs. *Journal of the American Academy of Audiology, 24*(5), 407–416.

 Human Resources in the Audiology Practice

Sarah Laughlin, MS

Introduction

The chapters within strategic practice management that discuss management of a healthcare practice and the story of human resources component within that practice have a thread that crosses several chapters in this book, especially Chapters 4, 8, 9, 12, 17, and 19. Throughout the other areas discussed within these chapters, there will be references to the roles and responsibilities of people that work within the practice. This chapter, however, not only focuses on the specifics of these roles and responsibilities but also presents the laws, regulations, and the process within the discipline of human resources that deal with the people within the practice. Few practitioners have the capacity, knowledge, and interest to be an expert in every area of running a business, and eventually, they will need to rely on others. This chapter will cover the various intersections that make up the field of human resources, which is humans acting as "resources" to affect outcomes in their business and community.

At its core, human resources is a set of staff attraction and retention activities, governmental regulations, and risk mitigation strategies that, when considered together, have the goal of producing a profit for the business and positive outcomes for patients (Figure 6–1). This chapter will discuss the many elements that owners, managers, and staff must be aware of to maximize the work experience for everyone.

Branding

The practice *brand* is a unique design, sign, symbol, words, or a combination of these that is brought together to create an image that identifies the business and, most importantly, differentiates the practice from its competitors (AMA, 2024). This is applicable not only to the patient's experience but to their employment experience as well. It also applies to the individual practitioner as a person, and as a professional. What is it that differentiates this practice from others competing for a successful position within the community? The practitioner's ability to articulate that difference will be key to success in practice and as a candidate for employment.

So, how is brand expressed in the workplace? In a word, it is "culture." The major elements of culture are symbols, language, norms, values, and artifacts (White, 2024). Culture in a practice can be expressed in many ways,

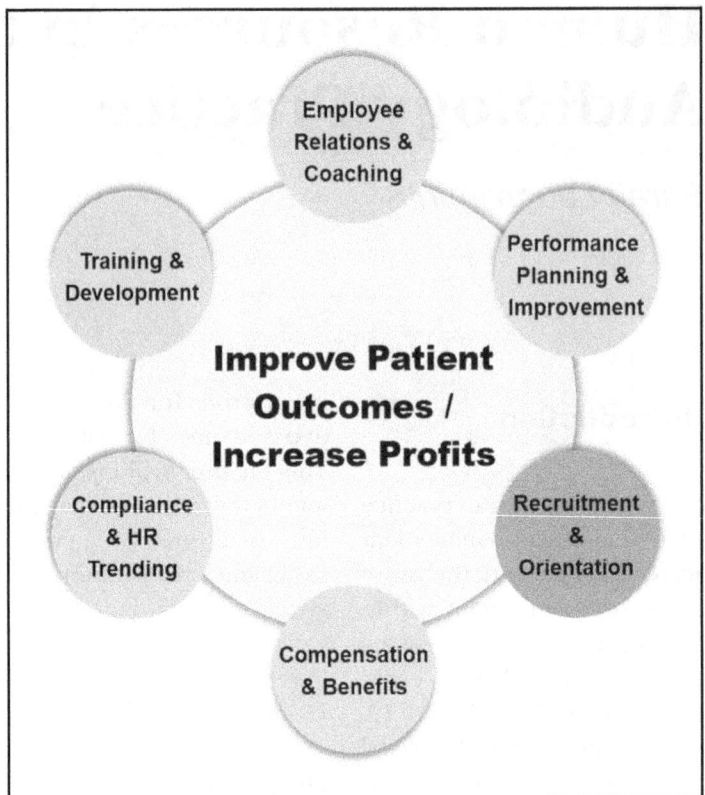

Figure 6–1. Improve patient outcomes/increase profits.

from shared history, funny anecdotes, types of patients seen, reputation in the community, to how often colleagues say "thank you" to each other. Congruence between the practice's culture and brand is fundamental to attraction and retention of the highest-level talented employees. It is the balance of what is said and what is done that cements the connection between brand and culture. If the practice presents that it is there to serve the community, but only markets to certain patients, the culture may suffer from a lack of clarity in what the practice is attempting to accomplish. If there is not alignment in language of the brand and emotion of the culture, then it will feel "off" and that will ultimately affect the success of the business negatively.

Crafting Mission, Vision, and Values

One method of crafting a shared language for the purposes of branding and then marketing the culture to prospective employees and patients is to identify the mission, vision, and values that describe the direction of the practice (Chapter 3). The process begins with articulating why the practitioner is in the business of hearing healthcare in the first place, whether as business owner or employee. The *mission* statement explains why the person is in business. The *vision* statement explains what the person hopes to accomplish. The *value* statement describes, in a few select words, how the person will achieve the practice's mission and vision. These should be short statements that people can actually remember, not aspirational paragraphs that are long and thereby long forgotten. For example, Peiper (2023) describes the Starbucks mission statement as "*To inspire and nurture the human spirit—one person, one cup and one neighborhood at a time.*" This is easy to remember, and each staff member's performance can be tied to this outcome.

The brand should permeate how a job opportunity will be marketed, from job ads to interview questions, so that prospective employees know what differentiates the practice from other employers. Terms such as diversity, inclusivity, and equity may sometimes feel like buzz words in the media, but when considered as points of building a team, they can be critical. The best teams include different viewpoints to connect with the widest array of patients.

Intrinsically, from the employee's standpoint, when looking at an employer, consider whether individual values align with the brand. Can it be determined what differentiates them from other employers? Does the practice website tell anything about working there? Similarly, as a prospective employee, has a personal brand been identified? How is this employee going to be different from others with the same credentials?

Employing a Team

Once an introspective analysis has been completed as to why the practice is in business and what differentiates it in the market, and if the revenue warrants the addition of staff, whether a front office patient care specialist or audiologist, then it is time to build a recruiting plan. The steps taken in preparing for the first or subsequent employees will include legal and cultural components in equal measure, which will span from the day the job is advertised to the day a person no longer works at the practice (Figure 6–2).

Prehire Assessment and Job Description

It can be useful to start the process of determining the scope of duties and the knowledge, skills, and abilities required by using a *Job Content Questionnaire*. This is a series of questions that consider both the qualities necessary to perform the job and the positions' stature within the hierarchy of the practice for the purposes of determining compensation. Key questions include:

- *Purpose.* Why does the job exist? How is success measured?
- *Organization of work activities.* What are the essential functions of the position and the knowledge, skills, and abilities (KSAs) required to perform those essential functions?
- *Job setting.* Where is the work performed? What are the physical requirements?
- *Level of responsibility for outcomes.* What is the reporting relationship? What is the risk if the task is not performed correctly or the end result is not achieved?

Once this information and the associated details are known, they can be

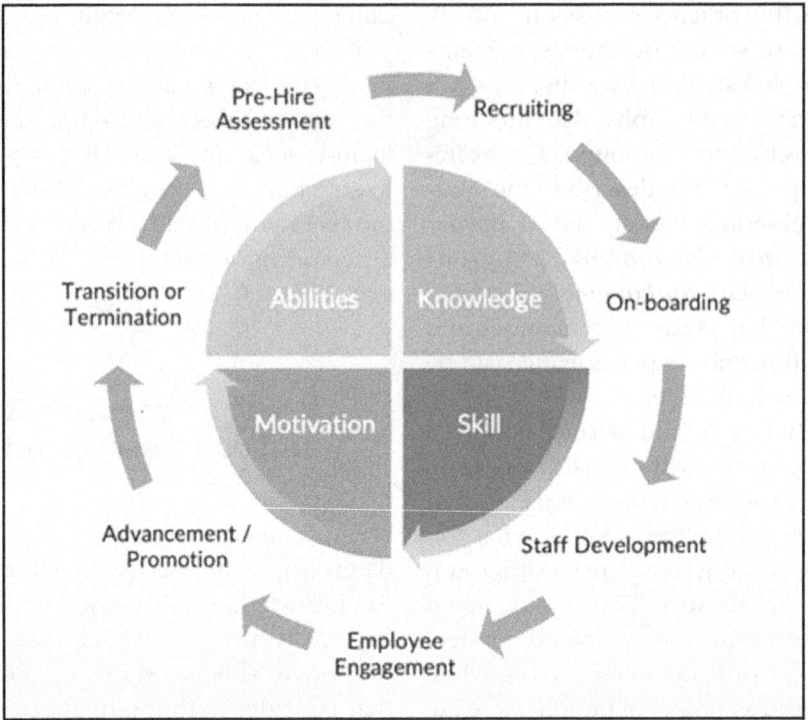

Figure 6–2. Employing a team.

combined into *a Job Description*. A job description is a format for gathering employment information. It is a tool that is helpful to have when considering performance as it gives a central point to discuss expectations for both the employer and employee. Consider it like a placemat at dinner; it is around which everything gets arranged and discussed.

Fair Labor Standards Act (FLSA)

From the information accumulated in the job description, it can be determined how this role should be categorized under the U.S. Department of Labor's Fair Labor Standards Act (FLSA) (FLSA, 2024). The FLSA is a set of laws that establish federal minimum wage,

regulation of overtime, recordkeeping for hours worked, and child labor. It is important to note that federal FLSA is the baseline for regulations. Many states have more generous labor laws, and those will supersede the federal laws and regulations. What is most beneficial to the employee will usually prevail.

The federal guidelines have established categories to determine who is exempt from both minimum wage and overtime pay and who is not. FLSA Documents (2024a) offers the following as *exempt categories*:

- *Executive*. To qualify for the *executive employee* exemption, all of the following tests must be met:
  - The employee must be compensated on a salary basis (as de-

fined in the regulations) at a rate not less than $684 per week.

- The employee's primary duty must be managing the enterprise or managing a customarily recognized department or subdivision of the enterprise.
- The employee must customarily and regularly direct the work of at least two or more other full-time employees or their equivalent.
- The employee must have the authority to hire or fire other employees, or the employee's suggestions and recommendations as to the hiring, firing, advancement, promotion, or any other change of status of other employees must be given particular weight.

- *Administrative.* To qualify for the *administrative employee* exemption, all of the following tests must be met:
  - The employee must be compensated on a salary or fee basis (as defined in the regulations) at a rate not less than $684 per week.
  - The employee's primary duty must be the performance of office or nonmanual work directly related to the management or general business operations of the employer or the employer's customers.
  - The employee's primary duty includes the exercise of discretion and independent judgment with respect to matters of significance.

- *Professional.* To qualify for the *learned professional* employee exemption, all of the following tests must be met:
  - The employee must be compensated on a salary or fee basis (as

defined in the regulations) at a rate not less than $684 per week.

- The employee's primary duty must be the performance of work requiring advanced knowledge, defined as work that is predominantly intellectual in character and includes work requiring the consistent exercise of discretion and judgment.
  - The advanced knowledge must be in a field of science or learning.
  - Advanced knowledge must be customarily acquired by a prolonged course of specialized intellectual instruction.
  - To qualify for the **creative professional** employee exemption, all of the following tests must be met:
    - The employee must be compensated on a salary or fee basis (as defined in the regulations) at a rate not less than $684 per week.
    - The employee's primary duty must be the performance of work requiring invention, imagination, originality, or talent in a recognized field of artistic or creative endeavor.

- *Outside sales.* To qualify for the *outside sales employee* exemption, all of the following tests must be met:
  - The employee's primary duty must be making sales (as defined in the FLSA), or obtaining orders or contracts for services or for the use of facilities for which a consideration will be paid by the client or customer.
  - The employee must be customarily and regularly engaged away

from the employer's place or places of business.

- *Highly Compensated Employees*
  - *Highly compensated employees* performing office or nonmanual work and paid total annual compensation of $107,432 or more (which must include at least $684 per week paid on a salary or fee basis) are exempt from the FLSA if they customarily and regularly perform at least one of the duties of an exempt executive, administrative, or professional employee identified in the standard tests for exemption.

Information about these categories and the exemptions for employees in certain computer-related categories can be found on the U.S. Department of Labor website.

US Department of Labor
Fact Sheet #17A

It is important to be aware of federal and state overtime regulations. Failure to properly categorize staff for the purposes of paying overtime, and thus either intentionally or unintentionally denying them these wages, is a violation of Wage and Hour laws and could make a practice subject to back pay, back interest, fines, and bad publicity.

Wage and Hour violations can also come from improperly designating someone doing work in the practice as an *independent contractor* when they should be categorized and paid as an employee. FLSA Documents (2024b) indicates that the Internal Revenue Service (IRS) provides guidance for those who need to review this distinction between employee and independent contractor. An assessment of the relationship will cover the following areas:

- Opportunity for profit or loss depending on managerial skill.
- Investments by the worker and the employer.
- Permanence of the work relationship.
- Nature and degree of control.
- Whether the work performed is integral to the employer's business.
- Skill and initiative.

Proper categorization of compensation for work being done is necessary to properly forecast and account for various expenses in the budget. An annual salary that is paid over the course of a year is easy to monitor in the budget as it is a consistent amount each month, but fluctuations over standard workweek hours for hourly, nonexempt, overtime eligible staff may require more thought in scheduling patients, or considerations for other office coverage, to keep expenses in check. It also impacts the employer-paid taxes that are associated with wage expenses.

Employers are responsible for various taxes to be paid on behalf of their staff. The most significant of these taxes is Taxes under the Federal Insurance Contributions Act (FICA). FICA is made up of a Social Security tax and a Medicare tax. The IRS (2024a) presents the tax rate for Social Security as 6.2% for the employer and 6.2% for the employee, or 12.4% total. The rate for Medicare is 1.45% for the employer and 1.45% for the employee, or 2.9% total. The employee's portion is deducted from their pay, and the employer remits their portion and the employee's portion to the federal government. Adjustments to wage base limits are made each year, and additional information can be found at IRS.gov.

States, cities, and other municipalities may have other employer- and employee-mandated employment taxes, most notably those for paid leaves of absence to care for oneself, sick family members, or birth and adoptions. To keep abreast of these important impacts to business expenses, most states have websites to register at to receive notices of changes to state laws and minimum wage updates.

While the FLSA only requires a minimum wage, it does not require vacation, sick leave, or holiday pay; in fact, most states do not. However, to be competitive in attracting talented staff, it is important to know what competitor businesses are offering in terms of monetary awards and benefits, what the budget allows, what the market potential is for growth, and how valuable a great culture can be for work-life balance.

Compensation Planning

Compensation for work performed will be most businesses' biggest expense. There are multiple factors that make up a compensation plan that is evaluated by both the employer and the employee in the employment relationship. *Direct pay* is the cash compensation that is seen in paychecks. *Indirect pay* is compensation that is paid by the employer on behalf of an employee for medical insurance, retirement plans, liability or malpractice insurance, licensure fees, life insurance policies, and other expenses.

There are three major categories of *direct pay*: base pay, incentive plans, and bonus plans.

Base Pay

Base pay is the salary or hourly wage that is accepted for the work that is regularly performed. Base pay is set by considering a combination of factors: knowledge, skills and abilities of the candidate, the prevailing wage in an area, what competitors are offering, and what the practice can afford. Understanding these factors will both assist the employer and employee to come to an agreement as to what the base pay will be at any point in time.

Calculating base pay is aided by salary surveys conducted by various professional organizations, such as ASHA, or AAA, but one of the best sources of wage data, and most consistently updated, is the Bureau of Labor Statistics (BLS). This source of total cash compensation is a benchmark, or a point of reference, from which employers and employees can compare where their pay falls in the market. However, it is important to remember that this is just one data point in determining compensation. Other factors within the culture of the practice will have a perceived value even if that does not translate into actual cash.

Below is an excerpt from the most recent update of Bureau of Labor Statistics data reporting national averages in the form of a *pay range*. Pay ranges are guidelines based on collected data. The *percentiles* represent where a person would typically be paid based on their knowledge, skills, and abilities at a point in time in their career (Figure 6–3). For example, a person in the 10th percentile would likely just be entering the profession of audiology. A person at the 50th percentile generally has 4 to 9 years of experience, and up from there.

The website will also show numbers by state of individuals employed in a profession, as well as pay ranges by state and locale. Keep in mind that because participation in salary surveys and the tabulation of data takes time, salary surveys are generally only updated every 2 to 3 years. In using any survey, data adjustments may need to be made due to inflation or other factors. It is best to try to get access to as many surveys as possible to look at trends to make decisions, to include looking at sample sizes to determine relevancy.

A new development in many states and cities is a requirement to post the job range when advertising for a job. This *transparency in pay* is actually helpful to those looking for a job to determine if their salary desires and those of the practice are close. It is also helping to close the wage gap that can exist between the pay of men and women doing similar jobs.

Incentive Plans

Incentive plans, sometimes called variable pay or commission plans, are those that are paid in addition to base wages and are generally tied to achievement of specific individual or team performance goals or *key performance indicators (KPIs)*. Incentive plans can be developed for any position. For example, for a billing manager, it may be paying a percentage of collections to ensure a steady cash flow, or for an audiologist, it may be based on net sales (gross sales less cost of goods, returns, etc.), to acknowledge their individual contribution above the baseline expectations (Figure 6–4). Incentive plans may be written to pay on monthly, quarterly, or annual schedules.

Percentile	10%	25%	50% (Median)	75%	90%
Hourly Wage	$ 26.97	$ 35.79	$ 42.19	$ 50.71	$ 60.00
Annual Wage (2)	$ 56,090	$ 74,440	$ 87,740	$ 105,480	$ 124,800

Figure 6–3. Percentile wage estimates for audiologists. *Source:* U.S. Bureau of Labor Statistics (2023).

Commission Plan Variables

Commission Plan Compenents		Model Variables
a)	Monthly Unit Goal	16
b)	Average Sale Price	$1,750
c)	Individual Commission	10%
d)	Est. Gross Margin %	60%

Commission Plan Examples

	Jan	Feb	Mar	Apr	May	5 Month Total	Annualized Total
Units	16	10	15	16	18	75	180
HA Sales	$28,000	$17,500	$26,250	$28,000	$31,500	$131,250	$315,000
Individual Commission Paid	$2,800	$1,750	$2,625	$2,800	$3,150	$13,125	$31,500
Total Base Salaries Paid	$7,290	$7,290	$7,290	$7,290	$7,290	$36,452	$87,485
TOTAL PROVIDER COMP	$10,090	$9,040	$9,915	$10,090	$10,440	$49,577	$118,985
Estimated Gross Margin	$16,800	$10,500	$15,750	$16,800	$18,900	$78,750	$189,000
Net Financial Gain for Practice	$6,710	$1,460	$5,835	$6,710	$8,460	$29,173	$70,015

Gross Margin/Total Comp:	1.6
Target:	1.5
+/- Target	106%

Figure 6–4. Example 1: Individual net sales incentive.

Bonus Pay

Another form of direct pay could be in the form of a *bonus*. This form of payment can be tied to the achievement of any goal, whether completing a project ahead of schedule or achieving a certain level of profit or revenue target. A common bonus that a practice might consider is called profit sharing. A profit-sharing plan is developed when a practice chooses to set aside a portion of its profits to share among the staff (Figure 6–5). This team-based bonus structure has the added benefit of allowing all staff to participate in the success of the practice, from the person who answers the phone, to the person who fits the hearing aid, to the person who puts the bill in the mail. It is a team effort.

It is important to remember that not all direct compensation has to be in the form of cash in a paycheck. It may be in the form of a fringe benefit such as a gift certificate or holiday gift. Be creative, but remember, the best incentive is one that the employee values.

When designing or giving a monetary benefit, it is important to keep in mind that according to IRS (2024c), the IRS monitors whether a gift or de minimus fringe benefit is taxable or not (irs.gov).

Indirect Pay

Indirect pay can take many forms, but the most common forms used by most businesses are health insurance, company-sponsored retirement plans also known as defined benefit and contribution plans, and paid time off (PTO). Private practices may have a limited budget, and sometimes budget limitations do not allow them to offer these plans, but they are common and often a necessity to attract the best personnel.

Health Insurance

The most common element in an *indirect pay program* is whether the employer has a *group health insurance plan* or if the employee needs to cover themselves with an *individual health*

YTD units		$ per HA	Total Team Bonus
0-250	x	$50	(250x$50) = $12,500
251-500	x	$75	(249x$75) = $18,675
501-750	x	$100	(249x$100) = $24,900
750-771	x	$125	(21x$125) = $2,625
		TOTAL =	$58,700
$58,700 / 9 audiologists = $6,522.00 each			

Figure 6–5. Example 2: Team threshold sales incentive.

insurance policy paid to an insurance provider. The benefit to a group health plan is that under Section 125 of the IRS tax code, there are tax benefits to the structure to consider (IRS, 2024d). However, for some small practices, a fully insured medical plan may be cost prohibitive. While a group policy is convenient, the lack of one should not dissuade a person from considering working for a small employer. There are several alternatives to assist employers and employees with their healthcare costs and needs.

The practice may offer the employee *a stipend*, an amount of cash to help defray the cost of their healthcare insurance premium. The federal government has developed Health Reimbursement Arrangements (HRAs) for small employers through individual marketplace plans or *Qualified Small Employer Health Reimbursement Arrangements (QSEHRAs)*. Health Care (2024) describes these plans as offering a tax benefit like those offered to IRS qualified group health plans. Other health benefits commonly considered are dental, vision, term life insurance, and accidental death and dismemberment.

Defined Benefit and Defined Contribution Programs

Once the big concern of medical insurance is covered, attention is turned to planning for retirement. There are two common forms of employer-sponsored retirement plans. *Defined benefit plans* (IRS, 2024e), such as a traditional pension plan, promise to pay a specified monthly benefit at retirement. These are less common and often found at universities or very large employers.

Defined contribution plans (IRS, 2024d), such as a 401(k) or 403(b) plan, are the most common form of employment-based retirement plans and are where the employee and/or the employer contribute to the employee's individual account under the plan. The IRS has created SIMPLE 401(k)s so that even small employers can help employees with their retirement goals and to be competitive (IRS, 2024f). An "employer match" is a common element of a Defined Contribution plan where the employer commits to contributing some amount to an employee's 401(k) retirement plan, usually a percentage of what the employee contributes. The employer match is dollar for dollar in the range of 3% to 6% of the employee's salary. It is basically money that would not be received if the employee was not participating in their own retirement planning. The employer match may be subject to "vesting," which is a time frame over which an employee must work in order to receive the employer's 401(k) match. For example, the employee would need to work 2 years in order to receive 20% of the match and additional years of employment for increases in the vesting percentage until they have reached 100% (IRS, 2024g). These are important details to look at when developing or assessing a benefit plan.

These types of qualified retirement plans are governed by ERISA (U.S. Department of Labor, 2024), the Employee Retirement Income Security Act of 1974. They require plans to provide participants with plan information, including plan features, enrollment, vesting, control of plan assets, and grievance procedures. If the practice has a plan and new employees want to start one, information about their plan should be readily available.

Paid Time Off (PTO)

As employees consider their various employment options and employers consider what they can afford to offer, *paid time off (PTO)* vacation and/or sick pay or a combination of both is usually very high on the list of considerations and should be clarified early in the employment process. It is still very common to see 3 weeks of PTO offered, or the equivalent of 2 weeks of vacation and 1 week of sick leave, but some employers will offer more or less paid time off. For some employees, it may be worth

negotiating more time off in lieu of base wage. Other benefit trends that can be very valuable include student loan payoff assistance, assistance with relocation costs, and sign-on bonuses. While the practice may offer these and more, others may not offer any of these benefits; nevertheless, it does not hurt to make the request.

Once the direct and indirect compensation and associated elements such as taxes are known, it can be useful to put it into the form of a *Total Compensation and Benefits Statement* to help visually educate current and prospective employees about the total compensation package that is often hidden from view.

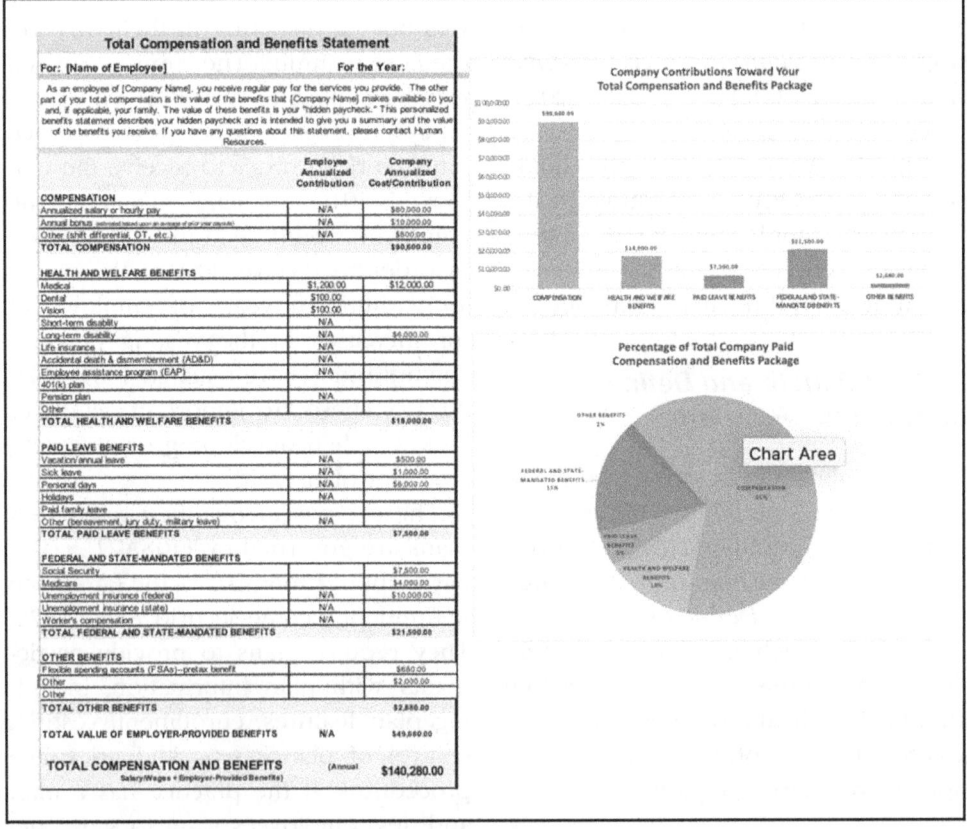

Figure 6–6. Total compensation and benefits statement.

A checklist, such as Figure 6–6, can be helpful to prospective employees comparing positions. Additionally, it can be helpful for a practice to show employees the many hidden expenses that make up the total of their compensation package for the work they perform. It is usually more than what current employees think.

Attracting Talent (Recruiting)

By preparing the foundation of identifying the brand and culture; the knowledge, skills, and abilities needed to run the practice; and the direct and indirect compensation available, the practice is ready to kick off the hunt for talent or be in position for adding a new role. See Figure 6–7 that outlines the job marketing pathways for attracting potential candidates. This is also where the marketing skills gained in other chapters become essential (Chapter 12).

From the job description, an advertisement is crafted for the job, the *job ad*. This should not be a cut and paste of the job description. As with any product ad, it should be about matching the practice culture with a candidate and be enticing enough to get someone to review it at least twice. A good recruiting ad should certainly describe what is required:

■ Minimal qualifications to do the job.
■ Describe the practice differentiation.

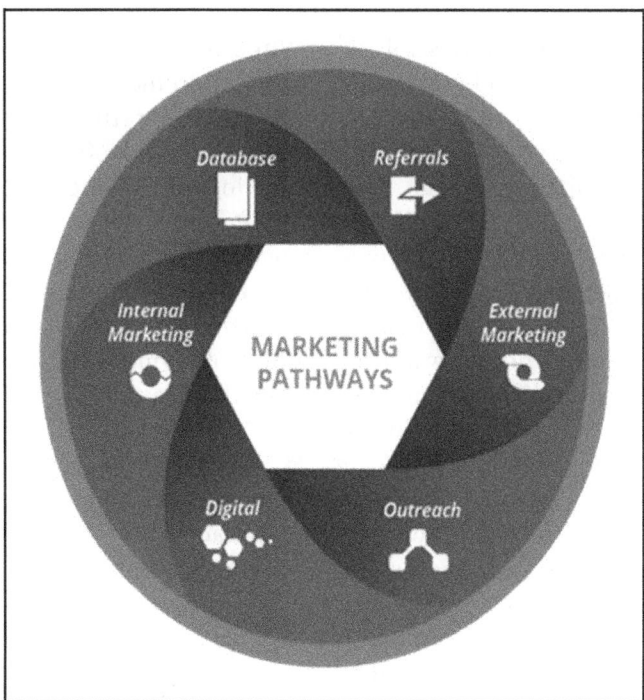

Figure 6–7. Job marketing pathways. *Source:* Fuel Medical Group.

- Unique opportunities for career growth.
- Generally, cover other factors that may come with employment such as healthcare or retirement plan.
- Items that would make this job opportunity stand out from those competing for the same pool of talent.

In addition to posting the job ad on career sites such as Audiology-on-Line or Indeed, the practice will want to prepare social media and other referral outreach plans to further spread the word about the position:

- Prospective employees and practices should have a LinkedIn profile that is frequently updated.
- Prepare an email for networking employee availability or the job opening and ask them for help in spreading the word.
- For hiring a front desk person or patient care coordinator, possibly create a printed flyer to hand out at community events.

Once the job opening(s) has been advertised and a pool of candidates has been chosen, it is time to prepare for interviews. Interview questions will fall into two categories: behavioral and technical. *Behavioral questions* are the ones that assist in understanding how a person will respond in certain circumstances or how aligned they are with the practice culture. *Technical questions* are posed to determine how well a person knows their profession. Behavioral-based interview questions are those that persuade a person to describe how they have or how they would handle a particular scenario. These types of questions often start with, "Tell me about a time when you . . ."

and then include "And describe what you learned from that experience." For example, "Tell me about a time when you had an issue with a coworker. Describe what it was and how you handled it, and what you learned from that or would do differently, if you had to go through it again." See Table 6–1 for questions to ask and not to ask during an interview.

Interview questions should be developed in advance of reaching out to any candidate. A consistent set of questions will assist in comparing candidates based on job-related factors, "apples to apples," as they say, but a set of established questions will also avoid asking random questions that could violate laws against discrimination.

How Should Job Candidates Prepare for Employment?

While the employer is preparing their job requirements and questions, it is also time for the prospective candidate to do their own research, which may include asking family and friends about their own interview experiences. This is helpful, especially when looking at a first professional position or when considering a job change. The following questions should be considered:

- What should applicants look for when considering a position within a practice?
- What are most employers looking for in a new employee?
- What was the most challenging interview question or experience?
- What is their advice about creating a resume and/or preparation for an interview?

Table 6–1. Interview Questions

Category	Objective	ASK	DON'T ASK or ANSWER
Technical	Understanding of and ability to administer diagnostic tests	What process do you find to be the most effective when administering a hearing test to children?	Do you have children of your own? (possible sex discrimination)
Behavioral	Professional development and continuing education	How do you keep yourself apprised of developments in the profession?	You got your degree a long time ago, you could be a bit rusty. (possible age discrimination)
Technical	Understanding of and ability to manage hearing rehabilitation	We serve a diverse population. Give a recent example of your experience in this area.	We have a fast-paced environment. Do you think you could keep up? (possible age discrimination)
Behavioral	Work/life balance	We have a very busy practice and are open on Saturdays. Are you available to work Saturdays?	We'd like to have someone stick with our practice. When do you plan to have children? (sex discrimination)

The Cover Letter and Resume

In the preparation of cover letter and resume, consider the purpose of each document and the reader audience. The *cover letter* is a one-page narrative that introduces the candidate's skills and, hopefully, shares something about the applicant's personality and what connects them to the position. The resume delineates experiences highlighting special expertise and how and where job-related knowledge, skills, and abilities have been obtained.

When crafting a resume from the job posting or advertisement, there are key words placed in the ad by employers regarding the job requirements. In the cover letter, a table may be created that says in one column, "this is what you're looking for" and, in the next column, "this is what I've done." It would go something like this:

- ■ *Intro:* I am applying for . . . .
- ■ *Body:* I would be a great choice for this job because . . . . Perhaps include a table as shown in Figure 6–8.
- ■ *Close:* Thank you for considering me . . . here is my contact info . . . look forward to hearing from you.
- ■ *Proofread:* Do not skip this step! Have someone else proofread these documents for spelling errors. Imagine the embarrassment when presenting a skill such as "great attention to detail" but there are

Job Ad/Description says you are looking for:	I have done that and more...
High patient volume	20 minute audiograms are no problem
Team player	Worked in small private practice where everyone had to pitch in to cover for vacations, phones, etc
Cochlear Implant interest/exposure	Worked alongside ENT Physician and Audiologist in performing 1-2 surgeries per month
Aural rehabilitation program coordination	Took classes in Speech Therapy and led 3-5 volunteers in small group sessions 2x week

Figure 6–8. Cover letter table for job resume.

misspelled word(s) in the resume or cover letter. Don't let that happen.

The resume is an opportunity to specify knowledge, skills, and abilities that create an equation of previous work and the outcomes from that work. This is where the possibility arises to separate this application from those that may have a similar educational background. Suggestions for the resume are as follows:

■ *Responsibilities* (the state of being accountable for something)
  ■ This is what has been done as part of a current position.
  ■ This is an opportunity to showcase previous successes as compared to the employer's needs for the advertised position.
■ *Accomplishments* (the successful achievement of a task)
  ■ These are examples that demonstrate success as a responsible employee.
  ■ The documentation should be concrete and include numbers, percentages, and dollar amounts.

Even if there is only babysitting experience, connection with pediatric patients can still be demonstrated. As an example of responsibility: Identified areas of interest for each individual child and organized safe and fun games that focused on each of those areas. As an example of accomplishment: Played Eye Spy game with street signs because they contain both colors and words to allow improvement of spelling skills.

The Application Process

Once the cover letter and resume have been proofread, it's time to apply for the position. Follow the application instructions in the ad and *think about the key words* that a recruiter or hiring manager may be using in social media outreach to find the appropriate candidate for the position. Also, plan on how to inform the network of friends and professional colleagues of interest in positions within the profession. Consider reaching out to any contacts that may know someone at the practice or someone who worked there in the past. Ask for a brief introductory meeting or "informational interview" to learn more about the culture, learning environment, and hiring process. This is a great way to become prepared and less nervous should there be a selection for a job interview.

Interviewing Applicants for Audiology Positions

The first phase of interviewing is generally a set of *screening questions* asked over the phone (*could also be Zoom or Teams*) in a 20- to 30-minute interview to determine if the candidate meets the basic requirements of the job, seems aligned with the culture, and meets the compensation requirements. Before investing a lot of time organizing an onsite visit, the phone screen can help both the employer and the candidate know if investing more time together is worth it.

Sample screening questions may include:

- What do you know about our practice?
- Why are you pursuing a new role right now and why are you interested in this particular role?
- What relevant education or experience do you feel will help you with the skills needed for this position?
- What other positions are you pursuing right now?
- Tell me about an interpersonal issue that you had with a coworker/team member. What was the issue and describe how you resolved it?
- Give an example of a time when you really blew it. What steps did you take to correct the mistake and what did you learn from it?
- How many patients do you typically see in a day? In a week? What is a comfortable patient load for you?
- What are your salary expectations? Have you ever worked in a variable pay environment? What was the structure?

- If you were selected for this position, when could you start? *Note: it's useful to ask this question to make sure your timeline and the other person's match.*

Follow-up or clarifying questions may be asked if either the candidate or the interviewers want more detailed information, for example, by asking, "Can you be more specific?" or "Tell me more about that."

Round Two—Formal Interviews

While the phone screening is usually conducted by one person, the next round of interviews should include two or more people to gain a more objective view. Additionally, if both interviewers agree, with justifiable reason, that the candidate should not move forward in the interview process, it is easier to defend the decision. This round of interviews should be done in person or some virtual-visual form such as on Zoom, Teams, and so on. Another option is also an in-person interview, depending on where the candidate and the practice are located.

Some practices will conduct more than one round of interviews. Candidates should always visit the practice and meet staff, including the front office and others with whom they may work. This is a helpful step to see how the prospective employee interacts with the team. If the candidate is not local, then a decision needs to be made as to who pays for the flight and hotel and for what period of time. Generally, the practice pays for the flight and hotel, or it is split between the practice and the candidate. The decision as to what costs to cover or reimburse should be communicated *upfront* so that there are no surprises by either party.

When assembling the interview team, consider their knowledge, skills, and abilities. If hiring a front office or patient care coordinator, include the hiring manager, but also consider including someone on the team that is already performing the job. It is also a good experience for them as they will be working together. Or, if adding a new role into the practice, consider asking someone outside the practice who is familiar with the position. Their technical expertise in assessing the candidate could complement the expertise of those working within the practice.

As the candidate evaluation process proceeds, it may be useful to consider *skills or personality assessments* to help further evaluate candidate qualifications. Job sourcing sites such as Indeed and other recruiting companies offer many skills and tests to prescreen candidates such as aptitude toward keyboarding, administrative tasks, and other assessments that can be purchased for implementation in the office during the on-site interview.

Personality assessments such as the Myers Briggs (MBTI, 2024), Keirsey (2024), or DISC (2024) can be useful in understanding how a person may structure their work and/or their communication preferences. A benefit of these personality profiles is that they will also generate interview questions to help probe more into how a person has or would respond to a situation. While these assessments can be used independent of whether anyone else in the practice has taken the assessment, it is useful for the purposes of understanding team dynamics if the rest of the team has completed the same assessments. Note that if a personality assessment is used, ensure that it has been validated for test-retest reliability and to avoid discriminatory biases.

Finalizing the Candidates

Once the top candidates are selected, the next step is to complete the reference checks. *References* are those individuals with whom the candidate has worked or volunteered that can discuss what it is like to work with them and where there may be opportunities for future growth and development. If possible, references should include at least one supervisor and a coworker. It is common to ask and provide three references as that helps assess trends in responses, and it is helpful when a hiring manager may only hear back from two of the three. If references are not responding, it is acceptable to ask the candidate either to call their references to encourage their participation or to ask for additional references. It is also acceptable to contact people known to the practice or the interviewers who may have knowledge of this person's work history even if they were not listed by the candidate. Keep in mind the goal is to gain more perspective on working with this person, not reconstructing their entire history.

In conjunction with the references, for some positions, it may be necessary to conduct a professional *background check*. There are several firms that for a fee will delve into criminal history, confirm credentials and licensure, and verify driving history. There are various state laws about how far back in someone's history criminal convictions may factor in the employment decision, so it is best to use a background check company familiar with the state laws. This extends to requests about criminal convictions on the practice's employment application. It is also important to understand the rules around conducting credit checks (Indeed, 2024) under the Fair Credit Reporting Act (FCRA) (FTC, 2024) and what communication plans need to be in place to use the information obtained.

The Offer

Getting ready to make the *job offer* is the exciting end to a long process. By now, the practice should be close in terms of compensation. Questions of base pay only, base pay plus incentive or other bonus structures, paid time off, health insurance needs, and an enthusiasm to work together should all have been answered by this time. Making a *verbal offer* outlining the terms of the employment arrangement is useful to surface any lingering questions or areas that may require some last-minute negotiation. Once this back and forth is concluded, the terms of the job offer should be written into an *offer letter*. So that everyone is clear as to what was agreed upon, this letter should outline:

- Position title.
- Work location.
- Date of hire.
- Pay.
- Pay periods.
- Benefits.
- Paid time off.
- Who is paying for licensure and/or conferences.
- Cell phone and/or car allowances.
- Other factors that may be pertinent to the job.

The offer letter is where it would also be noted if the role is "at will" or if it is a position with a specified contract. Muhl (2001) describes *employment at-will* as a situation where an employee without a contract usually can be fired for good cause, bad cause, or no cause at all. It is useful to note in the offer letter if the position is "at will" to clarify that there is no contractual agreement being made or considered should the employment relationship end, either by the employer or the employee. Not to be confused with an independent contractor, *an employment agreement or contract* may be required for professionals who have a critical role in the practice, such as those that see patients or oversee financial or administrative outcomes. Contracts can be negotiation tools and will cover terms such as term of employment, process for giving notice to end employment, if separation or severance pay will be offered when employment ends, and who covers tail insurance for those claims made after employment or a policy cancellation. Other concerns are those regarding competitive entities within a "noncompete" clause, confidentiality, disparagement, solicitation of patients or staff, and how disputes related to any of those elements will be resolved. Just because an employment agreement is presented *does not mean that terms cannot be negotiated.* For current and future reference for *noncompete*, an important aspect may be what constitutes the radius of identified competitors with whom they say you cannot work. If the radius appears unreasonably far, it is acceptable to call that out and negotiate something more reasonable. Or, in some states, the *"noncompete" clause* may have to be removed entirely.

Once an opening is filled, federal law requires businesses to retain hiring records for a minimum of 1 year from the date the job is closed. This includes but is not limited to all applications, resumes, reference checks, background checks, or credit checks (SHRM, 2024).

Considering the hiring process and outcomes, consider the following hiring mistakes that can cause both the candidate and the practice frustration and sometimes legal difficulties:

The Process:

- Did not review/update job descriptions and qualifications prior to launching the search.
- Set unrealistic/excessive requirements.
- Did not engage in broad enough recruitment outreach strategy or cast a wide net.
- Posted a vague/nondescriptive job advertisement.
- Did not check candidate's references.
- Did not establish a thorough training and onboarding process.

The Interview:

- Asked non-job-related questions during the interview.
- Did not craft appropriate interview questions.
- Did not review the resume/application before the interview.
- Too quick to judge/short interview based on non-job-related qualities.

The Candidate:

- Failed to confirm availability/forgot to ask about ability to work weekends or overtime.

- Overly impressed with an applicant's education.
- The individual was persistent.
- Did not take into consideration transferable skills.

The Regrets:

- Hired for image and not for experience.
- Hired individual because they are friends or have family members working for the practice.
- Hired individual because they were a great patient/customer.
- Hired an individual who was desperate for a job.
- Hired someone less qualified to save money.
- Hired someone overqualified, and now they're bored.

Retention of Talent Begins With Onboarding

The ability to retain talent starts with a solid plan for educating a person about how they can be successful in the practice. This should be thoughtfully developed before the person's first day of employment. This is generally called an *onboarding plan*, and it's more than showing a person the bathroom and taking them to lunch on their first day of employment.

On the first day of employment, there are required forms to be completed, which include:

- Form I-9 Employment Eligibility Verification (USCIS, 2024), which must be completed within 3 business days of employment.

- W-4, Employee's Withholding Certificate (IRS, 2024h), related to federal and state income tax.
- Notification to applicable state employment security departments, which assists with child support collection and unemployment-insurance fraud.
- Other forms may include direct deposit and emergency contact information as well as an acknowledgment of the practice's policies and procedures regarding anti-harassment or antidiscrimination, which may or may not be contained in an employee handbook.

See Appendix 6–A for a sample onboarding checklist plan.

At this point, it is in the interests of both the manager and the employee to quickly establish a successful working relationship. This is also the point where the manager assists the new employee in understanding the practice culture and the norms of working in the clinic that build the foundation for answering "here's how things are done here." The best way to begin that process is to commit to both a training plan for achieving the outcomes listed in the job description and a process for giving and receiving performance feedback.

Weekly meetings should be established to review key performance indicators (KPIs) and milestones for how success will be measured. These meetings do not need to be long, and they should not be missed. While everyone is busy, skipping scheduled weekly meetings is a sure way to miss an opportunity for course correction before it becomes a big problem.

The meeting can be 15 minutes and as simple as consistently asking a few key questions:

- What new things were learned this week, and how is it being applied?
- What challenges are being presented and how is that impacting performance?
- What can be done to assist in these issues for contemplating success?

While considering how to assist a person in learning to be productive in the practice, remember to use all available tools that can address various learning styles, and the best one is the cell phone that everyone has at their disposal these days.

- *Visual and auditory learners.* Use a cell phone to record training topics that can be reviewed by new employees. These do not need to be high-production videos. They are meant for reference.
- *Read/write learners.* Have a notebook ready for these employees and encourage notetaking and time to create checklists and printed job aids. Offer to review their checklists.
- *Kinesthetic learners.* As hands-on learners, allow time to watch them do the task, providing feedback along the way.

Daily, Weekly, or Monthly Meetings

Because it is important to keep everyone informed of practice goals and objectives, it is also useful to conduct daily or weekly "standup" meetings and/or monthly or quarterly all-staff meetings. If employees are in multiple locations, consider recording the meetings and sending them via email to all staff.

Vitasek (2022) offers a 1597 quote from Sir Francis Bacon, "Knowledge is Power." Giving the staff the power to connect patient experience and business goals is the best way to reinforce the mission, vision, and values of the practice.

- Inviting patients to tell their hearing healthcare journey.
- Grand rounds, including nonclinical staff.

Guidelines:

- Assignments for topics should be made consistently, so the employee knows what they are responsible for each month.
- Peer-to-peer acknowledgments (sometimes referred to as kudos): before each meeting, send a message to all staff asking for ideas; if none, insert observations of teamwork or great patient service.
- Monthly focus: Could be anything from patient greetings, to cleaning the fridge.
- Each month, ask staff what they would like to have covered.

Working Remotely

The dissemination of information with staff in various formats now allows an opportunity to view changes in the workplace that may require adaptation. Before COVID-19, there were some remote workers, but most businesses required their workers to be at the office all the time. This was the customary method of working, and managers felt that it was the best way to serve their customers. However, efforts to keep workers during the tough pandemic times caused more people to work remotely than ever before.

From a human resource perspective, it has been necessary to reconsider those positions that work very well with a remote worker and others where workers must be physically in the office. These remote positions have now become a significant component of the workforce in various businesses, offering flexibility to members of the team but conducting services that, with today's technology, do not require a physical presence within the clinic, such as billing or customer service. The positions conducted remotely will likely grow substantially in the future as AI and technology continue to make working virtually realistic and profitable for the business. Clinical positions, however, generally require a physical presence within the clinic but because of COVID-19 many now have a telehealth component (Chapter 21) that will likely grow in the future.

Therefore, some positions within the clinic may lend themselves to remote work. In larger multispecialty, multilocation practices, hospitals, and other major facilities, remote workers can do billing, customer service, and other valuable positions that do not have direct patient contact. Positions such as patient check in/out and direct clinical service provision do not lend themselves to working remotely.

Outsourcing

Practices may choose to *outsource* certain services such as external billing services or customer services to a local

SAMPLE MEETING AGENDA

■ **BUSINESS UPDATES**
  ■ Any changes that the team should be aware of?
    ▪ Provide an open opportunity to ask/encourage questions.

■ **FINANCIALS TO GOAL (KPIs)**
  ■ How is the practice measuring patient engagement?
  ■ Targets: year, quarter, or week (as appropriate)

■ **MARKETING**
  ■ What promotions are coming up?
  ■ What is being said about the practice on the Internet?
    ▪ From this, what have we learned, changed, or should we pay attention to?
  ■ What events are on the horizon?
  ■ How did the last marketing event do?
  ■ Recommendations for future events or changes to the current plan?

■ **IN THE NEWS . . .**
  ■ Interesting news events in insurance, otolaryngology, audiology, general healthcare, and so on

■ **MONTHLY FOCUS**
  ■ What is "one" thing that that should be focused on by everyone?
  ■ Next month—review practice performance and pick a new focus area.

■ **CELEBRATIONS OF SERVICE**
  ■ Customer service excellence
    ▪ New online reviews
    ▪ In-office patient successes
    ▪ Thank you from one staff person to another fellow staff member
    ▪ Community support

■ **MILESTONES**
  ■ Anniversaries of employment
  ■ Birthdays

■ **OTHER**
  ■ Guest speakers

company rather than provide those services internally. Webb (2017) suggests that *offshoring*, outside the United States (Philippines, India, or others), is another method for operations to obtain some of these nonpatient care services at reasonable costs.

Job Sharing

In this new workforce, work/life balance is extremely important. An option might be to take one job and split the hours or days to create a *job-sharing* arrangement with two people who want to work only part-time. In the new working world, the practice could consider a workweek of four 10-hour days or other *flexible work hours arrangement* that allows a productive employee to attend after-school events and other activities. Any of these trends in the workforce will require adjustments in culture, techniques in monitoring performance, and, significantly, changes in work expectations of each other. The challenge for everyone is to be and stay open to these new ideas and evaluate them as dispassionately as possible to determine what is in the best interest of the patient and the practice.

Performance Goals in the Workplace

Determining when objectives are on track or if course corrections need to be made is aided by developing goals that can be measured and tracked. Some commonly used formats for developing, identifying, and communicating objectives that are worth delving into more include:

- *SOAR* for strategic planning based on what you already do best: Strengths, Opportunities, Aspirations, and Results (Zaluski, 2023).
- *SMART* for being specific with goals: Specific, Measurable, Attainable, Realistic, and Timely (SMART, 2014).
- *RASCI* for identifying roles and responsibilities on goals and projects by identifying who is: Responsible, Accountable, Supportive, Consulted, and Informed (RACI, 2024).

If it is possible to be specifically and deliberately ahead of goals, Capelli and Tavis (2016) indicate that businesses may be able to eliminate the *annual review*. Instead of the annual review, businesses could consider opting for more frequent and less formal feedback opportunities, whether peer to peer, manager to employee, or employee to manager. Creating and engaging in this more open way of sharing expectations is helpful to both the top performer and the individual who may be struggling in their job.

Coaching, Counseling, and Mentoring

As employees learn new skills or adjust to new performance measures, they benefit from being supported through *coaching* (O'Connell, 2020). This is different from performing the actual training itself or managing the end results. Coaching is identifying and engaging together in the processes that work best for the person to achieve a goal or increase performance. Unfortunately, there are times when a coaching approach stops working and it is necessary to begin *counseling* the employee

(Mitchell, 2016). This is a more short-term strategy directed at improving performance and outlining what could happen if changes in performance do not occur. When someone says that they were "written up" in business, this is the process of documenting that counseling has occurred. This is documentation in the worker's record that expectations are not being met and that the consequences of failure have been discussed, such as termination of employment. It is important to remember that not every job is for every person, so the counseling steps are tracked and documented. The situation might be signaling that it is time for this employment relationship to end. While that may mean moving a person into another better-suited role, it could also mean that they leave the practice.

As coaching or counseling may be taking place, it is also useful to pursue a *mentoring* relationship with someone more experienced in a desired area of growth. D'Angelo (2023) presents that a mentor can be in the workplace, but often it is one or more people outside of the practice. Mentors are people who give advice and guidance based on their practical knowledge throughout life. They are extremely valuable to professional development. There are mentors available around the profession, such as the ADA Mentor program, pairing seasoned audiology professionals with new clinicians and directing them to a successful future.

The Employee Handbook

Another essential tool to assist both clerical and professional staff understand expectations is an *Employee Handbook* (Chapter 9), although there is no legal requirement to have a "handbook." It is a useful mechanism, however, for grouping together in one place the policies and procedures that govern the cultural, practical, and legal aspects of employment within the practice that all staff can easily access. Written policies provide consistency and ease for managers and staff when the inevitable questions come up such as, "What holidays do we have off?" Some of the important legal requirements that should be contained in an employee handbook and communicated to staff include:

- Non-Discrimination Practices under Title VII (EEOC, 2024)
  - Applies to businesses with 15 or more employees
  - It is illegal to discriminate in employment practices based on the basis of race, color, sexual orientation, gender/pregnancy, religion, national origin, disability, or genetic information. (States and local jurisdictions may include other criteria.)
  - Governed by the Equal Employment Opportunity Commission (EEOC)
- Age Discrimination in Employment Act (ADEA) (ADEA, 2024)
  - Applies to businesses with 20 or more employees
  - May not discriminate based on age. At the federal level, that is 40 years or older and is lower in some states, such as Oregon.
  - Consider following the "Platinum Rule" to treat others as they would like to be treated, which is

not the same as your opinion on the subject.

■ Americans With Disabilities Act (ADA) (ADA, 2024)
  ■ Applies to businesses with 15 or more employees
  ■ Many people can perform jobs with a little help. To ensure candidates can do the job you've specified, hiring managers can ask, "Would you be able to perform the essential functions of this job with or without accommodation?" This may mean a larger monitor for someone that needs larger font to see or close-captioned phones for someone at the front desk with hearing loss.

■ Antiharassment
  ■ Takes a stand that harassing and bullying behavior, to include sexual harassment, is counterproductive to a good culture and working environment.
  ■ Spells out the consequences of noncompliance.

■ Leaves of Absence
  ■ Federal Family Medical Leave Act (FMLA) (FMLA, 2024)
    ▪ Governed by the Department of Labor.
    ▪ Provides 12 weeks of unpaid job-protected time off.
    ▪ Applies to businesses with 50 or more employees in a 75-mile radius.
    ▪ Many states have similar or more generous laws that must be followed and run concurrently with the federal leave of absence law.
  ■ Many states now have paid leave of absence programs that may run concurrently with the federal and state unpaid job-protected laws.
  ■ Medical Leave of Absence: While small practices may not be required to offer the same job-protected leaves of absence as federal or state laws, it is useful to have a consistent policy if some unpaid time off can be provided, even if it is not the full 12 weeks of FMLA.
  ■ Pregnancy Disability Leave: Many states have laws that distinguish time off to recover from pregnancy separately from the bonding leave under the federal Family Medical Leave Act (FMLA).

■ PUMP Act: Returning to Work & Lactation Accommodations (CAA, 2022)
  ■ Under the FLSA, nursing mothers are entitled to reasonable breaks and private space to pump at work for up to 1 year after their child's birth.

■ Uniformed Services Employment and Reemployment Rights Act (USERRA) (CREW Act, 2022)
  ■ Protects civilian job rights and benefits for those serving in uniformed service.

■ Breaks for rest and meals
  ■ State and federal laws govern and specify periods of paid and unpaid time off that must be provided to staff working in the practice.

■ Consolidated Omnibus Budget Reconciliation Act (COBRA) (COBRA, 2024)
  ■ Applies to businesses with 20 or more employees who offer group health insurance policies.
  ■ Allows terminating employees to extend their healthcare through the group policy for 18 months

and, in certain circumstances, longer.

- Employees pay the full cost of the insurance, in addition to a 2% administration fee.
- Health Insurance Portability and Accountability Act (HIPAA) (HIPPA, 2017)
  - Addresses national standards for the protection of individually identifiable health information by three types of covered entities: health plans, healthcare clearinghouses, and healthcare providers who conduct the standard healthcare transactions electronically.
- Health Information for Economic and Clinical Health (HITECH) Act (HITECH, 2009)
  - Addresses the privacy and security concerns associated with the electronic transmission of health information.
- Occupational Safety and Health Administration (OSHA) (OSHA, 2024)
  - Ensures a safe and healthy work environment for staff.
  - Covers posting notices, holding safety meetings, and logging incidents.
- Use of company property, electronic communication, ChatGPT, et al.
  - While for the most part, any electronic communication generated on company equipment, such as email, is owned by the practice, it is important to be aware that various laws and regulations govern surveillance cameras, recording conversations, and social media posts outside of work.

Federal and state laws require posting in common areas of the practice, such as a break room, notices about topics such as employment laws, minimum wage, and employee rights to various paid and unpaid leaves of absence. Required postings can be found at the federal and state department of labor sites, or combined posters can be purchased annually from various sources who compile this information. Organizations such as the Society for Human Resources Management can also be helpful resources to keep on top of changes in employment law.

Employee Resignation or Termination

As employees learn new skills and develop new knowledge, it may be time to move into a new role (Chapter 7) or to voluntarily leave the organization to further professional goals. In some cases where counseling to improve performance is not working, it may be time to involuntarily terminate the employment relationship. If there is a contract, then the terms of a "just cause" separation will be spelled out in the documentation. If the employment relationship is "at will," then the parameters of termination are more flexible.

Voluntary Resignation

In terms of *voluntary termination or a resignation*, the usual minimum notice period is *2 weeks before the last date of employment*. This time period tries to allow for the time it takes to recruit and train a new person in that employee's duties. Since this often takes longer than 2 weeks to obtain new people in an office or professional setting, more notice is appreciated by most employers. The requested terms of notice will usually be spelled out in the employee handbook.

As valuable as the interview process is when someone comes into the organization, it is also useful to conduct *exit interviews* when someone voluntarily leaves the organization so that management can better understand if there are changes or improvements that can be made to the employment experience for those working in the practice. The owner-manager should be looking for themes and analyzing why turnover in staff is occurring. Not all turnover is bad; sometimes it is the right thing. Questions may include:

■ What is the main reason for leaving?
■ Is compensation or benefits not on par with competitors?
■ What did you like about working here?
■ What did you like least about working here?
■ Would you recommend the practice to a friend or relative as a place to work or as a patient?
■ What areas could your manager do a better job?

As a manager, you may be evaluated by these same types of questions, so again, it's useful to consider how culture plays into the employment experience.

Involuntary Employment Termination

When a person is involuntarily terminated from their job, either from being fired or position elimination, they may be eligible for *unemployment insur-ance* payments while they look for other suitable work. This is another tax paid by employers to help employees who lose their jobs. The decision to grant unemployment insurance is made by the applicable state jurisdiction.

In addition to unemployment insurance, some employees, whether by contract or through an arrangement with the employer, may be offered a *separation or severance agreement*. This is a legally binding document that offers an additional amount of money to the departing person, worth between 2 weeks or multiple months of base pay and/or insurance payments to cover COBRA costs. In return for these monetary benefits, the employee agrees to certain terms, including that they will not sue the practice for various perceived discriminatory practices or not be employed by a competitor, similar terms to those outlined in an employment agreement.

Keep in mind that there are many jobs in the world and each workplace has its own culture, meaning that not every job is right for every person. However, if leaving a professional position, be respectful of the patients and coworkers by giving plenty of advance notice.

Communication of Changes in Employment, Benefits, etc.

While a practice may have the best branding, culture, employment practices, and adherence to the law, changes can happen in employees' lives, the marketplace, or the legal landscape. To that end, it is best to be prepared with a communication plan that can be dusted off when required, whether for a small change in benefits or to a major business crisis. Remember that "Knowledge is Power" and people perform best when they feel included in what is happening. Below are general considerations for a good communication plan:

- Be clear and honest.
  - Explain "*WHY*" the practice is conducting this change or activity.
- Consider the emotional impact: Knowing that people will react emotionally first—think fight or flight—people will ask themselves:
  - Will this change be relatively hard or easy?
  - Will I keep my job?
  - What will I tell my family, friends, patients?
- Tell people what is in this change for them.
  - Is there anything positive in the process?
- Explain the process.
  - Think of detailed steps that will allow the message to be easily shared with people who are not in the meeting, such as those on vacation on that day.
  - Remind the meeting attendees to be open to questions because it improves the process. It also lets people vent and get the negative emotions out.
- Tell people what they need to do next.
  - What is the action?
  - Will calls be answered differently?
  - What is the new process?
- Consider who will be delivering the message and how.

- Would the practice owner or the employee's manager be a better spokesperson for the change?
- Does the message need to be tailored to different audiences?
  - Marketing activity means different things to different staff members.
  - Process change may be better accepted if it comes from someone high up in management.
- Create two-way communication channels.
  - Questions, questions, questions . . .
  - Who is the go-to practice leader for questions regarding the change?
  - Is there an open door to a practice leader, or is there a chain of management that should be followed?

Summary

Regardless of personal work experience, there is an opportunity to model the desired practice culture. As a clerical or professional employee, there are many opportunities to shape the work experience, such as:

- Becoming a mentor and a coach assisting the development of coworkers.
- Asking questions that clarify situations and add new professional experiences to the resume.
- Becoming involved in the practice of marketing to gain a deeper understanding of the business.
- Learning employment laws and keeping abreast of changes in fed-

eral and state regulations to help manage risks in the practice.

- Choosing to communicate the expectations for compensation and recognition in a way that demonstrates an understanding of the KPIs, the revenue, and expenses that flow through the practice.

In short, audiologists can actively engage in a professional career that will ultimately offer substantial financial and personal satisfaction.

References

ADA. (2024). The Americans With Disabilities Act (ADA) protects people with disabilities from discrimination. ADA.gov. https://www.eeoc.gov/prohibited-employment-policiespractices#:~:text=Under%20the%20laws%20enforced%20by,)%2C%20disability%20or%20genetic%20information

ADEA. (2024). The Age Discrimination in Employment Act of 1967. U.S. Equal Opportunity Commission. https://www.eeoc.gov/prohibited-employment-policiespractices#:~:text=Under%20the%20laws%20enforced%20by,)%2C%20disability%20or%20genetic%20information

AMA. (2024). Branding. American Marketing Association. https://ama.org/topics/branding

CAA. (2022). FLSA protections to pump at work. U.S. Department of Labor, Wage and Hour Division. https://www.dol.gov/agencies/whd/pump-at-work#:~:text=Employees%20are%20entitled%20to%20a,Appropriations%20Act%2C%202023%20into%20law

Capelli, P., & Tavis, A. (2016). The performance management revolution. *Harvard Business Review.* https://hbr.org/2016/10/the-performance-management-revolution

COBRA. (2024). Continuation of health coverage (COBRA). U.S. Department of Labor. https://www.dol.gov/general/topic/health-plans/cobra

CREW Act. (2022). USERRA—Uniformed Services Employment and Reemployment Rights Act. U.S. Department of Labor, Veterans' Employment and Training Service. https://www.dol.gov/agencies/vets/programs/userra

D'Angelo, M. (2023). How to find a mentor. *Business News Daily.* https://www.businessnewsdaily.com/6248-how-to-find-mentor.html

DISC. (2024). DISC profile. Personality Profile Solutions, LLC. https://www.discprofile.com/

EEOC. (2024). Prohibited employment policies/practices. U.S. Equal Opportunity Commission. https://www.eeoc.gov/prohibited-employment-policiespractices#:~:text=Under%20the%20laws%20enforced%20by,)%2C%20disability%20or%20genetic%20information

FLSA. (2024). Digital reference guide to the fair labor standards act. https://www.dol.gov/sites/dolgov/files/WHD/legacy/files/Digital_Reference_Guide_FLSA.pdf

FLSA Documents. (2024a). Fact Sheet 13: Employee or independent contractor classification Under the Fair Labor Standards Act (FLSA). https://www.dol.gov/agencies/whd/fact-sheets/13-flsa-employment-relationship

FLSA Documents. (2024b). De minimis fringe benefits. https://www.irs.gov/government-entities/federal-state-local-governments/de-minimis-fringe-benefits

FMLA. (2024). Family and Medical Leave Act. U.S. Department of Labor, Wage and Hour Division. https://www.dol.gov/agencies/whd/fmla

FTC. (2024). Fair Credit Reporting Act. Federal Trade Commission. https://www.ftc.gov/legal-library/browse/statutes/fair-credit-reporting-act

Health Care. (2024). Exploring coverage options for small businesses: Health Reimbursement Arrangements (HRAs) for small employers. https://www.healthcare.gov/small-businesses/learn-more/qsehra/

HIPPA. (2017). HIPAA for Individuals. U.S. Department of Health and Human Services. https://www.hhs.gov/hipaa/for-individuals/index.html

HITECH. (2009). HITECH Act Enforcement Interim Final Rule. U.S. Department of Health and Human Services. https://www.hhs.gov/hipaa/for-professionals/special-topics/hitech-act-enforcement-interim-final-rule/index.html

Indeed. (2024). FAQ: What is a credit check on an employee? Indeed.com. https://www.indeed.com/career-advice/career-development/credit-check-on-employee

IRS. (2024a). Topic no. 751, Social Security and Medicare withholding rates. U.S. Internal Revenue Service. https://www.irs.gov/taxtopics/tc751

IRS. (2024b). Sections 125 and 223—Cafeteria plans, flexible spending arrangements, and health savings accounts—elections and reimbursements for same-sex spouses following the Windsor Supreme Court decision. U.S. Internal Revenue Service. https://www.irs.gov/pub/irs-drop/n-14-01.pdf

IRS. (2024c). Defined benefit plan. U.S. Internal Revenue Service. https://www.irs.gov/retirement-plans/defined-benefit-plan

IRS. (2024d). Definitions. U.S. Internal Revenue Service. https://www.irs.gov/retirement-plans/plan-participant-employee/definitions#:~:text=Defined%20Contribution%20Plan%20is%20a,any%20investmen%20and%20administrative%20fees

IRS. (2024e). Defined benefit plan. U.S. Internal Revenue Service. https://www.irs.gov/retirement-plans/defined-benefit-plan

IRS. (2024f). Choosing a retirement plan: SIMPLE 401(k) plan. U.S. Internal Revenue Service. https://www.irs.gov/retirement-plans/choosing-a-retirement-plan-simple-401k-plan

IRS. (2024g). 401(k) plan overview. https://www.irs.gov/retirement-plans/plan-sponsor/401k-plan-overview

IRS. (2024h). W-4: Employee's withholding certificate. U.S. Internal Revenue Service. https://www.irs.gov/pub/irs-pdf/fw4.pdf

Keirsey. (2024). Keirsey Temperament Sorter. https://keirsey.com/

MBTI. (2024). Myers-Briggs Personality Test. Consulting Psychologists, Inc. https://www.mbtionline.com/?gclid=Cj0KCQjwqdqvBhCPARIsANrmZhPLzXe2dwYYRqqRhN2DqQuRh4WJ2-lqK6IDTtNzbG3Rq_bB_YwmGhMaAktEEALw_wcB

Mitchell, B. (2016). Ask the Expert Career Blog. ASAE. https://www.asaecenter.org/association-careerhq/career/articles/talent-management/coaching-vs-counseling-whats-the-difference

Muhl, C. (2001). The employment-at-will doctrine: three major exceptions. *Monthly Labor Review*. https://www.bls.gov/opub/mlr/2001/01/art1full.pdf

O'Connell, B. (2020). Coaching in the workplace: It's different from traditional managing. Society of Human Resource Management. https://www.shrm.org/topics-tools/news/managing-smart/coaching-workplace-different-traditional-managing

OSHA. (2024). Job safety and health: It's the law workplace poster. Department of Labor, Occupational Safety and Health Administration. https://www.osha.gov/publications/poster

Peiper, H. (2023). A new mission for Starbucks. https://stories.starbucks.com/stories/2023/a-new-mission-for-starbucks/

RACI. (2024). What is RACI? An introduction. RACI Solutions. https://www.racisolutions.com/blog/what-is-raci-an-introduction

SMART. (2014). SMART goals. https://www.projectsmart.co.uk/smart-goals/brief-history-of-smart-goals.php

SHRM. (2024). What are the federal retention guidelines for applications and resumes that we do not select? Society for Human Resource Management. https://www.shrm.org/topics-tools/tools/hr-answers/federal-record-retention-guidelines-applications-resumes-candidates-not-select

U.S. Bureau of Labor Statistics. (2024). Occupational employment and wages, May 2022 29-1181 Audiologists. https://www.bls.gov/oes/current/oes291181.htm

U.S. Department of Labor. (2024). ERISA. U.S. Department of Labor. https://www.dol.gov/general/topic/health-plans/erisa#:~:text=The%20Employee%20Retirement%20Income%20Security,for%20individuals%20in%20these%20plans

USCIS. (2024). I-9, employment eligibility verification. U.S. Citizenship and Immigration Service. https://www.uscis.gov/i-9

Vitasek, K. (2022). Knowledge is power—and why you should share it? *Forbes.* https://www.forbes.com/sites/katevitasek/2022/05/17/knowledge-is-powerand-why-you-should-share-it/?sh=7cfe74fb5c7c

Webb, J. (2017). What is offshoring? What is outsourcing? Are they different? *Forbes.* https://www.forbes.com/sites/jwebb/2017/07/28/what-is-offshoring-what-is-outsourcing-are-they-different/?sh=1f267ac12a2e

White, L. (2024). Culture. Encyclopædia Britannica, Inc. https://www.britanica.com/topics/culture

Zaluski, A. (2023). Using a SOAR analysis to enhance your strategic planning. Notion. https://www.notion.so/blog/soar-analysis

Appendix 6–A
Sample Onboarding Plan

Office Onboarding Checklist			
Office Onboarding Checklist	Party responsible	Date completed	Notes/comments
PRE HIRE			
Return offer letter or employment agreement and set up new employee file			
Send welcome letter to employee explaining parking, start time, what to wear on first day, etc.			
Initiate internal announcement about new staff so colleagues are prepared			
Prepare press announcement for external/internal purpose			
Notify credentialing coordinator (hospital)			
Post website page announcement/welcome			
Make photo arrangements if needed to update website			
Develop new employee's profile for web			
Assign training partner			
Schedule orientation time and develop and distribute orientation schedule			
Provide copy of first and second week schedule			

continues

Host welcome reception or lunch for new employee (provide cake or other refreshments)			
ORIENTATION			
Give tour and introduce to all colleagues, show location of bathroom, lunch, etc.			
COMPLETE I-9, W-4, benefit enrollment forms, security			
Salary/payroll—set up in payroll system			
Complete benefits review			
Do confidentiality agreement			
Assign name/security badge (if required)			
Give copy of handbook and review key policies			
Give copy and review job description			
Document performance expectations and timeline for job proficiency			
Review roles for other positions in office and how this position interacts with them			
LICENSURE/CREDENTIALING			
Initiate licensure and create process for performance feedback			
Meet with and/or coordinate completion of third-party payer applications			
Notify malpractice			
Process third-party payer applications			

Set up accounts for billing			
Notify electronic billing vendor			
Follow up on all hospital and third-party payer applications			
CLINIC			
Assign rooms			
Assign workstation			
Determine office hours/on call schedule if applicable			
Review break and lunch schedules			
Order scrubs or lab coats, if applicable			
Order business cards			
Revise letterhead			
Orient to HIPAA protocols in office			
SYSTEMS			
Set up passwords			
Install and set up computer access			
Assign phone number			
Assign email name			
Develop schedule template (include staffing needs, scheduling preferences, reviewed with provider)			
Enter master schedule in PM system or appropriate system			
Assign provider schedule			
Notify answering service			
Install/change signage (lobby, rooms, wall, etc.)			

Assign email name			
Install computer			
TRAINING TOPICS			
Overview of various internal roles—who to go to for what and what you are expected to handle on your own			
Procedures for walk-ins			
Infection control			
KPIs (key performance indicators) for audiologist: % returns, average selling price, binaural rate, conversion rate, units sold per month			
ALDs—what's offered, what does the audiologist recommend to be added			
Computer software: how to make appts, receive payments, check in and check out			
Expectations for effectively collecting patient history and charting			
Emergency plans—patients, staff, building, etc.			
Opening the practice: how to turn things on, ensure ready for the day			

7 Essential Business Principles for Audiologists as Clinical Managers

Brian Taylor, AuD

Introduction

To be business oriented when seeing a full caseload of patients requires certain skills that may not be immediately evident. Therefore, whether assuming the title of clinical manager or director, or a recent graduate aspiring to hold one of these titles, this chapter may become a trusted companion. Its content represents 30-plus years of practical experience balancing the roles of clinical audiologist and business manager. By bringing the skills outlined here to life in a clinic, the manager and their team can be more productive, and life will be less stressful by successfully juggling the dual responsibilities. Although these principles do not guarantee success in this dual role, it is hoped they offer the capability for more effectiveness as they are applied to daily work procedure.

Audiologists have a greater than 50/50 chance of practicing with at least one other audiologist under the same roof. For example, one of the most common employers of audiologists is otolaryngology practices. There are more than 10,000 otolaryngologists in clinical practice, and

survey data, collected in 2014 by the American Academy of Otolaryngology, indicate the typical ENT medical practice employs four full-time audiologists. Additionally, it is common for other clinical entities, such as Veterans Administration (VA) hospitals, private practices, and even a growing number of retail chains to employ more than one audiologist or other credentialed hearing care professional in their business. In fact, it is the exception, rather than the rule, that a sole audiologist would be working alone, completely independent, in any type of business or clinical setting. Even if they do not work under the same roof, a growing number of audiologists comprise virtual teams, scattered around a large geographic area and interacting on the Internet and Zoom or Skype. Why does this matter? Because when people work in groups, there tends to be a natural hierarchy or pecking order. For individuals under the age of, say, 40, the notion of hierarchy might seem outdated. After all, society is much less hierarchical today than it was in the 1980s, and that is surely a positive development. However, for more than a hundred years, American businesses have relied on hierarchy to get things done. Today, organizations have much flatter organizational structures, but some degree of hierarchy in business is needed to avoid chaos. Sometimes these hierarchies are formal, others flatter or more informal, but as the esteemed business management expert Peter Drucker once said, "If two or more people are working together in an organization there will be conflict."

Relying on hierarchy and an organizational chart is used to minimize conflict and chaos. As a clinician aspiring to work as a manager, it is critical to accept the reality of working in an organization that has some amount of hierarchy. Once this reality is accepted, working within the organizational structure to accomplish things benefits both the business and patients seeking assistance and guidance. Of course, there are perks associated with being near the top of a business's organizational chart. The title, usually manager or director, is loftier and, of course, the pay is usually better. Higher pay and a status title, however, come with greater responsibility.

This chapter will provide guidance on how to juggle the everyday responsibilities of clinical practice with the strategic work of being an effective manager or director. Further, there is evidence to suggest a growing number of audiologists, especially those under the age of 40, will assume, just a few short years after graduation, a managerial role within a clinic or business. This is driven largely by an impending shortage of audiologists (Windmill & Freeman, 2013). Many of these audiologists will be expected to fill a dual role in which they manage a team of others while continuing to see patients at least a day per week.

Amlani (2018) indicates a mounting student loan debt for recent AuD graduates will create a greater incentive to accept a higher-paying role with managerial responsibilities. Together, these factors indicate a need for audiologists to become better versed at basic management principles and skills.

You Have Been Promoted, Now What?

Samantha graduated with a doctorate in audiology in 2020, with more than $100,000 in student loan debt. She has been employed at a reputable, rapidly growing, corporate-owned medical practice since graduation 5 or so years ago with an annual salary just under $85,000. The clinic manager, an audiologist with more than 20 years of clinical experience, recently left the practice to accept a more lucrative role as training manager for a hearing aid manufacturer. Samantha, given her experience and performance in the clinic, is a prime candidate to step into her former boss's managerial role. Sam is eager for promotion and to assume the role that bears the title, clinical director. The promotion provides a sizable bump in annual salary to over $95,000 and allows the capability to continue to see patients, something that Samantha loves.

The catch, there is always a catch, is that Samantha now has some added responsibilities: The other three audiologists will report directly to the clinical director on the organizational chart, so there will be the responsibility to conduct annual performance reviews and monitor their productivity. Since the clinic is growing, another audiologist or perhaps an audiology assistant might be hired, something Samantha needs to anticipate and plan. Additionally, Samantha will be the person who meets with the clinic CFO each month to review the financial performance of the audiology department. Part of that conversation, at some point soon, is likely to be how the audiology department plans to adopt several new clinic initiatives that are concerns of the board of directors, including over-the-counter hearing aid sales, and the acceptance of more managed care third-party contracts with a hearing aid benefit. Unlike clinical work, which involves providing responsive and immediate service to the patients seen each day, as manager, Samantha must think about the future and plan for it. This new dual role requires two divergent skill sets to be successful:

- Respond to the immediate daily needs of patients in the clinic.
- Anticipate and plan for the future needs of the clinic.

Unfortunately, academic training and real-world experience have only provided expertise in clinical audiology, not how to keep seeing patients and manage the Department of Audiology. Hopefully, this chapter will serve as a guide for the new clinical director or manager by presenting the expectations and solutions associated with the title's responsibilities.

The Professional Landscape

According to the U.S. Bureau of Labor Statistics (2023), employment of audi-ologists is projected to grow 21% from 2016 to 2026, much faster than the average for all occupations. However, because it is a small occupation, the fast growth will result in only about 3,100 new jobs over this 10-year period. In practical terms, these numbers, especially when combined with the growing number of audiologists graduating with substantial student loan debt, mean that more and more audiologists will be assuming the role of clinician-manager. These clinician-managers will need to be proficient multitaskers, as they continue to provide patient care while building infrastructure and improve the productivity of a team, comprising fellow audiologists, audiology assistants, and front office staff. Audiologists assuming the role of clinician-manager will be expected to multitask by providing patient care while managing the day-to-day operation of their clinic and a staff who might be working in other locations. Many of these burgeoning clinician-managers have scant formal business or management training, yet they are expected to perform all the essential duties of a director of a business entity. Left to their own devices, a lack of training in basic management skills, paired with the dual role of clinician, leads to frustration, cynicism, and burnout.

The objective of this chapter is to provide time-tested, practical tips and tools for the clinician-manager who finds themselves in this dual role for the first time. One of the central ironies of life as an audiologist in the second decade of the 21st century is that as diagnostic technology and amplification devices become more sophisticated, the human connection, inherently a messy and imperfect interaction between people, becomes even more critical to long-term success. The ability to relate to other people transcends the provider-patient relationship and influences all relationships in the practice.

If practicing audiology prior to 2004, there has been a dramatic change in how audiology is practiced. What was once considered more of a small, backwater profession filled with small independent practices has, in less than 20 years, transitioned into big businesses with several large corporate entities that rely on standardized forms, written procedure manuals, and fine-tuned financial dashboards with several key performance indicators (KPIs) to assist in making administrative decisions. Simultaneously, hearing aid technology and diagnostic testing have gained in sophistication and complexity at a dizzying pace. Plus, there is now the rise of telecare.

Even as the technical capacity of hearing aids and the ability to collect data about the human auditory system grows exponentially, the need for someone to apply human judgments to decisions will never go away. These human judgments, of course, will be needed in our diagnostic and rehabilitation work as clinically trained licensed professionals. How those important skills evolved in the era of Big Data and artificial intelligence is yet to be determined. Facilitating, enhancing, and improving the human connection in the workplace hierarchy leads to less stress in patient care and more success as a manager. Known as managers or directors, these are the individuals tasked with using data to make human judgments about the interworking of the clinic or business.

The Peter Principle (Peter, 1969) states that workers get promoted until they reach their level of incompetence. That is, as workers get better at their job, they continue to rise up the career ladder until they reach a point where their career stalls. Samantha, described above, by virtue of a recent promotion, is exposed to new responsibilities outside of patient care. While working with extreme competence, there is the risk of becoming yet another casualty of the Peter Principle.

Worse still, Samantha could be the victim of something far more common than the Peter Principle. Like many clinical audiologists who have gained a high level of competence delivering patient care that get promoted, Samantha is more at risk for despising her job, casting a continual pall of negativity around the entire staff and eventually leaving clinical work all together, a tremendous loss for her medical center and the patients they serve. The anecdote to negativity and cynicism in the workplace starts with the ability to understand the basic economics of audiology that keeps it a sustainable profession.

Understanding the Business Dynamics of the Profession

The modern practice of audiology requires clinicians to understand the business dynamics of their profession. This is especially true in a modern economy that prizes efficiency, where more and more small "mom-and-pop" shops are rolled up under a large corporate entity. For less experienced professionals, like Samantha, this means becoming a student of the economics of the profession. Knowing the economic models that underlie the generation of revenue inside a clinic rests at the heart of understanding the business dynamics of audiology.

Becoming a student of the economics of audiology means understanding how revenue is consistently generated in a practice and knowing what levers can be pulled to optimize it without compromising the quality of patient care.

Even though audiology is facing some disruptors to its current economic engine, including over-the-counter hearing aid sales and rising third-party contract business, the retail sale of hearing aids is likely to remain a core part of the business. For newly minted clinical directors/managers, audiologists, like Samantha, understanding the business dynamics of the profession starts with building your knowledge of the metrics associated with dispensing hearing aids and how these metrics can be influenced by the execution of sound management principles. To become a better student of the economics of audiology, clinician-managers can learn and apply three basic, yet universal business management principles to provide them with nine repeatable actionable skills. This allows the new manager to incorporate, no matter the clinical setting, techniques to improve the productivity of the modern audiology practice. By learning and applying these skills to the first 100 days as a clinician-manager, it is believed that the result can be higher productivity.

Regardless of how many hours are devoted to direct patient care over the course of the week (less than a half day or more than four days per week), the principles and skills outlined here are designed to assist in avoiding the Peter Principle or its dastardly cousin: promotion to a position that is quickly hated. Let's begin with a simple premise. Carrying the title of Clinician Manager or Clinical Director means that there is the additional responsibility of being the con-

duit between staff and the owners or executives of the clinic. Although there is a love of seeing patients, there is the additional responsibility of management representing the interests of the owners and executives to the other audiologists and individuals who are part of the department. In a sense, the manager or director is the glue who holds the organization together, communicating up the organizational hierarchy expressing the needs and wishes of rank-and-file staff, while communicating down the hierarchy, expressing the strategy and expectations of executives and owners.

The term "communicating down" is not meant to pejoratively imply that you are condescending to staff. Rather the term is meant to describe how you communicate in a hierarchical organization—remember all organizations, by definition, are hierarchical. Clinician-managers or directors are uniquely qualified to be the "glue person" as they understand the needs of both ends of the organization's hierarchy. Like an orchestra conductor, the manager's role is to ensure everyone is performing to their capability and working seamlessly together. It is to instill in staff the organization's mission and values to enable productivity.

By definition, clinic managers or directors represent the organization to colleagues for which they are responsible. It is imperative not only to set a good example but also perform the essential duties of someone who ensures the performance of a group of people within the organization.

Productivity is a term that can be a little fuzzy. In any business, productivity will be defined in economic terms. In audiology practice, that means that productivity will be judged by how much revenue is generated or how many hearing aids are dispensed or tests are conducted. Since time is a resource, economic output has a time component. Therefore, productivity is usually defined as some economic output over the course of an hour, a day, a month, or a year. Although productivity takes on many forms, it is the responsibility of the manager to ensure productivity is being optimized by each member of the team. If a clinician, being productive could mean spending ample time with each patient and successfully identifying hearing aid candidates and fitting them with amplification devices. For front office professionals, productivity might mean optimizing the number of patients who booked and showed up for appointments. For a clinician-manager or director, productivity is likely to be defined as the ability to create an infrastructure within the team than enables each person to be more productive.

Another important concern with a promotion to the clinician-manager is that there is role power. Role power simply means that as part of management, there is the ability to make life-altering decisions for those within your department. Typically, managers can hire and fire people, and thus role power is something that requires great responsibility to wield. Do not take this power lightly. Role power, however, on its own is not enough to lead a team. Clinician-managers or directors must strive to support their inherent role power with the ability to influence others. The ability to influence other people starts with the ability to be an effective communicator. Stated differently, role power is inherited because of the title, but the power to influence is earned. The remainder of this chapter shows how to embrace the dual role of clinician and manager, earn the ability to be an influencer, and

incrementally improve the productivity of the clinical team.

One last comment before addressing the key business principles and skills. It is a common stereotype of anyone that carries the title of manager or director to be labeled a micromanager. Why are so many managers derogatively referred to as micromanagers? Likely because there is a lack of management skills training and many people on staff receive minimal direction from their current manager. They have been conditioned to have very little asked of them. That is, even if there is a formal organizational chart, the managers who have people reporting to them are not participating in any formal management of the procedures. While the manager might conduct an occasional staff meeting or annual performance review, many of the daily activities associated with active management are seldom completed. When a manager with more formal training or a willingness to be more directive in leading a team assumes the role of manager, anything besides the bare minimum of running an occasion staff meeting or conducting annual performance reviews is perceived as micromanaging.

The micromanaging stereotype may be overcome by gaining the trust and respect of staff. This begins with clearly communicating the role of management in a productive organization, which is to guide a team toward higher levels of performance. In short, while carrying the title of manager or director on the organizational chart, it is imperative that those within the department know expectations related to their performance. Effectiveness as a manager essentially boils down to how you ask for incrementally improved performance and results. That process starts with building trust and rapport.

The Three-Legged Stool of Productivity

The term productivity has been presented a few times in this discussion. Since it is a common business term, here is a definition. Perhaps the most critical role for any clinician-manager is the ability to continue to devote some time to direct patient care while simultaneously trying to improve the overall productivity of the team. Regardless of how productivity is defined in the organization, the definition of productivity is likely to change over time; there are three interlocking principles that, when the clinician-manager methodically focuses on them, are likely to produce positive results. Like a three-legged stool in Figure 7–1, these three areas of the organization are interconnected and require diligent oversight and planning. The three components listed below do not work in isolation. It is the responsibility of the clinician-manager to ensure each component is used to build the infrastructure of their team.

- Principle 1: Develop people, grow relationships.
- Principle 2: Make a profit, ethically.
- Principle 3: Have a plan, work the plan.

Each of these three legs of the stool has a corresponding business principle that is outlined below. It is the responsibility of the clinician-manager to understand each business principle and bring it to life within their functional area of the organization. For each of the three principles, there is also listed three corresponding skills that demonstrate how the principle is implemented in daily practice.

Principle 1: Develop People, Grow Relationships

Samantha has been offered the role of clinic director and accepted the promotion. At Samantha's first meeting with the CEO of the clinic, a sheet is handed out that shows the clinic director's position

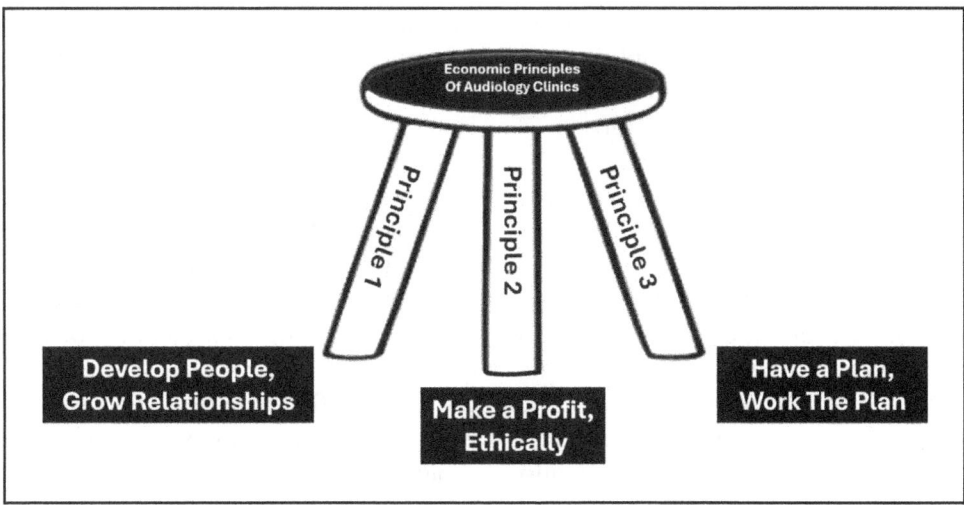

Figure 7–1. The three-legged stool economic principles of audiology clinics.

SUNDAY NIGHT

Sunday night sets the tone for the entire week. Take 15 minutes on Sunday night of quiet time to think about the most important priorities for the week ahead. Jot down these items (keep the list to 10 or fewer) on a to-do list. Writing them down helps prioritize what's most critical to getting down in the week ahead and it helps set the tone for a productive week.

---

on the organizational chart. There are four audiologists who report directly to the clinic manager. Additionally, the three front office professionals who work at the front desk and, according to the organizational chart, report to an off-site clinical manager have a "dotted line" to Samantha as well. Samantha is proud of her accomplishment as her name is near the top of the organizational chart, just below the CEO of the clinic. After all, there is a sizable pay raise, plus the nice sounding title, Clinical Director. Intuitively, Samantha knows that with greater role power comes greater role responsibility. Instead of basking in the glory of her promotion, it is time for Samantha to get to work. What are the new priorities and how will they be implemented? The plan starts with *Principle 1*: Develop people, grow relationships.

Culture Counts

Culture is an integral part of any organization, and its effects filter throughout the organization. Thus, culture is the backbone of any productive team. The questions are what a positive workplace culture is and how is it built. It is difficult to find a good definition of a positive work culture, but it is obvious when it is present. A positive workplace culture is built on mutual respect and trust among staff, regardless of where they fall on the organizational chart. It exists when a problem occurs during a typical day at the office and no one is blamed for the problem; rather, the staff works together to resolve the problem proactively and quickly. In the case of an audiology clinic, it could be a patient having to wait too long to see the audiologist or a patient unhappy about the performance of their hearing aids. In a negative culture, someone usually behind the scenes is blamed for the problem. Or a staff member, who can usually fix the problem, gets defensive or fails to take any action. Discussions with experienced clinicians present that a positive culture is one based on mutual respect and trust among all staff working together as a team each day. Without a positive culture, many staff members will struggle to find the real value in their work, which often ends in a variety of negative consequences for the bottom line of the practice. If a positive or negative issue can be identified when it is obvious, the next logical question is, how does a clinician-manager create a positive workplace culture? A big part of that answer

---

THE FIRST 100 DAYS

Much of a newly promoted manager's success is based on their first 100 or so days on the job. It is when there is a blank slate from which to build a reputation as an authentic leader within the organization. It is a time to advance and foster professional relationships, set the tone for how results are achieved by members of the team, and paint a vivid picture of success. The three principles and their accompanying nine skills outlined here can be put into place during the first 90 to 120 days within the new managerial role, or if the manager has been in the role for a while, it's not too late to start the process of adding these skills.

---

lies with the ability of the clinician-manager to develop people and grow relationships. The three skills listed below will assist managers in the development of people and grow relationships that directly affect workplace culture. These skills include:

■ Conducting one-on-ones and staff meetings.
■ Coaching and delegating.
■ Providing feedback, including annual performance reviews.

Skill 1: Conducting One-on-Ones and Staff Meetings

The ability to build a workplace culture centered on mutual respect and trust starts with the ability of the clinician-manager to have a solid relationship with members of their team. This trusting relationship is built on a foundation of clear, consistent communication and knowing each person of the team. The best way to get to know each person on the team is to spend time with them, and this occurs with scheduled one-on-one meetings. It might seem rather formal to schedule periodic one-on-one meetings with each member of your team, but it's a proven approach to building a long-term professional relationship. When scheduled for 15 to 30 minutes either weekly or every other week, the one-on-one is the cornerstone to developing people and growing relationships. Held in the manager's office or a semi-private area, this is time devoted exclusively to the person you are meeting with where projects, challenges, tasks, and so on can be discussed. The beauty of the scheduled one-on-one that has been conducted with each member of the team over time is that trust and mutual respect increase and the content of subsequent one-on-one meetings becomes more open and honest; therefore, the office culture becomes more positive and productivity improves. It is at the discretion of the clinician-manager if a tracking form should be used to record the agenda of the one-on-one meeting. Although it makes the meeting a little more formal, one advantage of the form is that when items are recorded on the form before or during the one-on-one meeting, both parties are more likely to remember the key parts of the discussion and refer back to prior meeting notes when necessary. Some of the key items discussed during a one-on-one meeting are listed below. Clinician-managers are encouraged to include these questions in their dialogue during these meetings:

■ How were your family/weekend/ activities?
■ How was your week—what has it been like?
■ What have you been working on?
■ Is there anything I can do to help, and if so by when?
■ How are you going to approach this (challenge or problem)?
■ What are the plans for reaching the departmental goals?
■ What can we do differently next time?
■ What did (Name) say about this?
■ Any ideas or suggested improvements?

Effective managers communicate with individuals throughout the organization. An offshoot of the one-on-one meeting is the staff meeting. Now, before delving into the topics of these meetings, consider that most organizations have far too many meetings. Often, these meetings are too long, they have too many people attending them, and they lack a focused agenda. Considering all the wasted productivity resulting from too many meetings, it's tempting to not have *any* meetings. However, a few focused meetings with a limited number of attendees are better than never having meetings. This is because well-orchestrated meetings are another communication tool that develops people and grows relationships.

A team is defined as the group of individuals who report to the manager's line of responsible people on the organizational chart. As a general rule, if there are 10 or fewer people on the team, staff meetings should be conducted once per month. The purpose of the monthly staff meeting is to carve out 60 to 90 minutes so that projects, initiatives, and strategies can be discussed with everyone on the team. Unlike the one-on-one, where each person shares the past week's business activities so the staff meeting has a broader focus, the monthly staff meeting is where larger business initiatives or plans are shared with the team and brainstorming can occur. To ensure that progress is made during monthly staff meetings, it is imperative that an agenda for the meeting be established and shared with all attendees prior to the meeting. If the monthly staff meeting is 60 minutes, there is enough time to cover two or three agenda items. These meetings keep the staff involved in critical business initiatives, helping them develop the ability to recognize and solve problems and actively voice their opinions on important topics. Here is a suggested cadence for the monthly staff meeting:

1. For each of the next 12 months, put time on the schedule each month for a 1-hour staff meeting.
2. Invite all members of the team to these meetings using Outlook or another company calendar.
3. One week prior to each meeting, ask each person on the team to provide discussion items for the upcoming meeting.
4. Create the agenda for the meeting by focusing on the two to three most critical topics. It is also helpful to leave some open time at the end for a more informal discussion. For each agenda item, desig-

---

AVOIDING MEANDERING MEETINGS

In larger organizations with more than a few dozen employees, or more than 10 people reporting to the clinician-manager, short weekly staff meetings can be used to keep everyone abreast of the latest developments within the organization. If these meetings are needed, keep them to an hour or less, with a highly focused agenda. Like monthly staff meetings, where more direct participation is expected, weekly staff updates are another tool to keep people informed.

---

nate one person who will lead the discussion on that item.

5. A day or two before the meeting, email the agenda to all members of the team.

6. Start the meeting on time and keep the meeting moving on time. If the group gets stuck on a point that causes agenda delays, ask the team to table the discussion and designate key team members to take the discussion offline and report back to the group at the next monthly meeting.

7. Designate one person to record meeting minutes and summarize key points.

8. One to 2 days following the meeting, email the meeting summary to all attendees.

9. Repeat Steps 3 to 8 each month.

Skill 2: Coaching and Delegating

Besides following up on key initiatives affecting the business, another important use of one-on-one meetings is coaching and delegating. Coaching and delegating are two sides of the same coin; both are used to improve the skills of people on the team but differ slightly in how each is implemented.

The purpose of coaching is to help members of your team reach higher levels of performance or master a new skill. Coaching is not conducted by the manager; rather, the manager guides the staff member through the process of improvement by identifying areas in their skill set that need improvement and identifying coaching resources. Effective coaching starts with the premise that everyone on the team, including the manager, is always aiming to improve in some area of work or acquire a new skill. This mindset not only builds a great workplace culture but also contributes to better productivity over the long haul.

Part of the time spent during one-on-one meetings can be devoted to coaching. Begin with the mindset that it will take 90 to 180 days to improve or develop a skill. Once the timeline is established, coaching can be broken down into four steps:

1. Collaborate on a goal. Examples: Improve conversion rate of hearing aid candidates coming in for a hearing aid evaluation by 25% or improve overall satisfaction as measured on an outcome report by a specific amount.

2. Collaborate on educational resources that will help reach the goal. Examples: Take a course on Audiology Online or identify a mentor within the organization that has the requisite skills to help the staff member improve and is willing to teach that person.

3. Collaborate on a plan using these resources. Example: Formalize the timelines, usually 3 to 6 months, and steps needed to improve the skills designated.

4. Follow up or check in on the progress. Over the agreed-upon timeline, periodically check in to see if the plan is working or in need of some tweaking.

Effective managers use one-on-one coaching to improve the productivity and skills of every person on their team. This process starts with the attitude that everyone has the motivation and capacity to improve or learn something new. It's the job of the manager to ensure that every one of their team has a plan. The role of the clinician-manager is to periodically follow up and ensure progress is being made.

An offshoot of coaching is delegating certain tasks to other people on your staff. Most everyone has worked with a manager in their career that wanted to do everything and refused to offload any tasks to others on their team. This is a huge mistake for at least two reasons. One, managers who refuse to delegate end up with too many tasks and become overwhelmed, and thus many of the tasks do not get done. Two, delegating tasks to others on the team is a great way to build their skills in new areas. Additionally, taking some important tasks off the manager's plate is a way to groom

less experienced staff members to be effective managers in the future. In a sense, delegating is a way to groom a successor or to help someone gain a promotion in another organization by giving that person opportunities to take on more challenging tasks. Perhaps because professionals who get promoted tend to take on many challenges with success, it is easy for them to simply do many of the tasks associated with management and not rely on other people. This is a lost opportunity to mentor someone to become a manager in the future. Delegation is about stretching the capacity of others by allowing them to do new tasks, some of which might be outside their comfort zone. For this reason, the ability to delegate is an underappreciated skill.

Skill 3: Feedback—Providing Annual Performance Reviews

The purpose of feedback is to communicate directly to staff about their performance. Feedback can be either positive ("Hey, great job") or correcting ("Hey, when you're late it puts everyone in the office behind schedule"). It is also the most challenging aspect of communication and the one that can derail a relationship when it is done incorrectly. It is listed here as the last essential skill because it takes the most time to become comfortable doing and it is advisable to build trust with staff through the execution of one-on-one meetings and coaching before jumping into providing a lot of feedback meant to improve performance. That does not mean that this stage cannot be early with staff. During the initial stages as a manager, it is helpful to remind the staff that part of providing feedback is to assist them in reaching higher levels of performance or mastering new skills. Further, part of feedback management responsibility is to observe and discuss performance. Once a new manager has set the stage and built some trust, the process of systematically talking about performance can begin. Accountability is the name of the game! The goal of feedback is to encourage effective future performance. With that in mind, it is a big mistake to observe some action or behavior from staff that needs correction and wait until the more formal review process to talk about it. Instead, effective feedback occurs almost immediately after the action is observed. Prior to being scared off about providing feedback on something that needs correcting, it is important to know that 90% plus of feedback should be positive in nature. In fact, any time something positive happens in your clinic, it should be noticed and discussed.

An example might be, "Hey, Mary, I loved how you good-naturedly addressed that patient when they got agitated about the long wait. Great job!" Assuming the positive feedback is de-served, everyone needs to hear that they are doing a good job. Another consideration about delivering feedback is that the clinic, with due respect, is not a fast-food joint. In other words, most of the people who are employed in a clinic have previous professional work experience and know how to conduct themselves in a professional manner. They show up on time, dress appropriately, and know how to politely interact with other people. Thus, they have earned the right to be given the benefit of the doubt when it comes to basic workplace interactions with patients and other staff. So, you seldom must be on the lookout for opportunities to correct people.

On relatively rare occasions, something is observed that needs to be corrected. Rectify it immediately and in a matter-of-fact, unemotional manner.

- First, ask the staff person if it is okay to share something with them.
- Second, state the observed behavior that needs to be corrected.
- Third, mention the impact of that behavior.

YOUR WAY IS NOT THE ONLY WAY

It is a very diverse world. No two people act or behave in the same way. In fact, diversity ought to be encouraged because often a range of insights and opinions helps us ferret out the best way of accomplishing goals. There is an array of human experience, and if the world works well for some, it does not mean that it works the same for others. There is more than one way, and it may be different from ways that are familiar. There is more than one right way to conduct business, interact with people, or solve a problem. Respect the diversity of opinions, personalities, and social styles in the workplace, and know there is no one correct way of solving problems or orchestrating a plan.

■ Fourth, encourage effective behavior in the future.

Sticking with the prior example:

■ Step 1: "Mary, can I share something with you?"
■ Step 2: "When you're 20 minutes late in the morning, the patients get agitated and it puts everyone on the staff behind all morning and they get upset, too."
■ Step 3: "What can I do to help you get to work on time?"

This type of direct, correcting feedback can only be delivered effectively once trust and rapport with the staff member have been established. That is why one-on-ones, conducted weekly, are so important. If there is not a trusting relationship with the person, this approach will be ineffective. For fellow clinicians in whom trust and respect are lacking, such a direct approach is perceived often as intimidating. With that in mind, a softer approach would involve using some of the phrases listed below when trying to correct some behavior associated with clinical practice, for instance, taking too much time to complete an audiological assessment, rushing through an appointment, using poor testing technique, or having poor report writing skills. First say, "I noticed when you do (state procedure or behavior), this (state consequences of action) happens." Then say one of the following:

■ "Have you thought about doing it this way . . . ?"
■ "What would happen if you tried this . . . ?"
■ "What could you have done differently?"

■ "Maybe try it this other way and let me know what you think?"
■ "Let's take a look at best practices in this area and see how it compares to your approach."
■ "I am interested in learning your rationale behind the approach you are using . . . tell me more about that."

Providing feedback and talking about performance are essential duties of the clinician-manager. The critical point is how it is conducted. Too often, because it is uncomfortable to do, many clinician-managers completely ignore giving feedback and do not do it at all. This is the easy way out and a lost opportunity to improve productivity or help staff develop new skills. By waiting until the formal annual performance review to talk about procedures and behaviors that need some correction, the business is not operating to its fullest potential. Instead of waiting and eventually becoming enraged about a procedure or behavior that is incorrect, intervene in a relaxed, unemotional, but direct manner. Talking about performance in a nonjudgmental way takes time to master, but its rewards are worth it.

Before moving to the next section, a word of caution about how feedback is delivered is warranted. Psychologists use the term negative bias to describe the innate human tendency to dwell on negative events. That is, a person can be involved in several pleasant experiences throughout the day, and one, even small, negative experience, such as your boss suggesting a behavioral correction, can ruin the entire day. To avoid negative bias, always deliver correcting feedback in a pleasant tone. Never make the correction personal; rather, focus on the behavior that needs to be improved or corrected in a matter-of-fact manner. While this is more difficult, setting the stage early with direct reports will set the tone for minimizing negative bias. The first principle of business management, developing people and growing relationships, is the cornerstone of a productive office culture. The role of clinician-managers is to utilize the three foundational communication skills outlined here for building a culture based on mutual trust and respect, all aimed at improving the productivity of everyone on the team.

Although the three communication skills are humanistic in nature, when practiced day in and day out, better productivity will be the result. Productivity, of course, is an economic term, and to achieve better productivity, it takes more than developing people and growing relationships. As Principle 2 describes, for any business, including a hearing care clinic, to be sustainable, the people who work in it must be able to generate enough revenue to ensure they stay in operation.

Principle 2: Make a Profit, Ethically

During the first week in the new role as clinical director, the CFO of Samantha's clinic emails several spreadsheets and reports. Samantha opens the Excel files, stares at the numbers, and wishes for more education in accounting. The new clinic director is unfamiliar with many of the terms and overwhelmed by all the numbers. Instead of pretending to know what the reports mean, Samantha reaches out to the CFO and asks for a meeting to better understand the numbers. Samantha learns from these 45 minutes with the CFO that one does not have to be in love with the idea that human performance can be reduced to financial data to appreciate how using these financial data can help with becoming a more effective manager. The key to succeeding in a business environment where human interactions are reduced to financial data is figuring out what the numbers say about performance. This begins with the clinician-manager defining successful performance in the clinic and working backward.

For example, if successful performance in the clinic is defined as each provider dispensing 20 hearing aids per month with zero returns for credit and 90% of all patients seen in the clinic being satisfied or highly satisfied with their service, then these metrics may be used as a starting point to relate the financial numbers with successful performance. In this example, 20 hearing aids per month might translate to $38,000 in gross revenue per month per full-time provider. As you will see below, other metrics on the profit and loss statement (P/L) flow from that gross revenue figure. It's up to the clinician-manager (with some guidance from the CFO or accountant) to ensure those numbers that define success in the clinic are realistically achievable and translate into a profitable business. There are three basic analytical skills needed to analyze financial reports and KPI dashboards, and in turn, use this information to shape performance in the clinic to make a profit, ethically. They are:

- Reading a Profit and Loss Statement
- Using financial data to influence or shape behavior
- Manage cash collected

Skill 1: How to Read a Profit and Loss Statement

There are several reports with financial information that are generated by accountants. The one, however, that has the most meaningful information and the one in which the eventual outcome can be controlled is the P/L. The ability to use financial data to make decisions that influence the operation of the clinic starts with the ability to understand how to read and profit and loss statements. Known as the P/L, the profit and loss statement is a cornerstone of any business. Although the various lines on a P/L vary across businesses, there are some items on it that are standard. It is up to the new manager to learn what the numbers on the P&L mean and how to influence them. Once familiar with the standard lines on the P/L, the differences in the clinic are usually easy to understand.

Beginning with the basics. If there is money flowing in and out of an organization, a P/L can be used to organize it. Perhaps the simplest example is personal household finances. If there are funds coming in and bills being paid, there is money moving in and out of the bank account. Consider the personal bank account as a business. To be solvent (or in the black), there needs to be more money coming in than going out. Figure 7–2 is an example of how a dual-income household might organize their monthly budget using a P/L report.

Start at the top of Figure 7–2 and work down. First, notice the top line is the total amount of income that is coming into the household, labeled gross revenue. Second, that really big number of $500K is whittled down considerably. Almost 40% of the gross revenue is never put into the bank account of the household because it is used to pay taxes, with a small per-

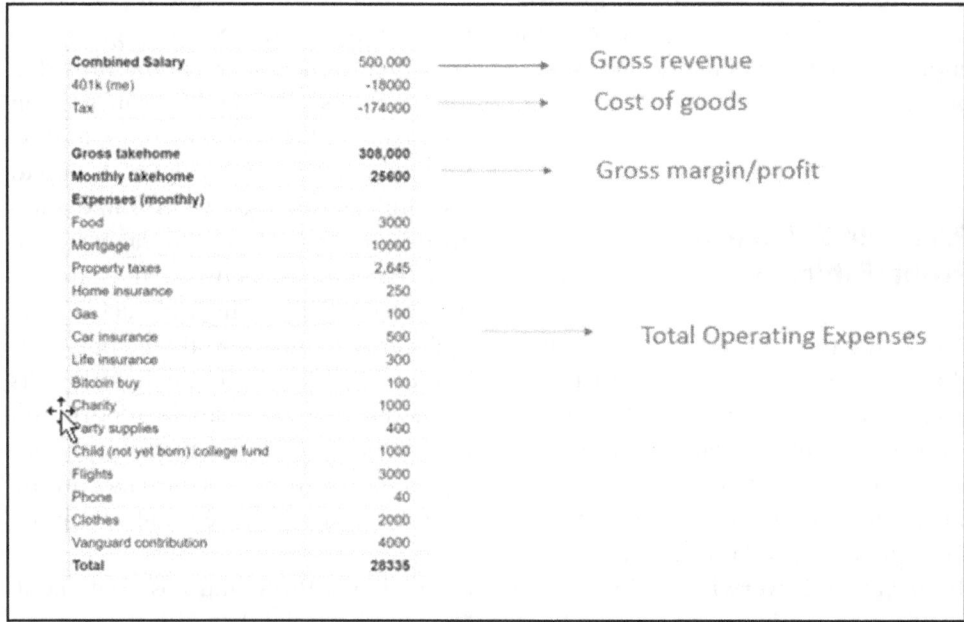

Figure 7–2. An example of a dual-income household organizing their monthly budget using a P/L statement.

centage going into a 401K retirement account. This money, taken out before it goes into the bank account, is similar to the cost of goods line on a P/L used by most clinics. (Later on it will be shown that upward of 40% of gross revenue in a hearing aid dispensing goes immediately to the manufacturer, and it is not used to cover any other expenses.) Even though the household is earning a substantial amount of money, it is not available to cover any day-to-day expenses. Third, the money left after taxes and the 401K are covered is referred to as the gross margin (or gross profit) of the household. This is the money the household lives on month to month. It is used to cover daily living expenses. Notice the daily operating expenses of the household. Everything from the mortgage to groceries and gasoline is included in the operating expenses. As the term implies, these are the expenses that allow the household to stay in operation each month. Finally, any remaining gross profit not used to cover operating expenses would be considered net profit. In a household, the net profit may be used to take a nice trip, make a home improvement, or invest in the stock market. Similarly, a clinic would use net profits as an investment or bonus.

Now apply these financial fundamentals to the clinic. For a manager or director of a clinic, a major responsibility is the generation of revenue. And, when generating revenue, it is necessary to know not only how much revenue is generated but also something about the expenses and profit that result from the generation of that income, which is where the P/L comes into play. The P/L is usually compiled by someone in the business with a background in accounting. A P/L, no matter how complex it looks,

consists of numbers that reveal how the business performed in the past. Most P/Ls have numerous lines of data on them, all important for the accountants and the CFO in the practice, but for the clinician-manager, there are five broad categories on the P/L that should be of concern. Since each practice's P/L is going to be different, the clinician-manager is encouraged to sit down with the person in the organization who completes the P&L to better understand the nuances. The five categories and what they mean are as follows:

- *Revenue.* This is the money generated through the sale of goods and services. In a hearing aid dispensing or audiology clinic, revenue is usually confined to two categories: sale of hearing aids and tests.
- *Cost of goods (COGs).* These are the items the business buys at a wholesale price and resells at a retail price. Hearing aids, assistive listening devices, and other various accessories that are resold in a clinic are tallied on the COGs line.
- *Gross margin.* Gross margin, sometimes called gross profit, is the difference between gross revenue and cost of goods. It is the margin that remains after the hearing aid or equipment manufacturer has been paid for the device sold.
- *Operating expenses.* Commonly known as overhead, there are usually several lines on a P/L that represent operating costs. Although each practice may call them different things or break them out on a P/L a little differently, everything from salary, rent, utilities, and marketing expenses is in the operating expense category. Operating

	Monthly Budget	Benchmark (% of total gross revenue)
Gross Revenue	$100,000	100%
Cost of Goods (COGs)	$35,000	35%
Gross Margin	$65,000	65%
Operating Expenses	$55,250	55%
Profit	$9750	10%

Figure 7–3. Examples of five essential lines on a P/L statement with corresponding benchmarks expressed as a percentage of total gross revenue rounded to the nearest whole number.

expenses is a large category, comprising both variable and fixed expenses. Another thing to remember about operating expenses is that these are the items that need to be paid just to keep the business open before any net profits are generated.

■ *Net profit.* This is the line representing profit after all operating expenses, taxes, and other items are deducted.

Now that there is a better understanding of the five broad categories on a P/L, the next topic is benchmarks. A benchmark is nothing more than a predetermined target, or what others might call "expected performance." In most organizations, the executive team, with a tremendous amount of input from staff, determines the benchmarks shown on the P/L. Clinician-managers certainly have a role in establishing those benchmarks for the business, but ultimately others within the organizations often have the final decision. In Samantha's example,

cited above, the CFO shared the benchmarks. So, in a sense, it is the CFO that is the referee of the P/L. The CFO oversees the process and enforces the rules. Like the actual lines on a P/L statement, benchmarks vary across organizations. Even though you might have a say in the development of future benchmarks, most new clinician-managers inherit benchmarks that they need to observe. Figure 7–3 shows the benchmark for 1 month of business, expressed as a percentage of gross revenue for each of the five broad categories on the P&L.

Figure 7–3 presents examples of five essential lines on a P/L statement with corresponding benchmarks expressed as a percentage of total gross revenue rounded to the nearest whole number.

In the example, for 1 month of business, $100,000 in gross revenue was generated. We can assume this was a traditional hearing aid dispensing business that bundled all their testing with the sale of devices; thus, almost all the gross revenue was generated from hearing aid sales. (Some practices choose to break out hearing aid sales revenue from testing revenue and have separate lines for each on their P&L.) Next, $35,000 was paid to hearing aid manufacturers for devices that were resold to patients. The benchmark (or target) was 35%. After the cost of goods is deducted from gross revenue, what remains is the gross margin to cover all expenses and (hopefully) with some left over as a net profit. In this example, notice that there is $55,250 (or 85% of the gross margin) used to cover all overhead or operating expenses, which leaves $9,750 left over at the of the month for profit. Fifty-five percent of gross revenue used to cover operating expenses might seem like a big number, but there are many bills to pay before a business sells anything. In an actual business, items such as salaries, wages, utilities, and marketing expenses would have their own line on the P/L and the cost of each item would be presented.

To Budget Is to Plan

Now familiar with the five broad categories on a P/L, those benchmarks shown are never perfectly aligned with what actually happens in a business. When the CFO in Samantha's business created the P/L for an entire year, he made some educated guesses about how much money would go into each category based on prior year performance and some other variables. These numbers represent the budget. A budget is nothing more than an educated guess or forecast of how each month will play out. Because CFOs and other people responsible for paying salaries and bills do not like uncertainty, they need budget forecasts to be as precise as possible. After all, they are the folks that must make sure all the bills are

paid each month and they want things to run as smoothly as possible. The budgeted numbers on a P/L represent a target, and there is always some degree of variability between a budgeted number and the actual number. A primary responsibility of any manager is to know how they can influence this variability and match the targeted (or budgeted) number on the P/L.

Consider the simplified P/L that compares budgeted numbers to the actual numbers for 1 month. It is this comparison on the P/L—budget versus actual—that requires vigilance from the clinician-manager. As the example in Figure 7–4 shows, for this 1 month, the practice underperformed relative to the benchmarks, seen in the far-right column representing the variance from the benchmark expressed as a percentage. Note that a negative percentage represents a variance below the established benchmark.

Remember, the numbers on a P/L reflect the past. You cannot change the past, but past numbers shape future behavior. To do this effectively, it helps to understand what numbers can change over the short term, and what numbers are "baked" into the P/L. For example, many operating expenses, like salaries, rent, and utilities are baked into the P/L for an entire year and are difficult for the clinician-manager to change over the short term. (We refer to the short term as 6 months or less.) Oftentimes, numbers that are baked into the P/L are fixed expenses that cannot be avoided and remain consistent each month.

Skill 2: Using Financial Data to Influence Behavior

In contrast to fixed expenses, there are some numbers that can be affected in a

	Monthly Budget	Actual Performance	Benchmark	Variance from Benchmark (%)
Gross Revenue	$100,000	$93,000	100%	-7%
Cost of Goods (COGs)	$35,000	$31,000	35%	-1.5%
Gross Margin	$65,000	$65,000	65%	0%
Operating Expenses	$55,250	$55,250	55%	0%
Profit	$9750	$6750	10%	-4%

Figure 7–4. Actual versus budgeted numbers on a simplified P/L.

big way by the manager over the short term. The next skill will be to examine and determine what numbers on the P/L can be quickly influenced by the manager.

To better understand how a clinician-manager can use P/L information, it is necessary to take a step back and look at how any audiology clinic can generate more revenue. In simple terms, there are just two ways for the clinician-manager to generate more revenue in an audiology clinic:

- See more patients.
- Dispense more hearing aids.

Influencing gross revenue boils down to the ability to do more of something over a designated period of time. Thus,

if gross revenue is below the benchmark, especially over the course of 2 or more consecutive months, the clinician-manager needs to identify some tactics that will bring more patients into the clinic or find a way to dispense more hearing aids. (Another tactic that can be used to improve overall revenue is raising retail prices, but this is usually a tactic reserved for senior-level executives and thus usually cannot be accomplished over the short term.) There might be occasions when gross revenue targets on the P/L are being achieved, but gross margins are lower than expected. This is the case when the cost of goods should be targeted for improvement. Remember, cost of goods and gross margin are two more lines on the P/L that can be influenced by the clinician-manager. Note these two lines on the P/L are interconnected. That is, lowering the cost of goods results in a greater gross margin.

There are two ways to improve gross margins. The first is raising retail prices, which is a tactic, usually reserved for senior executive involvement and is completed over the long term. That tactic is negotiating more favorable terms with the manufacturer, which usually means the clinic is committed to buying a higher number of units in exchange for a lower wholesale price. The second tactic is one that the clinician-manager has more direct control over. That tactic is identifying hearing aids that have a favorable cost of goods and dispensing more of those products. This requires the clinician-manager to look at the established retail price and compare it to the wholesale and, thus, gaining an agreement with the audiology staff to dispense (when appropriate) hearing aids that have the cost of goods in alignment with the benchmark. Another tactic that clinician-managers can use to control the cost of goods is monitoring discount rates.

Policies, along with processes that educate staff on why these policies are implemented, are an integral part of using financial data to influence behavior. And, it is a great reason to remember why Principle 1, developing people and growing relationships, is so critical in making financial decisions, when a buy-in and support from everyone are crucial. With respect to the skill of using financial data to influence behavior and policies in the clinic, the ability of managers to set aside at least 1 to 2 hours per week to methodically review the P/L, with an emphasis on gross margins, and COGs of each device dispensed over the course of a week will enable for an actionable plan to be implemented that can move the needle in a positive direction when required.

Another type of report that usually takes data from the P/L statement and organizes it into a more actionable form is called a dashboard. A dashboard, which can be created by a person skilled in finance, is a useful way to digest a lot of important information quickly. Figure 7–5 is an example of a dashboard used to monitor some KPIs related to hearing aid revenue. Like many dashboards, the number in Figure 7–5 shows the manager how two KPIs, per unit average selling price and per unit gross margins, have been influenced by management intervention. In this example, the dashboard was created to track a weakness that was uncovered during routine monitoring of the monthly P/L. The dashboard in Figure 7–5 shows how much of a financial impact the intervention had on revenue and profit. The main point to remember is that a dashboard can be created for any financial metric that enables managers to track results over time and compare them to past performance. If working in a large organization, someone in the finance department can assist in the creation of dashboards for the department from P/L reports.

Skill 3: Managing Cash Collected

If the P/L statement represents what has happened in the clinic in the past, the cash flow statement represents the future, because without cash coming into the business, it will not stay afloat. When we talk about cash, it doesn't necessarily mean people are paying cash for services. It simply means that people are paying all or most of their bill upon the receipt of services. Being good at collecting cash means that there is a solid cash collection policy in place and that staff, who must ask patients for payment,

Key Weakness – Low ASP ($1,541)

Metric	Before	After	Improvement
Total Units / Month	80	80	-
ASP	$1,541	$2,076	+ $535
Gross Margin / Unit	$848	$1,246	+ $398

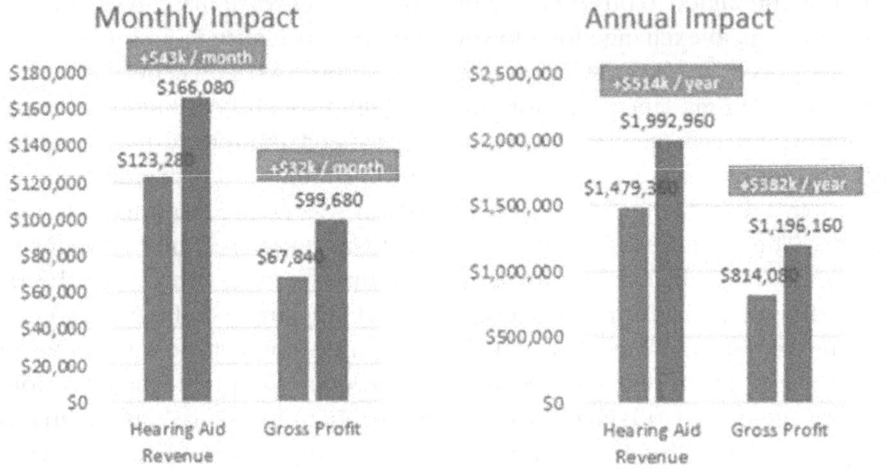

Figure 7–5. An example of a dashboard used to monitor some key performance indicators.

SHORT-TERM VERSUS LONG-TERM THINKING: YOU NEED BOTH

Managers plan for the long term and influence the short term. For an audiology clinic, this usually means that budgets, expenses, and other projects are planned or forecasted in advance. When planning and budgeting for a full calendar year, that's long-term planning. Clinician-managers have a lot of control over the short term. This means that their immediate actions, based on data from a financial report or dashboard, can influence results over the next few months.

clearly understand the policy and that the policy is followed by everyone. Although someone in the accounting department is collecting detailed information on cash received, the role of the clinician-manager is to make sure that the department is securing payments from patients when services are rendered.

This can be accomplished by putting a couple of simple rules in place, monitoring cash that is collected, and following up with staff as needed. The key point about cash flow is to have a workable plan, train staff to the plan, and closely monitor the execution of the plan. Although each practice varies in how cash is collected for services, the following are some standard rules that apply to most practices:

■ Verify insurance information prior to the visit. Clearly and accurately inform the patient what their out-of-pocket expenses will be prior to the visit. Collect these out-of-pocket fees when patients arrive for their appointment.

■ Collect payment for out-of-pocket hearing aid expenses at the time the hearing aids are dispensed. Have a policy in place that requires the patient to pay half the balance when the hearing aids are ordered

and the second half at the time the hearing aids are dispensed.

■ Use a third-party financing company (e.g., Care Credit) when necessary and prequalify patients. Avoid payment plans in which patients pay you directly over time.

■ Allow patients to use credit cards and make it easy for them to pay their bill.

■ Ensure that all staff who engage in billing and collecting processes understand the policies and know how to talk about them with patients. Provide training when needed.

■ Monitor cash collected each week. Use the three skills corresponding with the first principle to infuse the importance of good cash collection practices into the clinic. In most clinics, there are personnel on staff who are trained to perform these cash collection tasks. The role as a manager will be to make sure the tasks are completed.

The second principle is to make a profit, *ethically*. As a healthcare provider, it is critical to follow the ethical guidelines of professional organizations. As a clinician-manager, it is an essential responsibility to balance the needs of

BILLING THE PATIENT VERSUS PAYING AT THE TIME OF THE VISIT

There is a difference between billing someone for a service and that person paying for the service. It is easy to bill but more challenging to collect a payment. The clinician-manager must have policies in place that collect payment for services.

the business with the needs of patients. And, when the priorities of these two constituents come into opposition, err on the side of the patient. Luckily, in most situations, doing what is right for patients will result in positive outcomes for the business. After all, everyone benefits from a stellar reputation for delivering quality care and service. Being able to make a profit ethically is underpinned by the mindset that you believe the services you provide people in your community have value and ought to be paid for at the time service is rendered. The business of audiology is not a charity, and to be around to serve patients another day, it is essential to be paid fairly and on time. When clinician-managers implement clear, commonsense policies around billing and cash collection, it allows frontline staff, responsible for asking patients to pay their bill, to be able to conduct their job without guesswork. Perhaps the best way to summarize the importance of ethics in the business world is to quote the economist Milton Friedman, who is one of the pioneers of modern commerce. In 1962, about 15 years before he won the Nobel Prize in economics, he said, "There is one and only one social responsibility of business—to use its resources and engage in activities designed to increase its profits so long as the business stays within the rules of the game, which is to say, engages in open and free competition without deception or fraud."

Principle 3: Have a Plan, Work Your Plan

The first two principles and their corresponding skills are related directly to the day-to-day management of the clinic. By communicating with staff and using financial data to influence behavior, clinician-managers can improve productivity over a 3- to 6-month time window. Now consider strategic initiatives in which the clinician-manager, usually with some guidance or input from other senior-level staff, uses past performance and knowledge about consumers as well as industry trends to create and execute future plans. The three skills covered in this section build on the first two principles and enable clinician-managers to solve problems, close gaps in performance, or orchestrate business strategies over the long run.

Skill 1: Implementing a Clinical Protocol

If there is more than one person working in the clinic, it is essential that everyone is working in synchrony. Even though it might sound like a term that comes from Henry Ford's 1930s assembly line, devising and executing a clinical protocol is a good way to ensure all members of a clinical staff are working harmoniously and efficiently. A clinical protocol is nothing more than a series of behaviors or procedures conducted by staff as they provide care to patients. When staff conducts their work in some organized and consistent manner, and that process has been formalized, it is a protocol. Now, just because patient care is referred to as organized, consistent, and formalized does not mean, by any stretch of the imagination, that everyone must robotically interact with patient the same way. Because patient care is conducted between two human beings (a patient and a provider), there is always some inherent disorderliness in that process that must be respected. After all, no two people are alike, and we cannot expect everyone to interact the same way with their patients (see Chapter 20).

The good news is that as the clinician-manager, there is major influence in how any clinical protocol is created and implemented. Consider a clinical protocol as a monogram on handmade garments. Although each handmade sweater looks exactly alike from a distance, upon closer inspection, there are unique characteristics with each monogram on a sweater. Look closer still and find some of the nuanced differences in the stitching each garment indicates that it has been handmade. No two are the same. That analogy applies to patients you might see in your clinic. In general, each patient goes through the same procedures, but upon closer inspection, we know there are many subtle differences, based mainly on the personality, outlook, and motivations of both the patient and the provider. The benefit of a clinical protocol is threefold.

■ *Consistency in workflow processes leads to greater efficiency.* When all the tasks are mapped out and defined from an initial phone call to scheduling an appointment to routine follow-up care, staff are more apt to focus on their responsibilities and how they mesh with others on the staff. Having familiarity with how you conduct specific tasks in the patient journey leads to getting more work done in less time, which is the definition of efficiency.

■ *Clinical protocol in which all members of the staff agree to conduct-*
ing similar procedures helps build a consistent brand or reputation. Patients can expect similar treatment and results no matter who they see. When staff are using the same forms and similar assessment methods, it builds a consistent level of care. Consistent care by everyone on the staff is a cornerstone of generating excellent patient outcomes.

■ *Attract and bring on board new staff more effectively.* When staff buys in to a predefined approach for delivering patient care based on fundamental philosophy, the orientation of a new hire into the practice will certainly be streamlined (see Chapter 6).

The real skill in creating and implementing any clinical protocol is balancing the need for some common procedures (ways of doing things), while maintaining respect for the individual differences in how each procedure is conducted by each provider. One way to get this balance right is for clinical staff to agree on conducting a few standard procedures consistently and recording that information on a common clinical form. What follows is a proven way to launch a clinical protocol within a group of audiologists with divergent backgrounds. A typical launch protocol is presented below:

■ Set a timeline for completion of protocol implementation and explain to staff why a clinical protocol is important to their success. Cite the three reasons listed above to support your rationale for establishing a clinical protocol.

Appointment Type	Time Allotment
Hearing aid evaluation	60 minutes
Diagnostic hearing test	30 minutes
Hearing aid check (2-week follow up)	30 minutes
Hearing aid fitting	60 minutes

Figure 7–6. Time allotments for various appointment types.

- Ask the group, What do they want to be known for? This is an aspirational question intended to get staff thinking about how they want to shape or influence their own reputation in the community. Give the staff a week or two to ponder the question, talk about the value of a stellar reputation, and convene a staff meeting to discuss the staff's response to this question.
- After the group has come to some consensus on their response to the question of what they want to be known for, scope out the appointment types that require a clinical protocol and the recommended time for an average visit. This might look like Figure 7–6. Next, the group comes to some consensus on minimal standards of care for each visit. That is, what must the provider do at each visit to ensure patient results are optimized?
- Once providers agree on what optimal patient results look like at the end of each appointment, the next step is the toughest: Providers

come to agree on how these results are achieved. From this discussion needs to spring a consensus on what tests, procedures, and forms will be used by all providers in the group. The role of the manager is to ensure that everyone on the staff has input and that each provider can defend their stance with reasonable clinical evidence.
- The result of this discussion will be the creation of a written protocol and a common form that everyone agrees to use. Through this discussion process, for example, the clinical staff might come to an agreement on using the Client Oriented Scale of Improvement (COSI) as part of the intake and outcome measurement process. They might even take it one step further and require that several questions from the Characteristics of Amplification Tool (COAT) are added to the intake form and that this form needs to be completed with every first-time patient during the hearing aid evaluation. Following these six

steps will get clinical staff one step closer to getting any clinical protocol or best-practice process off the ground. The role of the manager is not to control the process and see that their agenda gets fulfilled. Rather, once trust and rapport have been established, effective managers enable everyone to have a say in creating the protocol, find a consensus, and ensure these six steps are completed in a timely manner.

Skill 2: Creating and Executing a Strategic Plan

Working with people is inherently messy; clinician-managers must learn to live with some ambiguity and uncertainty. However, trusting and respecting the staff and keeping the best interests of the patients the top priority, even the biggest obstacles can be overcome—if there is a plan. The second skill to support Principle 3 is creating and executing a strategic plan.

A strategic plan is business jargon for a set of goals that are used to improve the organization or to change course to overcome obstacles in the business cycle (see Chapter 1). Strategic plans can differ in their content and structure, but they have one commonality: strategic plans focus on the future. Considering the dual role of clinician-managers, a big challenge associated with creating and executing any strategic plan is taking attention away from the daily bustle of the clinic and focusing attention on addressing future needs of the business. It is so easy to get caught up in the daily needs of running a clinic where it seems there is always something that requires immediate attention that strategic planning can be neglected.

Businesspeople with some formal training know that a strategic plan is a management activity used to determine organizational priorities, close an operational gap, ensure that staff is working toward a common goal, establish agreement around intended outcomes, and adjust the organization's direction in response to a changing marketplace. It is a deliberate and disciplined effort that produces fundamental decisions and actions that shape and guide what an organization is, who it serves, what it does, and why it does it, with a focus on the future. Effective strategic planning articulates not only where an organization is going and the actions needed to make progress but also how it will be successful. Similar to the first skill in this section, the role of the clinician-manager is to ensure everyone on the staff is involved in the process, a consensus is reached, and the plan is executed. Creating a strategic plan requires careful and deliberate attention. There are three basic steps to creating and implementing any strategic plan. It is up to the clinician-manager to oversee that each of these three steps is completed in a timely manner.

SWOT Analysis

SWOT stands for strengths, weaknesses, opportunities, and threats (see Chapter 4). A SWOT analysis serves as a template for trying to understand the performance of the organization within the context of the competition and other changes that might be occurring within a certain profession or industry (Figure 7–7).

■ *Strengths:* factors that give the clinic an edge over its competitors.

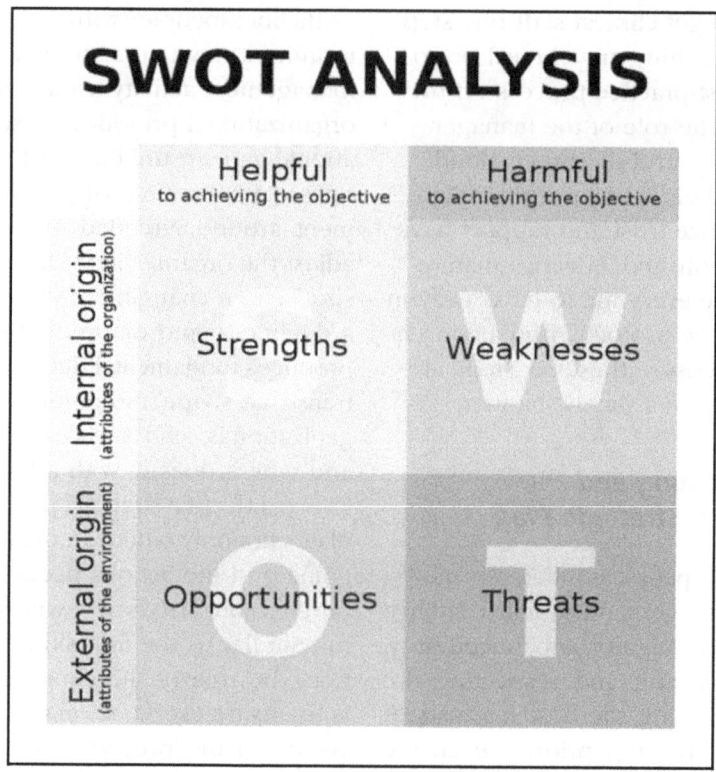

Figure 7–7. SWOT 4-Box Matrix. *Source:* Xhienne (https://commons.wikimedia.org/wiki/File:SWOT_en.svg), "SWOT en," https://creativecommons.org/licenses/by-sa/2.5/legalcode

■ *Weaknesses:* factors that can be harmful to the clinic, which could be exploited by competitors.

■ *Opportunities:* favorable situations that can bring a competitive advantage to the clinic.

■ *Threats:* unfavorable situations that can negatively affect the clinic.

Often, strengths and weaknesses are internal to a company and can be directly managed by it, while the opportunities and threats are external, and the company can only anticipate and react to them. A SWOT analysis is usually plotted on a four-box matrix (Chapter 5).

Before the group convenes to create the SWOT analysis, it is essential for everyone to do some homework in preparation. Homework can take on several forms, including learning more about how competitors are conducting business, trends in the industry, and changes in consumer behavior. If you were conducting a SWOT analysis on the clinic in 2024, some of the external threats would be over-the-counter hearing aids, changes in managed care, or the rising popularity of Medicare Advantage programs. The ability to leverage an internal strength to address these threats could, quite possibly, turn these threats into opportunities. The ability to conduct an honest and accurate SWOT analysis is directly related to the mutual respect and trust that has been developed within the team. Without respect and trust of the team, it is almost impossible to conduct a SWOT that reflects the reality of your business. For this reason, clinician-managers need to earn the privilege of conducting a SWOT analysis after they have established goodwill among their staff. If you are a new clinician-manager, it is helpful to wait 90 to 120 days to conduct your first SWOT and allow some time to build some trust and rapport.

Identify a Target and Formulate a Plan

After the SWOT analysis, the next step is to formulate a strategic plan. The strategic plan must have a clear goal that moves the needle in the business. That is, after the plan has been created, targets that have been identified in need of improvement and the measurement milestones that will demonstrate success. Usually, a strategic plan reflects more than one priority within the business than needs to be executed in the short, medium, and long term. Short-term priorities are typically 90 days or less, medium term are 3 to 9 months, and long term are over the course of a year or more. For example, if the clinic needs to improve the overall profit margin from 5% to 10%, after conducting a SWOT analysis, the team could begin brainstorming ways to improve profitability over the short, medium, and long terms. Short-term priorities are those that are quick to implement and have little cost or risk, while on the other end of the spectrum, long-term priorities need more time to plan and execute,

plus they often require the most investment or more risk.

In addition to short-, medium-, and long-term goals, the planning process needs to include a breakdown of the steps needed to achieve each goal, along with the person who is responsible for executing each step.

Executing the Plan

The key to executing a strategic plan comes down to a single word: *discipline.* Executing a strategy plan with several goals is like following an exercise or diet regime. Some days progress toward the goal seems futile, but perseverance is the key when obstacles get in the way. Once short-, medium-, and long-term goals have been targeted, the next step is to ensure that the plan will be executed. This is a critical step because many managers fall in love with their plan but lack the persistence to execute it. Executing the plan comes down to the ability to utilize the skills that develop people and grow relationships to ensure that the strategic plan put into place gets done. Weekly one-on-one meetings are an excellent opportunity to monitor progress toward a goal. Figure 7–8 demonstrates a medium-term goal and how it has been broken down into smaller steps with each step delegated to a person on the team to oversee its progress. Note that each step outlined below has a person delegated as the responsible person, charged with completing that step. The role of the manager is to ensure that each of these individual tasks is getting done and that progress toward the larger goal is occurring incrementally. Oftentimes, the process moves in fits and stops, but the manager needs to keep the big picture

Steps Toward Goal	Responsible Person
Review current clinical hearing aid evaluation and fitting protocols	Clinical manager
Review return rates of each audiologist and ask each for ways to improve it	Clinical manager
Investigate returns across manufacturers – look for patterns in returns related to manufacturer, report out to team in 1 month	Audiologist 1
At next staff meeting, review all ways to improve return rate	Team

Figure 7–8. Example of breaking down medium-range goals as part of a strategic plan.

in mind and ensure that progress toward the goal is being made. Note in Figure 7–8 the steps are outlined to accomplish one principle goal: Reduce hearing aid return rate by 50%.

Regardless of the type of strategic plan, there are a few simple rules to remember about executing it.

1. Break the plan into smaller action items, like those shown in Figure 7–8.
2. Delegate a responsible person to complete or oversee each action item.
3. Make sure each action item has a timeline or an agreed-upon due date for completion by the delegated to complete the task.
4. Follow up on progress toward the final goal and modify action items and timelines as needed.

Skill 3: Learning to Juggle Various Projects by Exercising Judgment and Flexibility

One of the key points for this skill is that successful managers must learn to live with some ambiguity and uncertainty in their dual roles of clinicians and managers. Although the role of clinician has a considerable amount of certainty associated with conducting routine assessments, the role of manager requires the ability to make trade-offs. Thus, this final skill is more of a mindset than a learnable, replicable skill. Much of effective management is carefully examining several options using the best information available at the time and determining the correct course of action. Using the other eight skills outlined in this chapter, it should be apparent that any strategic imperative or obstacle can be addressed through the practice of making firm decisions based on solid information and sound judgment. In the role of clinician-manager, there are three strategic goals that need to be balanced. These three variables are:

- Cost of the service/devices.
- Quality of the service/devices.
- Customer satisfaction.

Be aware that if too much time and attention is focused on just one of these variables, it will be at the detriment of the other two. For example, if too much effort is concentrated on providing the lowest cost service and product, quality and customer satisfaction will suffer. On the other side of the equation, if the focus is quality, it may be at the expense of costs charged to the consumer.

The bottom-line message is that it is the responsibility of the clinician-manager to acknowledge the trade-offs among these three goals and ensure that time, attention, and resources are balanced for all three goals as others on the team do not necessarily pay attention to the big picture.

Creating Esprit de Corps

Esprit de corps is French for spirit of body. Spirit of body refers not to the human body but rather to a body of multiple people—for example, a military unit, a business, or a sports team. To have esprit de corps is to have high regard and pride for the organization or team to which one belongs. In the dual role of clinician and manager but also engaged in the daily work of seeing patients, you are uniquely equipped to demonstrate "do as I do, not as I say behavior."

Communicating by one's actions can be very powerful. An effective method to set the right tone for your team is stepping in and lending a hand during the daily operation of clinical activity, sometimes in unexpected ways. This shows the team that the manager does what is expected of each member of the team. Demonstration through actions that "whatever it takes" to successfully operate the clinic will ultimately leave an indelible impression on everyone within the organization.

Working With a Mentor or Trusted Advisor

The primary objective of this chapter is to provide inexperienced managers with a roadmap of how to be successful in the dual role of clinician and manager. Having some concrete skills from application to this dual role goes a long way, but what has been covered here is really "just the tip of the iceberg." There are many nuances and complexities associated with juggling the role of clinician with manager. Beyond reading a P&L and creating a dashboard for use to influence the team performance, managers need to be proficient at creating and managing annual budgets, hiring (and probably at some point) discharging (firing) employees, and strategic plan modification. To overcome the complexities of difficult situations, the final skill is finding a mentor.

One of the most impactful things an inexperienced manager can do is to identify a person of trust to be a mentor. Mentors do not need to be a person who works side-by-side in the clinic or organization; it is okay to have them on "speed dial" so that when advice or another opinion is required, they are there to assist. When looking for a mentor, it should be a person who has played the dual role of clinician and manager themselves and shows a willingness to assist when required. A mentor needs to be honest, someone willing to provide unvarnished opinions, and available at a moment's notice. Importantly, a mentor needs to have a scheduled meeting with their mentee at least once per month. Like the one-on-one meetings, this time should be scheduled with a specific agenda to cover key points. Also, these scheduled meetings, which typically take an hour each month, are the ideal time to review financial data and how this information can be used to influence behavior and performance in the clinic. After all, to improve financial results in the clinic, there will need to be a plan for influencing behavior and performance of all contributors to the clinical operation.

A mentor, simply stated, is a person who can assist in the orchestration of a plan that affects behavior, performance, and the overall results in the clinic. A good place to find a mentor is through the state professional organization, preferably a person who practices in another location that does not compete directly with the clinician-manager's business. Another great place to find a mentor is at the Academy of Doctors of Audiology (ADA). Because it comprises many clinicians who are business savvy, ADA is ideally suited to seeking a mentor. Once rapport has been established with the mentor, set up a time to chat on the phone or Zoom/Skype once a month. In whatever the method used for working with the mentor, it is a relationship well worth establishing.

If a mentor is not available, the next best option is to cement a relationship with someone who can be a trusted advisor. There is no shortage of individuals, often with a business background that could qualify them as a trusted advisor. Buying groups and practice development specialists inside the hearing aid industry are two other places to possibly find a trusted advisor. Like a mentor, a trusted advisor must be willing to meet at least once per month to review all aspects of your business and be willing to share their candid opinion, be it positive or negative. These meetings need to utilize financial data in the decision-making process. Regardless of their status, mentor or trusted advisor, the main objective of either role is to provide an open forum in which ideas, tactics, and strategies are exchanged.

Be a Better Boss: Other Intangible Skills for the Aspiring Manager

Since the winddown of COVID-19 restrictions, a growing number of people continue to work from home. It is common these days to manage a group of people who either work from home or work in other offices. Whatever the specifics, having a group of employees all working in different locations is now the norm. The rise of the remote workforce places new challenges on managers as they are tasked with getting workers with disparate interests while residing in different physical locations during the workday and for the purpose of achieving a common goal. For these reasons, it is believed that the following skills are important in leveraging better results from the team.

■ *Establish etiquette for virtual meetings.* Because so much critical information is communicated during remote or virtual Zoom, Teams, or Webex meetings these days, it is crucial that a clear understanding of what background should be used. All attendees should be informed of a few etiquette details, such as camera on the entire time, what background should they use, who created and distributed, and if attendance is mandatory and how long the meeting will last. A detailed agenda should be distributed prior to the meeting and indicate the attendees and the role they will play in the meeting.

■ *Ensure that all staff know how they contribute to the financial success of the business.* Regardless of role, each employee on your team is entitled to know how their daily tasks contribute to the financial success of the entire organization. For employees who interact directly with customers (e.g., clinical audiologists), the discussion can center on the amount of revenue that can be generated through assessments and dispensing of hearing aids. For employees who may not directly interact with customers (e.g., custodians or accountants), the conversation can focus on how their expertise frees up time for the manager so they can use their time more effectively. The bottom line is everyone on the team needs to know how their role synchs with others on the team, so that financial success has a better shot at being optimized.

■ *Instill a sense of purpose.* Just as important as knowing how they each contribute to the financial success of the company, employees need to know they are making a positive difference in the lives of customers. Given the quality-of-life improvements that come from better hearing and balance, instilling a sense of purpose in the staff of an audiology-related business should be easy.

■ *Overcommunicate but avoid micromanaging.* It should not be a surprise that a critical component to being a successful boss is knowing how to effectively communicate. After all, as a boss, you need to hire and discharge (fire) people, develop people, articulate expectations and strategies, and oversee both financial and clinical success. As a boss, the plate is full, and it is easy to be perceived as a micromanager. No one likes to feel like they are being monitored all the time. Everyone likes to have a sense of autonomy as to how they perform their job. To avoid the reputation of a micromanager, it can help to reframe your style as overcommunication. When you inform your team that you like overcommunication, it invites them to be more open. This is why weekly one-on-one meetings and other informal chats with staff are so essential. Assuming trust has been developed, getting the team to overcommunicate has many benefits. It keeps the clinician-manager "in the loop" on important developments that ordinarily "fly under the radar" and it empowers the team to maintain an open line of communication.

■ *Being a good boss takes a lot of patience.* Many of the skills that were necessary to be a good clinician may not transfer to being a good boss. At the heart of being a good clinician and a good boss is the ability to communicate. The objective of this chapter has been to provide some foundational skills that assist in being a better boss.

Building on these Basic Principles, Developing Habits, and Routines

By hueing closely to the principles and skills outlined here, Samantha was successfully able to make the transition from a full-time clinician to the dual role of clinician-manager. This successful transition has renewed Samantha's enthusiasm for audiology and challenged her to learn some new skills. These new skills allow greater managerial responsibility, either within the current organization or another one, if a different challenge is assumed elsewhere. Even if there is a move to another organization at some point in the future, with some of the management principles outlined here, a successor has been successfully groomed for the next clinician-manager. With time, patience, and some attention to detail, any clinician excelling at patient care can also become an effective manager. Samantha is still at heart a clinician but now understands that managers need to carve out at least a couple days per week

to manage. By mastering these nine skills discussed in this chapter, Samantha can build on her initial successes and develop in her role of clinical manager/director to assume even greater leadership roles within any organization. With the skills outlined here, both hats can be worn successfully. To quote the cattle rancher, cyberlibertarian, and Grateful Dead lyricist—a true Renaissance man, the late John Perry Barlow: "Avoid the pursuit of happiness. Define your mission and purpose and pursue that." There is no better place to pursue that ideal than as a clinical audiologist who is leading a team, all rowing in the same direction, making the world a better place.

References

Amlani, A. (2018). A comparative analysis of repaying the AuD student loan debt. http://hearinghealthmatters.org

Horstman, M. (2016). *The effective manager.* Wiley Press.

Peter, L. (1969). *The Peter principle.* William Morrow & Co Inc.

U.S. Bureau of Labor Statistics. (2023). Occupational outlook: Audiologists. https://www.bls.gov/ooh/healthcare/audiologists.htm

Windmill, I. M., & Freeman, B. A. (2013). Demand for audiology services: 30-yr projections and impact on academic programs. *Journal of the American Academy of Audiology, 24,* 407–416.

8 Employee Compensation Strategies

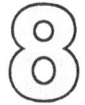

Robert M. Traynor, EdD, MBA, and Brian Taylor, AuD

Introduction

Many believe the most challenging aspect of practice management is fair and equitable compensation for employees, the goal of which is to pay employees, compensating them enough to be motivated and excited to go to work each day. While at the same time, the employer must be able to compensate employees without going into debt. Most practices are small without a human resources department, where the owner of the practice also becomes the human resources director. Consequently, audiologists have generally maintained an ambivalent relationship with compensation since the 1970s, when the profession first began dispensing hearing aids. At that time, audiologists were compensated by a salary with a benefits package that was paid mostly by hospitals, physicians, universities, or government agencies. At the time, the profession typically provided services, evaluations, and other non-product-related functions that created difficulty making a decent living in the field. In these situations, the way in which audiologists were compensated was shrouded in mystery: Clinicians merely showed up at work, saw their patients, and received a paycheck every 2 weeks.

One of the most significant changes since these halcyon days is that today's compensation packages are more complex. The methods by which audiologists are paid today is much more likely to be based, at least in part, on a variable pay structure. As this chapter outlines, variable pay structures are based on a percentage of total revenue generated in the practice where a significant part of total revenue in most practices is related to hearing aid sales. This change in compensation to a variable pay structure has tended to yield more lucrative compensation packages for audiologists who dispense hearing aids, but it does leave the door open to potential ethical breaches, as covered in this chapter.

The objective of this chapter is to examine how audiologists receive compensation. It offers a better understanding of the various ways audiologists are compensated and why audiologists are compensated for the dollar amounts they receive. In brief, audiologists and their support staff do not simply show up for work each day and magically receive a paycheck every month. Certain economic principles, such as supply and demand, underpin how much audiologists are compensated. Additionally, audiologists must generate and collect a certain amount of revenue through their work to receive a specific amount of compensation. That is, the more revenue audiologists generate, the more likely they are to receive higher compensation.

Before delving into the nuts and bolts of compensation, however, it is helpful to examine compensation strategies more broadly. Carrison and Walsh (2004) suggest that businesses, especially for human resource issues, should be maintained by the principles and techniques of the United States Marine Corps (USMC), building motivation for the mission and esprit de corps rather than merely a compensation package. They indicate that for all the differences between the military and the profit-driven corporations, these enterprises share the same key goal: to create a high-performance organization filled with committed, motivated personnel. Unfortunately, many of today's professionals are unlike the military and look to the compensation package first and motivation, esprit de corps, and the mission of the practice second. At the end of 8 years of study in a university program and the beginning of the career, audiologists should feel well compensated for the expenditure of time, energy, effort, and funds spent for school gaining the background, credentials, and experience to serve their patients.

This anxious relationship with compensation becomes complicated when there is a balancing act between fair compensation methods for clinicians, ethical standards created by the profession, and fairness to patients. On one hand, the profession and many clinicians

are *not comfortable* with variable compensation methods, but typical salary compensation systems lead to less motivation, less overall compensation for professionals, and, as a result, less efficiency in the use of revenue by the practice. Audiologist employees within a practice should be compensated to allow a good living commensurate with their credentials and experience and, possibly, an opportunity to buy into the practice or clinic of their own over time. Clerical employees should receive salary, benefits, and other compensation based upon their experience, longevity, and contributions to the practice.

Strategies for compensation are not straightforward; they are compounded not only by ethics and historical methods but also by annual reviews, raise procedures, profit participation, incentives, rewards, and other frustrating but necessary complexities. Therefore, the purpose of this chapter is to present perspectives into various intangible and tangible components of compensation packages for an audiology practice with special emphasis on payment arrangements for practice owners, their professional audiologist employees, and clerical staff.

The Nature of Compensation

Compensating people is a complex task requiring organizational systems and practices. Compensation systems have influences both inside and outside the organization. In today's world, there are new outside influences on compensation expectations, such as Internet searches for salaries in different geographic locations, analyses of what is expected for years of experience and education for a particular profession, and online chat rooms that discuss these issues. There are two sides to a compensation coin. One side represents income to employees and, the other, the cost to the employer. The term compensation is used to indicate the various forms of pay such as money, benefits, and nonfinancial rewards. Compensation packages for any size business have two components, intangible and tangible, and, according to Elsdon (2003), the key to obtaining and keeping good employees, particularly professionals, is to create an environment where employees want to stay and grow professionally with the practice. Although compensation packages in audiology practices are generally less than in large firms, providing expertise and contributions to a small company has definite advantages for the employees. Shwiff (2009) indicates that these advantages include:

- An opportunity to be more "hands on."
- The need to wear multiple hats resulting in a wider range of experiences and enhanced audiological and business skills.
- Greater chance for recognition for contributions.
- The "big frog/small pond" factor that results in speedier promotions and greater personal benefits.
- A stronger sense of ownership for ideas and concepts generated as well as work completed.
- Participating in a culture more geared toward fulfilling employee needs.
- A job that better utilizes employee's aptitudes and interests.
- Flextime.

- Remote working—telehealth.
- A chance to buy stock options and benefit financially from personal contributions to the practice.

Three Classes of Employees in an Audiology Practice

Generally, there are three classes of individuals within an audiology practice with different compensation packages: the *owner, employee audiologists, and the clerical staff.* Audiology practice owners are entrepreneurs, investing in a business to offer private clinical services to the public. For the practice owner, their monthly salary is sustenance. The perquisites (perks) of ownership can provide special benefits, the hope to sell the practice for a retirement income, independence, and, one hopes, the satisfaction of watching their small business grow into a thriving practice. Mathis et al. (2016) present three common elements of employment compensation packages: the psychological contract, job satisfaction, and loyalty and commitment. A portion of the package offered by the employee and paid for by the employer includes these factors, which may be an exceptional value or a substantial problem, depending upon the practice situation and the employee.

The Psychological Contract

Mackenzie (2016) suggests that an employee's psychological contract with a practice can be understood as a "deal" between employer and employee concerning "the perception of the two parties, employer and employee, of what their mutual obligations are toward each other." Lavelle (2003) formally defines a psychological contract as an unwritten expectation between employees and employers regarding the nature of their work relationship that is, to some degree, based upon past experiences of both parties. This psychological contract is a direct result of the downsizing of companies over the past few years and the resulting "free agent" nature of employees. In the past, employees may have given their loyalty and commitment to a company and been disappointed as the company had minimal commitment to them, cutting their pay, or involuntarily modifying their work relationship. When a company (or a practice) has a minimal commitment to their employees, they often become free agents offering their services to the highest bidder with no particular commitments beyond the contract dates.

Recently, employees have questioned if a company (or a practice) is worth their loyalty and commitment. Konrad (2006) suggests that when individuals feel they have some control and perceived rights in the organization, they are more likely to be committed to the organization. Audiology practices working toward a better quality of life for their patients are very likely to obtain a psychological commitment from both the employer and the employee since they both firmly believe in the cause. Clerical employees also feel a sense of belonging to the process and usually become psychologically involved, working toward the common goal of better hearing for the patients.

Job Satisfaction

Mathis et al. (2016) broadly define job satisfaction as a positive emotional state resulting from evaluating one's job experience. Conversely, job dissatisfaction occurs when expectations are not met for either the employee or the employer. Figure 8–1 offers factors that affect job satisfaction. For an audiology practice, the satisfaction of the employees with their position in the organization is very important to success since often it is the employees that represent the owner practitioner to the patients.

Performance should never be of concern if the employee is a fully educated, licensed audiologist or an experienced clerical employee. Although an employee may have the training and the experience, sometimes motivation to provide the evaluations, products, or support services could possibly be lacking. Motivational difficulties may include but are not limited to:

- Illness.
- A fight with a spouse that morning.
- A bad day.
- Low or reduced respect for the boss.
- Disagreement with the policies and procedures of the practice.
- General laziness.

Whatever the motivational problem, it is essential that these difficulties be rectified as soon as possible as they will only get worse, creating more concern for the practice owner, the other employees, and, ultimately, the patients.

Job satisfaction also is part of the job itself. Although employees expect to be able to perform in the position for which they are hired, a clerical employee may not expect to clean hearing aids as part of their position, or an employee audiologist may not expect that they will need to answer the phone or clean the office as these activities may

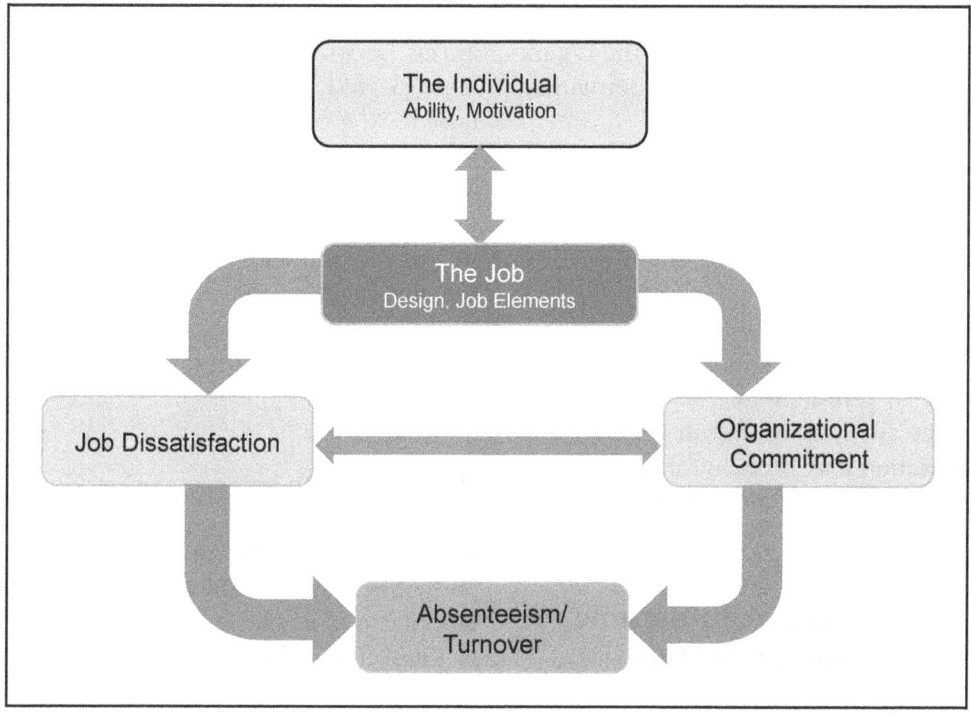

Figure 8–1. Factors affecting job satisfaction and organizational commitment (Mathis et al., 2016).

have not been part of their former positions. Part of creating satisfaction is the explanation of the position so the employee knows, upfront, the practice owner's expectations. Job satisfaction is greatly enhanced by openness in the job interview, presenting the specifics of each position in the practice along with expected extra duties. This "upfront" presentation of expectations leads to high overall job satisfaction, resulting in the employee's commitment to the organization. Motivated, committed employees have less absenteeism and are less likely to be looking elsewhere for employment. In tight labor markets or where audiologists are not readily available, job satisfaction and loyalty to the organization are clear factors in turnover.

Organizational Commitment

According to Mathis et al. (2016), organizational commitment is the degree to which the employees believe in and accept the organizational goals and desire to remain with the organization. Their data suggest that employees with a minimal commitment to the organization are not as satisfied with their jobs and are more likely to withdraw from the organization. Susanto et al (2022) offer that the relationship between job satisfaction and commitment with absenteeism and turnover has been affirmed across cultures, in both full- and part-time employees, genders, and occupations. Findings demonstrate that absenteeism and turnover are related as both involve withdrawal from the organization: absenteeism being a temporary withdrawal from the organization, whereas turnover is permanent.

Types and Philosophies of Compensation

In a comparison of the human resource literature, philosophical differences exist in terminology for various types of reward systems, but in general, compensation may be either intrinsic or extrinsic (Mathis et al., 2016).

Intrinsic or Intangible Compensation

Intrinsic rewards are intangible and may include praise or expressions of appreciation for a job well done or meeting performance objectives. Other psychological and social forms of compensation, such as paid time off, social status, travel opportunities, and retirement plans, are also intrinsic forms of employee rewards.

For many employees, the most valuable part of a compensation package is the intangible benefits offered by the position. Studies have found that intrinsic factors, such as professional growth and having a work environment in line with personal values, are more significant in predicting career satisfaction than extrinsic factors such as pay and continuing education. According to Ford (2024), balancing lives has become more important than ever, allowing flexible schedules, relaxed atmospheres, childcare, and other lifestyle benefits are almost as important as salaries, especially to Millennials. Their study of Millenni-

als indicates that 77% prioritize a balanced personal life over advancement at work and 52% would be willing to take a 20% pay cut to prioritize quality of life. Although a mainstay among Millennials, this is not just a recent concern among professional and clerical workers as this trend has been increasing for 25 years by employees in the United States, Europe, Russia, and Japan relative to qualities. The trend has been toward:

- The ability to balance work and personal life.
- Work that is truly enjoyable.
- Security for the future.
- Good pay or salary.
- Enjoyable coworkers.

Tangible compensation appeared as a distant fourth on their list of reasons for leaving positions, suggesting the importance of intangible benefits. More than two-thirds indicated that they would be willing to leave their company for such opportunities. Obringer (2024) indicated that 90% of 1,000 workers felt work/life balance was as important as health insurance and more than one-fourth of those surveyed considered the balance of work and family was more important than a competitive salary, job security, or support for an advanced degree.

In a study supporting the importance of indirect or intangible benefits of employment, 30% of all employees planned to quit their jobs in the next 2 years. Their concerns were not necessarily due to their cash compensation package but rather a function of the following reasons presented here in order of importance.

- Dissatisfaction with the manager.
- Lack of career opportunities.
- Job not "stretching" enough.
- Personal reasons (spouse, partner moving on, maternity, etc.).
- Cash compensation.

In the past few years, consistent research findings have been that cash compensation has been at the bottom of the list relative to the reasons workers were quitting their jobs, suggesting intangibles have become substantially more important than actual cash. Thus, the literature indicates that it is usually intrinsic compensation, not salary dissatisfaction, that leads employees to explore alternative job prospects.

Extrinsic or Tangible Compensation

Extrinsic rewards are tangible and may be both monetary and nonmonetary. Tangible rewards are of two types.

- Direct compensation.
- Indirect compensation.

Direct compensation is the money that changes hands in the form of base pay and variable pay offered by the employer to the employee in exchange for the work performed. Indirect compensation usually refers to employee benefits, such as health insurance, offered to all employees as part of employment in the organization. Figure 8–2 clarifies and details direct (tangible) and indirect (intangible) compensation for employees and represents the system by which most practice employees are compensated (Jensen et al., 2007).

Compensation Philosophies

Professional employees can be compensated in a variety of arrangements. Shwiff (2009) offers some business models for paying professional employees that are not unlike those offered to physicians, dentists, chiropractors, and other healthcare professionals. Audiology practices must decide what type of compensation system they want to offer. The system will be based upon the philosophy of the practice owner, the job market, economic conditions, and regional compensation figures.

Entitlement-Based Programs

Entitlement programs are those that assume all employees who have worked another year are entitled to pay increases with little or no regard for performance. Organizations that use an entitlement philosophy will commonly refer to these yearly increases as "cost of living" increases and they may or may not be tied to actual economic indicators. The net result of using an entitlement philosophy is that the employer will pay more for their employees each year, no matter what the performance of the business, since raises and bonuses become income to which employees feel entitled. Characteristics of entitlement compensation programs are as follows:

- Seniority bases.
- Across-the-board rises.
- Pay scales raised annually.
- Holiday or "Santa Claus" bonuses.

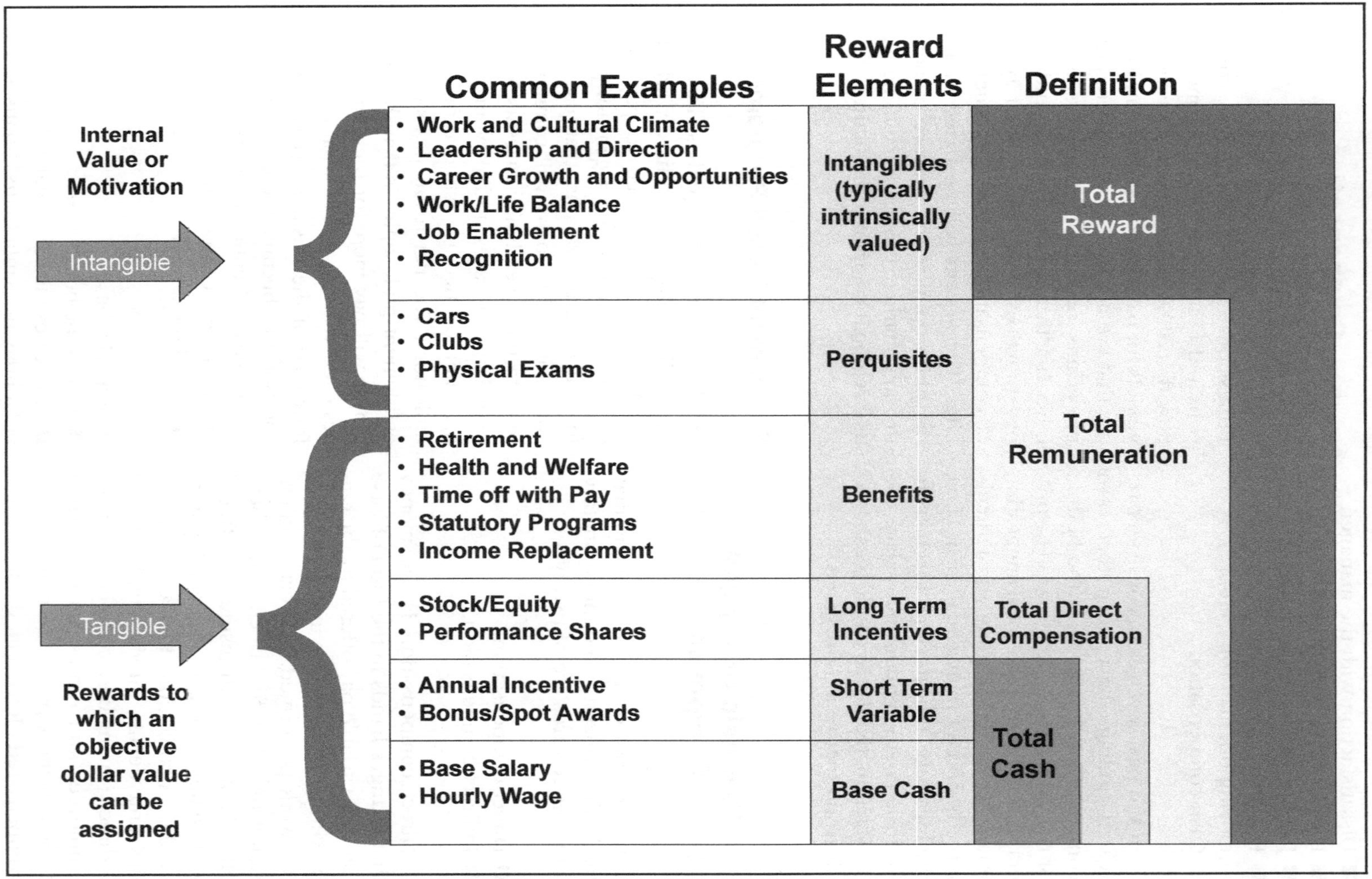

Definition	Reward Elements	Common Examples
Total Reward	Intangibles (typically intrinsically valued)	• Work and Cultural Climate • Leadership and Direction • Career Growth and Opportunities • Work/Life Balance • Job Enablement • Recognition
Total Remuneration	Perquisites	• Cars • Clubs • Physical Exams
	Benefits	• Retirement • Health and Welfare • Time off with Pay • Statutory Programs • Income Replacement
Total Direct Compensation	Long Term Incentives	• Stock/Equity • Performance Shares
Total Cash	Short Term Variable	• Annual Incentive • Bonus/Spot Awards
	Base Cash	• Base Salary • Hourly Wage

Internal Value or Motivation — Intangible

Rewards to which an objective dollar value can be assigned — Tangible

Figure 8–2. Direct (tangible) and indirect (intangible) compensation (Jensen et al., 2007).

Performance-Based Programs

Kyeremanteng et al. (2019) indicate that there is a trend to offer pay-for-performance in healthcare companies. Pay-for-performance is an umbrella term for initiatives aimed at improving the quality, efficiency, and overall value of healthcare. These arrangements provide financial incentives to hospitals, physicians, and other healthcare providers to carry out such improvements and achieve optimal outcomes for patients.

In a performance-based compensation philosophy, pay changes reflect the true differences among employees. Employees who perform satisfactorily or better than their coworkers advance in their positions, whereas those who are poor or marginal performers fall behind in the pay scale. These performance-based systems award bonuses and incentives according to the performance of an individual, the team, or the organization. Characteristics of performance-based compensation systems typically are:

- No raises for length of service.
- No raises for longer-service poor performers.

- Job market–adjusted pay structures.
- Broader compensation comparisons across the industry.
- Bonuses tied to performance results.

A comparison of the advantages and disadvantages of each compensation system is presented in Table 8–1 and described in detail in the following sections.

Straight Salary Model

According to Shwiff (2009), employees often prefer the straight salary approach, whereas more and more companies and professional practices are moving toward the alternative methods of compensation to incentivize their employees and spread their human resource costs across good and bad business seasons. Straight salary compensation systems are the traditional method of payment where the professional audiologist works in the clinic for a certain number of hours per week and is compensated with a salary. In this model, the employee obtains the same amount of salary each month for

Table 8–1. Comparison of Compensation Philosophies

	Straight Salary	Variable Pay	Skill Based
Advantages	1. Easy 2. Dependable for employees	1. Incentives 2. Rewards 3. Motivating 4. Variable cost	1. Incentive to learn new skills 2. Training for the employee 3. Higher trained staff
Disadvantages	1. No incentive 2. No rewards 3. Fixed cost	1. Ethical concern 2. Pay varies	1. Base pay begins lower 2. Must build skills to advance base pay 3. Training costs

the work provided if the clinic is active or slow. The individual will actually be contracted for all the work they can possibly do within the confines of the practice schedule. These systems usually offer no rewards for extra effort, hard work, cross-training, and/or overtime, and there is usually none exerted. Although experience suggests that straight salaries work relatively well for clerical individuals and part-time employees, this system usually fails to provide sufficient motivation for a full-time audiologist. A straight salary compensation method does not consider:

■ The practice cash flow situations.
■ Incentives for the employee.
■ Rewards for extra work or creativity.

Practices generally are susceptible to seasonal highs and lows. Many patients return to spend the summer in climates they have left due to the cold in winter months. In extremely slow periods, it would not be beneficial for the employer to pay a salary when the opportunity to produce revenue is at a low ebb. Conversely, when these "snowbirds" return, the audiologist employee will be working extremely hard.

Variable Compensation Model

The variable compensation model, sometimes referred to as "pay at risk," places a portion of the compensation contingent upon performance. This model provides incentives for employees by allowing them to share the profit that is generated by their increased contributions to the productivity of the practice. A variable pay program not only ensures a healthy bottom line for the clinic but,

according to Leapsome (2024), can be a solution for disengagement and poor performance. In many fields, surveys point out that employees are not motivated by their current compensation system and, in fact, do not even believe their performance has any influence on compensation. A variable compensation program should include the following components:

■ *Profit sharing.* Profit-sharing programs are employee incentives wherein a portion of the practice's profits will be set aside at year end and distributed to the employees.
■ *Group incentive.* Group incentives are given for participation in a group project or an overall goal of the practice.
■ *Recognition.* Individual incentive, or key contributor awards. These awards are for the individual achievement by a particular employee, such as the completion of an AuD, obtaining skills that will be useful to the practice, high sales, or other individual contribution to the practice that results in benefit to the practice. These awards may take the form of a lump-sum bonus, awards of stock or equity in the practice, or simply a restaurant coupon or a plaque but are meant to recognize the individual contribution.
■ *Project/team incentive.* Group awards involving a team of individuals that work together to further the goals of the practice. These awards are for group efforts that contribute to the success of the practice, such as a busy month, learning a new office management system, or other group effort that makes the practice more efficient.

■ *Participative peer award.* Nominations of an employee by another employee for a job well done may not be obvious to the practice owner. These are also individual awards that may take almost any form but are usually reserved for small rewards such as lunch or dinner, plaques, or some other simple recognition.

Designing a variable compensation program is no small task. An incentive program that rewards an employee for diligent, hard work for providing excellent patient-centric care will go a long way toward motivation. Leapsome (2024) also indicates that exceptional care should be taken into consideration by the practitioner in the design of a variable pay program offering the following:

Employers must create a work environment that inspires, engages, and empowers employees. From fostering a culture of recognition to providing opportunities for growth and autonomy, the following are some methods that motivate employees and drive the practice to success:

Validate and Appreciate

Recognition acknowledges efforts, contributions, and achievements, and it shows that peers, managers, and the organization value the employee's work. Feeling appreciated fosters an emotional connection with work, boosting job motivation and self-esteem. This could be via a kudos wall or virtual platform for shout-outs and gratitude for hard work. It is important to recognize everyone who has interacted with a project, not just those who took it to the finish line.

Provide Training

Practices that provide training assist their employees in acquiring new skills, knowledge, and competencies. By developing their capabilities, employees feel more competent and confident in their roles, which can boost motivation and increase loyalty. These increased skills may be used to provide new services and increase the practice revenue.

Offer Mentorship

Mentorship programs that create opportunities for both professional and clerical colleagues to establish meaningful relationships with mentors who are genuinely invested in their future can be a powerful employee motivation strategy. The presence of both formal and informal mentors can enhance job motivation and growth, providing skills that increase potential for increasing their value to the practice.

Encourage Autonomy

Autonomy provides employees with a sense of ownership and control over their work and allows them to provide services that are in line with their personal style as well as clinical strengths. They feel empowered to make decisions, set goals, and determine how to approach their tasks and clinical endeavors. This sense of ownership provides a stronger sense of loyalty, responsibility, and commitment, motivating employees to take initiative and be accountable for their successes and those situations that require improvement.

Provide Career Development Opportunities

Career development is another important consideration when deciding how to motivate both the clerical and professional teams. This goes beyond promotions. Skills training, workshops, and courses help employees acquire new knowledge relevant to their roles, learn new practice techniques, and prepare for future career aspirations. Offering opportunities for continuous learning and professional development demonstrates an investment in the growth of the employee as well as enhances the practice. Career development boosts motivation in the practice as it offers both clerical and professional personnel a stronger sense of clarity and most of all a future.

Offer Comprehensive Benefits

A survey by Glassdoor (2015) found that 79% of employees would prefer additional benefits over raises in pay, and this preference was 10% to 15% higher among younger employees. Comprehensive benefits, such as high-quality mental health benefits, retirement plans, and health insurance, may motivate an employee by providing a sense of security. These days, this can involve quite an investment from the practice, but even some benefits in this direction make a statement toward how valuable employees are and the difference they make to the patients within the practice.

Provide Useful Resources

Ensuring that workers have the resources they need to do their jobs is crucial for employee motivation. When professional employees have access to sophisticated tools, such as the latest equipment, rehabilitative treatment technology, and other treatment resources, they can work more effectively, provide better diagnoses, have more successful rehabilitative outcomes, and support the overall vision of the practice. Clerical employees supplied with the latest computers and programs and advanced accounting capabilities will give them the ability to provide the very best services. This increased efficiency and productivity not only breeds a sense of accomplishment but also fuels workers' motivation as they have the resources they need to meet their goals.

Improve Processes

Having well-established systems in place, such as clear workflows and transparent communication, can also positively affect employee motivation in both groups (Chapters 6, 7, 9, 15). When employees know how to navigate their tasks and where to seek guidance, it creates a sense of empowerment and enables them to perform at their best. Conversely, a lack of transparency and unclear processes can be demotivating, leaving individuals feeling uncertain and hindered in their work.

Skill-Based Compensation (SBC)

Specifically, Dierdoff and Surface (2008) define skill-based compensation (SBC) as a nontraditional pay system that ties base wages of the employee to knowledge and skills obtained rather than simply the job to which they are assigned. The philosophy is that both professional and clerical employees will be proactive in obtaining new, job-related skills if they are compensated for such efforts. For example, a clerical person may have an aspiration to become an audiology assistant (Chapter 10), requiring substantially more skills and becoming more valuable to the practice, generating a salary increase. Or, an audiologist may want to learn how to assess central auditory disorders or program cochlear implants, also becoming more valuable to the practice. This is a basic principle of behavioral psychology: Actions that lead to rewards will be repeated. Thus, the underlying concept behind a skill-based pay system is relatively simple: Increase an employee's compensation as they acquire skills and become more valuable to the practice. There are four types of SBC plans, which can be categorized by the type of skills tracked and rewarded as follows:

- Vertical skill plans measure the acquisition of input/output skills (e.g., being able to calibrate audiometric equipment without the assistance of a technician or successfully troubleshooting computer problems).
- Horizontal skill plans reward the acquisition of complementary skills (e.g., individual learns how to do both accounts payable and accounts receivables) across several jobs.
- Depth skill plans reward skill specialization (e.g., developing a specialized skill in pediatric assessment and management or running the front desk and developing skills in hearing aid troubleshooting and cleaning).
- Combination plans reward any of the skills of the above.

Shwiff (2009) presents that skill-based programs reward individuals for acquiring certain work-related skills or additional technical proficiencies. It contributes to job enlargement and enrichment by breaking down narrow job classifications. Specifically, the benefits of a skill-based compensation program are as follows:

- Flexibility is increased by encouraging the performance of multiple tasks. It enables job rotation and contributes to a leaner workforce.
- It enhances productivity and quality through better use of human resources.
- It facilitates technological change.
- The higher pay levels, continuous training, and job enlargement through the broadening of skills tend to reduce staff turnover.
- Elimination of unnecessary jobs can result from a workplace having broad, rather than narrow, skills. It also reduces the need for supervision.
- Broadening of skills leads employees to develop a better perspective of practice and how it operates.
- It is an incentive for self-development.
- It provides employment security through skills enhancement.
- Since the reward flows from the application of a skill and it does not reduce opportunities for others to similarly increase their skills and earnings, there is likely to be less competition among individuals.
- Since the pay increases because skills are linked to a measurable standard, the criticism of subjectivity often associated with performance appraisals and

individual-based performance-related pay is avoided.

Skill-based compensation could be also applied to audiologists who seek and attain specialty certification in cochlear implants or pediatrics or advanced training that would enable the practice to expand or add new diagnostic or treatment protocols. Furthermore, practices often hire new audiologists directly out of school, and these individuals are not initially able to conduct all evaluations on all populations in a timely manner. Skill-based compensation works well for these new clinicians as they will get familiar with the equipment and specifics of the practice's procedures in a shorter time. Thus, the base starting pay for a new clinician may need to be lower and increased as the skills and capability to work independently increase. Clerical employees hired to greet patients and set up files could also learn how to keep books, conduct superficial hearing aid cleaning, order products, send products out for repairs, and so on. Generally, human resource professionals agree that skill-based compensation programs:

- Encourage skill development.
- Reward learning.
- Increase individual productivity.
- Encourage more flexible staffing.

Computing a Tangible Base Salary and Salary Range for Employees

A crucial step in a compensation program for a practice is setting the base pay and salary ranges for all employees. This should be part of the job description for every position. Obringer (2024) describes a procedure for establishing a standard base pay program and offers fixed salary ranges for employees performing the standard duties of their jobs. Applying this system, an audiologist who has only conducted diagnostics for 5 years or a new audiologist directly out of school might be on the lower end of the scale, whereas a veteran clinician able to see a full range of patients would be at the top of the compensation range. Although setting a base pay structure can be challenging, the following points should be considered:

- Determine where your practice falls relative to competitive compensation packages within the region.
- Set up your base pay levels to be competitive with other practices in the area.
- Use the Internet to review salaries, nationally and regionally. An invaluable resource for determining salaries is membership in the Academy of Doctors of Audiology, where numerous resources are available to determine compensation structures geared specifically for audiology practices.

Market Banding

Mathis et al. (2016) offer a method called "market banding" used by human resources professionals to establish base pay and salary ranges. Market banding is used for smaller groups and classifications of employees and is ideal for use by audiology practice owners to compute base salary and salary ranges. The straightforward steps to tangible salary and salary ranges using the market banding approach are outlined in the following sections.

Step 1—Job Families

In most audiology practices, three distinct job families will surface: the practice owner, audiologist employees, and the clerical assistants. Designating these families is Step 1 of the process.

Step 2—Salary Review Surveys

The second step is to launch a regional survey that reviews salaries for the various job families. Determine the median salaries and the highest to lowest salaries from the median in percentages. For example, if the median base salary for an employee audiologist with 10 years' experience is $80,000 and a 13% adjustment up and down is noted between the highest and lowest salaries survey, then the raw survey result would be $80,000 ± 13%.

Step 3—Adjustment for Practice Personnel Expenditure

In this example, once obtained, the median salary ($80,000) must be adjusted according to the practice budget for overall personnel expenditure. This adjustment amount is found as the result of calculations on the personnel budget by the practice owner and the accountant's input of revenue relative to the overall expenditure for personnel. From the $80,000 figure (obtained from survey information), a negative personnel expenditure adjustment of $6,000 (suggested by the practice accountant) is needed to adjust the median base salary to $74,000.

Step 4—Figuring the Salary Range

In the example presented here, $74,000 would be the median salary adjusted for practice personnel budget limitations. The survey also indicated that there was a 3% salary range from the adjusted median salary. Thus, the base salary range for an audiologist employee in this practice would be ± $7,215 or a salary range of $64,380 to $83,620. The practice owner may use this information to adjust the salary offering slightly up or down according to the quality of the application.

Step 5—Figuring the Hourly Rates for Clerical Employees

The same "market banding" procedure can be applied to hourly employees using a survey to determine median hourly rates for clerical employees. For example, if the survey indicated a median salary for a qualified receptionist with 5 years' experience and computer skills was $16.00 per hour, according to the practice owner's philosophy and the accountant's personnel budget, a recommendation of $1.00 per hour reduction would bring the hourly wage to $15.00. If the survey indicated an hourly wage variation of ± 10% for employees with these qualifications, then the hourly wage range for the practice clerical staff would be $13.50 to $16.50 per hour. There are Internet sites for a fee that will present average salaries for audiology employees and clerical assistants. Although often not as regionally accurate as market banding, these sites can be valuable in the determination of salaries and salary ranges when it is difficult to obtain information from surveys and local sources.

Benefits for Employees

Audiologist employees and clerical staff may be offered a number of other tangible benefits included in a package. The practice owner may decide to include all of those listed here or compile another list with their accountant and/or human resource consultant. This list of benefits for employees is modified from that offered by Jensen et al. (2007) in Figure 8–3. After the base salary, the tangible benefits of the position are incentives to provide a comfortable situation for the employee so that they will be able to concentrate on their work each day as well as feel well rewarded for their labor and expertise.

Bonus or Spot Rewards

These are bonuses offered for an individual's job well done, teamwork on a specific project, or simply meeting the goals of the practice. Specifically, these rewards could be for meeting a sales goal for a particular number of assessments forauditory brainstem response (ABR) and videonystagmography (VNG) or hearing instruments for a particular month and might take the form of a restaurant certificate, expenses to a meeting, or cash. Usually this is a small amount that simply serves to acknowledge the extra effort and encourage it in other employees.

Performance Shares in the Company

As an incentive or reward, the practice owner may choose to offer shares in the company for a job well done. The practice owner recognizes that the extra effort to meet a goal demonstrates interest in the success of the practice.

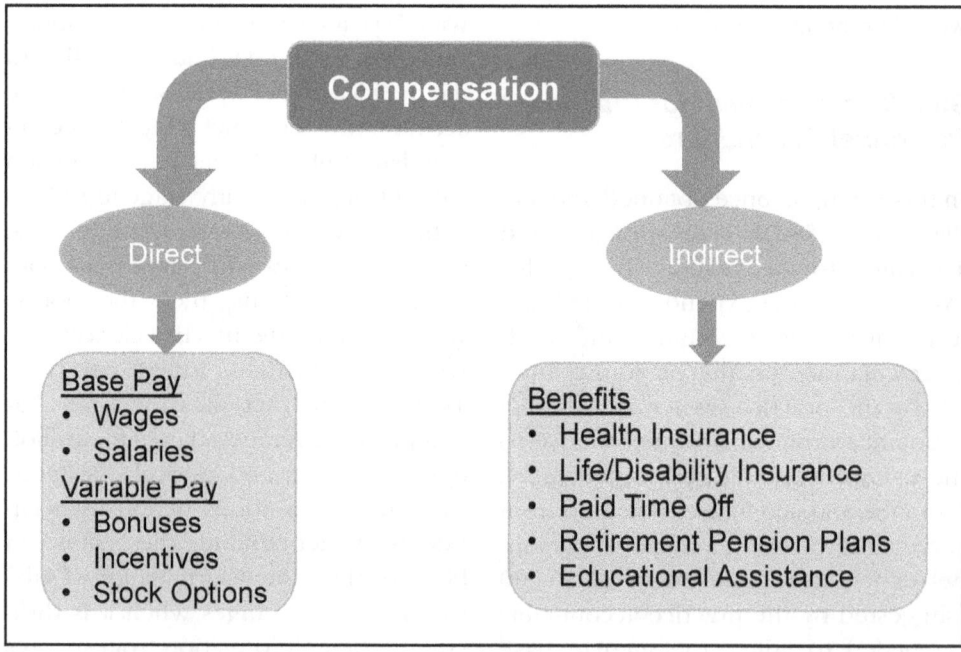

Figure 8–3. Employee compensation (Jensen et al., 2007).

Therefore, shares in the company can be a method to reward loyalty.

Annual Employee Incentive or Bonus Program

These programs reward the employee for meeting sales and/or marketing goals over the year. Usually based on targets for the year, if the practice meets the targets, the bonus is offered. Annual bonuses can be given during the holidays, the anniversary of employment, or at the discretion of the practice owner. It is important that annual incentives and bonuses are presented as rewards for a job "well done" and not given frequently and in the same amounts. If given incorrectly, these incentives will typically be perceived by the employees as not a bonus but as part of their usual and customary compensation, defeating the incentive purpose of the bonus program.

Income Replacement (Disability Insurance)

Short-term disabilities, such as broken ankles or hospital stays, can be part of the overall employment package or simply handled internally by the practice owner according to the policies and procedures manual. Income replacement or long-term disability insurance is not a common benefit of employment but may be offered by some practices for long-term disabilities. Long-term disabilities are considered serious injuries that cause major life changes, such as confinement to a wheelchair, brain injuries, or other physical modifications that affect the employee's capability to be productive. Long-term disability insurance is a must for the audiology prac-

tice owner but usually not part of the employee's package. When offered as a benefit to the employees, these benefits are usually presented as an optional insurance that may be purchased by the employees through private funds.

Statutory Programs (Workers' Compensation)

In all states, it is mandatory that employers purchase workers' compensation insurance. Employees are never required to pay any part of the premium for this coverage since it is the employer that is covered by these policies. The purpose of these policies is to protect the practice and the practice owner from damages that could be awarded in lawsuits that could conceivably put them out of business. For example, a faulty infection control program in an audiology clinic could be grounds for a workers' compensation claim.

Paid Time Off (PTO)

Specific types of time off are usually presented in the policies and procedures manual, but special time off with pay can be awarded to employees as an incentive or reward for extra work on a specific project or reaching a goal.

Health and Welfare Insurance

While health insurance has always been part of a benefits package for employees, at this writing, health insurance benefits are in a state of flux. Due to the passage of the Affordable Care Act in 2010 and now the probable repeal and replacement of this legislation that is currently before Congress, it is difficult to determine how regulations and incentives will apply to clerical and professional positions in audiology clinics. Currently, regulations fluctuate according to the state, insurance plans now come and go, government websites do not work, and a myriad of other issues make businesses hesitant to hire offering health and welfare insurance. Of course, these benefits provide security for the employee and their family and ensure that health difficulties can be taken care of expeditiously at reasonable cost. Health insurance, discussed in detail later, is usually available through insurance brokers, specialists in the insurance business offering a variety of policies to the practice and its employees. Currently, it is best to consult these professionals that follow health insurance programs to obtain the latest information on how to provide these benefits or if the clinic can afford to offer these benefits at all.

Retirement Program

Programs for retirement, though beneficial and necessary for employees, have been significantly reduced in the past few years. Practice managers may choose to offer these programs, offer them with modifications, or not offer them at all, especially in light of new regulations for Social Security and discussions if these government programs will exist in the future. When offered, retirement programs can take on many different forms, such as stock option programs, 401(k) plans, and simple savings plans. It is best to discuss these programs with financial advisors, the practice accountant, or the practice attorney as regulations for these programs can be quite complicated and vary from state to state.

Physical Exams

Some practices offer wellness exams in their clinic or at an outside office. These wellness exams are considered a nice benefit but are usually not included in the usual benefit package.

Clubs

Dues to a country, fitness, social, or golf club are usually reserved for the practice owner. Occasionally, the employee audiologist may be invited to become a member as part of an incentive or a benefits package. When offered to employees, there is usually a marketing reason to provide such a benefit. For example, a club where referral sources gather may result in patients for the practice.

Automobiles

Transportation benefits are not part of the usual tangible package for employee audiologists or clerical personnel. There may be special circumstances, however, where travel is required that makes this benefit necessary for employees. Rather than supplying a vehicle for employees, it makes more sense to provide transportation or pay mileage and expenses according to procedures outlined in the policies and procedures manual (Chapter 9) if the employees are required to travel distances to maintain clinics in other cities.

Education Benefits for Employees

Most practice owners consider their employees an important investment. Practices want to hire the best and the brightest and then give them the experience and continuing education they need to stay current in their profession or, for clerical personnel, to further their education and/or increase office skills. As part of their benefit package, the employer may choose to offer an education benefit to enhance the package. Particularly in these times of changing tax regulations, it is best to consult the practice's accountant before offering these benefits to employees so that the legal implications and seen and unseen costs are covered.

Insurance Benefits

Insurance benefits are essential to any business operation, and the audiology practice is no exception. To attract and retain high-quality employees, the practice must offer competitive insurance benefit programs. The specific programs offered are determined by the regional employment market, the needs of the employees, and the companies that offer policies in the area.

Health Insurance

Health insurance is an important benefit for every employee, including the practice owner. As indicated earlier in this chapter, the whole health insurance industry is in total disarray at this writing. The unsuccessful Affordable Care Act of 2010 has been a complete disaster nationally and disrupted the whole health insurance industry. Currently, there is a movement to repeal and replace this unsuccessful legislation with a more "user-friendly" program. While this new program will most likely be more readily available and cover necessary health concerns at a substantial

savings to employers, these programs are subject to drastic change over the next few years. How small business will handle these new programs has yet to be determined, but if these programs return to methods of consideration used in the past, there are several questions a practice owner must ask when considering healthcare insurance for the practice employees:

- What coverage plans are available in the area?
- Does my insurance broker carry health insurance?
- Should I use an HMO or a PPO to save costs?
- Should I pay all of the policy for the employee or only a portion of the premium?
- What other ancillary services, such as vision and dental care, should I offer in addition to standard health insurance?
- How will government regulation of the provision of health insurance change what the practice needs to do for their employees in the next 5 years?

The above questions are answered by health insurance brokers that have studied all the various policies and providers in the area. Insurance is their business, and they are eager to present a proposal to the practice considering several companies with the costs versus benefits presented. The broker typically has analyzed these programs and will make recommendations depending upon the needs of the practice. It is recommended to invite the health insurance broker to the practice to discuss insurance options at least once a year with the entire staff. All employees should participate in the discussion of this important benefit as it facilitates an understanding of the advantages and disadvantages of the various health insurance options and the rationale for the choice of a particular program. The provision of health insurance will be precarious for quite some time.

Disability and Life Insurance

The offering of disability and life insurance to the employee is not normally part of a regular compensation package for employees of a small audiology practice but is, as presented earlier, essential for the practice owner. Depending on the size of the practice group, life insurance can be offered to employees for as little as 5 cents per $1,000 worth of coverage. The practice employees and prospective employees appreciate this benefit as they do not usually need a physical before they are covered by the policy and can often convert the plan to an individual life insurance plan, if and when they leave the practice. The actual amount of this policy should be discussed and decided by the practice owner and accountant. Additionally, if the practice pays for the benefit, it is considered taxable income, whereas if the employee pays for the benefit, it is considered insurance and is nontaxable.

Vacations, Holidays, and Personal Time Off

Generally, practitioners will spend about 10% of their payroll on paid time off for their employees, but it is a highly rated employee benefit. Employees attempt to balance work, family time, and life experiences. An established policy for paid time off (PTO) should be written and included in the policies and procedures manual. It should include the number of days granted relative to years of service, specifying lunch and break times as well as holidays paid and unpaid. Practices usually provide paid holidays for their employees. Although the specific holidays offered to the employees vary according to the individual practice owner based on philosophy, religion, regions, and state, the typical holidays include:

- New Year's Day.
- President's Day.
- Memorial Day.
- Independence Day.
- Labor Day.
- Thanksgiving Day and the day after.
- Christmas Eve and Christmas Day.

In addition to standard holidays, the practice may also choose to provide one to two floating holidays or personal days. These days can be used whenever the employee would like to use them and often make up for religious holidays that are not part of the practice's standard paid holiday schedule.

Obringer (2024) indicates that the average number of vacation days provided by businesses for new employees is 10 per year, with increases to 15 after 5 years and 20 after 10 to 15 years. Vacation time is usually accrued on a monthly or quarterly basis, and most practices use a calendar year to make their recordkeeping easier. Obringer indicates that the business standard for a practice is to provide 6 to 9 sick days per year. Unlike vacation time, the number of sick days offered typically does not increase with increasing years of service and unused sick leave does not carry over to the following year. Another necessary decision for the practice owner is if employees will be allowed to use their paid sick days to take care of the illnesses of family members. Most audiology practices have fewer than 75 people and do not fall under the Family Medical Leave requirement, and thus the practice owner is not required to provide time off for employee family illnesses (Burrows, 2006; Ellison, 1999).

Stock Options

Sometimes used as a tool to retain employees, a stock options benefit has some appeal in today's job market. Doctors of Audiology are not merely looking for work but a *long-term position within a practice.* Stock options represent an attractive incentive in the hiring and retention of quality professional and administrative personnel. These programs are under the control of the U.S. Securities and Exchange Commission. Consultation with the practice's accountant and a licensed securities broker is imperative before stock options are offered. The plan must also be viewed by the attorney of record for the practice.

Retirement Programs

Retirement may seem like a long way off, but it is an important item to consider in attracting and retaining employees. There are several types of plans to choose from for retirement programs. The practice should consider this benefit only through the advice of the accountant, financial advisor, and

the practice's attorney regarding the specific advantages and disadvantages of each type.

Cash, Deferred Profit-Sharing Plans, and 401(k) Programs

Some companies offer profit-sharing programs. Profit-sharing programs require establishing a formula for distribution of the company profits. These plans are usually based on a distribution percentage of the employee's salary but require the employee to be in their position for a specified period before the profit-sharing programs are available to them. This vesting period makes profit-sharing programs primarily an incentive to retain employees.

Cash Profit-Sharing Plans

Cash profit-sharing plans pay benefits directly to the employees in cash, check, or stock as soon as profits are determined. Profit sharing allows the practice owner to decide if a contribution will be affordable and, if affordable, how much the company will contribute to the plan. Learner (2012) indicates that a designated profit level should be established as a goal to achieve, which allows the program to automatically go into effect when profits of a certain amount are reached for the year. The percentage of profits or the arbitrary level at which the program initiates action is usually shared by the employees and is normally established and articulated in advance. For example, the practice owner may say that 10% of all profits over $50,000 will be set aside for the profit-sharing program. In corporations, profit-sharing contributions are usually made by a fixed formula, or an amount decided by the Board of Directors (BOD) (often the BOD is simply the practice owner). In high profit years, contributions are made, and during less profitable years, contributions can be deferred. Profit-sharing plans also allow the practice owner to control how the money is invested. This plan is not as expensive to administer as other plans that require administrative professionals for management. The major drawback to a cash profit-sharing program is that these programs do not qualify as a retirement plan since they are difficult to predict contribution schedules and are at the discretion of the practice owner.

Deferred Profit-Sharing Plans

Deferred profit-sharing plans are designed to provide benefits for retirement. The benefits for retirement are based on the total of the contributions and the results of the investments made over time. The difference between cash and deferred plans is that a deferred plan must provide a definite predetermined formula. The benefits at retirement are based strictly upon the sum total of the contributions made according to the formula and the quality of the resulting investments.

401(k) Programs

U.S. Legal (2024) defines a 401(k) program as a contribution plan that enables employees to choose between receiving current compensation and making pretax contributions to an account through a salary reduction agreement. Employers may but are not required to make matching contributions to employees'

accounts. These plans defer federal income taxes and, in most cases, state income taxes as 401(k) contributions are made before payroll tax deductions. This is conducted to effectively reduce the employee's income before the taxes are figured, allowing them to invest with before-tax dollars and pay taxes on the income later when their incomes are lower during retirement. As part of the process, the employee receives an investment return on their money, occasionally with the practice matching their contributions. This use of "before-tax dollars" to defer taxes allows the employee to simplify their investment decision and contribute through a payroll deduction. The U.S. Department of Labor (2024) states that when the practice owner establishes a 401(k) plan, there are certain basic preparations that must be conducted:

- Find an administrator or service provider for the plan.
- Decide if the practice will make contributions to the plan.
- Inform the employees that there is a 401(k) plan.
- Arrange for a trust fund or other account to receive the proceeds from the 401(k) program.
- Submit a written plan to the IRS that describes the type of 401(k) plan and how it operates. Most of the administrators, such as banks or mutual funds, can assist with this requirement.
- Learn about the fiduciary responsibility, reporting, and disclosure requirements that are a part of managing a 401(k) plan.

The 401(k) plan is a major commitment to employees. Although there may be years when there are no contributions, the employees still have their own contributions, and they are making money with before-tax dollars that allow them to benefit greatly from the program. For the practice owner, there is a significant amount of paperwork and administrative monitoring that goes along with these programs, but once organized, the day-to-day operation of the plan will be handled by the administrator who works out the payroll deductions and makes the appropriate deposits of practice profits to the appropriate accounts.

Base Salary, Benefits, and Perquisites for the Practice Owner

There must be tangible and generous monetary rewards for the practice owner to offset the risk assumed in the initial and continuous investment in the practice. Market banding works very well to figure base salaries and salary ranges for employees but not for practice owners. Most practice owners do not readily offer their salary and benefits to others in a survey and, therefore, these market banding ranges are difficult to obtain for practice owners. A good "rule of thumb" is for the practice owner to set their salary about the same or slightly above the employee audiologists and then use the perks and management skills to offset the difference.

In close consultation with the practice accountant, the perks of practice ownership can be used to glean other forms of direct and indirect compensation that generally go along with business ownership or executive-level employment. Increased perks will sometimes work to the practice's advantage as they are often partially or fully deductible.

Virtually all tangible and intangible rewards presented previously in Figure 8–2 and possibly others not listed may be available as compensation to the practice owner. Compensation of the owner of the practice, who is often the chairperson of the board of directors for the practice's corporation, may require a formal discussion and a resolution at a corporate board meeting to allow the practice owner certain perks. The board of directors of these small corporations usually consists of the owner's accountant, attorney, and relatives so they will likely vote for a liberal salary and benefits. Most states allow the practice owner that is chairperson of the board of directors to have compensation for their service on the board, which may consist of extra perks or an actual tangible salary. Although the practitioner may choose a salary that is virtually unlimited, their base salary should follow some logical compensation sequence like the other audiologist employees of the practice.

Benefits and rewards of being in business belong to the practice owner. Bank prizes for depositing money, benefits from suppliers (if the ethical choice is to accept them), and other incentives normally available to business owners are a tangible benefit of entrepreneurship. For example, it is quite common for audiology practices to pay many of their supplier accounts payables on credit cards. The benefits of the credit cards, such as airline miles, cash rebates, points for merchandise, and other benefits, are usually a tangible reward for the owner of the practice.

When business is profitable, the practice owner can award themselves a handsome bonus, a reward, an incentive, extra retirement contribution, time off, or other benefit, provided that all legal, corporate, and tax regulations are observed. Additionally, benefits such as travel to meetings, books, continuing education, and country club memberships for themselves and their families may be written off as legitimate business expenses.

Disability and Life Insurance

Insure.com (2024) indicates that nearly one third of all Americans will suffer a serious disability between the ages of 35 and 65. Practice owners need to consider these statistics and consider disability and life insurance as an essential part of their compensation package. Disability and life insurance policies allow an income cushion to continue practice operations in the event of the disability or death of the owner. These benefits are not necessarily just for the practice owner but also for the good of the employees, the owner's family, and the patients.

Short-term disability, in the United States, is not provided by many employers and certainly not by most private practices, even for owners. Short-term disability insurance, however, is designed to replace an employee's income on a short-term basis as a result of a disability. Short-term disability (STD) pays a percentage of the practice owner's salary if temporarily disabled. Temporarily disabled is defined by Insure.com (2024) as not able to work for a short period of time due to sickness or injury (excluding on-the-job injuries, which are covered by work-ers' compensation insurance). Short-term disability policies typically provide a weekly portion of the practice owner's salary, usually 50% or 60%, or 66% for 13 to 26 weeks, depending on the program selected. If the practice owner has enough in savings to meet personal and practice needs for a 3-month period without working, then short-term disability insurance is not necessary. However, if there is not much in savings or the practice is a solo operation, a short-term disability policy is essential.

Long-term disability is not required by law, but it should be considered as an essential benefit for the practice owner. Long-term disability insurance helps recover about 60% of the insured income for an extended period of time, usually ending after 5 years or when the disabled person turns 65, when Social Security benefits usually pick up the disability benefit. There is usually a period of time before the long-term disability policy will pay benefits, usually 30 to 180 days or when the short-term disability policies end. As a practice owner, audiologists in self-supporting private practice must consider long-term disability insurance. The economic security of the practice and, therefore, the practitioner, all the employees, and their families are at risk when illness or injury strikes the practice owner.

Although some degree of protection is secured automatically from Social Security Disability through FICA deductions, Social Security only guards against catastrophic loss of all work capability. When dealing with the government, there are specific rules and regulations that must be adhered to by these agencies. Qualification for Social Security disability requires that a claimant must be unable to perform any gainful work at all. There is no partial or percentage disability under the Social Security Act.

Private insurers, however, offer income protection in the event of a disability over a wide range of disability types and levels, including temporary disruption of capability (short-term disability) to perform, permanent or long-term disability, and partial disability coverage. Qualifying for private disability benefits is not as demanding and, in some cases, not as demeaning as meeting the requirements of Social Security. Less demanding qualification does not mean that an assessment of ability to perform duties will not be evaluated. Private insurers will assess the capabilities of the insured and cover needs relative to that assessment.

Thus, disability income insurance is an important benefit that should be paid with after-tax dollars, especially for the practice owner. As there are many variables in the selection of these policies, it makes sense to use an insurance broker to assist in the selection. These policies are often handled by the same broker as the practice's health insurance, and their job is to present an insurance package that includes the state minimums as well as some optional program that meets the needs of the practice. Some of the variables of these policies include everything from the exclusion period, which can be based on different time periods if it is an injury or illness, to preexisting condition limitations, self-reported claim limitations, own-occupation protection, and rate guarantee. The specifics of the amount of income replacement and the benefits to the practice should be discussed in detail with the practice ac-

countant to ensure adequate cash flow to the practice as well as to the practice owner.

As with disability insurance, life insurance for the practice owner is essential. Proceeds of the policy ensure the survival of the practice in the event of death of the owner. While the proceeds of the policy will pay necessary practice expenses until arrangements for its disposition are finalized, the actual amount of life insurance should be discussed with the practice accountant.

Automobiles

The practice may lease or purchase a vehicle for use by the practice owner. This vehicle is technically for the purpose of making deliveries, providing transportation to peripheral clinics during the day, and other places required for business. Any other use of the vehicle is personal use and is usually taxable to the practice owner. Thus, most practices provide the practice owner with a company vehicle (either leased or purchased) and declare a percentage (85% to 95%) to be used for business purposes and another percentage (5% to 15%) to be used for personal purposes. The practice owner may deduct all the acquisition costs and maintenance expenses.

Country Club Dues

Along with practice ownership is the ability to become a member of exclusive clubs in the area and to deduct some of the expense as marketing. As with other incentives such as automobiles, the wise practitioner pays a portion of the dues themselves. This allows most of the expense to be considered as a business deduction, but also a portion is paid by the owner with the taxable income to ensure there are no questions about the personal or business use of the club.

Putting It All Together: Insights Hiring Another Employee

Knowing when to hire another person for the practice is one of the most critical decisions an owner or manager will ever make. This is largely because the price of labor is high and relatively fixed. Even the lowest-paid employees come at an annual cost of more than $30,000 when wages and benefits are calculated. Experts generally agree that a business' pretax profit needs to be at least 10% of total annual revenue before hiring another person on the staff. In other words, if 10% or higher pretax profit has not been generated in the last year, you probably need to keep your labor costs constant. However, if pretax profit is 10% or more of total revenue, then you can begin the process of hiring another person.

The two major reasons for bringing another person on board is generating more revenue (and profit) or lessening the practitioner's workload. The former represents a challenge surrounding the division of labor, while the latter signifies a change in the owner's role within the organization akin to shareholder status rather than practitioner/owner status. Regardless of the specific reason, it is important that the efficiency of the labor has been carefully evaluated and how much revenue, calculated

in dollars per hour, you generate with your time.

Once it is known that the practice can afford to hire another person, a decision must be made on how this new staff member will contribute to the profitability of the business. Broadly speaking, there are three ways to divide the labor force. First, there are staff who bring more patients into the practice through marketing. These are the "finders" within the practice. Second, there are staff who take care of the patients through their counseling and clinical efforts. These are the "minders" in the practice. Third, there are staff who take care of the essential back-office activities, such as phone scheduling, billing, and coding. These are the "grinders" in the practice. Of course, in many smaller private practices, the same person may play two or even all three "finder-minder-grinder" roles simultaneously. The laws of supply and demand determine how much each of these roles—finders, minders, and grinders—will be compensated. For example, no special credentials beyond sound bookkeeping skills, phone rapport, and jovial service skills are needed for many of the "grinder" roles. Yes, these roles are essential to the practice, but they don't often require higher post–high school education or a special credential. Therefore, the role of "grinder" is typically easier to fill, and the take-home pay is commensurate to the relative ease of filling the position. In contrast, "minders" often require special training or credentials such as a license to practice audiology; therefore, these roles are harder to fill and are compensated at a higher level.

Therefore, the decision to hire another person for the practice is a consequential one that needs to be carefully weighed. At a minimum, the practice must have sufficient revenue to justify any new hire. The owner or manager needs to ask themselves practical questions before adding to the head count:

■ Will the new hire result in more time to market services and expand business?
■ Will bringing a new person on board result in more products being dispensed or serving more patients?
■ Will patients be provided more efficient service or quicker delivery, with the result that higher quality would lead to additional patients?

The bottom line is that the cost of hiring a new employee must be offset by the added revenue and profit of having additional labor available that improves overall office efficiency and/or quality of care. Unfortunately, there are few resources that offer guidance on when to hire and how to divide labor within a practice in order to improve productivity. The purpose of this section is to offer some insight and guidance on these important topics.

Believe it or not, running a profitable audiology practice has more in common with the National Football League (NFL) than is obvious to the practice owner. For about 30 years, the NFL has operated under a salary cap. The main objective of the salary cap is to control the costs of labor and ensure league parity (competitiveness) by requiring all teams to spend the same amount of money on their labor force, the football players. In 2024, each NFL team had about $255.4 million that they could spend on a roster of 53 players. If each player on the 53-man roster was paid equally, each would receive about $4.818 million per year. Of course, each player does not receive equal pay, as some positions are considered much more valuable, and thus a considerably higher salary is warranted. The salary cap forces teams to control costs. The intent of the cap is to stoke competition by forcing all teams to have the same pool of financial resources. An added benefit of a salary cap is that it helps prevent situations in which a club will sign a high-cost player in order to reap the immediate rewards of success now, only to later find themselves in financial difficulty because of those high costs as the player's skills diminish over time. Without caps, there is a risk that teams will overspend to win now at the expense of long-term stability.

Additionally, salary caps incentivize teams to develop talent over time. This is more likely to lead to team stability, which is important for fans. No one wants to see their teams lose year after year or, worse yet, go completely out of business because they went on a crazy spending spree. Like most other professional sports, a salary cap is something that is mandated by the NFL commissioner. Teams cannot choose to ignore it. For teams that exceed the salary cap, there are severe penalties that could jeopardize the competitiveness of the team in future years.

Private businesses, on the other hand, do not have the luxury of following a mandated salary cap to keep their labor costs in check. Even though they are not required to hold their costs under a salary cap, using "salary cap thinking" is an effective way to know when you can bring a new employee into the business and at what approximate pay grade.

Case Study: Hiring Decisions and Salary Caps

As a general statement, labor productivity is what powers sustainable businesses. This means that business owners must find the proper balance between what tasks the staff performs during the workday and what dollar amount the staff is paid to perform those tasks. In other words, the practice must be busy, but the owner must be busy doing the things that lead to optimizing revenue for the business over the course of a day, month, and year.

Regardless of how labor efficiency is measured in the office, the idea of a salary cap is a great way to achieve business goals without overspending on the costs of labor. Consider a simple example of how a practice owner might determine their salary cap using a couple of assumptions. As mentioned, most experts suggest that a business needs at least 10% pretax profit to be sustainable. This pretax profit is not used to pay salaries but is set aside to reinvest in the infrastructure of the business or to cover expenses for a particularly poor month of low sales or high returns. In addition, the combination of hearing aid cost-of-goods and other expenses, including marketing, rent, and utilities, needs to be around 50% of gross revenue. These assumptions are shown in Table 8–2 for a practice that has been in existence for more than 10 years. (We chose $1 million because it is a nice round number, not because it represents any type of benchmark.)

In this example, the owner, who happens to be an AuD-trained audiologist, has toiled for more than a decade building a practice from scratch and is faced with the knotty decision of whether to hire a recent AuD graduate from the local university, an experienced clinical audiologist with sales experience, another lesser credentialled assistant, or perhaps not hire anyone.

By accounting for a pretax profit of 10% and all direct costs (excluding labor), a clear idea is evident of how much the practice can afford for labor before making any hiring decision. In Table 8–2, the salary cap is $400,000, which represents 40% of the total annual revenue of this practice. This is the amount of money the practice can spend on labor, including the salary of the audiologist/owner. Note that the costs of labor (salary, wages, and other

Table 8–2. Hypothetical Financials for a Private Practice

Revenue	$1,000,000
Direct costs (costs of goods, marketing, building expenses, utilities, etc.)	($500,000)
Gross profit	$500,000
Salary cap (40% of total revenue)	($400,000)
Total expenses	($900,000)
Pretax profit	$100,000

Table 8–3. Key Variables for the Hypothetical Private Practice

	Salary + Benefits (total compensation)
Audiologist/owner	$199,500
Assistant 1	$77,000
Assistant 2	$57,000
Total	$333,500
Cap space (available labor costs)	**$66,500**

fringe benefits) are typically the largest fixed costs associated with operating a practice. In this example, labor costs are labeled as the salary cap.

Another important point gleaned from the example outlined in Table 8–2 is this: The costs of labor, labeled salary cap, can be expressed as a percentage of total gross revenue. In this example, that percentage is 40%. This serves as a reasonable benchmark for how much revenue is allocated to cover all the costs of labor. Although 40% is the benchmark in this example, other practices could have a lower, say 30%, or higher benchmark. These benchmarks are often projected by financial analysts who can model labor costs as part of the overall cost structure and profitability needs of the practice.

Consider the example in Table 8–2. In the ideal world, it may be tempting to bring on one or two more "star performers" (e.g., experienced, audiologists) to maintain this half-million dollars in gross profit, along with the expectation that the business will experience double-digit growth over time. The reality, however, is much different since each of those proven star performers is likely

to command a premium salary of about $150,000 annually, plus benefits. (If the usual 33%-of-the-salary is for benefits, that brings the total compensation to $199,500 per star.) The math in Table 8–2 indicates that the owner must be extremely cautious in hiring decisions. That is, the salary cap figure of 40% of total gross annual revenue cannot be exceeded.

Consider a more careful look at the salary cap if this practice employs one audiologist/owner (a "minder") and two full-time assistants responsible for billing, coding, marketing, and answering the phone, among other necessary activities (two "finders" and "grinders"). Remember, according to Table 8–2, its annual salary cap is $400,000. This figure represents how much money is available for compensating employees while maintaining profitability.

Table 8–3 provides a breakdown of labor expenses relative to the salary cap. The available cap space presents that the practice has $66,500 to spend on another staff member. Using the salary cap as the primary guide in making the decision to hire another professional, it may be realized that for this practice, there is a stark choice between three hiring possibilities.

Considering the NFL analogy, there are points to remember about these three hiring options.

1. *The first-round draft choice.* Hire that new AuD graduate who is a potential star performer at well below the market value. Under this scenario, the star performer would accept a salary + benefits of $66,500 with the expectation of growing the business over a finite period. This choice may be most appropriate, if the current audiologist/owner wants to continue with their current workload while continuing to grow the practice and eventually transition out of the business.

2. *The proven free agent with a high-performance track record.* Hire an existing star performer at current market value. Under this scenario, the proven star performer would command compensation of roughly $200,000 (salary + benefits). Since this is well over the salary cap, the audiologist/owner could choose to stop actively seeing patients or drop to part-time status and receive a dividend from pretax profits rather than a high salary + benefits. Alternatively, the owner could decide to exceed their salary cap and hire this person with the expectation that they will grow revenue in a fashion commensurate with their salary. In this example, given their total compensation of $200,000 and a labor cost benchmark of 40%, this new hire should be expected to generate $500,000 in total annual revenue. If the owner decides to exceed their salary cap in this manner, a detailed plan on how the new hire will be expected to generate half a million dollars in revenue during their first 12 months of employment must be agreed upon.

3. *The free agent utility person.* The third choice would be for the audiologist/owner to continue with their current workload and bring in an assistant that could conduct some of the testing, follow up with repairs, and other front office and back-office duties. This person would likely be an audiology assistant who may also be eligible to obtain a state license to dispense hearing aids. The numbers may be worked backward to see how much labor is going to be needed to service patients in the practice's database, which generated $500,000 in annual gross profit over the past year.

To know which hiring choice is best, consider some other data from this practice, depicted in Table 8–4.

The real question is how many workers are needed to service 100 new patients and 220 experienced patients who repurchased, in addition to taking care of hundreds more of existing patients you are likely to see over the course of the few years. Assume that it takes an average of 4.5 hours of time over the course of 1 year to service new patients and an average of 3 hours of time to service an experienced patient fitted with new hearing aids. For the 220 patients fitted with hearing aids, that's 690 cumulative hours of the audiologist/owner's time. Now compare

Table 8–4. Table of Key Variables for the Hypothetical Private Practice

Revenue from the sale of hearing aids	$850,000
Revenue from testing and service contracts	$150,000
Total number of patients in database	4,000
Total number of patients who purchased hearing aids last year	220
New patients who purchased last year	100
Total units dispensed last year	380

those numbers to the capacity of each professional in your practice, applying a couple of other important concepts:

The Division of Labor

The key to staying under the salary cap is the judicious use of support personnel. After all, it is often the middling utility player who bails the star out of an ineffective performance by delivering a hit in crunch time! With a salary cap, the practice must rely on the utility person to deliver in the clutch. Support personnel or an audiology assistant (the free-agent utility player) must accept the role of "jack-of-all-trades" within the organization. In addition to conducting the essential work of scheduling appointments, other duties may include hearing aid cleaning/ troubleshooting, conducting hearing aid orientation classes, and facilitating physician marketing campaigns. It is imperative, of course, that before any work is allocated to a nonaudiologist, the owner or manager must check with the state licensing board to see what licenses and credentials are required to complete some of the patient-facing tasks outlined above.

According to the foregoing calculations, each clinician and support staff has approximately 1,840 hours available for the year to contribute to generating revenue by serving patients in various capacities. A primary objective of the owner or manager is to ensure that as many hours as possible of those available for the year (in this example, 1,840 hours) are applied toward direct patient interaction that generates revenue. This is known as *labor efficiency*. Labor efficiency is basically ensuring each patient-facing employee is spending their time on activities that maximize the generation of revenue for the practice. For example, in a primary physician's practice, physicians do not weigh patients, take their blood pressure, or even draw blood. Lesser credentialled, qualified staff would be doing those essential activities, freeing up the physician to conduct physical examinations. The same type of labor division should occur in audiology practice (Chapter 10). Today's audiologists can employ audiology assistants to conduct some of the less complex, yet essential work, thus freeing up time to see more new patients. The basic principles of labor efficiency state that the most credentialed staff should be spending their time doing activities that generate the highest revenue per hour rates. This concept is also known as *practicing at the top of your scope*. This means spending as much time as possible doing work in the practice that no one (except other licensed audiologists) else can do and delegating more routine tasks to others who are credentialed to complete them.

Considering these basic principles of labor efficiency, recall the daily workload of the star performer. Owners or managers might be wondering, "What is the maximum volume that the star performer can handle, or even should handle, before work quality starts deteriorating?" The answer to that question is not an easy one because it depends on the staff member. However, after more than 45 years of working with many different practitioners that have various years of experience, audiologists can suffer burnout if scheduled for more than 6 or 7 hours of direct patient contact per day during a 5-day workweek. In a typical setting, after vacations, sick time, and "administration" time are taken into consideration, an audiologist has, at maximum, 1,380 hours of clinical time per year to see patients (about 6 hours per business day).

In the above scenario, the audiologist/owner is using 50% of their clinical time to fit patients with hearing devices (1,380 total clinical hours/690 hours). Since the audiologist/owner still has about half of their time available to see existing patients for annual follow-ups, hearing screenings, and so on, it probably does not make sense to hire another star performer, unless the current owner is wanting to transition out of the business over the next year or two. Fortunately, the practice presented in this scenario has two ambitious support staff who can play the role of utility person by providing a range of services for the practice. Therefore, this audiologist needs to be efficient with time, rather than hire another star performer, even if that star decides to work for less than market value. Assuming the audiologist/owner wants to continue to see patients on a full-time basis, the decision to bring in a first-round draft choice or star free agent should be delayed until the practice is at 80% or more of full capacity seeing new and existing patients for hearing aid fittings.

Support personnel and audiology assistants are being used successfully in a variety of practice settings, including the military, the VA, educational institutions, hospitals, industrial settings, and private practices. History has shown that the use of support personnel can be a tremendous asset to an audiology practice, both by improving productivity and by increasing profitability and patient satisfaction. Delegating tasks that do not require the education and expertise of an audiologist to support personnel would allow the audiologist to see more patients, potentially generating more revenue, which can lead to increased profitability.

Just imagine how many more patients could be seen if the owner or manager did not have to clean hearing aids, complete order and repair forms, set up testing procedures, troubleshoot equipment, and teach patients how to clean, insert, and remove hearing aids. Not to mention demonstrating how to use Bluetooth streaming, remote controls, t-coils, loop systems, and other assistive devices. They could actually spend more time providing vitally needed services, such as family counseling, outlining realistic expectations, performing speech-in-noise testing, assessing central processing function, and developing relationships with patients, as well as marketing to potential referring physicians (Chapter 10).

Revenue-Generating Hours

The decision to hire another staff member is never a capricious one. Regardless of the status of the employee being considered, a star free agent, a first-round draft pick, or a utility person, both a salary cap and a calculation of labor efficiency can be used to make a data-driven decision. Of course, the supply and demand of the local labor market and the overall pretax profitability of the practice contribute to any hiring decision. Generally, the audiologist/owner should work to maximize the overall productivity of their existing staff before hiring another person. There is also another vitally important lesson that can be gleaned from this salary cap exercise: The use of projections to model financial performance. In this example, several variables were used to conduct some primitive modeling of expected future performance. Those projections included the following variables, which were used to make some basic hiring decisions:

- Total possible full-time workdays/year 260 (2,080 work hours).
- Vacation days per year: 10.
- Professional leave (continuing education) per year: 5.
- Sick days per year: 5.
- National/state holidays: 7.
- Personal time (emergencies): 3.
- (Total nonwork time): 30 days.

- **Total days available for work: 230 days.**
- 2 hours per day set aside for "administration time" for each audiologist.
- Available time = 230 days = **1,840 hours/year.**
- Billable hours/day = 6 hours per 8-hour workday = 1,380 hours/year for audiologist.
- For the support staff, the number of days available for work is also 230 days.
- Available time = **1,840 hours/year for each support staff.**

A key lesson here is that any hiring decision must be made after projecting how many possible revenue-generating hours are available per customer-facing employee, along with how many patients they need to see to generate sufficient revenue to cover their labor costs and the unmet demand for hearing care services in the local community served by the practice.

The Road to a $100,000-Plus Annual Salary

The exercise outlined above also serves as a good lesson for how to earn a salary exceeding $100,000 annually. The unvarnished reality is that new audiologists do not enter the labor force with a brand-new clinical doctorate in audiology and magically begin earning a six-figure salary. The new clinician must generate ample revenue with their time to earn any salary, and the more desired earnings are predicated by how each clinic day is spent. The good news is that applying some simple math to how time is spent each clinic day can provide valuable insights into compensation. By knowing the benchmark for total labor costs, in this case it is 40%, the audiologist can determine how much total gross revenue they must generate annually to keep all other costs aligned. In this example, that figure is $500,000 in annual revenue to align with a labor cost benchmark of 40%. The next question is, how does an audiologist who desires an annual salary exceeding $100,000 spend their time in the clinic?

The audiologist who desires a $100,000 salary wants to spend all their clinical time conducting hearing assessments in a busy medical practice. This means that the audiologist wants to spend their time conducting comprehensive audiological assessments, hearing rechecks, and other basic tests done in medical practice. The amount of revenue generated in a practice depends on the reimbursement rate of each test as well as the total number of assessments conducted each day or week (Chapter 17). In this example, assume the reimbursement rate for comprehensive audiometry on a new patient is $90, and reimbursement for the various types of recheck procedures ranges from $25 to $50 per patient. Also assume that an audiologist can see six new patients per day (6 × $90 = $540) and 12 recheck appointments per day (12 × $35 = $420). At capacity, working diligently with little or no breaks, seeing 18 patients per day, those values equate to $960 of revenue per day conducting basic assessments like the types found in most otolaryngology practices. That figure of $960 projected over an entire year (48 weeks) equates to roughly $46,080. A gross revenue figure well below 500,000,

and certainly nowhere close to what is needed to pay the "going rate" for an audiologist working full-time. As you can see, knowing the reimbursement rate of each procedure conducted in the clinic, along with how long it takes to complete each procedure and the total number of procedures completed over the course of a given period (day, week, month, year), determines how much revenue is generated.

Before newly graduated audiologists get discouraged, remember that reimbursement from basic testing is quite low and that audiologists must see an extraordinary number of patients to generate ample amounts of revenue from it to cover all the costs of running a clinic. What can be done? The answer is this: Spend more time doing things that generate higher sums of revenue. Here is a simple exercise that can help newly graduated audiologists better understand how to spend their clinical time doing the "right" things that contribute to optimizing revenue generated per hour:

1. Make a list of all the clinical testing procedures conducted in the clinic. Ask the clinical manager what the top 10 most popular CPT codes used by audiologists is for the practice. The fees on this list should range from between $150 to less than $50 per procedure.

2. Find out how much time, on average, it takes to complete each procedure in the top 10 list. The range should be between an hour and 15 minutes.

3. Find the average gross margin for hearing aids dispensed to patients who pay out-of-pocket for their hearing aids. The gross margin is

the retail price paid by the patient minus the wholesale price (cost of goods) paid to the hearing aid manufacturer. For the private pay market, the average gross margin should be around $1,500 to $2,000 per patient. This represents the per patient fitting fee for the private pay market.

4. Find the fitting fee paid per new hearing aid patient for those who acquire hearing aids through a managed care contract. That number should be between around $800 and $1,500. Now, rank order all the procedures and fitting fees. Develop a clinic schedule that allows maximization of time with those procedures that generate the highest per patient fees.

Dispensing hearing aids or conducting so-called special testing like balance assessments that get reimbursed at higher rates is the pathway to a more lucrative salary. Consider the example of dispensing hearing aids. Both the fitting fee from a managed care contract and the private pay gross margin received from dispensing a pair of hearing aids are likely to exceed $1,500 per patient. Using this figure of $1,500, even if five patients are fit with hearing aids per week, that equates to $360,000 in annual gross revenue. When the five fittings per week are combined with six to eight basic assessments every week, that $500,000 annual revenue figure gets closer to what is needed to pay the $100,000 salary.

The same principle applies to balance assessments, which typically get reimbursed at $300 to $400 per hour. The more of those assessments conducted at a higher rate, the more annualized re-venue generated. The lesson here is this: Spend as much time as possible on the activities that generate the most revenue. Given the current reimbursement rates, the most bang-for-the-buck comes from dispensing hearing aids to adults.

Negotiating Your Compensation in the Real World

As this chapter draws to a close, it is a good time to provide some insight into how many audiologists are reimbursed in the real world by variable or blended compensation plans. Variable or blended compensation means that audiologists receive a weekly salary along with a bonus that is paid on a monthly, quarterly, or annual basis. As the name implies, the variable component of the compensation package changes depending on the revenue generated or the profit yielded for the time frame in which it is calculated. For example, in many variable components of a compensation plan, the audiologist receives a specific percentage (e.g., 10%) of all revenue generated on hearing aid sales. The variable component of the compensation package is paired with a salary, which is typically the same dollar amount paid to the employee every 2 weeks. Compensation that is structured this way ensures that the employee receives a competitive salary for their work with the added incentive of earning more by qualifying for a bonus. Owners tend to prefer variable compensation strategies like this because it keeps the high fixed costs of the salary more manageable while at the same time allowing for higher, more competitive compensation when the practice generates additional revenue. In other words, the more revenue or the better the profit, the higher the variable pay for the employee. The potential downside to a variable compensation plan based on hearing aid sales is that it incentivizes audiologists to unnecessarily pressure people into buying hearing aids. If owners and business managers that make compensation plan decisions are concerned about ethical breaches due to variable compensation strategies, they can structure compensation plans so that salaries are higher. Given the ebb and flow of hearing aid sales throughout the calendar year in many audiology practices, however, a compensation plan that is 100% salary is more challenging to manage.

In 2024, the median salary in the United States for a newly graduated audiologist was around $70,000. Of course, there is wide variability depending on the location of the practice. If a practice dispenses hearing aids or conducts balance testing, there is probably an ample opportunity to earn more as part of a variable pay compensation strategy. New audiologists need to ask about variable pay strategies in the clinic and to embrace the possibility of earning a bonus based on dispensing hearing aids or conducting balance assessments. Compensation should always be a win-win situation. The audiologist employee earns a competitive salary and has incentive to earn more with a productivity bonus, while the employer wins by having a loyal employee who takes great care of patients and brings in revenue that sustains the practice. This win-win situation is established by knowing how revenue is generated, how time is spent in the clinic by every person who works there, and how labor is divided there.

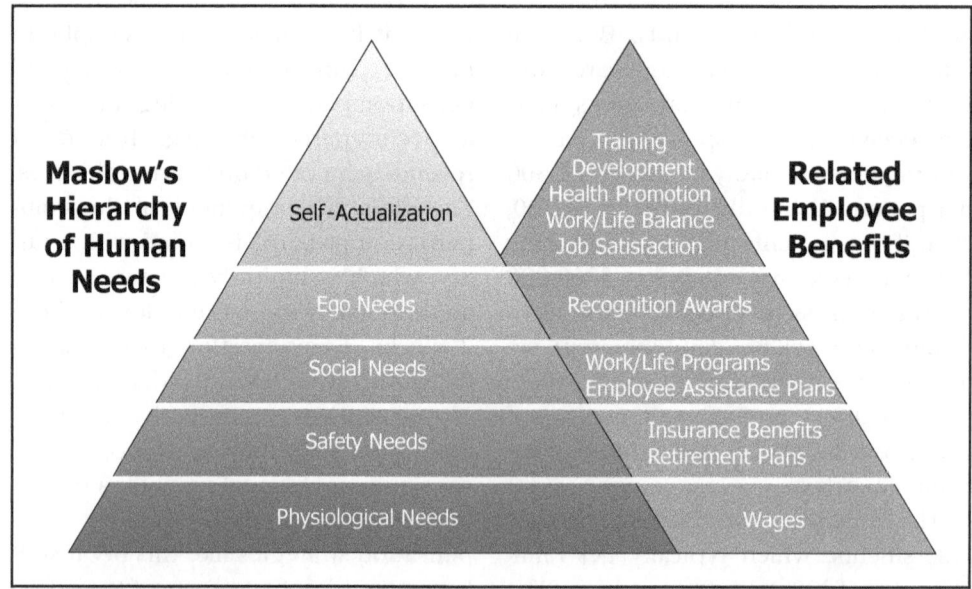

Figure 8–4. Maslow's Hierarchy of Needs applied to human resources (Jensen et al., 2007).

Summary

In summary, compensation is an analogy offered by Jensen et al. (2007), who draw a parallel between employment compensation and the hierarchy of needs theory (Maslow, 1943) illustrated in Figure 8–4.

According to Maslow's theory, once a person has satisfied their basic physiological and safety needs, attention is then focused on social and ego needs with self-actualization being the pinnacle of achievement. The correlation between components of compensation packages and Maslow's theory suggests that self-actualization or job satisfaction will only exist if there is a fair salary that meets physiological needs, health benefits and safety needs, work/life programs and social needs, recognition to feed the ego, and training and employee development. The road to self-actualization or job satisfaction seems to follow a clear progression from tangible compensation components to the intangible, and once the tangible needs are met, it appears that intangibles become extremely important to job satisfaction and ultimately retention of good employees.

References

Anderson, K., & Zhu, G. (2002). *Organizational climate technical manual*. Hay Group.

Burrows, D. (2006). Human resource issues: Managing, hiring, firing, and evaluating employees. *Seminars in Hearing, 27*(1), 5–17.

Carrison, D., & Walsh, R. (2004). *Semper Fi: Business leadership the Marine Corps way*. American Management Association.

Dierdoff, E. C., & Surface, E. A. (2008). If you pay for skills, will they learn? Skill change and maintenance under a skill-based pay system. *Journal of Management, 34*(4), 721–743.

Ellison, K. (1999). *Managing employees*. Lectures for CAS 7803, Business and Professional Issues, University of Florida Working Professional Doctor of Audiology Program, University of Florida, Gainesville, FL.

Elsdon, R. (2003). *Affiliation in the workplace: Value creation in the new organization*. Praeger Publications.

Ford. (2024). Working for balance. https://corporate.ford.com/microsites/ford-trends-2024/working-for-balance.html

Glassdoor (2015). 4 in 5 Employees Want Benefits or Perks More Than a Pay Raise; Glassdoor Employment Confidence Survey (Q3 2015). https://www.glassdoor.com/blog/ecs-q3-2015/

Insure.com. (2024). The basics of short-term disability insurance. Insure.com. http://www.insure.com/disability-insurance/short-term-disability.html

Jensen, D., McMullen, T., & Stark, M. (2007). *The manager's guide to rewards*. American Management Association.

Konrad, A. (2006). Engaging employees through high involvement work practices. [PDF] Engaging employees through high involvement work practices. Semantic Scholar.

Kyeremanteng, K., Robidoux, R., D'Egidio, G., Fernando, S., & Neilipovitz, D. (2019). An analysis of pay-for-performance schemes and their potential impacts on health systems and outcomes for patients. https://www.ncbi.nlm.nih.gov/pmc/articles/PMC6607710/

Lavelle, L. (2003, September 29). Coming next: A war for talent. *Business Week* (p. 1).

Leapsome. (2024). Variable compensation: Definition, types, pros and cons. https://

www.leapsome.com/blog/variable-com
pensation

Learner (2012). Profit Sharing Plans: One way
to share the pie. David Learner & Associates. https://www.davidlerner.com/?s
=sharing+the+pie

Mackenzie, B. (2016). What is a psychological contract? Alchemy Performance
Assistant. https://www.alchemyforman
agers.co.uk/topics/6ixdhhPwDvZFjsZc
.html

Maslow, A. (1943). The Theory of Motivation. *Psychological Review*, 50, 370–396.

Mathis, R., Jackson, J., Valentine, S., & Meg-
lich, P. (2016). *Human resource management* (15th ed.). Cengage.

Obringer, L. (2024). How employee compensation works. How Stuff Works. http://
money.howstuffworks.com/benefits1.htm

Shwiff, K. (2009). *Best practices: Hiring
people, recruit and keep the best people.*
Hylas Publishing.

Susanto, P., Hoque, M., Jannat, T., Emely, B.,
Zona, M., & Islam, M. (2022). Work-life
balance, job satisfaction, and job performance of SMEs employees: The moderat-
ing role of family-supportive supervisor
behaviors. *Frontiers in Psychology Section of Organizational Psychology, 13.*
https://www.frontiersin.org/journals
/psychology/articles/10.3389/fpsyg
.2022.906876/full

U.S. Department of Labor. (2024). 401(k)
business plans for small business,. Employee Benefits and Security Administration. https://www.dol.gov/agencies/ebsa
/key-topics/retirement/401k-plans

U.S. Legal. (2024). 401(k) Law and legal
definitions. USlegal.com. https://defini
tions.uslegal.com/4/401-k-plans/

 # Policy and Procedures Manual

Robert G. Glaser, PhD

Introduction

Policy and Procedures Manual, Employee Handbook, and Employee Manual are titles to documents created to communicate the expectations of employers to their employees and what employees can expect from their employers. In some practice venues, there may be two sets of documents that serve as operational guides.

The Policy and Procedures Manual (P&P Manual) may serve as the informational source developed for a specific individual or group of employees. Although the Policy and Procedures Manual serves as the basis for employee manuals or handbooks, it may also be reserved solely for the use of specific managers or directors within an organization. Employee Manuals or Handbooks may be developed from the P&P Manual for specific employees depending on their informational needs. An Employee Manual or Handbook for an audiologist may differ greatly from those generated for administrative staff despite the fact there will be operational issues common to all employees. No matter the title of the document, employee manuals or handbooks are critically important to optimize consistent operations in both small and large practices.

Policies Versus Procedures

Policies establish the rules of the practice; procedures clarify operational issues. Policies provide the rules of engagement around which employees operate. They commonly include rules for paid time off (PTO), sick leave, jury duty, covered holidays, dress code, confidentiality, and a host of other parameters that set forth the character and tone of the practice. For example, PTO must be readily delineated so that both new hires and long-term employees understand the rules of computation and acquisition of time off, the nature and definition of various types of PTO (personal leave, military leave, sick leave), the process to request PTO, whether it is cumulative or needs to be used or lost, and so on.

Procedures prescribe and substantiate operational topics such as how the practice defines a comprehensive audiologic examination, delineating the acquisition of clinical information and data from the patient to come to an appropriate diagnosis. Although the procedure establishes the clinical components of what constitutes the examination in the practice (history, pure tone, speech threshold, and recognition testing, otoacoustic emissions testing, speech in noise, extended high frequency audiometry, central auditory processing etc.), it should not be so detailed that it includes specific instructions of the technical components of the procedures. It is not so much how an audiologist gets to the data as much as the quality of the data gleaned from the clinical test battery that has been chosen to constitute the comprehensive audiologic examination as a procedure for the practice. The decision to select a procedure for the comprehensive audiologic examination was determined based on the best methods to arrive at an accurate and valid diagnosis.

The Need for a Policy and Procedures Manual

The P&P Manual establishes operational and personnel characteristics necessary to provide professional services in accord with the mission statement or philosophy of the practice. It enables the practice owner or manager to establish these parameters in concert with their vision of how the practice is to operate and the manner and types of services to be provided.

Beyond systematizing administrative and operational aspects of the practice, the Policy and Procedures Manual provides rules and guidance for decision-making and appropriate actions to be taken throughout the practice at every level of involvement: owner, director, department head, and clinical and administrative staff. It should be considered the ultimate resource document for an audiology practice whether the venue of service delivery is an autonomous audiology practice, a hospital department, an educational resource center, an ENT department in a medi-

cal school, or a private ENT/audiology practice.

Each employee must agree with and abide by these "rules of engagement," which clarifies what the employer should expect from the employee and what the employee can expect from the employer. An employee's acceptance of these rules and procedural guidelines is critical to their becoming "stakeholders" in the practice. Additionally, employees who fail to comply with the tenets and principles in the P&P Manual do so under a stipulated understanding that they are jeopardizing their continued employment. That stipulation is completed by the employee signing and dating an acknowledgment form indicating their agreement to the tenets set forth in the P&P Manual.

The P&P Manual can serve as a tutorial document for potential new hires and the basis for their orientation to the practice. Each person considered for employment must be able to follow the established rules and procedural guidelines. They should be encouraged to ask for clarification if they do not understand or have differing views on policies or procedures. If a potential employee is unable to agree with the tenets of the practice as set forth in the P&P Manual, they should seek employment elsewhere.

The P&P Manual sets the tone of the practice, including how it feels and looks to patients and/or referral sources—employee dress and demeanor in the office or on the telephone; the structure, brevity, content, and turnaround time of reports; front office staff interactions with the referral source's office staff; and response to the number of rings on an incoming call. Many if not all of the policies and procedures are geared to devel-

---

POLICY AND PROCEDURES MANUAL
ACKNOWLEDGMENT FORM

I have read the Policy and Procedures Manual for (*insert the practice or specific practice venue*). By acceptance of the Policy and Procedures Manual (P&P Manual), I acknowledge notice and agree to abide by and provide services or interact with patients, referral sources, and others in accordance with all policies and procedures set forth in the P&P Manual. I recognize the need and agree to maintain patient health information in a secure fashion such that each patient's health information is protected and secured in accordance with current HIPAA regulations. I understand that changes may be made from time to time and that (*insert the practice or specific practice venue*) has the right and authority to make any representations contrary to the statements set forth in the P&P Manual. I also acknowledge that no one employed by, or acting on behalf of (*insert the practice or specific practice venue*), is authorized to make oral statements to change the at-will employment relationship between (*insert the practice or specific venue)* and its employees. I understand that (*insert the practice or specific practice venue)* or I may terminate my employment at any time for any reason.

Signature _____ Date _____

---

oping patient satisfaction and loyalty, which have been identified as critical elements in securing the long-term success of any practice.

Legal Considerations in Developing a Policy and Procedures Manual

As indicated in Chapter 3, a Policy and Procedures Manual is important no matter the number of employees. It establishes a basis for many otherwise unstated, ambiguous, and/or misunderstood aspects of the employment relationship. Critically important to that re-

lationship is the confirmation of the "at-will" status of the employee and the right of the employer to terminate employment for any or no reason.

Some argue that a P&P Manual will not prevent an employee from filing a suit against the practice and its owner(s). Although it will not prevent a legal encounter by an employee, it may give them pause to do so. Having the rules of engagement set forth and the terms of employment stipulated by the employee may serve as an adequate defense against employee-related legal claims. A written document is the practice's best chance of not having a court case centering on the owner or practice manager's word against that of the employee. The remedy is to develop a well-written document that has been reviewed and approved by the attorney-of-record for the practice.

When preparing the P&P Manual, it is best to assume that it may be viewed as a legally binding contract. For that reason, among many, the legal counsel for the practice must evaluate the entire document. They will ensure that appropriately worded disclaimers are in place and that the language in the document is in accordance with the employer-employee relationship. Miller and Jentz (2006) aptly point out that employers have learned hard lessons from court decisions about what is said in P&P Manuals. They indicate that promises made in an employment manual may create an implied-in-fact contract. They suggest that employers make it clear to employees that the policies expressed in the P&P Manual must not be interpreted as a contractual promise and that the manual is not intended as a contract. They suggest the following disclaimer, appropriately adapted to the needs of the workplace venue, be set off and prominent from the surrounding text by using larger type, all capital letters, or some other device that calls the reader's attention to it:

This policy manual describes the basic personnel policies and practices of our Practice. You should understand that the manual does not modify our Company's "at-will" employment doctrine or provide employees with any kind of contractual rights.

An All-Encompassing Compliance Document

In the important arena of establishing the "rules of engagement" between an employer and an employee, consideration should be given to establishing a general compliance document. The employee signs the document upon employment agreeing to a variety of appropriate stipulations, including records of protection and confidentiality, information important to the practice, forms, electronic and hard copy files, and so on. The employee, therefore, agrees to these stipulations on an a priori basis before their resignation or termination as an "at-will" employee.

OUTLINE OF A POLICY AND PROCEDURES MANUAL

Policy and Procedure Manual
 INTRODUCTION TO THE
  PRACTICE
 MANUAL AS ULTIMATE RE-
  SOURCE DOCUMENT;
  WHAT IT IS AND IS NOT
  (DISCLAIMERS)

THE MISSION OF THE
  PRACTICE
PRACTICE PHILOSOPHY
MANAGEMENT RIGHTS
ACKNOWLEDGMENT FORM(S)
 ACKNOWLEDGES HAVING
  READ AND WILLINGNESS

continued on next page

continued from previous page

TO ABIDE BY POLICIES
WITHIN P&P
COMPLIANCE DOCUMENT
REGARDING CONFIDEN-
TIAL AND PROPRIETARY
INFORMATION
Policies
ADMINISTRATIVE STAFF
PRIORITIES
BILLING-COLLECTION POLICY
CERTIFICATION vs LICENSES
COLLECTION POLICY
CONFIDENTIALITY
CONFLICTS OF COMMITMENT:
CONFLICTS OF INTEREST
CONSENT FORMS FOR PROCE-
DURES AUDIOLOGY
CONSENT TO PERFORM
EMI-CERUMEN REMOVAL
CONVENTION AND WORK-
SHOP POLICY
CUSTOMER SATISFACTION &
COMPLAINT RESOLUTION
DISASTER POLICY
DISCIPLINARY POLICY
DISCRIMINATION AND
HARRASSMENT IN THE
WORKPLACE
DRUG AND ALCOHOL
POLICY
EQUAL EMPLOYMENT
OPPORTUNITY
EMERGENCY MEDICAL ASSIS-
TANCE PROTOCOL
EMPLOYEE ACCESS TO BUSI-
NESS DATA
EMPLOYEE EVALUATION/
PERFORMANCE REVIEW

EMPLOYEE STANDARDS OF
CONDUCT
DRESS
DEMEANOR
COLLEGIALITY
SUBSTANCE ABUSE
SMOKING
HARASSMENT OF STAFF,
COLLEAGUES, PATIENTS
REVIEW P&P MANUAL
ANNUALLY
EQUIPMENT CALIBRATION &
REPLACEMENT
HEARING INSTRUMENT LOST
HEARING INSTRUMENT
REPAIR
HEARING INSTRUMENT
RETURN
INCIDENT REPORT
INFECTION CONTROL
INTERNET USAGE
LEAVE
LIABILITY INSURANCE: MAL-
PRACTICE INSURANCE
OUTSIDE EMPLOYMENT
PATIENTS WITH PRIOR COL-
LECTION ACTION
REFERRING PATIENTS TO
OTHER PRACTITIONERS
RELEASE OF PATIENT
INFORMATION
TUITION ASSISTANCE
WEATHER
Clinical Procedures
Personnel: Position Descriptions
Documentation
Reimbursement Capture by Coding
Optimization

Overview of a P&P Manual for an Audiology Practice

There is little uniformity across the tables of content for P&P Manuals and Employee Handbooks. Content varies with the practice venue, the practitioner/owner, and the extent of clinical services offered in the practice. There is no set rule, order, or list that might signal completeness of information. The spectrum of details in P&P Manuals ranges from minimalist statements to extensive descriptions of issues with definitions, footnotes, and comprehensive legal precedents. It is important that the scope of issues in the P&P Manual be well met and adequately conveyed so that the document is clear and concise, leaving little question in the mind of the reader.

The best judge of completeness of information and topics covered relative to the venue of the practice is the attorney-of-record. They must review the document to ensure completeness, correctness, and accuracy relative to current laws established in the state wherein the practice is located and according to federal guidelines. An attorney's view of the P&P Manual will be grounded in employment law and compliance as well as the best interests and protection of their client.

Each practice venue has unique needs. If the practice is in a hospital department, most of the P&P Manual will likely have been completed at the corporate level. It may be left to you as the director or head of audiology to complete those sections pertaining specifically to the clinical services offered and the personnel delivering those services in your department. The completed document will be reviewed by the hospital's legal staff as well as the administrator charged with oversight of your department. If you are in a university setting, clinical oversight as well as oversight of research activities will likely have to review the P&P Manual. As with corporate oversight in hospitals, universities may have greater numbers of reviewers and personnel in oversight capacities with the final oversight commonly resting with the office of the provost.

The outline that follows may not appear logical to some, incomplete to others, and overextended by those who adhere to the "less is better" philosophy. It is offered as a guide more than an all-inclusive document. Each section should be given weight appropriate to departmental needs. Selected examples will be offered for your consideration, and in some cases, more than one option will be offered. Developing a comprehensive P&P Manual is beyond the scope of this text, but this outline should enable practice owners and program directors to get a good start and create a document that can be reviewed and edited by your attorney, accountant, and others with experience and knowledge in developing similar documents.

NOTE: The proposed text of the P&P Manual will appear in *italics* with commentary and suggestions in regular font.

Policy and Procedures Manual for Audiology Associates

Introduction

This Policy and Procedures Manual (P&P Manual) contains the policies, practices, and procedures of Audiology Associ-

ates. *This P&P Manual is not intended to be all-inclusive. Audiology Associates reserves the right to make final decisions regarding the interpretation and application of its policies, practices, and procedures, whether or not identified in the P&P Manual, and to change or discontinue them at any time. The Manual also contains general information about the benefits that are available to you.*

Audiology Associates is concerned not only with your job performance but also with you as an individual. If you have a question about work or any material in this Manual, contact the practice manager. Remember that a question can be answered only if it is raised, and conditions with which you are dissatisfied can be improved only if you bring the dilemma to management's attention.

Audiology Associates maintains an open, honest, and cooperative work environment. This work environment gives us an opportunity to get to know you and encourage you to understand and share the goals of Audiology Associates.

This manual is not intended to create or constitute an employment contract between you and Audiology Associates. Because the P&P Manual is not contractually binding, you have the right to terminate our employment relationship at any time, with or without any notice or reason, and Audiology Associates retains the same right, unless specified differently by contract. Our employment relationship can be defined as employment "at will." Audiology Associates may have to make decisions without prior consultation with its employees. As such, Audiology Associates maintains exclusive discretion to select, hire, promote, suspend, dismiss, assign, supervise, and disci-

pline employees; to establish, change, or abolish policies, procedures, rules, and regulations; to determine and modify job descriptions; and to assign duties to employees in accordance with the needs and requirements determined by Audiology Associates.

Purpose of the Policy and Procedures Manual

The P&P Manual was developed to provide you with guidelines and policies regarding your employment with Audiology Associates. This manual is an important guidebook to be used as a resource regarding policies, employee guidelines, and our practice standards. We hope that this manual will be beneficial in establishing the responsibilities of both the employer and employee to each other and eliminate any misunderstanding that may occur due to misinterpreted communications. These policies have been developed to serve current needs and may be adjusted periodically. Management employees are encouraged to recommend revisions they feel appropriate.

Practice Philosophy: A Mission of Commitment to Patients

- *We pledge to always make decisions in favor of the patient and referral source at every opportunity knowing that we cannot be wrong if we are trying to be right for those whom we serve.*
- *We are professionally, ethically, and personally committed to providing excellent care in a timely and car-*

ing manner to all members of the communities we serve.

■ *Our audiologists represent the finest professional resource for hearing and balance evaluations, tinnitus assessment and management, hearing instrument evaluation, fitting, and follow-up care in the communities we serve.*

■ *The entire staff of Audiology Associates recognizes and appreciates the importance of all healthcare providers and their staff who refer patients to us for our specialized care and consideration. We strive to maintain their trust by issuing timely, concise, and accurate reports and by maintaining an active liaison between our referral sources and their patients.*

■ *Each member of our practice subscribes to the following Patient's Bill of Rights:*

Patients in our practice should . . .

1. *Expect more from Audiology Associates than any other provider in our community.*
2. *Know that each patient will be respected by everyone in our practice.*
3. *Expect us to answer your phone call in a timely, friendly, and welcoming manner.*
4. *Upon arrival, expect to be greeted in a friendly and appreciative manner by everyone in our practice.*
5. *Know that we recognize the importance of their time.*
6. *Expect a quick response and immediate action all the time by every member of our practice.*
7. *Require excellent communication from us.*
8. *Know that we will listen and understand their concerns.*
9. *Expect quick and accurate resolution of questions or concerns about your account.*
10. *Receive an apology if we are in error.*

Management Rights

It is important that a manual for employees have a clear statement of the rights of practice managers to conduct business in an appropriate and professional manner according to their terms. The statement need not be lengthy. It must clarify the roles, obligations, and expectations that management considers important to the continued operation of the practice as a business. Likewise, the employee should understand clearly where they fit in relative to management. The wording is commonly straightforward and must leave little room for conjecture as to the roles of management and the intent to operate the practice as a business.

Rights of Management

Audiology Associates has and will always consider the opinions of each member of the practice about working conditions, ways and means to accomplish all tasks important to the success of our practice, and other matters of importance to the members of our team. From time to time, Audiology Associates must make decisions without input from the members of the team. As such, Audiology Associates retains all managerial and administrative rights referred to inherently and by law. These rights include, but are not limited to, the right to exercise judgment in establishing and administering policies and procedures, and to make changes in them; the right to take whatever action is necessary, in management's judgment, to operate the practice; and the right to set standards of productivity and services to be rendered. The management of business and the direction of those working in the practice including, but not limited to, the responsibility to hire, promote, transfer, suspend, or discharge, and the responsibility to relieve employees from duty because of lack of work, or other reasons, are vested exclusively in the management of Audiology Associates. In addition, Audiology Associates has the right to amend, modify, or delete provisions of this manual with or without prior notice.

Acknowledgment Forms

Critically important to any P&P Manual is a statement, signed and dated by the employee indicating that they have read the document and agree with its content and implied or actual actions, which may be put into effect by the owner or manager of the practice. Any document that stipulates specific compliance, duties, rules or expected actions, or response by an employee must be signed and dated during the earliest stages of employment. It is difficult to get documents signed immediately prior to or after an employee has been discharged.

Two examples follow. The first is an acknowledgment form that commits the signer to the tenets of the P&P Manual. It underscores the need for confidentiality and compliance with HIPAA regulations. The second is an equally

---

ACKNOWLEDGMENT FORM

I have reviewed a current copy of Audiology Associates Policy & Procedure Manual. By acceptance of the manual, I acknowledge notice of all policies contained therein. I agree to maintain patient information in a secure fashion such that each patient's health information is protected and secured, in accord with current HIPAA regulations. I understand that changes may be made from time to time and that Audiology Associates has authority to make any representations contrary to the statements set forth in the manual. I also acknowledge that no one employed by or acting on behalf of Audiology Associates is authorized to make oral statements that change the at-will employment relationship between Audiology Associates and its employees.

I further understand that Audiology Associates or I may terminate my employment at any time for any reason.

Signature   *Date*

GENERAL COMPLIANCE DOCUMENT
AUDIOLOGY ASSOCIATES

In accord with my resignation or discharge as an at-will employee, I submit and agree to and with the following statements in compliance with office policies and HIPAA regulations:

- *Patient records, notes, and/or other information pertaining to the patients of Audiology Associates will remain confidential and will not be removed physically or electronically.*
- *Financial information about individual patients and/or any fiscal information pertaining to Audiology Associates will remain confidential and may not be removed physically or electronically.*
- *Information important to Audiology Associates including, but not limited to, personnel information, supplier information, and any/all statistics pertaining to the operations of Audiology Associates will remain confidential and will not be removed physically or electronically.*
- *Information about the current status, future plans, and other information deemed important to current and future operations of Audiology Associates will remain confidential and will not be removed physically or electronically.*
- *Forms, computer programs, equipment manuals, patient protocols, or other documents regarding operational and patient-related matters pertaining to Audiology Associates shall remain at the office in physical and electronic forms, and information contained therein must remain confidential.*
- *Books, journals, and related materials not purchased by personal funds will remain the property of Audiology Associates.*
- *All forms developed for use at Audiology Associates are hereby copyrighted and remain the intellectual property of Audiology Associates. As such, none may be removed or used in whole or in part for any reason except when permission has been granted in writing.*
- *All physical and electronic files used in the execution of duties as an employee of Audiology Associates remain the property of Audiology Associates and may not be removed in any form.*
- *In the interests of the patients served and the continuity of their care, all charts and related correspondence will be completed by noon of the day immediately prior to the last day of employment.*

_____ *Date*_____

important acknowledgment document specifying the proprietary rights of the practice. Although it will not prevent theft of documents, forms, and the like, the courts have taken a dim view of individuals leaving a business or practice with proprietary or trade information after they have affixed their signature to a compliance document describing specific proprietary items and information that must be left at the workplace. Of course, these documents can be combined, but by having two separate forms, the underlying reasons and differing content are made clearer. Each should be signed in the initial stages of employment, after the P&P Manual has been read and orientation to the practice has been completed. The second form advises the employee that in the event they decide to leave the practice or is terminated, there are specific rules regarding confidentiality, pirating forms, and removing items considered important to the practice.

Policies

Policies represent the rules of the practice. The following alphabetic list of policies with examples will not represent a comprehensive list for every practice. Each will provide a starting point to develop an appropriately written document for your practice venue. To enable both comments and instructions on the language to be considered in these policy sections, two different fonts will be used: italics for policy language and regular font for instructional comments.

NOTE: The proposed policy language will appear in *italics* with commentary and suggestions in regular font.

Administrative Staff Priorities

1. *Booking patients into the office: We cannot help if they are not here.*
2. *Take care of referral sources: They and their support staff members are our partners in caring for THEIR patients: Courtesy, respect, and an abundance of assistance are critical to providing excellent service that will sustain referrals. If you take care of them, they assume their patients will be well cared for in our practice.*
3. *Smooth the process of every visit: Take the appointment from the hands of the referral source staff to our hands—let them get back to work while we book the appointment and get preliminary information from the patient.*
4. *Take great care of each phone call. Consider the caller your boss, since we all work for the patients coming to our practice. Always make decisions in favor of the patients and the referral sources.*
5. *To schedule follow-up visits, call twice before leaving a voice message; if no response to voice message, send postcard asking them to call us.*
6. *Send handwritten thank you notes to those patients who have referred patients to our practice—they have entrusted their friend or relative to our care and they deserve our thanks and appreciation.*
7. *Call newly fitted patients or those with recently repaired instruments within 3 to 5 days of the (re)fitting to check their status before their return visit—if they are struggling, get them on the schedule PRIOR to their scheduled follow-up visit.*

8. *When a patient calls or presents a hearing instrument for repair, obtain their description of the problem, when and how often the problem occurs. If the instrument is dead, check for occlusion and battery problems. Advise need to return for repair, turnaround time, and costs if applicable.*

9. *Hearing instrument repairs, accessories and batteries, out-of-warranty adjustments, or modifications are to be paid same day of service.*

AUDIOLOGY ASSOCIATES FINANCIAL AGREEMENT

Payment is expected at the time of service unless other arrangements have been made. We accept cash, checks, MasterCard, Visa, American Express, and Discover Card.

■ *We will submit charges directly to your insurance carrier as a courtesy. Submitting the charges is no guarantee they will be paid.*

■ *Insurance policies may or may not pay for the services you receive in our office. Coverage varies with each insurance carrier; a few plans cover all charges, some cover 80%, and others cover less than 50%. The amount your insurance company pays for the services you receive is between you and your insurance carrier.*

■ *YOU ARE RESPONSIBLE FOR PAYING ALL CHARGES INCLUDING DEDUCTIBLES, COINSURANCE AND SERVICES, DEVICES, AND RELATED ITEMS NOT COVERED BY INSURANCE. ACCOUNTS NOT PAID WITHIN 45 DAYS MAY GO TO A COLLECTION AGENT.*

■ *HEARING INSTRUMENTS ORDERED AND NOT PICKED UP WILL BE SUBJECT TO RESTOCKING AND HANDLING FEES WHEN RETURNED TO THE MANUFACTURER.*

■ *EARMOLDS AND/OR IMPRESSION COSTS ARE NONREFUNDABLE AND MUST BE PAID IN FULL.*

I have read and understand the above and agree to pay all charges. I authorize my insurance company to make direct payment for all services rendered. Release is hereby granted to send records by any means appropriate to healthcare providers or others deemed necessary by Audiology Associates.

Signature:_____Date: _____

Witness:_____Date: _____

Billing and Collection Policy

Every patient in our practice has signed an agreement indicating they are responsible for paying all charges incurred during their care in our practice. The billing cycle for Audiology Associates is 45 days. Accounts with unpaid balances will be sent to collection if, in that time, payment in full or scheduled payment arrangements have not been established. There must be a written agreement on the method and dates of payment if balances are to be carried beyond the billing cycle.

Each patient must receive notification by phone or letter 15 days prior to our sending their account to collection. Once the account has been placed with the collection agent, all payments must be made to that agency. No attempt should be made to discuss accounts in collection since the account is no longer with our practice. They must be referred to the collection agency if they have questions or concerns.

Confidentiality

All information pertaining to the patients we serve must remain confidential. Conversations about patients entrusted to our care must be completed such that those in waiting or treatment rooms will not overhear the conversation. Patient charts and other information, including the appointment book should be secured from view. At no time should a patient be discussed outside office with anyone, including another staff member.

Since all patient information obtained by Audiology Associates is confidential, it may not be released to an insurance company or any other party without the patient's written permission on file: Breach of confidentiality of patient information will result in immediate termination of employment.

Conflicts of Commitment and Conflicts of Interest

A conflict of commitment exists when an employee assumes obligations external to the practice, which interferes with the employee's properly discharging their obligations and commitment to Audiology Associates. Full-time employees must make full-time commitments to Audiology Associates. Part-time employees with obligations external to the practice must ensure they are fully committed to Audiology Associates when discharging their duties on behalf of our practice. Full disclosure of any obligation external to Audiology Associates is expected regardless of the numbers of hours of employment.

Obligations external to Audiology Associates that represent direct competition for similar patients, referral sources, or care contracts constitute a conflict of interest. A conflict of interest must be disclosed by the employee and a determination made as to the course of action that will resolve the issue. Expeditious disclosure and resolution of such conflicts are in the interests of all involved. Failure to resolve conflicts may result in termination of employment.

Consent Forms for Specific Procedures

Consent forms will not prevent legal action. They exist as an acknowledgment that the procedure has been explained, risks have been discussed, and

---

**CONSENT TO PERFORM CERUMEN REMOVAL
AND/OR EARMOLD IMPRESSION**

Cerumen removal and/or earmold impression procedures involve the introduction of instruments and/or material into your ear canal(s). The audiologist will use accepted procedures to avoid adverse results. Cerumen removal and earmold impression involve the risks of discomfort, bleeding from the ear canal, puncture of or damage to the eardrum, and ear infection.

I, the undersigned patient, hereby acknowledge that I have read and understand the important notice printed above. I understand that no guarantee has been made to me as to the results. I recognize the risks of receiving the procedure(s) described. I hereby request and consent to the procedure(s).

*Patient Name*_____ *Signature*_____

Audiologist Name_____ Signature_____

Date_____

---

the patient acknowledges having been advised of the risks.

Patient Satisfaction and Complaint Resolution

Every practice must ensure that the patient has a voice in their care. If the patient feels as though they have been treated inappropriately, unfairly or otherwise ill-treated, the patient should have a means to address the issues with the owner or practice manager. The simpler the policy, the more expedient the result. Complaint resolution is as much about the speed with which you reply as it is with the resolution of the complaint. The policy can be as simple as having all patients with unresolved complaints referred directly to the practice manager for resolution within 24 to 48 hours. They can deal with the situation directly after discussing the situation with members of the administrative and professional staffs involved in the complaint. The goal is to resolve conflict in favor of the patient at every opportunity. That does not mean, however, that the practice manager needs to roll over every time a patient lodges a complaint. If the complaint exceeds limits set forth in procedural guidelines and is beyond appropriate reasonability, resolution completely in favor of the patient might jeopardize the validity of the policies and procedures of the practice. Flexibility in favor of the patient is expected. Not responding favorably to a patient's unreasonable demand must not be construed as inflexibility. Every business needs to draw the line somewhere, especially those operating in the arena of healthcare.

Disciplinary Actions

Audiology Associates enjoys a fine reputation as a healthcare provider. That reputation in no small part is directly related to employees who take pride in the services they provide. Employees are expected to conduct themselves in a courteous and professional manner toward patients, referral sources, and their fellow employees at all times. Policies and guidelines are to be followed to maintain the integrity of the practice and the standards of care we have established in the communities we serve. When difficulties affecting your performance or the performance of others dictate disciplinary considerations, the following disciplinary guideline represents the progressive steps that will be taken:

1. *A verbal warning*
2. *A written warning*
3. *Final warning*
4. *Termination*

Management will consider all the facts surrounding an employee's misconduct in determining appropriate discipline. Generally, however, a verbal warning may be given for initial, minor violations of practice policies or procedures. The written warning is given for repeated violations or initial violations of a more serious nature. A final warning, which is always in writing, is given

for the most serious offenses other than those calling for immediate discharge or for continued repetition of the type of violations for which one or more written warnings have been given.

Management reserves the right to bypass any of the progressive steps of discipline depending upon the facts and severity of the offense. Management may give an employee a written or final warning as the first warning. Management can also terminate an employee without warning: When misconduct is of a very serious nature, an employee will be discharged immediately. The following acts are examples of serious misconduct and not intended to be an all-inclusive list:

1. *Conviction of a felony*
2. *Theft or misappropriation of funds*
3. *Possession, use, or sale of an alcoholic beverage or nonprescribed or illicit drugs while on Audiology Associates premises or while on duty at another practice site*
4. *Reporting to work under the influence of intoxicants, including alcohol, nonprescribed drugs, or illicit drugs*
5. *Possession of firearms, knives, or other weapons while on the premises or while on duty at another practice site*
6. *Fighting or attempting to injure another person while on practice premises or while on duty at another practice site*
7. *Engaging in horseplay or using abusive, threatening, or provocative language toward another person while on the premises or while on duty at another practice site*
8. *Engaging in sexual harassment*

9. *Insubordination (e.g., refusal to promptly obey a work instruction or job assignment from a supervisor or the practice manager)*
10. *Dishonesty, including falsification of records (e.g., payroll, insurance, and personnel records)*
11. *Failure to report unexcused absences*
12. *Immoral or indecent conduct on premises or while on duty at another practice site*
13. *Gambling on premises or while on duty at another site*
14. *Willful destruction of practice property*
15. *Unlawful possession, use, manufacture, distribution, or dispensing of illicit drugs, controlled substances, or alcoholic beverages during the employee's work period, whether on the premises of Audiology Associates or at site(s) where the employee is carrying out duties on behalf of Audiology Associates*

Each employee is responsible for knowing the rules of expected conduct, as well as the procedures outlined in this manual. Should you have any questions about the application of any rule or any discipline you have received, discuss it with the practice manager.

Drug and Alcohol Policy

Audiology Associates maintains a safe and healthy environment for its employees and the patients and referring healthcare providers whom we serve. The use or trafficking of illicit drugs, on or off the job, has an adverse impact on our practice and will not be tolerated.

Possession of prescription drugs while on practice premises or representing Audiology Associates at a related site is permissible only if:

■ *The drug is kept in the original container with both the employee's name and prescribing doctor's name on it*
■ *The drug was dispensed within 12 months*
■ *Written permission is submitted from the prescribing doctor who certifies the employee can work while taking the indicated dosage*

Audiology Associates reserves the right to have a second physician determine whether the drug might adversely affect performance.

If an employee appears to be impaired or there is reason to believe that he or she may be in possession of alcohol or drugs, the employee may be ordered to undergo a drug and alcohol screen at the expense of Audiology Associates. Employees who are directed to undergo a drug or alcohol test will be suspended pending laboratory analysis of the sample. If the test is positive, the employee will be disciplined, up to and including termination of employment. If the test is negative, the employee will be paid for any lost work time. Employees are permitted to have the same sample retested at their own expense.

Educational Allowances

Audiology Associates provides a minimum of 3 days for CEU eligible educational training at an approved meeting with approval of the practice manager. Registration, economy class airfare, ac-

commodations, and reasonable expenses will be paid upon submission and approval of receipts. Additional funding for other CEU eligible educational meetings may be approved as needed by the practice manager.

Equal Employment Opportunity (EEO) Policy

In accordance with applicable local, state, and federal law, Audiology Associates is committed to a policy of nondiscrimination and equal employment opportunity. All employment decisions will be made without regard to sex, sexual preference, race, color, religious creed, national origin, ancestry, age, non-job-related handicap, disability, HIV AIDS, or HIV AIDS-related conditions.

Emergency Medical Assistance Protocol

Every practice must have a plan to respond to emergency situations. In the event an individual in the practice becomes ill and requires emergency medical care, every member of the administrative and professional staffs must follow a set of steps to secure the situation and engage emergency personnel as soon as possible. The protocol should be practiced at least twice a year. Every telephone in the practice should have the office address and cross streets listed on the phone cradle—a handy reminder in the fast-paced confusion of an emergency. The steps in the protocol will vary from setting-to-setting. At the minimum, a basic plan should include the following steps:

Emergency Medical Assistance Protocol

1. *Upon determining a patient or guest is in distress, call out to other practice personnel for help.*
2. *Dial 911 and notify the operator of the situation and give the address of the practice.*
3. *Do not leave the individual; however, you must make sure that emergency personnel can access your location.*
4. *Another staff member should go outside to direct emergency personnel.*
5. *The practice manager should follow the individual to the hospital and make sure the family is contacted.*
6. *If the individual requiring removal from your practice has been referred by their physician, contact the referring physician immediately and apprise them of the situation.*
7. *Follow-up with the patient or the family the next day.*

Access to Operational Information of the Practice

Information in any form pertaining to the business operations of Audiology Associates is confidential. Daily business and professional operations such as, but not limited to, patient care visits, numbers of hearing instruments dispensed, billing and coding information, fiscal information, patient and referral source databases, contracts to provide services, and any similar information are considered confidential, and access to these and other operational data is restricted to the practice manager and their designees on a need-to-know basis. Failure to comply with this policy will result in termination.

Performance Review

The first performance review for all personnel will be completed by the practice manager within the first 90 days of employment and at least annually thereafter.

The purpose of a review is to provide each employee with an opportunity to voice their concerns and to express thoughts about how their participation in the practice enhances patient care. They should take the opportunity to discuss items of interest or concern with the practice manager.

The practice manager will review the employee's performance and provide suggestions to improve specific areas. If significant resolution of deficiencies is considered necessary, additional training and reassessment of performance may be established in a defined time frame. The performance evaluation will be summarized by the practice manager in writing for the employee's personnel file and a copy will be provided the employee.

Professional Appearance and Dress Code

A professional image is important to our patients and helps solidify their positive attitudes about our professionalism and their perceptions of the quality of

services we provide. Good grooming and a professional appearance are expected of all employees. Employees are required to wear white lab coats with their names embroidered or on a name tag. The practice will supply appropriate lab coats to all personnel. Dress shirts and ties with dress slacks or khakis and appropriate shoes and socks are expected for men. Skirts and slacks with appropriate blouses or sweaters and appropriate shoes are expected for women. Athletic shoes, jeans, sweatshirts, tank tops, and blouses displaying the midriff are prohibited. Additionally, professional attire is expected to be worn when attending professional meetings as a representative of Audiology Associates.

Replacement of Lost Hearing Instrument Under Warranty

If a hearing instrument is lost while under warranty, a replacement instrument will be secured for the patient under the manufacturer's terms of replacement. There will be no charge for the replacement instrument. There will be an inclusive $375.00 fee for earmold impression, programming, and placement of the replacement instrument, including all adjustments necessary during three follow-up visits available for 1 year following the replacement.

Hearing Instrument Repairs

Hearing instrument repairs completed after the warranty period must be paid in full on the day the instrument is replaced. The cost of the repair may not include charges for reprogramming if the instrument has not been reprogrammed to the original settings.

Return of Hearing Instrument Within 4 Weeks Postfitting

Should a patient return a hearing instrument or instruments within the allotted trial period, the patient will be required to pay restocking charges as stipulated in the hearing instrument receipt booklet. Returns and restocking charges after the postfitting period will be decided on a case-by-case basis.

Internet Usage

Information contained in Audiology Associate's computer and information systems (all of which shall be referred to as "information systems") are the property of the Audiology Associates.

Email Procedures

1. All email correspondence is the property of Audiology Associates and is for business purposes only.
2. Employee email communications are not considered private despite any such designation either by the sender or the recipient.
3. Messages sent to recipients outside of Audiology Associates, if sent over the Internet and not encrypted, are not secure. Encryption requires prior approval by Audiology Associates.
4. Audiology Associates will monitor its email system—including an employee's mailbox—at its discretion in the ordinary course of busi-

ness. Please note that in certain situations, Audiology Associates may access and disclose messages sent over its email system.

5. The existence of passwords and "message delete" functions do not restrict or eliminate Audiology Associate's ability or right to access electronic communications. The delete function does not eliminate the message from the system.
6. Employees shall not share an email password, provide email access to an unauthorized user, or access another user's email box without authorization.
7. Offensive, demeaning, or disruptive messages are prohibited. This includes, but is not limited to, messages that are inconsistent with Audiology Associate's policies concerning "Equal Employment Opportunity" and "Sexual Harassment."

General Internet Procedures

1. Audiology Associate's network, including its connection to the Internet, is to be used for business-related purposes only and not for personal use. Any unauthorized use of the Internet is strictly prohibited. Unauthorized use includes accessing personal accounts or any form of social media, posting or downloading pornographic materials, engaging in computer "hacking," and other related activities attempting to disable or compromise the security of information contained on Audiology Associate's computers (or otherwise using Audiology Associate's computers for personal use).

2. *Because postings placed on the Internet may display Audiology Associate's address, make certain before posting information on the Internet that the information reflects the standard policies of our practice. Under no circumstances shall information of a confidential, sensitive, or otherwise proprietary nature be placed on the Internet.*

3. *Subscriptions to news groups and mailing lists are permitted when the subscription is for a work-related purpose. Any other subscriptions are prohibited.*

4. *Unless the prior approval of management has been obtained, users may not establish Internet or other external network connections that could allow unauthorized persons to gain access to Audiology Associate's systems and information. These connections include the establishment of hosts with public modem dial-ins, World Wide Web homepages, and File Transfer Protocol (FTP).*

5. *All files downloaded from the Internet must be checked for possible computer viruses.*

6. *Any data on any computer hard drives or electronic media (discs, etc.) that pertain to Audiology Associates, its patients, or staff are considered the property of Audiology Associates and must be kept in confidence following the guidelines set forth in the Confidentiality Statement. Upon termination of employment, all data must be returned to Audiology Associates intact and any copies must be deleted from hard drives and/or electronic media.*

7. *No software or peripheral device is to be installed on Audiology Associate's system without prior authorization.*

8. *Any employee who violates this policy shall be subject to disciplinary actions, including termination of employment.*

Paid Time Off (PTO)

Employees are asked to schedule their vacation at least 1 or 2 months in advance of the time they desire to be away.

If two employees ask for the same PTO dates and a conflict is deemed important and unavoidable, the individual who submitted their Request for Leave form first will be granted the PTO requested.

"Request for Leave" forms can be obtained from the practice manager.

All Requests for Leave forms must be competed and submitted to the practice manager. Emergency PTO will be considered accordingly, but we expect a phone call regarding the situation and an estimate of time away from your responsibilities.

Paid Time Off Schedule

Full Time: (5 days a week; 32–40 hours and up; 50 consecutive weeks)

1st year	*7 days*
2nd & 3rd years	*15 days*
4th, 5th, & 6th years	*20 days*
7th, 8th, & 9th years	*25 days*
10th year and above	*25 days*

Part Time: (3 days per week; 30 hours and up; 50 consecutive weeks)

1st year	*5 days*
2nd & 3rd years	*7 days*
4th, 5th, & 6th years	*10 days*
7th, 8th, & 9th years	*12 days*
10th year and above	*14 days*

- *Above PTO must be used in 1-hour increments.*
- *PTO earned but not taken during the calendar year is not cumulative from year to year and will be forfeited if not taken by December 31 (Use or lose policy).*
- *In the unfortunate event of a long-term illness, the employee will meet with the practice manager to discuss their PTO status.*

Patients With Prior Collection Actions

Individuals returning to our practice for reassessment, hearing instrument repairs, or follow-up visits with a history of having been placed in collections must pay for all services on a cash or credit card basis only. Exceptions to this policy may be considered on a case-by-case basis.

Position Descriptions

Every position of employment within a practice requires a written description of general and specific duties, management responsibilities if appropriate, oversight and reporting responsibilities, and spe-cific areas of data handling and access. Qualifications for each position should be made clear, including specific degree or training requirements. Patient care responsibilities should be delineated relative to the expected clinical proficiencies necessary to provide specific services. An example of a position description for a receptionist follows:

Position Description for Receptionist

<u>*Reports to:*</u> *Practice manager*

<u>*Managerial Responsibilities:*</u> *None or as directed by the practice manager*

<u>*Qualifications:*</u> *Associate's or bachelor's degree in business or related field preferred. Past work experience should include healthcare or related field as front office receptionist or position that included patient or practitioner interactions.*

<u>*Hours:*</u> *40 plus hours per week (flexible as needed)*

<u>*Responsibilities:*</u>

1. *Opening and closing the office*
2. *Confirming all appointments for the next business day and pulling charts*
3. *Ordering supplies for the audiology department*
4. *Coordinates audiologists' schedules*
5. *Schedules patient and vendor appointments*
6. *Greets patients and gathers billing information*
7. *Answers telephone, screens and directs calls, takes messages*
8. *Enters selected charges and payments in the computer*

9. *Prepares daily bank deposit*
10. *Organizes and files patients' charts*
11. *Obtains medical concurrences*
12. *Performs receptionist duties at satellite offices*
13. *Researches and enters new patient data into the computer*
14. *Assists in the orientation and training of new employees as needed*
15. *Has joint responsibility for office maintenance*
16. *Faxing/mailing report results to primary care physicians and others*
17. *Other responsibilities as directed by the practice manager*

Referring Patients to Other Practitioners

Patients may be referred to other healthcare providers when needed, if they have come to our practice on a self-referred basis, independent of a physician or other healthcare provider's referral. If the patient has been referred to our practice by a primary care provider or other healthcare practitioner and there is a definitive need for referral to another specialist or healthcare entity for additional evaluation or treatment, the patient must be returned to the original referring source for disposition and management with suggestions.

Tuition Assistance

Tuition assistance may be provided for completion of an AuD or PhD on a case-by-case basis. According to the Federal Tax Codes, up to $5,250.00 of payments received by an employee for tui-

tion, fees, books, supplies, etc. under an employer's educational assistance program may be excluded from gross income (Code Sec. 127; Reg. 1.127-1).

Inclement Weather

When forecasts indicate inclement weather that may result in school closings due to impassible road conditions, the practice manager (or designee) will take a copy of the schedule home (patient phone numbers should be listed) the night before threatening weather. The practice owner and/or practice manager will decide on the following course(s) of action:

- *If conditions are obvious, scheduled patients may be cancelled and rescheduled the afternoon or evening prior to the anticipated weather situation.*
- *If severe, inclement conditions arise in the early morning, the patients may be cancelled and rescheduled before 8:30 a.m.*
- *The practice owner and/or manager will contact each member of the staff to determine their ability to arrive at the office(s) or service sites. Depending on the response, patients may be cancelled and the workday may be considered cancelled.*

Clinical Procedures

Each clinical procedure offered in the practice should be delineated. Every CPT code employed in the practice constitutes a procedure; each should be well described with approximate times to complete the procedure with cooperative patients.

Summary

A P&P Manual is an essential part of communication within the practice. It stands as the rulebook, the reference book, and a reminder of why patients and referral sources are the focus of the practice. Regardless of the number of people employed by the practice, the P&P Manual should be updated on an annual basis. There are no hard-and-fast rules about what should or should not be available to the readers of the manual. An outline of a P&P Manual for an audiology practice follows for your consideration. It can be easily adjusted to include speech-language pathologists, psychologists, physical therapists, or other healthcare providers and counselors with appropriate position descriptions and minor changes in language specific to each discipline included in the practice. Regardless of the numbers of employees and their relative contributions to the practice, the wise practice manager or owner will solicit as much input from every member of the practice team in the preparatory stages of the manual. After all, the P&P Manual is about the services and the contributions provided as members of the team that is the practice.

References

Burrows, D. L. (2006). Human resource issues: Managing, hiring, firing, and evaluating employees. *Seminars in Hearing, 27*(1), 5–17.

Miller, R. L., & Jentz, G. A. (2006). *Business law today.* Thomson Higher Education.

10 The Effective Incorporation of Assistants in Audiology Practice

A. Nichole Kingham, AuD, ABA

Welcome to the Real World of Audiology

Imagine—after years of rigorous education, relentless effort, and unwavering determination, the long-awaited opportunity to assume a full-time role as a staff audiologist finally materializes—a testament to the dedication and perseverance needed to obtain a doctorate in audiology. This coveted position represents the pinnacle of professional achievement, offering the chance to deploy acquired skills in the practice of audiology and service to the community. Every interaction with patients on a full schedule brings a feeling of accomplishment and satisfaction that lives are being changed for the better. But then reality sets in. The sense of pride and accomplishment is soon replaced with the realization that work hours frequently extend past 5 o'clock. Chart notes and calls to manufacturers to check the status of an order must be completed during lunch hours. Trips to FedEx to drop off repairs and new orders are not an uncommon experience.

Training on new products, protocols, and equipment must be completed on weekends because the schedule is too full to complete the requirements of the job within an 8-hour workday. Burnout begins to set in. Time with friends and family seems to be dwindling, and satisfaction with the "dream job" may be called into question. In fact, Zimmer et al. (2022) showed that this is not an uncommon experience for new professionals. They may have the highest rate of burnout. Severn et al. (2012) found that burnout stemmed from one or more of six factors: time demands, audiological management, patient contact, clinical protocols, accountability, and administration or equipment (Figure 10–1).

The reality is that practicing at the full scope of audiology requires grace, fortitude, and astute management of time and resources. It also requires finding ways to practice audiology effectively but efficiently. Dr. Diana C. Emanuel, professor in the Department of Speech-Language Pathology & Audiology at Towson University in Maryland, published data in 2021 relating to an

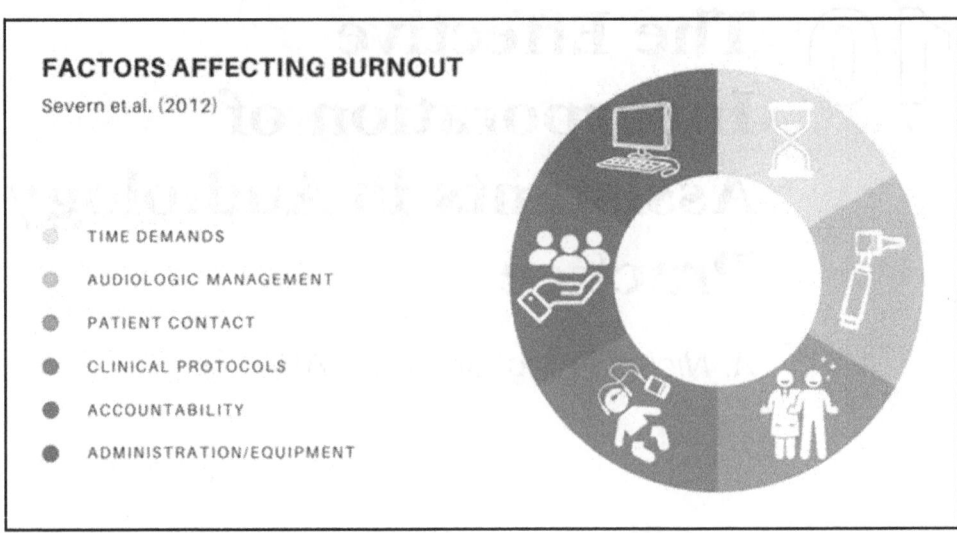

Figure 10–1. Factors affecting burnout (Severn et al., 2012).

interview study conducted that showed stress is common in audiology. In an interview with Gus Mueller, PhD, she noted the reasons why:

> Relative to my interview research, I often heard audiologists describe acceptance, and resentment, of the dual-level roles that some audiologists have. While all employees have myriad tasks at work, logic dictates a division of labor for efficient operations, with roles associated with credentials, expertise, salary, and so forth. What I found interesting was that many audiologists described serving as both a professional healthcare provider and as their own assistant and that many of the duties expected of audiologists were not expected of other doctoral-level healthcare providers. (Mueller & Emanuel, 2022)

The demand for hearing and balance healthcare services increases as the population increases. However, more professionals need to enter the field of audiology to meet the demand (Figure 10–2) (Windmill & Freeman, 2013).

This demographic trend places additional pressure on audiologists to see more patients in a shorter period of time while audiology managers stress revenue generation, efficiency in productivity, and increased help rates, all the while requiring that audiologists maintain high standards of patient-centered care. Furthermore, the evolving landscape of healthcare delivery, including the introduction of over-the-counter (OTC) hearing aids, changes in reimbursement policies, advancements in technology, and shifts in patient preferences, can further compound these pressures. Audiologists may feel compelled to continuously adapt to these changes while grappling with the demands of their families, professional aspirations, and clinical responsibilities, leading to feelings of frustration or disillusionment with their profession.

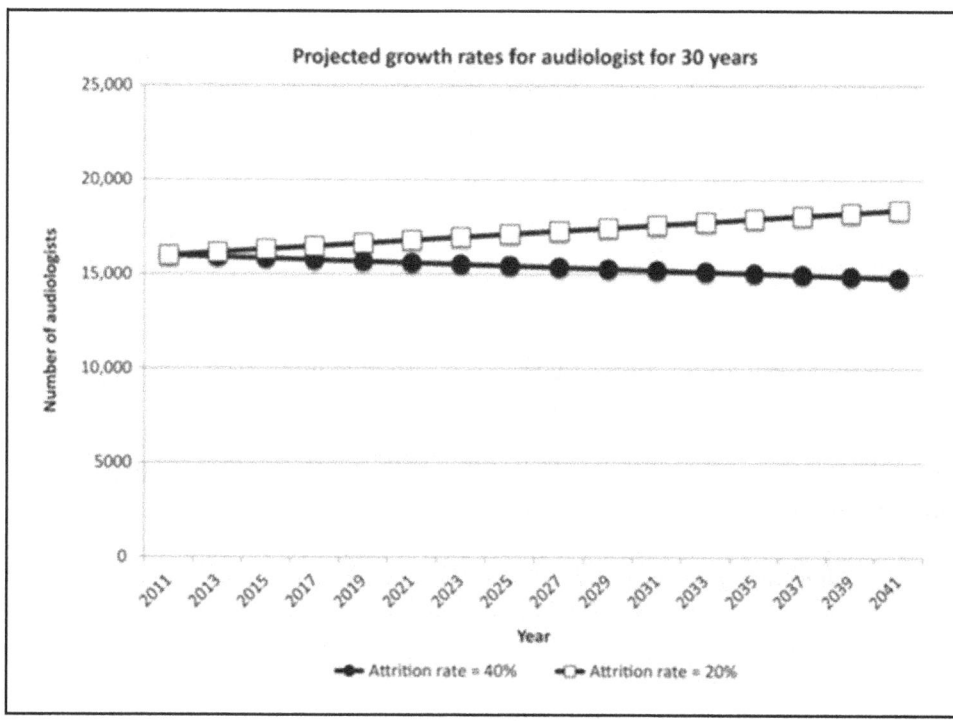

Figure 10–2. Projected growth rates for audiologists for 30 years (Windmill & Freeman, 2013).

HELP RATE

Key performance indicators, or KPIs, are often used in business to determine how successful team members are at meeting the goals that the business owners or managers have set for them individually or as a whole for the business to be profitable or for it to meet a target of some kind. One of the more common KPIs is the help rate. The help rate is the number of patients a clinician can help move forward with a proposed solution: hearing aids, tinnitus treatment, or an extended service plan, for example. If 100 patients came to the clinic and all 100 had hearing loss that would benefit from amplification, but the clinician can only help 45 of them move forward with a treatment plan, the clinician's help rate is 45%.

Addressing these challenges and reducing the likelihood of burnout requires a multifaceted approach that includes open communication, mentorship, ongoing professional development opportunities, and support systems within the clinic itself. One of the most effective support systems is the use of allied staff who can assist in providing the excellent care that patients are searching for without requiring the full measure of that care to rest on the audiologist. Although dreadfully underutilized (Andrews & Hammill, 2017; Wince et al., 2022), the audiology assistant is one such staff member. These trained professionals provide valuable assistance in various aspects of clinical practice. By effectively utilizing audiology assistants, hearing healthcare practices can optimize their workflow, improve patient access to care, and enhance the overall quality of services provided in the audiology clinic. This chapter will explore the history and role of audiology assistants, strategies for their effective utilization, and best practices for maximizing their contributions to the practice.

The History of Audiology Assistants

Audiology assistants have been involved in audiologic care for many years. Before the role was defined, the audiologist's assistant was the person staffing the front desk who often took on tasks to assist when patients required immediate help. The Veterans Administration has utilized assistants since World War II due to increased hearing loss in service members with combat-related noise ex-

posure (Karzon et al., 2018). Professor Jerry Northern, PhD, a founding member of the American Academy of Audiology who served as its third president, reported on the use of support personnel in 1972 (Northern & Suter, 1972). Northern noted, "Supportive personnel will allow the certified audiologist to make a better contribution toward fulfilling the community's need for services and provide more time to perform those activities for which his extensive education has prepared him." There would be many more years of discussion and debate before the national audiology organizations would support a scope of practice for audiology assistants. And utilization of the audiology assistant has been slow to take hold.

Utilization of Audiology Assistants

Since audiology assistants have been discussed and defined by industry professionals for more than 40 years, most clinics would utilize assistants on a day-to-day basis. Research shows, however, that audiology assistants are, in actuality, vastly underutilized. Hammill and Freeman (2001) conducted a survey that revealed that, at that time, 24% of audiologists employed or supervised an assistant in their clinics. More recent surveys by Andrews and Hammill (2017) and Wince et al. (2022) showed that the number had risen from just 10% to 34% of audiologists surveyed. Why, over two decades, has the profession of audiology failed to realize the benefits that the utilization of audiology assistants can bring to both clinics and clinicians? The reasons are multifaceted and, until recently, the national audiology organizations did not define the scope of practice for audiology assistants, leading to a lack of clarity and overall confusion about what an audiology assistant can and cannot do in a hearing and balance clinic (Nemes, 2001). Other reasons include few training programs for audiology assistants, which then requires the staff or supervising audiologist to become the trainer, leading to another draw on the clinician's time. Lastly, multiple research studies have found that many audiologists fear that training an audiology assistant may actually be a case of training their competition or allowing the audiology scope of practice to be undermined (Duran, 2002; Hamill & Freeman, 2001).

Audiology Assistant Scope of Practice

Over the years, the national audiology organizations, the American Speech-Language-Hearing Association (ASHA) and the American Academy of Audiology (AAA), have discussed the definition and scope of practice for audiology assistants. AAA created a position statement in 2021 defining the assistant as "a person who, after appropriate training and demonstration of competency, performs duties and responsibilities that are delegated, directed, and supervised by an audiologist. The assistant's role is to support the audiologist in performing routine tasks and duties so that the audiologist is available for the more complex evaluative, diagnostic, management, and treatment services that require the education and training of a licensed audiologist." In general, audiology assistants increase the pro-

ductivity and efficiency of a clinic by completing tasks related to direct and indirect patient care that are essential to the practice but do not necessarily require the audiologist's expertise. They, in effect, free up time for the audiologist to do the work of audiology.

As one of the primary contacts for patients, be it by phone or in person, the audiology assistant position, at its core, is designed to ensure that every contact with the clinic is a positive one and that each experience helps in the differentiation of the clinic from other experiences the patient may have had with other similar businesses. It is evident in both the ASHA and AAA scope of practice that the assistant position *is not meant to be autonomous*. The audiology assistant should instead be *under the direct supervision of an audiologist.*

Defining the Role of Audiology Assistants

What does an audiology assistant actually do? The answer is complicated. It will depend on the type of clinic and its exact needs, the patients' demographics, and the state licensure rules and regulations for hearing healthcare professionals.

The Type of Clinic and Their Demographics

While the core responsibilities of the audiology assistant may be similar across clinic types, the exact tasks an audiology assistant performs and the patient population they serve will differ according to the setting.

Hospitals

In a hospital setting, audiology assistants may be called an "audiology technician." They will work alongside audiologists to assist in diagnostic testing and readying patients for vestibular exams. In some instances, audiology technicians are able to perform a full test battery that a physician supervises. They are likely to be involved in administrative tasks such as scheduling appointments, managing patient records, and coordinating with other health professionals for continuity of care with other healthcare professionals. Due to the diversity in patient populations in the hospital setting, audiology assistants will likely encounter a broader range of hearing-related issues and work with patients of all ages and abilities.

Private Practice

In private practice, audiology assistants are likelier to have a more hands-on role in everyday patient care. The main goal in a private practice setting is to assist the audiologist and to provide support during hearing aid fittings and regular hearing aid checks. They will also play an integral role in the continuity of care and creating excellent patient experiences. In some cases, they also assist in marketing efforts and outreach to physicians and the local community.

Pediatric Clinics

In pediatric clinics, audiology assistants may be involved in conducting hearing screenings for infants and young children, as well as assisting with specialized diagnostic tests tailored to pediatric patients. Communication with parents and caregivers is a specialized skill that requires specific training for this population of patients.

State Licensure Laws

State licensure laws for audiology assistants vary across the United States. The majority of states do not have specific licensing requirements for audiology assistants, while others require certification, and some only require registration of the assistant. In states where licensure is written into state law, the requirements to obtain licensure differ significantly. These requirements can include a specific education level of the applicant, continuing education requirements, limitations in the scope of practice, specialty certification requirements through ASHA or the Council for Accreditation in Occupational Hearing Conservation (CAOHC), or a specified number of hours of training under the supervision of a licensed audiologist. The ASHA website has a resource list that links each state's licensure requirements (or lack thereof) for audiology assistants. To get the most accurate, up-to-date information on state licensure requirements, it is always best to consult the state licensing board in the state where the clinic resides.

The Most Common Tasks

Ultimately, the audiology assistant role will be defined by the audiologist directly supervising the assistant. The most common tasks fall under the following categories:

- Patient Intake and Support
- Administrative Tasks
- Child Testing and Nondiagnostic Screening
- Patient Education and Counseling
- Hearing Aid and Hearing Accessory Support

Patient Intake and Support

Audiology assistants are crucial in supporting an audiologist through patient intake and support tasks. They welcome patients warmly, ensuring they feel comfortable and valued from the moment they arrive. Additionally, audiology assistants obtain and update patient medical histories, ensure accurate recordkeeping, and administer questionnaires. They offer support and information regarding appointments and procedures, alleviating patient concerns and ensuring a smooth experience. They will also assist in coordinating patient care services, guaranteeing seamless transitions, continuous connections, and continuity of care.

Administrative Tasks

Audiology assistants should be cross-trained to help with administrative tasks. They will help to keep the clinic running smoothly and can help to manage appointment schedules and calendars, optimizing clinician time and ensuring patients are seen in a timely manner. Their involvement in billing and insurance processing can facilitate financial transactions with accuracy and professionalism. Audiology assistants will also maintain meticulous patient records and documentation, ensuring compliance with regulatory standards and facilitating communication among healthcare

providers. Additionally, they oversee inventory and supplies, ensuring essential resources are available when needed, thus optimizing, improving, and ensuring clinic efficiency.

Child Testing and Nondiagnostic Screenings

Audiology assistants contribute to the hearing evaluation of small children and those patients who cannot participate in the standard hearing evaluation due to mental or physical conditions. They can assist the audiologist in the sound booth during visual reinforcement (VRA) and play audiometry. In clinics without audiology assistants, VRA and play audiometry may require a second audiologist to assist in obtaining reliable test results. In general, it is not cost-effective to have two doctorate-level audiologists complete a single diagnostic evaluation. Instead, an audiology assistant can easily be taught the intricacies of being just interesting enough to keep the patient's head pointed forward, while not so interesting as to distract the patient from hearing novel sounds during VRA or by teaching the patient the task of participating in play audiometry. Audiologists are best equipped to teach assistants ways to interact with difficult-to-test patients to assist in obtaining reliable results on these essential diagnostic tests.

Audiology assistants can also provide nondiagnostic hearing screenings and immittance measures without interpretation to identify the potential need for further testing. Performing screenings is a simple way to provide exceptional patient care. For example, if a patient returns to the clinic with a complaint of not hearing well, the audiology assistant should first check the hearing aid(s) for function. If the hearing aids are found to be in good working order, there must be another reason the patient is feeling they are not hearing well. Training the assistant to perform a simple hearing screening of pure-tone thresholds at 500, 1000, 2000, and 4000 Hz and allowing them to refer to the audiologist for a complete diagnostic evaluation if changes are noted is excellent patient care and a great way to show patients that they are cared for. The goal should always be to offer patients a solution to the issue at hand. If the patient notes not hearing well and the answer is, "Well, your hearing aids are fine," the clinic is not offering best patient care.

State regulations permitting, audiology assistants can perform otoscopy and ear canal inspections to assist clinicians in assessing ear health and identifying abnormalities. It should be standard practice to check patient ear canals at each appointment to ensure that debris is not interfering with hearing.

Patient Education and Counseling

Audiology assistants can support patients by providing valuable information regarding hearing aids, assistive devices, and hearing conservation practices, empowering patients to make informed decisions about their hearing health. Additionally, audiology assistants can assist patients in developing communication strategies and coping mechanisms for managing hearing loss, offering support and guidance throughout their journey toward better hearing.

One of the more common tasks an audiology assistant will perform is the counseling portion of the hearing aid delivery. This task alone can decrease the time the audiologist spends with the patient, increasing the clinic's efficiency as a whole. In general, it makes good business sense to have audiologists spend their time in revenue-generating activities such as diagnostic hearing evaluations and hearing aid evaluations.

The counseling a patient receives during the hearing aid delivery includes a review of contracts, teaching the patient about battery insertion or use of the charger, cleaning and maintaining their instruments, telling left from right, insertion and removal techniques, Bluetooth® pairing, and phone app instruction, and it often concludes with completion of paperwork and taking payment. Assistants can also support the audiologist by readying equipment for such an appointment, such as setting up for conducting real ear measures. This initial counseling can also be a great time to educate patients about the expectations for continuing care and about accessories that are available to patients to assist in better hearing on a daily basis.

Hearing Aid and Hearing Accessory Support

The most common tasks an audiology assistant will complete are related to the care and maintenance of hearing aids. Cleaning, completing minor in-house repairs, sending and receiving repairs and new orders, tracking shipments, and testing for function, as well as readying instruments for delivery, are arguably the most time-intensive tasks in an audiology clinic. The time savings alone for the clinic by having

Hearing Aid Quality-Control Checklist	
CONFIRM	**EXECUTE**
☐ Style/type	☐ Listening check
☐ Technology level	☐ Visual check
☐ Color	☐ Electroacoustic analysis
☐ Receiver strength/length	☐ Compare to manufacturer specifications sheets
☐ Serial number(s)	☐ Directional microphone check
☐ Earmold	

Figure 10–3. Quality control checklist. *Source:* Adapted from Jorgensen and Gellhaus (2022).

an audiology assistant complete these tasks on a regular basis is likely the most beneficial reason to have an audiology assistant on staff and adds most to the efficiency of the practice.

Under supervision, they also aid in setting hearing aids to first fit[1] and checking the function of hearing aids in the hearing instrument test box, ensuring patients receive optimal support for their hearing needs. Numerous studies by Jorgensen and colleagues discuss the need to verify hearing aids when they arrive in the clinic—new or repaired (Jorgensen, 2016; Jorgensen & Gellhaus, 2022; Jorgensen & Novak, 2022). Jorgensen states in these publications, "It May Meet Your Standards, but Does It Meet Mine?" "By checking the devices when they arrive in the clinic, audiologists can focus on the

concerns of the patient, knowing that the aids are not contributing to the difficulties." It is good patient care to ensure the hearing aid(s) are functioning properly before delivering them to the patient. Nothing is worse than placing an instrument on a patient only to find that it is malfunctioning somehow. Jorgensen suggests using an in-house protocol to ensure that hearing aids are checked consistently, and by using a checklist, patients will consistently receive instruments that function as expected (Figure 10–3).

Hearing Aid Checklists

Having multiple providers involved with the care of patients and the maintenance of their hearing devices can increase the possibility of mistakes in management of the patient's needs. It is the old adage, "There are too many cooks in the kitchen." As providers move about their day, it can be challenging to maintain

---

[1]State law dictates what an audiology assistant can or cannot do regarding programming hearing aids. Please consult with State Department of Health regulations.

lines of communication about the patient care being provided. Using checklists is a critical component of providing the best possible care by decreasing miscommunication and involving all parties to complete essential tasks. The following checklists will be helpful to improve communication:

■ Hearing Aid Delivery Checklist
■ Hearing Aid Service Checklist
■ Walk-in/Drop-off Checklist
■ Earmold Order Checklist
■ End-of-Month Checklist

Hearing Aid Delivery Checklist

Involving the audiology assistant in the hearing aid delivery process can significantly decrease the time required for the audiologist to spend with the patient. Many of the tasks completed during a hearing aid delivery do not require the expertise of an audiologist. However, this appointment is arguably one of the more important in the journey for the patient with hearing loss. During this appointment, the patient is taught how to use and clean their new hearing aids, how to connect the hearing aids to accessories or apps, and how to insert and remove the devices, among other things. They are also given appropriate expectations about the level of service they will receive from the clinic. The hearing aid delivery appointment is an excellent opportunity to allow patients to create a connection with the audiology assistant, establishing them as an important part of the care team. The use of a checklist gives the audiologist insight into what the audiology assistant covered with the patient (Figure 10–4). This has the added benefit of documenting what was covered for future reference in the in-

stance that a patient comments, "I was never told that"—a comment that is unfortunately a common one.

Hearing Aid Service Checklist

Hearing aid services are an essential aspect of excellent patient care. Not only is it the responsibility of the clinic to provide ongoing care to patients who purchase hearing aids, but doing so can create lifelong patients who return again and again to purchase new products. In an article about creating "customer delight," Taylor and Rogen (2011) noted, "In our experience, we have found that a practice needs between 20 and 25 patient contacts over a 4- to 5-year period between hearing aid purchases. Using a combination of semi-annual patient check-up appointments and newsletters is a proven strategy to retain patients."

During hearing aid check appointments, the patient's hearing aids are checked for function, cleaned, and debris removed, and patients will pick up any spare parts (i.e., filters, domes, and batteries) and receive any firmware updates on their hearing aids (Figure 10– 5). It is also appropriate for the audiology assistant to check the patient's ear canal for excessive earwax via an otoscopic inspection.

Walk-in/Drop-off Checklist

For audiologists with a full schedule, walk-in patients can drastically change the flow of the day and can easily cause delays in seeing scheduled patients. To both lessen the disruption in the schedule that walk-in patients can create *and* help every patient feel important, the audiology assistant should be responsible for seeing walk-in patients

EASTSIDE AUDIOLOGY

Hearing Aid Delivery Checklist

Patient Name: _____ Date: _____

Provider Name: _____

Hearing aids set to first fit: ☐	Review beep indicators ☐
Hearing aids set to previous fit: ☐	
Tested for Directionality: ☐	**Connectivity:**
Tested in HIT box: ☐	Aids paired to phone ☐
	App reviewed ☐
Review of Systems:	
Insertion and Removal ☐	**Warranty:**
Use of VC ☐	Service ☐
Use of Push Button ☐	Loss/Damage and deductible ☐
Use of Battery door on/off ☐	
Use of Battery door standby ☐	**Fitting Verification:**
	Real Ear ☐
Care of Aid:	Other ☐
Cleaning ☐	
Turn off when not in use ☐	**Reasonable Expectations:**
Avoid water, hairspray, humidity ☐	Noise ☐
Use of dry-aid-kit ☐	Own voice ☐
EM tubing or dome change (circle 1) ☐	Difficult settings ☐
Receiver Length: _____	Hours of Use ☐
Dome size: _____	Accommodation time ☐
Battery:	**Accessories:**
Size: _____ ☐	Use Review ☐
Toxicity ☐	Warranty expiration ☐
How to change ☐	
Battery Supply ☐	**Auditory Training:**
Low battery indicator ☐	5 Keys ☐
Battery life in hours: _____	"Cheat Sheet" given ☐
Battery Life in days: _____	"Tip Sheet" given ☐
Program use:	**Follow-up:**
Review of Programs ☐	6-month checkup reviewed ☐
Automatic only ☐	Patient scheduled for next appt ☐
P1:_____ R/L	
P2:_____ R/L	**Comments/Issues to resolve at next visit:**
P3:_____ R/L	
When to use programs ☐	_____
Telephone use ☐	
Automatic program ☐	_____

Developed by Nichole Kingham, Au.D.
www.AudiologyAcademy.com
Version 2.2 2024

Figure 10–4. Hearing aid delivery checklist. *Source:* Created by Kingham, N. Eastside Audiology, Nichole Kingham (2024).

EASTSIDE AUDIOLOGY
HEARING EXPERTS. SOUND ADVICE.

Audiology Assistant Checklist

Patient Name: _____ Date: _____

Provider Initials: _____ Make/Model: _____

Date Fit: _____ Service Warranty End Date: _____

Hearing aids in and on correctly: ☐	**Batteries Given**	☐
Clean and check complete:	**Review of Warranty:**	
_____ ☐	Repair Warranty	☐
_____ ☐	Loss and Damage Warranty	☐
	Service "Warranty"	☐
_____ ☐		
	Review of System:	
	Use Review	☐
Review of Patient Concerns:	Care Review	☐
_____ ☐	Battery Review	☐
_____ ☐	User Programs Review	☐
_____ ☐	Follow-up Care Review	☐
Does patient feel hearing has changed?	Discussion of HAT	☐
☐ Yes ☐ No	Discuss 5 Keys	☐
	Next check up appt set	☐
Hearing Screening Performed: ☐	Friends/Family Referral Program	☐
	Patient Testimonial requested	☐
Diagnostic HT scheduled? ☐		
Otoscopic Check ☐		

Comments/Issues to be resolved and Plan of Action:

_____

_____

_____

Developed by Nichole Kingham, Au.D.
www.AudiologyAcademy.com
Version 2.2 2024

Figure 10–5. Audiology assistant checklist. *Source:* Created by Kingham, N. Eastside Audiology, Nichole Kingham (2024).

whenever possible. By leveraging the skills and capabilities of audiology assistants, clinics can optimize their capacity to care for drop-in patients while maintaining high standards of patient care and operational efficiency. A checklist specifically for walk-ins can help the patient communicate what is happening with the hearing aid without directly explaining the issue to the audiology assistant (Figure 10–6). This removes the responsibility from the patient care coordinator or front desk manager to communicate what the patient is experiencing, increasing efficiency. The walk-in/drop-off form can also act to communicate important information between the front desk and the audiology assistant, such as the time of walk-in, whether the patient requires a callback, or whether the patient dropped off one or two hearing aids, among other information that might otherwise be forgotten due to experiencing a busy clinic schedule.

Earmold Order Checklist

A well-trained audiology assistant can support the audiologist in sending out orders and repairs. However, having an audiology assistant involved in ordering earmolds can be complex due to the many different styles, configurations, and materials. While verbally explaining these order details would be inefficient, an earmold order checklist decreases the time the audiologist needs to spend readying the order and allows for the efficient support of the ordering process (Figure 10–7).

End-of-Month Checklist

An end-of-month checklist can be instrumental in ensuring that audiology assistants diligently complete tasks regularly. This systematic approach promotes efficiency and accuracy in managing various responsibilities within the clinic that are under the prevue of the assistant. The checklist should include a comprehensive range of duties, including patient appointment scheduling, equipment maintenance, inventory management, and administrative tasks. By consistently reviewing each item on the checklist, audiology assistants can verify that all essential tasks have been accomplished, thereby maintaining smooth clinic operations. Additionally, the checklist serves as a valuable tool for supervisors to monitor performance and provide constructive feedback, facilitating continuous improvement in service delivery. Overall, the disciplined use of a monthly checklist guarantees that the audiology assistant completes their essential job functions and upholds the high standards of patient care set out by the clinic administrators. An Essential Job Functions Worksheet can be helpful in creating the list of duties and responsibilities listed on the End-of-Month Checklist (Figure 10–8).

Essential Job Functions

Although the state may define the Scope of Practice for an audiology assistant, often there are no rules and the audiologist defines their role within the practice. Determining essential job functions can bring clarity to the task of defining what duties and responsibilities will be assigned to the audiology assistant.

A simple method is to have staff audiologists develop a list of daily duties and tasks. Within this list, the audiologists determine which of those tasks require licensure as an audiologist or

Place your logo here

Place your tag line here

Drop-In Hearing Instrument Service

Patient Name: _____

Phone Number: _____

Date: _____   Time: _____

Description of Problem:

	Right	**Left**
Shell cracked/broken	☐	☐
Needs Tubing	☐	☐
Intermittent (on or off)	☐	☐
Fades in or out	☐	☐
Batteries are dying quickly	☐	☐
Poor sound quality Describe:	☐	☐

_____

Other Describe: ☐   ☐

_____

If anything happened that may have caused the instruments to malfunction, please describe. For example, were they exposed to moisture or dropped?

_____

_____

Drop-In Service Policy

Thank you for coming in today! We do not want to discourage you from dropping by, however, a staff member may not be available to service your instrument right away. We will make every attempt to have your instrument back to you or to update you on the status of your instrument within 24 hours. In the future, the best way to make sure that someone is available to work on your instruments would be to make an appointment with one of our Doctors of Audiology, the Hearing Specialist or our Audiology Assistant. All will be happy to help you!

Thank you for placing your trust in us!

Figure 10–6. Walk-in/drop-off checklist. *Source:* Created by Kingham, N. Eastside Audiology, Nichole Kingham (2024).

EAR MOLD ORDERING INFO			

Manuf: EmTech   Westone   Microsonic

EAR: Left   Right   Both

New Order   Remake

New User   Old User

Helix Curl On   Helix Curl Off

Ear Texture Soft   Normal   Firm

Hrng loss: _____

Canal Length: Short/Med/Long/Cut to mark

EARMOLD STYLE: _____
#2 skeleton, #3 canal, #3W canal w/ hook, #5 full shell
STA- open fit canal style, STC- open fit canal w/ lock

Material: _____

Mold Color: _____

Venting:	No vent	Pressure	Small
	Medium	Large	IROS
	OPEN	Small SAV	Lrg SAV

Tubing: _____

Need in house by: _____

Special instructions: _____

_____
_____
_____
_____
_____

Developed by Nichole Kingham, Au.D. v2.2 2024

Figure 10–7. Earmold order checklist. *Source:* Created by Kingham, N. Eastside Audiology, Nichole Kingham (2024).

hearing instrument specialist. If licensure, certification, or registration is not required for the task, it is likely a task that could be completed by an audiology assistant. Essential job function worksheets are a tool that can be helpful in organizing the different aspects of clinical and administrative tasks that are completed on a regular basis in the clinic. These job function worksheets can be found with a simple Internet search. They serve several purposes:

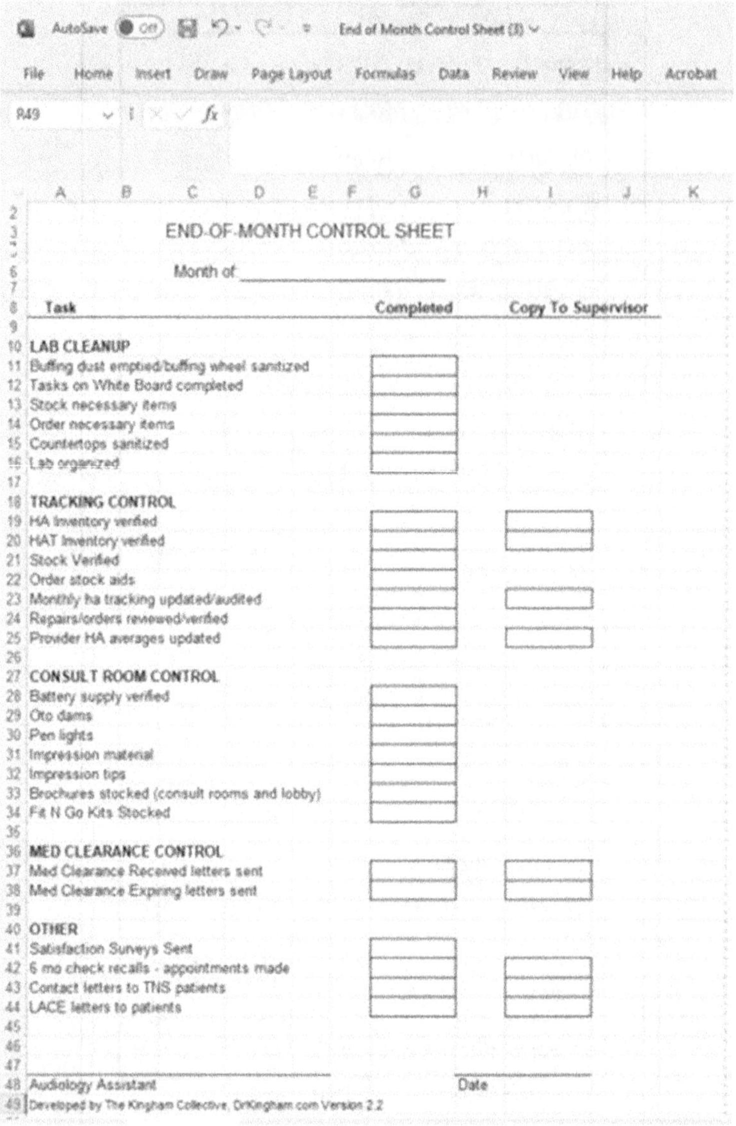

Figure 10–8. End of the month checklist, spreadsheet. *Source:* Created by Kingham, N. Eastside Audiology, Nichole Kingham (2024).

1. *Clarity:* Essential job function worksheets provide clarity to clinic management as well as to both audiologists and audiology assistants about the expectations surrounding the core responsibilities associated with the role an audiology assistant will play within the clinic, ensuring alignment with the clinic's mission and goals.

2. *Recruitment:* These worksheets are instrumental during the re-

cruitment and selection process, enabling the clinic to effectively communicate job expectations to potential candidates and ensure the selection of individuals who have the necessary skills and qualifications.

3. *ADA compliance:* Essential job function worksheets can help ensure compliance with the Americans with Disabilities Act (ADA). Employers must be able to identify the essential functions of a job to reasonably accommodate a qualified individual with a disability.

4. *Communication:* These worksheets also serve as a reference point for discussing overall performance during evaluations, allowing the employer or supervisor to assess the audiology assistant's performance based on the essential functions of the position.

5. *Training and development:* The development of training systems within the clinic ensures that audiology assistants will continually gain knowledge and skills on the job. An essential job function worksheet can assist clinic owners and managers in the development of an audiology assistant training regimen.

See Appendix 10–A for the Essential and Marginal Job Functions Worksheet.

Training an Audiology Assistant

To set an audiology assistant up for success and ensure that they are well prepared to carry out their responsibilities, the training an audiology assistant re-

ceives must be consistent and ongoing. Training programs for audiology assistants, whether in-house, online, or in a classroom, should cover topics such as:

- Basic anatomy and physiology of the auditory and vestibular systems
- Audiometric testing procedures and equipment function
- Infection control
- Safety protocols
- HIPAA requirements
- Patient care and counseling and customer service skills
- Practice management software
- Administrative tasks
- Hearing aids and hearing aid programming
- Hearing aid servicing
- Use of the Hearing Instrument Test Box

Currently, there are no accredited degree programs specifically for audiology assisting. Audiology assistants can receive formal education by pursuing an undergraduate Speech and Hearing Science degree. Otherwise, three programs in existence are certificate of completion programs. These are Florida's Nova Southeastern University online certificate of completion program, the Audiology Academy online certificate of completion program, and the Georgia State University hybrid online and in-person certificate program.

The best portion of the training experience is within the clinic itself. This hands-on experience guided by the supervising audiologist offers the audiology assistant an opportunity to gain insight into patient care but also to learn the protocols and procedures that are specific to the clinic.

The key to great outcomes in training an audiology assistant is to prepare a training plan. The supervising audiologist should schedule a specific time that focuses on a specific topic or skill. This means that the schedule may initially be inefficient for the audiologist doing the training in the first few weeks after the audiology assistant joins the practice. This focused training requires extra time from the supervising audiologist to explain processes and procedures and/or the demonstration of practice skills. Flexibility in this training schedule will ensure that the audiology assistant has time to ask questions and dive deeper into topics if needed. Taking extra time in the beginning may decrease the overall length of time required to get the audiology assistant fully integrated into patient care.

Best Practices for Audiology Assistants

Best practices for an audiology assistant in a hearing clinic can be a roadmap for effective utilization. Several best practices can assist the clinic to maximize the contributions of their assistants:

Quality Assurance

Implementing regular quality assurance measures protects the best interests of patients and the clinic. Quality assurance measures also protect the audiology assistant. New employees do not often know what they do not know. Monitoring the performance of audiology assistants and ensuring adherence to established protocols and procedures makes good business as well as clinical sense. Common quality assurance measures may include chart audits, case reviews, and proficiency evaluations.

Patient-Centered Care

The audiology assistant should feel empowered by their supervisors and coworkers to engage in patient-centered care. Best practices should include training in the necessary skills and resources to support patients in understanding their hearing health and treatment options.

Continuity of Care

Establishing continuity in patient care fosters trust among patients. If patients lack clarity regarding the responsibilities of each member of their care team, they may experience uncertainty about whom to rely on for support or guidance. Supervisors should promote continuity of care by ensuring audiology assistants are thoroughly acquainted with patients' specific needs and treatment strategies. This approach aids in maintaining uniformity and improving the overall patient journey.

Professional Boundaries

Supervisors should establish clear professional boundaries for audiology assistants to ensure that they understand the limitations of their roles and responsibilities. Best practices relating to professional boundaries will encourage open communication with audiologists in cases where additional guidance or oversight may be needed.

ESTABLISHING PROFESSIONAL BOUNDARIES

Professional boundaries are crucial to maintaining ethical standards and professionalism in the hearing healthcare clinic. Audiology assistants, especially when new to the field, may need training on professional boundaries. Below are some best practices related to professional boundaries for an audiology assistant:

1. *Understanding scope of practice:* Audiology assistants should be familiar with their job description and the limitations of their role in the clinic. Audiology assistants should be familiar with what tasks they are allowed to perform and when to defer to the audiologist.
2. *Maintaining confidentiality:* Audiology assistants should always respect a patient's confidentiality and privacy. Specific training should be given on the Health Insurance Portability and Accountability Act (HIPAA) and when it is appropriate and inappropriate to discuss patient information.
3. *Establish clear communication:* Audiology assistants should wear a nametag that communicates their role to patients, and they should be able to clearly communicate the role they play in patient care. Patients should understand the limitations of the role and when they can expect to see an audiologist.
4. *Seek supervision:* Audiology assistants are not autonomous. They will work under the direct supervision of an audiologist. Audiology assistants should consult with audiologists regularly, especially in situations that fall outside the scope of practice for an audiology assistant or require the use of clinical judgment.
5. *Establish appropriate patient boundaries:* Audiology assistants should not engage in personal relationships with patients or their family members. Maintaining professionalism and focusing solely on providing excellent patient care should be the gold standard.
6. *Establish professional boundaries with colleagues:* Audiology assistants should respect their roles and responsibilities within the healthcare team.
7. *Document carefully:* Audiology assistants should be taught appropriate documentation and should practice documenting all patient interactions accurately and objectively.
8. *Practice self-*care: Teaching employees to care for their own well-being to prevent burnout and decrease stress is good for the whole team. Encourage and empower the audiology assistant to seek supervisor support if they experience stress or emotional challenges in their role.

Professional Ethics

Supervisors should provide guidance and training on ethical considerations related to patient confidentiality, informed consent, and professional conduct. Upholding ethical standards in the audiology clinic is essential for maintaining trust and integrity in patient care.

Paying an Audiology Assistant Well

The typical pay rate for an audiology assistant depends largely on three factors:

■ The education and experience level of the applicant
■ The geographic area of the clinic
■ The type of clinic

Checking websites like Indeed.com and Payscale.com can be helpful in determining a starting wage for an audiology assistant. In considering what an audiology assistant should be paid, investigate the current pay rate for medical assistants in the area. Given the scope of practice of a medical assistant, audiology assistants are similar enough to grant comparisons between these two occupations.

Consider placing the audiology assistant on a graduated scale for a pay rate that increases as their experience increases (Figure 10–9). Tying a graduated scale into training goals will motivate the assistant to meet those goals and keep training on track.

After the audiology assistant has completed training, consider adding key performance indicators (KPIs) to the job description. Key performance indicators

---

ETHICS DEFINITIONS

Business Ethics: "Business ethics are principles that guide decision-making" (Boyles, 2023).

Patient Confidentiality: "Confidentiality is the right of an individual to have personal, identifiable medical information kept private" (Encyclopedia.com).

Informed Consent: "The process in which a health care provider educates a patient about the risks, benefits, and alternatives of a given procedure or intervention" (Shah et al., 2023).

Professional Conduct: According to the American Academy of Audiology code of ethics, "Members shall provide professional services and conduct research with honesty and compassion, and shall respect the dignity, worth, and rights of those served" (AAA, 2019).

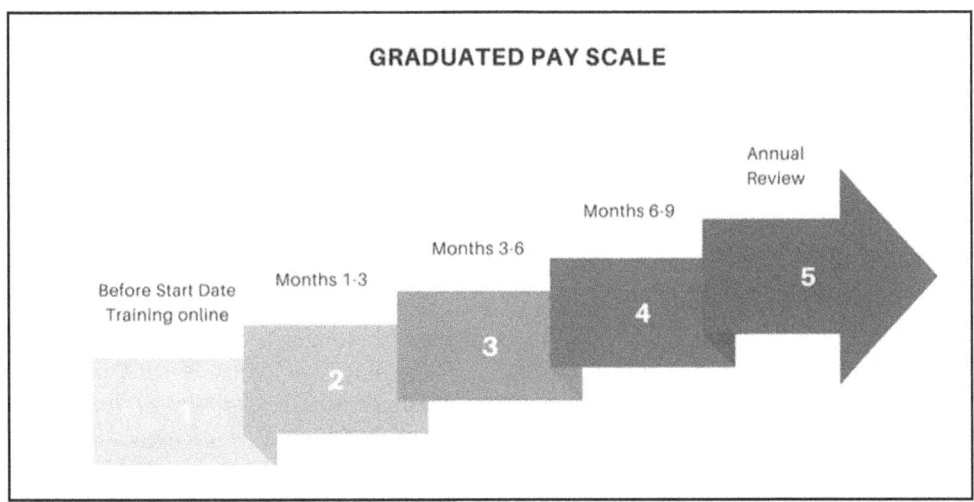

GRADUATED PAY SCALE

Figure 10–9. Graduated pay scale for audiology assistants. *Source:* Eastside Audiology, Nichole Kingham (2024).

are tasks that are above and beyond the general scope of practice that, if completed, benefit both patients and the practice. By reaching KPI goals, the audiology assistant can increase their monthly pay and increase the revenue of the practice. Some examples of KPI for audiology assistants include:

- Calling x number of established patients to have them return to the clinic.
- Calling x number of patients who have expired warranties or service plans to discuss a new coverage or service plan extension.
- Calling x number of patients regarding new technology advancements.
- Creating a monthly point-of-sale goal for accessories.
- Creating a Friends and Family referral goal.
- Creating a patient online review goal.

Summary

As clinic owners, managers, and audiologists consider methods to see more patients in less time, the use of support staff such as audiology assistants should be an integral part of that consideration. In addition, the use of audiology assistants can *decrease burnout* clinicians feel when they must be their own assistant. As the number of patients with hearing loss increases, decisions regarding the scope of practice, licensure versus certification or registration, and the role audiology assistants should play in the audiology clinic will become more important. Providing excellent patient care while facilitating work-life balance and decreasing stress in the workplace for audiologists, the audiology assistant must be an integral component of the audiology team. This chapter provides the history, scope of practice, and best practice considerations that are needed to evaluate and develop the competitive strategies for successfully incorporating an audiology assistant into any practice.

References

American Academy of Audiology. (2019). Code of Ethics of the American Academy of Audiology. https://www.audiology.org/wp-content/uploads/2021/05/201910-CodeOfEthicsOf-AAA.pdf

American Academy of Audiology. (2021). Position Statement, Audiology Assistants. https://www.audiology.org/academy-publishes-audiology-assistants-position-statement/

Andrews, J., & Hammill, T. (2017). Audiology assistant scope of practice and utilization. *Audiology Today*, *29*(4), 48–55.

Boyles, M. (2023). What are business ethics and why are they important? Harvard Business School Online. https://online.hbs.edu/blog/post/business-ethics

Duran, J. (2002). The role of audiology assistants in a clinical setting. Doctoral dissertation, University of South Florida. http://scholarcommons.usf.edu/etd/1519.

Emanuel, D. C. (2021). Occupational stress in U.S. audiologists. *American Journal of Audiology*, *30*(4), 1010–1022. https://10.1044/2021_AJA-20-00211

Encyclopedia.com. (n.d.). Definition of patient confidentiality. https://www.encyclopedia.com/medicine/encyclopedias-almanacs-transcripts-and-maps/patient-confidentiality-0

Hammill, T., & Freeman, B. (2001). Scope of practice for audiologists' assistants: Survey results. *Audiology Today*, *13*(6), 34–36.

Jorgensen, L. E. (2016). Verification and validation of hearing aids: Opportunity not an obstacle. *Journal of Otology*, *11*(2), 57–62.

Jorgensen, L. E., & Gellhaus, J. M. (2022). It may meet your standards, but does it meet mine? *Audiology Today*, *34*(4), 46–52. https://www.audiology.org/news-and-publications/audiology-today/articles/it-may-meet-your-standards-but-does-it-meet-mine/

Jorgensen, L. E., & Novak, M. (2022). Verification and validation: Just the standards. *Seminars in Hearing*, *43*(2), 85–93.

Karzon, R., Hunter, L., & Steuerwald, W. (2018). Audiology assistants: Results of a multicenter survey. *Journal of the American Academy of Audiology*, *29*(5), 405–416.

Mueller, G., & Emanuel, D. C. (2022, April 11). 20Q: Occupational stress and audiologists. *Audiology Online*. https://www.audiologyonline.com/articles/20q-occupational-stress-and-audiologists-28159

Nemes, J. (2001). What should be the role of audiologic technicians? It's debatable. *The Hearing Journal*, *54*(8), 23–31. https://journals.lww.com/thehearingjournal/fulltext/2001/08000/what_should_be_the_role_of_audiologic_technicians_.5.aspx

Northern, J. L., & Suter, A. H. (1972). Supportive personnel in audiology. *ASHA*, *14*(7), 354–357.

Severn, M. S., Searchfield, G. D., & Huggard, P. (2012). Occupational stress amongst audiologists: Compassion satisfaction, compassion fatigue, and burnout. *International Journal of Audiology*, *51*(1), 3–9.

Shah, P., Thornton, I., Turrin, D., & Hipskind, J. H. (2023). Informed consent. StatPearls Publishing. https://www.ncbi.nlm.nih.gov/books/NBK430827/

Taylor, B., & Rogin, C. (2011). The top-10 ways to create consumer delight with hearing aids. *The Hearing Review*. https://hearingreview.com/hearing-products/the-top-10-ways-to-create-consumer-delight-with-hearing-aids

Wince, J., Emanuel, D. C., Hendy, N., & Reed, N. (2022). Change resistance and clinical practice strategies in audiology. *Journal of the American Academy of Audiology, 33*(5), 293–300.

Windmill, I. M., & Freeman, B. A. (2013). Demand for audiology services: 30-Yr projections and impact on academic pro-

grams. *Journal of the American Academy of Audiology, 24*(5), 407–416.

Zimmer, M., Emanuel, D., & Reed, N. S. (2022). Burnout in U.S. audiologists. *Journal of the American Academy of Audiology, 33*(1), 36–44.

Appendix 10–A
Essential and Marginal Job Functions Worksheet

This worksheet will help audiology clinics determine the essential and marginal functions of the audiology assistant position. The worksheet should be completed or reviewed before (1) beginning the hiring process, (2) requesting a fitness for duty under the FMLA, (3) initiating the reasonable accommodations process, and (4) completing an annual review. The essential and marginal functions worksheet should accompany the job description to determine whether an applicant can perform the essential duties of a position.

When completing the worksheet, consider these important questions:

- Would eliminating this function from the audiologist's required duties substantially improve the clinic's efficiency?
- Would there be significant consequences if the audiologist did not perform this function?
- Can other employees complete this function if necessary?
- What equipment is used to complete this function? How frequently is the equipment used?
- What are the physical and mental requirements of this function?
- What critical skills, experience, training, education, and/or license are needed?
- How much time per week is spent by an audiologist doing this function?
- Could this function be performed in another way?

Employee Name:

Employee Position:

Date:

Instructions:

1. Review the job description for the position.
2. Identify the essential functions of the job—those duties that are funda-mental to the position.
3. Define marginal functions—duties that are secondary or noncritical to the role.
4. Rate each function based on its importance to the position and to the clinic as a whole.

Function	Essential (E) / Marginal (M)	Importance Rating (1–5)*
Conducting hearing screenings	E	
Conducting immittance measures without interpretation	E	
Handling patient complaints and respond-ing to patient requests	E	
Generating reports	E	
Facilitating patient questionnaires	E	
Performing earmold impressions	M	
Assisting with administrative tasks	M	
Participating in company events	M	
Conducting recalls to established patients	E	
Providing technical support to patients	E	
Provide support and comfort to patients during examinations and procedures	E	
Handling customer complaints	E	
Handling phone inquiries, managing emails, and assisting with general adminis-trative tasks as needed.	E	

continues

Appendix 6–A. *continued*

Function	Essential (E) / Marginal (M)	Importance Rating (1–5)*
Creating and reviewing hearing aid sales contracts	E	
Completing supply orders	E	
Updating company website	M	
Attending industry conferences	M	
Cleaning, calibrating, and maintaining audiometric equipment and testing rooms to ensure proper functionality	E	
Maintaining accurate patient records, including test results, medical history, and treatment plans	E	
Ensuring confidentiality and compliance with HIPAA regulations in handling patient information	E	
Assisting audiologists in fitting hearing aids and other assistive listening devices	E	
Instructing patients on how to use and maintain their hearing aids effectively	E	
Scheduling appointments and managing patient appointment calendars	E	
Conducting routine checks on patients' hearing aids and assisting with in-house repairs as necessary	E	
Other (specify)		

*Importance rating.

1. Not important
2. Somewhat important
3. Important
4. Very important
5. Critical

Notes:

- Essential functions are those duties that, if not performed by an audiology assistant, would affect the efficiency of the clinic.
- Marginal functions are those duties that may enhance the effectiveness of the clinic but are not vital or could be completed by another employee.
- Ensure that each function is rated accurately based on its relevance to the position and its significance in improving the efficiency of the role of the audiologist in the clinic.

Review and Approval:

Audiology Assistant Signature: _____ Date: _____

Supervisor Signature: _____ Date: _____

11 Accounting and Fiscal Management

Robert M. Traynor, EdD, MBA

Introduction

Accounting principles are defined rules that ensure businesses follow the same financial practices. By using these guidelines to standardize how the clinic tracks and interprets accounting data, accurate comparisons of financials from different time periods can present a clear understanding of the health of a practice. Accountants are trained in bookkeeping procedure and in the preparation, audit, and analysis of accounts (Grigg & Lane, 2023).

Audiologists are practitioners, not accountants, and do not need to know the specifics of preparing asset, liability, and

---

AN OVERVIEW OF ECONOMIC EXCHANGES IN AN AUDIOLOGY PRACTICE

In a perfect world, a transaction would simply be between the patient and the audiologist. Tracy (2001) describes six basic types of economic exchanges for which accountants ensure correct business interaction (Figure 11–1). Generally, these economic exchanges involve many others who are part of necessary interactions in daily operations of the practice:

- Patients.
- Government.
- Equity sources of capital.
- Debt sources of capital.
- Suppliers and vendors.
- Employees.

These basic exchanges are how the practice interacts with the real world of daily operations.

continued on next page

---

continued from previous page

The practice deals with the patients through employees, office and clinical supplies, and hearing instruments and support items purchased from suppliers, vendors, and hearing instrument manufacturers and repair facilities.

If cash reserves are unavailable to purchase these products or pay the employees and other expenses, the practitioner may have to obtain an interest-bearing loan or establish a credit line through their banker. Another option available to the practice owner is to add partners or stock-

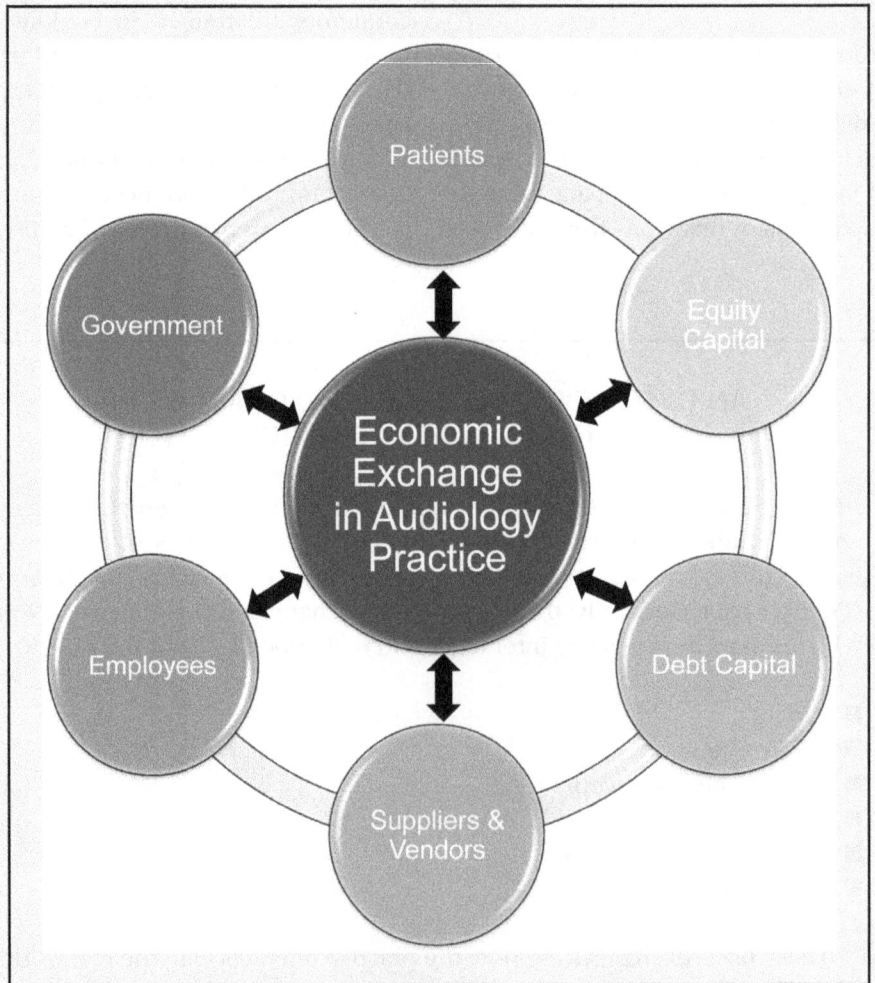

Figure 11–1. Economic exchanges in audiology practice.

continued on next page

continued from previous page

holders who can bring additional financial opportunities in exchange for shares in the practice. These partners or stockholders will own a percentage of the practice and appropriately expect a return on their investment. Additionally, as they are financial stakeholders in the practice, they will likely want a say in the day-to-day operations and management of the business segment of the practice. The attorney for the practice will be involved in document preparation to establish the most appropriate method for adding partner/stockholders. The accountant for the practice will reconfigure the books to include allowances for the partner/stockholders and to make sure the practice meets its financial obligations to them.

capital account entry reports and accounting theory, but a business owner should be familiar with the terminology and have a general knowledge of the procedures. This not only is essential for monitoring the success of the practice but also allows for intelligent conversation with the professionals that *do* understand accounting concepts. Knowledge of accounting principles will:

■ *Facilitate communication:* Allows for effective communication with bookkeepers and accountants.
■ *Assess practice health:* Helps demonstrate the health of an audiology practice.
■ *Evaluate profitability:* Enables the evaluation of profitability for locations, employees, and procedures.
■ *Inform management:* Offers the practitioner valuable knowledge for decisive management.

The more a practitioner knows about appropriate accounting methods, the better their capability to understand and execute professional business recommendations for adjustments in procedures and/or policies to ensure profitability.

Business Costs

Before beginning a discussion of fiscal management and accounting, it is necessary to address business costs. Accountants and bookkeepers compile and document revenues and costs to accurately reflect how the practice is performing and whether financial actions are needed. A major concern for a practice manager is controlling costs, a major step toward profitability. Costs that must be accounted for in any business are as follows:

Opportunity Costs

There are procedures in audiology practice that generate profit and those that do not generate much profit due to required equipment, space, expertise, labor, and other resources. Fernando et al. (2024) discuss the fundamental economic concept of *opportunity cost* as the forgone business benefit that would have been derived from an option other than the one that was chosen. The business concept of opportunity cost is based upon the fact that the practice has limited resources that should be used efficiently to generate profit. Good business sense suggests that the expenditure of those resources should only go to profitable procedures, sometimes generating a trade-off of one product, procedure, or service in favor of those more profitable. Thus, the efficient use of business resources to generate income becomes the question.

Consider auditory brainstem response (ABR) testing in audiology private practice. In the 1980s, 1990s, and early 2000s, this procedure was an integral component of most audiology clinics for ruling out acoustic tumors, assessing children and babies, and evaluating the difficult-to-test and developmentally disabled. With the advent of magnetic resonance imaging (MRI), otoacoustic emissions (OAEs), and other audiological procedures, declining reimbursements, insurance discounts, equipment maintenance, and the need for continuing education, many private practices have dispensed with this unprofitable procedure. For survival of the business, when a procedure becomes unprofitable, such as in the case of ABR, the practice owner/manager and the accountant must analyze the practice resources required to offer the procedure that could be used to generate profit more efficiently by instituting new more profitable procedures and discontinuing the ABR procedure. The question became, when the ABR procedure lost its profitability, would the business be better off by using the clinic space, funds for the equipment and updates, time conducting the procedure, and continuing education to conduct a more profitable procedure? While there may be other benefits to offering the ABR procedure other than profit (stature in the community, referral source

needs, marketing, and others) that must be weighed relative to discontinuation of the procedure, the owner/manager, in conjunction with their accountant, must continually weigh the opportunity costs of clinic offerings to maintain profitability.

Fixed Costs

Fixed costs, sometimes known as overhead, are those incurred each month. Examples of fixed costs include bank loans, rent, telephone, utilities, salaries, and payroll taxes that must be paid even if there is no business conducted. These expenses must be paid each month before any profit is created. In the break-even analysis presented in Figure 11–2, the practice must dispense 10 hearing instruments to cover fixed expenses each month, before moving on to paying the variable expenses that lead to profitability.

High fixed expenses commonly generate cash flow issues that can, if left unchecked, become a primary cause of financial collapse resulting in failure of the practice.

Incremental or Variable Costs

Incremental or variable costs are the increase in total costs resulting from an increase in the amount of business conducted. The greater the amount of business transacted, the higher the incremental/variable costs. Incremental/variable costs include the costs of hearing instruments, commissions to employees, warranty support, and materials costs (electrodes, probe tips, disposable headphone tips, earmold impression material and other items), which will vary relative to the number of hearing instruments dis-

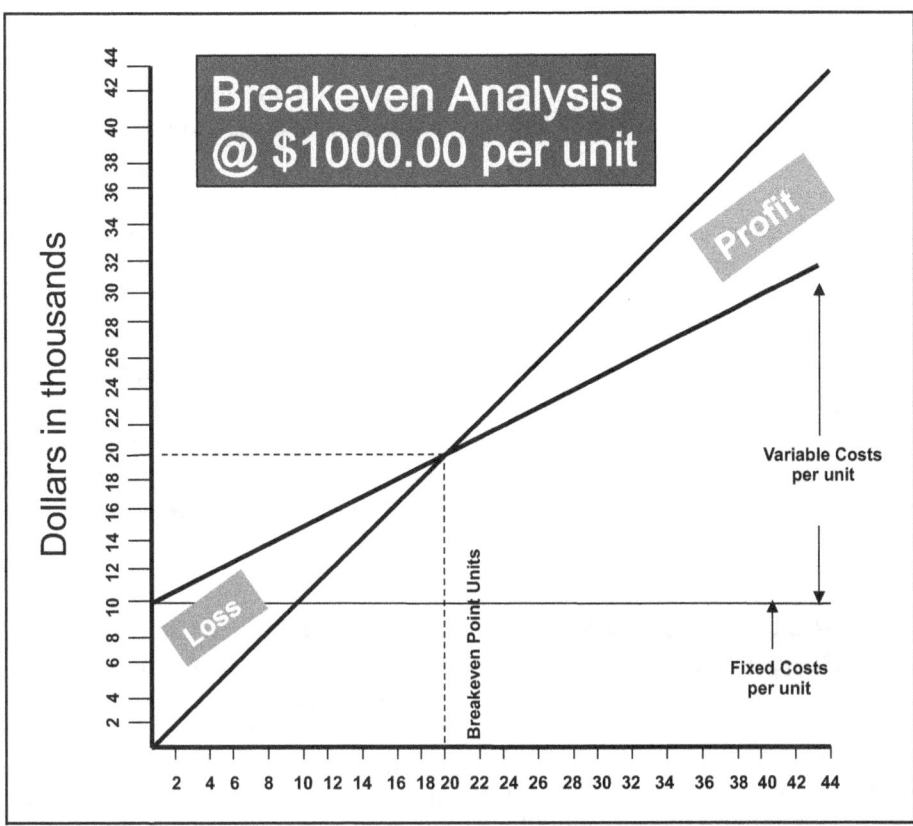

Figure 11–2. Sample of breakeven analysis.

pensed, procedures conducted, or services provided. The owner/manager, in conjunction with the accountant, must calculate and be on top of these incremental costs as they have an effect on the overall profit generated by the business conducted.

Avoidable Costs

Avoidable costs are those that have not yet been incurred or can be reversed. In all businesses, there are methods to reduce costs by simply incurring less expense. For example, sometimes it is better to have the employees clean the office than to hire a janitorial service, to use a less expensive brand of equip-

ment that performs the same function as the expensive brand, to have employees pay a percentage of their health insurance costs, to not upgrade the mobile phones, and/or to carefully observe the opportunity costs involved in offering new procedures and products. Although these are only a few examples of how to cut costs, more inventive methods may be practical for different practice venues.

Sunk Costs

According to Tuovila et al. (2024), *sunk costs* are basically the opposite of avoidable costs in that they are expenses to which the practice is irreversibly committed and, once incurred, will not be recovered. In audiology practices, these are costs for equipment, such as audiometers, ABR/OAE and videonystagmography (VNG) units, computers, software, and peripheral systems. While these items substantially depreciate when purchased, the classic example of a sunk cost is a new sign that marks and brands the practice. Although it can be used for years and is certainly worth its initial cost, it is not likely that another audiology practice will want to purchase it. Similar to other business expenses, once the sign is obtained, it is a sunk cost that will never be recovered.

Accounting in an Audiology Private Practice

Accountants provide the practitioner with internal and external methods for monitoring theft and embezzlement, as well as honest bookkeeping errors by performing internal audits. Simultaneously, accountants may also offer personal and business financial planning services and business valuations. Accountants not only ensure funds are deposited in the appropriate accounts but also advise the practitioner about the fiscal health of the practice. They provide information about cash flow and retained earnings relative to the adequacy of funding required to conduct day-to-day business transactions. It is also the responsibility of the accountant (in association with the practice bookkeeper) to ensure that expenses are paid on time and that transactions for these payments are recorded properly. In addition, property such as sound rooms, audiometers, VNG equipment, paper, printers, pens,

and so on should be inventoried and accounted for to control their use and assess real value for property tax purposes and business expense deductions.

Accountants prepare reports for practitioners to assist in evidence-based decisions regarding the success or failure of daily operations, specific procedures, or a new market offering. These reports are fundamental to understanding the reasons for positive or negative changes in the bottom-line performance of the practice. An accountant's primary responsibilities vary from one practice to another, but common areas include, but are not limited to:

- Cash into the practice (receivables).
- Cash payments from the practice (payables).
- Inventory and purchases.
- Property accounting.
- Tax accounting methods: cash or accrual.
- Payroll preparation.
- Assistance in monitoring the bookkeeper/financial manager.

Just as audiologists are licensed to practice in their respective states, accountants are licensed by the State Boards of Accountancy. Similar to audiologists who choose to seek certification, accountants may seek certification from the American Institute of Certified Public Accountants (AICPA). Their certification title is Certified Public Accountant (CPA) (AICPA, 2024). Just as all audiologists are now doctors of audiology (AuD), not all audiologists are board certified; all certified public accountants are accountants, but not all accountants are CPAs. While American Board Certification

(ABA) and/or the Certificate of Clinical Competence in Audiology from the American Speech-Language-Hearing Association (ASHA) certification is voluntary for audiologists, so is the certification process for accountants.

Audiologists have specialty certification opportunities through the ABA and ASHA, and CPAs have specialty certification available to those seeking advanced credentials as well. For example, the AICPA offers specialty certification for CPAs in the conduct of business valuations. The Accreditation in Business Valuation (ABV) identifies those CPAs with advanced training and certification in assessing and issuing valuations of various businesses, including healthcare practices.

Cash and Accrual Methods of Accounting

The *cash method* and the *accrual method* (sometimes called cash basis and accrual basis) are the two principal methods of keeping track of a business's income and expenses. Typically, if a business is very small, the cash method is chosen to keep things simple. As the business grows, it may be necessary to use the more complex accrual basis of accounting as it provides a better picture of a company's profits during an accounting period. Further, the accrual basis of accounting will also provide a better picture of a company's financial position at a moment or point in time. Fishman (2024) sums up the differences between the two methods by indicating that the differences between a cash basis and an accrual basis are simply the timing of when transactions,

including sales and purchases, are credited or debited to the accounts. Whichever method is used, it is important to realize that either method only presents a partial picture of the financial status of the business. Whether the practice is inclined to choose either the cash or the accrual basis, the accountant of record must be involved in the decision process. They can clarify the two accounting methods and recommend the best course of action for the practice circumstances and venue (Figure 11–3).

The Cash Method

The core of the cash method of accounting is the flow of cash in and out of the practice. Income is recorded when received and expenses are paid when they occur: Both income and expenses are put on the books and charged to the period in which they are received, and taxes are paid based on actual revenue in hand. Historically, accountants have recommended the cash basis for small businesses with minimal inventory, less complex business structure, and only one or two partner/owners involved. Although the cash method provides a more accurate picture of how much actual cash the business has, it may offer a misleading picture of longer-term profitability. Under the cash method, for instance, the books may show one month to be spectacularly profitable, when actual sales have been slow and, by coincidence, a lot of credit customers paid their bills in that month. From a tax perspective, it is sometimes beneficial for a new business to use the cash basis of accounting so that recording income can be put off until the next tax year and expenses can be claimed immediately.

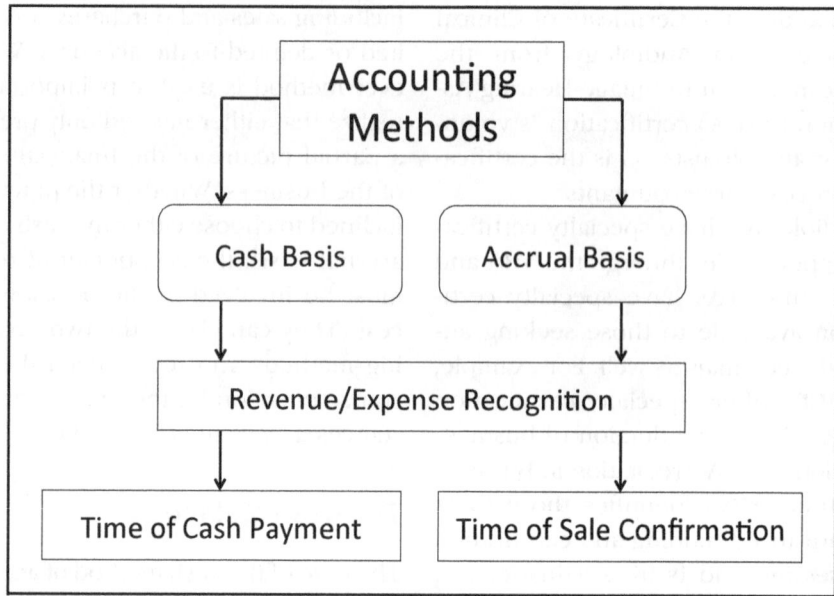

Figure 11–3. Cash and accrual accounting.

The Accrual Method

The accrual basis of accounting requires that income and expenses be entered into the ledger when a transaction occurs regardless of whether monies have been received for the services or products provided. Expenses are deductible when the practice is billed, not when the expenses are paid. Taxes are paid based on the revenue reported on the ledger with or without the revenue in hand.

The obvious downside to this method resides in the fact that the practice might have to pay income taxes on monies that have not been collected in part or in full. The owner or manager of the practice can minimize the downside of the accrual method by collecting revenue for services and hearing instruments as soon as possible, preferably at the time of service. That may or may not be a problem for hearing instruments; however, most patients rely on their insurance carriers

to pay their medical bills, including diagnostic studies common to the practice of audiology. Third-party payers who reimburse in a timely fashion aid in reducing the tax impact inherent in the accrual method of accounting. While the accrual method shows the ebb and flow of business income and debts more accurately, it may not accurately present the available cash reserves, which could result in a serious cash flow problem. For instance, the income ledger may show thousands of dollars in sales, while in reality, the bank account is empty because patients or insurance companies have not paid.

Generally Accepted Accounting Principles (GAAP)

General knowledge of accounting procedures and good communication skills

1. **Principle of Regularity:** GAAP-compliant accountants strictly adhere to established rules and regulations.

2. **Principle of Consistency:** Consistent standards are applied throughout the financial reporting process.

3. **Principle of Sincerity:** GAAP-compliant accountants are committed to accuracy and impartiality.

4. **Principle of Permanence of Methods:** Consistent procedures are used in the preparation of all financial reports.

5. **Principle of Non-Compensation:** All aspects of an organization's performance, whether positive or negative, are fully reported with no prospect of debt compensation.

6. **Principle of Prudence:** Speculation does not influence the reporting of financial data.

7. **Principle of Continuity:** Asset valuations assume the organization's operations will continue.

8. **Principle of Periodicity:** Reporting of revenues is divided by standard accounting periods, such as fiscal quarters or fiscal years.

9. **Principle of Materiality:** Financial reports fully disclose the organization's monetary situation.

10. **Principle of Utmost Good Faith:** All involved parties are assumed to be acting honestly.

Figure 11–4. Generally Accepted Accounting Principles (GAAP). *Source*: Account ing.com (2024).

can ensure an understanding of where and how the revenue is generated and the costs involved in the daily practice operation. Accountant reports and bookkeeping operations are prepared according to internationally accepted accounting rules called the Generally Accepted Accounting Principles (GAAP), a universal method of valuing profit and measuring assets and liabilities. While each of these principles has detailed and extensive descriptions, Accounting.com (2024) presents the GAAP principles in Figure 11–4.

Although GAAP procedures vary somewhat from one country to another, GAAP rules are used to conduct accounting in all businesses and strict adherence is required. GAAP describes how transactions for costs, profit, inventory, sales, and other business specifics are recorded and allows a comparison of one practice to another as businesses all use the same procedures for accounting. U.S. law requires businesses releasing financial statements to the public and

companies publicly traded on stock exchanges and indices to follow GAAP guidelines. Thus, most small businesses also record their transactions using this procedure.

The fundamental accounting rules vary slightly from one source to another, but Silbiger (2012) summarizes seven basic concepts that guide the policies relative to the principles underlying the GAAP rules in Figure 11–4. These fundamental concepts using GAAP include:

- *Economic entity assumption.* The accountant keeps all the business transactions of a sole proprietorship separate from the business owner's personal transactions. For legal purposes, a sole proprietorship and its owner are considered to be one entity, but for accounting purposes, they are considered to be separate entities.
- *Monetary unit assumption.* Economic activity is measured in U.S. dollars, and only transactions that

can be expressed in U.S. dollars are recorded. Since this is a basic accounting principle, it is assumed that the dollar's purchasing power has not changed over time. As a result, accountants ignore the effect of inflation on recorded amounts. For example, dollars from a 2012 transaction are combined (or shown with) dollars from a 2024 transaction.

■ *Time period assumption*. This accounting principle assumes that it is possible to report the complex and ongoing activities of a business in a relatively short, distinct time interval such as the 5 months ended May 31, 2023, or the 5 weeks ended May 1, 2023. The shorter the time interval, the higher the probability that an accountant needs to estimate amounts relevant to that period. For example, the property tax bill is received on December 15 of each year. On the income statement for the year ended December 31, 2023, the amount was known, but for the income statement for the 3 months ended March 31, 2024, the amount was not known, and an estimate had to be used. According to GAAP, it is imperative that the time interval (or period of time) be shown in the heading of each income statement, statement of stockholders' equity, and statement of cash flows. Labeling one of these financial statements with "December 31" is not good enough: The reader needs to know if the statement covers the 1 week ended December 31, 2023; the month ended December 31, 2023; the 3 months ended December 31, 2023; or the year ended December 31, 2023.

■ *Cost principle*. From an accountant's point of view, the term "cost" refers to the amount spent (cash or the cash equivalent) when an item was originally obtained, whether that purchase happened last year or 30 years ago. For this reason, the amounts shown on financial statements are often referred to as historical cost amounts. Due to this accounting principle, asset amounts are not adjusted upward for inflation. In fact, as a general rule, asset amounts are not adjusted to reflect any type of increase in value. Hence, an asset amount does not reflect the amount of money a company would receive if it were to sell the asset at today's market value.

■ *Full disclosure principle*. If certain information is important to an investor or lender using the financial statements, that information should be disclosed within the statement or in the notes to the statement. It is because of a basic accounting principle including numerous pages of "footnotes" that are often attached to financial statements. An example of this is if a company is named in a lawsuit that demands a significant amount of money. When the financial statements are prepared, it is not clear whether the company will be able to defend itself or whether it might lose the lawsuit. As a result of these conditions and because of the full disclosure principle, the lawsuit will be described in the notes to the financial statements. A company usually lists its significant accounting policies as the first note to its financial statements.

■ *Going concern principle*. This principle assumes that a company will continue to exist long enough to carry out its objectives and commitments and will not liquidate in the foreseeable future. If the company's financial situation is such that the accountant believes the company will not be able to continue, the accountant is required to disclose this assessment. The going concern principle allows the company to defer some of its prepaid expenses until future accounting periods.

■ *Matching principle.* This principle requires companies to use the accrual basis of accounting. The matching principle requires that expenses be matched to revenues. For example, sales commission expenses should be reported in the period when the sales were made (and not reported in the period when the commissions were paid). Wages to employees are reported as an expense in the week when the employees worked and not in the week when the employees are paid. If a company agrees to give its employees 1% of its 2023 revenues as a bonus on January 15, 2024, the company should report the bonus as an expense in 2023 and the amount unpaid at December 31, 2023, as a liability. As the future economic benefit of items such as advertisements cannot be measured (and thus the ad expense cannot be matched with related future revenues), the accountant charges the ad amount to expense in the period that the ad is run.

■ *Revenue recognition principle.* In an accrual-based accounting system (as opposed to the cash basis of accounting), revenues are recognized as soon as a product has been sold or a service has been performed, regardless of when the money is actually received. Under this basic accounting principle, a company could earn and report $20,000 of revenue in its first month of operation but receive $0 in actual cash in that month. For example, if ABC Audiology completes its service at an agreed price of $1,000, ABC should recognize $1,000 of revenue as soon as its work is done. It does not matter whether the patient pays the $1,000 immediately or in 30 days. Do not confuse revenue with a cash receipt.

■ *Materiality.* Due to this basic accounting principle or guideline, an accountant might be allowed to violate another accounting principle if an amount is insignificant. Professional judgment is needed to decide whether an amount is insignificant or immaterial. The principle of materiality also suggests that financial statements usually show amounts rounded to the nearest dollar, to the nearest thousand, or to the nearest million dollars depending on the size of the company.

■ *Conservatism.* If a situation arises where there are two acceptable alternatives for reporting an item, conservatism directs the accountant to choose the alternative that will result in less net income and/ or less asset amount. Accountants are expected to be unbiased and objective, and conservatism assists accountants in "breaking a tie" but does not direct accountants to be conservative. The principle of conservatism leads accountants to anticipate or disclose losses, but it does not allow a similar action for gains. For example, an accountant may write inventory down to an amount that is lower than the original cost but will not write inventory up to an amount higher than the original cost.

Types of Bookkeeping

Bookkeeping can be conducted in a single entry or double entry. *Single-entry* bookkeeping keeps track of revenue against the expenses and offers simplicity but not enough detail to track the sources and destinations of revenue and expenses. A system that offers detail is the double-entry bookkeeping system that is now the standard of accounting (Figure 11–5).

Pioneered by medieval Venetians, the *double-entry* system treats a transaction as an exchange between two accounts. The double-entry method has two characteristics in that each transaction is recorded in two accounts and each account has two columns. Double-entry systems have some distinct advantages over simple single-entry systems:

- Accurate calculation of profits and losses in complex organizations.
- Inclusion of assets and liabilities in the bookkeeping accounts.

- Preparation of financial statements directly from the accounts.
- Easier detection of accounting errors, fraud, and embezzlement.

The recording transactions in each account involve two significant items: debits and credits, with debits in the left column and credits in the right column. For each debit, there is an equal and opposite credit, and the sum of all debits must equal the sum of all credits. The debit/credit principle makes it easier to find errors, fraud, or embezzlement within the double-entry bookkeeping system. In the double-entry system, balanced entries are made that keep the accounting equation in balance so that:

$$\text{Assets} = \frac{\text{Liabilities} + \text{Owners}}{\text{Stockholders Equity}}$$

Receivables and Payables

The accountant will set up a *chart of accounts* depicting all transactions necessary to record incoming revenue (e.g., payments from patients or third-party payers) and pay bills necessary to satisfy vendors, landlords, and other providers of services or goods to the practice (e.g., rent, hearing instrument manufacturer). The chart of accounts represents an exhaustive list of important accounts

Date	Accounts	Debit	Credit
July 8	Cash	300.00	
	Hearing Aid Repairs		300.00

Figure 11–5. Double entry bookkeeping.

that must be monitored and carefully followed since it is the basis for the general ledger for the practice. The general ledger for the practice is the nuts and bolts of the financial monitoring system. This list of transaction categories is called the *chart of accounts*. Table 11–1 is a sample chart of accounts that presents some of the subaccounts that would be included in a typical audiology practice accounting system.

In this example, under the asset account, there are many subaccounts such as cash, accounts receivable, and diagnostic equipment. A typical audiology practice income account would include all the revenue sources broken down by each service and sales. Most revenue-generating services are associated with

Current Procedural Terminology (CPT) codes (Chapter 17), but it is not necessary to restrict the income accounts to services with CPT codes. Expense accounts will include utilities, payroll, cost of goods sold, office supplies, and so on. Every transaction will be assigned to an account, enabling the practice manager to analyze thousands of business transactions within the framework of a discrete number of categories.

As the sample in Table 11–1 presents, the chart of accounts has a short descriptive name of the account and a number. The numbers are somewhat arbitrary as any number may be assigned to individual accounts. Most accounting references suggest that it is wise to leave some available numbers for adding ad-

Table 11–1. Audiology Practice Example: Chart of Accounts

Account #	Description
1000.00	**ASSETS**
1001.00	Current Assets
1003.00	Cash
1004.00	Non-Refundable Deposits
1005.00	Accounts Receivable
1007.00	Total Current Assets
2000.00	Fixed Assets
2001.00	Office Equipment
2002.00	Diagnostic Equipment
2003.00	Building
2010.00	Total Fixed Assets
2015.00	Accumulated Depreciation
2050.00	TOTAL ASSETS

Table 11–1. *continued*

Account #	Description
3000.00	**LIABILITIES**
3005.00	Current Liabilities
3007.00	Property Taxes
3008.00	Property Insurance
3009.00	Accrued Wages
3011.00	Accounts Payable
3025.00	Total Current Liabilities
3030.00	Long Term Liabilities
3030.01	Bank Loan
3050.00	TOTAL LIABILITIES
4000.00	**EQUITY**
4001.00	Retained Earnings
4030.00	Total Equity
4050.00	TOTAL LIABILITIES AND EQUITY
5000.00	**INCOME**
5001.00	Sales
5001.01	Hearing Aids – Digital
5001.02	Hearing Aids – Other
5001.03	Assistive Devices
5001.04	Batteries
5002.00	Audiologic Diagnostics
5002.01	92552 – Pure Tone Audiometry
5002.02	92557 – Comprehensive Audiometry
5002.03	92587 – Evoked Acoustic Emissions
5003.00	Vestibular/Balance
5003.01	92541 – Spontaneous Nystagmus
5003.02	92543 – Caloric Vestibular Test

Table 11–1. *continued*

Account #	Description
5004.00	Rehabilitative Services
5004.01	92591 – Hearing Aid Selection, binaural
5004.02	92594 – Hearing Aid Selection, binaural
5050.00	TOTAL INCOME
6000.00	**EXPENSES**
6002.00	Rent
6015.00	Payroll
6020.00	Fringe Benefits
6021.00	Payroll Taxes
6022.00	Workers Compensation Insurance
6023.00	Health Insurance
6028.00	Utilities
6031.00	Postage/Mail Services
6035.00	Professional Fees
6035.01	ABA Dues
6035.02	AAA Dues
6036.00	Continuing Professional Education
6040.00	Total Professional Fees
6042.00	Magazine Subscriptions
6043.00	Professional Journal Subscriptions
6046.00	Coffee Service
6047.00	Safe Deposit Box
6050.00	Promotion and Advertising
6051.00	Referral Development
6061.00	Accounting Expense
6070.00	TOTAL EXPENSE

Source: Benn & Traynor, 2008; Traynor, 2017.

ditional accounts if needed at a future date. While most audiologists will never set up a new accounting system, it is beneficial to review a typical audiology practice's chart of accounts to identify the information being tracked by the system. This information can be essential to salary negotiations, budget requests, equipment justification, clinic expansion, and other critical business decisions. The chart of accounts is used in every business transaction, and it is essential that the bookkeeper enters the data and assigns various transactions properly. In practice, if a check is written to pay a balance due to a supplier on accounts payable (a liability account), the details of the transaction, including the amount, the supplier, and the expense account associated with the payment, are also recorded. To complete the transaction, the reduction in accounts payable (a liability account) is associated with a reduction in cash (an asset account). This two-part transaction is the basis of a "double-entry" bookkeeping system (Traynor, 2019).

Inventory Control and Property Tax Accounting

Recording purchases and related acquisition costs of items necessary for daily practice operations is important for a variety of reasons, not the least of which is to establish appropriate tax preparations and deductions. The accountant will establish appropriate guidelines to record all transactions that are important to the practice and will work with the of-

---

KEY QUALITIES IN A BOOKKEEPER/FINANCIAL MANAGER

As accounting for the incoming and outgoing funds is essential to a successful practice, special attention must be given to the person that handles the money. The first credential for bookkeepers and/or financial managers is honesty. Since the practitioner has patient, management, supervisory, marketing, and other responsibilities, there is no time to babysit, second guess, or follow up every transaction of the bookkeeper or financial manager. Practitioners, however, should be wise to the bookkeeping process as well as accounting methods to recognize when employees are being dishonest. If direct monitoring is not possible, then the practice accountant should monitor these transactions at least monthly to discourage and/or eliminate employee criminal activity. Although this monitoring is costly in accounting fees, the result of embezzlement is likely substantially higher and can not only affect the office cash flow for paying the bills but also threaten the very existence of the practice as well as the practitioner's valuable professional and financial reputation.

continued on next page

continued from previous page

Pedneault et al. (2012) suggests that any person hired in this position will represent the practice and its owners to suppliers, bankers, and patients; therefore, a special person is required that must be screened in more detail during the hiring process. Special due diligence for the authenticity of the applicant's resume, letters of reference, military records, and copies of diplomas and transcripts are important. In today's world of identity theft and impersonation, each of these documents must be checked for reality as well as accuracy. Pedneault and colleagues further recommend that for individuals in such powerful positions, credit and criminal records checks are also important. While these checks are not for every candidate for the position of bookkeeper, they are certainly necessary for the one that ultimately becomes the top applicant.

Believe it or not, bookkeepers and financial managers stealing funds from practitioners is extremely common and, according to law enforcement, becoming routine with all the methods of identity theft available (Traynor et al., 2014; Traynor, 2016). If the practice does have an issue with embezzlement, it is very difficult to obtain cooperation from the police or district attorney for prosecution without specific evidence, and only one in nine of these cases are ever prosecuted. Embezzlement is a problem for not only audiologists but also physicians, dentists, chiropractors, and other professionals that have significant cash flow in their practice. The practice manager or chief executive officer (CEO) must watch for changes in the accounting process or procedures, illogical business expenses, spending habits of the person involved, capricious movement, and/or disappearance of funds in bank accounts. *Do not use* a signature stamp for checks as the stamp can easily be used by the unauthorized, duplicated by others, or set as a signature for computerized checks. Additionally, guard the practice of debit and credit cards as once someone knows the pin, they can actually pull funds from the practice at the ATM. Daily monitoring of the bank accounts and questions to the bookkeeper/financial manager as to any suspicious expenditure are essential to wise practice management. If possible, the practice accountant should monitor their work and audit the accounts at least semiannually to reduce the possibility of embezzlement.

Bookkeepers and financial managers should be knowledgeable of business with a basic understanding of the essential differences among the five basic types of accounts (assets, liabilities, equity, income, and expenses) so that transactions are organized properly. The practice owner or CEO is ultimately responsible for all that happens with the books, ensuring that

continued on next page

continued from previous page

expenses, employees, payables, and taxes are paid, but a good, honest bookkeeper or financial manager can make life much easier. Bookkeepers and financial managers should also clearly understand that the three basic financial statements include the balance sheet, the income statement (profit/loss statement), and the cash flow statements are fundamental to tracking the costs by item and procedural detail.

The days of manual bookkeeping systems are gone forever, making it essential to find a bookkeeper with a knowledge of the basics of bookkeeping software, Word, Excel, email, and the Internet. They should be committed to enhancing their skills with additional classes or self-study to ensure that they're staying up to date with the accounting skills the business demands.

AIPB (2024) suggests general factors to be considered when hiring the bookkeeper:

- *Organizational skills.* Able to maintain orderly and up-to-date financial records.
- *Reliability.* Consistent and dependable in meeting deadlines and completing tasks.
- *Integrity.* Trustworthy and ethical in handling financial data and transactions.
- *Communication skills.* Able to effectively communicate financial information.
- *Analytical skills.* Capable of analyzing financial data and identifying discrepancies.
- *Adaptability.* Able to learn new software and adapt to changing requirements.
- *Experience and knowledge.* Proficient in accounting principles and bookkeeping practices.

Since an audiology practice is somewhat unique in that there are procedures and techniques specific to the practice of audiology, such as various office management systems, Medicare regulations, other insurance technicalities, as well as the general concerns of the psychological overlay that accompanies hearing and balance disorders. Familiarity with these other issues can assist the bookkeeper in putting a rationale with the situation to explain certain issues with cash flow and accounting categories that may not be part of other businesses. These special concerns when bookkeeping for an audiology practice are in addition to the general considerations:

continued on next page

continued from previous page

■ An understanding of the big picture of audiology practice within the community.

■ The knowledge and capability of the office management system (Chapter 15).

■ Since the audiology clinic runs on computers, good computer skills are essential.

■ An interest in continuing their education into the finer points of Medicare, other health insurance, and updates in their profession as well as audiology office management systems.

■ A willingness to make a strong commitment to the business.

fice manager/bookkeeper to optimize tax reporting, credits, and deductions. Although accountants can issue quarterly reports, semiannual reporting is less costly. As long as the practitioner is paying attention to fiscal details, semiannual reporting is usually adequate. A single end-of-year report is not adequate to monitor the overall fiscal health of any healthcare practice. It is one thing to make up for an error or initiate needed changes in reporting at the midyear point; however, it is another to have to retread the path of a full year of business transactions.

Payroll Preparation

Appropriate federal, state, and local payroll taxes such as Social Security, Medicare, city taxes, and other deductions must be accurately calculated, applied, and recorded. The practice accountant should establish levels of deductions and review the first two or three sets of payroll checks for accuracy. Although these deductions used to be deposited at the practice's bank each month in a special account reserved for government tax collection, it is now necessary for the practice to deposit these funds at a special website reserved for this purpose by the Internal Revenue Service (IRS) and other collection agencies. Failure to deduct and deposit these taxes has severe penalties for the practice owner and possible liabilities for the individual within the practice designated responsible for developing the payroll and depositing the taxes. It is the practice owner, however, who bears the ultimate responsibility of ensuring all taxes are deducted and that these funds have been directed to the appropriate depository. Even if the practice is a corporation, a tax liability can still be assessed against the owner or anyone individually that has control over dispersing funds for the practice.

It is cost prohibitive for most practices to have the accountant complete the payroll. A reasonable solution is to secure the services of a payroll company. There are several companies operating on a national basis specializing in payroll preparation, such as Paycom (2024) or ADP (2024). Their clients include large and small companies and a variety of healthcare providers. Payroll preparation companies follow specific tax guidelines for state (varies from state to state) and federal reporting and will calculate deductions as directed, issue payroll documentation, and print payroll checks drawn on the practice bank account. Practitioners should consult with the accountant about payroll services available in their area.

Financial Statements

There are two primary objectives of every business: *profitability and solvency*. Financial statements are documents typically prepared by the practice accountant that reflect the business's solvency (*the balance sheet*), its profitability (*the income statement*), and a view of its financial health (*the cash flow statement*). Bankers and other lenders depend on the financial statements to support their decisions to grant credit opportunities. Additionally, the figures on financial statements are the basis of the calculations for business ratios that offer important, informative metrics and milestones about activity, liquidity, profitability, and debt of the practice.

The Balance Sheet

The *balance sheet* contains the elemental fiscal components of the practice such as assets and liabilities and the owner's or stockholder's equity. Stobierski (2020)

indicates that a balance sheet provides a summary of a business at a given point in time. It is a snapshot of a company's financial position, as broken down into assets, liabilities, and equity. Balance sheets quickly present a view of the financial strength and capabilities of the business as well as answer important questions such as:

- Is the business able to expand?
- Can the business easily withstand the normal financial ebbs and flows of revenues and expenses?
- Should the business take immediate steps to strengthen cash reserves?
- Do the numbers make sense?

When a balance sheet is reviewed externally by someone interested in a company, it is designed to give insight into what resources are available to a business and how they were financed. Based on this information, potential investors can decide whether it would be wise to invest in a company. Similarly, it's possible to leverage the information in a balance sheet to calculate important metrics, such as liquidity, profitability, and debt-to-equity ratio. It is designed to give insight into whether a company is succeeding or failing. Based on this information, an internal audience can shift their policies and approach by:

- Doubling down on successes.
- Correcting failures and pivoting toward new opportunities.

By its very nature, a balance sheet is always based upon *past data*. While investors and stakeholders may use a balance sheet to predict future performance, past performance is no guarantee of future results.

The balance sheet gets its name from the fact that the two sides of the statement must numerically balance. Assets are recorded on the left side of the balance sheet, and liabilities and owner's (or stockholder's) equity are recorded on the right side of the balance sheet, as presented in Table 11–2.

Total assets are set to equal 100%, with all other assets listed as a percentage of the total assets. On the right side of the balance sheet, total liabilities and equity are also set equal to 100%. Entries of all liabilities and owner's equity accounts are represented as the appropriate percent of the total liabilities and equity. The balance sheet must contain all of the practice's financial accounts and should be generated at least once a month. Monthly review of the balance sheet provides a comprehensive overview of the practice's financial position at that point in time.

Assets

Assets, presented on the left side of the balance sheet, are items of value and represent the financial resources of the practice. Accounts listed on the balance sheet are placed in order of their relative degree of liquidity (ease of convertibility of assets into cash); therefore, cash is always listed first as it does not require an action or an agent to convert cash into cash. Accounts receivable is listed second since it represents cash but must be "converted" into cash by collection. Assets are commonly differentiated into two classes: current assets and fixed or long-term assets.

Table 11–2. Balance Sheet

Audiology Associates, Inc. Balance Sheet December 31, 2023			
Assets		**Liabilities & Owners' Equity**	
Current Assets:		Current Liabilities:	
Cash	34,000.	Short-Term Debt	20,000.
Accounts Receivable	80,000.	Accounts Payable	35,000.
Merchandise Inventory	170,000.	Other Accrued Liabilities	12,000.
Total Current Assets	284,000.	Total Current Liabilities	67,000.
Property, Plant and Equipment (Fixed Assets):		Long-Term Debt	50,000.
		Total Liabilities	117,000.
Equipment	40,000.		
		Owners' Equity	203,000.
Less Accumulated Depreciation	4,000).		
		Total Liabilities and	
Total Assets	**320,000.**	Owners' Equity	**320,000.**

Source: Adapted from Viele et al. (2016).

Current assets are short lived and expected to be converted into cash or to be used up in the operations of the practice within a short period of time, usually within a fiscal year. Current assets include cash, accounts receivable, hearing instruments, assistive listening devices, and accessories in inventory and prepaid expenses, such as insurance.

Long-term or fixed assets are assets that will not be turned into cash within the practice's fiscal year. Examples of long-term or fixed assets include audiometric and other equipment used in the practice, office equipment and computers, purchased vehicles, purchased buildings, leasehold improvements, and telephone systems. These assets are found in the balance sheet listed as "Property, Plant, and Equipment" or "Fixed Assets." To best conceptualize long-term or fixed assets, consider that most fixed assets are purchased over time and must be in place over a long period of time to foster the day-to-day clinical and business operations of the practice. As equipment ages, it is said to depreciate. This depreciation of the equipment is an expense and can be claimed as a tax deduction. The accountant for the practice will evaluate the appropriate method for calculation and the extent of deductions available for every fixed asset listed on the balance sheet.

Liabilities

Liabilities include all obligations the practice has acquired through daily operations. Liabilities include accounts payable (e.g., hearing instrument acquisition costs), accrued business expenses or interest owed on loans, and other obligations. Owner's or stockholder's equity includes financial investment by

the owner or shareholders and the earned profits that are retained in the business. Presented on the right side of the balance sheet (see Table 11–2), current liabilities are listed as amounts owed to lenders and suppliers and are usually separated by those that are due in the short term and long term. As with the asset categories, current liabilities are delineated into subcategories such as short-term debt, accounts payable, and accrued liabilities. These are referred to as current liabilities since they are due to be paid within a short period of time, usually within the fiscal year. A separate category is for long-term debt, such as bank or other loans payable over a much longer period, usually longer than the fiscal year. All current and long-term liability amounts are then totaled collectively to reflect the total liability of the practice. Owner/stockholder equity is also listed on the right side of the balance sheet. This represents funds that were initially invested by the owners/stockholders as well as the profit that was earned and retained in the practice.

The Income Statement

Income statements, sometimes called *profit and loss statements* or "P&L" statements, depict the status of overall profits. Averkamp (2024a) indicates that the income statement is important because it shows the *profitability* of a company during the time interval specified in the heading (Table 11–3).

The period of time that the statement covers is chosen by the practice accountant and will vary according to the purpose of the review. Profitability of a practice is important for many reasons. If a practice was not able to operate profitably, the bottom line of the income statement indicates a net loss and a banker/lender/creditor may be hesitant to extend any or additional credit. On the other hand, a practice that has operated profitably where the bottom line of the income statement indicates a net income has demonstrated its ability to use borrowed and invested funds in a successful manner. A practice's ability to operate profitably is important to current lenders and investors, potential lenders and investors, management, competitors, government agencies, labor unions, and others.

The format of the income statement or the profit and loss statement will vary according to the complexity of the business activities. The income statement simply includes information as to how much money has been earned (revenue) and subtracts how much has been spent (expenses), resulting in how much has been made (profits) or how much has been lost (deficits). Basically, the statement includes total sales minus total expenses. In an audiology practice, revenues are defined as the inflow of funds from providing patient care or the dispensing of products. Expenses can be considered the sacrifices made or the costs incurred to produce these revenues. If revenues exceed expenses, net earnings result, whereas if expenses exceed net revenue, a loss is recorded.

As with other financial statements, the income statement, presented in Table 11–3, may be prepared for any financial reporting period and is used to track revenues and expenses for the evaluation of the operating performance of the practice. Averkamp (2024a) suggests that managers can use income statements to find areas of practice that are over bud-

Table 11–3. Income Statement

Audiology Associates, Inc. Income Statement Year the Ended December 31, 2023	
Net Sales	1,200,000.
Costs of Goods Sold	850,000.
Net Profit	350,000.
Selling, General and Administrative Expenses	311,000.
Income from Operations (EBIT)	39,000.
Interest Expense	9,000.
Income before Taxes (EBT)	30,000.
Income Taxes	12,000.
Net Income	**18,000.**

Source: Adapted from Viele et al. (2016).

get or under budget and areas that cause unexpected expenditures. Additionally, income statements track increases or decreases in product returns and cost of goods sold as a percentage of sales. It also offers some indication of the extent of income tax liability. The format of an income statement is structured according to the type of business being conducted; therefore, income statements may vary from one practice to another depending on the particular mix of diagnostics, hearing products, and rehabilitative services. The practice accountant will design the income statement to best represent the business.

Net sales on the income statement consist of sales figures representing the actual revenue generated by the business. Viele et al. (2016) state that the net sales entry represents the total amount of all sales less product returns and sales discounts. Directly below the net sales in Table 11–3 is the cost of goods sold (COGS). COGS are costs directly associated with making and/or acquiring the products. These costs include the acquisition of products, such as hearing aids or assistive devices provided by outside suppliers. If hearing instruments are repaired or manufactured by the practice, COGS could also be materials, parts, and internal expenses related to the manufacturing or repair process, such as faceplates, shells, microphones, receivers, and components. Net profit, sometimes called gross profit, is derived by subtracting the cost of goods sold from net sales. Net profit, however, does not include any operating, interest, or income tax expenses.

Just below the net profit entry in Table 11–3 is a category for selling and general administrative expenses. This subcategory is described by Viele et al.

(2016) as a broad "catch-all" category for all expenses except those reported elsewhere in the income statement. Examples of selling and general administrative expenses that are recorded here are legal expenses, the owner's salary, advertising, travel and entertainment, and other similar costs. The actual income from operations, sometimes called *earnings before interest and taxes* (EBIT), is the result of deducting the selling and general administrative expenses from the net profit. The earnings before interest and taxes (EBIT) is the net revenue generated by the practice, but there are still interest expenses and taxes that must be recorded. At this point, the interest expense is deducted and then tax amounts are subtracted to arrive at the net income (or loss).

Account Balancing

Account balancing is primarily for the bookkeepers in the practice, but it is beneficial for the practitioner to know how the procedure works. Simple accounting programs specifically designed for small businesses, such as QuickBooks, have revolutionized bookkeeping tasks. These relatively inexpensive programs, some of which are now incorporated into office management systems such as CounselEar, Sycle.net, Blueprint, and others, substantially reduce or virtually eliminate many of the common accounting mistakes that have plagued bookkeepers for decades (Chapter 15).

One of the common bookkeeping tasks is the trial balance. The trial balance of the books is usually conducted at the end of the month, quarter, or year but could be done at any time. The purpose of the trial balance is to determine if the total debits and the total credits balance for all of the asset and liability accounts. Occasionally, these accounts do not balance, and it is necessary to find errors and determine how to reverse them. Although accounting software programs have safeguards and special routines that will assist in finding these errors, it may be necessary to check for the following common causes of trial balance errors:

- Errors in the recording of a transaction.
- Posting errors.
- Computation of account balances.
- Copying balances to the trial balance.

The Statement of Cash Flows

The official name for the cash flow statement is *the Statement of Cash Flows*. Since the income statement is often prepared under an accrual basis of accounting, the revenues reported may not have been collected. Similarly, the expenses reported on the income statement might not have been paid. The balance sheet could be reviewed to determine these facts, but the cash flow statement has already integrated all that information. As a result, savvy practice managers and investors utilize this important financial statement. The cash flow statement reflects the cash position of the practice as well as the sources and uses of cash in the practice during a specified business cycle. It presents how cash flows in and out of the practice. Monthly cash flow statements are useful, but quarterly statements of cash flow provide a look at trends that might be developing in the overall cash flow picture.

Profit and cash flow are intimately related. A practice can be highly profitable yet on the verge of bankruptcy if the profits are sequestered in accounts receivables: *high profit, low cash flow*. This situation results in limited cash to pay the practitioner and other employees and to service the accounts payable. Conversely, if there is substantial cash inflow to a practice with excessive overhead costs strangling profitability, financial difficulties will ensue: *low profit, high cash flow*. This is a situation in which the practice owner has overextended available resources with ill-conceived equipment purchases, exceptional leasehold costs, or extraneous staff salaries and other questionable business decisions.

To illustrate how cash flows in and out of the practice, Viele et al. (2016) indicate that the statement of cash flows is used to identify the sources and uses of cash over time and can be compared to the current period for analysis. In Table 11–4, the cash flow statement is divided into three general sections, cash flow from operating activities, cash flow from investment activities, and cash flow from financing activities.

The operating activity section begins with the net income (taken from the income statement, Table 11–3) and includes all transactions and events that are normally entered to determine the operating income. These entries include cash receipts from selling goods or providing services, as well as income earned as interest and dividends, if the practice has investments. Cash flow from operating activities also includes cash payments such as inventory, payroll, taxes, interest, utilities, and rent. The net amount of cash provided (or used) by practice operating activities is the key figure on a statement of cash flows. The operations

Table 11–4. Statement of Cash Flows

Audiology Associates, Inc. Statement of Cash Flows Year the Ended December 31, 2023	
Cash Flows From Operating Activities:	
Net Income	$18,000.
Add (Deduct) Items Not Affecting Cash:	
Depreciation Expense	4,000.
Increase in Accounts Receivable	80,000).
Increase in Merchandise Inventory	170,000).
Increase in Current Liabilities	67,000.
Net Cash Used by Operating Activities	$(161,000).
Cash Flows From Investment Activities:	
Cash Paid for Equipment	$(40,000).
Cash Flows From Financing Activities:	
Cash Received From Issues of Long-Term Debt	$50,000.
Cash Received From Sale of Common Stock	190,000.
Net Cash Provided by Financing Activities	$240,000.
Net Cash Increase for the Year	**$39,000.**

Source: Adapted from Viele et al. (2016).

section is of the most interest as it presents the specific areas of the practice where cash was consumed.

The second section of a statement of cash flows reviews income generated from investing activities. This section includes transactions and events involving the purchase and sale of securities, land, buildings, equipment, and other assets not generally held in the practice for resale. This area of the statement also covers making and collecting loans, if the practice internally finances products and services these loans to consumers. Investing activities are not classified as operating activities as they have an indirect relationship to the central, ongoing operation of the practice.

Transactions in the third section record cash flows from financing activities and deal with the flow of cash between the practice, the owners (stockholders), and creditors as well as the cash proceeds from issuing capital stock or bonds. For example, if there was a need to transfer profit from the practice to the owners or from the owners (or creditors) into the practice, it would be reflected in the financing activities section. The statement of cash flows is used for the following purposes:

1. The cash from operating activities is compared to the company's net income. If the cash from operating activities is consistently greater than the net income, the company's net income or earnings are said to be of "high quality." If the cash from operating activities is

less than net income, a red flag is raised as to why the reported net income is not turning into cash.

2. Some investors believe that "cash is king." The cash flow statement identifies the cash that is flowing in and out of the company. If a company is consistently generating more cash than it is using, the company will be able to increase its dividend, buy back some of its stock, reduce debt, or acquire another company. All of these are perceived to be good for stockholder value.

3. Some financial models are based upon cash flow. Careful review of the Statement of Cash Flows can present valuable information to the practitioner as to where the cash generated goes and presents an invaluable opportunity to make adjustments in practice operations for management purposes.

Types of Practice Analysis

Analyst Notes (2024) describes these comparisons as *cross-sectional analysis* and *time-series analysis.*

Cross-Sectional Analysis

Cross-sectional analysis involves the calculation of financial ratios and compares them to an industry standard usually compiled by a trade organization. Although cross-sectional analysis facilitates a comparison of a small two-person practice with a large corporate conglomerate in many areas, these cross-sectional analyses are not readily available to practices in audiology except possibly to a few practice appraisers and audiology

franchises or huge buying groups such as Audigy, Pivot, American Hearing Aid Associates, and others.

Time-Series Analysis

Since it is difficult to obtain data for a realistic comparison of practice performance to an industry standard, the time-series analysisis of the most value to a practitioner. A time-series analysis compares the practice's performance to itself over various periods of time, usually month to month, quarter to quarter, or year to year. This type of analysis involves conducting calculations on financial statements to determine financial ratios. These ratios from other points in time compared to current totals can reveal a wealth of information to the practitioner or other stakeholders. More specifically, Viele et al. (2016) offer that these ratio calculations can assist in the determination of a practice's financial position as well as the overall practice operations in terms of liquidity, activity, debt, and profitability. These relatively simple measures can be calculated and tracked by spreadsheets to be reviewed over time to demonstrate the health of the practice for obtaining loans, supplier credit, reviewing success and failure for management decisions, or simply general information. Ratios calculated on these statements also provide information regarding the practice's capability to meet its obligations regarding supplier expenses, employee salaries, product returns, loans, leases, and a multitude of other miscellaneous expenses that become apparent in the balance sheet calculations. Most buying groups such as Audigy, American Hearing Aid Associates, Pivot Hearing, and the various office management systems now offer "dashboards" to assist in monitoring the analysis of the practice on a monthly, quarterly, or yearly basis.

Financial Accounting Ratios

Until the financial data are used to track information about the practice, the *balance sheet, income statement*, and *statement of cash flows* are just numbers. Financial accounting unlocks the real information within these statements by conducting some simple calculations on the balance sheet and income statement data. Many of these calculations are now offered within the various financial information "dashboards" offered by buying groups or office management systems. This section, however, presents a description and calculation of the popular ratios to facilitate an understanding of how the measurements are derived and their purpose.

These ratios are calculations on the various totals primarily from the balance sheet (Table 11–2) and the income statement (Table 11–3). While the practice accountant may decide to calculate ratios from the statement of cash flows (Table 11–4), they will not be discussed here as they are not as common as those represented in this discussion. Ratio calculations offer the practitioner the capability to track specific information for management purposes. These calculations, called *financial accounting ratios*, are used in business to compare the practice to other practices or to compare the practice to itself at different points in time.

Balance Sheet Calculations

There are four general types of financial ratios that are used to analyze the balance sheet. These ratios demonstrate the strengths and weaknesses of a practice regarding:

- Liquidity.
- Activity.
- Debt or leverage.
- Profitability.

Although liquidity ratios are used to measure the short-term ability of a practice to generate enough cash to pay currently maturing obligations, activity ratios measure how effectively the organization is using its assets by specifically analyzing how quickly some assets can be turned into cash. Debt or leverage ratios reflect the long-term solvency or overall liquidity of the practice and are typically of interest to the investors and/or the bankers that have loaned money to the practice. Profitability ratios are an indication of practice performance and look at the adequacy of the practice's net income, the rate of return, and profit margin as a percentage of sales.

Liquidity Ratios

There are two general types of liquidity ratios used routinely: the *current ratio* and the *quick ratio*.

Current Ratio

The *current ratio (CR)* is sometimes called a working capital ratio. The CR is a calculation of how many times the practice's current assets cover its current liabilities. Averkamp (2024b) describes the current ratio as the proportion of current assets to current liabilities where a large amount of current assets in relationship to a small amount of current liabilities provides some assurance that the obligations coming due will be paid. Put another way, the current ratio asks the question, Can the practice pay its bills?

The current ratio is figured as follows:

$$\text{Current Ratio} = \frac{\text{Current Assets}}{\text{Current Liabilities}}$$

If the result of a CR calculation is less than 1, the practice will not be able to meet its current liabilities, whereas if the CR is 2 or more, the practice can pay its bills with money left over. Usually, most bankers and practice managers like to see this ratio at least between 1 and 2. The CR calculation includes prepaid expenses, such as insurance and inventory, and sometimes presents a cloudy, overoptimistic view of the real capability to meet expenses.

If the inventory and other prepaid expenses are included in the calculation, it increases the CR, offering a higher ratio than if these prepaid expenses are not included. Thus, the current ratio can sometimes present an unrealistic picture of the practices' capability to pay its expenses. This may be especially true as audiology practices move from mostly ordering hearing instruments to stocking open fit products.

COMPUTATION OF THE CURRENT RATIO AND QUICK RATIO (ACID TEST RATIO)

The current ratio and quick ratio are activity ratios calculated on balance sheet totals useful in the determination of if the practice can pay its expenses (Table 11–2). The current ratio formula is as follows:

$$\text{Current Ratio} = \frac{\text{Current Assets}}{\text{Current Liabilities}}$$

Referring to Table 11–2, find the total current assets of $284,000 and the current liabilities of $67,000. Once these figures are found, put them into the formula as presented below:

$$\text{Current Ratio} = \frac{\$284,000}{\$67,000} = 4.2$$

continued on next page

continued from previous page

In this example, this practice has 4.2 times the amount of funds necessary to pay its expenses. Stocked items, or inventory, including the CR can often present an overestimate of the practice's expense-paying capability. If the inventory is included in the calculation, it increases the CR, offering a higher ratio than if the inventory is not included. To correct for this, the QR is used and calculated with following formula:

$$\text{Quick Ratio} = \frac{\text{Cash + Marketable Securities + Accounts Receivable}}{\text{Current Liabilities}}$$

To compute the QR from the balance sheet offered in Table 8–2, add the cash to the accounts receivable to obtain the current assets (there are no marketable securities) to obtain the total current assets of $114,000.

$$\text{Quick Ratio} = \frac{\$114,000}{\$67,000} = 1.7$$

Once obtained, divide $114,000 by the total current liabilities of $67,000 and obtain a quick ratio of 1.7. Since the QR must be over 1 to pay its bills, this practice has enough funds to pay their current expenses. In this example, the QR offers a more realistic picture of the practice's capability to pay expenses.

To figure activity without considering the inventory and prepaid expenses, the *quick ratio (QR)*, also known as the *acid test ratio (ATR)*, can be used. The QR or ATR evaluates the practice's liquidity without considering the inventory and prepaid expenses and, in doing so, often presents a more accurate assessment. The QR is figured as follows:

$$\text{Quick Ratio} =$$
$$\frac{\text{Cash + Marketable Securities} + \text{Accounts Receivable}}{\text{Current Liabilities}}$$

As with the CR, quick ratio values less than 1 demonstrate that the practice has serious difficulty meeting everyday expenses. Creditors and practice managers also prefer to see this ratio between 1 and 2.

Defensive Interval Measure

Another useful liquidity calculation is the *defensive interval measure (DIM)*. The DIM is a ratio that measures the time for which a practice can operate without any external cash flow or, simply, how long the practice can operate if there is no business. DIM is determined by the amount of cash or assets on hand that could be used to keep an otherwise healthy practice open if there are unforeseen problems, such as hurricanes, major snowstorms, a pandemic, or other situations where business ceases or drastically slows down. In accounting, emergency funds used to keep a business going during these tough times are called defensive assets (DAs). By definition, the DAs are those assets that can be turned into cash within 3 months or less, such as cash (savings), marketable securities, or accounts receivable. To figure the DIM, based on a specific amount of DAs, it is first necessary to know the projected daily operating expenses (PDOE) of the practice or how much it costs to keep the practice open each day. To find the PDOE, simply go to the income statement and find the selling and administrative expenses for the year and divide by 365:

CALCULATION OF THE DEFENSE INTERVAL MEASURE (DIM)

Although natural and other disasters are rare and often do not create difficulties beyond 2 to 3 weeks, there are some that can create issues for a much longer time, such as Hurricane Katrina, wildfires, floods, snowstorms, and other disasters. The possibility of issues that can cause the absence of business for a period of time makes it essential to know how long the business can sustain itself with no income. The defense interval measure (DIM) is a ratio that determines the time for which a practice can operate without any external cash flow or how long the practice can operate if there is no business. The DIM is determined by the amount of cash or assets that can be liquidated to keep the practice open if there are uncontrollable situations where business ceases or drastically slows down. The formula for the DIM is as follows:

$$\text{Defense Interval Measure} = \frac{\text{Defensive Assets}}{\text{Projected Daily Operating Expenses}}$$

To compute the DIM, however, there are some things that must be known. First, the practice must know the amount of funds that can be used for defense purposes. In accounting, these funds are called DAs and can consist of many different types of assets, but they must, by definition, have the capability to be turned into cash within 3 months. The amount

continued on next page

continued from previous page

of the DAs necessary will vary from practice to practice, but it is suggested that somewhere between a 90- and 120-day capability should be available. To calculate the DIM to determine the length of time that the practice can open its doors in an emergency, it is necessary to consider the PDOE. The PDOE is calculated by the following formula:

$$\text{Projected Daily Operating Expenses} = \frac{\text{Total Yearly Expenses}}{365}$$

To arrive at the PDOE, simply go to the selling and general and administrative expenses located on the income statement in Table 11–2 and find the total yearly expenses of $311,000. Then divide the total yearly expenses of $311,000 by 365 as presented below:

$$\text{Projected Daily Operating Expenses} = \frac{\$311,000}{365} = \$852.00$$

In this example, it costs the practitioner $852 per day to stay open each day. This is if the practice is open 365 days per year and most practices are only open Monday through Friday, and thus, the divisor should be much less, on the order of [365 – 104 (days closed)] or 261, and in this case, the PDOE would be much higher at about $1,191 per day. If the practitioner has $50,000 available for DAs, then the practice's defensive interval measure would be 58.6 days or, with the more conservative measure, 41.9 days. To meet the recommended DIM of a minimum of 90 days, the practitioner in this example would need $76,680 for the first example of $107,190 for the more conservative example.

Projected Daily Operating Expenses =

$$\frac{\text{Total Yearly Expenses}}{365}$$

Once the projected daily operating expenses (PDOE) are known, the DIM is found by dividing the DAs by the PDOE:

Defense Interval Measure =

$$\frac{\text{Defensive Assets}}{\text{Projected Daily Operating Expenses}}$$

The DIM calculation gives the practice manager the length of time the business could survive if revenue was substantially reduced or absent.

Activity Ratios

Activity ratios are calculations that allow the manager to review how efficiently the practice uses its assets to generate cash. Although there are a number of activity ratios that can present the efficiency of the practice, the *accounts receivable turnover ratio (ART)*, the *inventory turnover ratio (IT)*, and the *total assets turnover ratio (TAT)* are quite useful to practice managers (refer to box for calculation examples).

Accounts Receivable Turnover Ratio (ART)

Ideally, all patients should pay when services are completed, but in reality, a good portion of patients have insurance, and it is well known that insurance companies pay slowly, sometimes 60 to 120 days after the services are rendered, and may often not pay the first time the claim is submitted. Additionally, some patients use credit to pay for the goods and services such as hearing aids, batteries, and repairs. Managers need to monitor the accounts receivable to determine how much is due to the practice and how long, on average, it will take to receive payment. The *accounts receivable turnover ratio (ART)* reveals how many times the receivable account is turned into cash each year. To obtain the ART ratio, it is necessary to first find the average amount that is due the practice from the receivable account or average accounts receivable (AR) balance. This is obtained by adding the accounts receivable balance at the end of last year (or other period) to the balance of the accounts receivable at the end of the current year (or another period) and divide by 2 (see box on next page):

$$\text{Average Accounts Receivable} = \frac{\text{AR (Year 1)} + \text{AR (Year 2)}}{2}$$

Once the average AR is computed, the ART ratio, or the time it takes to convert this account into cash, can be obtained by taking the net sales (sales after returns and discounts are subtracted) and dividing that amount by the average accounts receivable balance:

$$\text{Accounts Receivable Turnover Ratio} = \frac{\text{Net Sales}}{\text{Average Accounts Receivable}}$$

Once known, the ART can alert the practice manager how long it takes, on average, to collect the amounts in the accounts receivable. In this calculation, the higher the ratio, the better; for example, if the ART ratio is = 5.3, the practice turns over the accounts receivable 5.3 times per year or every 2.26 months, which is about average. To obtain more detail, the calculation of the number of days it takes to turn the accounts receivable can be obtained by simply dividing the average accounts receivable into 365, in this case 68.86 days. The box on the next page offers a calculation example where the accounts receivable is turned 21 times per year, about every 17 days.

In the above example, the accounts receivable turnover time is very short, but it can often take much longer to receive cash from those that have been extended credit. If the accounts receivable only turns two or three times per year, it may make some sense to consider factoring accounts receivable. Factoring is a process specially designed to

AVERAGE ACCOUNTS RECEIVABLE (AAR) AND ACCOUNTS RECEIVABLE TURNOVER RATIO (ART)

Managers need to monitor the accounts receivable to determine how much is due to the practice and how long, on average, it takes to collect these credit sales. The accounts receivable turnover ratio (ART) reveals how many times the receivable account is turned into cash each year (Figure 11–2). To obtain the ART ratio, it is necessary to first find the average amount that is due the practice from the receivable account or average accounts receivable (AAR) balance. This is obtained by adding the accounts receivable balance at the end of last period to the balance of the accounts receivable at the end of the current period and divide by 2. In this example, our interest is in the average accounts receivable balance from the past 2 years. To calculate this AAR, use the following formula:

$$\text{Average Accounts Receivable} = \frac{\text{AR (Year 1)} + \text{AR (Year 2)}}{2}$$

The calculation of the average accounts receivable (AAR) balance comes from the balance sheet. Referring to Table 11–1 (balance sheet), find the current AR balance of $80,000 and assume that last year's AR balance from last year's balance sheet was $31,000. Using these figures, the AAR would calculate as follows:

$$\text{Average Accounts Receivable} = \frac{\$31,000 + \$80,000}{2} = \$55,000$$

Once the AAR is determined, then the accounts receivable turnover ratio (ART) can be calculated using the formula presented below:

$$\text{Accounts Receivable Turnover Ratio} = \frac{\text{Net Sales}}{\text{Average Accounts Receivable}}$$

From the income statement (Table 11–3), the net sales are $1,200,000, which is divided by $55,000, the average accounts receivable, as follows:

$$\text{Accounts Receivable Turnover Ratio} = \frac{\$1,200,000}{\$55,000} = 21$$

The example above demonstrates that the accounts receivable turns over about 21 times per year of about every 17 days.

turn over the accounts receivable and is used in many other professions, including medicine, dentistry, chiropractic, and optometry. Factoring companies can give the practice quick cash infusion by purchasing the receivables at a discount. Although this process is a way to increase cash flow without increasing debt, it largely depends on the creditworthiness of the patients and the insurance companies with which the practice interacts as well as the amount of monthly invoices.

For example, if the monthly accounts receivable regularly totals at least $8,000 to $10,000, factoring firms will act as a collection agency for the practice. Although some of these companies have some upfront fees, it is recommended to shop around, as many simply take a percentage of the receivables and often immediately advance as much as 80% to 90% or more of the confirmed amount of the receivables. The factoring firm later collects from patients and companies that owed when the account is due. If accounts receivable totals $60,000 or more and it runs 90 to 120 days, it may make sense to pay a factoring company to collect it. If there is a 10% fee on the $60,000 it would cost $6,000. In this situation, they would pay the practice $54,000 in cash immediately. If the fee is more or less than the costs, the benefits of factoring need to be weighed by the practitioner. Certainly, the accounts receivable is often a tremendous source of cash and if handled correctly can keep the practice from actually needing a loan during business downturns.

AVERAGE INVENTORY AND INVENTORY TURNOVER RATIO

The IT ratio is a calculation that measures how fast the inventory is sold. As in the measurement of the accounts receivable turnover ratio, before figuring the inventory turnover ratio, it is necessary to obtain the value of the average inventory on hand in the practice. Thus, the average inventory (AI) is found by adding the beginning inventory for the period to the ending inventory previous period, such as year, and dividing by 2.

$$\text{Average Inventory} = \frac{\text{Beginning Inventory} + \text{Ending Inventory}}{2}$$

The calculation of the AI balance comes from the balance sheet. Although the practitioner could look at any period, in this case, the consideration is in looking at how many times the inventory will turn each year. Referring to Table 11–2 (balance sheet), find the current merchandise inventory balance of $170,000 and assume that last year's merchandise

continued on next page

continued from previous page

inventory from last year's balance sheet was $111,000. Using these balance sheet figures, the AI would be calculated as follows:

$$\frac{\$170,000 + \$111,000}{2} = \$140,000$$

Once the AI is determined, the inventory turnover ratio can be calculated to determine how many times the stock will turn during the year. Inventory turnover ratio is calculated as follows:

$$\text{Inventory Turnover Ratio} = \frac{\text{Cost of Goods Sold}}{\text{Average Inventory}}$$

To arrive at the inventory turnover ratio, it is necessary to refer to the income statement (Table 11–4) and find the cost of goods sold, $850,000. This is the total amount of goods that were sold during this 1-year period. The $850,000 cost of goods sold is divided by the average inventory of $140,000 obtained earlier to present a calculated inventory turnover ratio of 6.

$$\text{Inventory Turnover Ratio} = \frac{\$850,000}{\$140,000} = 6$$

An IT of 6 indicates that the inventory in this practice turns over six times per year, every 2 months, or 60 days. This calculation is useful in ordering stock, such as batteries or stock RIC or open-fit hearing instruments in that it is necessary to have a 60-day supply of goods on hand to ensure that the goods will not sell out before another shipment can be obtained.

Inventory Turnover Ratio

With the advent of receiver-in-the-canal (RIC) hearing instruments and the recent addition of over the counter (OTC) devices into hearing care practices, clinics may have more inventory than in the past. Additionally, there are likely other stock products such loaners, demonstration instruments, batteries, accessories, assistive devices, and other items. When inventory exists in the practice, it is important to understand how fast the inventory turns so that plans can be made for restocking. The *inventory turnover (IT)* ratio is a calculation that measures how fast the inventory is sold. Prior to figuring the inventory turnover ratio, it is necessary to obtain the value of the average inventory on hand in the practice. Thus, the average inventory is found by adding the beginning inventory for the year (or period) to the ending inventory for the previous year (or period) and dividing by 2 (see box on previous page).

Once the average inventory is known, the IT ratio is computed by dividing the cost of the goods sold by the average inventory. If, for the year, the IT ratio was 5.9, the inventory will turn almost six times each year.

$$\text{Inventory Turnover Ratio} = \frac{\text{Cost of Goods Sold}}{\text{Average Inventory}}$$

As with other activity ratios, the turning of the inventory can be further delineated to reflect how long it takes the inventory to sell out in days by simply dividing 365 by the IT ratio. In this example, if the inventory turns about six times per year, then it takes about 61 days for the inventory to sell out. These data assist the manager in planning product orders efficiently throughout the year, ensuring that there is always a fresh, sufficient supply as well as taking advantage of a discount.

Total Assets Turnover Ratio

An activity measure that presents how effectively the practice assets are turned

---

TOTAL ASSETS TURNOVER RATIO

An activity measure that presents how effectively the practice assets are turned into cash is the total assets turnover (TAT) ratio. The TAT ratio looks at the sales for goods and services and is divided by the total assets to arrive at how many times the practices assets turnover per year.

$$\text{Total Asset Turnover Ratio} = \frac{\text{Total Assets}}{\text{Net Sales}}$$

To calculate the total assets turnover ratio, it is necessary to obtain information for both the balance sheet (Table 11–2) and the income statement (Table 11–3). From the balance sheet, the total assets are obtained at $320,000, while the net sales of 1,200,000 are obtained from the income statement. The calculation is simply dividing the total assets into the net sales to determine how many times the practice assets are turned into cash each year. A total asset turnover ratio of 3.75 offered in this example suggests that this practice is efficient in that it will turn its assets into cash 3.75 times per year or about every 94 days:

$$\text{Total Asset Turnover Ratio} = \frac{\$1,200,000}{\$320,000} = 3.75$$

into cash is the *total assets turnover (TAT)* ratio. In practice, the TAT ratio looks at the use of assets, such as employees, materials, space, and equipment, and then calculates how effectively these assets are turned into cash. The TAT ratio takes the sales for goods and services and divides that by the total assets to arrive at how many times the practice assets turnover per year.

$$\text{Total Asset Turnover Ratio} = \frac{\text{Net Sales}}{\text{Total Assets}}$$

Of course, the higher the TAT value, the better, as this is an indication that the assets of the practice turn over more times during the year and suggests that the assets are used efficiently.

Debt or Leverage Ratios

Two ratios that are beneficial to the practitioner in presenting how much debt the practice has relative to its assets are the *debt to assets (DA)* ratio and the *times interest earned (TIE)* ratio. These ratios give indications whether the practice has the capability to support more debt for purposes such as loans, adding equipment, or opening another location.

The Debt to Assets Ratio

The *debt to assets (DA)* ratio is expressed in percentages and offers an indication of how much liability the practice has for every dollar of assets. Creditors can review the debt to assets ratio and obtain insight as to the ability of the practice to withstand losses without impairing the interest of the creditors. Although good and bad debt to asset ratios are different for each industry, the general goal for most practices should be to keep the percentage as low as possible as a high the number indicates that the practice is more dependent on borrowed money in order to sustain itself. Similar to the personal debt to asset ratios familiar for personal loans, Hayes (2024) indicates that business lenders are concerned

---

DEBT TO ASSETS (DA) AND THE TIMES INTEREST EARNED (TIE) RATIOS

The DA presents how much liability the practice has for every dollar of assets and provides the creditors with information about the ability of the practice to withstand losses. The DA is simply the total liabilities divided by the total assets from the balance sheet.

$$\text{Debt to Assets Ratio} = \frac{\text{Total Liabilities}}{\text{Total Assets}} =$$

continued on next page

continued from previous page

In this example review of the balance sheet, Table 11–2 will find the total liabilities of $117,000 and total assets of $320,000. Dividing the total liabilities by the total assets yields 36.5%, suggesting that for every dollar of assets, the practice has 36.5 cents of debt. Although not serious debt, in practice, the debt to assets ratio should be as low as possible.

$$\text{Debt to Assets Ratio} = \frac{\$117,000}{\$320,000} = 36.5\%$$

The times interest earned (TIE) ratio is an indication of how many times the practice earns the amount of interest charged on the money that it has borrowed. The TIE is computed by taking the earnings before interest and taxes (EBIT) and dividing it by the interest expense; both values are obtained from the income statement (see Table 11-3).

$$\text{Times Interest Earned Ratio} = \frac{\$39,000}{\$9,000} = 4.3$$

In the example, the EBIT is $39,000, divided by the interest expense of $9,000 for a times interest earned ratio of 4.3. These ratios should be between 3 and 5 and a TIE less than 1 is an indication that the practice cannot pay its bills.

if the DA is high, as this suggests that small changes in cash flow might cause serious difficulties in the capability to repay debt. The DA computation is simply the total liabilities divided by the total assets.

Times Interest Earned Ratio (TIE)

The *times interest earned (TIE)* ratio is an indication of how many times the practice would be able to pay its interest using its earnings. The TIE provides lenders additional information as to the success of the company and its capability to repay loans for expansion projects, or other activities. The TIE is computed by taking the earnings before interest and taxes (EBIT) and dividing it by the interest charges.

$$\text{Times Interest Earned Ratio} = \frac{\text{Earning Before Interest and Taxes}}{\text{Interest Charges}}$$

Audiology practices should have a TIE should be somewhere between 3 and 5, indicating that the earnings are at least three to five times greater than the interest payments. A TIE that is less than 1 is evidence that the practice cannot pay its interest commitments.

Profitability Ratios

Although most of the routine calculations presented so far are utilized with the balance sheet, sometimes the ratios that may tell the most about a practice are the profitability ratios. These profitability ratios are clues as to how well the practice has performed and looks at whether the practice's net income is adequate, the rate of return achieved, and profit margin as a percentage of sales is satisfactory. The ratios routinely considered in this group are the *profit margin on sales (PMOS)* using information from the income statement and the *asset turnover (AT)* ratio that uses information from both the income statement and the balance sheet discussed earlier in this chapter.

Profit Margin on Sales

The *profit margin on sales (PMOS)* presents what is achieved after all of the expenses are subtracted and calculates how much of every dollar of sales are profit. This calculation can establish if the margins are adequate from one period to another to sustain the practice. To compute the PMOS, net profit is divided by sales:

$$\text{Profit Margin on Sales} = \frac{\text{Net Profit}}{\text{Sales}}$$

PMOS results are represented in a percentage that reflects the amount of each dollar that is profit. For example, if the calculation yields 20%, then $0.20 cents of every dollar collected is profit. These values can be tracked to determine up or down changes during the year.

PROFIT MARGIN ON SALES

The profit margin on sales (PMOS) presents the profit margin achieved after all of the expenses are subtracted and presents how much of every dollar of sales is profit. To compute the profit margin on sales, net profit is divided by the net sales. For example, refer to the income statement, Table 11–3, and find the net profit of $350,000 and the net sales of $1,200,000.

$$\text{Profit Margin on Sales} = \frac{\$350,000}{\$1,200,000} = .29$$

To arrive at the PMOS, simply divide the net sales into the net profit and obtain .29. This figure refers to the fact that 29 cents of every dollar is profit from this practice. This figure can be tracked to determine if there are changes that require attention.

Tying It Together

A fundamental monitoring of the financial health of the practice is essential through the use of the ratios discussed previously. The ratios described are certainly not an exhaustive list, and the practice accountant may recommend other ratios be monitored in addition for special purposes. Knowledge of how fast the accounts receivable turns into cash is important to the cash flow into the practice and essential for paying the bills. A look at the debt structure, operating costs, and profitability offers a simultaneous sense of reality and security to the practitioner.

Knowledge of these ratios and what they are today, however, is not enough. Ratios must be tracked and compared to other months, quarters, or years before they unlock the important information essential for management modifications. Tracking or monitoring ratios allows the practitioner to evaluate the liquidity, activity, debt, and profitability over time to investigate the reasons for successes or failures and make appropriate adjustments.

A classic example of how tracking can be of assistance in the explanation of difficulties in a practice is presented in Figure 11–6. This figure presents quick ratios for Audiology Associates, Inc. for the years 2019 to 2023. A review of the quick ratio histogram for the years 2019, 2020, 2022, and 2023 demonstrates that the quick ratios are greater than 1, indicating that the practice could pay its bills with money left over during those years. In 2021, however, the quick ratio was less than 1, suggesting that there were problems paying business bills and thus had to borrow funds to meet expenses that year.

Although this information is of great benefit, it must be remembered that all financial statements and the subsequent ratios generated represent specific informational snapshots in a specified window of time. These data reflect how business has been in the past and, due to competition, market pressures and other significant factors may or may not be predictors of the health of the business in the future.

Ratios can be very helpful in the evaluation of a practice, but Viele et al. (2016) offer caution on the use of ratio analyses. They indicate the best information about a company's financial health is determined from comparisons and analyses of a group of ratios, not a single ratio, and that these comparisons need to be made at similar times of the year to arrive at accurate data on the practice's performance. In the example presented in Figure 11–6, simply tracking the quick ratio across the years provided information as to what the quick ratio was during the good and bad years, but it is necessary to review other ratios to explain *why* the quick ratio was less than 1 during 2021.

Tracking a number of ratios allows the practitioner to search further for differences between 2021 and other years to ensure that these difficulties are not repeated. By tracking other ratios and comparing them to the quick ratios from 2019 to 2023, the answer to the problem experienced by Audiology Associates, Inc. becomes evident. Figure 11–7 presents the tracking of the accounts receivable turnover ratio (ART) for Audiology Associates, Inc. for the same period 2019 to 2023. Recall that the ART pres-

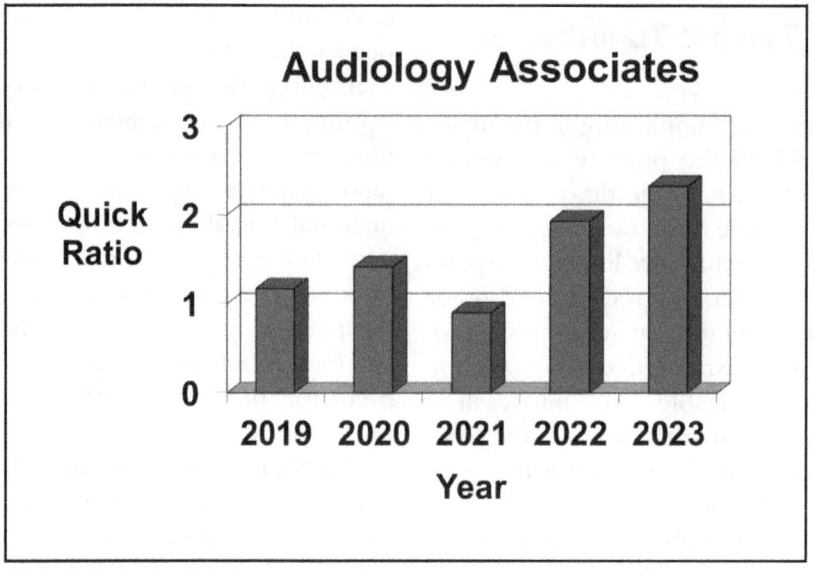

Figure 11–6. Sample quick ratios, Audiology Associates years 2019–2023.

ents how long (in days) it takes for the practice to turn the accounts receivable or credit sales into cash. Figure 11–7 demonstrates that in most years, it only takes 40 to 50 days to turn the accounts receivable into cash. In 2021, however, it took over 90 days to clear the accounts receivable.

By reviewing Figures 11–6 and 11–7 together, the practitioner can see at a glance one possible reason for the problems in 2021. In 2021, when the quick ratio documented that it was difficult to pay the bills, the accounts receivable turnover ratio indicated that it took over 90 days to turn credit sales into cash. When compared to the other years, it took almost twice as long to be paid for products and services in 2021 than the other years, offering a possible explanation for the financial difficulties. Obviously, tracking the various ratios and reviewing them over time greatly eases the management burden on practition-

ers and provides a mirror to reflect the problems in the practice and to fix them before they have had too much impact. In current times, it is rather easy to obtain software or set up a spreadsheet that can easily track ratios and apprise the manager instantly of the difficulties or successes to make decisions.

The development of an assessment technique most appropriate to the venue and demographics of a particular practice should be through the guidance of the practice's accountant. Managing the practice with the clarity that data provide represents the highest form of evidence-based practice management.

Finance for Audiologists

Generally defined, finance is a discipline that studies and addresses the way in which individuals, businesses, and orga-

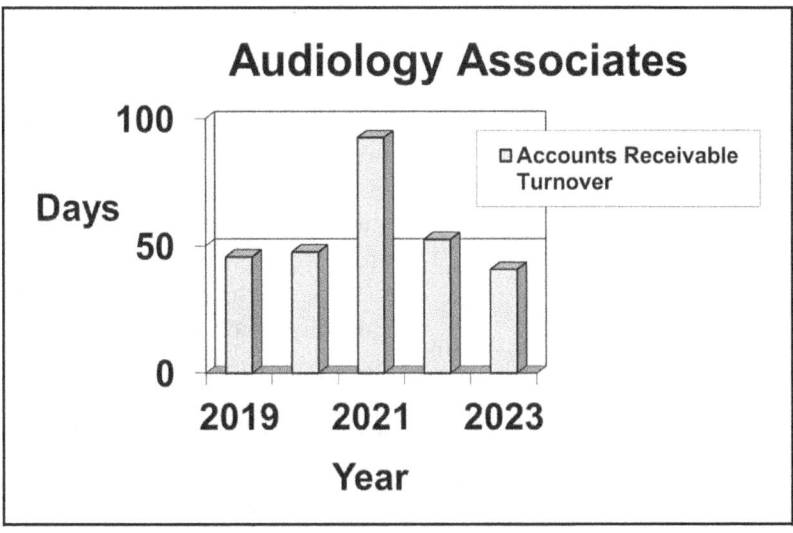

Figure 11–7. Accounts receivable turnover ratio, audiology associates years 2019–2023.

nizations raise, allocate, and use monetary resources over time, taking into account the risks entailed in projects that create wealth. Finance is used by individuals (personal finance), governments (public finance), businesses (corporate finance), and a wide variety of organizations, including schools and nonprofit organizations. The goals of each of the above activities are achieved through the use of appropriate financial instruments, with special consideration to their institutional setting. Finance is one of the most important aspects of practice management for without proper financial planning, a new practice cannot even start, let alone be successful. As cash is the single most powerful liquid asset, managing cash is essential to ensure a secure future and developing wealth for both for an individual practitioner as well as the practice. For audiology practice management purposes, the term finance incorporates:

- The management and control of assets.
- Profiling and managing project risks.
- Finding funds for the generation and maintenance of business.

When considering the financial operations of the practice, a special set of techniques are used to manage financial affairs, particularly the differences between income and expenditure while monitoring the risks of their investments. In a profitable practice where income exceeds expenditure, the practitioner can lend or invest the excess income. Excess profit must be invested to build defensive assets for the practice or for funding expansions, equipment, or other projects that lead to more profit. On the other hand, in an unprofitable practice where income is less than expenditure, the practitioner may need to raise capital by borrowing, selling shares in the company, decreasing its expenses, or increasing its income.

Investing the Profit

When the practice is profitable, the profit should be invested to provide security for the practice when business is slow. These savings and investments for the practice are, as presented above, called defensive assets to be used when times are difficult to pay employees, accounts payable, and other expenses. Typically, a certain portion of these assets will be kept in a place where they can be rather liquid such as a certificate of deposit or a mutual fund that allows for transfers to the business account as necessary. The best method of securing and sustaining the investments to be used as defensive assets is to consult with the practice's accountant and/or an experienced financial planner.

Borrowing Money for the Practice

Although the practitioner would rather not need to borrow money, there is usually a time when this is necessary to pay suppliers, employees, and other monthly expenses. Most practitioners are aware of borrowing for personal loans, auto loans, and educational loans, and loans for the practice work very much the same.

One of the three most important individuals to the practice is a good banker. Without the financial advice and assistance of an experienced financial advisor, the practice will have difficulties. The practitioner should not just shop for a bank, but should shop for the *banker*,

who knows the individual and the practice. The correct banker will be willing to review the business plan more readily and can help with the investment of profits or supply cash infusions as necessary, but it is the individual relationship that makes the difference. There are always risks involved in borrowing money, so the business owner should carefully analyze the need for it first. Bankrate.com (2024) indicates that the practice's place in the business life cycle will help determine the type of loan needed. There are three basic phases in a company's early years: seed, startup, and growth.

- *Seed money* is used for initial planning. These funds sustain during the time that market research is conducted and are also used to create a business plan. Few small-business owners require a lot of cash for organizing and planning, so this step is typically self-funded.
- *Startup funds* used to get the business started can vary greatly. This phase may be financed by the owner or a commercial lender. The credibility for the lenders is based on the practitioner's business plan (see Chapter 3). Even though the practitioner is a doctor, banks and commercial finance companies are less likely to lend money to startups unless there is a significant amount of collateral pledged by the owner. If collateral doesn't meet the standards of a conventional loan offered by a bank, the next consideration should be the Small Business Administration (SBA). The bank may be a preferred lender with the SBA and can approve a loan under the SBA-guaranteed loan program

where the bank's risk is minimized because the government guarantees payment.

■ *Growth financing* is used when the practitioner has a successful practice and wants or needs to expand. This growth point is when practitioners look to banks or large investors for cash to fund new locations, equipment, and other cash need during this growth phase of the practice.

When money is borrowed for a company, the lender (bank) receives interest and the practice will pay a higher interest rate than the lender pays for the money from the Federal Reserve and pockets the profit (see Chapter 1). The bank charges the interest at a rate that reflects their risk in the transaction. Thus, if a loan is considered for a startup practice with little or no track record, the practitioner will usually pay a higher rate than an established practice that has an established clientele and solid financial history. The purpose of the business plan (see Chapter 3) is to convince the lenders that the risk for this specific practice is minimal so that the correct amount of funds can be obtained at a reasonable interest rate. As borrowing money is expensive, Bankrate.com (2024) suggests some points to consider when deciding whether a loan is needed:

■ Make sure it's capital lacking, not good cash flow management.
■ Borrow in expectation of needs, not in desperation—or due to the risk, expensive terms may need to be accepted.

■ If the business is in transition to its next life stage, probably there is a need for cash to foster growth.
■ The purpose needs to be specific and outlined in a solid business plan.
■ The health of the industry must be in the business plan as it will make a difference in how favorably the loan proposal is viewed.
■ Establish a good credit relationship with a banker by opening accounts or taking out small lines of credit, but be cautious to not get into debt without a plan for paying it back.

There are two basic kinds of loans available, *short term* and *long term*. Short-term loans generally reach maturity in 1 year or less and can carry the business through the doldrum months in a seasonal practice. For example, if the practice is in Arizona and there are no patients in the summer or if in northern Minnesota and there are no patients in the winter, lines of credit, working capital loans, and accounts receivable loans that are repaid in a short term can be essential to survival. Long-term loans usually mature in 1 to 7 years but can be longer for real estate or equipment. These loans are used for major business expenses such as vehicles, purchasing facilities, construction, and furnishings. They also can be used to carry the practice through a depressed business cycle.

Recently graduated Doctors of Audiology who want to create a startup practice on their own will have an uphill struggle, despite the accuracy of their well-developed business plan and accurate projections for profitability. Traditional lending institutions will consider the practice, the demographics, and letters of recommendation but, in the end, likely not fund the venture completely. The bank might provide startup funding and create a flexible line of credit at specific times in the practices' first 3 years but even that is a weak assumption. Glaser (2006) refers to the realities of securing conventional financing for new AuD graduates with substantial debt from their education. He states that the note (bank loan) must be secured with assets, not promises of future income, or the note must be cosigned by an individual with the means to repay the note. Especially in a very slow economy and after the recent overhaul of the financial regulations, debt load (the amount of indebtedness) plays heavily in determining loan eligibility.

Couple the above with the fact that bankers, by nature, are conservative and skeptical of practitioners with little or no track record or experience in managing a practice. Bankers are in business to lend money but well aware that often startup businesses, even medically based healthcare practices, are often unsuccessful, especially when those requesting these startup funds have little training or experience in business and practice management.

Basic Financial Management

Managing a business is no small feat, as it requires an adept understanding of financial systems and processes. Knowing the basics of business finance management can feel overwhelming to many business owners, but it is essential for the success of any business. Without careful and responsible fiscal control, businesses often find themselves in trouble and heading toward bankruptcy.

Ensuring that expenses are tracked, overspending is avoided, and income is effectively managed allows companies to increase their profits and allow for future growth.

Budgeting

A major error in the financial management of a practice is not planning for the future. One such plan may involve building a budget to use as a guideline for the expenditure of funds. Budgeting is the process of developing and adopting a profit and financial plan with definite goals for the coming period. Budgets are financial plans that include forecasting expenses, revenues, assets, liabilities, and cash flows based upon a plan that is guided by the goals of the practice manager for a particular period, usually a year. Once the budget is determined, the actual performance of the practice can be compared to the budgeted goals to determine progress or the lack of it.

First, the budget allows for an understanding of the profit dynamics and financial structure of the practice, and second, it becomes the plan for changes in the coming period. The preparation of a budget forces the practice manager to focus on the factors that must improve in order to increase profit. In most audiology practices, it is rare to see a budget planned for more than a year in advance. Although budget preparation can be time-consuming, if not devised, the practice may be at risk of paying higher taxes, overpaying for products, and/or making bad investment choices in equipment and/or in office expansions.

Although budgets for major corporations can be quite complex and take months to complete, for a small audiology practice, the process can be relatively simple. There are many different sources for budgeting software that can be easily obtained online. Before beginning the budget, the practice manager needs to make some assumptions about the industry, the local economy, and other factors such as increased competition that will affect the business. These decisions will drive the budget for its optimism or conservatism, depending upon the outlook. The budgeting process should be conducted with the assistance of an accountant or other business professional by examining expenditures from the previous year and allotting an amount for each category based upon the expected increase or decrease in revenue. If it is a new practice, the business plan can be a good source for the budget for the first 1 to 3 years. Existing practices may begin budgeting a six-step plan:

1. *Examine the practice revenue.* One of the first steps in any budgeting exercise is to review the existing business and revenue sources. Add all those income sources together to determine how much money comes into the practice monthly. It's important to do at least the previous 12 months. Notice the practice's monthly income changes over time and look for seasonal patterns. Understand the seasonal changes to allow the practice to prepare for the leaner months. These historic data and observed trends allow revenue projections for future months. At this point, ensure that calculations are for *revenue, not profit.*

2. *Subtract fixed costs.* Add the practice's historic fixed costs and use them to predict future costs. Fixed costs might occur daily, weekly, monthly, or yearly, so make sure to get as much data as possible. The practice's fixed costs are then subtracted from the revenue.

3. *Subtract variable expenses.* Certain expenses fluctuate over time as well as increase or decrease according to the amount of business conducted. Use the expense data and the seasonal adjustments to estimate these future variable costs. During lean months, attempt to lower the practice's variable expenses. During profitable months when there's extra income, it may be possible to spend on variable expenses in anticipation of these expenses later in the year.

4. *Set aside a contingency fund for unexpected costs.* When creating a practice budget, ensure there is extra cash and plan for contingencies. During the good times, the practice should save defensive assets in the event of an emergency.

5. *Determine the profit.* Add the projected revenue and expenses for each month. Then, subtract expenses from revenue and the resulting number referred to as net income. If you end up with a positive number, you can expect to make a profit. If not, there will be a loss. Compare the projected profits to past profits to determine if the result is realistic.

6. *Finalize the practice budget.* Are the resulting profits enough to work with, or is there too big of a loss? Practice overspending? Regularly compare the actual numbers to the budget to determine whether the practice is meeting those goals, and course

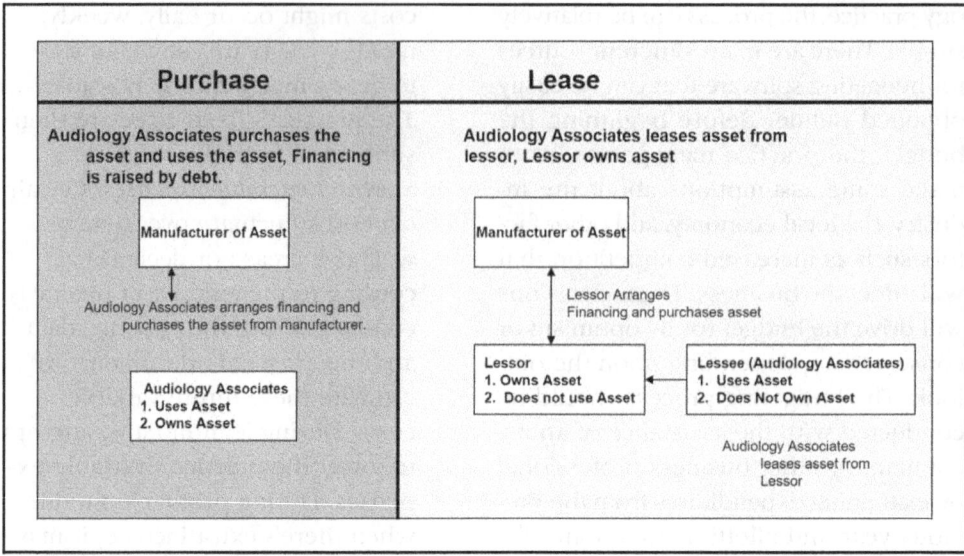

Figure 11–8. Lease versus purchase of equipment.

correct if necessary. It may be necessary to adjust the estimated numbers.

Lease Versus Purchase of Equipment

In general, the purchase of items that appreciate makes sense because the dollar is worth less each day. Items that depreciate, however, are usually better paid for with today's dollars because they will continue to devalue from the date of purchase until the value reaches zero over time. Thus, it may be wise financial management to purchase the office space, as it does not usually depreciate and may appreciate over time, and to rent or lease equipment such as the real ear, OAE, VNG, or ABR unit and audiometer and avoid the use of working capital to pay for a depreciating asset.

What is a lease? Basically, it is the renting of equipment and, depending upon how the lease is set up, can also

be used as a method to purchase. In a purchase, the equipment is obtained directly from the manufacturer or their representative and is funded by the use of capital or by incurring debt. The example in Figure 11–8 compares the options of purchase or lease.

In a lease, Audiology Associates (lessee) agrees to lease a new piece of equipment from a leasing company (lessor). An application is made to the leasing company and, upon approval, the leasing company purchases the equipment from the manufacturer or their representative. In this situation, the leasing company owns the equipment. The general positive and negatives of lease versus purchase are presented in Table 11–5 but are subject to interpretation by the practice manager based on the financial situation of the practice.

Leases often have a lower investment at the beginning, as compared to loans that usually require a down payment of 15% to 20%; however, at the end of

Table 11–5. Equipment Acquisition: Lease v. Purchase

Lease	Purchase
Conserves Capital No down payment	**Consumes Capital** Down payment required
Flexibility of Payments Lease payments are fixed and do not change with interest rate fluctuation	**Specified Payments** According to interest rate, term of loan may change with interest rate fluctuation
Convenience On the spot financing and immediate delivery	**Inconvenience** Apply for loan, credit application, counts against debt of the practice
Protection Against Obsolescence A lease can be structured to include upgrades and partial or complete equipment swaps either at mid-term or at lease-end	**Cannot Turn in for Upgrades** What you bought is what you got . . . forever
Eliminates Risk At the end of the lease it is turned in or bought for $1.00	**More Risk** Must junk it, use it, or sell it at the end of the loan
Off Balance Sheet Financing Can potentially increase borrowing capacity while easing the budgeting process and preserving key financial ratios	**On Balance Sheet Financing** Uses up precious capital and causes debt ratio to be higher
Improved Return on Assets (ROA)	**Less Return on Assets (ROA)**
Paid with BEFORE Tax Dollars	**Paid with AFTER Tax Dollars**

the lease payment program, the clinic will not own the equipment. It must be turned in or the practice may choose to pay a slightly higher payment and be able to purchase the item at fair market value, sometimes only $1.00, at the end of the lease. For office equipment or audiologic equipment, technology constantly evolves, and thus the capability of the instrumentation that was pur-chased today will change over the next 3 to 4 years, possibly outdating it. Obsolescence is part of the audiology profession just as it is part of many other professions that utilize equipment for analysis and rehabilitative treatment of various physiologic difficulties. The goal, then, for rapidly changing equipment is to simply have the right to use it for a specified period of time since it will eventually be worthless. On the other hand, if the equipment is a sound room that is less sensitive to technology changes, it makes sense to purchase it and then use the room as long as the practice exists without a monthly expense. Various companies offer Excel spreadsheets that assist in the calculation of the lease purchase decision. These preprepared analysis systems can assist practitioners when the decision is not obvious.

Types of Leases

There are several different lease products on the market that apply to various situations and types of equipment. Two types that are often used in audiology practices are the *operating lease* and the *long-term or capital lease*.

Operating leases are relatively short-term contracts for the use of an item. As the term of the contract is relatively short, the payments are lower to the leasing company and usually not enough to allow the lessor to fully recover the cost of the asset. As the term of the lease may be less than the economic life of the asset, the remaining value of the item is called a residual value. For example, if a car is leased for 2 years, the car will have a substantial residual value (or left-over value) at the end of the lease, and the lease payments made will pay off only a fraction of the original cost of the car. The lessor, in an operating lease, expects the lessee to either lease the car again, purchase it for the residual value, or turn it in. If turned in, the lessor will either lease or sell the car (or equipment) again. Sometimes, in operating leases, the lessor is responsible for taxes, insurance, and maintenance of the item,

which is usually passed on to the lessee in the form of higher payments.

Another defining characteristic of the operating lease is that the lessee may have the right to cancel the lease with very short notice by turning in the item and ceasing payments, although this option usually requires a higher payment for the cancellation option. Although practices have these operating leases for the automobiles, hearing conservation vans, and other very large items that they will never pay off, there are other types of leases more appropriate for leasing audiometric equipment, computers, and office furniture.

Long-term leases are also referred to as capital leases, lease purchase, $1 buy-out, or full-payout leases and are usually for longer terms involving equipment. Lease Crunch (2024) describes a financial lease as being similar to a loan, with the lessee building equity in the equipment as they make each payment. Because of this, the lessee has to account for the asset as a conditional sale and must depreciate the equipment as a capital asset. At lease termination, the lessee may purchase the item at fair market value or fixed price, or for some items, such as equipment or software, a $1 purchase option is usually available for a slightly higher payment. The term for these financial leases must exceed 75% of the estimated economic life of the leased property and the value of all the lease payments must be equal to 90% or more of the cost of the leased property.

As with all financial decisions, lease versus purchase options should be considered with the assistance of the practice's accountant, who appreciates the balance sheet implications of each option as well as the profitability of the procedure that will be conducted.

Capital Investment

Expansion to a new location and lucrative market is a viable consideration when a practice is prospering. This venture will not likely be funded internally; therefore, the practice manager will find it necessary to go to a bank, credit union, or other financial lender for a loan to secure appropriate space, develop needed tenant improvements, and obtain requi-site business and clinical equipment for the new office.

The lender will need to know if there is a high likelihood of success in this new venture to ensure consistent payments on the loan. As presented in Chapter 3, the practitioner must present a sound business plan and realistic financial projections for profitability. There are several methods that can be used to figure the rate of return on the project, but two methods commonly used are the breakeven analysis (BA) and/or the net present value (NPV).

NET PRESENT VALUE (NPV) CALCULATION

Probably the most accurate technique to use in the estimation of the payoff for a remodeling or expansion project is one that considers the initial investment in addition to the everyday operation expenses and the interest rate at which the funds were borrowed. One method is to look at a calculation of the net present value or NPV often used by corporations to describe a number of project proposals allowing the manager to choose the project that will have the highest return and a positive NPV value. All projects, according to Tuovila (2021), that carry a negative NPV will most likely fail and should not be attempted. A simple definition of the NPV of a project or investment is that it presents the sum of the present values of the annual cash flows minus the initial investment. In a new clinic site, these annual cash flows are the net benefits (revenues minus costs) generated from new clinic site during its lifetime. In the NPV calculation, these cash flows are discounted or adjusted by incorporating the uncertainty or risk of the success of the clinic and time value of money. In financial literature, the NPV offers the most robust financial evaluation to estimate the overall value of an investment.

Although there are Internet calculators for NPV, Colernick (2024) states that the calculation of NPV involves three simple yet nontrivial steps. The first step is to identify the size and timing of the expected future cash flows generated by the project or investment. The second step is to de-

continued on next page

continued from previous page

termine the discount rate or the estimated rate of return for the project. The third step is to calculate the NPV using the equations shown below:

$$NPV = Co + \frac{\text{Cash Flow Year 1}}{(1 + r)} + \frac{\text{Cash Flow Year 2}}{(1 + r)^2}$$

$$+ \frac{\text{Cash Flow Year 3}}{(1 + r)^3}$$

Consider the following example in Table 11–6, where the cost to remodel the space for the new diagnostic audiology center at the hospital is $27,000. The clinic can borrow the funds for this project at 6.5% for the project.

This $27,000 includes items such as furniture, carpet, lighting, creating treatment rooms, reception area, wall coverings, art, and other appointments. The clinic also has some extra equipment that will be used in the new facility so there is not equipment cost. Cash flow estimates have been estimated by the accountant with input from the practitioner at $25,000 for year 1, $40,000 for year 3, and $75,000 at year 3. It is expected that after 3 years of operation, the new clinic could be worth $75,000.

$$NPV = \$27,000 + \frac{\$25,000}{1.065} + \frac{\$40,000}{1.134} + \frac{\$75,000}{1.207}$$

$$NPV = \$27,000 + \$23,474.17 + \$35,273.36 + \$62,137.53$$

$$NPV = \$93,885.06$$

As this is a highly positive NPV, the project should be conducted.

Table 11–6. Costs for Diagnostic Center NPV

Audiology Associates, Inc. Diagnostic Center
Initial Investment   Remodel Space (Borrowed at 6.5% Interest Rate..............................$27,000

Estimated Dash Flows
        Year 1..$25,000
        Year 2..$40,000
        Year 3..$75,000

Future Value of Practice if Successful...$75,000

Breakeven Analysis (BA)

According to the SBA (2017), the *breakeven analysis* is used to determine when the practice will be able to cover all its expenses and begin to make a profit. It is important to include startup costs in the analysis to assist in the determination of the sales revenue needed to pay the ongoing business expenses. Basically, the breakeven analysis is the level of sales at which profits are zero or the point at which total revenues equal total costs. The calculation of a breakeven analysis involves the use of the formula:

$$\text{Breakeven (B)} = \frac{\text{Fixed}}{(\text{Gross Profit per Unit} - \text{Variable Costs})}$$

BREAKEVEN ANALYSIS

The breakeven analysis is a determination of what needs to be sold, monthly or annually, to cover the costs of doing business, or the breakeven point. The breakeven analysis is not the best analysis because:

■ It is frequently mistaken for the payback period or the time it takes to recover an investment.
■ It depends on the concept of fixed costs. Technically, a breakeven analysis defines fixed costs as those costs that would continue even if the business went broke. It is best, however, to use the regular running fixed costs, including payroll and normal expenses, which offers better insight regarding financial health.
■ It depends on averaging the per-unit variable cost and per-unit revenue over the whole business.

The purpose of the breakeven analysis formula is to calculate the amount of sales that equates revenues to expenses and the amount of excess revenues, *also known as profits*, after the fixed and variable costs are met. The calculation of a breakeven analysis involves the use of the formula:

$$\text{Breakeven (B)} = \frac{\text{Fixed}}{(\text{Gross Profit per Unit} - \text{Variable Costs})}$$

For example, Audiology Associates wants to open a new location for its hearing aid sales at the local hospital accepting referrals from local physicians for amplification products. The fixed costs are $20,000 per month and the variable costs are $250 per unit. At a sales price of $2,250, each unit will have a gross profit of $2,000 over and above the fixed and vari-

continued on next page

---

continued from previous page

able costs. Therefore, the question to the practitioner that owns Audiology Associates is how many units must be sold each month to break even?

Using the breakeven analysis calculation, simply take the fixed expenses of $20,000 divided by the gross profit per unit ($2,250) minus the variable costs ($250).

$$\text{Breakeven (B)} = \frac{\$20,000}{(\$2,250 - \$250)}$$

$$\text{Breakeven (B)} = \frac{\$20,000}{\$2,000} \, BA = 20$$

From this analysis, the clinic must sell 20 hearing aids each month to just break even (Figure 11–2). Of course, as this is only the point where the clinic breaks even, hopefully there will be substantially more than 20 units sold each month so that the new hearing aid center can stay in business (Prakash & Aebisher, 2022).

In the calculation of a breakeven analysis, the fixed expenses are simply divided by the gross profit minus expenses. This will result in the number of sales (or audiometric procedures or hearing aids) needed to break even. Of course, the practitioner is in business to make a profit and hopes to see many more procedures sold than simply enough to break even.

Kenton (2023) indicates that any expenditure made in the hope of generating more cash later can be called a capital investment project. For these large capital investment projects, it is best to incorporate a calculation that considers the initial investment, everyday operation expenses, and the interest rate of the loan. Although there are a number of financial calculations that attempt to predict the success of capital investment projects, a relatively simple calculation is the net present value (NPV).

The key to understanding the NPV calculation is, as indicated previously, the concept that the value of money is less tomorrow than it is today. This is why banks and other financial institutions charge interest. The value of the money may be less tomorrow, but also the use of this money means that it cannot be used for another purpose.

In capital investment projects, it is often necessary to know if there is a possibility that the project will be successful while still in the planning stages. This allows the practitioner to choose the most successful project among a number of proposals based upon the calculated NPV. The chosen project is the one that has the highest return and a positive NPV value. Tuovila offers a straightforward

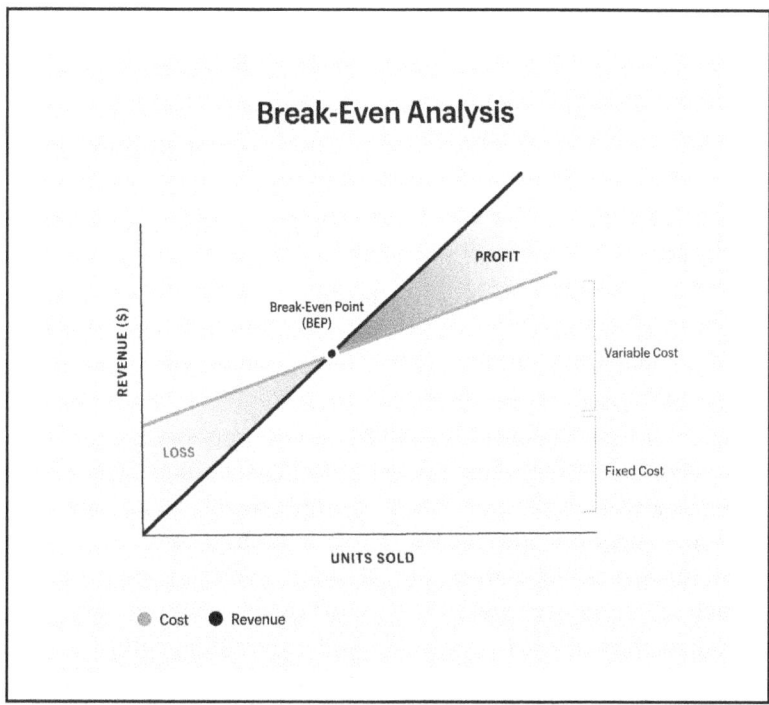

Figure 11–9. Breakeven Analysis.

statement about negative NPV that all projects that carry a negative NPV are losers and should not be attempted. The rules for the use of NPV indicate that the value of the practice will be increased by conducting those capital investment projects that are worth more than they cost—projects with a positive NPV. Capital investment calculations, such as NPV and other project evaluations, should be conducted with the assistance of the practice accountant to ensure accuracy of the cash flow predictions.

Embezzlement

If a financial advisor is used, they should not have access to the practice finances,

bank accounts, or books as these individuals can create extreme difficulty for practice managers if they are dishonest. Their credentials should be checked, rechecked, and police records investigated before they have access to any accounts or financial information. In this new century, all a dishonest person needs are the business tax ID number or a personal Social Security number along with a birthdate and other minimal information to facilitate a major fraud. These frauds can have severe tax implication for the practice, the practice manager, and even other employees that may have had control over funds. Stated earlier, the fact that the practice is a corporation does not shelter its owners and others against mismanagement of tax filing responsibilities. The advice is to be very careful as to who has access to financial accounts and sensitive information for the company and the employees.

Can You Tell Who Is an Embezzler?

In an early investigation into the crime of embezzlement, Peterson (1947) observed that the embezzler is an anomaly in the field of crime. Previous arrest and/or prison records are frequently not available to act as a warning of possible dishonest conduct. Steady work records often conceal the psychological or financial instability that may be present in the person. Pedneault et al. (2012) states that no one has yet to discover a "surefire" method of avoiding the employment of potential embezzlers as they follow no pattern and offer no outward signs. They may be 18 or 80, work for a firm for 4 months or 40 years, be paid $1,800 or $18,000, and steal anywhere from a few hundred dollars to many hundreds of thousands. Pedneault and colleagues further state that for the most part, embezzlements are committed by individuals who have no previous criminal records and whose business and personal background are beyond reproach. While there are many methods embezzlers can use to hide their crimes, there are often warning signs evident in the employee's behavior long before the theft is uncovered. These warning signs can have legitimate explanations individually, but several red flags together could signify an embezzlement problem. Generally, there are a number of behaviors that might offer clues:

- An overly enthusiastic employee who consistently asks questions about business processes and procedures.
- Employees who make major lifestyle changes, living beyond the means afforded by their salary.
- Employees with excessive debt created by divorce, an affair, drug abuse, or ongoing financial or legal issues.
- Gambling debts are a major cause of embezzlement. Be suspicious if employees visit casinos routinely or gamble heavily.
- Employees refusing to take time off or not wanting someone else to take over their duties.
- Beware of employees who want to work when no one is around, such as after hours or on weekends.
- A hostile attitude toward reasonable questions, particularly about financial transactions.
- A disgruntled employee dissatisfied with the practice or the practice owner.

Why do these people break the bond of trust with their employers? Sometimes these employees are even the practice owner's relatives. What causes them to not only break the trust of their employer, but create insurmountable issues within families?

Cressey (1973) describes the "triangle of fraud" and that all three factors must be present before a person will commit fraud or embezzlement (Figure 11–10):

- Need.
- Opportunity.
- Rationalization.

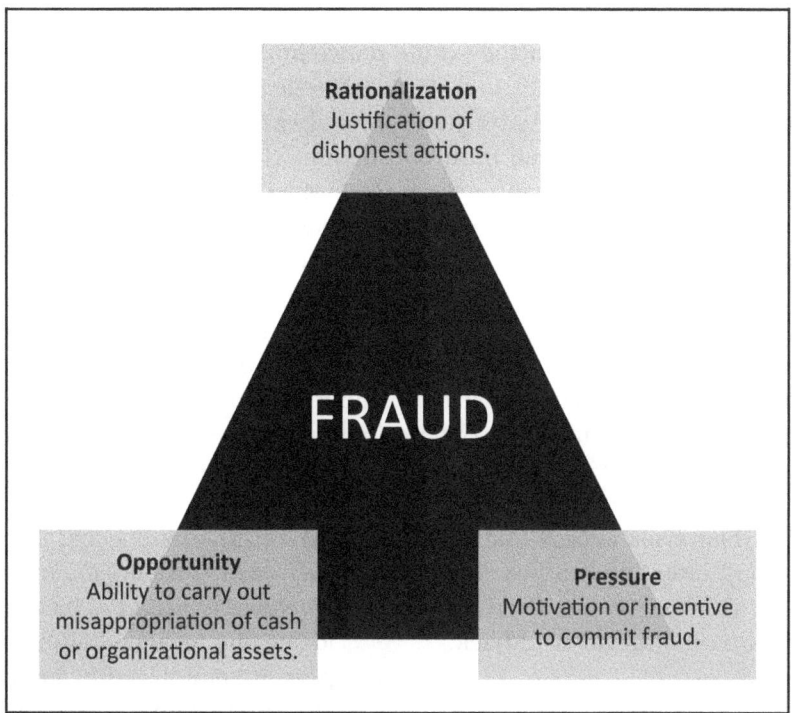

Figure 11–10. The Fraud Triangle. *Source*: Cressey, D. (1973). *Other peoples' money* (p. 30). Reprinted with permission, Patterson Smith, Montclair, New Jersey.

Need involves stealing to resolve a desperate financial problem such as an addiction to drugs, alcohol, gambling, shopping, or an extramarital affair. Embezzlers may simply be attempting to keep up with their peers financially or motivated by the pressure created by the loss of a job, a spouse, divorce, or just drowning in debt.

Opportunity is defined as a perception that there is a low probability of being caught. In accounting, the descriptive word for this is "poor internal controls." For some employees, the opportunity to steal is very difficult to resist. The combination of being the trusted individual in the practice who conducts the business, handles the funds, writes the checks, makes deposits, and reconciles the bank statements combined with a busy, possibly absent practice owner is opening the door to theft.

Zeune (2015) discusses rationalization as the employee's mental process of making their illegal action fit within a personal code of conduct or ethics. In other words, the dishonest employee must be able to "talk himself into the action." Rationalization often results in what he refers to as "situational fraud." An employee's propensity to steal or embezzle can be predicted based on a widely accepted formula:

- 5% to 10% of employees would never—ever—do anything wrong.

- 5% to 10% of employees are always scheming to steal whatever they can obtain.
- 80% to 90% of remaining employees who will commit "situational fraud" results from being in a position to steal and easily rationalize the illegal deed.

There is also rationalization of the theft with thoughts such as, "I deserve a raise or who are these people to make all this money and I cannot?" or other such issues. Often there are good intentions of borrowing the funds and a desire to pay them back later. While there may be good intentions to just take a loan, while the theft is not discovered, the funds are often never paid back.

Tips for Embezzlement Prevention

While there is no surefire method of preventing embezzlement, there are some precautions that can be taken by practice owners to lessen their chances of be targeted. First, set a good example for employees. An employer who dips into petty cash, fudges on an expense account, uses company funds for personal items, or sets other examples of loose business behavior will find employees rationalizing dishonest actions. A second discouragement for embezzlement is establishing a climate of accountability. Employees should know their jobs and feel trusted to do them but should also realize that they are held accountable for their actions. It is important for busy audiology practice managers to examine the financial procedures within the clinic and determine what controls can be added to forestall dishonesty. The system should be designed to provide documented evidence in the event someone does try to embezzle funds. A major legal problem in embezzlement claims is proving the amount that was stolen. If embezzlement does occur, the practice owner will be expected to support the loss with evidence, documented facts, and figures obtained from the books.

While most professional accountants and CPAs offer similar suggestions to minimize embezzlement, here are nine longtime tips that can control embezzlement in the practice:

1. *Do an extensive background check before hiring the final employee candidate.* It's a good idea to be informed about the person being hired *before* they are hired. Do not simply rely on recommendations, interviews, and their resume. It is necessary to conduct a criminal record check and a credit check before the final candidate is hired into positions where they are expected to handle funds, such as bookkeepers, office managers, and others who are involved with the day-to-day cash flow transactions.

2. *Keep track of the practice's checks.* Purchase and use prenumbered checks and periodically look for missing check numbers by using the *Missing Check* report. Have a written "voided check" procedure that requires all voided checks to be coded to an expense account called *"Voided Checks."* Never sign a blank check, *NEVER* use a signature stamp, and do not insert a graphic of a signature to be printed on each check.

3. *Sign and verify all checks, especially payroll checks*. It is a good idea to sign all checks personally, even the small ones. The benefit of signing all checks is that the signature will be a requirement for money to leave the business.

4. *Make bank deposits nightly*. The practice owner should make the nightly bank deposits. While there is not usually much cash in the clinic, this is especially true for cash payments as they are often large, and it is tempting and easy to steal.

5. *Understand the books*. Embezzlement is easy to miss and difficult to prove if bookkeeping is sloppy or unsupervised. Practice owners need to be educated in financial statements and know how to evaluate them. The more that is understood about accounting and the particular accounting software, the easier it is to pick up irregularities.

6. *The bank and credit card statements should be reconciled by the practice manager.* It should be a practice policy that the owner is the one who is responsible for reconciling the monthly bank and credit card accounts. This way, the practice owner can ensure that no one is forging signatures by simply reviewing the checks and the statements.

7. *Separate the mailroom from Bank Deposit & Reconciliation*. As mentioned earlier, one of the most common ways to embezzle money from an employer is called "lapping." To lap, an embezzler skims a little bit of the cash that comes in each month and then adjusts the books to hide the skimming. As long as the person skimming the cash also maintains the checkbook and reconciles the bank accounts, it's easy for the theft to go unnoticed. By reviewing the mail, conducting daily bank deposits, and performing the reconciliation, the practice manager discourages "lapping" schemes.

8. *Protect other valuable assets.* From an embezzler's perspective, cash is the most convenient item to steal as it is portable, easy to store, and easy to convert. While cash is watched closely by embezzlers, they often steal other items of value, such as office equipment, inventory, supplies, and sometimes even patient files.

9. *Require vacations.* There is a final embezzlement prevention tool that many big businesses use and should be considered by small audiology practices as well. Require regular vacations of a week or two. Some embezzlement schemes are so clever that they're almost impossible to catch, but one typical weakness in most of them is that they usually require ongoing maintenance on the part of the embezzler. By mandating employee vacations, the practice owner can observe what happens if the employee is absent for a few days.

Those handling funds in the clinic need to be closely and routinely monitored to ensure that all of the profits stay within the practice and not in someone else's pocket. When embezzlement does occur, the practice and its owner and often their family become victims.

Embezzlement can not only have a profound effect on the success or failure of the practice but also cause psychological effects on the owner and cast a dark shadow on their business and personal reputations.

Epilogue

Fiscal management is fundamentally the practitioner or practice manager's accountability for the practice. A fiscally responsible manager not only knows where the funds are, who needs payment, and when bills need to be paid but also stays current on ever-changing costs. The practice owner must routinely review expenses, financial statements, and ratios as well as track monthly, quarterly, and yearly changes to be able to adjust to the external and internal fluctuations of the business cycle.

Finance is an area in which most audiologists have no interest or background. A chief financial officer (CFO) is the main financial policymaker in the company with duties often extending into many other areas, including accounting, budgeting, and capital investment. Wise practice CFOs borrow smartly, expand cautiously, and invest in sound projects that will bring future success to the practice. Good financial investment may even counteract business problems, such as equipment breakdowns, slow business, unforeseen emergencies, and embezzlement, providing a source of unencumbered cash to augment income as the situation changes. Since the practitioner is usually the CFO of the practice, the goal of this chapter was to stress the necessity of understanding the accounting process, how to review and track financial statements, the importance of preparing budgets for the efficient use of funds, and how to calculate the benefits and realities of expenditure projects.

References

Accounting.com. (2024). General Accepted Accounting Principles. https://www.accounting.com/resources/gaap/

ADP. (2024). ADP Payroll. https://www.adp.com/

AICPA. (2024). American Institute of Certified Public Accountants. https://www.aicpa-cima.com/home

AIPB. (2024) American Association of Professional bookkeepers: Website. https://aipb.org/

Analyst Notes. (2024). Time series and cross sectional data. CFA Study notes. http://analystnotes.com/cfa-study-notes-distinguish-between-time-series-and-cross-sectional-data.html

Averkamp, H. (2024a). Introduction to the income statement. The Accounting Coach. https://www.accountingcoach.com/income-statement/explanation

Averkamp, H. (2024b). The quick ratio (acid test ratio). The Accounting Coach. https://www.accountingcoach.com/blog/quick-ratio-acid-test

Bankrate.com. (2024). Website. https://www.bankrate.com/

Colernick, K. (2024). How to calculate the net present value. Calculate Stuff. https://www.calculatestuff.com/financial/npv-calculator

Cressey, D. (1973). *Other people's money*. Patterson Smith.

Fernando, J., Drury, A., & Rathburn, P. (2024). Opportunity cost: Definition, formula, and examples. Investopeia. https://www.investopedia.com/terms/o/opportunitycost.asp

Fishman, S. (2024). Cash vs. accrual accounting. Nolo. http://www.nolo.com/legal-encyclopedia/cash-vs-accrual-accounting-29513.html

Grigg, B., & Lane, R. (2023). Accounting principles: Basic definitions, why they're important. https://www.nerdwallet.com/article/small-business/basic-accounting-concepts

Glaser, R. (2006, September). Financial components of audiology practice, The Business of Audiology, Sonic Innovations Business Series Workshops, Phoenix, AZ

Hayes, A. (2024). Total debt-to-total assets ratio: Meaning, formula, and what's good. Investopedia. https://www.investopedia.com/terms/t/totaldebttototalassets.asp

Kenton, W. (2023). Capital investment: Types, example, and how it works. Investopedia. https://www.investopedia.com/terms/c/capital-investment.asp#:~:text=Capital%20investment%20is%20the%20expenditure,assets%20and%20most%20are%20depreciated

Laurence, B. (2024). Business equipment: Buying vs. leasing. Nolo. https://www.nolo.com/legal-encyclopedia/business-equipment-buying-vs-leasing-29714.html#:~:text=The%20answer%20depends%20on%20your,has%20a%20long%20usable%20life

Lease Crunch. (2024). Operating lease vs. finance lease: What's the difference? Lease Crunch. https://www.leasecrunch.com/blog/finance-leases-vs-operating-lease

Paycom. (2024). Paycom payroll. https://www.paycom.com/

Pedneault, S., Rudewicz, F., Sheetz, M., & Silverstone, H. (2012). *Forensic accounting and fraud investigation* (3rd ed.). CPE Store.

Peterson, V. W. (1947). Why honest people steal. *Journal of Criminal Law and Criminology*, *32*(2), 94–103. http://scholarlycommons.law.northwestern.edu/cgi/viewcontent.cgi?article=3463&context=jclc

Prakash, P., & Aebisher, C. (2022). Break-even analysis: What it is and how to calculate. Nerdwallet. https://www.fundera.com/blog/break-even-analysis

Silbiger, S. (2012). *The 10-day MBA*. Harper Collins Publishers.

Small Business Administration (SBA). (2017). Breakeven analysis. Business financials. https://www.sba.gov/starting-business/business-financials/breakeven-analysis

Stobierski, T. (2020). How to read and understand a balance sheet. Harvard Business School. https://online.hbs.edu/blog/post/how-to-read-a-balance-sheet

Tracy, J. (2001). *Accounting for dummies* (2nd ed.). Wiley Publishing.

Traynor, R. M. (2016). Embezzlement—could it really happen to you? *Audiology Today, 28*(4), 42–52.

Traynor, R. M. (2019). Accounting for audiologists. In B. Taylor (Ed.), *Audiology practice management* (3rd ed.). Thieme.

Traynor, R. M., Wooten, A., & Allison, P. (2014, June). *Embezzlement in audiology*. Panel presentation at the 30th Scott Haug Audiology Retreat, New Braunfels, TX.

Tuovila, A. (2021). Net present value (NPV) rule: Definition, use, and example. Investopedia. https://www.investopedia.com/terms/n/npv-rule.asp

Tuovila, A., Boyle, M., & Rosenston, M. (2024). What is a sunk cost—and the sunk cost fallacy? Investopedia. https://www.investopedia.com/terms/s/sunkcost.asp

Viele, D., Marshall, D., & McManus, W. (2016). *Accounting: What the numbers mean?* (11th ed.). McGraw-Hill.

Zeune, G. (2015). How to predict when people will embezzle . . . and how to stop them. White Collar Crime fighter. http://www.theprosandthecons.com/articles/How%20to%20Predict%20When%20People%20Will%20Embezzle%20WCCF.pdf

12 Fundamentals of Marketing an Audiology Practice

*Robert M. Traynor, EdD, MBA,
Brian Taylor, AuD, Nick Fitzgerald, BA,
and Kevin M. Liebe, AuD*

Introduction

Audiology has evolved into a fully accepted healthcare discipline, joining colleagues in optometry, dentistry, chiropractic, and other occupations as an independent doctoral-level profession. Since audiology has now achieved stature commensurate with other independent doctoral level professions, a reasonable question remains:

Why does a highly educated, fully credentialed, licensed, and board-certified audiology practitioner HAVE to market their practice

In private practice, audiology becomes a business. Marketing is ultimately an exercise in shaping people's attitudes toward a specific business. Get it wrong and, at best, people ignore the business and, at worst, they seek to avoid whatever the business has to offer. Get it right and people will usually follow whatever action is recommended. In the past, audiologists simply established a few referral sources and made a rather good living by conducting hear-ing or balance evaluations, dispensing a few hearing aids each month, offering expert and timely written reports, and providing personalized customer service. Today, intense competition from every direction dictates that marketing a specific audiology practice is essential for success. This fierce competition places a greater burden on audiologists to spend more time and funding on the development and execution of marketing strategies that shape people's attitudes toward doing business with them. As presented in Chapter 4, competition is no longer just from other audiology colleagues or traditional hearing aid dispensers within the local market; local practices are now bombarded from all angles. Today's competitors are statewide with telehealth, nationally with direct-to-consumer offerings, and international from Internet offerings. It is now part of a successful audiology practice, no matter where it is, to differentiate. And, that is why, now more than ever:

A highly educated, fully credentialed, licensed, and board-certified audiology practitioner HAS TO market their practice.

This process is no longer just a good idea for audiology practice owners or managers, but an essential component in the competitive game is differentiating their business from all the others.

The *goal* of marketing is to stand out from *all these competitors* by drawing attention to the practice's superior business techniques, expertise, people, products, and services.

Needs, Wants, and Demands

According to Kotler and Keller (2016), consumers are looking for products and services that fulfill their needs, wants, and demands. *Needs* are generally the basic human requirements such as air, food, water, clothing, and shelter. For the marketing of audiology products and services, the targeted fundamental need is hearing and balance. These human needs become *wants* when directed toward specific objects or services required to satisfy those needs. At this point, the consumer turns wants into *demands*. Consumer demands are described as wants for specific products with an ability to pay. As part of the marketing process, practices need to not only generate wants for their products and services but also ensure that the wants are backed up by the ability to pay, turning these wants into demands. Marketers have distinguished five types of needs:

1. Stated needs (The patient wants the best hearing care available at the lowest price possible).
2. Real needs (The patient wants a hearing aid that works in all situations).
3. Unstated needs (The patient expects good follow-up from the audiologist).
4. Delight needs (The patient would like the audiologist to include features such as TV streaming).
5. Secret needs (The patient wants their friends to think of them as a savvy consumer).

Many hearing care marketing messages seen on television, the Internet, and elsewhere only address the first of these needs and shortchange consumers. The marketing messages that meet only stated needs have led to confused consumers seeking hearing care.

The Confused Hearing Care Consumer

A further complication of this competitive landscape is that *consumers are totally confused*. The challenge to audiology practice owners and managers of differentiation is amplified every day by a market that intentionally causes consumer *confusion*. This confusion is presented every day on television, the Internet, newspapers, and other media reminding audiologists that their competition comes from not simply a local region but involves international competitors in every community across the world. It is unfortunate that a successful practice in the current hearing care market is not always the best-prepared hearing care professionals; it is often those that offer the best-prepared marketing message to these confused consumers. In short, confused consumers in the community must be convinced that this specific clinic offers unique services and products compared to the

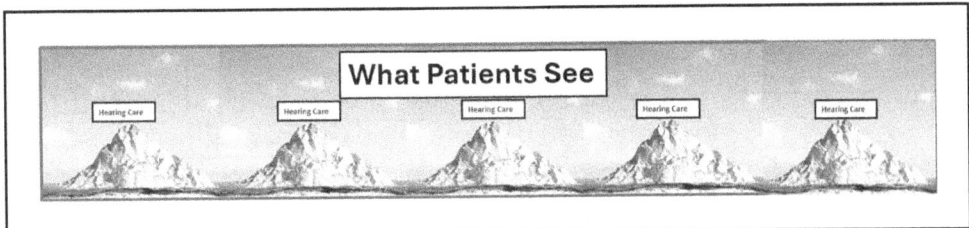

Figure 12–1. What patients SEE in the hearing care market. *Source:* Adapted from McClelland (1973).

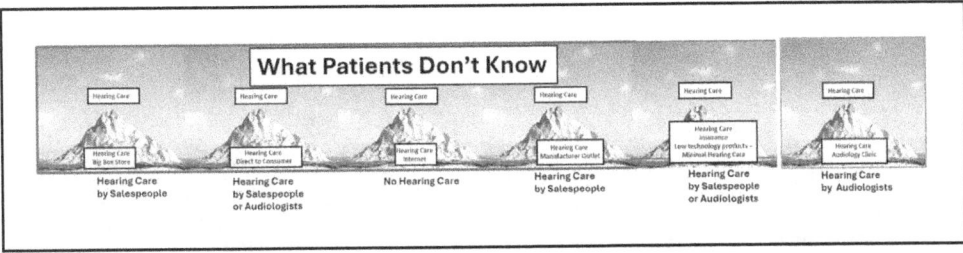

Figure 12–2. What patients DO NOT KNOW about the hearing care market. *Source:* Adapted from McClelland (1973).

local, statewide, national, and international competition.

To offer an understanding of the consumer confusion within the marketplace, McClelland (1973, 1985, 1987, 1989) presents the iceberg analogy. This concept reviews how consumers, the practice's prospective patients, currently see hearing care as it is presented through worldwide market offerings. It begins with the presentation offered in Figure 12–1.

As with an iceberg, all that consumers see is the *"tip of the iceberg"* projecting out of the water. The iceberg tip presents the concept, created by those in the market, that since all hearing care is essentially the same, the consumer's goal became just "get a good deal." While some consumers appreciate the differences offered within a full-service audiology clinic, it is up to the owners and managers of these clinics to

ethically point out differences in the types of hearing care offered, as seen in Figure 12–2. Generally, these differences are not presented in the marketing brochures sent out by the lesser-qualified operations.

These lesser-qualified businesses are simply sales operations, mostly staffed by hearing aid dispensers and not audiologists. While some consumers might see an audiologist, that audiologist is often compromised by their employer's ultimate goal of selling a product, not necessarily the process of aural rehabilitation. Therefore, it is up to the owner-managers of audiology clinics to market their products and services by presenting differentiation, as demonstrated in Figure 12–3.

In this analogy, the bottom portion of the McClelland's iceberg is the depth of offerings to consumers of hearing care from a full-service, patient-centric audi-

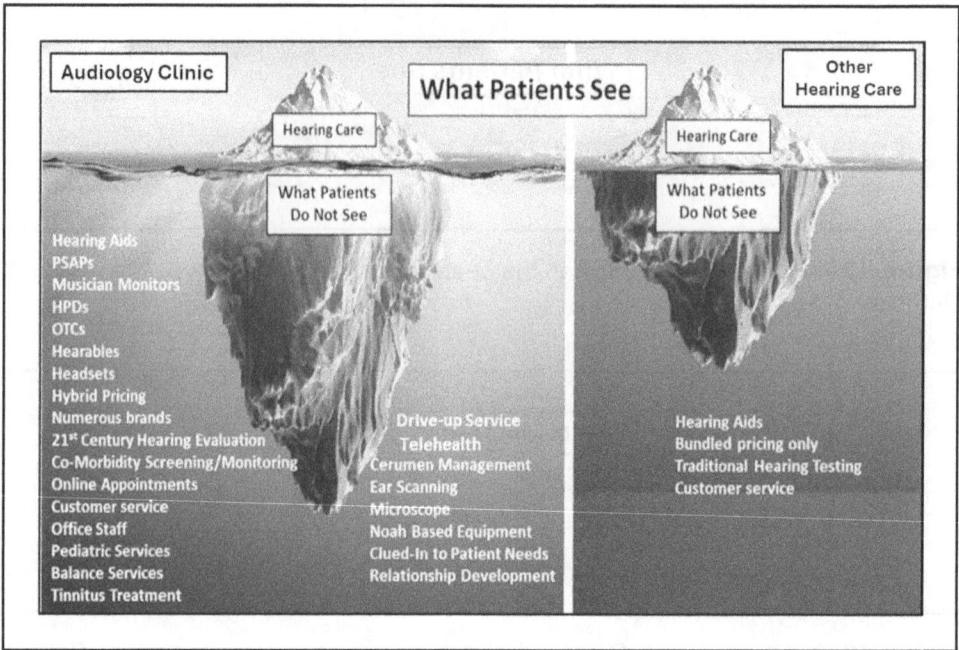

Figure 12–3. What patients DO NOT KNOW about hearing care providers. *Source:* Adapted from McClelland (1973).

ology clinic compared to other "clinics" in the market. It is obvious that the audiology clinic has many more services and products available with significantly more expertise than the other hearing care businesses, but *the confused consumer does not realize these differences*. The lesson to be learned from this analogy is that without marketing to these confused consumers, they may not realize the special benefits offered from a full-service practice.

Professional Marketing Defined

Kotler and Keller (2016) describe marketing as the science and art of exploring, creating, and delivering value to satisfy the needs of a target market at a profit. Marketing identifies unfulfilled needs and desires. It defines, measures, and quantifies the size of the identified market and the profit potential while pinpointing which segments the practice can serve best.

The American Marketing Association (2024) further defines marketing as the set of institutions and processes for creating, communicating, delivering, and exchanging offerings that have value for customers, clients, patients, partners, and society at large. Although it may have a social or managerial purpose, marketing is the creation of demand for a product or service by establishing public awareness. Additionally, marketing has been described as the process of planning and executing the conception, pricing, promotion, and distribution of ideas, goods, and services to

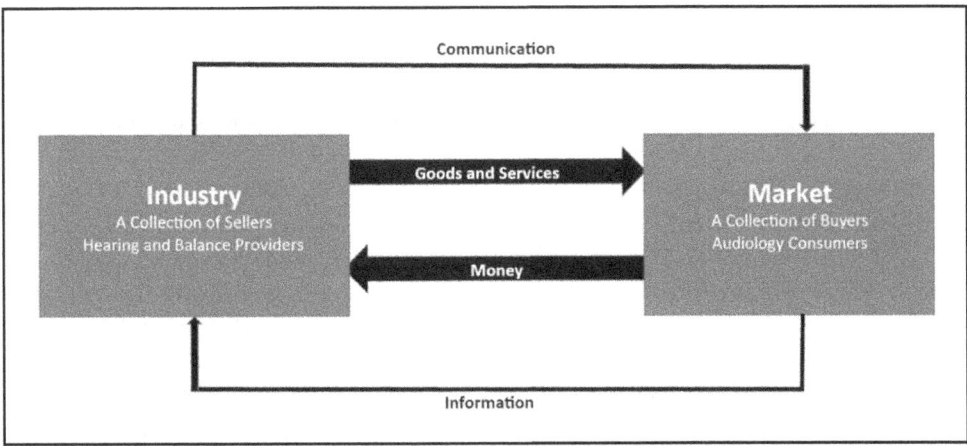

Figure 12–4. The relationship between providers and the market. *Source:* Adapted from Kotler and Keller (2016).

create exchanges that satisfy individual and organizational goals.

What do these definitions mean to audiologists? They mean that marketing encompasses everything necessary to generate awareness and desire to purchase a product or service by potential consumers. Put simply, marketing is basic communication between a collection of sellers (such as audiologists) and a collection of buyers of products and services (such as hearing/balance-impaired consumers), presented in Figure 12–4.

This collection of sellers offers products and services to the market that consists of a collection of buyers who pay money for those products and services. Although the concept in Figure 12–4 presents how the system works, the goal is to have this collection of buyers choose one seller over another. The information obtained from this collection of buyers is useful in how the marketing process is conducted. Marketing could also be described as dependent upon obtaining accurate information from the market so that the seller can correctly

communicate with the buyers. In the marketing of a profession, however, it is essential that marketing information is ethically presented.

Branding the Practice

One of the first marketing decisions that must be made when presenting an audiology practice to the collection of buyers is how it will be branded. Since branding is the key to the image presented to patients, it must be considered the first component of any marketing exercise.

The benefits of any product or service are communicated to potential customers by its brand. Every offering, from cleaning supplies to luxury cars, has a brand. There is just no escaping a brand.

In basic terms, the practice's brand is what people think of when the topic of hearing aids or hearing loss or any hearing or balance-related problem enters their mind. The moment the practice product or service is branded in a consumer's mind, it begins to exist as something that can be sold, typically at a higher price point than any generic alternative. (That is why more expensive items have a well-known brand associated with them and their generic equivalent—if there is one—is sold at a lesser price.) There are several factors in the modern world that make it extremely difficult to maintain the mystique associated with a premium brand.

In the hearing care industry, branding has evolved considerably over time. The following will review how much branding in audiology has changed over the past two decades. By most accounts, 2004 doesn't seem like a long time ago. The Internet, laptop computers, even smartphones were around then. Ironically, due to the rapid convergence of these technologies, there are some monumental changes in how audiologists acquire customers. Although there are many products and services that could be discussed in the branding of an audiology practice, hearing devices are currently the largest revenue source for audiology clinics, and thus, it makes sense to look at these products for this branding discussion.

To appreciate these changes, it is necessary to revisit the year 2004 and examine something that could be called the hearing aid value chain, which is a process by which hearing aids are manufactured, distributed, and resold to the end user. Manufacturers produced hearing devices and sold them to retail clinical providers. These retail clinical providers added an essential service component and resold the devices to their customers. The important point is that the end customer, the patient with hearing loss, does not have any direct contact with the manufacturer

of the device. The patient, even if they wanted to know, had no way to learn about the inner workings of the device supplier. The person with hearing loss was completely dependent on learning about hearing aids through their interaction with the audiologist.

Over the past 20 years, due to the myriad of changes in the marketplace, manufacturers have slowly unveiled the curtain; the inner workings of the manufacturing and distribution process are no longer shrouded in mystery as consumers (patients) have the capability of acquiring hearing aids directly from manufacturers. Today, through interactive websites and consumer advocacy reviews on social media, consumers have insight into the interworkings of the manufacturing process. Today's consumers can learn about the various hearing aid models and components used and can comparison shop using websites that the hearing aid device manufacturers have created and even through their facilities, such as Hearing Life or Connect Hearing. Additionally, customers can explore and purchase alternative technology options, such as over-the-counter hearing aids and personal sound amplification products (PSAPs) by going direct to the manufacturer's website. This abundance of product information from multiple sources changes the way in which independent providers need to brand their practice. Instead of focusing on the hearing aid as the driver of the brand, providers must now make their service and other unique audiological offerings the center of their brand.

Taken one step further, a few decades ago, consumers had limited information available to them prior to making a buying decision. Then, it was relatively easy to build a well-known brand through a few referral sources or minimal advertising. Branding was simply a part of the overall communications strategy. All a business had to do was create a logo image and brand "personality" to gain traction with consumers in the market. Prior to the information age, which arguably began about 2004, companies could methodically build their reputations and enjoy the spoils of this status for many years without the risk of a few saboteurs causing harm to their brand. Today, in this hyperconnected world, a few saboteurs, those few individuals who may have had a negative experience or interaction with a particular practice, are much more likely to cause irrevocable harm. For audiologists, this means that the process of building and maintaining a brand is ongoing. Audiologists must remain vigilant at all times of their brand reputation. Brand reputation, of course, is the overall perception that the public has of a company. This brand is shaped by a variety of factors, including the people and personality of the clerical and professional staff, products or professional services, customer service, marketing, and digital and social media presence. A good brand reputation can lead to increased sales, customer loyalty, and investor confidence.

Brand Reputation and Brand Promises

The brand presented to the market is what distinguishes one practice from another. Each day, brand promises are made to prospective patients. These promises are made through literature, signage, airwaves, print advertising, websites, social media, direct mail, and other means of communication. While prom-

ises are certainly easy to make, the key to winning new patients and keeping existing clientele loyal to the practice is the delivery of those promises. Promise delivery is exhibited through the practice by the attitude of the professional team as well as the products and services that accompany them. This connection between promises and their delivery is what leads the consumer to choose a particular practice or clinician from the crowd. A marketing program should distinguish the audiology practice (as a brand) from the other practices (other brands) with a primary goal of standing out from all other viable local, state, national, and worldwide options. For consumers to choose one specific practice over another involves "branding the practice" with a marketing campaign that establishes the practice as *the place* for them to receive hearing care.

D'Alessandro (2001), in his classic description of branding, presents that a brand is whatever the consumer thinks of when they see or hear a company's name. For example, what comes to mind when thinking of Mercedes-Benz, BMW, Apple, Hewlett-Packard, or Harley-Davidson? Some of the best products worldwide have built strong brands so that in consumers' minds, the thought is immediately of quality, image, reliability, and customer service. Audiology practitioners build their brand *every time* they see a patient, report back to a physician, present a market offering, participate in a public relations activity, or simply interact with the community. Branding a practice has very tangible rewards as people in general will happily pay more for a known brand than a generic alternative. Consider personal shopping habits. The consumer could save substantially by buying generic cola, beer, paper towels, wine, laundry detergent, and so on; however, most do not purchase these generic brands as they are unknown for quality, reliability, and general value for the money. Audiology consumers, either consciously or unconsciously, assume that the name brand is better. By creating a value-added brand, it will make the big-box stores, the Internet, manufacturers' clinics, insurance clinics, and other, less costly brands, less important, and often not considered.

Six Reasons for Developing a Solid Brand

Across the marketing literature, there are six basic reasons for developing a solid brand for the market. These are especially true in the market of 2024, where competitors are not just local but from everywhere in the world:

1. *People prefer to buy brands because they reduce perceived risk.* Consumers know that advertisers invest a lot of money in building their brands and hence have a lot to lose if they offer substandard products or services. Therefore, although patients (especially Baby Boomers) may be willing to try a new brand, they are more likely to stay with a brand if their experience has been positive.

2. *People buy brands for status.* Often consumers will spend more for a product because it is more expensive. Consider brands such as BMW, Mercedes, Rolex, or others. It is a special place to be if an audiology practice is considered the highest-level brand in the marketplace where consumers are willing to pay more for the status of being a patient in the preferred clinic.

3. *People refer to more often and more passionately a brand they like and trust.* A truly great brand will achieve near cult-level loyalty from patients to the point where consumers identify with their brands. Harley-Davidson is not just a motorcycle. Ferrari is not just a car and Audiology Associates is not just a hearing aid place. It is possible that good practice branding could lead to loyal patients if they considered an audiology clinic as a provider of not just hearing aids but improved hearing and quality of life.

4. *Practice branding builds and accelerates a practice reputation.* A brand must be molded and shaped by the patient's experience in the clinic. These experiences must be built into the branding of the practice by being consistent.

5. *Practice branding attracts the right type of patient.* Branding assists in attracting the desired type of patients to the practice. If the practice specializes in pediatric, auditory processing, balance, tinnitus, or hearing aid patients, branding will assist in appealing to the exact audience of interest.

6. *Practice branding offers a competitive advantage.* In the highly competitive 2024 market, a practice needs to stand out in a positive and highly distinctive way. Practice and providers are continuously being compared to all others in the marketplace via social media and review sites and

elsewhere. Therefore, identifying the practice's specific target market is one of the main factors to consider for branding in order to gain a competitive advantage. Note, however, that effective branding encompasses the entire experience and relationship that patients have with the entire team. When the practice communicates what makes it a special experience, expectations are set. It becomes a direct or implied promise that the patient will receive the benefit and that unexpected value, which will be anticipated upon each clinic visit.

Building a Unique and Powerful Brand

There are nine components in building a brand for a hearing care practice that are outlined in Figure 12–5. These are the essential components of a brand and are as follows:

■ *The Vision or Unique Selling Proposition (USP).* This component can be thought of as the vision the owner/manager sees as the personality of the company, communicated through an identifying mark, logo, name, tagline, voice, and tone.
■ *The Meaning.* The meaning describes the vision and USP for the company. The statement should portray the uniqueness of the practice and what sets the practice or professional apart from the competition. For Harley-Davidson, it is the consumer experience of becoming

part of a culture, not just a motorcycle. For BMW, it is the "Ultimate Driving Machine," not just a car. For Audiology Associates, it is not just a hearing aid, it is "Better Hearing for a Better Life." The USP is the one thing patients remember about a particular audiology practice among the 3,000 or so commercial marketing messages they receive every day.
■ *Coherence.* Refers to the consistency of the message communicated to the marketplace and the consistency in the fulfillment of the brand's promise each time it is accessed.
■ *Durability.* This relates to long-term strength or stability of the brand promise. Does this brand still meet the expectations that have been built during previous experiences? Is it still offering an unexpected experience for personal attention, expertise, costs, and other benefits the same as the last time the brand was accessed?
■ *Value.* Standing out from the competition by building a reputation for honoring the practice's core values can be very powerful. In today's market, consumers prefer to do business with brands that share their values, so the representation of your company to the patients' needs to be a clinician that can identify with the target audience.
■ *Commitment.* Commitment to the brand is brand loyalty, Thus, it is imperative that the USP statement reflects the patient experience in the practice.
■ *Flexibility.* Flexibility helps a brand stay relevant and engaging in a dynamic and diverse market. It also

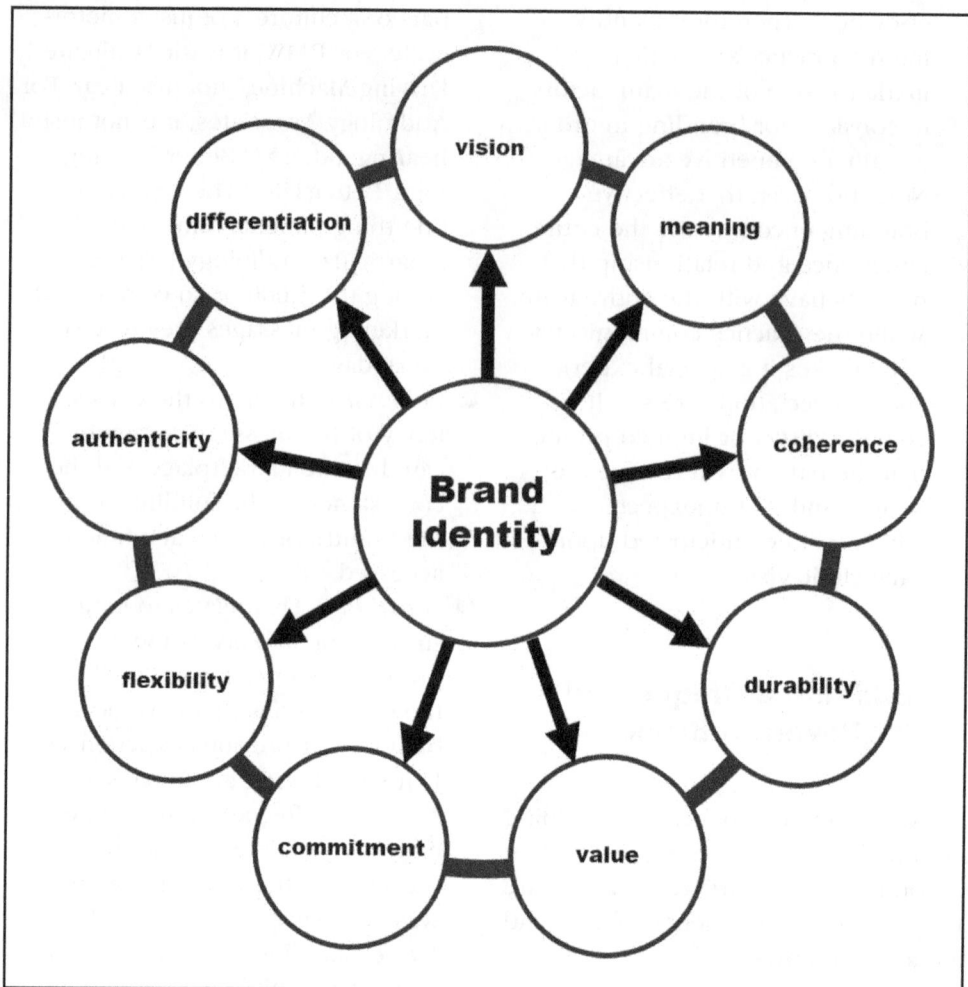

Figure 12–5. Components of brand identity for hearing care practice.

assists in a brand's expression, its creativity, and innovation.

- *Authenticity.* Brand authenticity refers to the degree to which a brand's marketing and messaging align with the reality of its products, values, and actions. An authentic brand is transparent, consistent, and genuine in its communication and behavior, which helps build trust and loyalty with customers.

- *Differentiation.* Brand differentiation is the process of distinguishing the practice's brand from the brand of competitors by emphasizing the unique aspects, attributes, or benefits the brand, service, or product offers. It is a critical component of the branding process as patients are often faced with multiple choices.

Positioning the Practice in the Marketplace

Positioning is the unique competitive advantage that influences the desired audience to view a practice and its professionals as the best choice. There are, however, ground rules in positioning that must be followed if the practice is to be successful. Positioning must be:

- True (what is claimed must be valid).
- Differentiating (present the practice with emphasis on distinctive features).
- Memorable (present an unforgettable market offering).
- Compelling (know the intended target audience and the tactics to be persuasive).

There is a difference between practice branding and positioning. The practice brand is the sum of experiences patients have with the practice, which is larger than the positioning statement alone. Positioning is a logical argument for the practice, while the practice brand is the emotional response and image being established.

Building the Patient Experience

As will be reviewed later, everything about the practice must tie together. This includes how the phone is answered, how long patients wait, the atmosphere, how the clinician and staff are dressed, the technology, manner of the clinical experience, location, signage, the building, furniture, color of the walls, and much more. All of these issues contribute to the shaping of the experience. Carbone (2004, 2016) indicates that offering products or services alone is no longer enough. Practices must provide their customers with a superb experience and orchestrate all "clues" that patients convey in the buying process into a personal interaction that results in a sale as well as patient loyalty. Carbone describes a process that is basic to any type of business but has specific applications to marketing an audiology practice as well as providing practice differentiation (Chapter 4). There are three types of clues that providers present to patients. Every time the person comes to the clinic, they are evaluating clues in each of these areas.

Carbone calls those that subscribe to these clues as "clued in" (Figure 12–6). These clues are:

- *Functional Clues.* These are obvious and rational patient perceptions of the staff, professionals, and all contacts before, during, and after the visit. These clues are the patient's perception of the functionality of the goods and services provided. In Carbone's example, he offers that patients will be evaluating issues such as the detail of the hearing evaluation, professionalism, expertise, and considering if they like the people in the clinic.
- *Mechanic Clues.* These are obvious clues from the patient's environment, such as sights, sounds, smells, and textures. Mechanic clues may also include the cleanliness of the clinic, rips in waiting room chairs, frayed carpets, lightbulbs that are out, and other maintenance concerns that the patient will draw

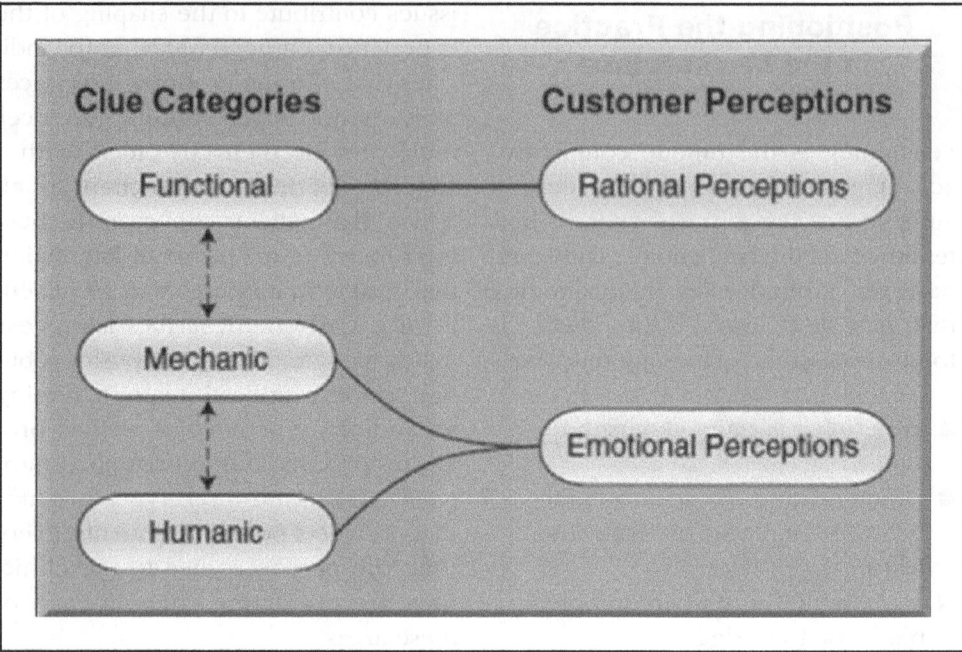

Figure 12–6. Carbone's "clued in" categories (Carbone, 2004, 2016). *Source:* Traynor (2019).

conclusions from of how the practice will take care of them based on the condition of the clinic.

- *Humanic Clues.* These are emotional clues from people, such as the loudness and tone of voice, body language, enthusiasm, gestures, and so on. Other humanic clues that patients take away from a clinic visit can also be:
  - The reception process.
  - The amount of paperwork.
  - Waiting time to see the audiologist.
  - The amount and quality of time spent with the clinician.
  - The details of the evaluation and counseling.
  - The fitting techniques, the exit, and follow-up.

Other well-known critical components of brand building include:

- *It starts with the patient's value system.* Audiologists (the sellers) are likely to think in terms of equipment (technical sophistication, hardware) or clinical quality (skill level, education/training, peer reputation), but the patients (the buyers) value service (access, amenities, ease of scheduling) and value-added items (product or service differentiation). Effective branding communicates to the tastes, attitudes, and sensibilities of the buyer, not the seller. The wants and needs of the patient (the buyer) are mainly rooted in results: better hearing, self-esteem, improved communication, and perhaps confidence in good interactive skills. Patients purchase benefits of the clinic or its products, not merely the features.

■ *Identification of a value-added edge over the competition.* Pinpoint what is highly unique about the practice that equates to value to the patient over and above the competition. Use this as the centerpiece for positioning the practice.

■ *The willingness to offend someone.* The practice position must be unique; however, it is impossible to be able to apply this to everyone. The challenge will be to appeal to many while recognizing that the positioning cannot be universal. Being everything to everyone is not unique; it's "stuck in the middle" (Chapter 4).

■ *The ability to deliver a consistent patient experience.* Patients expect a consistent high-quality experience with no surprises. It takes only a few negative occurrences to totally rupture brand credibility and betray the trust that has been so difficult to build.

■ *Being consistent in the delivery of branded communications.* In addition to delivering consistent in-office experiences, the practice manager must effectively communicate the brand message at every marketing opportunity.

Part of the patient experience is the office environment, location, and atmosphere. Marsh (2012) states that in today's audiology clinic, even the smell of the office can be part of the clinic's brand. Since purchase rates and satisfaction ratings are connected, negative in-office experiences can lead to a loss of 10% to 30% of a clinic's business and create negative branding within the community.

Professional and Product Types of Competition

To better understand the clinical competition within the marketplace, it is useful to understand the types of clinicians and how they stand up against today's audiologists. The following is an adaptation of D'Alessandro's (2001) four types of competition confronting audiology practices:

Brand Competition

This category represents all AuD audiologists offering hearing care in the same market area. These competitors are "branded" with the AuD and to consumers appear to be exactly alike. In the consumer's mind, without proper market offerings to differentiate a specific clinic from other hearing care offerings in the area, patients would presume that the same products and services could be obtained from any AuD branded professional. Thus, it is not enough to brand the credential; branding of the clinic and the individual audiologist is fundamental to success.

Industry Competition

This type encompasses all doctoral-level competitors offering hearing care to consumers other than those with the AuD. Pertaining to the field of audiology, this would include doctoral-level audiologists with a PhD, EdD, or ScD and physicians. While the AuD brands the clinicians, to consumers, these individuals are "doctors" also and appear to be the same in their capability to provide products and services to the hearing impaired. Prior to the AuD, this was the designation for the doctoral-level tier of the profession. Over the years, these doctoral-level individuals are being replaced by those that hold the AuD clinical credential. Although MDs will most likely be otolaryngologists focused on medical-surgical treatment of the audiovestibular system and the initial professional the consumer considers for hearing loss, tinnitus, or disequilibrium issues, they refer out for aural rehabilitative treatment those living with hearing loss, tinnitus, or disequilibrium issues. Therefore, regardless of the hearing care industry competition, it is essential in order to obtain those referrals to develop a unique branding of the clinic to stand out as the facility or audiology professional to be chosen.

Form Competition

These are all those remaining competitors that provide hearing care. This category would include master's degree audiologists, hearing aid dealers, drug stores, big-box stores (Walmart, Costco, Sam's Club), Internet offerings, insurance company or managed care offerings, over-the-counter hearing aids, personal sound amplifiers, or other establishments that offer hearing care and/or sell similar products. Form competitors are those where considerable diversity in products, services, and capability may exist in their ability to serve patients. Branding a practice with a tasteful and ethical market effort that presents the type of hearing care offered by an AuD can often provide the differentiation of hearing care providers desperately needed by consumers.

Generic Competition

All products that cost the same as hearing care are also a competitor. In this instance, patients weigh the costs of hearing care against other (possibly more desirable) recreational activities such as cars, vacations, cruises, appliances, or, on the service side, office visits, physical therapy, eye exams, dental reconstruction, and so forth. It can even be a choice between hearing care and life-sustaining medications. This is simply an application of the basic economic principle of "opportunity cost" (Chapters 1 and 11). This suggests that there is only a finite amount of funds and if the funds are utilized to purchase an item, then those funds are not available to use for another purpose. It is a simple fact that the prescription products sold in audiology practices, especially hearing instruments, are expensive for most patients and compete for attention with other products and services of similar value.

While marketing is what builds a particular brand of audiology in the consumers' minds, D'Alessandro (2001) indicates that it is not easy to build a great brand. He classically states that it takes an artistic sense of proportion and timing as well as a ruthless willingness to distinguish oneself from competing brands.

Branding Principles

When it comes to establishing and maintaining a brand, the bottom line is that a practice can never coast on past performance. Because independent audiology practices do not have economies of scale, they are especially vulnerable to a lack of brand identity. (Think about what is known about a chain restaurant compared to what you know and expect about a small mom-and-pop diner—you are much more likely to read reviews on Yelp before visiting a local independent restaurant than, say, buying dinner at Applebee's.) Here are four specific tactics that ensure small audiology practices are part of the conversation when a customer is deciding to make an appointment:

■ Given the importance of other people's opinions in the buying process, the clinic owner/manager must take the time to ensure three distinct members of their community (existing patients, other small businesses/service clubs, and primary care physicians) have a firm understanding of the business's value proposition and these three groups enthusiastically "toot your horn" when asked about better hearing and communication.

■ Make it easy for customers to comparison shop. Provide a link, preferably to an independent source, where customers can do some comparison shopping from the comforts of home. This comparison shopping should not be confined to devices. Providers are encouraged to have a presence of websites that allow customers to read reviews from others on the quality of service and attention they received.

■ Provide a memorable patient experience that is not centered on the device (Chapter 20). When the device is the center of attention, it is easy for consumers to compare. However, when the core focus becomes offering aural rehabilitation and other services that lead to patient behavior changes, the atten-

tion has successfully moved away from the device as the center of the transaction.

■ Decouple the fee for services from the products dispensed. Make it easier for patients to comparison shop by associating a specific price for services that may be different or unique to the practice. Take the time to devise high-value service packages that are unique to the practice.

■ The convergence of social media, Wi-Fi, and smartphones requires independent practitioners to rethink their marketing strategy and brand identity. It is no longer about running consistent advertising in the local newspaper. Independent practices would be wise to create and maintain their own memorable, high-quality brand.

Diffusion of Innovations (DI)

Another general theory of marketing deals with the diffusion of innovations (DI) originally offered by Rogers (2003). Still valid today, DI offers a perspective into how populations adopt new ideas and technologies. The DI five levels of adopting new technologies are presented in Figure 12–7 and listed below:

■ Innovators—2.5%—Venturesome
■ Early Adopters—13.5%—Respect
■ Early Majority—34%—Deliberate
■ Late Majority—34%—Skeptical
■ Laggards—16%—Traditional

When a technology is brand new, Rogers (2003) describes how a new idea or technology progresses from brand new

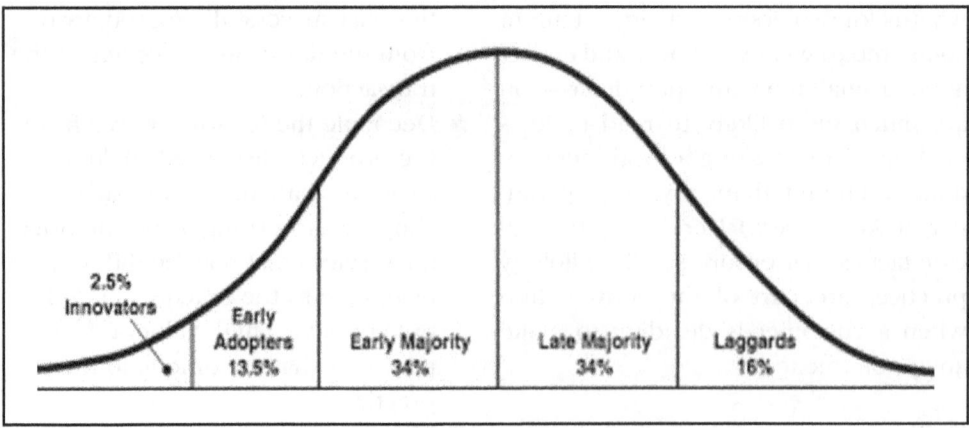

Figure 12–7. Diffusion of innovation. *Source:* Rogers (2003). *Diffusion of innovation.*

and used by no one to the mainstream. The five categories and the types of individuals who are usually part of each of these categories are described below:

Innovators—Venturesome

Innovators are venturesome and the very first to try the new technology. Reviewing and trying new technologies first is almost an obsession with these individuals, and thus they will be part of the first 2.5% of a social system to be involved with these concepts or devices. Innovators are the quickest to adopt an innovation, but they may be seen as fickle by other community members and are less likely to be trusted and copied. According to Rodgers, an innovator requires some prerequisites such as they:

■ Need to have access to financial resources for trial and error of new technologies.
■ Have the ability to understand and apply certain complex technical knowledge.

■ Are able to cope with a high degree of uncertainty for an innovation they adopt.

Early Adopters—Respect

The next level comprises 13.5% of a population identified as *early adopters*. These early adopters respect the concepts and innovations in a new idea and are generally thought to be the main portion of a social system that stimulates the critical mass into adopting the new idea. They are considered more mainstream within the social system than the innovators and are characterized by acceptance of innovation, as well as having the financial resources to be able to adopt the innovation. This group is considered by their peers as "the individuals to check with before adopting an innovation." As a respected member of their community, early adopters put their stamp of approval on a new idea, and thus others will consider the new idea seriously. Characteristics of an early adopter:

■ They conduct research on the various new technologies and make judicious yet innovative decisions on ideas and technologies that will allow them stand out.

■ To their peer group and interpersonal networks, they decrease uncertainty about new ideas and technologies by conveying their subjective opinions.

Early Majority—Deliberate

While the *early majority* component of the adoption process (the next 34%) adopt ideas and technologies just before the average member of the community, they are amenable to change and persuaded of the benefits offered from the innovation by observing. These individuals provide links to others that exponentially cause others to adopt. Early majority adopters are those that:

■ Seldom hold opinion leadership positions in their peer group or interpersonal network.

■ Early majority individuals tend to deliberate for some time before completely adopting the new idea or technology.

■ They have a deliberate willingness to adopt new innovations but seldom lead.

Late Majority—Skeptical

The *late majority* make up another 34% of a population. These adopters within the social system are skeptical and adopt new innovations after the average member of the group of adopters. It may be an economic necessity (such as a competitor using the innovation) or due to peer pressure as to why they have decided to adopt the new ideas. Late majority adopters are those that:

■ May have economic reasons for not adopting earlier.

■ Need peer pressure to motivate them into adoption.

■ Require that most of their uncertainty about a new idea or technology must be removed before they feel it is safe to adopt.

Laggards—Traditional

According to Rodgers (2003), *Laggards* are the last 16% to adopt an innovation within a social system. Rodgers indicates that these individuals are the near isolates in the social networks of their system. Generally, laggards tend to have these characteristics:

■ Laggards tend to be suspicious of new ideas and technologies.

■ They have no opinion leadership.

■ Peer pressure is necessary to motivate their adoption.

■ This group may never consider the innovation.

■ This category may have some economic concerns about adopting the new innovations.

Marketing Plans

A good marketer will communicate their brand to the market and receive feedback that can be used to stimulate demand for products and services. Planning a successful marketing program involves conducting marketing research to know how, when, and where to wisely expend that hard-earned marketing budget. A marketing plan is highly detailed, heavily researched, and written so that many inside and some outside the practice will be able to understand the concepts. Although there is no one format for the marketing plan, it is an exercise that essentially forces the practitioner to look internally into the practice. The box below offers a sample marketing plan for an independent audiology practice. As with business plans, marketing plans can be a key component in obtaining funds to pursue expansions, equipment, or other operational modifications but are gen-erally pursued for any of the following reasons:

- The plan is required as part of the yearly budget planning process.
- The plan is required for a specialized strategy to introduce new products, enter new markets, generate a new strategy to fix an existing problem, and other issues.
- The plan is a component within an overall business plan, such as a new business proposal for an existing practice to the financial community.

Marketing research is usually conducted for three distinct purposes: plan-

---

Marketing Plan

Based on business goals, marketing mission, and marketing strategy.

Goal: Increase annual hearing aid gross sales from $ to $$.

- *Assumption:* The clinic's convenient hours and exemplary professional services increase the likelihood of patient satisfaction over our competitors.
- *Assumption:* The clinic's satisfied hearing aid users will help increase our sales through positive word-of-mouth promotion and repeat sales.
- *Assumption:* Aural rehabilitation training increases user satisfaction with their hearing aids.

Objective:

Increase participation in the Aural Rehabilitation Workshop (ARW) by adding three new attendees each month for the next 12 months beginning January 1, 20XX.

continued on next page

continued from previous page

- *Tactic:* Use direct mail, personal contact, and affiliation with key referral sources to promote the ARW offered at a monthly evening program at ABC Audiology. The target market is all patients experiencing communication difficulties despite hearing aid use regardless of where they received their amplification and their significant others.
- *Action:* John's marketing company will develop an informational direct mail piece to be distributed quarterly to the target market of adults over age 70 in the target market area.
- *Action:* The clinic's front desk staff will call patients who scored 2 or lower on the Hearing Satisfaction Survey at their annual evaluation and invite them to participate in the ARW.
- *Action:* Audiology will contact the local HLAA chapter monthly, in person or by written communication, to inform/remind leaders of the ARW and provide copies of the informational direct mail piece for dissemination to their club members.
- *Action:* Front desk staff will keep a count of ARW attendees monthly and compare numbers to those obtained the year prior.

Objective:

Increase the annual number of word-of-mouth referrals as identified by new patient listing a "referred by" name on the initial intake sheet, from 113 identified in 20XX to 150 in 20XX beginning January 1, 20XX.

- *Tactic:* Use multimedia avenues and staff call to action to describe and promote the Patient Referral Program to existing patients, significant other support persons, family, and friends.
- *Action:* Have a marketing company develop a standard column for inclusion in the newsletters, describing the PRP program prior to the January publication.
- *Action:* Audiology and staff will remind patients of the PRP and ask them to make a referral if they have been satisfied with the clinic's services. This will be tracked by initialed designation on the patient visit checklist. This will be tracked for KPI goals.
- *Action:* The clinic's front desk staff will illicit response for "referred by:" on the New Patient Intake Form. This will be tracked for KPI goals.
- *Action:* Front desk staff will post information and benefits of PRP on Facebook once a month for 12 months beginning January 20XX.

ning, problem-solving, and control. Control-oriented marketing research assists the practice manager in the isolation of trouble spots within the practice and promotes knowledge of how the clinic is performing. Kotler and Keller (2016) define market research as the systematic design, collection, analysis, and reporting of data relevant to a specific marketing situation facing an organization. Clinics use marketing research in a variety of situations. For example, marketing research offers insights into patient motivations, purchasing behavior, and satisfaction. It can assist in the assessment of market potential and market share, as well as measure the effectiveness of pricing of product (Chapter 13), distribution, and promotional activities.

Market research is typically used for planning and deals largely with determining which market opportunities are viable for the practice. When a viable opportunity is uncovered, research can provide an estimate of the size and scope of the opportunity so it can be better managed. The use of market research for problem-solving focuses on making short and long-term decisions relative to the mixture of market communications to be used in presenting and branding the practice to the community. For example, one of the major problems for some audiology practices can be the rise and fall of demand for products and services. The example presented in Figure 12–8 summarizes the problem that a practice may have with the seasonal demands for products and services.

Although the demand for hearing aids and other audiological services varies by the part of the country in which they are offered, Figure 12–8 indicates that

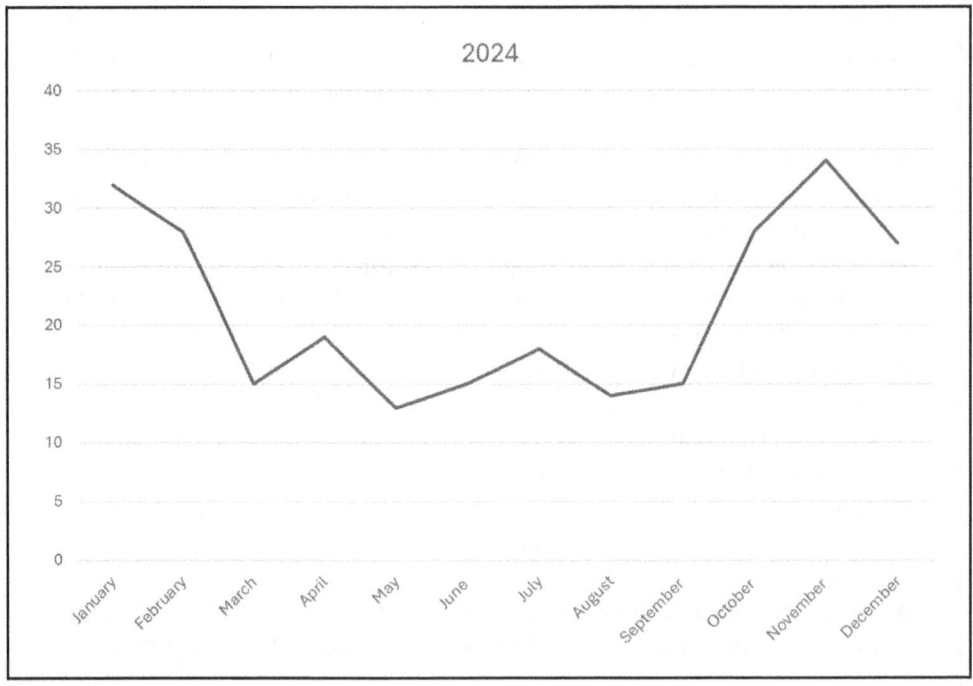

Figure 12–8. Hearing aid units sold by month.

for this example, there is more demand early or late in the year with a downturn in hearing aid units sold during the summer. Since the product demand changes throughout the year, it must be stimulated at certain times of the year by an organized marketing plan that is based upon sound market research. This pattern of demand, or demand analysis, suggests that the marketing plan requires more funds when the demand is low (midyear) and less funding when demand is high (October to January).

A demand analysis can be conducted for all products and services offered in the clinic, including hearing aids, routine audiometric evaluations, OAEs, ABRs, VNGs, operative monitoring, and ALDs as well as small accessories. Since marketing is an expensive process, successful practices spend their valuable funds presenting their brand of audiology to the community based upon their demand predictions and market research.

Market Segmentation

In the business world, the answers to many marketing questions are obtained using a concept called market segmentation. Market segmentation is the process of defining and subdividing a large homogeneous market into clearly identifiable segments having similar needs, wants, or demand characteristics. Its objective is to design a mixture of market offerings that precisely match the expectations of consumers (patients) in the targeted segment. Few practices are large enough to supply the needs of the entire consumer spectrum; therefore, a practice must break down the total demand for products and services into segments that can best be handled. Successful market segmentation involves four basic factors:

- A clear identification of the segment of the market to be approached.
- A measure of the segment's effective size.
- The accessibility of the segment through promotional efforts.
- The appropriateness of the market segmentation in relation to the policies and resources of the practice.

Market segments are broken down into major components:

- Geographic.
- Demographic.
- Psychographic.
- Behavioral.

These general categories of market segmentation should be further delineated and are often combined to identify specific target populations that are the most likely candidates for the market offering.

Geographic Market Segmentation

Geographic segmentation can be reduced from a large area, such as a state, to a region, a city, or a neighborhood or subdivided for seasonal offerings for various geographical settings, such as festivals, to offset the rise and fall of product or service demands. One of the first considerations is a geographic segmentation where the market is divided into segments relative to where the patients reside.

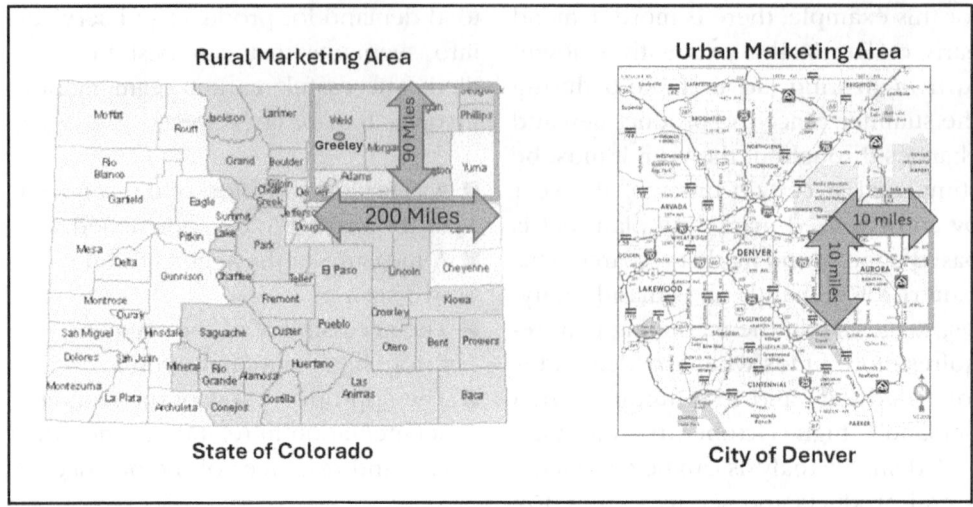

Figure 12–9. Rural and urban geographic marketing areas.

As seen in Figure 12–9, market areas can be quite different. To obtain the same number of responses to a rural market compared to an urban offering, the geographic area will need to be substantially larger, simply based upon the population differences between the two areas. Another geographic difference might be the culture of the rural community versus the urban community. For example, it might be that there would be a higher number of noise-induced losses in the rural areas than in the urban areas due to the use of farm equipment. Often relating a cultural issue with a geographic placement can increase the response to a market offering.

Demographic Market Segmentation

Demographic segmentation is a large category often utilized to target the product or service offering to different individuals within the market. These categories identify specific sectors of the market by age, income, race, family size, occupation, generation, family life cycle, education, nationality, religion, gender, and social class (Figure 12–10). For example, the demographic target market for an audiology practice that offers hearing aids is usually individuals above age 60, middle to upper incomes, any race, one or two in the family, retired or employed person, any occupation, without children at home, of any education level, any nationality, any religion, or gender from any socio-economic classification.

In 2024 and beyond, the generational focus demographic for marketing audiology products and services within a private practice includes *Baby Boomers and Generation X*. To most who are just beginning to learn marketing, the question becomes: Who are these people and where are they within the generation code used to describe the various age groups? To understand these generations and the interest in them from a business standpoint, they must be totally understood (Figure 12–11). Although these populations are discussed in Chapter 20, it is important to eval-

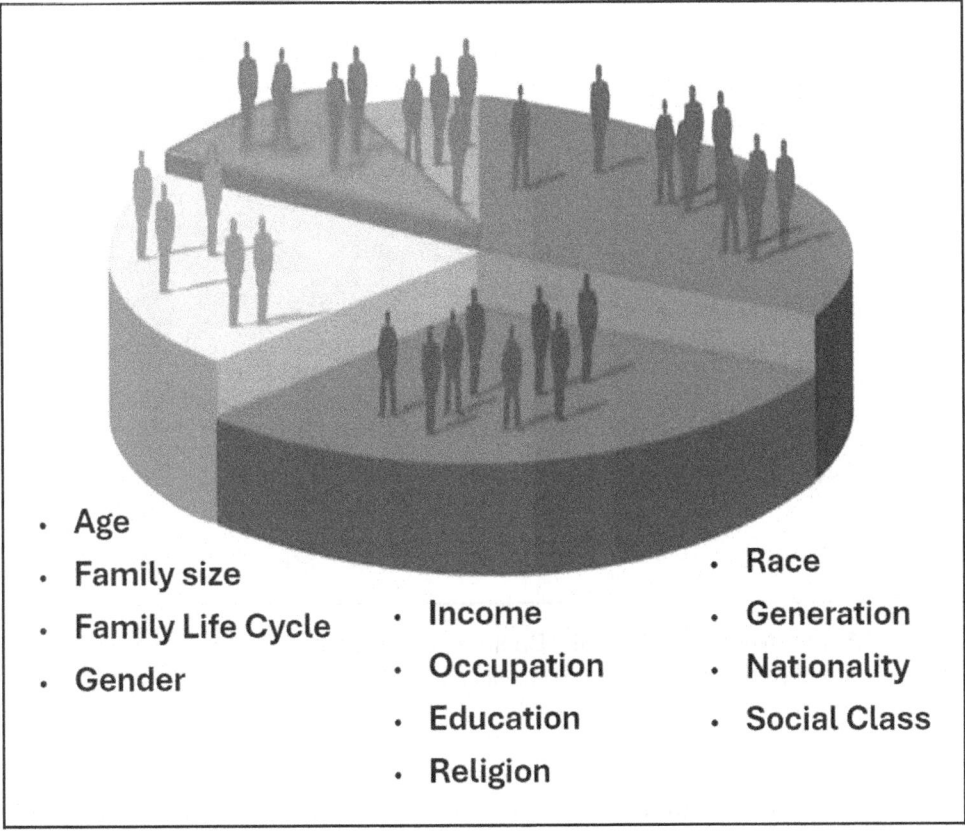

- Age
- Family size
- Family Life Cycle
- Gender

- Income
- Occupation
- Education
- Religion

- Race
- Generation
- Nationality
- Social Class

Figure 12–10. Demographic market segmentation.

uate each segment from a marketing perspective.

Baby Boomers

Baby Boomers are a group of individuals who emerged after the end of World War II, when birth rates around the world spiked. The explosion of new infants became known as the baby boom. During the boom, 76 million babies were born in the United States alone. PRB (2024) indicates that even though several million Baby Boomers have died in the decades since, immigration to the United States has helped replenish the supply. As of late 2019, the U.S. Census Bureau estimates (Pew Research Center, 2020) put the baby boom population at 71.6 million. Historians have concluded that the Baby Boomer phenomenon most likely involved a combination of factors:

- People wanting to start the families that they put off during World War II.
- The Great Depression of the 1930s that came before the war.
- A sense of confidence that the coming era would be peaceful and prosperous.

Clarke and Velasquez (2024) describe that the climate for Baby Boomers was formed in the late 1940s and 1950s, when generally wages increased, busi-

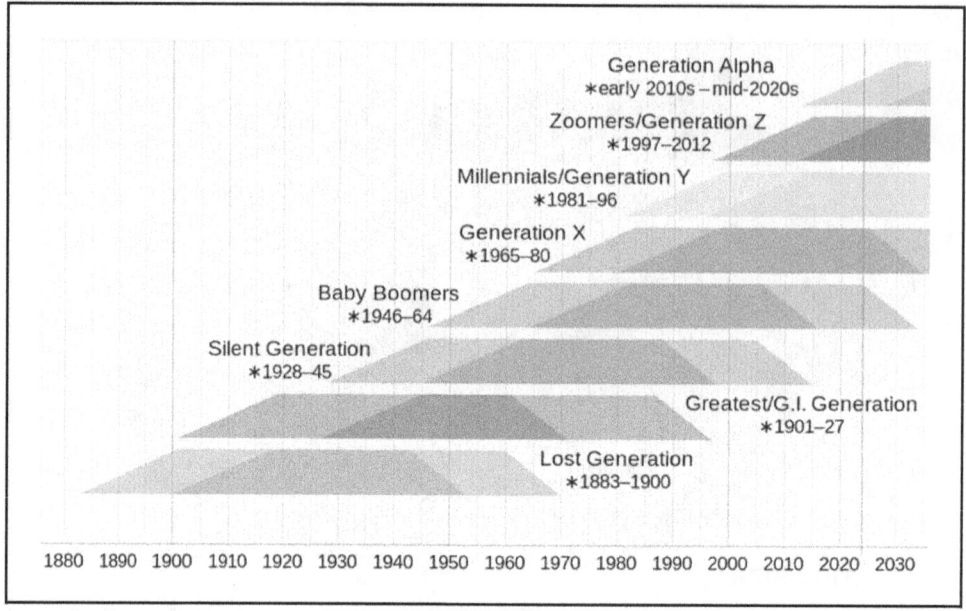

Figure 12–11. Where are the Baby Boomers and Generation X in the mix? *Source:* Cmglee (https://commons.wikimedia.org/wiki/File:Generation_timeline.svg), https://crea tivecommons.org/licenses/by-sa/4.0/legalcode

nesses were thriving, and there was an increase in the variety and quantity of products for consumers. Accompanying this new economic prosperity was a migration of young families from the cities to the suburbs. The GI Bill allowed many returning veterans to buy affordable homes in tracts around the edges of cities. This led to a suburban ethos of the ideal family consisting of the husband as the provider and the wife as a stay-at-home mom with their children. These suburban families began to use new forms of credit to purchase consumer goods such as cars, home appliances, television sets, and businesses. Businesses also targeted their children, the growing Boomer generation, with advertising and marketing efforts. As the Boomers approached adolescence, many became dissatisfied with this ethos and the consumer culture asso-

ciated with it, which fueled the youth counterculture movement of the 1960s.

As the longest-living generation in history so far, Baby Boomers are at the forefront of what has been called a longevity economy. Fengler (2021) reported that Baby Boomers spent about $8.7 trillion in 2020 on goods and services, and by 2030, these Baby Boomer expenditures are expected to increase to $15 trillion, an increase of 53.2%. These data, when combined with the known demographics for hearing loss, indicates that Baby Boomers should be the main focus of audiology clinic marketing efforts.

Generation X

The children of the Baby Boomers are Generation X, the name used to describe the generation of Americans born between 1965 and 1980, although some sources use slightly different ranges. In 2024, this puts Generation X at age 44 to 59 years (Figure 12–11). Thus, many may require audiology services currently and most will be ready to see an audiologist in the next 5 years. Some characteristics of Generation X are:

- Sometimes called Gen Xers, they grew up in a time when there were more dual-income families, single-parent households, and children of divorce than when Baby Boomers were growing up.
- Many were "latchkey kids," returning from school to an empty home while their parents were still at work.
- They were the first generation to grow up with personal computers to some extent, thus becoming tech-savvy.
- They were the first generation to grow up with cable television and MTV, the network that initially broadcast music videos 24 hours a day.
- They lived through the end of the Cold War with the fall of the Berlin Wall in 1989 and the collapse of the Soviet Union in 1991.
- They witnessed the tragic explosion of the space shuttle *Challenger* in 1986.
- They experienced shaky economic times as children and young adults, enduring the recessions of the 1970s, 1980s, and 1990s.
- They have more student loan debt than previous generations, which took its members many years and, for some, decades to pay off.
- Many were unemployed, or underemployed, and a number of Gen Xers as adults had to move back home to live with their parents.

In recent decades, they have experienced the economic fallout from the Great Recession (2007–2009) and the COVID-19 pandemic. On the whole, Generation X was likely to be the first generation whose members would not be more financially well off than their parents were. These conditions have made the Generation X individuals:

- Resourceful and independent.
- Keen on maintaining work-life balance.
- Often described as being cynical, attributed to the economic and societal tumult they experienced as children and young adults.

As compared with previous generations, members of Generation X are more ethnically diverse; some one-third of Gen Xers identify as non-White, are somewhat less likely to be involved in organized religion, and tend to be more liberal on social issues, such as same-sex marriage.

These and other characteristics make Generation X individuals different from their Baby Boomer parents but are still a market for audiology products and services. Therefore, when the Baby Boomers and Generation X are combined, the target market will be a huge but competitive market for audiology clinics.

Psychographic Market Segmentation

Psychographic segmentation refers to dividing the market up by religious beliefs, values, lifestyle, social status, activities, interests and opinions, lifestyle, personality, and other psychological criteria, presented in Figure 12–12. For

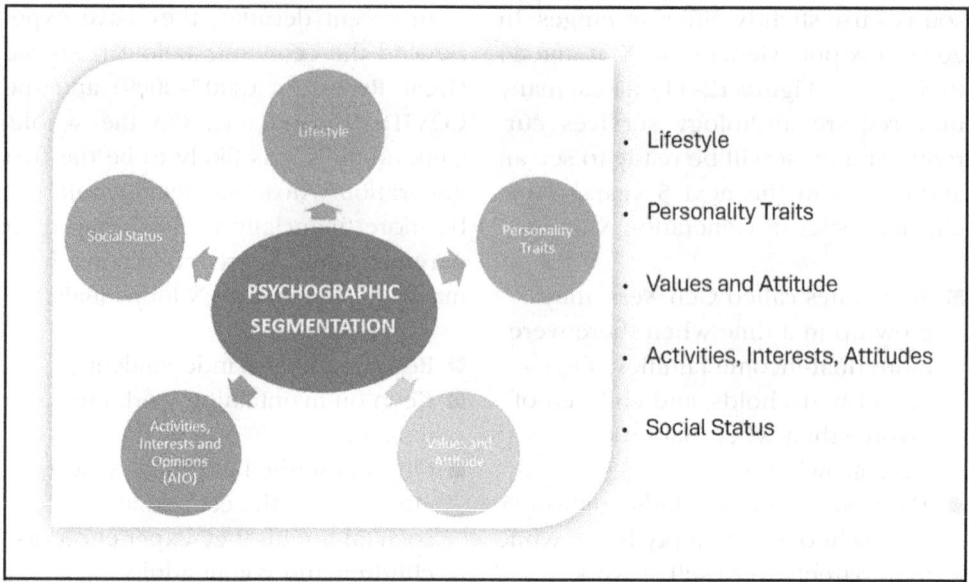

Figure 12–12. Psychographic market segmentation.

example, all those individuals at an assisted living center, musicians, or gun enthusiasts might be singled out for a specific marketing campaign targeted toward their lifestyle.

Behavioral Market Segmentation

Behavioral segmentation involves the areas of language, beliefs, priorities, values, and culture (Figure 12–13). Some communities communicate in their native language and continue their cultural customs and interactions. They are less likely to follow American culture and more likely to follow their native culture. For example, Dallas, Texas, has a Vietnamese population where they speak, interact, and do business in their native language. A similar community in Chicago is Hispanic, where Spanish is spoken more than English, and the culture is more Latin American.

They are special cultures with their own language, often with different beliefs, priorities, and values. Many of these unique population areas mandate marketing with linguistic and cultural sensitivity.

Behavioral segmentation can also involve everything from birthdays or anniversaries to involvement in special ethnic events.

In audiology practices, patients are often not at the readiness stage but later reach a certain hearing loss level that begins to affect their interactions with friends and family members, or their social life is reduced due to a hearing issue, although accessing a consumer in this stage is quite beneficial to the patients as well as for the practice. Patients who have been seen a year or so before can be targeted for access when they may be more psychologically ready for treatment. For amplification product sales, it is helpful to have segmentation within the clinic

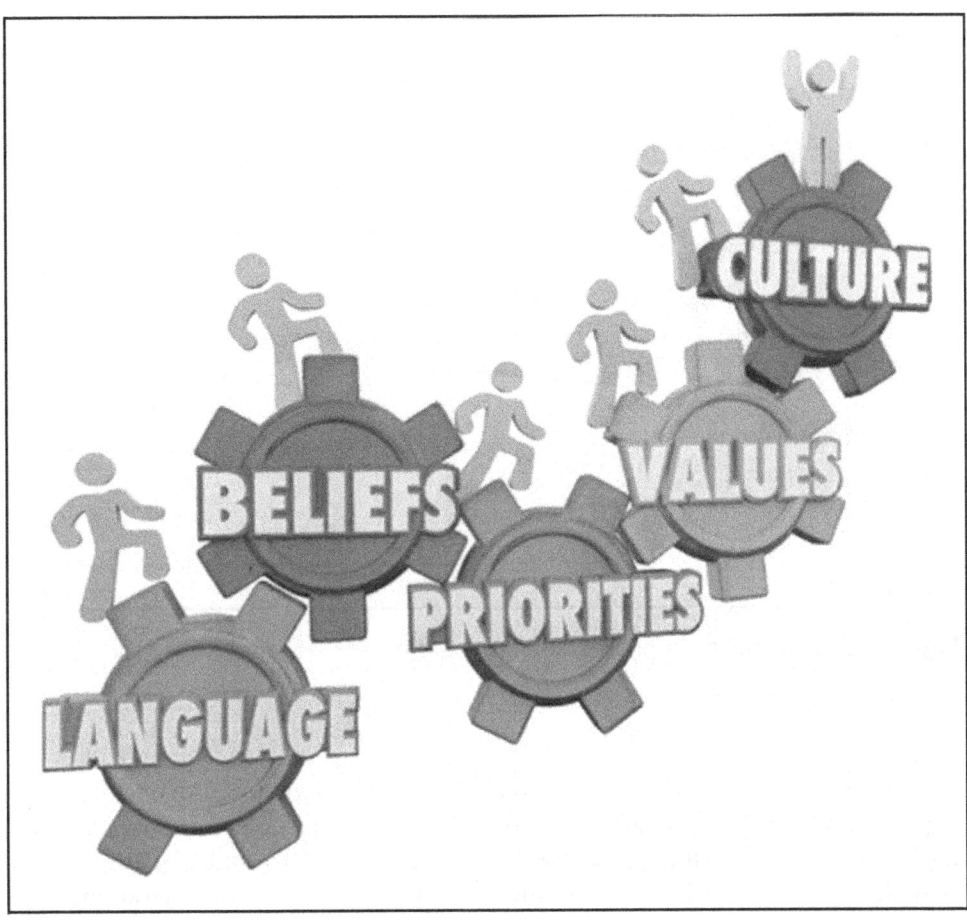

Figure 12–13. Behavioral market segmentation. *Source:* iqoncept/Depositphotos.com.

database for those patients who have been "tested, not treated" as these patients are likely to now know that they have a hearing impairment that needs attention and are likely to act given the right market offering.

Multisegmental Marketing

The real benefit of target marketing is when the general segments are further delineated and utilized together as multiattribute market segmentation. These multiattribute segmentations create a population composed of individuals who have a need and want for the products or services. Generally, the better the segmentation, the better the response to the market offering. Although it is necessary to find a portion of the segmentation that requires audiology goods and services, a common mistake is to identify too broad of a market. Thus, it is essential to be accurate in the target market segmentation as segmenting too broadly will minimize the efficiency of the marketing program while increasing costs, and too small of a market will reduce the number of individuals presented with the market offering. Figure 12–14 presents an example of ma-

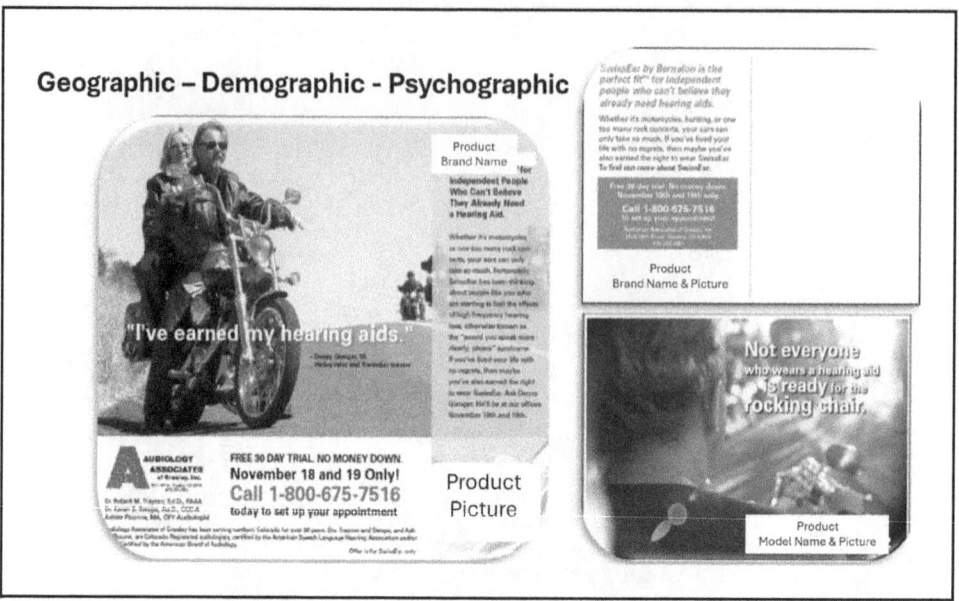

Figure 12–14. Multisegment marketing program.

terials from a successful direct mail program that was coupled with radio segments. While this was a few years ago, the message is that the same types of multisegments can be used to successfully target audiences.

This successful program used a combination of geographic, demographic, and psychographic information to target the 55-year-old and older motorcycle riders who were having difficulties hearing spouses and others. The tagline was "I earned my Hearing Loss." The radio component was a female voice that said, "Honey we have some *Bills* to pay?" and the male answer was, "I already took my *Pills* today!"

The Marketing Mix

The marketing mix is the specific combination of how the basic marketing elements are used to present the practice into a marketplace. Often called the Four Ps of marketing (McCarthy, 1960), product, price, place, and promotion are combined to make up the overall marketing plan. The marketing mix concept is presented in Figure 12–15.

Since the purpose of marketing is the creation of value for patients by presenting the benefits received from using the products and services relative to the costs incurred, patients are usually willing to make exchanges for value (usually money) when:

- The benefits of the exchange exceed their perception of the cost.
- The products and services offer a superior value compared with the alternatives.

Kotler and Keller (2016) amplify this purpose in a discussion of customer wants, needs, and demands. The most basic concept in marketing is that of human needs and, in their terms, re-

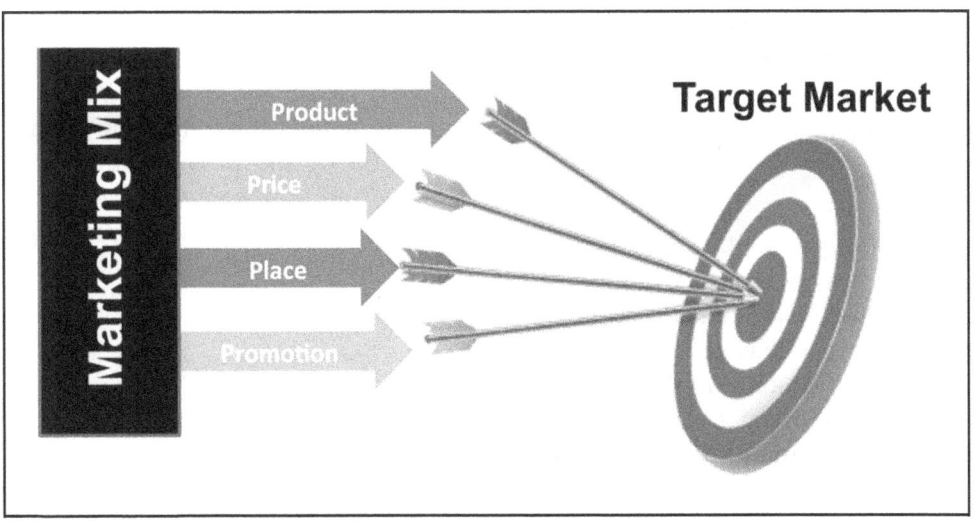

Figure 12–15. The marketing mix (McCarthy, 1960).

ferred to as states of "felt deprivation." These states include basic physical needs for food, clothing, warmth, safety, and hearing. Most audiologists realize that good hearing brings social needs for belonging and affection and provides for individuals' need for communication.

Wants are the form of human needs that take shape by the culture and individual personality. Patients *need* hearing aids, but *want* to go on a cruise, or *want* to obtain a new car. According to Kotler and Keller, wants are shaped by society and are described in terms of objects that will satisfy those wants. They feel that when these wants and needs are backed by buying power, they become demands. Given their wants/needs and resources, consumers demand products with benefits that add up to the most value and satisfaction.

Marketing managers, in their attempts to create consumer value and satisfaction, generally focus their efforts on the *Four Ps* (McCarthy, 1960), the *Product*, its *Price*, the *Place* provided,

and its *Promotion*, also called the *Marketing Mix*. These Four Ps are closely related to the four customer or patient-related variables that Lauterborn called the *Four Cs*. Beebe (2023) presents that the four Cs look at the marketing mix from the patient benefit point of view and suggests that products are *the customer solution*, price is the *customer cost*, place or *channel is the customer convenience*, and promotion is the *customer communication*. Thus, the Four Ps should be considered in light of the Four Cs to provide perspective to the marketing process. A further expansion of the Four Ps of marketing is often presented by authors in other publications, such as the 6Ps, 7Ps, and so on, but they are simply an extension and delineation of the four basics: product, price, place, and promotion.

Kotler and Keller (2016) indicate that marketers describe three characteristics of products and services that must be understood for effective marketing. These include durability, tangibility, and consumer use. Durability and tangibility include both nondurable and durable goods.

Durability and Tangibility

Nondurable goods are tangible goods normally consumed in one or a few uses, such as beer and shampoo. Kotler and Keller feel that because these goods are purchased frequently, the appropriate strategy is to make them available in many locations, charge only a small markup, and advertise heavily to induce trial and build brand loyalty and preference. This type of product would be the consumables for hearing aids, such as batteries (if any these days), possibly chargers, domes, disposable earplugs, and other consumable accessory, as well as comfort application products that go along with hearing instruments.

Durable goods are tangible goods that normally survive many uses, such as refrigerators, machine tools, and clothing. They normally require more personal selling and service, command a higher margin, and require more seller guarantees. For an audiology clinic, these products would be the hearing aids themselves and their hardware, such as earmolds. Other products could be assistive listening devices, custom earplugs, musician monitors, and so on. Since there is greater involvement in time and attention, the sale of durable goods requires a higher margin to offset the audiologist's education, research and development, and the necessary warranties.

Services

Services associated with the products are defined as intangible, inseparable, variable, and perishable products that normally require more quality control, supplier credibility, and adaptability. Thus, audiological services are highly influenced by the provider, their credentials, and how well they can adapt to human factors, disease issues, age aspects, and lifestyle variables.

Marketing Mix— The Product

Most audiology practices sell basically the same mix of products and services. They offer hearing instruments, nondurable goods in support of the hearing instruments, rehabilitative treatment, and a mix of other services, including specialized diagnostic hearing and balance assessment. Some practices offer additional items to the product mix such as cerumen management, intraoperative monitoring, cochlear implant adjustment, central auditory processing assessment, various levels of hearing conservation, and other procedures. When a consumer searches for a solution to their problem, it is the product component of the marketing mix, both goods and services, tangible and intangible, that will satisfy their needs and ultimately their demands.

Product offerings provide benefit or satisfaction to the target group, in this case audiology patients. Product mix becomes part of the practice's image and, therefore, it is important to be aware of the specific factors that will influence a consumer's choice of providers for certain audiological products. The following are some of the factors that influence the product mix:

■ Product variety.

- Quality, design, and features.
- Technology, brand name, packaging, and sizes.
- Services.
- Warranties.
- Return policy.

A hearing instrument manufacturer must have the correct technology mix in their product line to appeal to an audiology practice; however, there are peripheral factors such as packaging, utility of the fitting software, warranty, access to inside support personnel, low repair rates, quick repair turnaround time, and well-informed field representatives that are important components of the relationship (Chapter 19).

After many years of discussion among manufacturers, engineers, audiologists, government agencies, and consumer groups, with much fanfare, over-the-counter (OTC) hearing aids went on sale in late 2022 (OTC Act, 2017).

Although audiologists are mostly involved with prescription devices, it is essential that they choose two to three OTC brands to dispense as part of their product mix. This allows sales to be made to those that are not ready for prescription devices. These individuals may be offered follow-up care programs at a separate cost, another revenue-generating product offered by the clinic. Further, this process keeps these patients within the practice, and as the impairment worsens over time, they will be back to the clinic for prescription instruments. The marketing program should emphasize that the patient is purchasing the benefits of the product and the added value of the audiologist's expertise required to fit and maintain the device. This should be the emphasis for both over-the-counter and prescription products.

Marketing Mix—The Price

One of the secrets to business success is pricing products properly. A poor pricing strategy may create problems that are difficult to overcome. Nagle et al. (2011) indicate that setting correct pricing for products and services is a great challenge. It could be that pricing is one of the biggest keys to success as it has such an effect on profit. If the price is high, the number of sales is usually lower but with higher profit, while if the price is low, the number of sales is high with minimal profit. From a business standpoint, the goal is to price the product mix where the most products are sold for the highest price possible without discouraging the consumer.

Although this seems a simple process, the delicate balance between practice profit and the consumer willingness to pay is difficult to ascertain. Nagle et al. (2011) suggest that pricing is a game because success depends not only on a practice's own pricing decisions but also on how consumers and the competition react to them. They further present that pricing decisions should always be made as part of an overall long-term marketing strategy designed to generate and capture more profit. Otherwise, it is possible to win many individual battles for market share and still end up losing the war for profitability. For a comprehensive review of pricing fundamentals and procedures as they directly apply to the audiology practice, the reader should review Chapter 13.

Once the practice manager has followed the steps in calculating the product prices, the components of the "pricing mix" can then be established. These would include:

■ List price—Full retail price as determined by a pricing method.
■ Discounts—Discounts, if any, from the full retail price.
■ Allowances—Cash allowances on the trade-in of valuable products.
■ Payment period—Period of time allowed for the consumer to pay for the product considering the amount put down at the time of order and how much deposit is lost, if any, for return of the product.
■ Credit terms—Terms for financing of goods and services by internal and external financing programs.

Marketing Mix—The Place

The *place* is where the services are offered, the atmosphere, and the image where the product is provided. In any business, a product is anything that can be offered to a market to satisfy a want or a need. The product not only includes the physical goods and services but also the experiences, events, places, properties, organizations, information, and ideas that accompany it. It is important to remember that place is not confined to a physical location. A practice's website, Facebook, or any other virtual locations are considered place as well.

Indeed, part of the product that is presented to the market is also the practice's image and the patient's experience throughout the process. From the first phone call from the patient or a referral, the entire experience is part of the branding of the practice. Convenience is a necessity in today's world; therefore, central location in the community, as well as accessible

parking with several handicap spaces with wheelchair and walker accessibility, is important. If possible, a handicap door allowing easy access for those with disabilities is a plus. Although it is helpful to have a number of convenient locations, the viability of multiple locations must be weighed against expansion costs and applicable business opportunities.

The Physical Facility and the Clinic

The place of practice should offer a clinical but comfortable atmosphere to allow for relaxation and comfort, reinforcing that the patient is in the right place for their hearing care. That experience necessitates a neat, uncluttered waiting room with a tasteful upscale décor considering all details, even the smell of the area (Carbone, 2016; Marsh, 2012).

The Flow Through the Clinic

The front office staff begins setting the brand image on the phone by their demeanor while scheduling the appointment. Greetings upon arrival must be courteous, interactive, and sympathetic to the patient's hearing impairment and other possible comorbid conditions. The audiologist should dress appropriately to see patients by wearing a clean lab coat that presents a professional image. Simply dressing for image is a good beginning toward branding the product image that will coexist with the clinicians, their personality, and the quality of services offered by the practice. In the past, many doctoral-level audiologists did not use lab coats. These were the days before the profession was a doctoral-level profession, and this attire was considered unnecessary and inappropriate by some professionals. The profession has totally changed over the years. Given that more audiologists are in private practice and working for themselves and branding the practice, the use of a lab coat fosters the image of a doctor offering services in a professional environment. Further, it presents the audiologist as an individual with credentials to ethically recommend further testing and/or prescriptive rehabilitative products. Image is so important to success in practice that it is a good idea to check the brand that is being presented to the community. Clinicians need to check their brand by calling the office using the main number and trying to make an appointment, checking on the elements of the experience:

- How were they greeted?
- Was it easy to make an appointment?
- How long did they have to wait for an appointment?
- Were they put on hold?
- Were they advised of what to bring for the first appointment?
- Were they made to feel important?

Online methods may be used to prepare patients, such as intake forms, histories, and so on. The practitioners and clerical staff should all be familiar with the process, how long it takes, the usual mistakes made when filling out paperwork, and so forth. If these processes are cumbersome, the patient may not ever get as far as an appointment, and thus they should be checked periodically.

Other Place Concerns

The practice manager should assess where the patients park and observe the following:

- Is the signage easy to read?
- Is the entrance to the practice clearly designated?
- Is the parking lot clean?

Additionally, professionals should also walk into the practice through the front door and see the practice's first impression from the patient's eyes:

- Is the entrance easily marked?
- Is the entrance inviting?
- Is the waiting room pleasant and comfortable?

Further, the practice manager should check the brand presented to consumers by asking the patient a few good questions such as:

- How were they treated when they called in for an appointment?
- Did they visit the clinic website or the Facebook page? Was it helpful? If not, what can be done to make it better?

This will convey to the patient that these details are of concern to the practice and that their satisfaction is important. Product brands are built by "doing the homework" necessary to make a particular brand of audiology stand out from the other brands already offered in the community. Once it is established that the brand is known as the most competent, professional, relaxed, and convenient clinic, most of the marketing is already done and the goods and services almost sell themselves.

Marketing Mix—Promotion

Promotion is essential for a successful audiology private practice. Without promoting the practice, the market does not know that the business exists. To have a successful promotional program, practice owners must realize that there are four specific types of consumers that require promotional intervention:

- Referrals from medical colleagues.
- Referrals from allied health colleagues.
- Existing patients in the database.
- Patients recruited from the public.

Each of these types of referrals is very important to the practice as all add substantially to the overall revenue of the practice.

Physician Referrals

Patients who are referred by medical colleagues should be a priority for a new practice. While there may be other practices existing within the community, there are always existing referral sources that may be physicians unhappy with the services their patients are receiving from others within the community. This is fertile ground to recruit new business for the practice. The best source of patient referral for general diagnostic and rehabilitative audiology services is from family practice, internal medicine, and occupational medicine. General surgeons are a reliable source

of referral for operative monitoring. It has been known for quite some time (Kochkin, 2004, 2009, 2012) that the most important social influence in a patient's life is the family physician. Depending upon the study, a patient is five to eight times more likely to purchase amplification than if directed to the clinic by someone else. Since marketing to referral sources requires these medical colleagues to entrust their patients for services, this is a special relationship that must be cultivated. Within the past few years, otolaryngologists have had their own audiology service providers dispensing hearing instruments within their practice. While there are some that practice without dispensing hearing devices, otolaryngologists are not usually a good source of referrals for audiology private practice. In fact, independent audiology practitioners need to be careful as to who is used for their otolaryngology referrals to protect their cadre of patients.

In 2024, it is not the actual physician who usually makes the decisions as to where patients are referred for treatment outside of their practice. This task is usually delegated to a referral manager who knows all of the best referral sources in the area, including audiologists, and thus this is the person who should be contacted and sent marketing materials. There are also physician marketing companies that offer marketing to physicians, especially their designated referral specialist.

Other Allied Health Provider Referral Sources

While referrals from physicians are essential to the success of a practice, the practice manager should not limit themselves to physicians. Other health professionals, such as physician's assistants, nurse practitioners, chiropractors, psychologists, physical therapists, occupational therapists, and speech-language pathologists, are also very good referral sources. They may also be contacted by the same marketing companies as used for physicians. These colleagues are often interested in some cross-marketing where each practice markets the other. For example, there may be a dentist who places the practice's brochures in their clinic and the audiology clinic places their brochures in the dentist's clinic. These placements serve as each practice endorsing each other. Cross-marketing is usually very successful as it is one trusted professional endorsing another.

Marketing to Existing Clinic Patients

Unless the clinic is a startup, there will be patients in the database who can be used for marketing purposes. An established practice will benefit from patient knowledge of and exposure to the practice's brand of audiology from time to time. Since they know the practice and the professionals involved, minimal marketing to existing patients nets a rather large benefit. Marketing to existing or former patients can be as much as half or more of a year's business when conducted correctly. While the key for this group is not to market to them too often, existing patients always appreciate something that will be of benefit to them, such as a new type of hearing device. In established practices, ensuring the existing database is satisfied is extremely important as on average, 60% or more of new hearing instrument sales are to the existing database. Existing patients respond well to informational items in emails, website blogs, newsletters, or other communications. Tapping into this market segmentation through the practice database is greatly enhanced using a sophisticated office management system (Chapter 15). These systems and new automated artificial intelligence (AI) programs reduce the time and energy required for marketing as well as increase the efficiency of the marketing program.

Marketing to the General Public

The most expensive source of patients is recruiting consumers from the general public. St. Clergy (2013) estimated that it costs $250 to $300 to bring a new patient into the practice using market communications. In 2024, now inflated costs are estimated to be between $400 to $800 per new patient while *the cost to keep a patient in the clinic is still about $200*. Given that the lifetime value of each patient is about $40,000 to $60,000, it is obvious that a practitioner should be very diligent in keeping the existing patients within the practice.

To generate patients from the public, a well-known formula in business is that marketing costs should be about 8% to 10% of the business's gross revenue. Thus, these expensive market communications, called *market offerings*, are in many forms, such as newspaper advertising, radio, television, direct mail ads, newsletters, online ads, Facebook, pay per click, or search engine optimization. These communications require the purchase of space, time, special techniques, creative artwork, and other expensive commodities that can absorb large amounts of marketing funds. Any of these specific advertising mediums may be used in isolation, but the best result is usually achieved by an organized marketing effort that incorporates several of these modalities simultaneously. Coordinated market offerings allow multiple exposures that gain maximum interaction with the audience by stimulating many senses simultaneously. In addition to advertising to the general population, a marketing program should also include a coordinated public relations or awareness campaign such as conducting presentations to service groups, as well as interaction with physician offices. The demonstration of products, services, and professional expertise to these groups can be an effective (and inexpensive) source of new patients, either from the audiences themselves or their family and friends.

General Considerations in Promotional Activities

Promotions can easily be over or underused in marketing the practice; however, a practice with no promotions will have a tough time in competitive markets. No matter what specific promotional technique is incorporated, it is best to begin the discussion with some evidence based themes woven into the methods. Staab (1992) offered some classic tips that ensure success with promotional programs that are still important to a marketing program today:

- Try to add value such as more warranty or other benefit rather than discounting products.

- Put the practice's imprint on promotions to make them exclusive and identifiable.
- Focus on the future; look for repeat business, not just new business.
- Give promotions a theme to help reinforce other promotional efforts.
- Target promotions as specifically as possible to obtain measurable results.
- Attempt to find methods to reward the best patients.
- If the promotion does well, look for cross-promotional opportunities.
- Find ways to make the patient feel good about choosing this clinic.
- Promotions should be presented in a quality manner within an affordability range.
- If the sales staff is involved, the promotion should be exciting and rewarding for them to participate, or it will not perform as well.
- Make promotions fun and easy to execute.
- Keep testing different promotions, even if specific promotions are working well.
- Design the promotion with the question, "What do hearing-impaired patients want us to do for them?" or rephrased, the patient should be able to ask, "What is in it for me?"

Many general areas can be included in direct marketing efforts that differentiate the practice. These marketing efforts can achieve results by diversifying the message or offering into several specific areas such as goods, services, experiences, events, persons, places, organizations, information, ideas, or technology, and so forth. Kotler and Keller (2016) lead practitioners to believe that all these areas can be considered and varied in their marketing programs.

Marketing Through the Goods

These are products such as hearing aids, accessories, and other physical products for sale in the clinic. The selling of goods can use manufacturer-produced or practice-generated ads that discuss technology, product changes, and/or product features but should emphasize the benefits of these features/technologies to the patient, but the clinic's brand should always be prominent.

Marketing Through the Services

Depending upon the audience for the marketing campaign, evaluations and other services offered in the clinic can be presented as an alternative to the traditional testing services. Highlighting other services besides audiometric evaluations such as ABRs, OAEs, balance testing, speech-in-noise testing, extended high-frequency testing, tinnitus treatment, programming of hearing aids purchased elsewhere, aural rehabilitation classes, and cerumen removal presents the practice as a facility that can help the whole patient. Consumers often view the offering of these other services as an indication of a *"patient-oriented"* facility and may not only seek services at this clinic but may also be inclined to refer others.

Marketing Through the Experiences

Although audiologists are aware of how new products can change the quality of life for the hearing-impaired individual, the patient is most likely unaware of the broad range of benefits that they will receive from items such as new technology amplification, a special telephone, rechargeable devices, television connection devices, or simply reprogramming their current hearing aids. Offering services "beyond the basics" in the form of focus groups and aural rehabilitation classes can also set a practice apart from the competition. These unique offerings are, in fact, a form of informal marketing as it encourages the sharing of experiences among patients with similar problems. Good firsthand experiences are probably the best form of advertising, and testimonials from those satisfied patients are a good, inexpensive source not only for new hearing aid fittings but also for refits, reprogramming, and audiological services. Testimonials should be placed where they can be seen easily, such as on the practice website or Facebook page to obtain the full benefit from them.

Marketing Through Events

Sponsoring or offering screening services at special events, such as health fairs, will foster awareness of hearing loss and treatment and thus draw people into the practice. Additionally, offering community lectures on hearing impairment to service groups, such as the Lions Club, Rotary, Kiwanis, or Sertoma, is a good marketing tool for visibility. While "open houses" have been used way too often over the years, they can be successful if conducted at strategic times and coordinated with multimodality advertising to ensure success.

Marketing Through People

This can be the marketing of a special individual, the practice owner/audiologist, or other expert, such as a manufacturer's representative acting as a spokesperson for the practice. Events that market a specific individual are usually more successful when combined with a special market offering with a timed response.

Marketing the Place of Service

The promotion of a specific location, such as rural, conveniently located, accessible by public transportation, plenty of available parking, or other relevant aspects pertaining to the locale of the practice, can be a special marketing edge.

Marketing Through Organizations

It is possible to gain recognition by building a strong, favorable image relative to organizations such as senior centers, church groups, or other local groups for the elderly or hearing impaired.

Marketing With Information

Information, such as explanations about hearing loss, hearing instruments, assistive devices, middle ear disease, and so forth, can be disseminated in brochures made available in displays in the office or through direct mailings.

Marketing the Benefits

Consumers do not really care too much about the features of a product, but they are interested in the benefits that the features create for them. Benefits that are often utilized liberally relative to hearing aids are that they help with speech understanding, reduction of background noise, elimination of feedback, hearing with the brain, and comfort, among others. While these "catchphrases" are substantially overused, it is necessary to present the same ads as the competition on occasion so that the practice is seen as offering the same or more benefits as others in the market area.

There are many marketing firms that advertise in professional journals and online to develop specialized mailing lists for practices. Many of the Internet sites aid in the design of multiattribute market segmentations, allowing the practitioner to design a direct mail list targeted for their specific market at about one third the cost of a list generated by professional marketing services. Practitioners must be cautious, however, as these marketers may appear to be very knowledgeable, effective, and efficient, and the practitioner may know more about their market than these services.

Developing a Marketing Strategy

Marketing involves the act of influencing consumer choice by demonstrating the value of a product or service. These programs are most successful when priorities are established, and focus is sharpened toward specific targets. If there are too many priorities, it is a "stuck in the middle strategy" and the branding of the practice will never be accomplished (Chapter 5). The limited resources of audiology practice make it necessary to maximize the profit generated by the marketing effort. An example of this focus is the use of market segmentation. As presented earlier, an example of a market segmentation might consist of presenting an offering to a demographic of interest, a specific audiometric configuration, degree, or type of hearing loss that would benefit from the product or service in question. No matter what the media, the message must be presented to those who need the offering to develop a want and ultimately its demand.

Traditional Forms of Advertising

In a competitive world where there is overlap in the job descriptions of commercial hearing aid dealers, physicians, technicians, and audiologists, marketing is an exercise that educates consumers about the audiologist's unique qualifications as a hearing and balance expert who influences product or service purchase over someone else. While marketing is not just selling or advertising, it should take cues from purchasing patterns and consumer needs so that sales become a consequence of marketing efforts. Advertising is a marketing tactic. Traditional forms of advertising, as outlined in this chapter, are still one of the most essential marketing tactics available to audiologists. Audiologists may choose from several methods of advertising that are appropriate for the practice target market. The following are methods of traditional advertising that have been used effectively in audiology practices.

Advertising Specialty Items

Specialty items are often great awareness reminders for the practice. These can be issued after the hearing examination or included in promotional mailings. Specialty items include refrigerator magnets, coffee cups, and pens or pencils with logos and practice information.

Articles and Columns

Articles in the newspaper are more typically now in the online editions, and local magazines are important for image and brand awareness of the practice. The practice manager should take every opportunity to always place the name of the practice in front of the public. A method of obtaining this type of advertising is to offer routine press releases or confer with the newspaper advertising representative for insertion into the main body of the newspaper or in a special advertising section. Audiology practitioners have leverage with newspapers if a regular advertiser. Since *May Is Better Hearing and Speech Month*, newspapers are looking for articles about communication disorders and hearing loss in the months of April, May, and June. Other months or weeks are devoted to specific yet related topics.

Hearing and cognition are closely intertwined; National Alzheimer's Week would be a good opportunity for an article on the effects of hearing loss in dementia. Diabetes and hearing loss are closely aligned, and thus articles in Diabetes month (November) will be considered by newspapers and other media. Christmas time brings noisy toys and an article about noise-induced hearing loss and prevention would be appropriate.

Billboards

Although not for everyone, billboards represent an expensive but innovative, effective advertising opportunity. Billboards are most frequently used for building an awareness of a practice. Personalizing the billboard with staff pictured in white coats near equipment will lend to the branding of the practice as a professional and technologically advanced site for hearing and balance care. Strategically placed billboards can be very effective when presented correctly and in conjunction with other marketing efforts.

Brochures and Circulars

Practice brochures should form the advertising and public relations cornerstone of the practice. Brochures must be articulate and printed on high-quality, glossy paper. Although these can be done on the practice's computer, professional designers usually maximize the message and imagery to be included and weave these messages into the marketing mix offered by the practice. Practice brochures should be issued to every new patient coming into the office as they serve as calling cards and sources of information for potential patients and referral sources. They should be "high end" and displayed in as many referral sources and cross-referenced practices as possible throughout the market area. Many primary care providers or their surrogates will simply hand the brochure to their patients and instruct them to call the office for an appointment. Healthcare professionals and other referral sources will judge the practice on the brochure by its quality, making it extremely important for the marketing mix.

Classified Advertising

Although classified advertising sections are not usually the place that consum-

ers reference for audiological services, there is the possibility for retrieving a few hearing-impaired consumers for the trial of a specific product, or if the clinic is conducting a true research project. Classifieds may offer an inexpensive option; however, it is not generally a successful investment of a marketing budget relative to the return.

Coupons and Gift Cards

Clinics need to be careful when using coupons or gift cards to reduce the price of prescription hearing instruments, offer services, or attract first-time patients. Consumers may suspect that the original price was set too high so that the promotional coupons may be used; however, the prudent use of coupons can be effective. For example, if the goal is to have members of the practice's existing database return for a visit, coupons offering batteries, upgrades for a rechargeable system, or hearing instrument cleaning will likely produce surprising numbers of returnees. Since it is known that the use of OTC devices will eventually lead to the use of prescription instruments, these tools could be helpful for the sale of OTC products. For example, the carefully targeted use of gift cards or coupon specials directed at OTC devices where the offer is the inclusion of limited rehabilitative services may lead to a loyal new patient who eventually will need the higher-prescription products. To be optimally effective, however, coupons should be tied to a reasonable marketing goal and have an expiration date for the offer.

Gift cards, gift baskets, or incentives for patients that encourage friends, relatives, and others to consider the clinic for hearing instruments can be more successful than direct mail for many practices. The use of gift cards as part of a mail piece is thought by some to net a greater return than direct mail pieces without the offer. While the return may be greater, the image of the practice and the quality of the patients obtained from these offers can be substantially degraded.

Product Demonstrations

Demonstrations generally work best in a place where prospective patients are already gathered, such as trade shows or health fairs. This offers a chance for the patient to see what the device can do for them in a relaxed, social environment. Demonstrations within the practice, as in a trial period with amplification for a specified time period, are not uncommon and enable the patient and those around them to evaluate the efficacy and communication improvements expected with advanced hearing instrument technology.

Direct Mail

The key to direct mail solicitation is defining market segmentation and the offer to be presented in the direct mail piece. First, the correct demographic of 65 to 90 must be chosen; any other age demographic does not reach those with the highest probability of possessing a hearing impairment. Although direct mail has worked relatively well with the previous generation of patients, these tactics do not work as well with the Baby Boomer population as these offers are commonly in the mailbox each day. Boomers and their children, Generation X, are more highly educated than past generations. They tend to be skeptical of these mailers offering some "deal" for the day or week. They have seen these ads before and generally look to these mailings as from a "sales operation," more interested in selling product than providing aural rehabilitative treatment. Even when targeted to a well-segmented population with a unique mailing and a well-planned offer, direct mail marketing has a general response rate under 1% of the number mailed. In fact, an excellent rate of return is considered .02% to .03%, and a .04% to .05% response is considered an exceptional response. These issues notwithstanding, Romney (2017) suggests that there are seven principles of effective direct mail marketing:

1. *Consumers evolve, causing marketing procedures to change over time.* Here the concern is that what has worked well in the market to attract consumers in the past may not work as well in the current market because consumers evolve and become immune to certain messages. For example, an "Open House" used to have quite a draw for new patients, but it has been so overused that it does not result in scheduled appointments.

   Marketers now suggest the term "Special Event," "Hearing Class," or other terms for the offering, which will, in time, become overused as well. Practitioners should be aware that marketing techniques need to evolve with the generations, stay fresh, and continue to differentiate the practice (Chapter 5).

2. *Demands strategic targeting of consumers.* This section refers to sophistication of target market segmentations that can be applied to searches for specific types of

consumers. For additional audiological services, the age group to
target is considered to be 60 to
90; therefore, the messages and
market offerings should possibly
appeal more to golfers, those who
go on cruises, pet lovers, motorcycle riders, and so on, for example.
These specific segmentations allow
for the fine tuning of messages
that can be the incentive to motivate a consumer. The goal should
not merely be obtaining a consumer for a specific offering but to
capture and retain them for life.

3. *Be proactive rather than reactive
   in the market.* The average repurchase rate for new amplification
   products by consumers is every
   3.8 years (Romney, 2017). Some
   estimate that the time patients
   wait after they are hearing impaired until they actually purchase
   hearing devices is about 5 years.
   Kochkin (2012) reported that new
   consumers may wait as long as an
   average for 12.4 years (median =
   8 years) before they have considered amplification. Roughly 20%
   to 25% of new patients come from
   advertising and direct mail to the
   public. A 5,000-person mailing
   will yield on average 12 calls,
   8 confirmations of an appointment, 6 patients who actually show
   up, 4 candidates for hearing instruments, and 2 patients who will
   actually purchase. This is for a net
   sale of four units based upon the
   campaign. Newsletters, blogging,
   and other communications also
   allow for proactivity in the marketplace. Generally, it is best to be
   the clinic that the others respond
   to rather than being the clinic that

has to respond to innovative offers
by others.

4. *Frequent repetition of message
   and tactics.* Direct mail campaigns
   are substantially more successful
   if they are combined with other
   media that is repeated routinely
   such as print, web, Facebook,
   newsletters, and possibly radio
   and television. In today's highly
   competitive market, it is necessary
   to saturate the market with ethical,
   informative, and beneficial offerings or the clinic will be left out of
   consideration.

5. *A rich and believable message.*
   Offerings for free hearing tests,
   free consultations, free packs of
   batteries, $400 off on two hearing
   aids, and others are very much
   the same as has been offered for
   many years and thus not unique.
   On the other hand, advertisements
   such as buy one get one free, 50%
   off, and all hearing aids $295 are
   unrealistic offers and perceived
   by consumers as "too good to be
   true" and therefore not believable.
   Realistic offers such as life-time
   batteries or a free rechargeable system might be more believable for
   patients as part of an offering.

6. *Arrest the attention of our recipients.* Getting attention is a
   major concern in today's direct
   mailing programs. To present a
   good direct mail offering, it must
   be opened by the consumer first
   before the offer can be seen. What
   gets the consumer to even open
   the direct mail piece can almost
   be science within itself. Some of
   the details that can bet a direct
   mail piece is opened in today's
   market are hand addressing,

colored envelopes, raised printing, unusual sizes, large cards, and other tactics. While caution must be used not to compromise the credibility of the clinic, some suggest that a gift card offer can get the piece opened more often, generating a better response to the mailing.

7. *Messages should arrive on time for the promotion.* Most importantly, direct mail offerings should avoid all holidays. Consumers are preoccupied with the time of year and are not interested in an offering, no matter what is presented. The best times for office events are generally thought to be the first and third weeks of the month and, generally, dropping the mail two weeks before is the best option. Usually, a delay in the arrival of a direct mail piece can make or break an offering. While there is no control over the U.S. Postal Service, the best for bulk direct mailings, it is best to design the drop of the direct mail pieces according to when the clinic has the offering available. Other marketing promotions that should arrive on time are "batteries for the birthday" as well as other time-ordered marketing pieces.

Direct Hearing Aid Sales and Medicare Advantage

It is common today for patients to obtain hearing devices from direct-to-consumer sources, especially since the implementation of the OTC legislation in October 2022. Manufacturers offer not only prescription devices but also OTC devices in a direct sales presentation to the consumer, providing their products with video instruction and telephone support. Unfortunately, most of the telephone programming support is delivered by hearing aid dispensers. For those "easy-to-fit" hearing losses with the proper support and the cost reduction, many patients do quite well under these programs as, for the costs, their expectations of benefit are not as high. It is, therefore, highly recommended for private practice clinics to offer products and/or follow-up care if the patient has obtained the devices elsewhere as it will most likely lead to the use of higher technology devices in the future.

Another controversial program is Medicare Advantage that has seen a major increase in the past few years. Medicare Advantage allows patients to seek a group such as United Health Care, Aetna, Humana, and others to provide their medical care under Part C of the Medicare program. These programs offer not only medical care but dental, vision, fitness, transportation, home care, diabetic supplies, home-delivered meals, and, a big one for audiologists, *Hearing Services.* These programs lure audiologists as providers by contracting to send patients to their clinics, but their reimbursement rate reputation for these patients has been shown to be very low. In Chapter 16 in this volume, Tedeschi suggests that audiologists considering serving as a provider for these insurance companies should have the practice attorney read the contract to determine their obligations to each referred patient. This review should be done prior to entering into the provider relationship with any insurance company. Tedeschi also indicates that often these contracts can be negotiated to a more reasonable reimbursement level, especially in areas where audiologists are scarce (Chapters 16 and 17).

An additional controversial Internet/direct mail enterprise is offered by United Health Care (UHC). This semi-ethical scheme offers patients hearing instruments by mail as a benefit of their insurance program for a nominal cost. Patients send in their audiogram to UHC, and UHC then sends the patient a programmed hearing instrument with written instructions on how to use the device. Obviously, not exactly aural rehabilitation. UHC has also established a separate company, Hearing Innovators, to handle these fittings but offers only nominal reimbursement to audiologists to support these patients. While it is up to the audiologist and their office manager to decide if they will offer support to these frustrating new models of practice, many clinics have opted to not support this endeavor. In a private practice clinical situation, working with too many of these increasing numbers of high-maintenance managed care patients takes time away from full-fee patients who contribute significantly to the cash flow of the practice. The benefits of new patients to the practice and the low reimbursement schedules must be taken into consideration. (Chapters 16 and 17).

Television

Much less expensive than in the immediate past, television, especially local cable channels, offers an opportunity to visually engage potential patients. Additionally, talk show hosts are often looking for a professional they can invite to generate interest in their show. These invitations are almost always free, sometimes even paid, and well worth the time as they generate good questions from the listeners and offer great exposure for the clinician and the practice. While still expensive, local cable channels have become rather affordable in the past few years, and the station and their producers usually assist greatly in the production of the advertising. These programs tend to work best when they are incorporated with other media, such as direct mail and print media. Even with changes in the costs, if television is the medium, however, costs are generally high and often prohibitive without significant subsidies from manufacturers.

Exhibitions and Fairs

Exhibitions and fairs are a reliable source of prospective patients, but the selection of the correct, beneficial exhibition or health fair is critical and involves a review of the demographics of the attendees. The health fairs, garden shows, car shows, or farm shows are a cost-efficient place to offer hearing screenings, presentations on hearing, and product demonstrations that will advertise the practice and draw consumers to the booth. These events are an opportunity to present the professionalism of the practice to the public face-to-face.

Magazine Advertisements

Local magazines are a good place to present a high-end message. It is a good idea to try to publish an article in the magazine and place an ad near the article. This reinforces the fact that the practitioner wrote the article and presents the practice's brand of audiology to the consumers. While these ads do not usually send much business to the practice, they are part of the overall visibility of the clinic.

Newsletters

Newsletters are effective tools to communicate with established patients, prospective patients, and referral sources. They should contain updates on hearing instrument technology, highlight important regulatory issues and changes in insurance coverage, and provide information about the front office and professional staff. They are also a good place to present families and other personal items that might be of interest to patients. Some practices feature not only the practitioner and their family but the staff families as well. As presented above, marketing to existing patients is a major source of revenue and the newsletter is one of the most efficient methods of communication with that market. An offer to them relative to accessories, services, hearing aids, evaluations, and so on is usually well respected. It breeds not only good communication but also substantial word-of-mouth advertising. Some clinics offer a newsletter occasionally, others monthly, but quarterly newsletters tend to maximize the benefit for the costs involved. Some clinics prepare their newsletter "in house" and others use a newsletter service for the designing and preparation and execution of the newsletters. Although the results are usually similar, a newsletter designed in house and by the owner or a provider within the practice is typically perceived as more personal. However, personal newsletters take a lot of time to prepare; therefore, that is the attraction to a commercially prepared document.

Newspaper Advertisements

Long a staple in practice advertising, the focus of the newspaper ad has centered on two distinct topics: price and time-sensitive deadlines for a "call to action," but not all newspaper ads have those goals. Getting the practice branded in the community as a center of excellence, a location where professional services prevail, and where primary care providers send their patients will also have an impact on newspaper readers. Of course, price shoppers will respond to "special pricing offers," and if providers are interested in attracting them, then newspaper ads pushing price is the way to go. If, however, the practitioner would like to have patients coming to participate in a continuum of professional, rehabilitative care, advertising presence in the newspaper will look vastly different than price-based ads.

At least initially, it is good to have a marketing consultant assist in the generation of a few good ads that can be placed strategically, no matter the marketing strategy. Marketing consultants vary in their expertise in marketing hearing instruments and to older patients, so choose them carefully. These consultants can be very expensive and sometimes offer little expertise above what is known by the practice owner, the office manager, and the professionals within the clinic. Some newspapers have seen a substantial reduction in readership and are not as good of a patient source as in the past. This can be checked with the representative of these media for information to determine if newspaper advertising can still be beneficial in the community.

Personal Letters

Personal letters are appropriate to referral sources, prospective patients, and those previously evaluated but who have decided not to act on your recommendation to consider the use of amplification (the so-called "tested not sold"). The initial mailing should be accompanied by the practice brochure or specific brochure about hearing instruments and/or hearing rehabilitation. The letters must be brief, no longer than three short paragraphs, and topics may include, but not be limited to, new products, new patient evaluation procedures, special offers, relocation of the practice, and other timely and appropriate issues.

Radio Advertisements

The use of radio tends to be best for short-term ads for the clinic rather than long-term routine advertising, usually lasting 2 weeks to 30 days or for advertising a special event. Sponsorship of programs and spots on a single station or multiple stations within the same market area usually net the same results. Radio is still an expensive yet strong medium that can brand the practice in a very short time. However, prospective patients get tired of the ads rather easily, and the effectiveness of this expensive medium is usually short-lived. Using clever, humorous, and testimonial spots, the listener can develop an image of the practice and what to expect from a visit. Since consumers spend a lot of time in their cars and offices, the expense is sometimes worth the exposure. In radio, the station will usually assist the clinic in organizing a radio marketing program, preparing spots, and suggesting communication formats

that have worked in the past for other businesses. Testimonials work particularly well in radio advertising, where a locally prominent person discusses their experiences in the practice. These testimonials further brand the practice as the place to go for hearing care.

Educational Seminars

No-obligation seminars are another form of advertising that can be used effectively. The concern with this type of advertising is that it must be conducted in an environment conducive to presenting the material in a nonobligatory way, such as in a classroom-style arena. These can be organized seminars that are advertised to the public or to a segmented patient base audience, but should be in an upscale venue, a hospital, or other environment that offers an atmosphere of professionalism.

Signage

Sounds simple, but signs are a true form of advertising. Each time the consumer passes the practice or looks for a practice, visible, professional, and ethical signage is essential. The sign outside the practice is basic communication with a wide expanse of potential consumers. It presents what is practiced at that location and should be professional in the truest sense of the word to reinforce the professional "brand" of service delivery available at that location. Signs should be chosen carefully as they are the best example of a "sunk cost" (Chapter 11).

Telemarketing

Telemarketing is a form of direct marketing in which a person uses the phone or any other means of communication to contact potential patients. Potential patients are identified and classified by various means such as history of purchases, previous surveys, participation in contests, or other public or private list. The classification process serves to find those potential patients most likely to buy the products or services offered by the company in question. Although used in the hearing industry, it is typically incorporated in high-pressure sales operations. Telemarketing offers information by paid telemarketing professionals using a script about products or services offered in the practice via the telephone to special targeted lists of consumers. It is often considered an invasion of their privacy by most people and does not present a highly professional image of audiology or the specific practice. While it might create some debatable results, with increasing public resistance and the advent of "no-call" lists or blocking apps, *telemarketing is not a technique that should be considered* as a viable marketing alternative.

Yellow Pages

Thirty years ago, this form of traditional advertising was essential. Ten years ago, it was still available, and today, in 2024, some may never have heard of this concept. The term Yellow Pages is synonymous with the old-style landline telephone. Today, however, very few even have a landline telephone and Yellow Page phonebooks, though available from some private companies, are almost extinct. The Yellow Pages still exist online. Yellowpages.com is a U.S.-based website operated as "the Real Yellow Pages" that provides listings for local businesses. While this form of advertising still exists and may be effective in some environments, and it does provide a segue to the broader concepts of websites and online advertising, there are better, more professional places to invest the practice's marketing funds.

Digital Marketing—A Whole New World

Digital marketing is such a huge component of the brand visibility in 2024 and with AI and other progress, it will only become a greater factor. Daily online usage plays a significant role in the everyday lives of consumers worldwide. It has totally changed how businesses market their products and services. Just as the yellow has faded from phone books, the rise of the Internet has changed the way humans interact as well as reshaped traditional communications media such as film, television, music, and, of course, the telephone. The emergence of new digital technologies and websites has accelerated forms of human interaction through online forums, instant messaging, and social networking.

Online activity has fostered the rise of social media, the source of change of how individuals and groups communicate, dividing personal and public online space. The mainstreaming of Internet features, such as digital music and video, user-generated content, and digital media sales, have revolutionized marketing techniques. The Internet has also irrevocably impacted all types of business, retail, wholesale, and professional businesses such as audiology clinics. Love it, like it, or totally hate it, audiology clinics are now part of ecommerce growth for the sale of products but also the delivery of services such as teleaudiology. Progressive clinics are no longer limited by isolated locations and brick-and-mortar buildings but are now able to expand the reach of their services outside their local communities and, when allowed by licensure, across state lines.

Some of audiology's target markets were born before the Internet, and others have never known a day without it. Today it is difficult to imagine life without it. In 2024, the Internet has been around for 41 years since its official creation on January 1, 1983.

Pelchen and Allen (2024) state that we live in a time when Internet usage is an all-day, everyday occurrence. Many people in the United States (as well as other countries) require consistent access to the Internet, whether remotely working, scrolling, or streaming. Since it is continuously relied upon, it is crucial to examine the trends and preferences that are impacting this ever-evolving digital marketing terrain. While these facts are consistently changing, the following are some key facts relative to worldwide Internet use in 2024:

■ *Internet use.* Out of the nearly 8 billion people in the world, 5.35 billion, or around 66% of the world's population, have access to the Internet, and the number of worldwide Internet users is expected to reach 7.9 billion by 2029. In the United States, over 330 million individuals use the Internet (Figure 12–16).

The amount of time users spend on the Internet varies by age group, but on average, people spend 6.5 hours on the Internet every day. However, individuals between the ages of 16 and 24 spend an additional 2.5 hours more time online than those between the ages of 55 and 64.

■ *Social media.* With Facebook, Instagram, Reddit, and TikTok leading the way, the Internet is full of social media platforms that offer opportunities for individuals to share and build connections online. As of 2024, there are 5.04 billion social media users. There are 36.4 million Baby Boomers or 53.8% using social media, with Facebook as their most used app (Figure 12–17).

This indicates that social media advertising is essential to the target demographics of Generation X and Baby Boomers. Additionally, it suggests that the target market is active on the Internet with their impression of the clinic and its operation; thus, owners and managers must check these sites for reviews of the clinic.

■ *Mobile phones.* The use of mobile phones has increased exponentially over the past few years, and in the United States, virtually everyone has this technology in all age groups. Smartphones are used in 76% to 89% of the audiology target market (Figure 12–18). The implications here are that websites must be designed to work on mobile phones or the consumers will not see the clinic's message.

■ *Blog posts.* There are 7.5 million blogs posted every day. The Internet is a treasure trove for blogs for years of recipes, fashion, finance, home décor, and improvement. Many of these blogs involve hearing, aural rehabilitation, assessment, and other audio vestibular disorders, such as Hearing Health

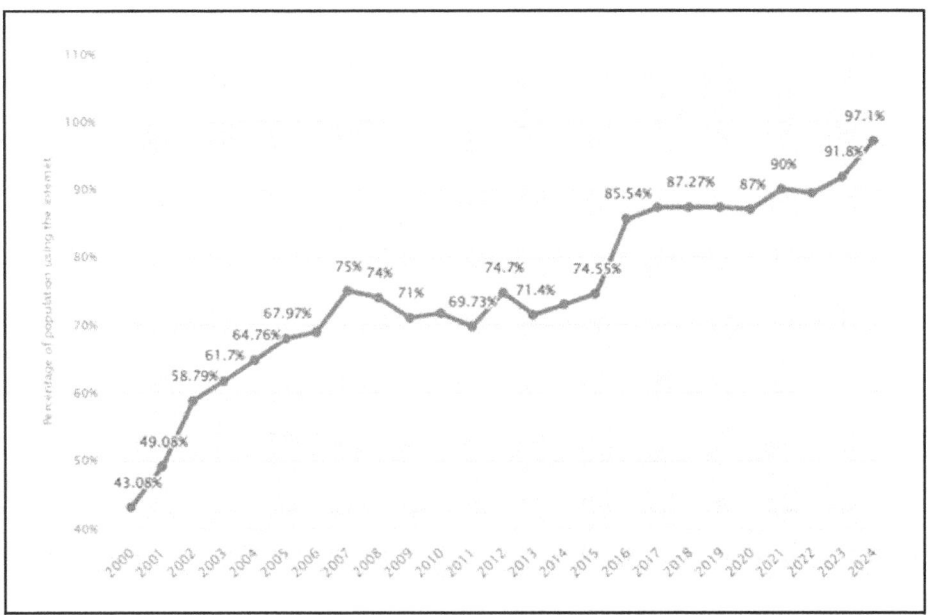

Figure 12–16. Internet users in the United States. *Source:* Statistica (2024).

Social Media Use in %			Target Market	
			Gen X	Baby Boomers
	Ages 18-29	30-49	50-64	65+
Facebook	67	75	69	58
Instagram	78	59	35	15
LinkedIn	32	40	31	12
Twitter (X)	42	27	17	6
Pinterest	45	40	33	21
Snapchat	65	30	13	4
YouTube	93	92	83	60
WhatsApp	32	38	29	16
Reddit	44	31	11	3
TikTok	62	39	24	10
BeReal	12	3	1	<1

Source: Survey of U.S. adults conducted May 19-Sept. 5, 2023.

Figure 12–17. General social media use. *Source:* Adapted from Pew Research Center (2014).

Mobile Phone Use in %			Target Market	
			Gen X	Baby Boomers
	Ages 18-29	30-49	50-64	65+
Cellphone	99	99	98	94
Smartphone	97	97	89	76
Cellphone, but not smartphone	1	2	8	17

Source: Survey of U.S. adults conducted May 19-Sept. 5, 2023.

Figure 12–18. Mobile phone use. *Source:* Adapted from Pew Research Center (2014).

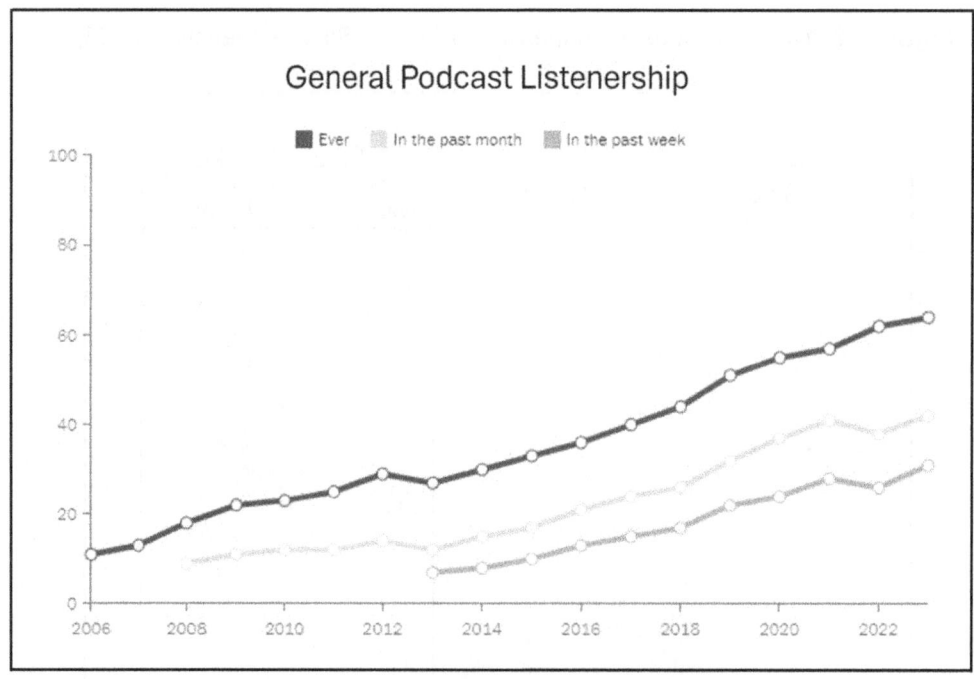

Figure 12–19. Percentage of Americans age 12+ that have listened to a podcast. *Source:* Pew Research Center (2023).

and Technology Matters, Hearing Tracker, and others.

■ *Podcasts.* A decade ago, in 2013, only 12% of Americans 12 and older said they had listened to a podcast in the past month. In 2023, 31% of those 12 and older said they had listened to a podcast in the last week, up from 26% in 2022 (Figure 12–19). This indicates that many of the audiology and consumer podcasts will be frequented by consumers.

The Practice Website

In today's digital age, a practice website is no longer just a supplementary tool; it has become an essential element for long-term success. St. Clergy (2013) calls a website "a window into the soul of the practice." *Websites are the telephone book of the 21st century.* As Generation X moves into the audiology clinic and the tech-savvy Baby Boomers move well beyond age 65, visibility on the Internet has become fundamental to success.

The practice website serves as the digital epicenter of the practice, representing the brand, engaging with patients, and fostering trust within the community. In the modern digital era, the practice's website and domain name are valuable assets, comparable to physical properties in the business world. Just like a physical location, these online assets become more valuable with use and promotion. Thus, it is crucial to secure ownership of them to maintain control over the practice's digital identity.

The website, however, is not a mere promotional tool; it is the heart of the online presence, serving as a platform for patient education, communication, and engagement. Although it is essential for the website to attract new patients, its uniqueness and appeal go well beyond marketing; it is also key to fostering trust and connection with patients.

Tailoring the Website for the Tech-Savvy Audience

Pew Research Center (2014) has revealed that Generation X enters the audiology clinic already tech-savvy, and Baby Boomers are far more tech-savvy than once considered, with 85% or more using the Internet. Additionally, new data indicate that 76% of Baby Boomers own smartphones, and 74% have broadband Internet access at home. These and other statistics highlight the need for practices to cater their websites to an increasingly digital-native audience.

To effectively appeal to these tech-savvy audiences, a practice's website must fulfill several key functions:

1. *User-friendly navigation and accessibility.* Ensuring that the website is intuitive and easy to navigate, with clear call to action and mobile responsiveness, is crucial for engaging visitors and providing a seamless user experience.
2. *Comprehensive patient education resources.* The website should serve as a valuable resource for patient education, offering informative content, frequently asked questions, and multimedia resources to empower patients with knowledge about their hearing health and potential treatment options.
3. *Online appointment, scheduling, and communication tools.* Enabling patients to schedule appointments and communicate with the practice through secure online portals can greatly enhance convenience and foster a stronger patient-provider relationship.

4. *Robust search engine optimization (SEO).* Implementing effective SEO strategies, including keyword optimization, local listings, and content marketing, can improve website visibility and help potential patients find the practice more easily.

Website Imagery

The main objective of a practice's website is to showcase potential patients and explain why they should choose to engage with this particular practice. To obtain the engagement, it is important to use personalized imagery. While stock images may be used, they are not helpful in connecting the practice with its audience. Visitors to the website are interested in knowing the clinicians, staff, and others associated with the practice. Staff images, office photos, or local landmarks can significantly enhance the visual connection between website visitors and the practice and its staff. Ultimately, it can be that these images are the deciding factors an individual considers when determining to make and keep an appointment with the clinic.

Calls to Action

The website should be designed to provide prospective patients with every possible opportunity to contact the office. A *call to action* (CTA) is a prompt that encourages website visitors to perform a specific action that is desired. These actions may include contacting the office via phone or filling out contact forms. It is important to strategically place multiple CTAs throughout the website to facilitate desired actions. For instance, there may be a button that says "Sched-

ule an Appointment" that links to an online calendar or contact form; this button is a call to action. Placing CTAs in the top header section or menu areas of the website ensures that they are easily visible to most visitors, thereby increasing the likelihood of receiving calls and inquiries for the practice.

Website Structure

The website's structure is paramount to long-term success. It is essential to include several basic elements to ensure effectiveness and functionality. These elements typically consist of:

- *Home page.* The main landing page provides an overview of the audiology practice's services and expertise, and it highlights key information about the practice.
- *Services page.* A dedicated page, or pages, should detail the range of services offered by the audiology practice, including diagnostic evaluations, hearing aid fittings, tinnitus management, and any other specialized treatments.
- *About us page.* This page offers insights into the audiology team, their qualifications, experience, and values. It helps build trust and rapport with potential patients.
- *Contact us page.* A page containing contact information, including the office address, phone number, email address, and a contact form for visitors to reach out for appointments or inquiries, needs to be included.
- *Location page (if applicable).* If the audiology practice has multiple locations, each location should have

its own page with specific address details and contact information.

- *Testimonials or reviews page.* Incorporating testimonials or reviews from satisfied patients can instill confidence in prospective patients and showcase the quality of service provided by the audiology practice.
- *Blog or news section.* A blog or news section allows the audiology practice to share informative content, hearing health tips, news updates, and promotions, enhancing engagement and attracting visitors to the website.
- *Legal notices.* Ensure compliance with legal requirements by including necessary notices such as privacy policies, terms of service, and HIPAA compliance statements.

By incorporating these basic elements into the website structure, a practice can effectively showcase its services, build credibility, and provide valuable information to potential patients.

Search Engine Optimization

Once the website is completed, it is important to use effective *search engine optimization (SEO)* to ensure good visibility on search engines like Google. Search engines use numerous factors to decide how high a website should appear in search results for specific keywords, and many of these factors are not directly related to the website itself. While SEO itself is an entire field of study, there are some simple strategies that a practice can use to improve its SEO and get started in the right direction.

Create Search Engine Listings

A practice's business profile on search engines will have a large impact on whether or not the website ranks locally. The ranking is how high the website actually is in the search with the goal of the site being at the top of the page, ranking number one. To assist in getting an optimum ranking, ensure the practice creates profiles for the practice such as Google Business Profile and Bing Local. Additionally, fill out the practice profile with accurate business information, complete and appropriate descriptions, categories, and photos. Google and Bing listings can be created at either of the websites below:

- Google Business Profile

- Bing Places for Business

Set Up a Process for Gathering Reviews

Currently, Google reviews are the primary reviews that influence the site's rankings in Google search results. Given that Google holds 86.58% of the search engine market share in the United States (Stat Counter, 2024), prioritizing Google Reviews is crucial for practices operating in the United States. While reviews on other platforms can still have an impact, only Google reviews directly affect Google rankings at present. It is important to adhere to applicable laws, website terms, and search engine guidelines when soliciting reviews. Increasing the number of online reviews will not only improve visibility in search engines but also enhance online reputation, ultimately attracting more patients to the practice.

Create Exceptional Content

Search engines value high-quality content, which includes written, visual, or multimedia material. This content aids search engines in understanding the relevance of a website to specific search queries. Without sufficient content, it becomes difficult for search engines to determine the topics for which a website should rank. Hence, it's crucial to have original and informative content on the website that accurately represents the practice's services and expertise. Consider starting a blog if practitioners have extensive knowledge to share and can commit to regular postings. A blog offers two key advantages:

■ A blog can attract online visitors searching for the topics that are written in the blog.

■ Writing consistent and frequent blog posts can cultivate a loyal readership over time. Posting consistently and frequently not only enhances brand awareness and authority but also SEO ranking, ultimately driving more traffic to the website.

Social Media

Social media is perhaps the most neglected element of a practice's online presence. This is because engaging with people on social media can be time-consuming and not always immediately rewarding. However, it is important to recognize the significant potential of social media in practice growth. Statistica (2024) has found that a notable 78% of Baby Boomers have a Facebook account that can be effectively targeted through social media marketing efforts.

Social media posts should strike a balance between being interesting and maintaining a professional tone. Occasionally, it is beneficial to include links to engaging articles or websites that would interest the followers of the practice's social media page. Moreover, it is crucial to humanize the practice by sharing "feel-good" posts about charity events, birthdays, or any other happy occasions involving the team. These "feel-good" posts are generally well received and encourage interaction from followers, making them an important component of the practice's social media strategy. The purpose of a social media page is ultimately to promote the practice and engage with prospective patients. So, while the practice should not be too aggressive and try to "sell" their social media followers, they should be referencing their own website and asking people to make an appointment or call at least from time to time.

Digital Marketing and Advertising

Digital advertising can be a potent tool for attracting new patients to the practice. However, the effectiveness of advertising campaigns can vary significantly based on factors such as who is managing the ads, the geographic location, and the cultural context.

It is vital to track the digital ad campaign success based on either cost per lead or cost per sale. This is crucial because digital advertisers often prioritize reporting metrics like "impressions" and "clicks" to the practice. Note that these metrics only indicate the number of times the ad was viewed or clicked on, providing limited insight into the ad's actual impact. Therefore, it is essential for the practice manager to be aware of the return on investment (ROI) of all ad campaigns, whether digital or otherwise, to make informed marketing decisions.

While a wide variety of advertising options are available in the digital space, the following sections outline the most popular.

Google and Search Ads

Search engine ads are highly relevant to users' searches, but they are mainly text based and lack visual appeal. On the other hand, Google display ads are visually striking but may not be as effective for small hearing practices. Google text ads, however, that appear on Google.com have been proven to be quite effective and are popular today with many hearing practices. With Google Ads, users can be targeted based on their location, search terms, and/or interests. This ensures that the practice's ads only appear on the most relevant searches.

One significant advantage of Google Ads, and other pay-per-click (PPC) ads, is that payment is required only when someone clicks on the ad. This ensures that the clinic's advertising budget is utilized efficiently and is not wasted on audiences uninterested in your ads.

Facebook Ads

Facebook offers various ad types, but the targeting is not as specific as Google Ads. Instead of focusing on context, Facebook targets are based on demographics or interests. This means that leads generated from Facebook ads may not always be as qualified as those from Google Ads, although quantity can compensate for quality in some cases. While Facebook ads may not be as contextually targeted as Google ads, they excel in visual appeal. A compelling visual campaign on Facebook can sometimes outshine Google ads. A digital marketing professional can offer advice on which type of digital ad is likely to provide the best return on investment and how to track its success effectively.

Email Marketing

Email marketing remains a popular and effective strategy for businesses across various industries, including hearing care. Despite the emergence of newer digital marketing channels and technologies, email marketing continues to offer several advantages:

■ *Direct communication.* Email allows businesses to communicate directly with their audience, delivering personalized messages tailored to individual preferences.

■ *Cost-effectiveness.* Compared to traditional marketing methods, email marketing is relatively inexpensive. It does not require printing or postage fees, making it accessible for businesses of all sizes.

■ *High ROI.* Email marketing often provides a high return on investment (ROI) when executed effectively. According to industry reports, the average ROI for email marketing is significantly higher than other marketing channels.

■ *Measurable results.* Email marketing platforms offer robust analytics, allowing businesses to track open rates, click-through rates, conversion rates, and other important metrics to measure the success of their campaigns.

■ *Segmentation and personalization.* Advanced email marketing tools enable businesses to segment their email lists based on demographics, behaviors, and preferences. This allows for more targeted and personalized messaging, which can improve engagement and conversion rates.

■ *Automation.* Automation features in email marketing platforms allow businesses to set up automated email sequences based on triggers such as user actions or specific time intervals. This helps streamline marketing efforts and maintain consistent communication with subscribers.

■ *Mobile compatibility.* With the increasing use of smartphones among all generations, emails are now more accessible than ever. Most email marketing campaigns are designed to be mobile-responsive, ensuring a seamless experience for users on various devices.

While newer marketing channels like social media and influencer marketing have gained prominence, email marketing remains a cornerstone of digital marketing strategies due to its effectiveness, affordability, and versatility. Practices considering the use of an email marketing program must make sure that the program does not violate spam laws such as the U.S. Controlling the Assault of Non-Solicited Pornography and Marketing Act (CAM-SPAM) (FTC, 2017).

Digital Marketing Automation

While office management systems (OMS) excel at scheduling appointments, their communication capabilities are often limited (Chapter 15). Typically, they send basic email appointment reminders to patients. Although some OMS systems offer more advanced automation, most marketing automation systems surpass them in this regard.

Marketing automation primarily aims to enhance practice efficiency by reducing staff time spent on repetitive tasks and utilizing technology to improve patient communication. This often leads to better outcomes for marketing efforts, such as website or digital advertising, by optimizing responses and streamlining related processes. Marketing automation platforms enable practices to automate a wide range of operations, sales, and marketing tasks. Essentially, these tools automatically track and engage patients, sometimes even intelligently, relieving office staff from manual intervention. This can result in economies of scale as the practice grows. Here are some examples of what these systems can do:

- *Voicemails.* Automatically send patients voicemails of the office singing "Happy Birthday" to them on their birthday, requiring no effort from the staff. This simple gesture enhances patient retention without any additional workload.
- *Text messages.* In instances where a call goes unanswered at the office, a marketing automation system can immediately send a text message offering to schedule an appointment, along with a calendar link, increasing convenience for patients.
- *Emails.* Marketing automation systems can be configured to send patients timely messages regarding their care automatically. This relevant and timely communication not only enhances patient satisfaction but also boosts sales.
- *Website chat.* Many marketing automation systems include a live chat feature that integrates seamlessly with the website. This live chat function can also be automated using chatbots or AI to attract more patients and facilitate appointment scheduling.

Marketing automation proves to be a highly effective tool for practice growth. With the advent of advanced language models like ChatGPT, marketing automation stands to benefit from full integration with AI, making it an even more powerful asset for practices.

Emergence of Artificial Intelligence and Marketing

While true artificial intelligence is still in development, the growing popularity of large language models (LLMs) like ChatGPT has led to widespread use of the term "AI." Although these tools aren't genuine artificial intelligence, they are capable of impressive feats and are advancing rapidly. Researchers at Neuroscience News (2023) have found that even expert linguists struggle to distinguish AI-generated content from human-written content. Additionally, AI platforms are continuing to expand beyond text generation, and some can generate images from textual descriptions or even create videos.

Businesses, including audiology practices, can benefit from utilizing AI in various ways. Whether it is drafting emails, generating blog topics, or crafting resumes, AI platforms can offer valuable assistance that save time and resources. As AI becomes more integrated into marketing automation systems, ad platforms, and websites, users can anticipate a surge in personalized online content. This integration is expected to boost staff efficiency by streamlining tasks, thereby enhancing efforts in advertising and communication efforts as well as yielding improved digital marketing results.

The Experience Economy

The experience economy is defined as "an economy in which many goods or services are sold by emphasizing the effect they can have on people's lives."

Experiences are their own category, just like "goods" and "services." Thus, an experience economy is the sale of memorable experiences to customers. The term was first used by Pine and Gilmore (1998) describing the next economy following the agrarian economy, the industrial economy, and the most recent service economy. As shown in Figure 12–20, the experience economy reflects what is called the progression of economic value. Note that experiences that are personalized to the individual customer warrant a higher price tag. Hearing Healthcare is an ideal application of the experience economy, where the primary role of the audiologist is to deliver life-changing experiences through treatment and remediations of hearing loss.

To fully appreciate how the experience economy concept works, it helps to provide some examples. Generally speaking, it takes a combination of goods or services to make an experience possible. For example, a skydiving trip bill could be broken down as:

■ The pilot for transport to a specific location and height.
■ The instructor's lesson.
■ All required gear.

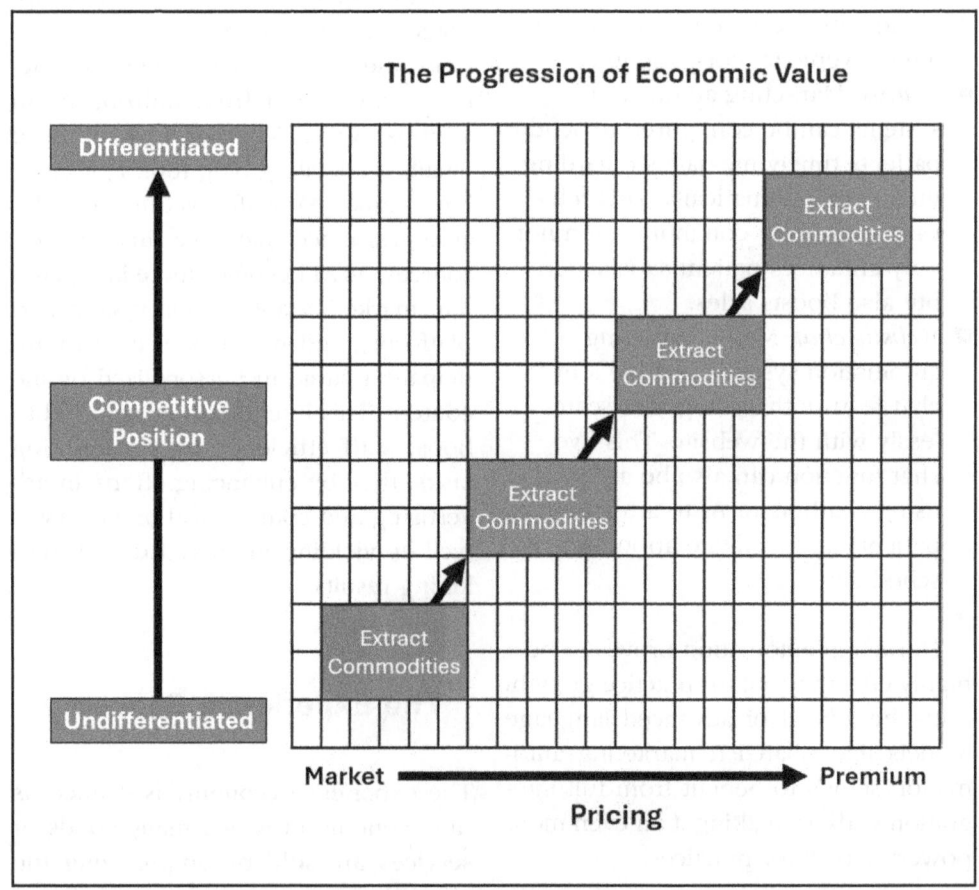

Figure 12–20. Economic value. *Source:* Adapted from Pine and Gilmore (1998).

- Transportation to and from the plane and landing zones.
- Insurance for the event.

It is the combination of all of those goods and services that results in an experience that is much more valuable than the simple sum of its parts.

The experience economy is a phenomenon since the 1990s where consumers recognize that there is more to life than just having stuff. The Internet has shown more people what is possible and how to do it. It has also shown that so many of our most valuable "things" are now freely available—music, movies, art, communication, education, and more. This concept could also be attributed to the longer hours most industries are adopting, now that everyone is accessible via their phones 24/7. Researchers have noted a trend that material goods are simply not as valued. That is why audiologists should think strategically and create meaningful (and memorable) patient experiences. As in the skydiving trip example, providers could break the patient experience in practices thusly:

- Appointment scheduling with the front desk professional.
- Parking and walking into the practice.
- Personal greeting from the front desk professional.
- Reception area wait time.
- Greeting by the audiologist.
- Case history and needs assessment.
- Hearing assessment.
- Explanation of results.
- Discussion of next steps.
- Closure of appointment, paying the bill.

When audiologists break down the patient's experience into a series of next steps, they can find methods to shape each "touchpoint" of the experience in a way that reflects their own personal brand.

Experiential Marketing

With knowledge of the experience economy and the progression of economic value, audiologists can create strategies that leverage experiential marketing. This is an innovative marketing concept that allows the consumer to experience the product before they take it home. For example, in the audiology practice, this would include a room that has the capability to project large images of a manufacturer's audio/video presentations that attempt to have the patient involved in the listening experience. These programs are readily available and can be utilized in conjunction with the mounted speakers and amplifiers to create a place where the patient can see and hear about products before they leave the practice.

Additionally, experiential marketing tactics include the use of memorabilia and themes. As the name implies, memorabilia are trinkets and tokens that can be given away to patients. They are intended to signify fond memories of the visit and create some positive emotions about their experience in the practice. Similarly, setting a theme for practice is a method to use a unifying concept to make the patient visit more memorable. For example, a memorable theme in an audiology practice would be the use of classic rock images and sounds anchoring the practice to fond memories of the 1950s to 1980s. Given the age of most patients seen in audiology practices, a classic rock theme using images and music is a way to conjure fond memories of the bygone past.

Summary

The aim of this chapter is to provide readers with an overview of all aspects of marketing and branding. No matter the scale and scope of the practice, no matter the location or target market, there are a few management core principles worthy of consideration. The most successful practices, those that have a sustainable business model with extremely happy and content employees and even happier, contented patients, implement the following four principles.

Have a Vision

A practice that clearly defines their mission and values is more likely to offer their community a unique service that stands apart from the competition. This process begins with the owner and other key stakeholders defining and defending a distinctive offering to the marketplace. This distinctive offering is likely to involve some combination of service delivery and professionalism that is attractive to a specific segment of the market. The function of marketing is matching a vision to a segment of the market that desires the practice's unique offering. This includes observing unfolding circumstances in a rapidly changing marketplace and possibly relying on some guidance and insights from independent consultants from outside the industry.

Create a Plan

Practices that take that vision and put into action with clear goals and priorities have a chance to stand out from the crowd. This requires the integration of information and respect for the culture of the clinic's organization. The function of a marketing plan is to ensure that the entire staff understands their role and responsibility for communicating the brand message and attracting patients to the practice.

Act, Even When Uncertain

The most thoughtful, meticulous plan is wasted if it is not put into action. The ability to take a specific course of action around a single initiative, focusing on that initiative until results are achieved, separates the cream of the crop from the mediocre. For many practitioners, it is relatively easy to set goals, but often there is not a thorough action plan. The most successful practices have the courage and discipline to see a plan through by taking a series of well-planned actions.

Measure Results and Modify Plans

Practices that carefully chose a handful of key metrics that are relevant for continuous improvement in both the patient care and financial part of business are often the most successful. In addition to utilizing just a few key metrics, data can be used to modify plans and actions to stay ahead of the competition and further fine-tune the day-to-day activities that define the business.

References

American Academy of Audiology. (2023). Code of Ethics. http://audiology.org

American Marketing Association. (2024). Definitions of marketing. https://www.ama.org/the-definition-of-marketing-what-is-marketing/

Beebe, M. (2023). Introducing the 4C Marketing Model and why you should follow it. Stevens & Tate Marketing Blog, https://stevens-tate.com/articles/introducing-the-4c-marketing-model-and-why-you-should-follow-it/

Carbone, L. (2004). *Clued in.* Pearson Education.

Carbone, L. (2016, July. *Creating an experience.* Workshop for Positioning Your Practice for Success, Unitron, New Orleans, LA.

Clarke, C., & Velasquez, V. (2024). Baby Boomer: Definition, age range, characteristics, and impact. Investopedia. https://www.investopedia.com/terms/b/baby_boomer.asp

D'Alessandro, D. (2001). *Brand warfare: 10 rules for building the killer brand.* McGrawHill.

Federal Trade Commission (FTC). (2017). CANSPAM Act: A compliance guide for business. https://www.ftc.gov/tipsadvice/businesscenter/guidance/canspamactcomplianceguidebusiness

Fengler, W. (2021). The silver economy is coming of age: A look at the growing spending power of seniors. Brookings. https://www.brookings.edu/articles/the-silver-economy-is-coming-of-age-a-look-at-the-growing-spending-power-of-seniors/

Getman, P. (2020). 7 reasons why brands matter to your consumers. https://tinybullyagency.com/7-reasons-why-brands-matter-to-your-consumers/

Kochkin, S. (2004). BHI physician program found to increase use of hearing healthcare. *Hearing Journal, 57*(8), 27–29.

Kochkin, S. (2009). MarketTrak VIII: 25--year trends in the hearing healthcare market. *Hearing Review, 16*(10), 11–19.

Kochkin, S. (2012). MarkeTrak VIII: The key influencing factors in hearing aid purchase intent. *Hearing Review, 19*(3), 12–25. http://www.betterhearing.org/sites/default/files/hearingpediaresources/MarkeTrak%20VIII%20The%20key%20influencing%20factors%20in%20hearing%20aid%20purchase%20intent.pdf

Kotler, P., & Keller, K. (2016). *Marketing management* (15th ed.). Pearson Prentice Hall.

Marsh, D. (2012, October). *Marketing to the mature marketplace.* Presentation to the Annual Convention of the Colorado Academy of Audiology, Vail, CO.

McCarthy, J. (1960). *Basic marketing: A managerial approach.* R.D. Irwin Co.

McClelland, D. C. (1973). Testing for competence rather than for "intelligence." *American Psychologist, 28*(1), 1–14.

McClelland, D. C. (1985). How motives, skills, and values determine what people do. *American Psychologist, 40,* 812–825.

McClelland, D. C. (1987). *Human motivation.* Cambridge University Press. https://psycnet.apa.org/record/1988-97516-000

McClelland, D. C. (1989). Motivational factors in health and disease. *American Psychologist, 44*(4), 675–683.

McKenna, A. (2024). Generation X demographic group. Britannica. https://www.britannica.com/topic/Generation-X

Nagle, T., Hogen, J., & Zale, J. (2011). *The strategy and tactics of pricing: A guide to growing more profitably* (5th ed.). Prentice Hall.

Neuroscience News. (2023). AI vs. human writing: Experts fooled almost 62% of the time. https://neurosciencenews.com/ai-human-writing-chatgpt-23892

OTC Act. (2017). S.670—Over-the-Counter Hearing Aid Act of 2017. United States Congress, Washington, DC. https://www.congress.gov/bill/115th-congress/senate-bill/670

Pelchen, L., & Allen. S. (2024). Internet use in 2024. Forbes Home. https://www.forbes.com/home-improvement/internet/internet-statistics/

Pew Research Center. (2014). Social Media Fact Center. https://www.pewresearch.org/internet/fact-sheet/social-media/?tabItem=4e4f05f3-58a4-4fc5-aab6-58b37a6dcb63

Pew Research Center. (2020). US Census Bureau estimates baby boomer population. https://www.pewresearch.org/short-reads/2020/04/28/millennials-overtake-baby-boomers-as-americas-largest-generation/#:~:text=Millennials%20have%20surpassed%20Baby%20Boomers,young%20immigrants%20expand%20its%20ranks

Pew Research Center. (2023, June 15). Audio and podcasting fact sheet. https://www.pewresearch.org/journalism/fact-sheet/audio-and-podcasting/

Pine, B. J., & Gilmore, J. (1998). Welcome to the experience economy. *Harvard Business Review*. https://hbr.org/1998/07/welcome-to-the-experience-economy

PRB. (2024). Just how many Baby Boomers are there? Population Reference Bureau. https://www.prb.org/resources/just-how-many-baby-boomers-are-there/

Rogers, E. (2003). *Diffusion of innovations* (5th ed.). Free Press/Simon & Shuster.

Romney, B. (2017, March). *Seven principles of effective marketing*. Presentation to One Retail Meeting, San Antonio, TX.

St. Clergy, K. (2013). Effective marketing: Developing and growing the practice. In R. Glaser & R. Traynor (Eds.), *Strategic practice management* (2nd ed.). Plural Publishing.

Staab, W. (1992). Sales promotion for office traffic control. In W. Staab (Ed.), *Applied hearing instrument marketing* (pp. 201–254). National Institute for Hearing Instrument Studies.

Statistica. (2024). Empowering people with data. Statistica. https://www.statista.com/statistics/309166/boomer-senior-social-networks/

Stat Counter. (2024). Search engine market share United States of America. https://gs.statcounter.com/search-engine-market-share/all/united-states-of-america

Traynor, R. (2019). Are you "clued-in" to offer the ultimate patient experience? *Hearing Review*, *26*(7), 25–27.

13 Fundamentals of Pricing Services and Products

Amyn M. Amlani, PhD, and
Robert M. Traynor, EdD, MBA

Introduction

In past editions of this text, the discussion of pricing in audiology practice has been comprehensive and comparable to other textbooks that present proven concepts and techniques across all types of businesses. As in several areas of audiology practice management, many traditional business concepts and techniques that apply to all general businesses are less ideal and pragmatic to audiology practices, while others must be discussed in greater detail. The topic of pricing falls into the category of heightened discussion, especially as it relates to the consumer who seeks audiology services.

Consumers of audiology services and products differ from the typical consumers who present themselves to other types of businesses. Due to their age, psychological readiness for services and products, and severity of their hearing issues, consumers in hearing healthcare are a special segment of the overall consumer population (Amlani, 2016). Consumers of audiology services and products are generally older individuals who are dealing with denial of their hearing problem and possess a distrust of professionals, hearing care clinics, and the products involved in the provision of the services. This segment of the population has lived long enough to understand the old Benjamin Franklin quote: "The bitterness of poor quality remains long after the sweetness of low price is forgotten."

Furthermore, the average consumer experiencing hearing difficulties is not familiar with audiologists—or the professional diagnostic and rehabilitative process—yet seeks interventions that restore their abilities to interact with family, friends, and their environment. The same consumers have, however, been predisposed to the uncompelling (and, sometimes, unethical) stories of not obtaining appropriate diagnostic or rehabilitative hearing care services and products. These and other factors require a special approach to pricing in audiology clinics to meet the needs of these special consumers. In pre-post, in-person, patient interactions with audiology providers, Amlani (2020) found that consumers expected *personal* hearing care service. Pricing decisions require audiologists to include the additional value of time-consuming, patient-centered interactions in their pricing. Amlani suggests that a pricing scheme should allow for adequate clinic time to consider not only a patient's hearing loss, age, and situation but also fundamental areas such as:

- Relationship building.
- An equal opportunity for patients to actively participate in their own hearing care treatment and management.
- Empathy when patients present their psychosocial concerns, especially when presented with a negative emotional stance.
- Family member input and participation as part of the overall hearing care treatment process.
- An acknowledgment of the consumer's emotional responses during the decision-making process to hearing cost options.
- Additional situational specific issues that arise during the treatment process.

It has been well established that, to patients, the price of hearing care *alone* is not the most important component in the process (Abrams & Kihm, 2015; Amlani, 2023; Amlani & De Silva, 2005; Picou, 2022). Since hearing care in an audiology setting provides value-added educational knowledge, experience, and clinical expertise, pricing must include the clinical costs for patient-centered hearing rehabilitation, as well as the cost of the bare products necessary to facilitate the process.

Business Basics

Price Elasticity

This chapter would be incomplete without a discussion on price sensitivity. *Price elasticity* (*E*) refers to how sensitive consumers are to changes in price and how their purchasing behavior is influenced by these changes (Amlani, 2009) and is mutually exclusive of the pricing orientation (i.e., business vs. consumer). Figure 13–1 represents a demand curve, with *price* (*P*) labeled along the *y*-axis and *quantity* (*Q*; i.e., units sold) labeled along the x-axis. In this figure, note that as *P* changes, there is a change in *Q*. For example, as *P* increases, there is a decrease in *Q*. Conversely, as *P* decreases, there is an increase in *Q*.

Next, there are two categories of classification with respect to price sensitivity. First, a service or product that is *not sensitive* to changes in price is termed *inelastic demand*, shown in Figure 13–2A. Panel A, on the left, shows a steep demand function (i.e., slope), where changes in price (*P1*), both increasing (*P2* relative to *P1*) or decreasing (*P3* relative to *P1*), yield small, incremental changes in quantity demanded (i.e., *Q1* relative to *Q2*, *Q1* relative to *Q3*).

Second, a service or product that is *sensitive* to changes in price is known to have an *elastic demand*, which is displayed in Figure 13–2B. Note that the demand function (i.e., slope) is flatter, where a change in price (*P1*), decreasing (*P3* relative to *P1*), yields a large, incremental change in quantity demanded (i.e., *Q1* relative to *Q3*).

Quantifying the sensitivity of price for a service or product is calculated as a

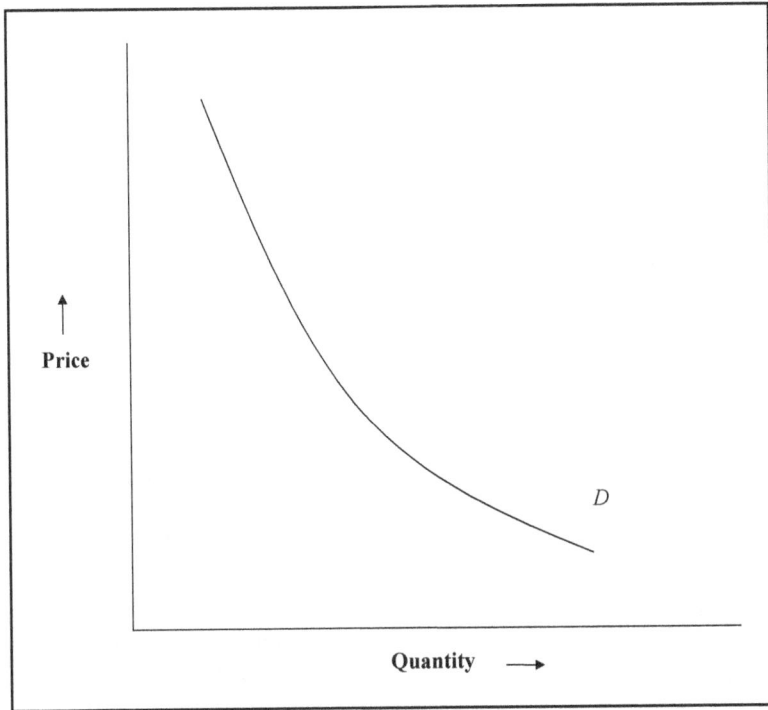

Figure 13–1. Relationship between price and quantity for a hypothetical demand function (D). *Source*: Amlani (2009).

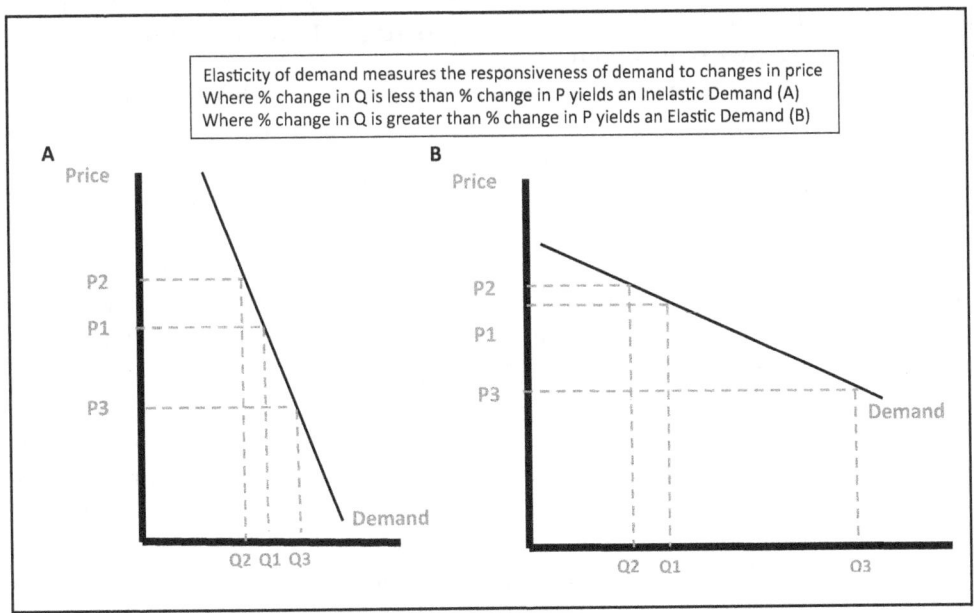

Figure 13–2. [Riley] Price elasticity of Demand. *Source*: Martin, F. (2016).

ratio of the percentage change in Q relative to the percentage change in P as expressed in the formula below:

$$\text{Price Elasticity of Demand } (E) = \frac{\% \text{ Change } Q}{\% \text{ Change } P}$$

The calculation for % Change Q is:

$$\frac{Q2 - Q1}{Qavg}$$

where $Q2 - Q1$ yields the difference between quantities at two points, and $Qavg$ is the average quantity between the same two points.

Similarly, the calculation for % Change P is

$$\frac{P2 - P1}{Pavg}$$

where $P2 - P1$ yields the difference between prices at two points, and $Pavg$ is the average price between the same two points.

The product of these calculations will yield a value (i.e., E), usually a negative number that is transformed to an absolute value. When the absolute value of E is $< |1|$, consumer demand is price insensitive (i.e., inelastic), meaning that changes in P will yield small, incremental changes in Q (i.e., units sold) of the service or product (i.e., Figure 13.2, Panel A). Conversely, when the absolute value of E is $> |1|$, consumer demand is price sensitive (i.e., elastic), meaning that changes in P will yield marked changes in Q (i.e., units sold) of the service or product (i.e., Figure 13.2, Panel B).

The demand function for the hearing aid industry is inelastic (Amlani, 2009, 2023; Amlani & De Silva, 2005). In other words, neither increasing nor decreasing price will grow nor reduce consumer demand. Instead, patient demand of service and product is dependent on universal availability—for example, the choice of over-the-counter (OTC) amplification products and remote care/telehealth, with the most important aspect being provider support.

Estimating Demand

There are two basic methods available for a business to measure the demand function. First, the demand function can be estimated retrospectively from historical records (i.e., price × quantity). Second, E can be estimated by sampling a group of consumers from the target market and polling them about different P and Q relationships.

Relationship Between Demand and Total Gross Revenue

Total gross (i.e., sales only) revenue (R) is calculated using:

$$R = P \times Q$$

where P represents price, and Q denotes quantity demanded. The reader should note that total revenue is impacted by the demand function E.

From a business standpoint, realizing the sensitivity of the local market demand plays a crucial role in gross revenue generation and, ultimately, profitability. Knowing the price elasticity for a specific type of service or product, the practitioner can arrive at an intelligent decision of how to price these services or products and when and how pricing changes will influence demand. In general, increasing R in an elastic market requires decreasing P, while increasing R in an inelastic market requires increasing P (for detailed examples, see Amlani, 2009). The latter statement is of importance to many practices that reduce or discount the price of lower-priced products. Given that lower-priced products tend to have an inelastic demand, reducing P does not yield marked increases in R. On the flip side, higher-priced products tend to have an elastic demand, and price reductions and discounts for these products will yield an increase in R.

Gross and Net Profit

According to Silbiger (2024), *gross* profit and *net* profit are two key financial metrics used to evaluate a practice's profitability, but they represent different stages in the profit calculation process. Gross profit is the amount the practice earns after subtracting the cost of goods (i.e., a category of expenses) from the total revenue (i.e., sales) generated.[1] In audiology practice, the costs of goods calculation will include expenses related to product acquisition costs and supplies, such as hearing aids, batteries, and assistive listening devices. Gross profit is calculated as:

$$\text{Revenue} - \text{Cost of Goods Sold (COGS)}$$

In business, this calculation indicates how efficiently a company is selling its services and products. It helps to assess the core profitability of a company's services and products before accounting for operating expenses (e.g., rent, utilities, and salaries), taxes, and other costs. For example, if Practice A has $1,000,000 in sales revenue (from services and products) and the cost of goods is $600,000, the *gross* profit yields $400,000.

Net profit, also known as net income or bottom line, which is the amount of money left after *all expenses* have been subtracted from total revenue, contrasts with gross profit. Net profit is calculated as:

$$\text{Gross Profit} - \\ \text{(Total Expenses + Interest + Taxes)}$$

Net profit is the overall measure of a practice's profitability and is a key indicator of overall financial health. Net profit is often used to determine profitability ratios, as well as assess company performance and reinvestment (Chapter 11).

Pricing

Pricing is one component of the marketing mix, a framework proposed by McCarthy (1960) that also includes three additional elements: place, product, and promotion (Chapter 12). Nagle et al. (2024) indicate that in a properly constructed pricing system, the last three elements of the marketing mix comprise a practice's effort to *create value*, while pricing equates to the *revenue* (i.e., money remaining after expenses have been subtracted) earned by the

---

[1]Gross revenue and gross profit are different terms. Gross revenue is the total amount of sales (i.e., revenue) generated by the business only. Gross profit is the difference between gross revenue and the cost of goods sold (COGS).

clinic from incorporating the value-added service component to the pricing structure. They conclude that if effective place, product, and promotion *sow the seeds* of business success, pricing can be considered the *harvest*. This "harvest" is essential to the financial success of any business. Thus, in a financially successful (i.e., high revenue yielding) audiological practice, clinical services promote the value-added elements of *product, promotion, and place*, while *price* signifies the threshold for the audiological services and products offered by the practice. A patient is only willing to engage in exchanging funds for services and products when their perceived value of what is being received is equal to or greater than price. The remainder of this chapter is dedicated solely to the topic of pricing.

Business-Oriented Pricing Strategies

The type of pricing strategy employed by a business must be consistent with its goals (i.e., generating sales that yield market share through high adoption rates and sustainable profitability). The pricing objective also reflects the practice's marketing, financial, strategic, and product goals, as well as the patient's expectations. Business-oriented pricing strategies are common in most audiology practices whose revenue emanates predominately from the sale of a product, namely, hearing aids. This model is depicted in Figure 13–3A.

There are several business-oriented strategies available (Kotler & Keller, 2016; Nagle et al., 2024), four of which are summarized below:

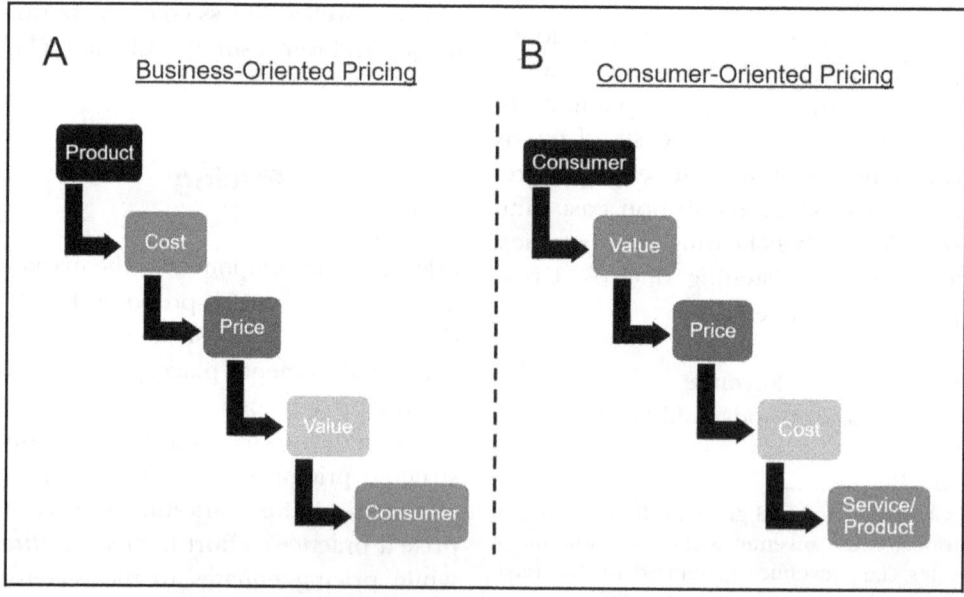

Figure 13–3. Business-oriented versus consumer-oriented pricing. *Source*: Adapted from Nagle et al. (2023).

- *Market skimming pricing.* Market skimming pricing is a strategy employed to maximize revenue (i.e., gross sales) from consumers who are less sensitive to price changes (i.e., inelastic demand) and are typically early adopters or affluent consumers. This concept assists the practice in the recovery of various expensive equipment costs, personnel, and other procedure offerings that are new to the market. This is commonly seen in the technology sector, where advanced services and products—such as balance and electrophysiology testing, or a new premium-tier hearing device—are initially sold for a high price. Market skimming offers high profit margins, recovers practice development expenses quickly, and, in affluent neighborhoods, can establish a practice with a premium brand image.

- *Market penetration pricing.* Market penetration pricing is levied when a business intends to build a strong customer base, discourage competition, and achieve economies of scale. This may be exemplified in audiology practice by offering alternative solutions (e.g., OTC products) that complement prescription products. A penetration strategy typically offers rapid adoption of the practice offerings while discouraging competitors from entering the market, increases brand awareness, and attracts consumers on a budget. This strategy is profitable (i.e., gross revenue minus operating expenses) *only* with a high volume of sales.

- *Neutral pricing.* The neutral pricing strategy is used in mature markets where competition is intense,

and price sensitivity is high in the market segment. The focus of this strategy is on differentiating services or products offered by a business through other means, such as quality or brand reputation. Profitability and success in this model are dependent on value-added product procedures and follow-up services. An added benefit of the neutral strategy is that once a business has matured, that business can maintain market stability by avoiding price wars with competitors. A limitation of this model is that it may be difficult for a business in a highly price-sensitive market to stand out as the market leader among the competition.

- *Cost-based pricing.* Cost-based pricing—formerly termed cost-plus pricing—is presented in Figure 13–3A. At first glance, the model offers an appearance of financial prudence (Nagle et al., 2024). Financial prudence is achieved by pricing every service or product to yield a fair return (i.e., revenue) relative to the overall fixed and incremental costs required to operate the business. Here, a business simply adds up the total cost of obtaining an item and tacks on a markup for its profit (i.e., revenue minus expenses), and the result is the final selling price. For example, a product that costs the business $1.00 (wholesale) to acquire and is marked up a weighting of 2.5 times would retail for $2.50. The cost-based pricing model works best—for both the practice and the consumer—when the local market is saturated with this strategy (Hart, 2021).

Consumer-Oriented Pricing Strategy

The reader will note that Figure 13–3B differs by 180 degrees from Figure 13–3A. The difference is a shift in priorities where Panel B prices, services, and products are based on consumer needs (i.e., value based), while Panel A is focused only on the sale of a product (i.e., profit based). The value-based strategy was founded on creating a relationship between the consumer and the business through *empathy, trust, and the valuation of treatment intervention* received with respect to the needs of the consumer. Here, the business focus is on delivering value to both returning consumers and those consumers entering the market for the first time. The current U.S. healthcare system has reformed, now concentrating on the principle of delivering value-based care—that is, focused on the needs of the consumer through an emphasis on quality of care, provider performance, and patient experience (Porter, 2010).

Amlani (2019) wrote, "Pricing objectives that do not pay attention to consumer needs and perspective are not a reliable long-term strategy. Consumer needs and values are constantly changing, and a business' pricing objective must be able to adapt to those changes to maximize revenue and profitability. In most cases, the business-oriented pricing strategies do not reach their potential annual revenue goals." The cogency of these statements is depicted in Figure 13–4, where consumer-oriented elements (left side) show higher revenue (i.e., height of the respective bars) compared to business-oriented elements (right side). The effect of this figure is termed the *value cascade* that highlights

a strategic approach known as value management. Value management provides businesses with outcomes and actions related to the evaluation and pricing of services and products. Nagle and colleagues (2024) remind the reader that price is linked to marketing through the creation of strategies of business goals, buyer personas, competitor differentiation, and value proposition that drive growth and, ultimately, profitability. The remainder of this chapter is devoted to assessing each stage of the value cascade shown in Figure 13–4.

Potential Value

Value management begins with the concept of potential value (left-most bar in Figure 13–4). In this initial stage, valuation for a service or product stems from brand recognition. To the consumer, brand recognition portrays the optimal functional, emotional, and psychological benefit, utility, and worth that the service or product can deliver in meeting their needs. Premium brand recognition service offerings and product offerings command high prices. Service offering examples include Ritz Carlton and Disney, and product offering examples include Golden Goose and Chanel.

Actual Value

A business's ability to deliver potential value is influenced by consumer behavior traits, such as personal preferences, purchasing power, functionality, and cultural and social acceptance. The outcome from the consumer behavior traits lead to actual value, and the relative difference to potential value is termed the

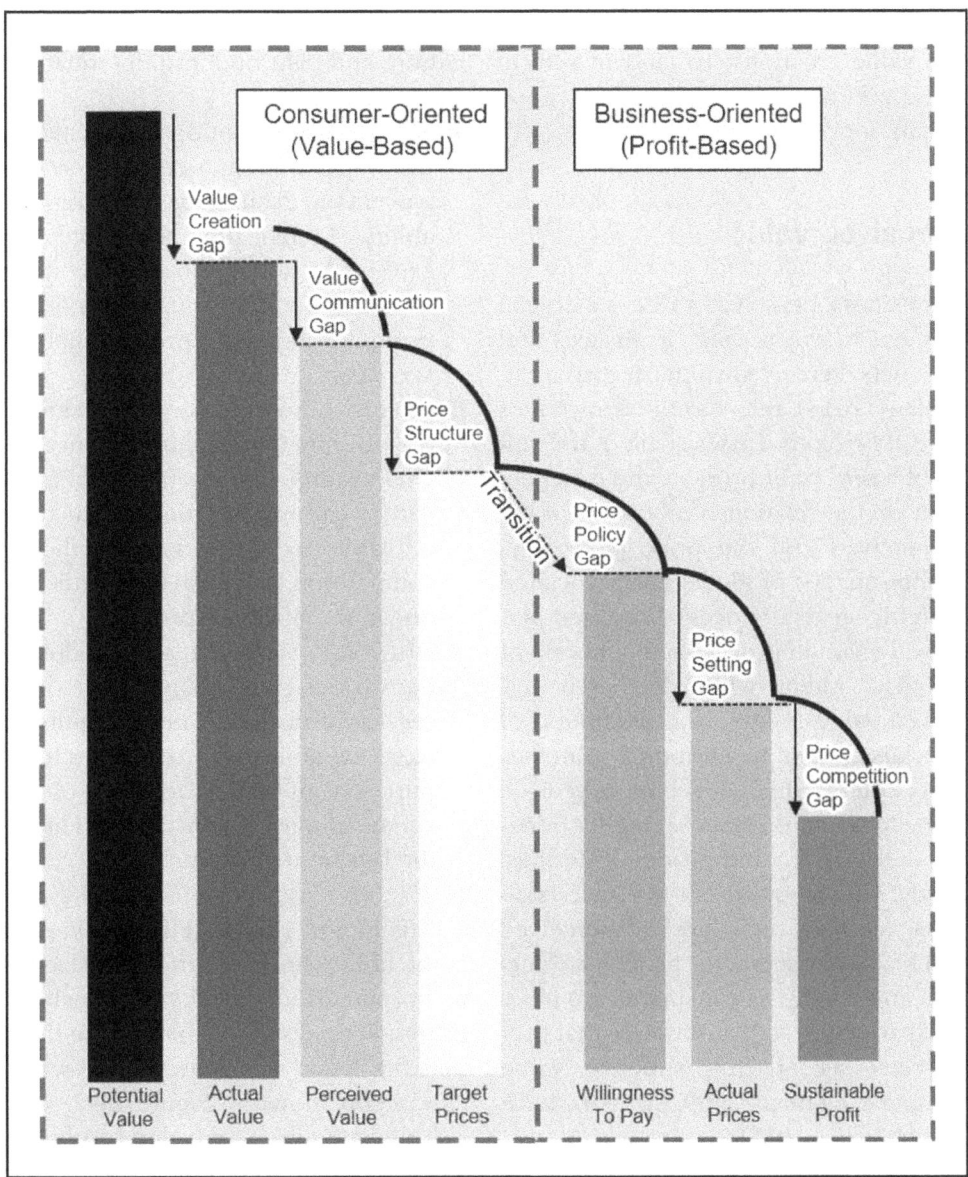

Figure 13–4. Value cascade. *Source*: Adapted from Nagle et al. (2023).

value creation gap (second left-most bar in Figure 13–4).

In business, actual value occurs organically, as exemplified by ease of use, effectiveness, speed, reliability, style, and the décor and demeanor of the office staff and practitioner during a clinical experience (Carbone, 2004). Shand

(2023) indicated actual value increases when consumers create a relationship with their providers. In addition, Preminger (2018) found that providers who took the time to listen to their patient's hearing healthcare needs were rewarded with increased trust by the patient. Enhancing the patient's experience through exemplary care will narrow (i.e., reduce) the value creation gap, and in return, these efforts generate a higher revenue stream for the business.

Perceived Value

In business, perceived value is a crucial element in the pricing of services and products. Perceived value, according to Amlani (2013), refers to the consumer's overall *perceptual* assessment of the utility of a service or product and is dependent on the relationship between what is received and the price paid (e.g., higher-quality products are associated with higher retail prices). Increased perceived value improves the likelihood of purchase intent, while decreased perceived value reduces the likelihood of purchase intent. In addition, businesses that foster a high level of perceived value to consumers can set higher prices for their service and product offerings. Lastly, the literature shows that businesses with a high level of perceived value also boast greater patient satisfaction and loyalty, as consumers are more likely to return to that business that they perceive as offering superior value (Gagné & Jennings, 2009; Kochkin, 2007; Valente et al., 2000).

This perception of value is influenced by various factors, including brand reputation, bare product features and benefits, quality, consumer experience, and marketing communications. *Differentiated offering* is one means by which to enhance perception. Here, a business develops a marketing strategy that encourages consumers to select their service or product over a similar service or product offered by competitor. There are several ways to differentiate, including service differentiation, product differentiation, and distribution differentiation.

■ Service differentiation can include the way the business offers assistance. One example is the availability of telehealth and remote care professional services to consumers when the competition only promotes in-person professional services.

■ Product differentiation can include the offering of a unique product. One example is the offering of a daily wear amplification product available to consumers when the competition only provides traditional amplification products.

■ Distribution differentiation includes the various channels in which a service or product can be acquired (e.g., the ability of a consumer to purchase an OTC hearing aid online versus in-person consumption at the business's location).

A common challenge for businesses is the ability to *communicate* these yet to be perceived benefits. The inability or unwillingness to communicate these benefits lends to the *value communication gap* shown in Figure 13–2.

The communication value gap is also influenced by the consumer's perception toward price. Research indicates that consumers do not evaluate price logically. Instead, consumers' perceptions of price are irrational and influenced by a variety of psychological factors, such as context, framing, price anchoring, and emotion rather than logical reasoning. These psychological factors are further confounded when one considers that hearing care is obfuscated by the perception of aging and the stigma related to hearing loss. Amlani (2020) further reports that patient readiness in seeking audiological rehabilitation was influenced negatively by the provider's behavior during a standard clinical evaluation.

Target Prices

Once a business has developed and communicated the appropriate communication of its services and products (i.e., perceived value), the next stage in the value cascade model is to establish target prices (white bar under the consumer-oriented strategy in Figure 13–4). The objective at this stage is to determine the price of a service or product that captures the maximum share in sales volume (the number of services or products sold).

Target pricing is determined using one of the business-oriented pricing approaches, based on competitive market research or, preferably, determined through data obtained during focus groups. Once the business determines the price of the service or product, the business then applies costs (e.g., cost of goods [COGS], operating, variable) to ensure profitability. The advantages of target pricing include:

- Market sensitivity to consumer behavior.
- Increased profitability through salient pricing determination.
- Understanding of resource and operational allocation as it relates to profitability.

The limitations of target pricing include the assumptions that:

- Pricing meets consumer perceived value (i.e., price structure gap shown in Figure 13–4).
- The demand of services or product is accurate.

In hearing healthcare, target pricing structures differ between consumers who pay privately versus consumers who are beneficiaries of insured contractual rates or third-party funding agencies. For the latter (i.e., insurance, third-party payer), the business has little, if any, ability to modify target pricing. Most third-party programs currently available constrict the business's potential value-added and differentiating service offerings by limiting the degree and frequency of professional services available to the consumer and through a limited offering of product options and types of technology.

Private Pay Segment

The remainder of the discussion in this section is directed toward the private pay segment. Consumers are heterogeneous when it comes to their purchasing behaviors and their perceptions toward a business, despite attempts demonstrated by the business to showcase perceived value (Kotler & Keller, 2016; Nagle et al., 2024). Given this variability in consumer behavior, it behooves a business to offer multiple pricing options. Figure 13–5 is an example of variable pricing segments for prescriptive and OTC amplification products. In this example, OTC devices— which are offered without value-added professional services—are priced less than prescription devices. In addition, it is worth noting that within prescription devices, pricing varies as a function of technology tiers.

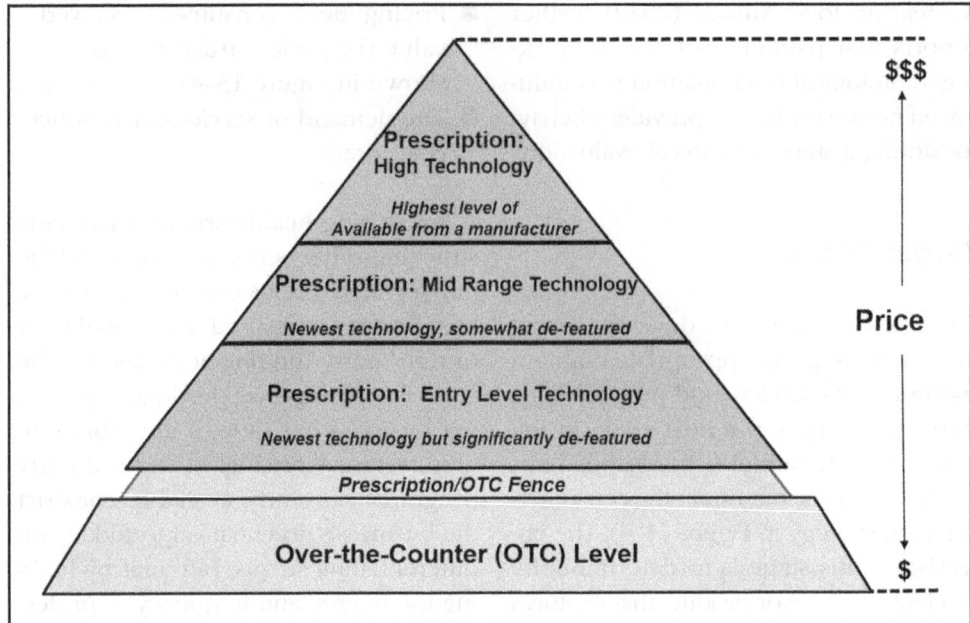

Figure 13–5. Price segments for prescriptive and over-the-counter (OTC) amplification products.

The rationale for a targeted pricing tiered system is illustrated in Figure 13–6. Panel A represents a scenario where a business offers only a single-tier pricing system. In this example, of the 100 people who sought out services or products from this business, only 50 individuals moved forward with the purchase while the other 50 individuals sought services and products elsewhere in the market. The reason for the low acquisition rate (i.e., 50%) stemmed from the business failing to meet the varying value perceptions of all consumers in this segment.

Panel B in Figure 13–6 offers consumers various tier options. From Panel A, we know that a single-tiered pricing strategy results in 50% acquisition of services or products. The addition of a second pricing tier increases consumer acquisition by 20%, and the addition of a third pricing tier increases consumer acqui-

sition by an additional 10%. In other words, a two-tiered system can result in as many as 70 individuals (out of a possible 100) consuming services or products, and that number increases to as many as 80 individuals (out of a possible 100) consuming services or products. Clearly, establishing a tiered, or fenced, system is important to ensuring revenue based on consumer perceived value.

Willingness to Pay

The objective for value-based pricing in the consumer-oriented pricing approach is grounded in the assumption that a consumer's relative willingness-to-pay (WTP) for one service or product versus another closely aligns with differences in the relative value of those services or products (Nagle et al., 2024). WTP rep-

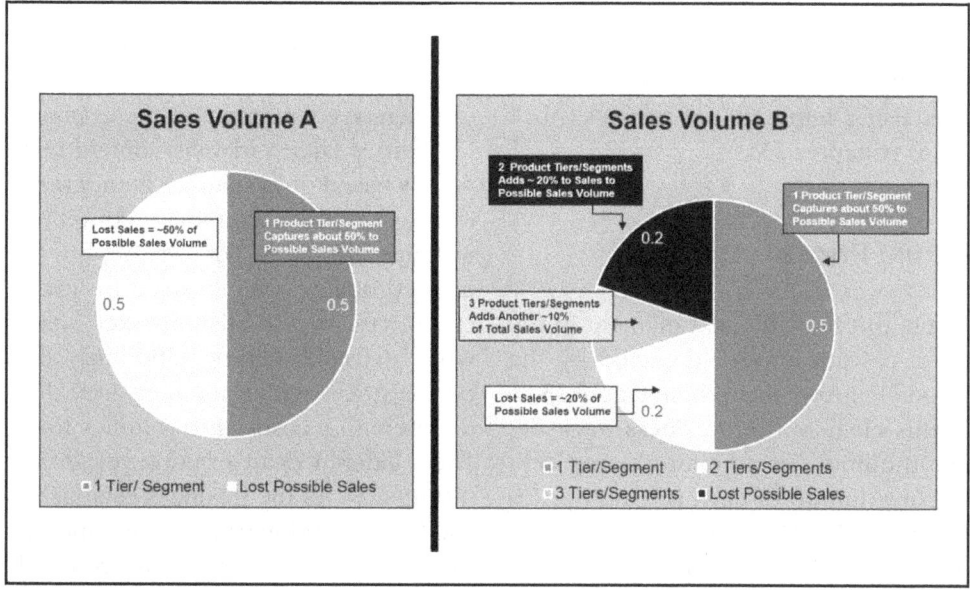

Figure 13–6. Effect of pricing tiers/segments on total sales (Kotler & Keller, 2016; Nagle et al., 2023).

resents the maximum amount of money consumers are willing to spend in exchange for a service or product based on its perceived value. Differences in target prices versus WTP result in a *price policy gap*, as shown in Figure 13–4.

A consumer's WTP is influenced by how the service or product, or both, is presented. The most common method of presenting perceived value is the bundled pricing approach. Here, the consumer is presented a total price that encompasses all of the services and products being purchased. Smith (2012) states that *price bundling* is a concept that benefits from the heterogeneity of demand. Specifically, bundled pricing posits that when there is consumer demand for two or more separate products, combining them into a single unit increases the added value and benefit of the purchase. Examples of the bundled approach include bundled fast-food meals,

automobiles, and all-inclusive travel packages. The bundled approach has been historically the most popular pricing system for hearing care services, in part, because of the lack of reimbursement provided to providers for rehabilitative services and technology sales.

Itemized, or unbundled, pricing is another method of conveying perceived value to the consumer. Itemized pricing is predicated on either providing the consumer with individual pricing for each service and product or providing packaged pricing for each set of services or products (Chapter 14). To date, this pricing strategy is preferred by consumers in the hearing care space because of the transparency it provides with respect to the perceived value it provides with respect to services rendered separately from the cost of the product (Amlani, 2013). At the provider level, however, this model has yet to be implemented on a national scale, despite the fact that insurance and third-party coding and reimbursement require that claims be filled using itemization of services (Abel, 2024) (Chapter 17).

Actual Prices

Actual prices is the next element in the value cascade model, depicted by the second bar from the right in Figure 13–4. In this element, the business must define the floor (i.e., minimum) and ceiling (maximum) of each pricing tier (in Figure 13–5). Much of these data will have been collected during the element phase of target prices. During the actual prices phase, the business must consider:

- Is the price point consistent with the clinic's overall practice marketing strategy?
- What are the nonvalue determinates of price sensitivity? This considers factors that influence how sensitive consumers are to changes in price, independent of the actual value or utility they perceive from the product or service.
- What are the *price-volume trade-offs* and the impact on profitability? Price-volume trade-offs refer to the relationship between the price of the value-added product and the volume of sales, and how changes in price can affect overall profitability. Understanding this trade-off is crucial as setting the right price is key to maximizing profits while maintaining or increasing sales volume.

At the end of the actual prices phase, prices generated (i.e., minimum, maxi-

mum) will reflect the value differences and maximize profitability within each pricing tier (in Figure 13–5). These values can then be communicated to consumers.

There is large variability among businesses based on consumer demographics, geographic economics, and business maturity phase. For instance, a newly opened business might need to undercut prices to establish market share, while an established operation may simply set prices within the tiers according to operating costs and volume goals. These differences are examples of a *price-setting gap*. As the business establishes itself in its local market, pricing modifications will be necessary for profitability purpose (i.e., narrow the price-setting gap). Any changes to prices must be communicated to the market.

Sustainable Profit

On the business side, there is a clinical cost per hour associated with treating patients that must be exceeded to remain profitable. This process involves determining the hourly rate for the clinic expenses, which is obtained by reviewing the total expenses for the previous year or, for startup clinics, an estimation of this expense. In an itemized system, the next step is to apply this rate to each of the services offered in the clinic, taking into consideration *the amount of time* it usually takes to perform this service. In Chapter 14, Sjoblad uses $200.00 per hour as an example, which converts each 15-minute interval to generate a $50.00 cost factor in an itemized pricing system seeing a walk-in patient for a 30-minute hearing aid check, and it would be necessary to collect at least $100.00 for that appointment. Thus, in either a bundled pricing scheme or itemization, *considering the amount of time a procedure takes is the first step in determining fees.* It is also important to realize this exercise in setting fees should be revisited annually, as overall clinic expenses and costs of goods to the practice change over time. Reviewing the hourly expense rate and reestablishing updated fee schedules on a regular basis will facilitate meeting the annual operating expenses and profit goals of the clinic.

It is likely ethical and reasonable to itemize each and every product, such as the audiologic evaluation, fitting, programming, and one to two follow-up visits. The bundled approach has, historically, been more accepted by both clinics and patients. At this writing, however, itemizing is beginning to catch on in many practices. With the possible changes that will come with the proposed practitioner status for audiologists, these changes may be essential. Whatever the clinical decision for bundling versus itemization, it is necessary to incorporate the concept into the overall pricing strategy and communicate the prices effectively to patients. The implementation and results of a contemporary program using an itemized structure are presented in Chapter 14, and the case for itemization is offered in Chapter 17.

Competition Pricing

Competition pricing is when practitioners lower their prices to gain market share with the idea that the increased volume in sales will offset the lowered prices. Lightspeed (2024) holds that prices should be lowered only when they are no longer justified by the value offered, in comparison to the value offered by the competition. Since a price cut can be so easily matched by the competition, it offers only a short-term competitive advantage at the expense of permanently lower margins. Additionally, price reductions result in reduced revenue (i.e., see Price Elasticity section of this chapter) and reduced value perception of business. Lowering prices is not a long-term solution to profitability.

Summary

Pricing in any business is a complex and critical aspect that impacts both the financial health of the practice and patient satisfaction. The pricing strategy must balance the need for profitability with accessibility and perceived value, while also navigating industry-specific challenges such as regulatory constraints, competition, and the high cost of service and products. General considerations for pricing include:

■ *Cost structure.* Consider the costs associated with providing services, including the cost of hearing devices and the value-added services provided to the patients. In setting prices, all costs must be considered, including the cost per hour of clinical services, which include diagnostic equipment, staff salaries, office overhead, and ongoing training. Pricing should cover these costs while allowing for a reasonable profit margin.

■ *Market demand and patient demographics.* The demand for services can vary based on factors such as the local population's age, income levels, and awareness of hearing care. Practices must tailor their pricing to the demographic and economic conditions of their specific market.

■ *Value perception.* Patients often perceive the value of services based on the effectiveness of the products, the quality of care, and overall experience. Communicating the benefits of professional care, such as improved quality of life and long-term hearing health, can justify higher prices and reduce price sensitivity.

■ *Competitive landscape.* Each business must consider the pricing strategies of competitors, including both local practices and larger retail chains. Offering differentiated services, such as personalized care, advanced technology, or itemized services, can assist in justifying premium pricing.

■ *Regulatory and ethical considerations.* Pricing is also influenced by ethical guidelines, particularly concerning transparency and fairness. Practices must ensure their pricing structures comply with legal standards and avoid practices like price gouging or misleading promotions.

■ *Tiered pricing.* Tiered pricing offers different levels of service or product features at varying price points, catering to different budget levels.

■ *Perceived fairness and trust.* The perception of pricing fairness is critical in maintaining consumer trust. Transparent pricing policies, where patients clearly understand what they are paying for and why, can enhance trust and satisfaction.

■ *Long-term relationship focus.* Every business must build long-term relationships with patients.

References

Abel, D. (2024, June). *Coding and reimbursement lecture.* Presented at the University of Arkansas for Medical Sciences, Little Rock.

Abrams, H., & Kihm, J. (2015). An introduction to Marketrak IX: A baseline for the hearing aid market. *Hearing Review, 22*(6), 16.

Amlani, A. M. (2009). It's not immoral to increase hearing aid prices in an inelastic market. *Hearing Review, 16*(1), 12, 14, 16. https://hearingreview.com/practice-build ing/marketing/its-not-immoral-to-increase -hearing-aid-prices-in-an-inelastic-market

Amlani, A. M. (2013). Influence of perceived value on hearing aid adoption and re-adoption intent. *Hearing Review Products, 20*(3), 8–12.

Amlani, A. M. (2016). Application of the consumer decision-making model in assessing hearing aid adoption intent in first-time users. *Seminars in Hearing, 37*(2), 103–119.

Amlani, A. M. (2019). Pricing strategies in audiology practice. In B. Taylor (Ed.), *Audiology practice management* (3rd ed., pp. 215–227). Thieme Medical Publishers.

Amlani, A. M. (2020). Influence of provider interaction on patient's need recognition towards audiological services and technology. *Journal of the American Academy of Audiology, 31*(5), 342–353.

Amlani, A. M. (2023, May 8). Audiology economics. Audiology Online: 20Q with Gus Mueller https://www.audiologyonline

.com/articles/20q-audiology-economics-28543

Amlani, A. M., & De Silva, D. G. (2005). Effect of economy and FDA intervention on the hearing aid industry. *American Journal of Audiology, 14*(1), 71–79.

Carbone, L. (2004). *Clued in: How to keep customers coming back again and again.* UPearson, Education.

Gagné, J. P., & Jennings, M. B. (2009). Factors influencing the perception of hearing aid benefit among older adults. *International Journal of Audiology, 48*(7), 399–407.

Hart, M. (2021). Cost-plus pricing: What it is and when to use it. https://blog.hubspot.com/sales/cost-plus-pricing

Kochkin, S. (2007). MarkeTrak VII: Obstacles to adult non-user adoption of hearing aids. *The Hearing Journal, 60*(4), 27–43.

Kotler, P. (2001). *Framework for marketing management.* Pearson Education Company.

Kotler, P., & Keller, K. (2016). *Marketing management* (15th ed.). Pearson Prentice Hall.

Lightspeed, J. (2024). Strategic pricing: When to lower prices in competitive markets. *Journal of Business Strategy, 58*(1), 34–47.

McCarthy, E. J. (1960). *Basic marketing: A managerial approach.* Richard D. Irwin.

Martin, F. (2016). [Riley] Price elasticity of demand. Slideshare. https://www.slideshare.net/slideshow/price-elascity-of-demand/69818778

Nagle, T., Hogan, J., & Zale, J. (2011). *The strategy and tactics of pricing* (5th ed.). Prentice Hall.

Nagle, T., Mueller, G., & Gruyaert, E. (2023). *The strategy and tactics of pricing* (7th ed.). Routledge, Taylor & Francis Group.

Picou, E. (2022). Hearing aid benefit and satisfaction results from the MarkeTrak 2022 survey: Applications of features and hearing care professionals. *Seminars in Hearing, 43*, 301–316.

Porter, M. (1998). *Competitive strategy.* Free Press. (Original work published 1980.)

Porter, M. (2008). *On competition.* Harvard Business Press.

Porter, M. (2010). What is value in health care? *New England Journal of Medicine, 363*(26), 2477–2481.

Preminger, J. (2018). Building trust and improving outcomes with family-centered hearing care. *ASHA Leader.* https://leader.pubs.asha.org/doi/10.1044/leader.OV.23012018.28

Shand, A. B. (2023). Core values in healthcare branding: The foundation of patient trust. *Journal of Healthcare Management, 45*(2), 123–134.

Silbiger, S. (2024). *The 10-day MBA, 5th edition: A step-by-step guide to mastering the skills taught in America's top business schools.* Harper Collins.

Smith, T. (2012). *Pricing strategy.* South-Western Cengage Learning.

Valente, M., Abrams, H., & Benson, D. (2000). *Audiology: Diagnosis, treatment strategies, and practice management.* Thieme Medical Publishers.

14 Itemizing Hearing Care in a University Clinic

Stephanie J. Sjoblad, AuD

Introduction

The profession of audiology has seen rapid changes in technology and new market distribution channels for hearing aids over the past several years. Over-the-counter (OTC) devices have been appearing online and in retail outlets. Developers of these new distribution channels often suggest the role of the audiologist is not necessary. These changes were driven in part by the President's Council of Advisors on Science and Technology (PCAST) report suggesting several recommendations for changes the federal government should make in the hopes it would decrease the cost of hearing aids, incentivize technology innovation, and provide more consumer choice when it comes to hearing care (PCAST, 2015). The National Academies of Science, Engineering, and Medicine issued 12 recommendations in their report "Hearing Health Care for Adults: Priorities for Improving Access and Affordability" (NASEM, 2016). One of the recommendations was that hearing healthcare professionals should improve transparency in their fee structure by *clearly itemizing the prices of technologies and related professional services* to enable consumers to make more informed decisions. These recommendations from the na-

tional level have brought more attention to the profession of audiology and are compelling a change in billing practices as the aim is to help make hearing care more accessible and affordable while keeping clinic doors open. This chapter was written to provide guidance to the audiologist regarding how to itemize professional hearing care services.

Definitions

When thinking about hearing aid pricing, for decades, the common practice has been to provide a bundled pricing structure. The hearing aids and all services to properly fit the devices, including follow-up in the future, were in one price, usually paid upfront. There is a growing trend of practices moving to unbundled billing models, especially more seasoned providers (Emanuel & Wince, 2024). Audiologists who offer more transparency in pricing should be competitive with online venues and big-box stores while ensuring that costs are being covered. To unbundle is to separate the charges for related products or services usually offered as a package (Dictionary.com, 2024a). While there are many benefits to unbundling, the most important is giving the patient the opportunity to

491

understand all facets of the hearing aid delivery process. In some instances, a bundled model may still make more sense, but there would still be an advantage to helping the patients understand what items make up the total fee. A term that may be preferable is to *itemize billing*. To itemize is to state by items, give the particulars, or list the individual units of the parts (Dictionary.com, 2024b).

Calculating the Hourly Rate and Assigning Fees on the Superbill

The most important part of the process of moving to an itemized billing model is to understand what it costs to run a clinic. The hourly rate of a fellow colleague or competitor down the street is not as important as what it costs to run a practice. Over the years, many audiologists have inquired what their fees should be and want to know what others are using for an hourly rate. If the practice does not calculate the rates and expenses for the practice, there is the risk of not covering costs (Chapter 13). Therefore, the first step in moving to an unbundled or itemized billing model is to determine what it costs per hour to keep the doors open. The breakeven hourly rate is the cost per hour that must be brought in to cover the fixed costs of the business. Once the hourly rate is determined, one can then create a superbill, utilizing existing Current Procedural Terminology (CPT) codes and Health Care Current Procedure Coding System (HCPCS) codes to set up a fee schedule (Chapters 16 and 17). An appropriate fee schedule cannot be created if the cost of doing business is unknown. Throughout this chapter, there are references to some of the most current codes that are relevant for the delivery of hearing care services.

In 2012, the American Academy of Audiology conducted a Hearing Aid Billing Practices Survey. In this survey, it was revealed that *less than half (49%)* of

---

CALCULATING THE COST OF DOING BUSINESS

The process of calculating the cost of doing business is straightforward if you have access to the clinic profit and loss statements (Foltner, 2009) (Chapter 11).

1. Determine the number of annual contact hours (Figure 14–1):
   - Determine how many hours per week one can see/bill patients. Keep in mind that even if a practice is open 40 hours per week, one must consider the time that is related to direct patient contact in determining this number.

continued on next page

continued from previous page

Determine how many hours (annually) you can bill for services provided

Patient contact hours per week: 30 hours

Number of weeks worked per year: 48 weeks

Number of providers: 2 providers

30 x 48 x 2 = 2880

Figure 14–1. Figuring out the breakeven hourly rate.

- Calculate the number of weeks per year that one actually sees patients (factor in vacation, holidays, sick days, and professional leave).
- Determine the number of providers in the practice.
- Multiply the hours per week by weeks per year by the number of providers.
2. Analyze the operating costs for the practice. Ideally, this would be broken down into several different expense categories, including:
   - Personnel (salary/benefits)
   - Clinic expenses (rent, utilities, phone, advertising, etc.)
   - Cost of goods (all things you buy for resale)
3. Calculate the breakeven hourly rate (Figure 14–2).
   - Subtract the cost of goods from total annual clinic expenses, and divide the remaining amount by the "annual contact hours" established in Step 1.
   - This is the breakeven hourly rate.
4. Add in desired profit (Figure 14–3).
   - Take annual expenses less cost of goods, add desired profit, and divide this number by the annual contact hours.
   - This is the hourly rate including the desired profit.

continued on next page

continued from previous page

$$\frac{\text{Annual Expenses}}{\text{Annual Contact Hours}} = \text{Hourly Rate}$$

UNBUNDLED MODEL (excludes Cost of Goods)

$$\frac{\$XXX,XXX.XX}{2880} = \$XXX.XX$$

Figure 14–2. Calculating the breakeven rate, excluding the cost of goods.

$$\frac{\text{Annual Expenses + Desired Profit}}{\text{Annual Contact Hours}} = \text{Hourly Rate}$$

Desired Profit (SAMPLE) = \$50,000

UNBUNDLED MODEL (excludes Cost of Goods)

$$\frac{\$XXX,XXX.XX + \$50,000}{2880} = \$XXX.XX$$

Figure 14–3. Calculation of the hourly rate including the desired profit.

One may wonder why the above calculations omit the "cost of goods" when calculating the hourly rate. It is expected that at a minimum, one would collect the manufacturer's invoice cost when dispensing the devices. This is not to say that one should use an actual manufacturer's invoice cost as the cost to the patient for the hearing aid. For many clinics, there will more than likely be a need to have an incremental markup over the manufacturer's invoice cost to help offset times when one cannot collect the hourly rate. A good example of this would be a Medicare patient who is seen for a comprehensive hearing evaluation (92557) as it is doubtful the reimbursement received from Medicare would cover the cost of doing business for the time allocated to see a patient for a comprehensive hearing evaluation.

Examples:

Hourly Rate	$ 100.00	$ 125.00	$ 150.00	$ 175.00	$ 200.00
HAC & Cleaning (20 min)	$ 33.33	$ 41.67	$ 50.00	$ 58.33	$ 66.67
HAC & EAA (30 min)	$ 50.00	$ 62.50	$ 75.00	$ 87.50	$ 100.00
Programming, EAA, and HAC (1 hour)	$ 100.00	$ 125.00	$ 150.00	$ 175.00	$ 200.00

The prices listed are for illustrative purposes only and are not to be construed as a recommendation of a given price for a given item or service. Audiologists should base their own prices on the results of their breakeven analysis, their third-party contractual commitments, and prevailing rates in their geographic area.

- HAC = Hearing aid Cleaning
- EAA = Electroacoustic Analysis

Figure 14–4. How to set clinic fees at an hourly rate.

audiologists surveyed understood how to calculate breakeven analysis and had done so to determine the costs of running the practice. The most common pricing strategies were arbitrarily choosing their rates or assessing the rates of their competitors to determine fees.

Setting Fees

After determining the hourly rate for the clinic, the next step is to apply this rate to each of the services offered in the clinic, taking into consideration the amount of time it usually takes to perform this service (Figure 14–4).

Using $200.00 per hour as an example, this converts each 15-minute interval to generate $50.00. Therefore, if seeing a walk-in patient for a 30-minute hearing aid check, it would be necessary to collect at least $100.00 for that appointment. *Considering the amount of time a procedure takes is the first step in determining fees.* It is also important to realize this exercise in setting fees should be revisited annually, as expenses and costs of goods to the practice change over time. Reviewing the hourly rate and re-

establishing an updated fee schedule on a regular basis will facilitate meeting the annual operating expenses of the clinic (Chapters 11, 13, and 24).

In-Network Versus Out-of-Network

If a clinic is an in-network provider for insurance coverage, which includes hearing aid services, make sure the fees are set *at or above the maximum amount the insurance company will reimburse.* To illustrate, assume the clinic is an in-network provider with the XYZ insurance company and it covers real-ear measurement services for $75.00; make sure billing is for all patients for at least $75.00 for real-ear measures (also known as conformity evaluation—V5020). If the billing is not at least $75.00, then money is left on the table. The best way to set fees is to consider the hourly rate as well as the maximum reimbursement received from any in-network insurance company. Request a copy of the fee schedule from all current "in-network" insurance plans to ascertain the maximum amount the insurance company will pay for a given service. If there are three companies and one will reimburse the above-mentioned procedure (V5020) at $65.00, another will reimburse $70.00, and the third one will reimburse $75.00, be sure the fee for that service is $75.00 or more billed to any one of the three providers. This would then be the usual and customary fee for all patients who are having this service. At least once a year, verify the fee schedule to determine where rates stand.

Fees for Hearing Aids

As discussed above, when considering how to price hearing aids for the clinic, keep in mind the invoice cost for the hearing aids is not the actual cost to the clinic. Other direct and indirect costs need to be factored into the price of the hearing aids. For example, if there is a payer mix that includes a high percentage of Medicare patients, then there may be a need to offset the poor reimbursement rates for diagnostic services in some other way. A markup on the manufacturer's invoice cost is one way to help offset those losses.

It is also advisable to review the manufacturer pricing multiple times throughout the year and negotiate the best discounts for the product. Audiology practices will continue to compete with sources that can get large-volume discounts for hearing aid purchases; therefore, this will be a crucial step to helping ensure the clinic can offer the lowest price possible to patients (even with a markup). The practice may want to consider joining a buying group or group purchasing organization, such as AuD-Net, Entheos Hearing, or others, to take advantage of potentially better volume discounts.

Establishing Value With Evidence-Based Practice

As audiologists, there are tools in the toolbox that big-box stores and online venues more than likely will not have. Striving to solidify the designation as experts in hearing loss diagnosis and treatment, more than ever as professionals, it is imperative that evidence-based practices are used with patients. The American Academy of Audiology established a task force to review this evidence and developed a very comprehensive guideline for the Audiologic Management of Adult Hearing Impairment (AAA, 2006). The reality is that many hearing care models relinquish these ideas by allowing self-evaluation and programming of hearing devices in the control of the patients. Therefore, more than ever, audiologists should be demonstrating what sets us apart and enables the delivery of exemplary hearing care.

A Model for Unbundled/ Itemized Hearing Care

One of the first questions asked might be, "Why do audiologists need to unbundle their fees for professional services and products?" After all, the professional has been providing these services in a bundled format almost since the inception of private practice. While this is true, there has been controversy on two fronts relative to fees for services, fairness to patients, and demonstrating the value of the audiologist in the provision of these services.

Background

A review of the literature on the topic of unbundling dates back close to 25 years. Gitles (1999a, 1999b) discussed that the consumer's view of the audiologist or hearing care professional is a view of a sales or service person, not a professional. Van Vliet (2003) stated, "Bundled pricing does not offer a full accounting of the clear scope of our services." Sweetow (2009a, 2009b) led an American Academy of Audiology Task Force to look at current hearing aid delivery models. The Task Force concluded in a two-part article, featured in *Audiology Today*, that there were advantages to unbundling that create the ability to use a fair and unbundled-only schedule to promote our specialized professional audiology services. The Task Force suggested that unbundling could also be used to argue for proper reimbursement, which would differentiate audiologists from nonaudiologists who dispense hearing aids. Further, the Task Force emphasized that audiologists *should never give away professional services* for the purpose of selling a product.

As these discussions were ongoing, the University of North Carolina at Chapel Hill–Hearing and Communication Center (UNC-HCC) decided to forge a new path and create an unbundled and itemized business model in 2005. The UNC-HCC audiology team was intrigued by audiologist Patricia Gans, who shared her clinic's unbundling success story in an article in the *Hearing Journal* (Nemes, 2004). The first cohort of doctoral students was in the midst of their training at UNC when this change was implemented. The audiology team was particularly attracted to the unbundling concept as it *placed more value on the skills of the audiologist and less on the device*. An equally strong motivation to change billing models was to help lower the upfront cost of hearing care and thus take steps to make hearing care more accessible and affordable. The UNC-HCC has managed to not only survive but thrive under this billing model for almost 20 years.

Disclaimer

It is important to note that the UNC-HCC is a community-based training clinic for doctoral students at the University of North Carolina in Chapel Hill. The clinic is funded entirely by clinical revenues and receives no state financial support; therefore, it functions as a private practice. However, as a university training clinic, the faculty audiologists have students training alongside them during each patient encounter. The following steps will help to outline the UNC-HCC clinic protocol for service delivery in an itemized business model.

Hearing Evaluation

The first step for most patients is a call to the office to schedule a hearing evaluation. The front office team gathers important demographic and insurance information when they are scheduling the patient. At the UNC-HCC, patients are scheduled for 1 hour for a hearing evaluation appointment, and sometimes it may be 1.5 hours if the front office team determines it is a more complex case. On the day of the appointment, the front desk team will get copies of all insurance cards and verify if they have received any physician referrals that may be necessary for submitting a claim for services. The audiologist conducts a review of the patient's intake form and then completes a comprehensive case history with the patient. After completing thorough diagnostic audiologic testing, the audiologist will review the test results and discuss next-step recommendations with the patient and their communication partner (if applicable). Patients who are motivated to pursue treatment are given a brief review of the process utilized at the UNC-HCC for candidates who would benefit from hearing aids, assistive technology, and/ or communication strategies training. Upon checking out, patients are given a hard copy of a link to the Characteristics of Amplification Tool (COAT) (Newman & Sandridge, 2006) assessment to complete. The UNC-HCC has a thorough description attached to this assessment that explains everything that will take place at the Hearing Aid Evaluation Appointment as well as outlining the cost of the next appointment. This helps ensure the patient is aware that most insurances do not cover the services in the next appointment and are prepared for the out-of-pocket fees. The audiologist writes a comprehensive report with all findings and recommendations, and this report is sent to the patient's referring physician. While the Food and Drug Administration (FDA) rescinded the requirement for medical clearance prior to hearing aid purchase (FDA News Release, 2016), the team at the UNC-HCC still believes a partnership with the primary care physician is in the patient's best interest. If the patient is self-referred, permission is obtained to send a comprehensive report to their physician. At a minimum, patients are encouraged to review their hearing evaluation results with their primary care physician.

Functional Communication Assessment

The UNC-HCC prefers the term "functional communication assessment" as opposed to hearing aid evaluation. There are two CPT codes that one can bill for this appointment.

- 92590: Hearing Aid Examination and Selection—Monaural.
- 92591: Hearing Aid Examination and Selection—Binaural.

The preference for the term functional communication assessment (FCA) allows a broader range of recommendations than just hearing aids. Some patients may only need to attend a class on communication management strategies or require a device to assist with listening to the television. Or perhaps, they may not be ready for hearing aids but would be interested in an OTC device. This appointment is *not* a free consultation to find solutions for patients. Long ago, the clinic would "bundle" this visit into the price of the hearing aids. However, if the patient chooses not to purchase hearing aids from the clinic, then the necessary hourly rate would not be recouped and there would be no demonstrated value for their expertise.

Subjective Assessments

Sweetow (2007) outlined an excellent method for gathering both objective and subjective information from the patient to form the basis for a treatment recommendation that takes the emphasis off the ears and looks at the whole person and their communication needs. The FCA appointment begins with a review of a prefitting assessment tool, such as the Characteristics of Amplification Tool (COAT) (Dillon et al., 1997), the Expected Consequences of Hearing Aid Ownership (ECHO) (Cox & Alexander, 2000), or the Abbreviated Profile of Hearing Aid Benefit (APHAB) (Cox & Alexander, 1995). Use of these assessment tools allows the audiologist to gather subjective information from the patient about their motivation to improve their hearing, as well as their expectations and their concerns. Gathering this information from the patient prior to the appointment can really help to guide the process and can assist in revealing the patient's personal reasons for pursuing help with their communication skills.

Objective Assessments

- Speech-in-noise testing is helpful to understand how a patient processes sound in the presence of background noise. The QUICKSIN test (Killian et al., 2004) is a very easy way to gain some useful information that allows the development of a treatment plan that goes beyond hearing aids.
- Gathering some objective information is also helpful in developing a treatment plan that will prove useful throughout the hearing aid fitting process. The UNC-HCC conducts Loudness Discomfort Level testing using the 7-point contour test developed by Cox et al. (1997).

- Other tests the audiologist may choose to conduct include the Acceptable Noise Level (ANL) test and the Performance Perceptual Test (PPT)
- Cox, R. M., & Alexander, G. C. (2000). Expectations about hearing aids and their relationship to fitting outcome. *Journal of the American Academy of Audiology, 11*(7), 368–382.
- Threshold Equalizing Noise (TEN) test to assess cochlear dead regions (Moore et al., 2000) (Moore, 2020).

Lifestyle Assessment

After gathering additional objective data about how the patient processes sound in more complex listening environments and understanding their preferences for loud sounds, the next step in the FCA appointment is to conduct a Lifestyle Assessment. The UNC-HCC developed a Lifestyle Assessment form that enables the audiologist to efficiently but thoroughly review the patient's day-to-day listening environments, as well as understand their phone needs, vision, dexterity, cosmetic concerns, and so on. After an in-depth interview of the patient's lifestyle and communication challenges, the audiologist and patient work together and develop some communication goals that the patient is particularly interested in improving by the end of the treatment process. The Client Oriented Scale of Improvement (COSI) is an easy tool to accomplish this goal (Dillon et al., 1997). The UNC-HCC uses a modified version of this to establish the patient's present abilities, expected abilities, and realistic abilities for each of their goals. Use of this assessment tool ensures the audiologist understands what the patient's main listening goals are, as well as confirming that the patient's expectations are appropriate considering their hearing loss and other test scores. Finally, the COSI then allows the audiologist to develop outcome measures that can then be revisited at the conclusion of the fitting period to see what progress has been made on the communication goals as a result of the treatment. The duration of the FCA could be upward of 1.5 hours, but at the end of this time, the patient has had a very comprehensive needs assessment and a customized treatment plan has been recommended. The treatment plan recommendation may include hearing aids, connectivity devices, FM/DM systems, custom earmolds, and audiologic rehabilitation such as auditory training, Better Hearing Workshop classes, and so on. The patient and audiologist will work together to determine which devices and tools will meet their needs and satisfy their budget. Earmold impressions would be taken at this appointment if custom earmolds or in-the-ear products are recommended.

The adoption of the FCA has demonstrated a very comprehensive approach to the selection of hearing technology and the development of a treatment plan far more complex than what patients would find at a big-box store or an online venue. The process of completing these assessments demonstrates the knowledge and skills of the audiologist as a key partner in the success of the treatment plan. The audiologist is viewed less as someone who sells hearing aids but rather as a professional who offers a comprehensive communication treatment plan.

There are two CPT codes (92590 Monaural Hearing Aid Evaluation, 92591 Binaural Hearing Aid Evaluation) that can be utilized for the FCA if the patient has insurance coverage and should be submitted after the appointment, regardless of whether the patient purchases hearing aids. The audiologist would benefit from charging for each earmold impression (V5275) and each earmold (V5264) ordered at the hearing aid evaluation (HAE) FCA appointment. Doing so ensures that should a patient elect to cancel the hearing aid order prior to their scheduled fitting, the fees for the services of taking the impression and the nonrefundable earmolds would already have been collected.

Hearing Aid Fitting Practice

The procedure for hearing aid fitting within the UNC-HHC clinic involves informing the patients at all steps through the process about the services rendered and their costs.

Hearing Aid Check

There is some behind-the-scenes work that happens before a patient is ever fitted with their hearing aids. At the UNC-HCC, the team believes these are essential procedures in an unbundled billing model as the audiologist can then be confident the devices are working properly when sent home with the patient. When the hearing aid(s)/earmold(s) first arrives from the manufacturer, a visual inspection is necessary to confirm that the product received is what was ordered. An audiology assistant could be utilized for these tasks, which includes confirmation with the order form, patient record, and the color, style, materials, and so on are the same as what was ordered. This can be followed by a listening check. The UNC-HCC presently utilizes graduate assistants and an audiology assistant for these tasks (Chapter 10).

Electro-Acoustic Analysis (EAA)

After verifying that the correct products have been received and passed a listening check, the next step is electro-acoustic analysis (EAA). All hearing aids (new and repaired) must undergo and pass this process. The AAA Task Force Guidelines for the Treatment of Adult Hearing Impairment (Valente et al., 2006) have strong evidence to support the importance of this procedure. As mentioned above, in an unbundled billing model, if one is charging for each visit, they must be confident that the devices are working and meeting ANSI standards prior to the patient leaving the clinic with them. The UNC-HCC completed a 1-year retrospective study of all hearing aid orders to ascertain what percentage of new hearing aid orders met ANSI standards upon delivery from the manufacturer. They discovered that 12% of brand-new hearing aids did not pass inspection; 18% of repairs also failed inspection (Sjoblad & Warren, 2011). At the UNC-HCC, it is an unusual day for a patient to return to the clinic after a fitting due to an ill-functioning hearing aid. Utilization of these CPT codes on a regular basis by all audiologists validates the importance of the service to both the patients and third-party payers.

Hearing Aid Fitting

On the day of the patient's fitting, the hearing test results and loudness discomfort levels (LDLs) are uploaded into the verification system prior to the patient's arrival in the fitting suite. The transfer of data from the audiometer to verification system and back has improved significantly over the years, and the transfer takes only a few seconds. At the start of the appointment, the patient is then seated in front of the verification system. The audiologist will show the patient their devices, inspect the ear canal, and check the fit/comfort of the devices in the patient's ear and then remove the hearing aid(s) to set up for real-ear probe microphone measures (REM).

The audiologist will discuss the purpose of the REM procedure with the patient to explain that the only way to have an accurate hearing aid fitting is to take their ear canal resonance into consideration while providing a customized fit using research-based prescriptive targets. The audiologist initially sets the adaptation level at maximum when running the initial REM curves. Three curves are usually completed (soft speech, average speech, and maximum power output (MPO). The audiologist will then adjust the software and continue to measure until targets are met throughout the speech range, which then maximizes the patient's audibility for speech. REM is an evidence-based procedure that demonstrates the audiologist's value and ensures that the devices are providing patient audibility without exceeding loudness preference levels. When one fails to use REM, they have failed to demonstrate what makes the services of an audiologist unique as opposed to just acquiring a hearing aid with the "first fit" settings (Bentler et al., 2016). As a revenue source, REM has the potential to become a revenue-leading source of income for audiology clinics, as this is a billable code and can be used for hearing aids regardless of where they are purchased. As new players enter the hearing aid market and offer devices at lower cost, knowing how to efficiently program hearing aids with a research-based tool is a method to reach customers who have not obtained an optimal fitting elsewhere.

Hearing Aid Adjustments

While the UNC-HCC recommends programming the hearing aids at maximum adaption levels, this may not be the level the patient prefers initially. Audiologists are educated that for maximum speech intelligibility, the goal is to be at 100% of targets, but sometimes, it is an incremental process to meet those targets. Patients with a long duration of hearing loss without amplification often cannot achieve this at the initial fitting. For those patients who do not leave the clinic at the most optimal settings for speech intelligibility at 100% of targets, at subsequent appointments, the audiologist will decide if they can inch back toward 100% of targets or if they need to give the patient more time at a reduced volume (Bentler et al., 2016). The audiologist may add a phone program or loop program and make a determination of any other necessary adjustments to enable the patient to have the best success at meeting their COSI goals prior to saving and disconnecting the hearing aids from the computer. Connectivity devices and pairing to the patient's phone may be conducted at the initial fitting, but often, they are added at the second appointment during the evaluation and adjustment period to enable patients to use the first week or two to

getting acclimated to just the hearing devices.

Counseling and Orientation

The UNC-HCC clinic usually devotes 1 hour to the initial hearing aid fitting and counseling appointment. Adding REM does not take any longer for the hearing aid fitting appointment; the first 15 to 20 minutes are programming with REM. The remainder of the appointment can then be spent reviewing care and use of the hearing instruments and discussion of communication management strategies. Prior to the patient being dismissed, the audiologist will review the purchase agreement with the patient and discuss all terms and conditions.

Purchase Agreement and Payment

The purchase agreement used should be developed in accordance with state law. It is recommended that each clinic check its licensing laws as it develops a purchase agreement as the requirements do vary from state to state. The UNC-HCC provides the patient with a purchase agreement and an invoice from the billing program. The first line on the purchase agreement outlines the fee for professional services and states that this fee is nonrefundable. Whether professional fees are nonrefundable can vary by state law. In North Carolina, the UNC-HCC can collect fees for services rendered. The purchase agreement also denotes the price for each device, as well as provides the warranty terms and clinic policies for services. The UNC-HCC *prefers the use of the term "evaluation and adjustment period" versus "trial period"* both when talking with patients and on the purchase agreement. After the audiologist has reviewed the purchase agreement and the patient signs the form, they are then sent to the front desk to check out. They have also been given a superbill, which has a detailed itemization of each of the services that was provided at the appointment and prior to the fitting, so their invoice will include a listing of all the services the audiologist provided for the hearing aid fitting appointment. The patient leaves the clinic with a copy of the purchase agreement as well as an invoice highlighting the services that were provided for their initial hearing aid fitting appointment. There are Healthcare Common Procedural Coding System (HCPCS) codes for services:

- V5020: Conformity evaluation and may include real-ear measures, validation, and functional gain measures.
- V5014: Repair/modification of a hearing aid
- V5011: Fitting/orientation/checking of the hearing aid

The audiology team is discouraged from accompanying the patient to the front checkout desk. All monetary transactions occur at the front desk with the practice manager or patient care coordinator. If a patient has an insurance benefit, this is verified prior to the FCA appointment, and at the time of the fitting, the UNC-HCC will collect whatever is the allowable patient responsibility and then process the claim. Whether private pay or third-party payer, the patient leaves the appointment with doc-umentation of all the services that were provided during their visit. Follow-up appointments are scheduled at the time the patient checks out.

Hearing Aid Fitting Follow-Up/ Audiologic Rehabilitation

Whether a clinic decides to completely unbundle and charge for all subsequent visits or package the fitting appointments into one nonrefundable fee is an individual choice. The UNC-HCC has used a 45-day period that is paid upfront for most purchases. This partially unbundled billing model for the fitting period ensures the patient has a successful fitting process. At each of the follow-up appointments in the 45-day period, the audiologist provides the front desk staff with a superbill of the services that were rendered but indicates that the patient "prepaid" for these services. This is often referred to as a "hybrid" billing model. For example, at the first follow-up visit, if the patient requested modification to the hearing aid programming to add an additional program and increase the experience level, the audiologist would circle the corresponding services on the superbill. When the patient checks out, they receive an invoice detailing the services of the day, but the invoice indicates the fees were prepaid. By doing so, the patient sees what services were performed and that the services were prepaid, not free.

Hearing Aid Fitting Final Follow-Up

When both the patient and audiologist agree that they have reached the final follow-up appointment of the 45-day service fitting period, the audiologist will go through a series of questions with the patient to ensure the patient is confident as to how to use their hearing aids and satisfied that their communication goals have been met. The UNC-HCC utilizes a checklist that assists with the training of students. The checklist includes a review of the following: proper insertion and removal of devices; verification the devices are comfortable; care and use, including how to properly clean the devices; and verification regarding the use of any program/volume control buttons and any accessories or connectivity devices. The audiologist reviews the client's original communication goals (COSI) and asks them to again "rank" each goal to see how it differs from their pretreatment ranking. Most patients at the UNC-HCC report significant improvement at the end of the treatment process, but in rare instances when a patient is not meeting their expected goals, further audiologic rehabilitation may be recommended. This could include attending a Better Hearing Webinar, participating in auditory training, and considering additional accessories and/or more counseling regarding expectations. The UNC-HCC highly recommends that all patients participate in the Better Hearing Webinars at some point during the first year after purchasing new hearing aids. Over the 20 years of utilizing evidence-based practices, the clinic return for credit rate is 1% to 2% annually, which is well below national averages. The process detailed in this chapter provides each client with a customized treatment plan based on evidence-based research while establishing that the audiologist contributed

valuable knowledge and skills to the successful outcomes.

Prior to the patient "graduating" from the 45-day evaluation period, there is a discussion about the clinic fee policies for future appointments. Some clinics may offer a service plan for those patients who want "peace of mind." The UNC-HCC patients most often elect to "pay as you go," so the clinic currently *does not offer service plans*. The fee for service model presently used helps to keep hearing care costs as low as possible as the patient is not paying upfront for appointments that may not be used. When the patient leaves for their final checkout appointment of their fitting process, the UNC-HCC provides them with an electronic version of the International Outcomes Inventory for Hearing Aids (IOI-HA) (Cox et al., 2003) to complete in an effort to gather some additional outcome data. The IOI-HA covers a set of seven core outcome items that are sufficiently general to apply to many different types of investigations carried out in different countries in the world. Additionally, patients receive a computer-generated satisfaction survey within 6 weeks of their final follow-up to ascertain some long-term outcomes and assess satisfaction with the procedures and services provided.

Routine Hearing Aid Checks and Maintenance

The UNC-HCC has a policy of scheduling patients for their follow-up appointments when they check out. Most patients will benefit from a minimum of two recheck appointments per year, at 6-month intervals. It is up to the individual audiologist to use their own discretion if a patient needs more frequent care. At the hearing aid check (HAC) appointment, the audiologist or audiology assistant will review the patient's case history to be sure there have not been any changes in hearing or other symptoms and discuss successes and/or disappointments. The visit includes an otoscopic inspection of the ear and discussion of findings with the patient. The patient's hearing aids are serviced with small parts replacement, such as tubing, filters, wax traps, mic covers, and so on. The devices are placed in a drying system and a listening check is completed. The audiologist or audiologist's assistant may also connect the devices to the computer to verify patient wear time with the device's data logging software, review experience level, complete firmware updates, and make programming adjustments as needed. If the device fails the listening check, the provider may replace receivers as needed and/or conduct electro-acoustic analyses. Occasionally, cerumen management by the audiologist may be needed and patients pay for this service, if needed. If the patient has Medicare, they sign an Advanced Beneficiary Agreement prior to service delivery. Patients check out with a superbill that has all the provided services circled. At the annual visit, the audiologist or audiologist's assistant will repeat the procedures listed above and may also recommend an updated EAA as needed. Even though the patient is "in warranty" with the manufacturer, they pay for the services the clinician provides in the office. It is important that this is plainly described when discussing the purchase agreement with the patient at the initial fitting and confirming the policy when the patient schedules the HAC appointment. Most patients understand the policy and expect to pay for services when they come in for an appointment. If the patient is reluctant to "pay as they go," the patient is reminded of the goal of keeping upfront costs as low as possible.

A La Carte Versus Service Plans

The UNC-HCC has favored the "pay as you go" model for the majority of patients, but there is certainly a place for these service plans in an audiology practice. In the past, the UNC-HCC policy was to outline the service plan option at the conclusion of the evaluation and adjustment period. An alternative business model would be to outline on the purchase order that service is covered for a certain time period, what it covers, and what the cost is for needed services. It is important in this new climate of hearing care that patients are making appropriate comparisons if they choose to price shop. If a clinic suggests that Brand X hearing aids cost $5,000/pair but does not provide an itemization of the cost of fitting, service, and devices, the patient will be comparing apples to oranges if they find the same Brand X hearing aids online or retail for a fraction of their cost. A practice may not necessarily have to unbundle to demonstrate value to their patients. Simply providing a detailed itemization of products and services will also demonstrate value and enable a more appropriate comparison for the price shopper.

Caring for Patients Who Purchased Elsewhere

Over the past 5 years, the UNC-HCC clinic has received more inquiries from patients who have purchased devices elsewhere, either moving away from their original provider or wanting another opinion. Occasionally, patients seek the university for services and not for device(s), and therefore, the clinic will not benefit from any markup on product. This scenario is far less of a concern if the clinic knows its hourly rate and bills at that rate for each and every patient visit. Every patient that comes to the UNC-HCC for service pays the same for the services rendered, without any consideration for where the devices were purchased. During an initial consultation with the patient, the audiologist will attempt to help the patient solve the problem that brought them in; sometimes it is just a good cleaning of their devices. Sometimes the case history and otoscopic inspection reveal a new hearing evaluation is needed, and other times, the patient may need the devices reprogrammed. UNC-HCC has programming software for most major manufacturers. When the patient has a device that is "locked" or proprietary, the clinic may be limited in how it can assist a patient that comes in, but that does not suggest the clinic should turn them away. It may be that after a good cleaning and real-ear measures, the patient can be reassured of a properly functioning device providing adequate speech audibility.

Over the years, the UNC-HCC has seen patients elect to pay for REM even when the audiologist cannot make any programming changes as the patient is then empowered to make more informed decisions going forward. Occasionally, after the visit, they will go back to their original provider, when possible, for adjustments. More frequently, however, patients decide to move forward with newer technology at the UNC-HCC because the audiologist has demonstrated their expertise during the course of the visit and made a good-faith effort to help them maximize their current technology. As more patients begin to purchase "starter" devices or less expensive devices elsewhere, there is always an opportunity to showcase skills as audiologists.

Varied Fitting Plans

During the 5-year window from the announcement that OTC devices would be forthcoming and the final rule (Federal Register Rule by the FDA, 2022), the UNC-HCC worked to establish offerings that would compete with OTC products. Utilizing value hearing devices, this university has set up a basic package that includes all services for the fitting and one follow-up visit. It is well known that there are patients not quite ready for hearing devices or desire a valuable option including the services of an audiologist. The UNC-HCC experience is that patients are most happy to pay for the provider's expertise, even if it costs them slightly more out of pocket. One way to help keep the overhead cost down for these fittings is to utilize the audiologist's assistant for as many of the tasks as allowed by state law. The aim is to educate every patient that the audiologist's assistants are qualified and a valuable team member in the hearing care process.

Summary

Itemizing professional services can benefit both the professional and the patients we serve. Itemizing establishes value while educating the patient that the device did not just work magically when it was taken out of the box. Should a practice choose not to unbundle, it would still be worthwhile to provide patients with details of services provided with a breakdown of the costs so that patients understand that they are not *just paying* for hearing aids. Audiologists must not fail to highlight that the "all-inclusive plan" also covers their knowledge and expertise.

HOW ITEMIZING MIGHT WORK IN OTHER CLINICS

As one contemplates how itemizing might work for your clinic, the following are some thoughts to ponder along with staff, to help begin to think about the value the audiologist brings to the table:

- At each patient visit, assess whether the services being provided are truly a prepaid service or whether consideration has been given to charging the patients for services.
- Utilize a superbill with each patient visit. If not using a superbill, it would be beneficial to the practice to create one to begin tracking patient encounters. Most of the needed codes are detailed in this chapter and the subsequent chapter on insurance billing (Chapter 17). Additionally, members of audiology professional organizations such as the Academy of Doctors of Audiology, the American Academy of Audiology, or the American Speech-Language-Hearing Association all may obtain access to sample billing sheets through those organizations. Once one has created a superbill, indicate which services were provided during the visit regardless of whether there is a charge and send the patient home with a detailed itemization of all services provided. If the service is part of a service plan, denote this on the invoice to dismiss the impression that the service(s) were free.
- If the clinic is not presently utilizing the AAA Task Force Guidelines for the Management of Adult Hearing Impairment when fitting amplification, consider how doing so could add value to the practice while justifying patient charges. The clinical practices outlined in these guidelines will set the clinic apart from the competition and demonstrate a higher value of the facility, with the added bonus of greater patient satisfaction.

continued on next page

continued from previous page

■ Continue to educate regarding itemizing of professional services at professional meetings offered by the Academy of Doctors of Audiology and the American Academy of Audiology, state professional meetings, and through journals articles as well as participating in online continuing education.

■ Stay current with best practice procedures as well as coding, billing, and insurance contracts (Chapters 16 and 17). One must stay well informed on what is happening not only within the profession but in all professions. There will always be a place for the open-minded audiologist to consider new ideas and those that deliver evidence-based care with compassion.

References

American Academy of Audiology. (2006). Guidelines for the audiologic management of adult hearing impairment. https://www .audiology.org/practice-guideline/guide lines-for-the-audiologic-management-of -adult-hearing-impairment/

Bentler, R., Mueller, H., & Ricketts, T. (2016). Probe microphone measures: Rational and procedures. In R. Bentler, H. Mueller, & T. Ricketts (Eds.), *Modern hearing aids, verification, outcome measures and follow up*. Plural Publishing.

Cox, R. M., & Alexander, G. C. (2000). Expectations about hearing aids and their relationship to fitting outcome. *Journal of the American Academy of Audiology, 11*(7), 368–382.

Cox, R. M., & Alexander, G. C. (1995). Abbreviated profile of hearing aid benefit. *Ear & Hearing, 16*(2), 176–186.

Cox, R. M., Alexander, G. C., & Beyer, C. M. (2003). Norms for the international outcome inventory for hearing aids. *Journal of the American Academy of Audiology, 14*(8), 403–413.

Cox, R. M., Alexander, G. C., Taylor, I. M., & Gray, G. A. (1997). The contour test of loudness perception. *Ear & Hearing, 18*(5), 388–400.

Dillon, H., James, A., & Ginis, J. (1997). The client-oriented scale of improvement (COSI) and its relationship to several other measures of benefit and satisfaction provided by hearing aids. *JAAA, 8*, 27–43.

Dictionary.com. (2024a). Unabridged. Itemize. http://dictionary.reference.com/browse /itemize

Dictionary.com. (2024b). Unabridged. http:// dictionary.reference.com/browse/un bundle.

Emanuel, D. C., & Wince, J. (2024). Do audiologists react well to change? *Audiology Today, 36*(2), 13–24.

FDA News Release. (2016, December 7). FDA takes steps to improve hearing aid accessibility. https://www.fda.gov/news events/newsroom/pressannouncements /ucm532005.htm

Federal Register Rule by the FDA. (2022, August 18). Food and Drug Administration. Medical devices; ear, nose, and throat devices; establishing over-the-counter hearing aids. https://www.federalregister.gov

/documents/2022/08/17/2022-17230/med
ical-devices-ear-nose-and-throat-devices
-establishing-over-the-counter-hearing-aids

Foltner, K. (2009). What's my time worth? Part 3: Breakeven analysis. *Advance for Audiologists, 11*(3), 44.

Gitles, T. (1999a). Re-inventing the profession: A new model of hearing care delivery (first of two parts). *Hearing Journal, 52*(9), 32–34.

Gitles, T. (1999b). Re-inventing the profession: A new model of hearing care delivery (second of two parts). *Hearing Journal, 52*(10), 53–55.

Killian, M. C., Niguette, P. A., Gudmunsen, G. I., Revitt, L. S., & Banerjee, S. (2004). Development of a quick speech-in-noise test for measuring signal to noise ratios loss in normal and hearing-impaired listeners. *Journal of the Acoustical Society of America, 116*(4), 2395–2405.

Moore, B. C. J., Huss, M., Vickers, D. A., Glasberg, B. R., & Alcántara, J. I. (2000). A test for the diagnosis of dead regions in the cochlea. *British Journal of Audiology, 34*, 205–224.

Moore, B. (2020). Testing for Cochlear Dead Regions: Audiometer Implementation of the TEN(HL) Test. Canadian Audiologist. Vol 7(4). https://canadianaudiologist.ca/moore-feature-11/

NASEM (National Academy of Sciences, Engineering, and Medicine). (2016). *Hearing health care for adults priorities for improving access.* National Academies Press.

Nemes, J. (2004). To bundle or not to bundle? That is the question. *Hearing Journal, 57*(4), 19–24.

Newman, C., & Sandridge, S. (2006, March 6). Improving the efficiency and accountability of the hearing aid selection process: Use of the COAT. *Audiology Online.*

President's Council of Advisors on Science and Technology (PCAST). (2015, October 26). Aging America & hearing loss: Imperative of improved hearing technologies [letter report to President Obama]. https://obamawhitehouse.archives.gov/sites/default/files/microsites/ostp/PCAST/pcast_hearing_tech_letterreport_final3.pdf

Saunders, G., & Forsline, A. (2006). The Performance-Perceptual Test (PPT) and its relationship to aided reported handicap and hearing aid satisfaction. *Ear and Hearing, 27*(3), 229–242.

Sjoblad, S., & Warren, B. (2011). Mythbusters: Can one unbundle and stay in business? *Audiology Today, 23*(5), 36–45.

Sweetow, R. (2007). Instead of a hearing aid evaluation, let's assess functional communication ability. *Hearing Journal, 60*(9), 26–31.

Sweetow, R. (2009a). Hearing aid delivery models: Part 1 of 2. *Audiology Today, 21*(5), 49–57.

Sweetow, R. (2009b). Hearing aid delivery models: Part 2 of 2. *Audiology Today, 21*(6), 33–37.

Valente, M., Abrams, H., Benson, D., Chisolm, T., Citron, D., Hampton, D., & Sweetow, R. (2006). Guidelines for the audiologic management of adult hearing impairment. *Audiology Today, 18*(5), 32–37.

Van Vliet, D. (2003). In praise of unbundling. *Hearing Journal, 56*(4), 36.

15 Office Management Systems

Brian Urban, AuD

Office Management System (OMS)?

For decades, a surprising number of hearing healthcare practices have monitored the ongoing success of their business by simply observing whether:

- Are there patients on the schedule?
- Is there enough money in the checking account?

While this fly-by-the-seat-of-your-pants method has never been the optimal method of measuring, tracking, and predicting business success, it has been employed because it is:

- Easy.
- Kind of, sort of, works most of the time.

Essentially, this method is the equivalent of addressing a patient's complaint of persistent feedback by just running the manufacturer's built-in feedback manager and sending them on their way. Sure, it might work, but the improvement is likely temporary (e.g., the feedback returns the next time the patient has a long conversation). What under-lying variables were automatically adjusted to negate the feedback (e.g., gain, compression ratios, knee points, etc.)? Did the sound clarity suffer as a result? And, most importantly, was follow-up completed with the patient to determine if the adjustment was effective?

As most providers realize, these quick fixes rarely result in satisfied patients. Without a systematic approach for truly understanding and managing the situation, these fly-by-the-seat-of-your-pants methods often hide the real issues while giving the impression that everything is fine.

Hearing healthcare is an amalgam of competing interests. It combines clinical services and federally mandated record-keeping with insurance submission and reimbursement with retail sales as well as tracking the business components of the practice. Consequently, routine, efficient methods for managing patient data are required to enhance quality patient care and prepare for the possible issues that may arise from simply conducting business. With the myriad of disruptions, influences, challenges, and opportunities facing the practice and the business of hearing healthcare, there is *no choice but to rely on data to succeed*. Whether in a private practice, ENT clinic, school system, hospital, or university setting, a consistent and rational approach to collecting and analyzing data is vital.

In the face of all this need for quality data, some business owners, administrators, and practice managers have been resistant to shred the paper, ditch the custom spreadsheets, and embrace a comprehensive, digital solution. If practitioners do make the switch, unfortunately some will still only view their office management system (OMS) as little more than an online schedule. While fear and complacency play a role, the real issue is a lack of understanding of the *true power of their clinic data*. The clinic is trying to tell its story—where it is weak or strong, vulnerable or bursting with potential, just waiting to be asked the right questions. As in many other healthy, fulfilling, and productive relationships, it is necessary to speak the same language to understand each other. An OMS is the translator that unlocks the clinic's full potential. To appreciate these systems to their fullest extent, it is necessary to understand the clinical, business, and regulatory factors that directly influence day-to-day clinical practice.

Clinical Factors

Frequently, the process of tracking a patient encounter is spread across a variety of different systems. This most commonly occurs when paper charts are being utilized and/or the current OMS does not support the entire patient workflow. This can result in providers and staff members being required to needlessly navigate between different systems (e.g., Microsoft Word, paper schedule, third-party biller, etc.) to document and bill for a single patient visit. This cumbersome process can lead to errors, missed opportunities, and unnecessary frustration among the staff. OMSs have the capability to integrate the entire patient workflow in a simple, intuitive fashion. As a result, the process of reviewing OMS programs begins with carefully examining the workflow as it currently exists (i.e., the good, the bad, and the ugly) as well as imagining the ideal design. Specifically, the following areas should be considered:

- Schedule—flexible and intuitive or restrictive and complicated?
  - Creating new appointments for existing versus new patients.
  - Recording referral sources.
  - Rescheduling appointments.
  - Block scheduling (creating and modifying blocks).
  - Tracking required physician referrals (e.g., required/not required for Medicare Part B recipients, requested, patient bringing, received, etc.?).
  - Adding patients to a waitlist.
  - Tracking companions (i.e., who will be joining the patient at the visit?).
  - Accessing the clinic schedule on different computers and devices.
  - Automatically sending notifications, confirmations, and reminders to patients via emails, text, and call messaging.
  - Transitioning between clinics, providers, and day/week/month/agenda views.
  - Monitoring multiple clinic schedules simultaneously.
  - Schedule options (e.g., general appearance, appointment type setup, etc.).

■ Patient administration—all-encompassing with rapid access to information or limited and clumsy?

  ■ Capturing and storing patient profile pictures.

  ■ Entering and reviewing patient demographics.

  ■ Sending on-demand emails and text messages.

  ■ Viewing interactive maps and providing patients with turn-by-turn directions.

  ■ Setting Do Not Call/Text/Mail/Email preferences and marketing opt-outs.

  ■ Recording contact information for other responsible parties.

  ■ Tracking referral sources and primary/referring providers.

  ■ Viewing preferred clinic and provider.

  ■ Recording patient notes.

  ■ Sending customized, online questionnaires and intake forms.

  ■ Entering insurance policy information (Payer/Payer IDs preset or manually maintained?).

  ■ Performing eligibility checks (i.e., determining in real time whether or not the policy details are valid).

  ■ Capturing and storing insurance card images.

  ■ Enabling patients to complete questionnaires and intake forms on tablet or computers.

  ■ Tracking appointments and patient visits.

  ■ Creating and viewing professional reports, patient counseling summaries, and chart notes.

  ■ Creating, viewing, and editing invoices.

  ■ Creating purchase agreements.

  ■ Tracking hearing instruments and accessories.

  ■ Creating repair forms.

  ■ Managing battery programs.

  ■ Uploading and viewing documents, images, spreadsheets, etc.

  ■ Tracking medications.

  ■ Activating and customizing a patient portal.

  ■ Tracking remaining authorized and no-charge visits related to third party administrators (TPA), services plans, and Medicaid.

  ■ Enabling marketing automation (email and direct mail) based on specific triggers and preferences.

Each of these activities can help make the workflow more efficient or be a source of confusion and frustration. Prior to committing to a system, the opportunity to perform realistic, on-demand testing should be made available and represent the full functionality of the OMS product. Thorough testing in a simulated clinic is vital for understanding how each system could benefit or hinder a practice.

Business Considerations

As noted at the opening of this chapter, "seat-of-your-pants" business management is no longer a reliable method to pay the bills or ensure practice growth. As a result, practice owners and managers need to rely upon ready access to their raw data as well as convenient summaries that help them make sense of their business. Beyond simply having a few canned business reports, the entire process of entering data through drawing conclusions must be considered in detail. In order avoid any unwanted surprises down the road, it is wise to ask:

- What data are being collected for each patient and encounter?
  - Referral sources.
  - Demographics.
  - Products and services provided (e.g., Superbill).
  - Diagnostic and service codes (ICD-10, CPT, HCPCS).
  - Hearing loss classification for each ear.
  - Patient tags (i.e., custom indicators such as Out for Medical Review, Memory Loss, Low Vision, Wheelchair, etc.).
  - Patient alerts.
  - Invoices.
  - Payments.
  - Claims.
  - Task reminders (manual and automated).
- How are the data entered?
  - Streamline, intuitive workflow.
  - Seamless transitions between different staff members.
  - Single data entry with applicable information automatically populating anywhere else in the system it is needed.
- What are the tools for viewing and interpreting the data on a routine basis? What are the methods for verifying that the data were entered in a complete and compliant fashion?
  - Real-time Dashboard.
  - Comprehensive Business Report Generators.
- Are those tools flexible or preset?
  - Built-in, customizable filters.
  - Options for taking action (e.g., downloading spreadsheets, printing letters, sending emails, etc.).

Reviewing these areas can highlight specific strengths and weaknesses of each OMS. Ultimately, understanding how they individually capture data and pro-vide analysis will be very important in determining how each system can support a clinic's needs going forward.

Healthcare Trends and Federal Requirements

The thought of a HIPAA breach or a Medicare audit can send most clinic managers into a cold sweat (Chapter 17). While clinics that observe best practices for data collection and management still have the same concerns, they can relax knowing that they are well prepared. The road to full compliance is rarely straight or typically smooth. However, in a "step-by-step fashion," clinics can learn how to navigate these twists and turns and enlist an OMS to help all along the way. To do so, it is best to begin by defining the basic terminology:

Electronic Medical Record (EMR)

The digital version of good ol' paper charts with the added ability to improve quality of care via patient tracking tools and access to aggregate data.

Electronic Health Record

An EMR that can share information between providers and departments in order to ensure coordination of patient care. EHRs enable patients to be seen by a variety of healthcare providers with their results and reports instantly available across the entire organization (Chapter 17).

Privacy Rule

As stated in the "HIPAA Privacy Rule" (2024), the "Privacy Rule" standards address the use and disclosure of individuals' health information—called "protected health information" by organizations subject to the Privacy Rule—called "covered entities," as well as standards for individuals' privacy rights to understand and control how their health information is used. Within the U.S. Department of Health and Human Services (HHS), the Office for Civil Rights (OCR) has responsibility for implementing and enforcing the Privacy Rule with respect to voluntary compliance activities and civil money penalties (Chapter 17).

A major goal of the Privacy Rule is to ensure that individuals' health information is properly protected while allowing the flow of health information needed to provide and promote high-quality healthcare and to protect the public's health and well-being. The Rule strikes a balance that permits important uses of information while protecting the privacy of people who seek care and healing. Given that the healthcare marketplace is diverse, the Rule is designed to be flexible and comprehensive to cover the variety of uses and disclosures that need to be addressed.

The Privacy Rule protects all "individually identifiable health information" held or transmitted by a covered entity or its business associate, in any form or media, whether electronic, paper, or oral. The Privacy Rule calls this information "protected health information (PHI)" (Chapter 17).

"Individually identifiable health information" is information, including demographic data, that relates to:

- The individual's past, present, or future physical or mental health or condition.
- The provision of healthcare to the individual.

- The past, present, or future payment for the provision of healthcare to the individual.

Basically, anything that identifies the individual or for which there is a reasonable basis to believe it can be used to identify the individual. Individually identifiable health information includes many common identifiers ("List of 18 Identifiers," 2024). Table 15–1 provides a list of all 18 PHI identifiers.

Security Rule

As stated in the "HIPAA Security Rule" (2024), "The Security Rule" requires covered entities to maintain reasonable and appropriate administrative, technical, and physical safeguards for protecting electronic protected health information (e-PHI).

Specifically, covered entities must:

- Ensure the confidentiality, integrity, and availability of all e-PHI they create, receive, maintain, or transmit.
- Identify and protect against reasonably anticipated threats to the security or integrity of the information.
- Protect against reasonably anticipated, impermissible uses or disclosures.
- Ensure compliance by their workforce.

The Security Rule defines "confidentiality" to mean that e-PHI is not available or disclosed to unauthorized persons. The Security Rule's confidentiality requirements support the Privacy Rule's prohibitions against improper uses and disclosures of PHI. The Security Rule also promotes the two additional goals

Table 15–1. HIPAA PHI: List of 18 Identifiers

1. Names

2. Address – All subdivisions smaller than a state

   - Includes Street address, city, county, precinct, ZIP code

3. Dates – Includes all elements (except for the year) of dates that are related to the patient

   - Birth date, visit date, fitting date, death date, etc
   - If patient is over 89 years old, year is also protected

4. Phone numbers

5. Fax numbers

6. Email addresses

7. Social Security numbers

8. Medical record numbers

9. Health plan beneficiary numbers

10. Account numbers

11. Certificate/license numbers

12. Vehicle identifiers and serial numbers

13. Device identifiers and serial numbers (e.g. hearing aids and accessories)

14. Web URLs (e.g. Patient's personal blog)

15. Internet Protocol (IP) address numbers

16. Biometric identifiers, including finger and voice prints

17. Photographs of the patient and any comparable images

18. Any other characteristic that could uniquely identify the patient

From CounselEAR, LLC. Reprinted with permission.

of maintaining the integrity and availability of e-PHI. Under the Security Rule, "integrity" means that e-PHI is not altered or destroyed in an unauthorized manner. "Availability" means that e-PHI is accessible and usable on demand by an authorized person.

HIPAA Breach

As described in the "HIPAA Breach Notification Rule" (2017), "a breach is, generally, an impermissible use or disclosure under the Privacy Rule that compromises the security or privacy of the protected health information." An impermissible use or disclosure of protected health information is presumed to be a breach unless the covered entity or business associate, as applicable, demonstrates that there is a low probability that the protected health information has been compromised based on a risk assessment of at least the following factors:

- The nature and extent of the protected health information involved, including the types of identifiers and the likelihood of reidentification.
- The unauthorized person who used the protected health information or to whom the disclosure was made.
- Whether the protected health information was actually acquired or viewed.
- The extent to which the risk to the protected health information has been mitigated.

Breaches can be as simple as one patient observing another patient's open file on a desk or as far reaching as someone stealing an entire patient database. Depending on the severity of the breach (e.g., number of patients, type of PHI), the clinic involved with the improper disclosure may be required to notify their entire patient database, HHS, and the media. These notifications must be provided promptly to individual patients for any size breach and, if over 500 patients are affected, the media as well (i.e., in no case later than 60 days following the discovery of a breach). The notifications must include:

- A brief description of the details surrounding the breach.

- A description of all of the types of information that were determined to be included in the breach.
- Steps that any affected patients should take to protect themselves from potential harm (e.g., activate a credit freeze, implement a fraud protection/monitoring program).
- A brief description of what the clinic is doing to investigate the breach, mitigate the harm, and prevent further breaches.
- Contact information for the clinic.

Medicare Audit

Through a process called "clawback" performed by Recovery Audit Contractors (RACs), Medicare providers can be required to supply documentation to justify individual claims. If the documentation for the billed services does not substantiate the physician's order as well as medical necessity, payments for those services can be reclaimed.

These contractors are paid a percentage of the amount that they help reclaim for Medicare. As a result, even if best practices for patient care are followed, if the documentation is not complete and compliant, the contractors are required (and incentivized) to recover any related payments to the clinic. The only way to ensure a successful audit is to utilize systems—whether they are paper charts or full OMSs—that are designed to support comprehensive, consistent documentation and claims submission.

Each of these topics has a direct effect on how patient data should be collected, stored, accessed, monitored, and reported upon. The single best way to maintain data security, breeze through an audit, and maximize the value of the patient data is to implement an OMS that employs best practices and supports the entire patient encounter (i.e., the clinical and business aspects). When the whole patient database is managed and utilized in a consistent, compliant fashion, risks regarding breaches and audits decrease dramatically. However, fortunately this process is not all about risk management. These same efforts will likely result in the value of the patient data (and inherently the practice) increasing.

The Search Starts at Home

The process of determining the correct OMS for a practice must begin with a deep and comprehensive analysis of what staff members need to succeed. Each staff member is presented with their own unique challenges and opportunities daily. Will an OMS help or hinder their ability to provide extraordinary patient care and support an efficient, thriving practice? The value of discussing with the entire staff regarding their wants, needs, and goals from an OMS cannot be overstated. Their input and buy-in will be essential for determining and implementing the best overall solution.

Workflow Evaluation

To begin, it is often best to review the entire workflow throughout a patient encounter. From scheduling to insurance verification, visit documentation to claim submission, and revenue tracking to monitoring marketing activities, each step introduces the potential for errors and omissions. Evaluating the patient life cycle from all perspectives

is crucial for detecting points of failure and determining if a particular OMS resolves or adds to these concerns.

So, how to approach such a broad topic? While it is easy to simply ask if a staff member likes or dislikes the current or proposed systems, unfortunately that type of approach may not produce any actionable intelligence. Instead, these questions must dive deeper, revealing the frustrations experienced by staff members on a regular basis. For example, regarding a current system:

- What tasks/activities routinely result in wasted time and/or effort?
  - Completing routine, tedious tasks (e.g., handwriting fax coversheets, repair forms, and purchase agreements).
  - Difficulty locating important information (e.g., device warranty dates, insurance policy details, patient notes, etc.).
  - Managing unnecessarily complicated tasks (e.g., creating/submitting claims).
  - Needing to reenter information (e.g., patient demographics, audiometric thresholds, QuickBooks data, claims remittance details, etc.).
  - Fixing errors (e.g., claims created incorrectly, documentation misfiled, etc.).
  - Duplicating effort (e.g., chart notes must be written/typed into multiple systems).
- What tasks/activities can result in miscommunications between staff?
  - Patient is not called to pick up their repaired hearing aid.
  - Superbill is not entered as an invoice.
  - Copay is not collected.

- The provider is not aware that their next patient is in the waiting room.
- Office manager does not know if the provider is on time or behind schedule.
- What tasks/activities can result in missed opportunities?
  - Tested-not-treated patients were not identified and tracked appropriately.
  - Cancelled/no-show appointments not followed up on consistently.
  - Patients with expiring warranties not being contacted proactively.

Imagining

How would those problematic tasks/activities be managed, and what specific features should be included in any new system? It is advisable to group the responses by job type and look for consistencies. Particular attention should be paid to the routine activities that are overly time intensive and prone to errors (e.g., coding and reimbursement) as they will often have the largest negative effect on productivity, revenue, and employee satisfaction. In addition, areas where workflow breakdowns occur can be a significant source of frustration for staff and hamper patient care. Once the hopes and concerns of the staff are fully understood, the focus can shift to the future of the practice.

Long-Term Needs Assessment

Beyond the immediate needs of the clinic and staff, any potential OMS should be seen as an integral part of the long-term success and, as a direct result,

value to the clinic. Having a sense of where the practice is headed will assist with this critical decision now. Ultimately, the OMS that is selected must be equipped to support the practice goals and growth outlook for all of the following:

- Adding additional staff and/or providers.
- Adding new location(s).
  - Acquisition or growing organically.
  - Integration of data from a different OMS into the current patient database.
- Adding new services (e.g., tinnitus, vestibular, electrophysiology, speech pathology, etc.).
  - Built-in features for documenting all applicable testing protocols.
  - Flexible coding/reimbursement to manage each service.
- Going paperless.
  - Tools for creating and completing documents without printing.
  - Convenient document storage.
  - Integrated fax/email features.
- Positioning for sale.
  - Easy access to the full database for generating the practice valuation.
  - Tools to demonstrate uniformity of data across patients.

Feature Review

Once the workflow and long-term needs assessments have been completed, the process of analyzing individual features within an OMS can begin. The availability and sophistication of those features will quickly start to differentiate which systems will help or hinder the practice now and in the future.

OMS Platform

While not specifically a feature, determining where the patient data will be stored and how it will be accessed are very important areas to consider. The basic descriptions of the three options are as follows. Also see Table 15–2 for a detailed comparison of the platforms and applicable OMSs for each.

- Standalone—database is stored locally (i.e., on the clinic's server computer).
- Standalone (hosted remotely)—database is hosted in a different location by the OMS and available via remote access (e.g., LogMeIn) over the Internet.
- Cloud based—database is stored in HIPAA-compliant data centers and available any time, anywhere online (i.e., data are accessed directly on the OMS' website).

Certain practice locations such as hospitals or universities may limit access to online systems and thereby require standalone OMS. However, these restrictions are increasingly being removed as cloud computing has become a widely accepted method for storing and accessing patient data in a HIPAA-compliant fashion.

Ease of Use

Not surprisingly, an intuitive, flexible system will be best accepted by the staff. This inherently reduces the startup challenges and encourages consistency from Day 1. As a result, paying attention to the "feel" of a system is crucial in the initial review. For example:

- Is the system patient-centric or schedule-centric?
- Do the steps in a typically patient encounter link together seamlessly or is the process disjointed?
- Can specific fields be modified to fit a clinic's preferences?

Once it has been established that the system "feels" good, areas regarding unique features, data security, ongoing access to data, integration partners, and business reporting can be reviewed.

Unique Features

Does the OMS go beyond the standard offerings and provide convenient methods for collecting, managing, and analyzing data? Here are some areas to consider:

Document Storage

- Enables uploading and direct scanning of files (e.g., pdf, gif, jpeg, xlxs, docx, etc.) and makes them available for preview or download as needed.

Professional Reporting (Figure 15–1)

- Assists with rapidly creating comprehensive, compliant official reports.

Table 15–2. Comparison of OMS Platforms

Standalone OMS	
Options: HearForm, TIMS, AuDBase	
Pros	**Cons**
• Complete control of OMS database • Ownership of the software license could be considered a practice asset • Data not transferred online (unless using Remote Desktop tools)	• Required to set up/manage server computer, database backups, and OMS software • Large, upfront expense • Annual maintenance/support fee typically required • Additional costs for upgrades and customizations • Only accessible from computers where the OMS software is installed • Potential for downtime if clinic's server malfunctions • May not be accessible from all types of devices (e.g., tablets, cellphones) • Can be challenging to setup/manage network of multiple offices
Cloud Based OMS	
Options: CounselEAR, Blueprint, Sycle, Auditdata, HearForm	
Pros	**Cons**
• Available 24/7 from any Internet-enabled device • Instantly connects all clinic locations • Data encryption and database backups completed automatically • No upfront costs to subscribe • New features and enhancements can be made available to all subscribers simultaneously	• Monthly subscription fee • Potential for downtime if clinic's internet or the OMS servers malfunction • No ownership of the software license

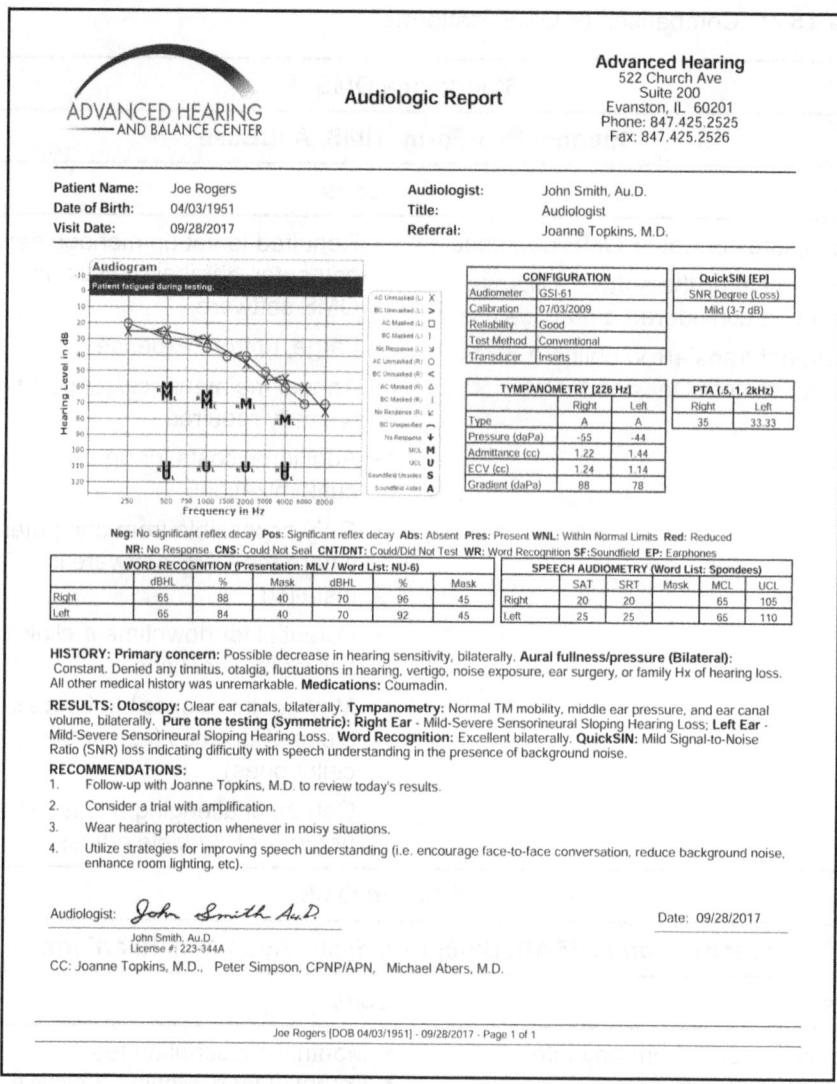

Figure 15–1. Example of a professional report. *Source:* From CounselEAR, LLC. Reprinted with permission.

Patient Counseling Tools (Figure 15–2)

■ Generates patient-friendly graphics and language designed to improve what patients remember.

■ Increases the likelihood that they will follow through with recommendations.

Patient Portal

■ Enables patients to log into their own portal to see approved content (e.g., reports, invoices, education materials, videos, etc.), ask questions, make payments, and schedule appointments.

■ Allows options to build the portal directly into a clinic's website.

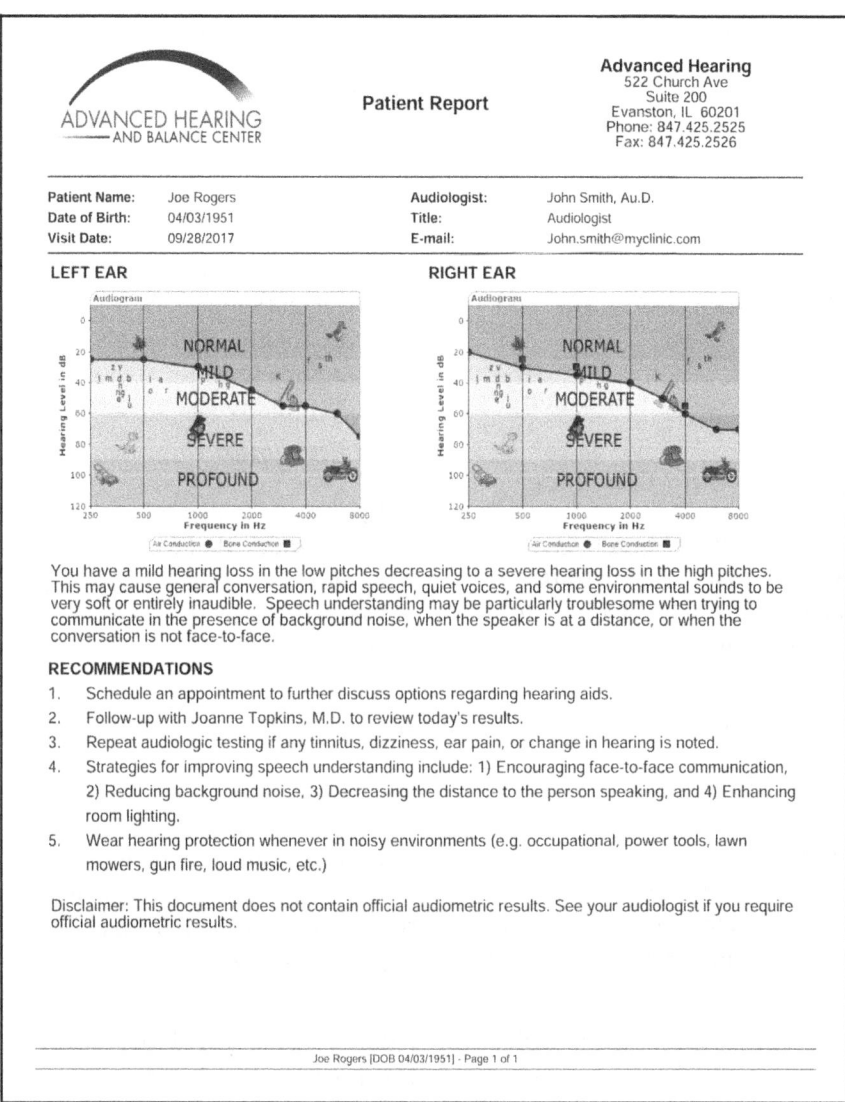

Figure 15–2. Example of a patient counseling summary. *Source:* From CounselEAR, LLC. Reprinted with permission.

Telehealth

■ Ability to conduct HIPAA-compliant telehealth sessions (scheduled or on demand) with patients or staff on any Internet-enabled device (Chapter 21).

Email, Text, and Fax Tools

■ Sends emails and texts automatically as well as on demand.

■ Sends professional reports, patient counseling summaries, and chart notes via fax and email.

Task Management

■ Manually or automatically creates tasks for specific staff members (or entire team).
■ Tracks tasks within a patient profile or across the clinic.

Real-Time Communication

■ Chat with staff members anytime via pop-up messages and alerts.

Billing and Coding Guidance

■ Comprehensive with a built-in superbill and a claims wizard.
■ Creates claims in CMS 1500 and ANSI 837p formats.
■ Supports outcomes-based reporting (MIPS).
■ All codes are kept up to date (e.g., annual changes: ICD-10 codes— October 1; CPT/HCPCS codes— January 1).
■ Enables direct import of claims remittance data (e.g., adjustments, payments, remittance codes, etc.).

Opportunity and Commission Tracking (Figure 15–3)

■ Monitors potential hearing aid fittings with high accuracy (i.e., on a visit-by-visit basis).
■ Calculates commission totals for individual providers.

Security and HIPAA Compliance

The HIPAA Privacy and Security Rules require clinics to take all reasonable measures to protect and limit access to patient data. Simply continuing the same practices that have always been in place may leave a clinic vulnerable to a HIPAA breach. In the event of a breach, ignorance does not count as a defense. As a result, it is necessary to understand how data are being managed and what security tools are available. Specifically, does the OMS follow best practices and provide a suite of controls for limiting access? For example:

Data Encryption

■ In transit (i.e., as information is transmitted online).
■ At rest (i.e., while sitting on a local server or in a cloud-based system).

Audit and Integrity Controls

■ Ability to monitor who has altered/ destroyed PHI and recover that information (e.g., patient profile, reports, and invoices/payments).
■ Ability to execute a Business Associates Agreement (BAA).

Routine Data Backups and System Redundancy

■ Ability to receive documentation that best practices are being followed.

Data Portability

■ Ability to download full records for individual patients or the entire database at any time.

Password Requirements

■ Ability to set timeouts, automatic lockouts with repeated login errors,

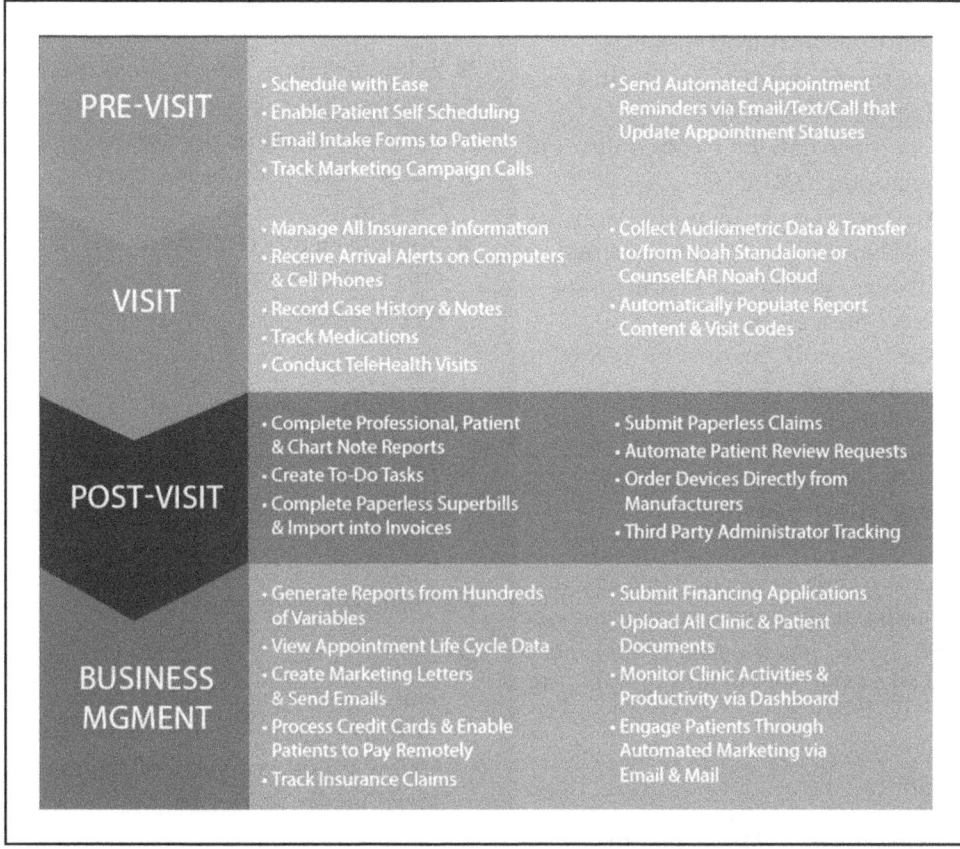

Figure 15–3. Capabilities of comprehensive office management systems. *Source:* From CounselEAR, LLC. Reprinted with permission.

and mandate periodic password updates.

■ Option to require multifactor authentication (MFA).

Discreet Access Levels

■ Ability to instantly set limits regarding what information each staff member can view and modify throughout the system.

Roaming Access

■ Ability to restrict access to a clinic's database to only computers physically located within that clinic (via IP filtering for cloud-based systems).

Ongoing Access to Data

Patient data should always be considered the sole property of the clinic, not the OMS. However, some systems restrict access to full downloads of patient data, documents, financials, and Noah files. As a result, it is important to ask whether complete backups are available on demand, by special request to the OMS, or not at all. Specific areas to review:

- What are the typical turnaround times for download requests?
- Are the file formats involved standard to the industry?
- Can these data be easily uploaded by another OMS?
- Are there any known omissions to the data set (e.g., appointments, invoices, payments, hearing aids, Noah files, etc.)?
- Are there any charges for receiving the backup?

Integration Partners

Does the OMS integrate with any/all of the following? If so, what are the software, setup, and training requirements, as well as the overall additional costs?

Noah

- Standalone—OMS communicates with and/or hosts the Noah database.
- Cloud based—Noah database is stored online and available within the OMS from anywhere.

QuickBooks

- Transfers invoices and payments from the OMS to QuickBooks.
- Avoids unnecessary double data entry and reduce errors.

Credit Card Processing

- Processes credit and debit card directly within the OMS.
- May enable remote payment for patients online.

Claims Clearinghouse

- Submits claims directly from the OMS to the claims clearinghouse.
- Receives real-time updates on claim status without leaving the OMS.
- Imports claims remittance details (e.g., adjustments, payments, etc.).

Patient Financing

- Completes and submits financing applications right within the OMS.

Patient Reviews

- Following appointments, automatically sends emails and texts to patients requesting that they leave a review on one or more of the major social media platforms.

Business Reporting

A patient database is only as good as the ability to turn it on its head and see what shakes out. As a result, tools throughout the system should encourage simple real-time analysis and comprehensive historical reviews. Specifically, it will be beneficial to verify the following:

Key Performance Indicators (KPIs)/Dashboards

- Can important, routine data be reviewed quickly?
- Are easy to understand tools provided for monitoring practice performance over time?

Marketing Tools

- Can the patient database be turned into a marketing treasure trove?
- What are the steps for (1) identifying patients to contact, (2) quickly taking action, and (3) tracking the outcomes?
- Can marketing automation be enabled?

Customizability

- Are all aspects of the system pre-defined or can specific features be modified at will?
- Are there potential charges for setting up templates or customizations?

Intangibles

One of the most enduring aspects of an OMS resides in its ability to support clinics while providing ongoing flexibility. In order to see the full picture and prevent any unwanted surprises, the following details should be examined:

Annual Contracts (Available/ Required/Optional)

- Locked into a contract or free to decide month-to-month?

Add-On Costs

- Are there any ala carte options available?
- What are the costs of the add-ons relative to purchasing equivalent services/systems independently?
- If there is direct integration, does it achieve the desired goal (e.g., enhanced staff productivity, patient satisfaction, or new referrals)?

Data Conversion (Table 15–3)

- What is the process for converting data from the current system to the new OMS?
  - What data can or cannot be converted (e.g., patient demographics, appointments, invoices/payments,

Table 15–3. Sample Conversion Guide

Sample Conversion Guide
Instructions: Check off each task as it is completed.
Step 1: Preparation & Training
☐ Schedule an OMS demonstration for staff and/or join the weekly scheduled overviews
☐ Practice in the test account/system and contact the OMS support with questions

Continues

Table 15–3. *Continued*

☐ Utilize the tutorial video library as a resource to review specific areas on demand
☐ Discuss the preferred timeline for the data conversion with the OMS support team
☐ Request/download Noah backup files and scanned documents, if applicable
☐ Review the following integration options, and if interested, contact the OMS support team for set-up procedures: ☐ Credit Card Processing ☐ Claim Clearinghouse ☐ Patient Financing ☐ Patient Reviews ☐ QuickBooks ☐ Noah ☐ Text Messaging ☐ Call Tracking
Step 2: Account Set-up
☐ Review areas to set-up within the OMS ☐ Clinic Profiles for all locations ☐ Advanced Settings (Clinic Staff, Schedule Settings, etc.) ☐ User Profiles for all staff ☐ Security Permissions (Clinics, Widgets, Business Reporting, etc.) ☐ Advanced Settings (Scanning, Notifications, Display Options, etc.) ☐ Insurance information for each provider, if applicable ☐ Tax Rates
☐ Send the following information to the OMS: ☐ Existing forms and questionnaires (e.g. intake, case history, purchase agreement, etc.) to be recreated within the system ☐ Provider signatures ☐ Clinic logo
Step 3: Conversion Day
☐ Follow the directions provided by the OMS support team to securely transfer the appropriate database files
☐ Track any changes made to the current OMS (e.g. chart notes, payments, etc.) during the conversion
☐ Once conversion is completed and verified, you will be notified as soon as possible

Table 15–3. *Continued*

☐ Verify conversion by comparing patient data between previous and new OMS (e.g. appointments, devices, invoices, etc.). Promptly, communicate any questions or concerns with the OMS support team.
☐ Areas to review and potentially make changes: 　☐ Line Item List 　☐ Referral Types ☐ Invoices (review Pending invoices)
☐ Enter any changes made during the conversion (e.g. chart notes, payments, etc) into the new OMS
Step 4: Implementation
☐ OMS support team will be in contact to provide any assistance the next business day after the conversion
☐ Utilize the new OMS and contact the support team via phone, email, or live chat with questions
☐ Schedule additional trainings as needed

Source: From CounselEAR, LLC. Reprinted with permission.

policies, devices, notes, documents, Noah data, etc.)?

- Can the OMS convert data from nonhearing healthcare-related or custom-built systems?
- How long will the process take?
- Will there be downtime during the conversion?
- Will the conversion be scheduled at a convenient day/time for the clinic or the OMS?

Customer Support

- What are the methods and availability? (e.g., phone, email, live chat, integrated ticketing system)

- Are video tutorials and live/recorded webinars available?

Responsiveness to Feedback

- Is there a general openness to critiques and suggestions?

Willingness/Ability to Create New Features

- Do ideas and suggestions simply drop into a bucket or do they result in new features and enhancements?
- How frequently is the system updated?

Summary

If staff members and patients are the lifeblood of a practice, the OMS is the heart that keeps everything connected and moving in harmony. From short-term gains to long-term goals, an OMS should propel a practice and put it on the cutting edge. The search for an OMS is one that should be taken with caution but viewed as a wonderful opportunity. Just begin with the right questions and the answers become clear.

References

HIPAA PHI: List of 18 identifiers and definition of PHI. (2024, April 5). http://cphs.berkeley.edu/hipaa/hipaa18.html

Summary of the HIPAA Breach Notification Rule. (2017, June 10). https://www.hhs.gov/hipaa/for-professionals/breach-notification

Summary of the HIPAA Privacy Rule. (2024, April 5). https://www.hhs.gov/hipaa/for-professionals/privacy/laws-regulations/

Summary of the HIPAA Security Rule. (2024, April 5). https://www.hhs.gov/hipaa/for-professionals/security/laws-regulations/

16 Audiology in the Insurance System

Thomas J. Tedeschi, AuD

Introduction

The audiology community in the last decade has seen an annual increased growth of third-party involvement in the hearing aid and hearing-related services reimbursement process. MarkeTrak 10 results showed that third-party funding for hearing aids through insurance had increased from 24% in 1989 to 55% in 2022 with 5% not sure if they had coverage (Powers & Carr, 2022). These programs are being offered by traditional commercial payers and their subsidiaries, Medicare and Medicaid contractors, government entities, workers' compensation programs, and third-party administrators. As a result, audiologists and hearing healthcare practices have numerous opportunities to become involved as providers of care in these programs. There are, however, many important aspects for the audiologist to understand and take into consideration when determining whether to participate in a contractual agreement and to determine if it is strategically a good decision for the practice.

An important point to recognize as one makes the decision to participate in a program is that each health plan is different and hearing aid coverage within a plan may vary according to a specific geographic location. It is therefore paramount to completely understand each and every aspect of the program prior to enrolling as a provider.

Additionally, the changing U.S. healthcare landscape has placed emphasis on improving the quality of patient care and reducing overall costs (NCQA, 2024). Regulators have taken a keen focus on making healthcare more affordable to the American people and hearing healthcare is not exempt from the discussions surrounding quality patient care and reduction in healthcare costs. Key stakeholders will often look to their largest spend on medical services. Most often this includes hospital, radiology, pharmaceutical, and specialty services. Hearing healthcare has gained greater visibility due to the fact the population is aging in the United States. The nation's 65-and-older population is projected to reach 88 million in 2050, double in size from the 2012 level of 43.1 million, according to two reports released from the U.S. Census Bureau (Ortman et al., 2014). The majority of the growth in the 65-and-older population is projected to occur between 2012 and 2030 as the Baby Boomers enter the older age group. Global life expectancy at birth is projected to increase by almost 8 years, climbing from 68.6 years in 2015 to 76.2 years in 2050 (Blackwell et al.,

2014). The health insurance industry is complex. The intent of this chapter is to present a basic understanding of its complexities, and what practititioners should keep in mind when dealing with these various groups.

Model and Programs Related to Hearing Health Care

Today there are a number of models and programs related to the reimbursement for hearing and hearing aid services. Each section will be covered in greater detail throughout this chapter (Baltazar, 2017).

Discount Programs

The implementation of the Patient Protection and Affordable Care Act's Essential Health Benefits provision shined a spotlight on the issue of hearing healthcare and hearing aid insurance, a benefit commonly left out of traditional commercial health plans and specifically excluded from Medicare. In (2023), Humana reported data from the Kaiser Family Foundation stating that 99% of all Medicare Advantage plans included a hearing benefit, which provided for hearing aids and hearing services (Ochieng et al., 2023).

When there is not a government or third-party payer contributing or paying for the services or hearing aids, a discount program may be available by the health plan and provides the health plan member with reduced or discounted pricing for hearing aids. A discount program is one where a Medicare Advantage plan provides its members discounted prices on hearing aids and related services (Rogin & Abrams). The plan creates partnerships with hearing care providers who, in turn, provide plan members with specific services and products at a reduced cost compared to the retail price. When there is not a health plan participation available, the patient is responsible for the entire purchase cost. This is commonly known as retail pricing for hearing services and hearing aids.

Per-Member, Per-Month Programs

Per-member, per-month (PMPM) programs are when an employer and/or insurance company sets up a PMPM for total coverage or specialty services for healthcare coverage for the employer or their membership. This PMPM generally will cover hospital, physician, and other specialty services. Hearing services and hearing aids are typically considered a noncovered service unless the health plan has a mandate from a regulatory agency, or an employer group wants to add coverage for hearing healthcare. To understand how much health costs are for a PMPM group, take the total yearly healthcare costs for a group, divide by the number of members, and then divide that number by 12. The low cost of the benefits is also similar to dental and vision programs. A fully insured hearing exam benefit through most programs costs employers only around 35 cents per employee per month, and a benefit that includes both hearing exams and devices can cost as little as $2 per employee per month. Under the PMPM, there are multiple plans that can be available. Most common are an allowance for services, which can range from $500 to

$2,000, or for a specific fee per ear for a hearing aid.

Government Administrated Programs

The U.S. government is directly accountable for Medicare and Medicaid programs. According to government data, Medicare covers approximately 66 million people, and approximately 81 million people were enrolled in Medicaid services. There are three types of programs: (1) Medicare, (2) Medicaid, and (3) dual eligible, combining both Medicare and Medicaid services. Medicare does not usually cover hearing aids, but there are options depending on the type of hearing loss and if an individual has a Medicare Advantage Plan. Medicare Advantage plans, sometimes called "Part C" or "MA plans," are offered by private companies and approved by Medicare. Medicare pays these companies to administer Medicare benefits. Medicare Advantage plans must include all Medicare services. Medicare Advantage plans may also offer additional benefits. However, each Medicare Advantage plan can charge separate out-of-pocket costs. Each plan can also have different rules for how services are delivered. Most Medicare Advantage plans require a referral for specialty care services and the provider must be a member of the plan's network.

Medicaid is a program that provides healthcare coverage for low-income families and individuals, for persons with disabilities, and in some cases the elderly. Medicaid coverage for hearing aids varies by state, and eligibility is subject to change. To determine if an individual qualifies for Medicaid coverage for hearing aid(s) and/or cochlear implants in

a state, the provider contacts the state's Medicaid program or visits Medicaid's national website at Medicaid.gov. These two sources provide the most current information. Medicaid services for hearing aids always require preauthorization from Medicaid. As a Medicaid provider, the provider agrees to accept the fees for services provided by the Medicaid agency.

Contracting With Commercial Insurance Companies

There are thousands of insurance companies throughout the United States. These are mostly regional health plans, but there are five major healthcare insurance companies, United Health Care, Aetna, Humana, Wellpoint Inc., and Cigna. There are many plans under the banner of these companies, and today, practice managers need to carefully examine the provisions of every contract before undertaking the commitment to abide by their terms. A good managed care contract, like any other form of business agreement, is clear, consistent, comprehensive, and concise. It will conform to both the intent of the parties, setting out their respective rights and responsibilities, and the requirements of state and federal law. It is extremely important to obtain a copy of the plan, know the restrictions and the reimbursements of each plan, and determine if being a provider under the plan is beneficial to the practice prior to seeing individuals who may seek services.

Commercial care contracts affect a provider's bottom line, yet many audiologists sign on the dotted line before reviewing the payer contracts carefully.

Why? Because they do not know how to spot the pitfalls that can put them at risk or cost them money. Understanding the language in commercial care contracts—even those already in place—can help the provider determine if certain benefits *are worth the risks*. And for new contracts, knowing the language can put the provider in *a better position to negotiate*. Unlike government contracts, a provider may be able to negotiate commercial care contracts.

It is also a good practice to review the contract with an attorney or business practice manager before enrolling as a provider for commercial contracts (Shaw, 2013). Information that is essential to a provider's practice is:

1. *Discounts*. Is this a discount plan? If so, what is the discount amount?
2. *Balance billing*. Are providers allowed to bill the individual any costs that are not reimbursed by the insurer?
3. *Reimbursement time*. What is the typical reimbursement time? A high rate of reimbursement may become less attractive when payment is *constantly overdue*. Care needs to be taken so that a practice's account receivables does not become too large. Also, the practice needs to pay the manufacturer for the cost of goods.
4. *Covered services*. Precisely what the "covered services" encompass is critical since the provider will agree to deliver them. Covered services should be listed explicitly in the contract.
5. *Medical necessity*. The contract will limit reimbursement to services that are not medically necessary. The key issue is who decides: the provider, or the group?

6. *Grievance process*. Is there a quick, fair grievance process or other review procedure?
7. *Termination process*. What are the termination provisions? May the insurer terminate the provider only for cause such as breach of contract or loss of license or without cause, that is, for no apparent reason? Does the contract afford the provider with due process rights and a hearing prior to the imposition of any corrective action?
8. *Payment*. The contract should state how, when, and what the provider will be paid. The provider's personnel should understand the claims' forms and processing procedures. Does the health plan have the right to change the fee schedule or capitation rate from time to time?
9. *Dispute resolution*. What dispute-resolution mechanisms are provided—arbitration, judicial review?
10. *Documents*. The service provider should obtain copies of, and analyze, all relevant documents, especially any documents that the contract incorporates by reference. These documents, whether actuarial data, policies, or procedures, can be integral parts of the health plan–provider relationship.

Pitfalls to avoid in commercial care contracts are presented in the box.

Credentialing

Provider credentialing is more than just another form to fill out or a minor nuisance; it is a complex, ongoing process

PITFALLS TO AVOID IN
COMMERCIAL CARE CONTRACTS:

1. *Contract reviews.* One of the most important tips is that requests can be made for a contract review at any time and most payers will comply.
2. *Arbitrary adjustments.* Avoid provisions that afford the payer the right to arbitrarily adjust and pay claims at a lower level than submitted. Incredibly, some contracts allow the payer to arbitrarily adjust claims and pay them at a lower level than submitted. The contract should stipulate that the audiologist has the right to appeal any payment not conforming to the payer's published edits.
3. *Takebacks.* Avoid provisions that allow for unlimited overpayment recovery or "takebacks." Periodically, audiologists receive letters from payers or independent vendors requesting refunds for claims that were paid as long as 3 years ago! An individual should never sign a contract that allows for unlimited overpayment recovery.
4. *Withhold provisions.* Withhold provisions represent an additional discount taken from the provider's reimbursement. No matter how the payer presents it, *withhold* is an additional discount taken from the provider's reimbursement to cover the commercial contractor's losses. Withhold language is usually found under *Payment and Reimbursement* or may be included as a separate addendum or attachment.
5. *Limited disclosure.* Limited disclosure of fee schedules does not allow for an accurate fee schedule evaluation. For a fee schedule evaluation to be accurate for the practice, you need to identify the frequency of all procedures performed and compare the fee schedule amounts to the practice's usual and customary fees.
6. *Appeal limitations.* Thirty-day appeal limitations put the burden of identifying claims issues on the audiologist. What is troublesome about appeal limitations, regardless of length, is that the responsibility falls on the audiologist to identify claim-processing errors.
7. *Unilateral changes.* Contracts that allow for unilateral changes give payers' carte blanche authority to do anything they want. It is very common to find provider agreements in which the payer grants itself the authority to make unilateral, mid-term changes to the provider agreement. Buried within the contract is a sentence stating the health plan may amend any portion of the contract at its sole discretion by giving the provider 30 days' notice. This means that the contract, in reality, is a 30-day contract and the plan can

continued on next page

---

continued from previous page

unilaterally decide to lower the reimbursement. A payer's unilateral right to amend mid-term is a deal breaker. This provision offers them carte blanche authority to do anything they want, and the practitioner is contractually obligated for the consequences. Any payer that refuses to remove such onerous provisions is revealing a dangerous clue to potential future problems.

8. *Vague contract language.* This is a less obvious method to obtain compliance with unilateral changes. Language provisions such as "As may be deemed necessary" and/or "from time to time" are less obvious ways to require acceptance of unilateral changes. Additionally, the use of "as may be established by the Payer" (especially if it occurs "from time to time") may create an obligation to policies and procedures that have not currently been established but may be in the future!

9. *Discounts.* The practitioner must watch out for discounts that are not obvious within the contract when they are extended to "affiliates." National payers and networks may include a statement that says that the agreement is entered into by itself and its affiliates. If the payer has affiliates, make sure that the contract includes an addendum that lists all affiliates.

---

and critically important. Without successful credentialing, provider reimbursement for services can be delayed and even denied. Given its many steps, critical deadlines, and lurking uncertainties, provider credentialing is business critical for your practice.

Credentialing, Licensing, Certifying—What's the Difference?

Credentialing is a broad term that can refer to a practitioner's license, certification, or education. Government agencies grant and monitor licenses; professional organizations certify practitioners. Certification can be either a prerequisite for licensure or, in some cases, an alternative to certification or licensure. Of course, being certified or licensed does not guarantee the provider is qualified and that practitioners must meet specific educational, training, or practice standards to qualify to provide certain services under a plan agreement.

The credentialing process includes reviewing qualifications and career history of licensed professionals, organizational members, or organizations. It may include reviewing and granting specific clinical privileges and allied health staff membership. As a hearing healthcare professional, there are requirements to be licensed and maintain continuing education in each state where the provider practices and to render this care to patients with fair and ethical standards. Many healthcare institutions and provider networks implement the credentialing process, generally through a credentialing team or credentialing verification organization, with review by a credentialing committee. Credentialing serves also to protect patient safety by ensuring the healthcare facility and professionals are of the highest quality.

When Is Credentialing Required?

Credentialing may be required at the time of hire, insurance enrollment, and/or licensing and *every 36 months* thereafter. Credentialing may also be required when changing jobs within an organization, including hospitals, nursing homes, and independent practices, or individually with a healthcare institution or provider network.

Why Must I Be Credentialed?

Credentialing, in general terms, is a verification of experience, expertise, interest, and willingness to provide care. In broad terms, credentialing encompasses obtaining privileges, as well as successfully enrolling in health plans as a participating provider. Even after submitting the myriad of documents and forms to a variety of third parties to verify credentials, the process may not be completely done. Even though most health plans do not require a full rehashing of the credentialing process, most oblige the

practitioner to submit annual updates. In other words, credentialing does not stop after the initial forms are submitted. This process consumes hours and hours each year, particularly if the practice has adopted an inefficient process. Credentialing is required for audiologists because they provide professional care to patients under healthcare laws. This is due, in part, to the increased educational requirements and service demand. Audiology is recognized as an independent medical profession rather than strictly rehabilitative in nature. Insurance payers use credentialing to select and retain qualified providers who will provide quality services to their members. Additionally, credentialing ensures insurance payers are protecting their members from fraud, waste, and abuse. Credentialing can be a maddening and time-consuming (therefore, costly) administrative process, but *the practice will not be paid until the provider is fully enrolled and credentialed* by the participating health plan.

Documentation Required for Credentialing

The following are the documents that will be required for credentialing:

- Driver's license/state identification card/passport.
- Social Security card.
- Professional license(s) to practice.
- Copy of highest level of educational degree.
- Board certification, if applicable.
- Resume (month/year required).
- Three peer references with similar professional background.

CREDENTIALING AGENCIES

The National Committee for Quality Assurance (NCQA) primarily governs health plans and independent and small group clinic settings that align to hearing healthcare organizations. NCQA's high standards enhance the quality of care while reducing various legal risks. Most healthcare insurance payers will recognize NCQA provider network accreditation, including Centers for Medicare & Medicaid Services (CMS).

A growing number of payers are now utilizing the services of the Council for Affordable Quality Health Care (CAQH, 2024). CAQH is a central repository allowing a provider to complete an online credentialing application. Insurance payers, who utilize CAQH, extract the provider information from CAQH, eliminating both paper and staff time completing the payer-specific application. The initial process of CAQH enrollment requires the provider to complete a one-time, online application.

- Name change documentation (if applicable).
- Type 1—National Provider Identifier (NPI). Required provider forms:
  - Attestation and Release of information.
  - Disclosure questionnaire.
  - Payer signature pages.

Prior to credentialing approval, most organizations are required to submit provider records to a credentialing committee for review and approval. In order to be fully credentialed, generally the provider must be approved by the committee. The credentialing committee is overseen by the medical director of the insurance payer. The committee reviews each provider to ensure they meet the quality-of-care expectations as set forth by their credentialing policies and allows providers to be approved to see patients. The credentialing committee reviews all providers at the time of initial credentialing, recredentialing, and upon notification of quality-of-care concerns.

There will be an ongoing monitoring of credentials. The payers may ask for updated documentation such as driver's license, license to practice, board certification, business license, and/or professional liability. At any time, the payer can conduct site visits to ensure assessment of quality, safety, security, and accessibility of office sites where patient care is rendered.

Credentialing is also necessary when enrolling in third-party contracts, and if done haphazardly or postponed, it can spell cash flow delays and scheduling nightmares. Fortunately, there are methods to minimize issues with credentialing. The following five steps are basic yet proven to simplify the process:

1. *Start early.* Though most credentialing can be completed within 90 days, allow at least 150 days. As payers have merged and supersized, a practice's ability to pull strings and expedite an application has shrunk. Practitioners are

working on the payer's timeline, and each payer has their own internal timeline for application processing. Give ample time to complete the process.

2. *Pay attention*. A recent notice from Anthem for Virginia says that 85% of applications are missing critical information that is required for processing. Missing, outdated, or incomplete information is most common in the following three areas:
   - Work history and current work status (include the effective date beginning with the practice).
   - Malpractice insurance.
   - Attestations.

3. *Stay current with CAQH*. CAQH started its uniform credentialing program about 20 years ago. Since then, many payers have adopted this program. Those entities who regularly update and attest with CAQH find credentialing and recredentialing much easier. Today, CAQH technology-enabled solutions, operating rules, and research help nearly 1,000 health plans, 1.6 million providers, government entities, and vendors connect, exchange information, and operate more efficiently.

4. *Link a provider's start date*. This one is a bit controversial—many practices are reluctant to possibly offend a new employee by badgering them to submit the requisite credentialing paperwork. Remember, the faster the employee becomes credentialed, the faster they can see patients from the enrolled plans.

5. *Know your state's regulations*. Several states have their own laws for timely credentialing, including reciprocity regulations and in-state credentialing. An individual moving from one practice to another within the same state does not go through the full credentialing process again.

Don't separate the credentialing process from contract negotiations. If new to practice or expanding the practice to include participation with a new payer, recognize the need to do more than just send in credentialing forms. The most effective business strategy is to first ensure the settlement on a satisfactory contract. Just signing on the dotted line and submitting paperwork is apt to bring only the payer's standard rate, which is likely lower than your expectations.

Essential Health Benefits

The Patient Protection and Affordable Care Act (ACA) was signed into law in March 2010 by President Barack Obama. According to the U.S. Department of Health and Human Services (HHS), the law's goal was to make health insurance available and affordable to people and small groups, such as employees of small businesses and organizations who are uninsured. Currently, the ACA requires nongrandfathered health plans in the individual and small group markets, to cover essential health benefits (EHBs), which include items and services in the following 10 benefit categories:

- Ambulatory patient services.
- Emergency services.
- Hospitalization maternity and newborn care.
- Mental health.

- Substance use disorder services, including behavioral health treatment.
- Prescription drugs.
- Rehabilitative and habilitative services and devices.
- Laboratory services.
- Preventive and wellness services and chronic disease management.
- Pediatric services, including oral and vision care (CMS website).

The ACA does not specifically exclude coverage for hearing aids. In fact, the ACA does not specifically exclude any coverage: It was written in a positive way, delineating several categories of benefits that must be included in insurance policies sold on the exchanges. While ACA does not exclude the coverage of hearing care as an essential health benefit, hearing care is also *not included* as an essential health benefit, and therefore exchange plans are not mandatorily required to cover hearing healthcare. States differ in their coverage of hearing aids. The Hearing Loss Association of American (HLAA) website includes a list of state exchanges and their specific hearing aid coverage (HLAA, 2024). Twenty states provide some coverage for hearing aids and related services but restrict the coverage to children and teenagers. As of 2024, only five states require coverage for adults: Arkansas, Connecticut, Illinois, New Hampshire, and Rhode Island.

Workers' Compensation

Worker's compensation is a form of insurance providing wage replacement and medical benefits to employees injured in the course of employment in exchange for mandatory relinquishment of the employee's right to sue their employer for the tort of negligence. Workers' compensation statutes are different in each state. Many states recognize hearing loss as a compensable work injury covered by workers' compensation. In some states, workers' compensation laws are more liberal and have greater coverage for hearing services and hearing aids if an employee's hearing loss is job related. The employee must show their injury occurred while performing their job duties, but it's not necessary to prove their employer was negligent. If an individual's hearing loss could be work related, it is recommended that the individual consult with an experienced workers' compensation attorney right away to evaluate a claim. Depending on the state where the provider is located, there are time limitations in which a claim can be made.

Veterans Affairs

The Department of Veterans Affairs (VA) is the second-largest cabinet department; the VA coordinates the distribution of benefits for veterans of the American Armed Forces and their dependents. The benefits include compensation for disabilities, the management of veterans' hospitals, and various insurance programs.

In October 1996, Congress passed the Veterans' Health Care Eligibility Reform Act of 1996. This legislation paved the way for the creation of a Medical Benefits Package—a standard enhanced health benefits plan generally available to all enrolled veterans. Like other standard healthcare plans, the Medical Benefits Package emphasizes preventive and primary care, offering a full range of outpatient and inpatient services. The VA is the largest employer of audiologists and speech-language pathologists in the United States with over 1,100 audiologists providing services across 400 sites of care. Assistance provided by the VA for hearing loss treatment depends on meeting general eligibility requirements. However, once met, veterans can receive benefits for hearing tests, examinations, and hearing aids. Veterans seeking information regarding eligibility should be directed to the local Veterans Administration office or Veterans Administration Medical Center.

within the first 12 months that you have Medicare Part B. The visit includes a thorough review of health, along with education and counseling about necessary preventive services. Hearing and balance disorders are addressed with two screening questionnaires: the Hearing Handicap Inventory for the Elderly (HHI-E) and the Dizziness Handicap Inventory (DHI).

Medicare consists of four parts: Part A (hospital insurance), Part B (medical outpatient services), Part C (Medicare Advantage plans), and Part D (prescription drug coverage) (Chapter 17).

Medicare

Medicare is a social insurance program that serves more than 65 million enrollees. It is the federal health insurance program for people who are 65 or older, certain younger people with disabilities, and people with end-stage renal disease (permanent kidney failure requiring dialysis or a transplant, sometimes called ESRD). Medicare was created when President Lyndon B. Johnson signed amendments to the Social Security Act on July 30, 1965.

Medicare Part B (medical outpatient insurance) covers diagnostic hearing and balance exams when performed by a qualified audiologist when a physician or other healthcare provider orders these tests to determine if the individual needs medical treatment. Medicare doesn't cover hearing exams, hearing aids, or exams for fitting hearing aids.

Medicare enrollees who are new to Medicare are entitled to the "Welcome to Medicare" program. This includes a physical exam, which is a one-time, preventive physical exam Medicare covers

Medicare Part A (Hospital Insurance)

Part A covers inpatient hospital stays, care in a skilled nursing facility, hospice care, and some home healthcare. As a Medicare Part A beneficiary, individuals receive coverage for hospital expenses that are critical to inpatient care, such as a semi-private room, meals, nursing services, medications that are part of inpatient treatment, and any other services and supplies from the hospital. Payment for audiology services in a hospital setting is included in the facility payment under Part A. Audiologists who work within these facilities have their charges billed under the hospital's billing.

Medicare Part B (Medical Outpatient Insurance)

Medicare Part B covers services and supplies that are medically necessary to treat health conditions. This generally includes outpatient care, preventive services, ambulance services, and durable medical equipment. It also covers part-time or intermittent home health and rehabilitative services, such as physical therapy, if they are ordered by a doctor to treat a condition. It covers hospital outpatient services and services usually provided in noninstitutional settings such as those rendered by physicians, diagnostic services such as those provided by audiologists, durable medical equipment, prosthetics and orthotics, and private practice speech-language pathology, physical therapy, and occupational therapy. Part B includes coverage of durable medical equipment (DME) and supplies. Under Part B, those services that are not provided directly by physicians must be obtained through a referral by a physician, physician assistant, or nurse practitioner (if allowed by state law). In the 2023 Physician Fee Schedule Final Rule, CMS finalized an exception to the physician order requirement for certain diagnostic testing services to broaden patient access to services furnished by audiologists. The finalized policy allows beneficiaries direct access (without an order from a physician or nurse practitioner provider) to an audiologist, but only for nonacute hearing conditions. For these directly accessed services, CMS established a new modifier for audiologists to use (Chapter 17). The direct access policy allows Medicare beneficiaries, once every 12 months, to receive care for nonacute hearing assessments that are unrelated to disequilibrium, hearing aids, or examinations for the purpose of prescribing, fitting, or changing hearing aids. A physician order is required for audiology services in all settings other than the exception noted above.

Audiology services under Part B have reimbursement rates established by the Medicare Physician Fee Schedule regardless of provider setting (private practice or otolaryngologist office), except for outpatient audiology services provided in hospitals. Payment is determined by the fee associated with a specific procedure code in those settings. Hospital outpatient audiology services are paid under the Outpatient Prospective Payment System (OOPS) and the fee schedule is updated annually. Hearing and balance assessment services are generally covered as "other diagnostic tests" and are payable under the physician fee schedule. Hearing and balance assessment services furnished to an outpatient of a hospital are covered as "diagnostic services" and are payable under the hospital OPPS or other payment methodology applicable to the provider furnishing the services. All audiological services require a physician referral based on medical necessity.

Medicare Part C (Medicare Advantage Plans)

This is a type of Medicare health plan offered and administered by a commercial health plan that contracts with Medicare to provide all Part A and Part B benefits (Original Medicare) and more. Medicare Advantage plans include:

- Health maintenance organizations (HMOs).
- Preferred provider organizations (PPOs).
- Private fee-for-service plans.
- Special needs plans and Medicare medical savings account plans.

Those individuals enrolled in a Medicare Advantage plan receive Medicare services that are covered through the plan and are not paid for under original Medicare. Most Medicare Advantage plans offer prescription drug coverage and can include annual audiological evaluations, hearing aids, and other hearing services. Medicare Advantage plans are offered by private insurance companies that are approved by Medicare and may cover benefits that go beyond original Medicare.

Medicare Part D (Prescription Drug Coverage)

Part D adds prescription drug coverage to original Medicare, some Medicare cost plans, some Medicare private fee-for-service plans, and Medicare medical savings account plans. These plans are offered by insurance companies and other private companies approved by Medicare. Medicare Advantage plans may also offer prescription drug coverage that follows the same rules as Medicare prescription drug plans.

Detailed information concerning Medicare reimbursements and billing can be found in Chapter 17 of this book, authored by Dr. Debra Abel.

Medicaid

Authorized by Title XIX of the Social Security Act, Medicaid was signed into law in 1965 alongside Medicare. All states, the District of Columbia, and the U.S. territories have Medicaid programs designed to provide health coverage for low-income people. Although the federal government establishes certain parameters for all states to follow, each state administers their Medicaid

program differently, resulting in variations in Medicaid coverage across the country. Beginning in 2014, the Affordable Care Act provided states with the authority to expand Medicaid eligibility to individuals under age 65 in families with incomes below 133% of the federal poverty level (FPL) and standardized the rules for determining eligibility and providing benefits through Medicaid, Children's Health Insurance Program (CHIP), and the Health Insurance Marketplace. To determine if an individual qualifies for Medicaid coverage for hearing aid(s) and/or cochlear implants in each state, the state's Medicaid program or Medicaid's national website at Medicaid.gov has the most current information.

Children's Health Insurance Program (CHIP)

The Children's Health Insurance Program (CHIP) was created by the Balanced Budget Act of 1997 and enacted Title XXI of the Social Security Act. CHIP is a joint state-federal partnership that provides health insurance to low-income children. In February 2009, President Obama signed the Children Health Insurance Program Reauthorization Act of 2009, extending CHIP through 2013. The Affordable Care Act (ACA) extended CHIP an additional 2 years through 2015. In 2015, the law was reauthorized again. Among many provisions, the laws extending the authorization continually have been renewed. States are prohibited from implementing eligibility standards, methodologies, or procedures that are more restrictive than those in place as of March 23, 2010, with the exception of waiting lists for enrolling children in CHIP.

States receive an enhanced federal match that exceeds the federal match for state Medicaid funding. In fiscal year 2022, CHIP expenditures were over $23 billion to help states insure low-income children who are ineligible for Medicaid but cannot afford private insurance.

Federal and state policymakers are currently balancing the need to address competing priorities and the need to provide program stability. In December 2016, the Medicaid and CHIP Payment Advisory Commission recommended a (5-year) extension, citing reductions in children's un-insurance rates and CHIP's recognition of states' role as laboratories for innovation. Today, CHIP services are financed through the fiscal year 2027. Individual state CHIP websites have the most current information on hearing aids and hearing services.

Basic Health Program

Section 1331 of the ACA gives states the option of creating a Basic Health Program (BHP), a health benefits coverage program for low-income residents who would otherwise be eligible to purchase coverage through the Health Insurance Marketplace. The Basic Health Program gives states the ability to provide more affordable coverage for these low-income residents and improve continuity of care for people whose income fluctuates above and below Medicaid and CHIP levels.

Through the Basic Health Program, states can provide coverage to individuals who are citizens or lawfully pres-

ent noncitizens, who do not qualify for Medicaid, CHIP, or other minimum essential coverage and have income between 133% and 200% of the federal poverty level (FPL). Individuals who are lawfully present noncitizens and who have income that does not exceed 133% of FPL but are unable to qualify for Medicaid due to such noncitizen status are also eligible to enroll in BHP.

Consistent with the statute, benefits will include at least the 10 essential health benefits specified in the Affordable Care Act. The monthly premium and cost sharing charged to eligible individuals will not exceed what an eligible individual would have paid if they were to receive coverage from a qualified health plan (QHP) through the Marketplace. A state that operates a Basic Health Program will receive federal funding equal to 95% of the amount of the premium tax credits and the cost-sharing reductions that would have otherwise been provided to (or on behalf of) eligible individuals if these individuals enrolled in QHPs through the Marketplace.

Commercial Payers

There are several different types of commercial payers, each with their own rules and regulations. This is a reason to pay special attention to their contracts as they can differ from one payer to another.

Health Maintenance Organization (HMO)

HMOs require the insured to select a primary care physician (PCP) who acts as gatekeeper. Think of the PCP as a personal health quarterback, providing for and strategically coordinating all of the individual's basic healthcare needs. When the need arises to see a specialist or require a diagnostic service, such as a hearing test, a referral is required from the PCP. The referral will always be to a provider within an HMO's network. If an individual should choose to see a provider outside of the network or without a referral, they will generally have to pay all costs out-of-pocket unless it is a true medical emergency or they have no other options. With an HMO, the physician network is local. To provide audiology services, the audiologist must be a participating provider. This requires contracting and credentialing.

Preferred Provider Organization (PPO)

A PPO is a health plan with a "preferred" network of providers in an area. An individual does not need to select a primary care physician, and a referral is not required to see a specialist. If an individual has services from a "preferred" (or "in-network") provider, they will only be responsible for paying a portion of the bill, according to the plan's coverage structure. If an individual should choose to see a specialist who is outside the preferred network, they will generally pay a larger portion of the bill than they would for an "in-network" provider, but most plans will still cover a portion of the bill. With a PPO, the individual will have access to out-of-state providers who are considered in-network. Audiology services require that the audiologist be a participating pro-

vider or network provider. This requires contracting and credentialing.

Exclusive Provider Network (EPO)

The exclusive provider network (EPO) is a network of individual medical care providers, or groups of medical care providers, who have entered into written agreements with an insurer to provide health insurance to subscribers. EPO is a bit like a hybrid of an HMO and a PPO. EPOs generally offer a little more flexibility than an HMO and are generally less expensive than a PPO. Like a PPO, an individual does not need a referral to obtain care from a specialist but, as with an HMO, patients are responsible for paying out-of-pocket costs if they receive care from a provider outside the plan's network. To provide audiology services as an in-network provider, contracting and credentialing is required.

Point of Service

A point-of-service (POS) plan is a type of managed care health insurance plan that combines characteristics of HMO and a PPO. The concept of the POS is based on the managed care foundation where there are lower medical costs in exchange for more limited choice. But POS health insurance does differ from other managed care plans. Enrollees in a POS plan are required to choose a primary care physician from within the healthcare network; this PCP becomes their point of service. The PCP may make referrals outside the network, but with lesser compensation offered by the patient's health insurance company. If an individual chooses to go outside the network, it is the individual's responsibility to fill out forms, send bills in for payment, and keep an accurate account of healthcare receipts.

The Big 5 Insurance Payers

There are thousands of individual payers in the United States. Those who have a major market share are referred to as the Big 5 payers (Tech Target, 2023). The Big 5 payers today are:

Elevance Health (Formerly Anthem)

Elevance Health, formerly known as Anthem before rebranding in June 2022, has maintained its presence as the nation's second-largest payer. Retaining some of its former branding, Anthem Blue Cross and Anthem Blue Cross and Blue Shield are the payer's brands that offer medical benefits. In 2022, total enrollment across 22 states was 47.5 million individuals with a net revenue of $156 billion.

Elevance and its affiliated brands offer traditional health plans and Medicare Advantage plans. Through continued simplification of offerings to address the key drivers of health, enhanced supplemental benefits, known as Essential Extras, provide consumers with the flexibility that will help them tailor their plan to their specific needs. Elevance offers hearing aid access by providing an allowance toward the purchase of prescription hearing aids and over-the-counter hearing aids on many plans. With Essential Extras, consumers have a choice among dental, vision, and hearing benefits.

Centene

Centene's membership primarily draws from government-sponsored lines of business, which includes Medicaid, Medicare, dual eligibles, and TRICARE. Enrollment in 2022 was 27 million individuals with annual net revenue of $144.5 billion. Centene has largely a government-sponsored portfolio. Centene owns seven companies, including WellCare Health Plans, Magellan Health, and Acariahealth, Inc. These subsidiaries are from the healthcare and pharmaceutical industries. The largest company with the highest revenue is WellCare Health Plans.

All plans under Centene's umbrella of companies offer hearing healthcare and hearing aid benefits. The hearing health plans vary among the different plans.

Aetna (CVS Health)

Aetna offers Medicare, Medicaid, Medicare Advantage, ACA, individual, and employer-sponsored health plans. Annual enrollment is 24.4 million individuals with revenue at $322.5 billion. Aetna became a CVS Health product in 2018.

Most Aetna benefit plans *exclude coverage of hearing aids*. Any applicable benefit plan exclusions and limitations for coverage of hearing aids apply to air conduction hearing aids, implantable hearing aids, and semi-implantable hearing aids. Plans that do not exclude hearing aids, either over-the-counter (OTC) or prescription hearing aids, are eligible for coverage if they are cleared by the U.S. Food and Drug Administration (FDA) and prescribed by a qualified healthcare provider and medical necessity criteria for hearing aids have been met.

Cigna

Formed by a merger in 1982 between the INA Corporation and Connecticut General Corporation, this global health service has been successful incorporating dental and Medicare verticals, offering Medicare prescription plans in all 50 states. Cigna has an enrollment of 18 million and net revenues of $180.5 billion.

Coverage for hearing aid devices varies across plans. Plan availability is limited to devices that are FDA-cleared hearing aids. Devices include air conduction hearing aids, partially implanted bone conduction hearing aids, and bone conduction hearing aids.

United Health Care

United Health Care is an operating division of UnitedHealth Group, the largest single health carrier in the United States, with an enrollment of 51 million and net revenues of $324.2 billion. The company was formed in 1977 through the reorganization of Charter Med Inc., which was established in 1974.

The company provides products and services to some 70 million Americans, and its pharmaceutical management programs provide more affordable access to drugs for 13 million people.

United Health Care has a number of divisions:

■ United Health Care Employer & Individual provides benefit plans and service solutions on a dedicated basis to large, multisite, and national employers and coordinates network-based healthcare benefits and services on behalf of small- to mid-sized employers, as well as individuals, students, and families.
■ United Health Care Medicare & Retirement is the largest business in the nation dedicated to meeting the growing needs of seniors.
■ United Health Care Community & State facilitates and manages healthcare services for state-sponsored public and Medicaid programs and their beneficiaries.

United Health Care Hearing

United Health Care Hearing, a subsidiary of United Health Care Group (UHG), provides hearing health benefits to its members and nonmembers. This benefit includes a direct-to-consumer option to purchase hearing aid devices online. This option is directed at the Medicare Advantage plan enrollees at a discounted rate per hearing aid, depending on the model selected. The concept of selling hearing aids direct to consumers via the Internet is not new, but United Health Care Hearing was the first model to provide an OTC model as an insurance benefit.

United Health Care Hearing does have contractual arrangements with hearing health professionals (audiologists and hearing instrument specialists) to evaluate patients when needed and offer fitting support. Their approach is intended "to increase access to hearing aids and the hearing health system for people who are not accessing the system today."

United Health Care Hearing has developed an online hearing test that, according to their marketing, is a user-friendly test that can be taken using standard computer equipment and earphones. The at-home test is one component of their overall hearing program and is offered free of charge for anyone who wishes to take a hearing test.

By leveraging the scale of United Health Care Group and bypassing supply chain intermediaries (audiologists), United Health Hearing feels they streamline the process and pass the savings to the consumer. Professional services are paid separately from the cost of the hearing devices.

Hearing Network Alliance

In today's highly competitive and ever-widening marketplace, insurance companies have started to look more and more at outsourcing as a valuable strategic management tool. Outsourcing can provide a company an "edge" over organizations that fall into the economic trap of "Jack-of-all-trades, master of none." Realistically, expertise is limited in the field of hearing healthcare for most insurance groups. It is virtually impossible to hire in-house "experts" in every field necessary to process and make determinations on specialty claims. Outsourcing, however, allows the company to utilize the experts while maintaining focus in its primary business. This, in turn, creates more flexibility and opportunity for the company to move forward

in providing more benefits for their enrollees. Insurance companies, especially the larger companies, do not want to negotiate individual contracts, provide credentialing, and hire additional personnel for hearing healthcare services, especially where there are many individual practitioners and very few large group practices. Since more and more programs are offering hearing healthcare benefits, companies are turning to third-party organizations to enroll providers, negotiate hearing aid contracts with manufacturers, recruit, train providers for the network, process claims, and perform other administrative services. More specifically, these third-party organizations are neither the insurer (provider) nor the insured (employees or plan participants), but they are administrators of the plan including processing, adjudication, negotiation of claims, recordkeeping, and maintenance of the plan.

There are a number of these specialty organizations that audiologists and hearing instrument specialists can participate in. These groups contract directly with the insurance companies. The groups offer the audiologist referrals that have insurance, and they process the claims for the professional. This streamlined process generally carries a reduced reimbursement, but the reimbursement is direct and faster with little administrative time for the audiologist.

The Hearing Network Alliance (HNA) is a network of third-party administrators that was created in January 2011 during the Board Meeting of the National Association of Specialty Health Organizations. HNA began with five founding members. Today the HNA brings together senior leaders from the majority of the hearing health networks.

HNA members share a common belief that hearing services are essential to good health and consumer quality of life. HNA as an organization is dedicated to increasing access to hearing health benefits and services. HNA and its member organizations work closely with health plans, employers, and insurance organizations to improve access to hearing healthcare, hearing aid benefits, and services. HNA members share a common interest in conveying the value of hearing and hearing healthcare as a health benefit, and all offer efficient products and networks that enable better consumer access to these services.

HNA's members are Amplifon Hearing Health Care, Birdsong Hearing Benefits, Demant Group Services/Your Hearing Network, Great Hearing Benefits, Start Hearing, TruHearing Inc., and United Health Care Hearing.

HNA's goals are as follows:

1. Increasing awareness of the value of hearing benefits to the public, health plans, and healthcare providers. They emphasize the important link between having a healthcare hearing benefit, being treated for hearing loss, and improving hearing outcomes. Hearing correction improves productivity, health, and quality of life.
2. Ensuring hearing benefit availability in insurance plans.
3. Demonstrating the contribution of hearing networks to access hearing benefits.
4. Ensuring efficient operations of hearing networks to enable these networks to be competitive in the marketplace and thus increase access to hearing health services.

5. Supporting hearing networks in improving and strengthening relationships with audiologists and other hearing care providers.
6. Serving as a primary informational resource on hearing care networks.

Hearing Network Participation

For many audiology practices, participation with third-party hearing network groups has become challenging due to the discounted prices and lower reimbursement rates for hearing aids provided through these groups. Some audiologists take issue with the fact that the audiologist provides the work and follow-up, but the HNA members are making a profit on their work. Each HNA network member has their own reimbursement structure; they also vary on products that can be dispensed. Some groups have offerings from all major manufacturers, some only a few specific manufacturers. There may also be different programs offered by the same organization. For example, TruHearing has the Choice program, which encompasses multiple manufacturers and their products, but they also have the Select program, which is limited to only two products. The audiologist may feel that the availability of only two products is too restrictive for the patient population. If you are a TruHearing provider, is it contractually required to participate in both programs? Is this contrary to the best practices policy for the practice? Whatever the policy, audiologists need to make informed decisions and use the many resources available to them when making the decision to become a participating provider (ASHA, 2024; Grimes &

Casey, 2014). Audiology organizations such as ASHA, AAA, and ADA strongly encourage their respective members to consider the following *before signing any agreement with a third-party payer:*

■ Calculate the breakeven hourly rate for your practice. This will help determine how much paying business is necessary to bring in each hour per full-time equivalent provider to break even. Most businesses cannot afford to accept reimbursement levels that fall below their breakeven rate except on a very limited basis. Additionally, consider desired profit and determine the minimum profit level the practice can afford to accept. The breakeven hourly rate plus the desired profit level are the figures that should be compared to the payer fee schedule to determine if it makes financial sense to participate with a payer.

■ Consider if the third-party contract will generate noncovered services and products. If so, also factor that into the financial analysis.

■ Read the entire agreement from the third-party payer and ensure that it includes a description of covered services and products plus a current fee schedule. Ideally, the fee schedule should include the procedure codes for all the services and products the practice provides, but it *must include* the procedure codes and expected reimbursement for all of the covered services and products. If a fee schedule is not included within the contract or was not otherwise shared with the practice, request a fee schedule from the payer before signing the contract. It is risky and not recommended that one sign a contract that does not

include a fee schedule. Also, check the contract for paragraphs that can restrict professional practice or the ability to collect reimbursement in a reasonable period of time. It is not uncommon for third-party payer contracts to include language that requires 24/7 care or limits billing for reimbursement to 60 days postservice. It is possible to modify these terms, as well as other contract terms, for the practice of audiology, but those changes must be made *before signing the contract, not after.*

■ Verify all contract terms and that the practice can meet those contract terms. Besides the fee schedule, consider infection control, licensing, quality assurance, site visit, and any other requirements that are stated in the contract. Violating the stated requirements can be grounds for lost reimbursement or contract termination.

■ Understand the type of contract that is being signed. Is it discounted fee-for-service, capitated, ancillary care, or some other type of contract? Each has its pros and cons and will impact reimbursement. Clarify covered and noncovered services and products as well as whether the payer allows for upgrades beyond covered services, as the provider's ability to upgrade beyond the covered service amount can be key for acceptable reimbursement, especially for those who dispense hearing aids.

■ It is important to utilize the services of an attorney who specializes in healthcare issues, including third-party contracting, and an accountant when legal, compliance, and/or financial questions arise when reading the agreement. Legal counsel is an important asset when negotiating a third-party payer agreement. Legal counsel can ultimately assist in protecting the practitioner and their practice from potential audit and financial risks and pitfalls, as well as help the practice maintain compliance with state and federal regulations (Chapter 2).

■ If, after reading the agreement and consulting with an attorney, there are still questions or concerns or if the fee schedule is missing any codes, address these questions to the payer, in writing, prior to signing the agreement. It is important to attempt to negotiate with the payer *prior to signing the agreement*; once that signature is affixed, the provider will be held to the fee schedules and requirements of that contract. Also determine if there is a penalty and what that penalty is if an individual with a health plan benefit buys a product direct and not through the third-party group.

■ Always secure an executed contract, meaning a contract that is signed and dated by both parties, and maintain that contract in a safe place for reference. Review and understand the expiration terms and make note of them. The contract may expire on some given date or automatically renew under some contract conditions. Either is fine, but an automatic renewal tends to be a bit easier in that it keeps the contract in place versus requiring an executed contract amendment to continue the contract, even under the same terms, beyond the stated expiration date. Throughout the year, make notes regarding any contract terms that require changes

at the renewal and bring those changes to the payer's attention at the conclusion of the contract term. Keep this fact sheet handy for assistance in the contract renewal negotiation as well.

Billing

Medical billing is a payment practice within the U.S. health system. It is the process that involves the audiologist to submit and follow up on claims with health insurance companies in order to receive payment for services rendered. The same process is used for most insurance companies, whether they are private companies or government-sponsored programs. Medical billers are encouraged, but not required by law, to become certified by taking an exam such as the Certified Medical Reimbursement Specialist (CMRS) exam, Registered Health Information Administrator (RHIA) exam, and others.

Current Procedural Terminology (CPT)

Code set is a medical code set maintained by the American Medical Association through the Current Procedural Terminology (CPT) Editorial Panel. The International Classification of Diseases, Tenth Edition (ICD-10) is a clinical cataloging system that went into effect for the U.S. healthcare industry on October 1, 2015, after a series of lengthy delays. Accounting for modern advances in clinical treatment and medical devices, ICD-11 codes were implemented in January 2022 and offer many more classification options compared to those found in the predecessor ICD-10 codes. ICD Diagnosis (Dx) codes are utilized today for all insurance claims and billings. The health Care Common Procedure Coding System (HCPCS) includes standardized code sets necessary for Medicare and other health insurance providers to provide healthcare claims that are managed consistently and in an orderly manner. HCPCS Level II coding system is one of several code sets used by healthcare professionals, including medical coders and billers. The Level I HCPCS code set includes CPT codes. Level II of the HCPCS is a standardized coding system that is used primarily to identify products, supplies, and services not included in the CPT codes, such as ambulance services and durable medical equipment, prosthetics, orthotics, and supplies (DMEPOS) when used outside a physician's office.

Today, Form 837P (Professional) is the standard format used by healthcare professionals and suppliers to transmit healthcare claims electronically. The Form CMS-1500 is the standard paper claim form to bill Medicare fee-for-service (FFS) contractors when a paper claim is allowed. The CMS-1500 form can only be utilized when a provider qualifies for a waiver from the Administrative Simplification Compliance Act (ASCA) requirement for electronic submission. In addition to billing Medicare, the 837P and Form CMS-1500 may be suitable for billing various government and some private insurers (Chapter 17).

Electronic Data Interchange (EDI)

Electronic Data Interchange (EDI) is the automated transfer of data in a specific format following specific data content rules between a healthcare provider and Medicare, or between Medicare and another healthcare plan. In some cases, that transfer may take place with the assistance of a clearinghouse or billing service that represents a provider of healthcare or another payer. EDI transactions are transferred via computer either to or from Medicare. Through use of EDI, both Medicare and healthcare providers can process transactions faster and at a lower cost. With Electronic Funds Transfer (EFT), Medicare can send payments directly to a provider's financial institution, whether claims are filed electronically or on paper. All Medicare providers may apply for EFT. All Medicare contractors include an EFT authorization form in the Medicare enrollment package, and providers can also request a copy of the form after they have enrolled. Providers simply need to complete the EFT enrollment process as directed by their contractor. Medicare payments will be made directly to the financial institution through EFT in as little as 2 weeks.

EFT Formats

Medicare contractors can use one of two formats to transmit provider electronic claim payments to financial institutions: Automatic Clearinghouse (ACH) format or Table 1 of the Accredited Standards Committee (ASC) X12 835 version 5010 implementation guide, which was adopted as a national standard under the Health Insurance Portability and Accountability Act (HIPAA) for electronic payment and remittance advice. Both of these formats are considered national standards. Further information on the use of EFT for provider payments is in the Medicare Claims Processing Manual (Pub.100-04), Chapter 24, Section 40.7.

Coordination of Benefits

Coordination of benefits (COB) is a term used when a patient has two or more health insurance plans. Certain rules apply to determine which health insurance plan pays primary (first), secondary (second), or tertiary (third). There are several guidelines to determine in what order the medical office must bill each health insurance plan.

Protected Health Information (PHI)

The HIPAA Privacy Rule provides federal protections for certain personal health information held by covered entities and gives patients an array of rights with respect to that information. The Privacy Rules are balanced so that it permits the disclosure of personal health information that is needed for patient care and other important purposes. To improve the efficiency and effectiveness of the healthcare system, HIPAA, Public Law 104-191, included Administrative Simplification provisions that required the Department of Health and Human Services (HHS) to adopt national standards for electronic healthcare transactions and code sets, unique health identifiers, and security. At the same time, Congress recognized that advances in electronic technology could erode the privacy of health information. Consequently, Congress incorporated into HIPAA provisions also known as Protected Health Information (PHI) (USDHHS (2024).

The following 18 items have been identified as Protected Health Information: names; all geographic subdivisions smaller than a state, including street address, city, county, precinct, zip code, and their equivalent geocodes; all elements of dates (except year) for dates directly related to an individual, including birth date, admission date, discharge date, and date of death; telephone numbers; fax numbers; electronic mail addresses; Social Security numbers; medical record numbers; health plan beneficiary numbers; account numbers; certificate and/or license numbers; vehicle identifiers and serial numbers; license plate numbers; device identifiers and serial numbers; web URLs; full face photos or comparable images; and any unique identification number, characteristic, or code (Chapter 17).

NATIONAL PROVIDER IDENTIFICATION (NPI)

The Health Insurance Portability and Accountability Act (HIPAA) of 1996 required the adoption of a standard unique identifier for healthcare

continued on next page

continued from previous page

providers. The NPI Final Rule, issued January 23, 2004, adopted the NPI as this standard.

The NPI is a 10-digit numeric identifier; the first 9-digit positions are the identifier, and the last digit is a "check" digit, which helps detect invalid NPIs. The NPI replaces other identifiers such as Medicare legacy IDs (UPIN, OSCAR, PIN, and National Supplier Clearinghouse or NSC).

All individual and organizational healthcare providers who are HIPAA-covered entities must obtain an NPI. An NPI number facilitates a simpler electronic transmission of HIPAA standard transactions, standard unique health identifiers for healthcare providers, health plans, and employers and a more efficient coordination of benefits transactions.

HITECH Act

The Health Information Technology for Economic and Clinical Health (HITECH) Act, enacted as part of the American Recovery and Reinvestment Act of 2009, was signed into law on February 17, 2009, to promote the adoption and meaningful use of health information technology. Subtitle D of the HITECH Act addresses the privacy and security concerns associated with the electronic transmission of health information, in part, through several provisions that strengthen the civil and criminal enforcement of the HIPAA rules. Because HITECH legislation results in an expansion in the exchange of electronic protected health information, it also widens the scope of privacy and security protections under the HITECH Act, which includes increasing legal liability for noncompliance.

Enforcement, historically, was not rigorously enforced, but the adoption of the final rule in 2013 clarified and strength-

ened enforcement activities. The enforcement of penalties and violations was to include covered entities and business associates.

HITECH imposes data breach notification requirements for unauthorized uses and disclosure of unsecured or unencrypted PHI. In audiology practices that have implemented an electronic health record system (EHR), individuals have a right to obtain their PHI in an electronic format. Only a fee equal to the labor cost can be charged for an electronic request. HITECH now applies HIPAA provisions to business associates, thus requiring business associates to comply with the HIPAA security rule. What does this mean for audiology practices? Most, if not all, software vendors providing EHR systems will clearly qualify as business associates. Business associates must report security breaches to covered entities consistent with notification requirements. Business associates are subject to civil and criminal penalties, just as the covered entities are subject to these penalties. Business associates and providers will now share more joint responsibilities than they have previously. There are additional requirements that modify HIPAA and affect HITECH. To stay informed, regular visits are recommended to the Department of Human and Health Services website at https//:www.hhs.gov/ocr/privacy.

FREQUENTLY USED TERMS

The following is a glossary of terms that will help you become familiar with the everyday vocabulary used by medical billing specialists and their peers. Because of the complexity of insurance, let this extensive glossary of key terms serve as a reference to help you get a better grasp on the language of this field.

A

Allowed Amount

The sum an insurance company will reimburse to cover a healthcare service or procedure. The patient typically pays the remaining balance if there is any amount left over after the allowed amount has been paid. This amount should not be confused with copay or deductibles owed by a patient.

American Medical Association (AMA)

The AMA is the largest organization of physicians in the United States dedicated to improving the quality of healthcare administered by providers across the country. The CPT code set is maintained and revised by the AMA in accordance with federal guidelines.

Aging

A formal medical billing term that refers to insurance claims that haven't been paid or balances owed by patients overdue by more than 30 days. Aging claims may be denied if they aren't filed in time with a health insurance company.

continued on next page

continued from previous page

Ancillary Services

Any service administered in a hospital or other healthcare facility other than room and board, including biometrics tests, physical therapy, and physician consultations, among other services.

Appeal

Appeal occurs when a patient or a provider requests that an insurance company reconsider its decision to pay for healthcare after denying a claim for services. Medical billing specialists deal with appeals after a claim has been denied or rejected by an insurance company.

Applied to Deductible (ATD)

This term refers to the amount of money a patient owes a provider that goes to paying their yearly deductible. A patient's deductible is determined by their insurance plan and can range in price.

Assignment of Benefits (AOB)

This term refers to insurance payments made directly to a healthcare provider for medical services received by the patient. Assignment of benefits occurs after a claim has been accepted and processed by an insurance company.

Application Service Provider (ASP)

ASP is a digital network that allows healthcare providers to access quality medical billing software and technologies without needing to purchase and maintain them themselves. Providers who use ASP typically pay a monthly fee to the company that maintains the billing software.

Authorization

This term refers to when a patient's health insurance plan requires them to get permission from their insurance providers before receiving certain healthcare services. A patient may be denied coverage if they see a pro-

continued on next page

continued from previous page

vider for a service that needed authorization without first consulting the insurance company.

B

Beneficiary

The beneficiary is the person who receives benefits and/or coverage under a healthcare plan. The beneficiary of an insurance plan may not be the person paying for the plan, as is the case for young children covered under their parents' plans.

Blue Cross Blue Shield

Blue Cross Blue Shield is a federation of 38 health insurance companies in the United States (some of which are nonprofit companies) that offer health insurance options to eligible persons in their area. Blue Cross Blue Shield offers healthcare plans to over 100 million people in the United States.

C

Capitation

A fixed payment that a patient makes to a health insurance company or provider to recoup costs incurred from various healthcare services. A capitation is different from a deductible or copay.

Civilian Health and Medical Program of Uniform Services (CHAMPUS)

CHAMPUS (now known as TRICARE) is the federal health insurance program for active and retired service members, their families, and the survivors of service members.

Charity Care

This type of care is administered at reduced or zero cost to patients who cannot afford healthcare. Providers may offer charity care at their discretion.

continued on next page

continued from previous page

Clean Claim

This refers to a medical claim filed with a health insurance company that is free of errors and processed in a timely manner. Some providers may send claims to organizations that specialize in producing clean claims, like clearinghouses. The Centers for Medicare & Medicaid Services (CMS) National Correct Coding Initiative (NCCI) promotes national correct coding methodologies and reduces improper coding, with the overall goal of reducing improper payments of Medicare Part B and Medicaid claims.

Clearinghouse

Clearinghouses are facilities that review and correct medical claims as necessary before sending them to insurance companies for final processing. This meticulous editing process for claims is known in the medical billing industry as "scrubbing."

Centers for Medicare & Medicaid Services (CMS)

The CMS is the federal entity that manages and administers healthcare coverage through Medicare and Medicaid. CMS coordinates with providers and enrollees to provide healthcare to over 100 million Americans.

CMS 1500

The CMS 1500 is a paper medical claim form used for transmitting claims based on coverage by Medicare and Medicaid plans. Commercial insurance providers often require that providers use CMS 1500 forms to process their own paper claims.

Coding

Coding is the process of translating a physician's documentation about a patient's medical condition and health services rendered into medical codes that are then entered into a claim for processing with an insurance company. Medical billing specialists must be familiar with many codes sets in order to perform their job duties.

continued on next page

continued from previous page

COBRA Insurance

A federal program that allows a person terminated from their employer to retain health insurance they had with that employer for up to 18 months, or 36 months if the former employee is disabled.

Coinsurance

The percentage of coverage that a patient is responsible for paying after an insurance company pays the portion agreed upon in a health plan. Coinsurance percentages vary depending on the health plan.

Collection Ratio

This refers to the ratio of payments received relative to the total amount owed to providers.

Contractual Adjustment

This refers to a binding agreement between a provider, patient, and insurance company wherein the provider agrees to charges that it will write off on behalf of the patient. Contractual adjustments may occur when there is a discrepancy between what a provider charges for healthcare services and what an insurance company has decided to pay for that service.

Coordination of Benefits (COB)

COB occurs when a patient is covered by more than one insurance plan. In this situation, one insurance company will become the primary carrier and all other companies will be considered secondary and tertiary carriers that may cover charges that remain after the primary carrier has paid.

Copay

A patient's copay is the amount that must be paid to a provider before they receive any treatment or services. Copays are separate from a deductible and will vary depending on a person's insurance plan.

continued on next page

continued from previous page

Current Procedural Technology (CPT) Code

CPT codes represent treatments and procedures performed by a physician in a five-digit format. CPT codes are entered together with ICD-11 codes that explain a patient's diagnosis. Medical billing specialists will enter CPT codes into claims, so insurance companies understand the nature of healthcare a patient received with a provider.

Credentialing

The application process for a provider to participate with an insurance company. Once providers have become credentialed with an insurance company, they have the opportunity to work with that company in providing affordable healthcare to patients.

Credit Balance

Refers to the sum shown in the "balance" column of a billing statement that reflects the amount due for services rendered.

Crossover Claim

When claim information is sent from a primary insurance carrier to a secondary insurance carrier or vice versa.

D

Date of Service (DOS)

The date when a provider performed healthcare services and procedures.

Day Sheet

A document that summarizes the services, treatments, payments, and charges that a patient received on a given day.

continued on next page

continued from previous page

Deductible

The amount a patient must pay before an insurance carrier starts their healthcare coverage. Deductibles range in price according to terms set in a person's health plan.

Demographics

The patient's information required for filing a claim, such as age, sex, address, and family information. An insurance company may deny a claim if it contains inaccurate demographics.

Durable Medical Equipment (DME)

This refers to medical implements that can be reused such as stretchers, wheelchairs, canes, crutches, and bedpans.

Date of Birth (DOB)

The exact date a patient was born.

Downcoding

Downcoding occurs when an insurance company finds there is insufficient evidence on a claim to prove that a provider performed coded medical services and so they reduce or remove those codes. Downcoding usually reduces the cost of a claim and reimbursement to the provider submitting the claim.

Duplicate Coverage Inquiry (DCI)

A formal request typically submitted by an insurance carrier to determine if other health coverage exists for a patient.

Dx

The abbreviation for diagnosis codes, also known as ICD-11 codes.

continued on next page

continued from previous page

E

Electronic Claim

A claim sent electronically to an insurance carrier from a provider's billing software. The format of electronic claims must adhere to medical billing regulations set forth by the federal government.

Electronic Funds Transfer

A method of transferring money electronically from one bank account to another bank account. This can be utilized by a patient, a provider, or an insurance carrier.

Evaluation and Management (E/M)

E/M refers to the section of CPT codes most used by healthcare personnel to describe a patient's medical needs.

Electronic Medical Record (EMR)

EMR is a digitized medical record for a patient managed by a provider onsite. EMRs may also be referred to as electronic health records (EHRs).

Enrollee

A person covered by a health insurance plan.

Explanation of Benefits (EOB)

A document attached to a processed medical claim wherein the insurance company explains the services they will cover for a patient's healthcare treatments. EOBs may also explain what is wrong with a claim if it's denied.

Electronic Remittance Advice (ERA)

The digital version of EOB, which specifies the details of payments made on a claim either by insurance company or required by the patient.

continued on next page

continued from previous page

ERISA

Stands for the Employee Retirement Income Security Act of 1974. This act established guidelines and requirements for health and life insurance policies, including appeals and disclosure of grievances.

F

Fee for Service

This refers to a type of health insurance wherein the provider is paid for every service they perform. People with fee-for-service plans typically can choose whatever hospitals and physicians they want to receive care in exchange for higher deductibles and copays.

Fee Schedule

A document that outlines the costs associated for each medical service designated by a CPT code or, for audiologists, the HCPCS code.

Financial Responsibility

Whoever owes the healthcare provider money has financial responsibility for the services rendered. Insurance companies or patients themselves may be financially responsible for the costs associated with care, and these responsibilities are typically outlined in a healthcare plan contract.

Fiscal Intermediary (FI)

The name for Medicare representatives who process Medicare claims.

Formulary

A table or list provided by an insurance carrier that explains what prescription drugs are covered under their health plans. Many health plans using third-party administrators have a hearing aid formulary.

continued on next page

continued from previous page

Fraud

Providers, patients, or insurance companies may be found fraudulent if they are deliberately achieving their ends through misrepresentation, dishonesty, and general illegal activity. Medical billing specialists who deliberately enter incorrect or misleading information on claims may be charged with fraud.

G

Group Health Plan (GPH)

A plan provided by an employer to provide healthcare options to a large group of employees.

Group Name

The name of the group, insurance carrier, or insurance plan that covers a patient.

Group Number

A number given to a patient by their insurance carrier that identifies the group or plan under which they are covered.

Guarantor

The party paying for an insurance plan who is not the patient. Parents, for example, would be the guarantors for their children's health insurance.

H

Health Care Financing Administration

The former name for what is now the CMS.

continued on next page

continued from previous page

Health Care Financing Administration Common Procedure Coding System (HCPCS)

HCPCS is a three-tier coding system used to explain services, devices, and diagnoses administered in the healthcare system. Medical billing specialists utilize codes in the HCPCS on a daily basis to file claims.

Health Care Insurance

This is insurance offered to a group or an individual to cover costs associated with medical care and treatment. Those covered by healthcare insurance typically must pay a premium for their plans in addition to various copays and/or deductibles.

Healthcare Provider

These are the entities that offer healthcare services to patients, including hospitals, physicians, private clinics, hospices, nursing homes, and other healthcare facilities.

Health Care Reform Act

The major healthcare legislation passed in 2010 designed to make healthcare accessible and less expensive for more Americans.

Health Insurance Claim

The unique number ascribed to an individual to identify them as a beneficiary of Medicare.

Health Insurance Portability and Accountability Act (HIPAA)

HIPAA was a law passed in 1996 with an aim to improve the scope of healthcare services and establish regulations for securing healthcare records from unwanted parties.

Health Maintenance Organization (HMO)

HMOs are networks of healthcare providers that offer healthcare plans to people for medical services exclusively in their network.

continued on next page

continued from previous page

Hospice

This refers to medical care and treatment for persons who are terminally ill.

I

ICD-10 Codes

ICD-10 codes are an international set of codes that represent diagnoses of patients' medical conditions as determined by physicians. Medical billing specialists may translate a physician's diagnoses into ICD-10 codes and then input those codes into a claim for processing.

ICD-11 Codes

ICD-11 codes are the updated international set of codes based on the preceding ICD-10 codes. ICD-11 became effective January 1, 2022.

Incremental Nursing Charge

A fee for nursing services a patient is charged during the course of receiving healthcare.

Indemnity

A type of health insurance plan whereby a patient can receive care with any provider in exchange for higher deductibles and copays. Indemnity is also known as fee-for-service insurance.

In-Network

This term refers to a provider's relationship with a health insurance company. A group of providers may contract with an insurance company to form a network of healthcare professionals that a person can choose from when enrolled in that insurance company's health plan.

continued on next page

continued from previous page

Inpatient

Inpatient care occurs when a person has a stay at a healthcare facility for more than 24 hours.

Independent Practice Association (IPA)

The IPA is a professional organization of physicians who have a contract with an HMO.

Intensive Care

Intensive care is the unit of a hospital reserved for patients who need immediate treatment and close monitoring by healthcare professionals for serious illnesses, conditions, and injuries.

M

Medicare Administrative Contractor (MAC)

MACs are private healthcare insurers that contract with the federal government to process Medicare claims.

Managed Care Plan

A health insurance plan whereby patients can only receive coverage if they see providers who operate in the insurance company's network.

Maximum Out-of-Pocket

The amount a patient is required to pay. After a patient reaches their maximum out-of-pocket, their healthcare costs should be covered by their plan.

Medical Assistant

An employee in the healthcare system such as a physician's assistant or a nurse practitioner who perform duties in administration, nursing, and other ancillary care.

continued on next page

continued from previous page

Medical Coder

A medical coder is responsible for assigning various medical codes to services and healthcare plans described by a physician on a patient's superbill.

Medical Billing Specialist

A medical billing specialist is responsible for using information regarding services and treatments performed by a healthcare provider to complete a claim for filing with an insurance company so the provider can be paid.

Medical Necessity

This term refers to healthcare services or treatments that a patient requires to treat a serious medical condition or illness that meets accepted standards of medical care. This does not include cosmetic or investigative services.

Medical Record Number

A unique number ascribed to a person's medical record so it can be differentiated from other medical records.

Medicare Secondary Payer

The insurance company that covers any remaining expenses after Medicare has paid for a patient's coverage.

Medical Savings Account (MSA)

An MSA is optional health insurance payments plan whereby a person apportions part of their untaxed earnings to an account reserved for healthcare expenses. A person with an MSA can only contribute a certain amount of their earnings per year. Any unused funds in an MSA at the end of the year will roll over to the next year.

Medical Transcription

The process of converting dictated or handwritten instructions, observations, and documentation into digital text formats.

continued on next page

continued from previous page

Medicare

Medicare is a government insurance program that started in 1965 to provide healthcare coverage for persons over 65 and eligible people with disabilities.

Medicare Coinsurance Days

Referring to days 61 to 90 of inpatient treatment, the law requires that patients pay for a portion of their healthcare during Medicare coinsurance days.

Medicare Donut Hole

This term refers to the discrepancy between the limits of healthcare insurance coverage and the Medicare Part D coverage limits for prescription drugs.

Medicaid

Medicaid is a joint federal and state assistance program that started in 1965 to provide health insurance to lower-income persons. Both state and federal governments fund Medicaid programs, but each state is responsible for running its own version of Medicaid within the minimum requirements established by federal law.

Medigap

Medigap is supplemental health insurance sold by private insurance companies to fill the "gaps" in original Medicare plan coverage. Medigap policies help pay some of the healthcare costs that the original Medicare plan doesn't cover.

Modifier

Modifiers are additions to CPT codes that explain alterations and modifications to an otherwise routine treatment, exam, or service.

continued on next page

continued from previous page

N

Noncovered Charge (N/C)

N/Cs are procedures and services not covered by a person's health insurance plan.

Not Elsewhere Classifiable (NEC)

A term used to describe a procedure or service that can't be described within the available code set.

Network Provider

A provider within a health insurance company's network that has contracted with the company to provide services to a patient covered under the company's plan.

Nonparticipation

This is when a provider refuses to accept Medicare payments as a sufficient amount for the services rendered to a patient.

Not Otherwise Specified (NOS)

This term is used in ICD-9 codes to describe conditions with unspecified diagnoses.

National Provider Identifier (NPI) Number

A unique 10-digit number ascribed to every healthcare provider in the United States as mandated by HIPAA.

No Surprise Act

A facility (such as a hospital or freestanding emergency room [ER]) or a provider may not bill you more than your in-network coinsurance,

continued on next page

continued from previous page

copays, or deductibles for emergency services, even if the facility or provider is out-of-network.

Office of Inspector General (OIG)

The organization responsible for establishing guidelines and investigating fraud and misinformation within the healthcare industry. The OIG is part of the Department of Health and Human Services.

Out-of-Network

Out-of-network refers to providers outside of an established network of providers who contract with an insurance company to offer patients healthcare at an established rate. People who go to out-of-network providers typically have to pay more money to receive care.

Outpatient

This term refers to healthcare treatment that doesn't require an overnight hospital stay, including a routine visit to a primary care doctor or a non-invasive surgery.

P

Palmetto GBA

A MAC based in Columbia, South Carolina, that is also a subsidiary of Blue Cross Blue Shield.

Patient Responsibility

This refers to the amount a patient owes a provider after an insurance company pays for their portion of the medical expenses.

Primary Care Physician (PCP)

The physician who provides the basic healthcare services for a patient and recommends additional care for more complex conditions as necessary.

continued on next page

continued from previous page

Point-of-Service Plans

A plan whereby patients pay less if they use doctors, hospitals, and other healthcare providers that belong to the plan's network. POS plans also require patients to get a referral from their primary care doctor in order to see a specialist.

Place of Service Code

A two-digit code used on claims to explain what type of provider performed healthcare services on a patient.

Preferred Provider Organization (PPO)

A plan similar to an HMO whereby a patient can receive healthcare from providers within an established network set up by an insurance company.

Practice Management Software

Software used for scheduling, billing, and recordkeeping at a provider's office.

Preauthorization

Some insurance plans require that a patient receive preauthorization from the insurance company prior to receiving certain medical services to make sure the company will cover expenses associated with those services.

Precertification

A process similar to preauthorization whereby patients must check with insurance companies to see if a desired healthcare treatment or service is deemed medically necessary (and thus covered) by the company.

Predetermination

A maximum sum as explained in a healthcare plan an insurance company will pay for certain services or treatments.

continued on next page

continued from previous page

Preexisting Condition (PEC)

PEC is a medical condition a patient had before receiving coverage from an insurance company. A person might become ineligible for certain healthcare plans depending on the severity and length of their PEC.

Preexisting Condition Exclusion

The existence of a PEC denies a person certain coverage in some health insurance plans.

Premium

The sum a person pays to an insurance company on a regular (usually monthly or yearly) basis to receive health insurance.

Privacy Rule

Standards for privacy regarding a patient's medical history and all related events, treatments, and data as outlined by HIPAA.

Provider

A provider is the healthcare facility that administered healthcare to an individual. Credentialed physicians, specialists, clinics, and hospitals are all considered providers.

Provider Transaction Access Number (PTAN)

This refers to a provider's current legacy provider number with Medicare.

R

Referral

This is when a provider recommends another provider to a patient to receive specialized treatment.

continued on next page

continued from previous page

Remittance Advice (R/A)

The R/A is also known as the EOB, which is the document attached to a processed claim that explains the information regarding coverage and payments on a claim.

Responsible Party

The person who pays for a patient's medical expenses, also known as the guarantor.

Revenue Code

A three-digit code used on medical bills that explains the kind of facility in which a patient received treatment.

Relative Value Amount (RVA)

The median amount Medicare will repay a provider for certain services and treatments.

S

Scrubbing

A process by which insurance claims are checked for errors before being sent to an insurance company for final processing. Providers scrub claims in an attempt to reduce the number of denied or rejected claims and comply with the National Coding Initiative.

Self-Referral

When a patient does their own research to find a provider and acts outside of their primary care physician's referral.

continued on next page

continued from previous page

Self-Pay

Payment made by the patient for healthcare at the time they receive it at a provider's facilities.

Secondary Insurance Claim

The claim filed with the secondary insurance company after the primary insurance company pays for their portion of healthcare costs.

Secondary Procedure

This is when provider performs another procedure on a patient covered by a CPT code after first performing a different CPT procedure on them.

Security Standard

The security standard serves as the guidelines for policies and practices necessary to reduce security risks within the healthcare system. The security standard policies work in concert with the security guidelines set in place with the passage of HIPAA.

Skilled Nursing Facility

These are facilities for the severely ill or elderly that provide specialized long-term care for recovering patients. Skilled nursing facilities are alternative healthcare establishments to extended hospital stays and may be covered by eligible patients' insurance policies.

Signature on File (SOF)

A patient's official signature on file for the purpose of billing and claims processing.

continued on next page

continued from previous page

Software as a Service (SAAS)

Medical billing software hosted offsite by another company and only accessible with Internet access. SAAS is useful for providers who don't want to maintain and update in-house medical billing software.

Specialist

A physician or other trained healthcare professional with expertise in a specific area of medicine. Oncologists, pediatricians, and neurologists are among the many specialists in the medical field.

Subscriber

The subscriber is the individual covered under a group policy. For instance, an employee of a company with a group health policy would be one of many subscribers on that policy.

Superbill

A document used by healthcare staff and physicians to record information about a patient receiving care. The superbill can contain demographic information, insurance information, and especially any diagnoses or healthcare plans written by the physician. A medical billing specialist inputs the information on a patient's superbill into a claim.

Supplemental Insurance

Supplemental insurance can be a secondary policy or another insurance company that covers a patient's healthcare costs after receiving coverage from their primary insurance. Supplemental insurance policies typically help patients cover expensive deductibles and copays.

continued on next page

continued from previous page

T

Treatment Authorization Request (TAR)

A unique number the insurance company gives the provider for billing purposes. A provider must receive the insurance company's TAR number before administering healthcare to a patient covered by the company.

Taxonomy Code

Medical billing specialists utilize this unique code set for identifying a healthcare provider's specialty field.

Term Date

The end date for an insurance policy contract, or the date after which a person no longer receives or is no longer eligible for health insurance with company. Term dates are typically determined on a case-by-case basis.

Tertiary Insurance Claim

A claim filed by a provider after they have filed claims for primary and secondary health insurance coverage on behalf of a patient. Tertiary insurance claims often cover the remaining healthcare costs such as deductibles and copays left over after the primary and secondary claims have been processed.

Third-Party Administrator (TPA)

The name for the organization or individual that manages healthcare group benefits, claims, and administrative duties on behalf of a group plan or a company with a group plan.

continued on next page

continued from previous page

Tax Identification Number (TIN)

A unique number a service provider or a company may have to produce for billing purposes in order to receive healthcare from a provider. The TIN is also known as the employment identification number (EIN).

Triple-Option Plan (TOP)

Also referred to as the cafeteria plan, this plan gives an enrolled individual the options to choose between an HMO, a PPO, or a traditional point-of-service plan for their health insurance. Some companies offer triple-option plans to their employees to accommodate the needs of a diverse staff.

Type of Service (TOS)

A field on a claim describing what kind of healthcare services or procedures a provider administered.

TRICARE

TRICARE is the federal health insurance plan for active service members, retired service members, and their families, in addition to survivors of service members. TRICARE was previously known as CHAMPUS.

U

UB04

A form used by providers for filing claims with insurance companies. The UB04 form has a format similar to that of the CMS 1500 form.

Unbundling

The submission of multiple procedure codes for a group of specific procedures that are components of a single comprehensive code.

continued on next page

continued from previous page

Untimely Submission

Claims have a specific timeframe in which they can be sent off to an insurance company for processing. If a provider fails to file a claim with an insurance company in that time frame, it is marked for untimely submission and will be denied by the company.

Upcoding

Upcoding is the fraudulent practice of ascribing a higher ICD-11 code to a healthcare procedure in an attempt to get more money than necessary from the insurance company or patient.

Unique Physician Identification Number (UPIN)

A unique six-digit identification number given to physicians and other healthcare personnel, which has subsequently been replaced by a National Provider Identifier (NPI) number.

Usual Customary and Reasonable (UCR)

The UCR is the amount of money stipulated in a contract that an insurance company agrees to pay for healthcare costs. After passing the UCR, a patient is typically responsible for covering their healthcare costs.

Utilization Limit

The limit per year for coverage under certain available healthcare services for Medicare enrollees. Once a patient passes the utilization limit for a service, Medicare may no longer cover them.

continued on next page

continued from previous page

Utilization Review (UR)

An investigation or audit performed to optimize the number of inpatient and outpatient services a provider performs.

V

V-Codes and Z Codes

A code set under ICD-11-CM used to organize healthcare services rendered for reasons other than illness or injury. V codes or Z codes report problems or factors that may influence present or future care. Appropriate V or Z code assignment is extremely important in terms of reporting, medical necessity, and avoiding inaccurate denials.

W

Workers' Compensation

Workers' compensation is paid by an employer when an employee becomes ill or injured while performing routine job duties. Most states have laws requiring that companies provide workers' compensation.

Write-Off

This term refers to the difference between a provider's fee for healthcare services and the amount that an insurance company is willing to pay for those services that a patient is not responsible for. The write-off amount may be categorized as "not covered" amounts for billing purposes.

References

Abrams, H. & Kilm, J. (2015, June). An introduction to MarkeTrak IX: A new baseline for the hearing aid market, *Hearing Review.*

ASHA. (2024). Important considerations for audiologists when reviewing third-party payer provider contracts. http://www.asha.org/Practice/reimbursement/private-plans/Important-Considerations-for-Audiologists-When-Reviewing-Third-Party-Payer-Provider-Contracts/

Blackwell, D. L., Lucas, J. W., & Clarke, T. C. (2014). Summary health statistics for U.S. adults: National Health Interview Survey, 2012. National Center for Health Statistics. https://www.cdc.gov/nchs/data/series/sr_10/sr10_260.pdf

CAQH. (2024). Council for Affordability in Healthcare. https://www.caqh.org/

FDA. (2024). Estimates based on manufacturers' voluntary reports of registered devices to the U.S. Food and Drug Administration. https://www.google.com/search?q=Estimates+based+on+manufacturers%E2%80%99+voluntary+reports+of+registered+devices+to+the+U.S.+Food+and+Drug+Administration%2C&oq=Estimates+based+on+manufacturers%E2%80%99+voluntary+reports+of+registered+devices+to+the+U.S.+Food+and+Drug+Administration%2C&gs_lcrp=EgZjaHJvbWUyBggAEEUYODIBBzkxNWowajeo AgiwAgE&sourceid=chrome&ie=UTF-8

Grimes, A., & Casey, P. (2014). Health insurance: Should hearing aids be included? Audiology Online. http://www.audiologyonline.com/articles/health-insurance-should-hearing-aids-1227

Hearing Loss Association of America. (2024). Communication access in health care. Affordable Care Act. Communication Access in Health Care - Hearing Loss Association of America

Humana. (2023). Understanding Medicare Advantage. Humana Health Policy Center. https://policy.humana.com/issue-area/understanding-medicare-advantage.html

NCQA. (2024). National Committee on Quality Assurance. http://www.ncqa.org/about-ncqa

Ochieng N., Biniek, J., Freed, M., Damico, A., & Neuman, T. (2023). Medicare advantage in 2023: Premiums, out-of-pocket limits, cost sharing, supplemental benefits, prior authorization, and star ratings. Kaiser Family Foundation. https://www.kff.org/medicare/issue-brief/medicare-advantage-in-2023-premiums-out-of-pocket-limits-cost-sharing-supplemental-benefits-prior-authorization-and-star-ratings/

Ortman, J. M., Velkoff, V. A., & Hogan, H. (2014). An aging nation: The older population in the United States. U.S. Department of Commerce Economics and Statistics Administration. https://www.census.gov/content/dam/Census/library/publications/2014/demo/p25-1140.pdf

Powers, T. A., Carr, K., & MarkeTrak (2022). Navigating the changing landscape of hearing healthcare. *Hearing Review, 29*(5), 12–17.

Shaw, G. (2013). Cover story: Negotiating third-party payments: Read between the lines. *Hearing Journal, 66*(9), 22–25. https://journals.lww.com/thehearingjournal/fulltext/2013/09000/cover_story__negotiating_third_party_payments_.1.aspx

Tech Target. (2023). Top 5 largest health insurance payers in the United States. Tech Target: Medicare, Medicaid and CHIP. https://www.techtarget.com/healthcarepayers/feature/Top-5-Largest-Health-Insurance-Payers-in-the-United-States

United Health Care Hearing. (2024). Explore prescription hearing aids. https://www.uhchearing.com/prescription

USDHHS. (2024). What is PHI? U.S. Department of Health & Human Services. What is PHI? https://www.hhs.gov/answers/hipaa/what-is-phi/

17 Coding Reimbursement and Compliance

Debra Abel, AuD

Introduction

Audiologists have historically experienced road bumps and roadblocks with coding, reimbursement, and the recognition by payers for the full cadre of services they provide. This is especially true given the explosion of third-party payers driven by the Medicare Advantage plans that may provide added services beyond those of traditional Part B Medicare, which may also include hearing aid benefits. It has been a long, arduous road of educating payers as to those services as well as defining "audiology" on a national and grass roots level. The road continues to unwind in an unprecedented, dynamic system on the cusp of different payment methodologies and device delivery models. Consequently, this education has also been conducted within the halls of Congress as well as the Centers for Medicare & Medicaid Services (CMS), viewed by some as the trend-setting gold standard for insurance reimbursement. Many third-party payers look to CMS, the Resource-Based Relative Value Scale (RBRVS), and the Medicare Physician Fee Schedule (MPFS) as the benchmark for establishing their own fee schedules, thereby perpetuating this inefficient system.

Understanding where audiology has been in the past and what the future holds for the profession in terms of autonomy and professionalism it is essential that a practice abides by established and mandated federal and state regulations. In addition to the reimbursement side, there are a plethora of issues and concerns to consider when contemplating the foray into independent practice, some legal and some practical, all of which will be touched upon here. This list of issues and concerns is not limited by any means. As such, federal, state, and local laws should be vetted prior to considering a private practice with an attorney versed in healthcare law, offering legal guidance and an accountant lending financial expertise.

At the time of the publication of this book, CMS continues to recognize audiologists only as *diagnosticians* and *not as providers of treatment of hearing and balance disorders*, yet it acknowledges that these areas are in an audiologist's scope of practice, which is determined by state licensure laws. However, effective January 1, 2023, a major change for audiologists enrolled in Medicare Part B occurred! Medicare changed its regulations regarding physician orders for non-acute and nonvestibular patients, only the second major change affecting audiologists since Medicare's inception in

1965! The first was in 2008 with the publication of Transmittal 84 that offered the guidance that the services of an audiologist must be billed with that audiologist's own National Provider Identifier (NPI). These 2023 changes will be detailed in the Medicare section of this chapter.

Many third-party payers have established their policies based on these Medicare-imposed requirements, but these diagnostic testing restrictions do not agree with state licensure laws, defining the scope of practice for audiology. State licensure laws recognize all services that audiologists are licensed to provide, and some payers do recognize and reimburse for all professional services. It is, however, important to remember that if a procedure is not recognized for payment by a third-party payer, that service may be considered a noncovered service and is the patient's responsibility to pay for that service if not contractually excluded. This needs to be confirmed for every patient as part of the hearing aid verification process.

With the movement to the doctoring profession and recognition of audiologists as service providers, evolution has occurred with most third-party payers and likely will continue. It is also incumbent upon audiologists to educate these payers on the profession, how the audiologists enhance the quality of life for patients, and the services that can be provided to their subscribers, including those not recognized by Medicare, but are recognized by state licensure laws and scopes of practice. On a grassroots level, it is encouraged that local audiology colleagues meet with the medical directors of insurance companies, or Medicaid, that do not recognize audiologists and/or all audiologic services.

While attending these meetings, be armed with the scopes of practice from the national audiology organizations, as well as redacted copies of several explanations of benefits (EOBs) from their competitors, to illustrate how audiology services have been successfully reimbursed. The intent of these meetings is to educate medical directors about audiology as well as the cost-savings benefits that the profession provides.

Code Creation and Valuation Processes

To understand coding, it is helpful to know how a code is valued and the resulting formula that determines Medicare reimbursement, which many third-party payers utilize as a basis for their own individual fee schedules. Medicare bases payments on the Resource-Based Relative Value Scale (RBRVS). There are three components that comprise the relative value unit (RVU). The first component is work or cognition and includes the time, physical effort, skill, and stress in providing the service. *Work* (RVUw) comprises approximately 50% of the total payment. The second component is the *practice expense* (RVUpe). This includes the overhead costs of operating and maintaining an office: the rent, the office's physical liability coverage, staff expenses, capital equipment purchases, as well as the disposables needed for the equipment utilized. Practice expense (PE) accounts for approximately 45% of the total payment of a CPT® code. The final component is *professional liability/malpractice* (RVUpli), which accounts for the remaining approximate 5% of the total payment.

Each of these three components (work, PE, and PLI) is multiplied by the *geographic price cost index* (GPCI) to reflect practice costs that differ across the country and considers the costs of maintaining a practice. For example, the costs of a metropolitan office will be higher in New York City than in a rural area found in the Midwest. Finally, all components are then multiplied by the *conversion factor* (CF), which changes on an annual basis as a result of congressional action. The final formula is:

$$RVUw \times GPCIw + RVUpe \times GPCIpe + RVUpli \times GPCIpli \times CF = Medicare\ Payment$$

What makes this situation additionally flawed is that this process is budget neutral; if the cost of one procedure is *increased*, another will be *decreased* somewhere in the payment system.

The Current Procedural Process of Code (CPT®) Evolution

New CPT® manuals are opened every fall to see if there are any new CPT® codes to implement in practices. The following will describe the process of how those codes appear. The American Medical Association (AMA) owns the 11,000 plus CPT® codes and has since 1966, about the time of Medicare's beginnings. The intent was to standardize codes for procedures performed for insurance submissions and for data collection. CPT® codes comprise one of the components of the transaction and code sets of the Health Information Portability and Accessibility Act (HIPAA),

which also includes the International Classification of Diseases (ICD), the diagnoses codes, and the Healthcare Common Procedures Coding System (HCPCS), which includes supplies, devices such as hearing aids, implantable and assistive listening devices, and several hearing aid–related procedures not addressed by the CPT® codes.

Utilization of CPT® codes is tracked by an organization referred to as "The RUC." The RUC database refers to the review of AMA's Specialty Society *R*elative Value Scale *U*pdate *C*ommittee. Prior to 2008, when the Centers for Medicare & Medicaid Services issued Transmittal 84, many physicians billed audiologic services to Medicare beneficiaries as *incident to.* The provision of "Incident to" services have requirements that did not include *other diagnostic tests* and is how audiologic tests are currently categorized. Therefore, this mistaken, pervasive practice of physicians filing claims for services performed by their audiologist-employee with the physician's NPI for the tests performed by that audiologist *should not have been done and should have ceased* in 2008 when the transmittal was issued, directing that audiologic services should be billed via *the NPI of the audiologist* who performed the audiologic and vestibular tests.

CPT® Code Requests

While a code request may be initiated by anyone, most of the code requests originate from interested parties such as professional organizations or societies. When a potential code will be utilized by several professions, often a code request is submitted by the organizations collaboratively. This coding request process has several requirements that need to be met:

■ All devices and drugs necessary for performance of the procedure or service have received Food and Drug Administration (FDA) clearance or approval when such is required for performance of the procedure or service.
■ The procedure or service is performed by many physicians or other qualified healthcare professionals across the United States.
■ The procedure or service is performed with frequency consistent with the intended clinical use (i.e., a service for a common condition should have high volume).
■ The procedure or service is consistent with current medical practice.
■ The clinical efficacy of the procedure or service is documented in literature that meets the requirements set forth in the CPT® code-change application (AMA, 2024a).

The CPT® Editorial Panel

The CPT® Editorial Panel is responsible for creating, revising, or updating the CPT® codes. This 21-member panel is composed of those physicians appointed by their national societies: two seats for members of the CPT® Health Care Professionals Advisory Committee (HCPAC), and 1 representative each from the Blue Cross and Blue Shield Association, America's Health Insurance Plans, the American Hospital Association; one seat for an at-large organizational member; one seat for an umbrella organization that represents private health insurers; and two non-voting liaisons from the Centers for Medicare & Medicaid Service (AMA, 2024b).

The CPT® Editorial Panel meets three times per calendar year, and it is at these meetings that new code requests are introduced or editorially revised. Of course, the code request can be tabled or rejected. If the code is accepted and then valued, the new code will appear in the next published CPT® manual, a year or two later. There are three categories of CPT® codes that reflect usage (I), performance measurement(s) (II), or emerging technology (III), and the code request must meet one of those category's descriptors. The traditional audiology codes are Category I codes and since the Category III codes are utilized for emerging technologies and services, automated audiometry codes can be found in this category.

The CPT® Code Valuation Process

In this complicated valuation process, there are two groups who are involved beyond the CPT® process: the RUC and the RUC HCPAC, who also meet three times per year shortly after the CPT® Editorial Panel meetings. The RUC comprises primarily physicians and there are a few additional seats that rotate on a 2-year basis: one for a primary care representative, two for a subspecialty of internal medicine, and one seat for a specialty society who is not a RUC member. The CPT® HCPAC reviews the code requests that are brought forth through their process, which includes creating new codes or editing existing codes. The HCPAC is vital to audiology as this represents limited license practitioners and other allied health professionals (AMA, 2024b) reviewing the two higher weighted components of the RVU: the work and practice expense components. The RUC HCPAC comprises 12 organizations to allow for nonphysician groups' representation, with the audiology seat alternated between ASHA and AAA. The recommendations on the RVUs are reviewed for nonphysician specialties' work and practice expenses and establish those values, the crux of the codes' values. Once a code has been created through the CPT® process, it goes through the RUC/HCPAC process. This includes a survey conducted to capture the components of the CPT® code and its worth. It is imperative that when the survey request is distributed, the specialist who performs that potential new procedure should weigh in with their data. This is the data pool for valuing the code by those who will perform it and will set that value for years to come. It takes a short amount of time but could yield a better gain in terms of payment if captured as accurately as possible.

This explanation may serve to assist audiologists to understand the process of a code coming to fruition, the journey it takes, and why there are not separate codes for every service performed. If that were the case, there would be a procedure code and a corresponding RVU that is likely to be less than palatable as evidenced in the last decade, not serving the profession or providers well. The time and process to take "codes to market" may take 24 to 36 months once the request is initially filed with the CPT® Editorial Panel for consideration until the RVU is assigned and published.

Billing Practices

As with any professional organization, by virtue of membership, audiologists subscribe to the code of ethics of our professional home. The American Academy of Audiology (AAA), the Academy of Doctors of Audiology (ADA), and the American Speech-Language-Hearing Association (ASHA) all have codes of ethics that can be located on their respective websites that direct professional behaviors. State licensure laws may also incorporate codes of ethics in either the statute or in the code. These codify acceptable practice for the profession. Not adhering to them may result in unethical and potentially illegal behaviors, potential punishments, and/or sanctions.

Audiologists and other healthcare providers utilize three coding structures, several mentioned above:

- Current Procedural Terminology (CPT®).
- International Compendium of Diseases 10th Revision Clinical Modification (ICD-10-CM and ICD-10-PCS).
- Healthcare Common Procedure Coding System (HCPCS).

These manuals should be in all audiology offices in the form of a printed manual, an app, or available online and ordered annually when they are published as these codes can change. The five-digit CPT® codes are the procedures that audiologists perform and are *owned by the American Medical Association (AMA)*. The ICD-10 codes are the disease codes with ICD-10-CM utilized in nonfacility settings such as independent private practices, otolaryngology offices, and other settings, while the ICD-10-PCS codes are utilized in facility settings such as hospitals. The HCPCS codes are the supply codes that include codes for the specific styles of hearing aids, implantable devices, professional fees, and assistive listening devices. All of these code families are utilized by other professionals, not just audiologists, but within each are codes that are commonly utilized by audiologists.

Third-party payers have a specific contract with the patient, the provider, and their company. Audiologists may have a general, boilerplate contract that applies to many of their subscribers and one that also specifies the "dos and don'ts" of their coverage, including disallowing "balance billing" for covered services. These contracts may include discounts, or if the patients are forced to wait for their reimbursement. It is vital to remember that this is only a vehicle for reimbursement, not for payment.

Third-Party Payers

There are many types of third-party payers:

- Medicare (Parts A, B, C, and D).
- Medicaid, Tricare, and health maintenance organizations (HMOs).
- Preferred provider organizations (PPOs).
- Point of service (POS).
- Fee for service (FFS).
- Workers' compensation.
- Disability.

To bill a patient, many offices have an encounter form, routing slip, or superbill, which is a list of the applicable and most widely utilized codes in

that facility, serving as the method of communication from the provider, identifying the services they performed and their diagnoses, to the billing personnel. Many offices have this process as a part of their office management system. The patient's name, date of service, and provider's name need to be included on an encounter form as well as the appropriate CPT®/HCPCS codes representing procedures, services, and/or devices that were provided as well as the diagnosis or diagnoses, so the claim can be submitted to the clearinghouse or insurance company that will bill on behalf of the clinic. It is not unusual for several appropriate and applicable ICD-10 codes to be affixed to a claim, including those addressing comorbidity. Most providers have an electronic healthcare system and/or office management system that has the capacity to bill as well as perform other tasks such as scheduling, inventory, appointment reminders, and so on.

For example, you perform 92557, the comprehensive audiometry code that includes pure-tone air and pure-tone bone conduction, speech reception thresholds, and word recognition on the patient who presents with decreased hearing acuity after an airplane flight. An air-bone gap is the result and is then confirmed with tympanometry and acoustic reflex thresholds (92550). The provider may elect to utilize H90.0, conductive hearing loss, bilateral, as the diagnosis. Continuing with this example, if the patient also complained of tinnitus in both ears, the provider could choose H93.13, tinnitus bilateral, as a secondary ICD-10 code. This should be documented in the chart along with the patient's case history, assessment results, and recommendations.

Documentation details are discussed later in this chapter. The clinic will also

---

MEDICAL NECESSITY

Medical necessity is defined in the Social Security Act, Title XVII, Section 1862 (a)(1)(a) as:

Those services that are reasonable and necessary for the diagnosis or treatment of illness or injury or to improve the functioning of a malformed body member.

Every payer requires that the services billed meet these requirements and can be thought of as the patient noting any change in hearing, balance, and/or tinnitus. This must be reflected in your documentation.

---

need to have the patient's permission to bill their insurer, which is often included on the facility's registration sheet or online portal. Also, often included on the same sheet or a separate sheet, if allowed by the payer, is the patient's signature on an insurance waiver, the statement that if their insurer does not cover the services, the patient understands they will then be financially responsible for those services.

To ensure the highest level of accuracy and reimbursement, the provider will need to choose the ICD-10 codes based on the greatest level of specificity and avoid the unspecified codes. There is no ICD-10 code for normal hearing and "rule-outs" are not acceptable submissions, but coding for the reason for the visit, for signs, symptoms, or the chief complaint the patient noted, is acceptable.

Medicare

Medicare, one of the largest insurers, has been in effect since the Lyndon Johnson years of the mid-1960s as a mechanism to supplement and provide health insurance for those aged 65 or older, blind individuals, individuals who have been on disability for at least 2 years, and those with end-stage renal disease (ESRD). Medicare is typically the patient's primary insurance, but with more people over the age of 65 continuing to be in the workforce, Medicare may be secondary to their employers' healthcare benefit, the primary payer.

CMS Program Memorandum AB-02-080 heralds "diagnostic testing, including hearing and balance assessment services, performed by a qualified audiologist is paid for as *'other diagnostic tests'* under §1861 (s)(3) of the Social Security Act (the Act) when a physician orders testing to obtain information as part of his/her diagnostic evaluation or to determine the appropriate medical or surgical treatment of a hearing deficit or related medical problem" (CMS, 2012). It further states, "Services are excluded by virtue of §1862 (a)(7) of the Act when the diagnostic information is already known to the physician, or the diagnostic services are performed *only to determine the need for or the appropriate type of hearing aid*" (CMS, 2012).

Since 2005, Medicare beneficiaries who are new to Medicare (within the first 12 months of enrollment) have been entitled to an initial preventative physical examination. Hearing and balance disorders are addressed with two screening questionnaires approved by several professional organizations, the Hearing Handicap Inventory for the Elderly (HHI-E) and the Dizziness Handicap Inventory (DHI). This is the opportunity for audiologists to be the diagnostic professional to address either or both of these health issues and to educate physicians of their importance by citing fall risk potential as well as the cognitive, self-esteem, and depression issues found in the elderly population as a result of hearing loss.

At this point in time, CMS devised the Medicare Administrative Contractors (MAC) jurisdictions to balance the allocation of workloads, account for integration of claims processing activities, and mitigate the risk to the Medicare program (CMS, 2024f). The jurisdictions reasonably balance the number of fee-for-service beneficiaries and providers and are substantially more alike in size than the previous fiscal intermediary and carrier jurisdictions. This restructuring was to promote much greater efficiency in processing Medicare's billion plus claims a year (CMS, 2024f).

The CMS issues National Coverage Determination (NCD) policies. Each MAC may create Local Coverage Determination (LCD) policies that are specific to those designated states for which a MAC has jurisdiction. As each MAC has the authority to interpret the Medicare statute independently, Medicare regula-

tions may not be the same from contractor to contractor. Providers need to have the most recent LCD policy issued by the MAC, as it or the Medicare Physician Fee Schedule (MPFS) is updated annually but can change at any time. There may not be an audiologic or vestibular procedure LCD for the practice area, but in this case, it is suggested to review one from another MAC. LCDs describe *medical necessity*, what CPT® and ICD-10-CM codes may be recognized for payment based on medical necessity and other parameters to which each Medicare provider needs familiarity. These can be obtained online at the Centers for Medicare & Medicaid Services website.

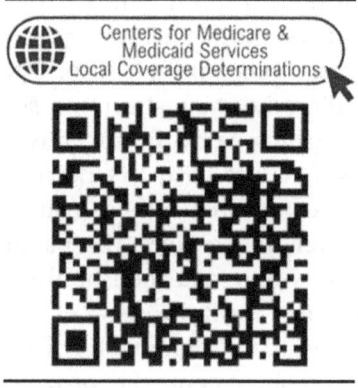

It may behoove providers to have a contact person in provider relations at your Medicare contractor's office to consult for guidance, as frontline staff is not likely to be familiar with the nuances specific to audiology requirements and Medicare. As a Medicare provider, it is essential to stay updated regarding the potential annual changes. Medicare comprises *four parts*:

■ Part A (hospital-based services).
■ Part B (typically outpatient services).

- Part C (Medicare Advantage plans, some of which have audiologic benefits for diagnosis, annual routine monitoring, and possibly a hearing aid benefit).
- Part D (medications).

Parts A and B will be discussed in detail in the following sections and how they pertain to audiology.

Part A

The components that comprise Medicare Part A are hospitalization, home healthcare, hospice care, and skilled nursing care after hospital discharge. Audiologists in inpatient hospital settings are considered Part A providers. All services provided in this setting are filed with the hospital's NPI and not of the provider, including audiologists. Those who bill independently will need to be contracted with the hospital, which then reimburses them for services provided, likely on a contractual basis. The Joint Commission for Accreditation of Healthcare Organizations (JCAHO) credentials hospitals and only those accredited hospitals will be reimbursed by Medicare.

Medicare Part A is funded by payroll taxes, self-employed individual contributions, and contributions from railroad workers and their employers. Payment to the hospital is via the patient's diagnostic related group (DRG), which is generally based on diagnosis, age, gender, and complications Beneficiaries can be enrolled in Medicare Part A and Part B, as well as Part A only for those who are still utilizing their employee benefits for healthcare. For those on Medicare Advantage plans, they are also enrolled in a Part C plan, which some consider a replacement plan as it replaces Medicare Part B and offers the "perks" that the Part C plan often offers that traditional Medicare Part B does not.

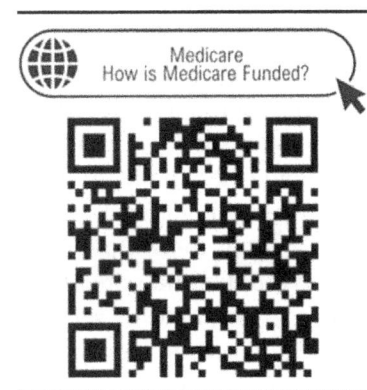

Part B

Medicare Part B recipients have outpatient services as their Medicare benefit, including physician office visits and related services as well as Part A benefits. Subscriber benefits for Part B audiology services would be found in the two most common outpatient settings: those in private practice who bill independently and those employed by otolaryngologists, with audiology services billed with the NPI of the audiologist when they perform the services and with the reassignment of benefits via filing the 855 R which triggers reimbursement to the practice. Part B services include the following:

- Medical expenses.
- Home healthcare.
- Laboratory services.
- Ambulatory surgical services.
- Outpatient medical services.

Part B Medicare is funded by premium payments, contribution from general revenues, and interest earned on the Part B Trust Fund.

All Medicare providers have the choice of changing their status once a year, traditionally in the fall, during open enrollment. If a change is not made during open enrollment, the previous year's status will remain in effect. In an economically challenged area, it is generally more beneficial for the patients if the clinician is a participating provider as it limits the patient's financial liability at the time of service; the majority of audiologists are participating providers. Medicare will pay the provider 80% of the Medicare Physician Fee Schedule (MPFS) allowed amount for allowed procedures performed and the patient pays their 20% coinsurance, or if the patient has a coordination of benefits in place, the claim is forwarded to their secondary insurance coverage.

Regardless of the participating or nonparticipating status, Medicare can only be billed for diagnostic audiologic services when *personally performed by an audiologist, a physician, and/or a nonphysician provider* such as a nurse practitioner and physician assistant and only *when there is a physician order* if there are vestibular and/or acute hearing loss complaints, based on medical

WHAT IS A PARTICIPATING AND NONPARTICIPATING PROVIDER?

When the clinician is a participating provider, the patient is responsible for paying copayments and unmet deductibles at the time of service. At the time of publication, audiologists were not one of the providers who Medicare recognizes to opt out; therefore, *all diagnostic services are to be filed to Medicare unless not enrolled in Medicare,* and then all diagnostic services are given away for free to all patients, not what a doctoring profession should consider.

With a more affluent demographic, patients may be receptive to pay their share at the time of service and reimbursed later. For nonparticipating or limiting charge enrolled providers, the claim is filed to Medicare, which reimburses the patient 80% of the allowable amount of the Medicare Physician Fee Schedule, which yields better cash flow for the provider as the patient pays the audiologist at the time of service. Secondary insurances often will pay the 20% coinsurance. A nonparticipating audiologist may not exceed the limiting charge. Nonparticipating providers receive 5% less than a participating provider. Limiting charge providers receive 10% more than a provider who is participating. In all cases, Medicare is billed for all eligible audiologic services (those that meet medical necessity and have a physician order for acute and/or vestibular complaints or once every 12 months based on medical necessity), and Medicare will reimburse the provider if they are par and will reimburse the patient if the provider is nonpar or limiting charge since the patient paid the provider.

necessity. If a CPT® code has a technical and professional component, a technician can perform the service under the direct supervision of the physician, who must be in the clinic and available. The professional component, which includes the interpretation and report of the same procedure, can only be completed by the audiologist, physician, or NPP and billed under their NPI.

As noted earlier, effective January 1, 2023, Medicare stated in the Medicare Physician Fee Schedule Final Rule that 36 audiologic tests would be reimbursed without a physician order for a medically necessary reason, once every 12 months, with the AB modifier for all tests performed. The AB modifier is defined as "audiology service furnished personally by an audiologist without a physician/NPP order for non-acute hearing assessment unrelated to disequilibrium, or hearing aids, or examinations for the purpose of prescribing, fitting, or changing hearing aids; service may be performed once every 12 months, per beneficiary" on 36 CPT® codes. There are no vestibular codes in the initial 36 codes, and in 2024, the two new osseointegrated device codes were added for a total of 38 procedures.

As a result of not needing a physician order for these specific tests once every 12 months, do not place a physician

THE CPT CODES THAT MEDICARE ALLOWS FOR USE WITH THE AB MODIFIER EVERY 12 MONTHS FOR NONACUTE, NONVESTIBULAR PATIENTS AS OF JANUARY 2025

92550	Tympanometry and reflex threshold measurements
92552	Pure-tone audiometry (threshold); air only
92553	Pure-tone audiometry air and bone
92555	Speech audiometry threshold
92556	Speech audiometry with speech recognition
92557	Comprehensive audiometry threshold evaluation and speech recognition
92562	Loudness balance test, alternate binaural or monaural
92563	Tone decay test
92565	Stenger test, pure tone
92567	Tympanometry (impedance testing)
92568	Acoustic reflex testing, threshold

continued on next page

continued from previous page

92570	Acoustic immittance testing, includes tympanometry, ART, and AR decay testing
92571	Filtered speech test
92572	Staggered spondaic word test
92575	Sensorineural acuity level test
92576	Synthetic sentence identification test
92577	Stenger test, speech
92579	Visual reinforcement audiometry (VRA)
92582	Conditioning play audiometry
92583	Select picture audiometry
92584	Electrocochleography
92587	DPOAEs; limited, 3–6 frequencies or TEOAEs, with interpretation and report
92588	Comprehensive diagnostic eval (minimum of 12 frequencies), with interp and report
92601	Diagnostic analysis of CI, patient younger than 7 years of age, with programming
92602	Subsequent reprogramming
92603	Diagnostic analysis of CI, age 7 years or older, with programming
92604	Subsequent reprogramming
92620	Evaluation of central auditory function, with report, initial 60 minutes
92621	Each additional 15 minutes (list separately in addition to code for primary procedure)
92622	Diagnostic analysis, programming, and verification of an auditory osseointegrated sound processor, any type; first 60 minutes
92623	Each additional 15 minutes (list separately in addition to primary code)

continued on next page

continued from previous page

92625 Assessment of tinnitus (includes pitch, loudness matching, and masking)

92626 Evaluation of auditory function for surgically implanted device(s) candidacy or postoperative status of a surgically implanted device(s); first hour

92627 Each additional 15 minutes (list separately in addition to code for primary procedure)

92640 Diagnostic analysis with programming of auditory brainstem implant, per hour

92651 Auditory evoked potentials; for hearing status determination, broadband stimuli, with interpretation and report

92652 For threshold estimation at multiple frequencies, with interpretation and report

92653 Neurodiagnostic, with interpretation and report

name or NPI in Box 17 or 17a on the CMS 1500 form or in those fields when billing electronically through an office management system.

Part C

Medicare Advantage plans were created in the 1997 Balance Budget Act to afford Medicare beneficiaries choices in their healthcare. This is accomplished via a coverage plan that provides services not traditionally covered by traditional Part B Medicare but for which the patient pays a higher premium. Annual audiograms and hearing aids, which are statutorily excluded in traditional Part B, may be included as benefits in Part C. At this writing in 2024, there were many large networks providing hearing aid benefit options, including discount options directly, or via a provider network, of varying requirements in terms of the number of office visits, the types of devices provided, and the processes of device ordering and payment (Chapter 16). Medicare Advantage plans may take the form of a preferred provider organization (PPO), a health maintenance organization (HMO), a point of service (POS), or a fee for service (FFS), similar to the private sector. With the large influx of Medicare beneficiaries, these third-party plans are on the rise and have been since 2014.

Part D

In effect since January 2006 as a component of the Medicare Modernization

Act, beneficiaries may be eligible for a prescription drug plan. Monthly premiums and deductibles may apply (Congress.gov, 2003). At this writing in 2024, there were no audiology benefits via Medicare Part D.

Advanced Beneficiary Notice

The alerting notice required for Medicare beneficiaries, the Advanced Beneficiary Notice (ABN), is a component of the Beneficiary Notices Initiative (BNI) and is presented in Appendix 17–A.

These statutory mandates are to ensure that the patient understands that all their healthcare may not be a statutorily covered service, to advise them of their expected out-of-pocket payment prior to the service being provided and to enable them to be more active participants in their healthcare decisions.

"Medicare does not cover everything. If you need services that Part A or Part B does not cover, you will have to pay for them yourself unless you have other coverage (including Medicaid) to cover the costs or you're in a Medicare Advantage Plan or Medicare Cost Plan that covers these services. Medicare Advantage Plans and Medicare Cost Plans may cover some extra benefits, like fitness programs and vision, hearing, and dental services" (Medicare.gov).

Beneficiaries are then expected to pay for those non-Medicare-reimbursed services that are listed on the ABN (Figure 17–1). In other words, if there is doubt that the procedure will be paid for by Medicare, it is mandatory that the Advanced Beneficiary Notice must be used and signed by the patient. It must also be dated with the procedure to be performed, an estimate for the cost of the anticipated services noted, and a copy given to the patient. Also on the form is the reason the procedure may be denied or partially paid. If Medicare does not pay, the patient may then be billed. A signature should be maintained on file and the modifier GA appended to the claim so that Medicare is aware that the ABN was given to the patient. Further, if the provider is in doubt of meeting medical necessity, this is also a mandatory use of the ABN. If an ABN is not issued to the patient and the service is denied, the provider is liable and *cannot seek payment* from the Medicare beneficiary. The ABN is *not required* to be issued for noncovered services, known as voluntary use, but may be suggested in some occurrences for the patient to understand their fiscal responsibility. The ABN is suggested when an audiologist performs never-covered audiology Medicare procedures, but those same procedures are reimbursed by Medicare when performed by other providers (e.g., cerumen management and vestibular rehabilitation) and also when a Local Coverage Determination (LCD) policy is in effect.

Although it may be reasonable to protect the patients and the practice, it is ill-advised to have every patient complete an ABN as this could be considered blanket utilization and is *not* a recommended policy. If the patient's visit is to perform a routine annual hearing test, for example, this is statutorily excluded, and a voluntary ABN may be offered to the patient *before* any services are provided as it notifies them that Medicare will *not* pay for that particular service for that reason. A voluntary ABN could be given to the patient if the visit was due to anything related to hearing aids, for example, because of statutory exclusion. Medicare is not billed for any of these services; therefore, the patient is financially responsible. If the patient has a secondary payer that requires a denial from Medicare, you can file the claim to Medicare to obtain the denial with the GY and/or GX modifiers (see Medicare modifiers listed later in this chapter).

It is necessary to contact the local Medicare carrier as local policies differ and therefore contractors may differ in their guidance. The ABN form, number CMS-R-131, can be located on the CMS website.

Centers for Medicare & Medicaid Services
Advance Beneficiary Notice

Medicare Participating Provider Status

This Medicare category is the most common among Medicare providers, which indicates that you accept Medicare assignment for covered Part B services for eligible Medicare beneficiaries. The assignment is 80% of the noted allowed amount on the Medicare Physician Fee Schedule for the region

and is paid to the practice. The patient then pays the practice their 20% coinsurance at the time of service. If they have a secondary insurance, it is then automatically forwarded and submitted to that secondary by Medicare if a coordination of benefits is in place. This category allows the provider a 5% higher fee allowance than a nonparticipating provider, but 10% lower than a limiting charge provider.

At this writing in 2024, medical necessity and a physician order are required when billing Medicare for diagnostic audiologic services if the patient has an acute hearing loss or vestibular complaints. If neither of these complaints are noted, the audiologist can bill Medicare once every 12 months for the medically necessary diagnostic tests completed with the AB modifier, and in Box 17, no physician name or NPI is necessary in this scenario. This modifier was created in 2023 for this purpose as "*audiology service furnished personally by an audiologist without a physician/ NPP order for non-acute hearing assessment unrelated to disequilibrium, or hearing aids, or examinations for the purpose of prescribing, fitting, or changing hearing aids; service may be performed once every 12 months, per beneficiary*" on 36 CPT® codes. The two new osseointegrated device codes that were effective as of January 1, 2024, were added to the list.

If an overpayment occurs, when Medicare pays more than the correct amount, the refund must be sent to the MAC as soon as it is discovered. If Medicare requests an overpayment, it must be refunded or a notification of discovery served within 60 days, or it may be considered a false claim, carrying a stiff penalty. Of course, there is the right to appeal if in disagreement.

Medicare Nonparticipating Status

This category indicates that the provider does not accept assignment, but you are enrolled in Medicare. Two subcategories are found within nonparticipating status, the first of which is nonparticipating provider, which is reimbursed at 5% less than a participating provider, and the second is limiting charge and allows 10% more than participating, the highest level of payment from Medicare to a provider. *The benefit of nonpar and limiting charge is an increase in cash flow for the practice since the patient pays the provider at the time of service and the patient is then reimbursed by Medicare.* The limiting charge is the maximum amount a nonparticipating provider may charge a Medicare beneficiary for a nonpar claim. As with all types of participation, medical necessity and a physician order are the two requirements when billing Medicare for diagnostic audiologic services when the beneficiary presents with acute hearing loss and/or vestibular complaints. For other patients, diagnostic services can be billed once every 12 months with the AB modifier for those 38 codes based on medical necessity.

Opting Out—Not an Option for Audiologists

Audiologists are not one of the professions allowed to opt out of Medicare; therefore, audiologists must be enrolled in Medicare or, if not, provide all di-

agnostic services at no charge to all patients. If a Medicare beneficiary requests their claim be filed to Medicare, the Social Security Act (Section 1848(g) (4) requires that claims be submitted for services rendered to Medicare beneficiaries on or after September 1, 1990; CMS, 2011). The only way that can be accomplished is to be enrolled in Medicare, which can be completed online via Provider Enrollment, Chain, and Ownership System (PECOS) or by filing the 855I enrollment form for an individual or for a group, the 855B. The 855R, the reassignment of benefits form, may also need to be completed for employees of a physician practice, assigning the benefits to the employer. For those who contract their services, the 855R is to

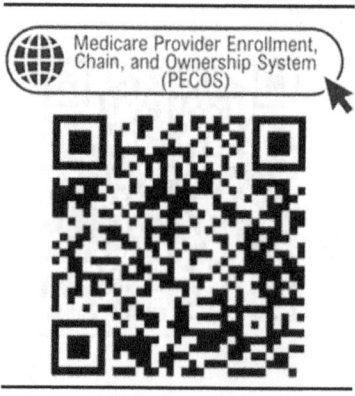

Medicare Provider Enrollment, Chain, and Ownership System (PECOS)

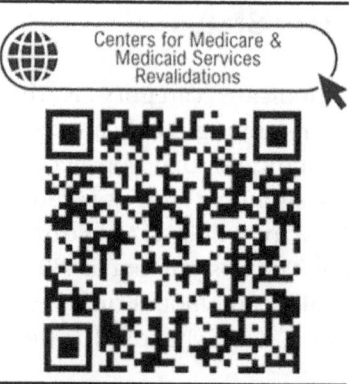

Centers for Medicare & Medicaid Services Revalidations

be filed for each facility where the audiologist provides services. Once initially enrolled, revalidation is to occur every 5 years.

Medicare Compliance

Compliance with mandatory claim filing requirements is monitored by CMS. Violations of the requirement may be subject to a civil monetary penalty of up to $2,000 for each violation and/or Medicare program exclusion. Medicare beneficiaries may not be charged for preparing or filing a Medicare claim (CMS, 2013).

Another aspect of Medicare compliance may require a chart review, known as an audit, if there is concern about questionable billing patterns and/or the potential of overutilization. This may be to confirm that services were rendered, to ensure that services were coded correctly, and/or to confirm those services met the definition of medical necessity. The reviewer/auditor may specify patient files for review. If the audit results in identified errors, penalties may be assessed, and if in disagreement, an appeal may be instituted by the provider. MACs conduct Comprehensive Error Rate Testing (CERT), another mechanism to identify problems via random claims review, which determines if potential billing issues exist and how those issues are to be addressed (CMS, 2017b).

According to CMS (2017a), there are five levels of appeal:

- Redetermination by the Medicare Administrative Contractor.
- Reconsideration by the Qualified Independent Contractor.
- A hearing before the administrative law judge.
- Departmental appeals board.
- Judicial review in U.S. federal court.

"Incident to" Billing

Historically, "Incident to" billing was and unfortunately continues to be the vehicle for physicians to incorrectly bill Medicare for the diagnostic services performed by audiology employees with the physician's National Provider Identifier (NPI). Diagnostic audiology services reside in a category known as "other diagnostic services" and, as such, are not to be billed "Incident to" a physician's NPI but are to be billed with the audiologist's NPI. "Incident to" billing dilutes the work audiologists do within the RUC data bank, a proprietary repository of services performed on Medicare beneficiaries that tracks the number of Medicare procedures performed and by what provider type. In other words, the profession does not receive recognition for the number of audiologic procedures performed if not filed under the NPI of the audiologist within this database. This erroneous practice persists in physicians' offices when filing

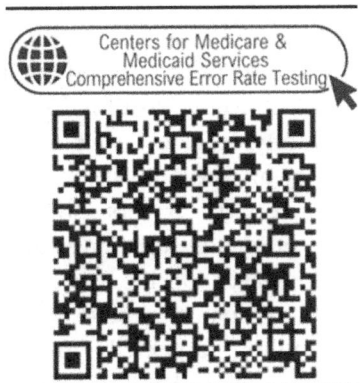
Centers for Medicare & Medicaid Services Comprehensive Error Rate Testing

Medicare claims, and if discovered, it is likely that paybacks, penalties, and interest will be assessed. This occurred in December 2014 when a Texas otolaryngology practice was fined nearly a quarter of a million dollars for incorrectly billing Medicare for hearing assessments performed by unqualified technicians (OIG, 2024).

CMS has established the following requirements in order to correctly bill "incident to":

■ An integral part of the patient's normal treatment when the physician or other listed practitioner personally performed an initial service and remains actively involved in the course of treatment.
■ Services commonly provided without charge or included in the physician's or other listed practitioner's bill.
■ An expense to the physician or other listed practitioner commonly provided in the physician's or other listed practitioner's office or clinic.
■ Physician or other listed practitioner provides direct supervision for the "incident to" services.
■ Only the physician or other listed practitioner who supervises the incident to services may bill them.

Again, this final point is the reason why this billing methodology should not be filed by way of the physician's NPI when performed by any licensed, enrolled audiologist due to the existence of their own provider category, "other diagnostic tests"; "incident to" services does not apply to the "other diagnostic tests" category.

While Medicare's "Incident to" billing rules address services performed by technicians employed by physicians in addition to other services, there are audiologic tests (CPT® codes 92537-92546, 92548, 92549, 92587, and 92588) that do have a technical component, the portion of the code that can be performed by a technician under the direct supervision of a physician (who must be in the facility and available for assistance), and are then allowed to be filed under that physician's NPI with the TC modifier. The other portion of these particular codes, the professional component, allows for another professional, including audiologists, to perform the interpretation and report. For the services performed by an audiologist, Medicare requires those procedures be filed under the NPI of the Medicare-enrolled audiologist who performed those diagnostic procedures with the -26 modifier for the professional component of the codes performed. Audiologists *cannot bill "incident to" to another professional*, such as a technician, another audiologist, and/or a hearing instrument specialist for services provided to Medicare beneficiaries. Fourth-year students are required to have 100% line of supervision with their audiology preceptor/supervisor to file those performed services to Medicare via the preceptor/supervisor's NPI and may participate in creating the report to the ordering provider and others involved in the patient's care. Other payers need to be consulted for their guidance as some disallow students providing any services, even when supervised by an audiologist.

For third-party payers other than Medicare, guidance regarding "incident to" billing is payer specific, and each payer's specific guidance should be sought prior to billing, especially given that many payers follow Medicare policies.

CPT® Codes With Technical and Professional Components

Due to the technical component (TC)/professional component (PC) split noted above, two families of CPT® codes utilized by audiologists have three options for payment. These include the technical component if the audiologist was the one who performed the test, the professional component if the audiologist only did the interpretation and report, or the global code that includes both the technical and professional components, resulting in the audiologist performing the test, interpreting the results and writing the report. The codes that have the TC/PC split include the vestibular codes 92537–92546, 92548, and 92549 and the otoacoustic emissions codes 92587 and 92588. If the test was performed by two different providers, the TC modifier is affixed to the claim next to the CPT® codes that were split between the technician and the professional component. This is indicated by modifier -26 that will be added according to the CPT® codes on the claim when the audiologist or physician performed the interpretation and report for the same tests. An example would be the otoacoustic emissions code 92587. If the technician performed only the test under direct supervision of a physician, that physician would bill 92587-TC and the audiologist who did the interpretation and report would bill 92587-26. If the audiologist performed the test and did the interpretation and report, it would be filed under the NPI of the audiologist with 92587. An audiologist cannot file a claim with the TC component if an audiology tech or assistant performed the test in a nonphysician setting, such as an independent private practice, as the audiologist must have personally performed the tests.

Medicare Payment Models

CMS has stated in the last few years that they will be converting fee-for-service payment into "pay for performance" or "value-based purchasing." These methodologies are based on a merit system to encourage excellence while trimming costs and are likely to be based on successful outcome measure reporting and quality of care results as well as care coordination. The Medicare Part B Physician Quality Reporting System (PQRS) was a likely step to this end, but was sunsetted on December 31, 2016, in order to transition to the two-track system, the Merit-Based Incentive Payment System (MIPS) and the Alternative Payment Models (APM) created by the Medicare Access and CHIP Reauthorization Act of 2015 (MACRA). At the time of this writing in 2024, MD/DO providers were required to report on measures beginning in 2017, but for nonphysician providers such as audiologists, it is not clear what the requirements for mandatory reporting for audiologists will be or the effective date. It is this author's belief that there will continue to be cross-cutting measures required of all providers as seen in PQRS with the documentation of current patient medications, depression screenings for tinnitus patients, and tobacco and alcohol cessation and intervention that were transitioned to MIPS. Because PQRS was a new methodology in its time, a short review of the past may provide some perspective for the future as the process of delivering healthcare evolves.

The Physician Quality Reporting System (PQRS)

An outcome measures reporting system originally known as the Physician Quality Reporting Initiative (PQRI) began as a voluntary program created to improve the quality of care to Medicare beneficiaries. In the early years of voluntary PQRI/S participation, a small percentage incentive was paid to providers, based on successful reporting for all eligible Medicare claims. This amount of the incentive decreased each year and then morphed into a penalty, also a percentage, in the last few years of PQRS. For example, if you failed to meet the measure specifications for correct reporting in 2014, your 2016 claims were paid at a negative 2% reduction in 2016. Beginning in 2010, audiologists were recognized as an eligible provider for PQRS, which resulted in greater recognition of the profession by CMS. In response, the Audiology Quality Consortium (AQC), a coalition of 10 audiology organizations, began to collaborate and support the audiology quality measures and provide their respective members with educative resources addressing these measures. At the time of this publication, there were 12 measures on which audiologists could report that are included in the audiology specialty set, with 6 of them required if classified as a mandatory reporter.

Other Third-Party Payers and Differences With Medicare

Although many third-party payers look to Medicare to set their policies and fee schedules, there are other entities that also need to be discussed when dealing with insurance companies as this is integral to audiology practice, especially given the advent of Medicare Advantage plans and insurance payers providing hearing aids directly or indirectly to patients. This alphabet soup of HMO, PPO, FFS, and POS is overwhelming but has been in existence for many years (Chapter 16).

Health Maintenance Organizations (HMOs)

In the HMO, the gatekeeper or primary care physician (PCP) is the conductor of healthcare for the patient. This may also be a pediatrician, an internal medicine physician, an obstetrician/gynecologist, and a family practitioner. Referrals to other healthcare providers are required, directed, and sanctioned by those listed above to control healthcare costs. Payment will not occur if a referral was not obtained.

Preferred Provider Organization (PPO)

Although it may be more of an out-of-pocket expense and a higher copay for an out-of-network provider, the patient does not need a referral and, in general, may see the provider of their choice. An in-network provider is one who is contracted directly with the PPO and an out-of-network provider is therefore one who is not contracted with that third-party payer. Patient costs are minimized with an in-network provider as the patient's responsibilities and the reimbursement percentages are typically less (e.g., 80% of the costs reimbursed by the payer, patient pays the remaining 20%) versus out-of-network that may have greater patient responsibility as well as greater exposure (70% of the costs reimbursed by the payer, e.g., patient pays the remaining 30%).

Point of Service (POS)

Considered to be a "step-down" from an HMO, POS patients have more out-of-network options. A physician referral is required, but there are greater financial benefits for staying in-network as is the case for most of these healthcare structures. Higher copays or coinsurances are disincentives when utilizing a non-network provider.

Basic Coding Tidbits

There are three coding systems that are pertinent to healthcare providers, including audiologists. The first of these are the CPT® codes (Current Procedural Terminology). CPT® codes are the intellectual, copyrighted property of the American Medical Association, and as such, the descriptions and other CPT® code information and associated publications must be purchased, as this information is not found in the public domain. The other two coding systems, the ICD-10s and the HCPCS codes, can be readily located on the Internet, in purchased codebooks, online, and via mobile applications.

The ICD-10s have two subgroups, the ICD-10-CM and the ICD-10-PCS. The ICD-10-CMs are the disease codes found in nonfacilities such as private in-

dependent audiology practices and otolaryngology/audiology practices. The ICD-10-PCS are the disease codes utilized by facilities such as hospitals.

Finally, the last of the three coding systems, the Healthcare Common Procedure Coding System (HCPCS), is utilized to file claims for hearing aids, some procedures (such as conformity evaluation), and assistive listening devices, including FM systems. For the staff/coders to know what was performed for payment to occur, especially if a provider is not utilizing any clearinghouse or office management system that allows for direct claims submission, the CPT® and ICD-10s are placed on a superbill or encounter form. The HCPCS codes are also assigned to the claim along with, at minimum, one ICD-10 code and any CPT® codes performed.

The next step in the process is to indicate the CPT® code(s) on the claim and then select a minimum of one supportive ICD code, the disease code. The reason the patient presented to the practice is likely the chief complaint and "signs and symptoms" are often the mantra noted by many coding experts to complete this diagnostic process. Patient symptoms, comorbidities, and the outcome of the testing are also all legitimate reasons to choose a diagnosis or diagnoses. For example, if a patient presents with bilateral tinnitus, ICD-10-CM code H93.13 can be utilized. If one also has a bilateral sensorineural hearing loss, H90.3 can also be claimed for the same CPT® code(s). It is extremely possible to have more than one ICD-10 code per patient encounter, describing the reason for the visit, the result of the outcome of the tests, and associated comorbidities (e.g., infections that were treated with aminoglycosides that resulted in the need for ototoxic monitoring; diabetes; family history of hearing loss, etc.). It may be necessary to contact the patient's provider(s) such as the primary care physician, the oncologist, and/or the endocrinologist for the most specific ICD-10 code describing the comorbidity situation. Given the large number of choices for these conditions and that choice of the codes for diagnosing comorbid conditions are not often included in the scope of practice of an audiologist, it is permissible to include if received from the appropriate provider and documented in the patient's chart notes.

The most specific ICD-10-CM codes are less likely to result in a denial. That said, avoid those codes that end with a nine or zero as they typically do not provide sufficient specificity. For example, H91.9, hearing loss, unspecified, is likely not the best choice for sensorineural hearing loss and is likely to elicit a denial.

Modifiers

Modifiers are important for ensuring accurate and appropriate reimbursement for services. CMS asserts that a modifier offers the ability to record or denote that a service or operation has been carried out and modified by a particular circumstance without changing its definition. There are several modifiers commonly utilized by audiologists.

Numeric Modifiers

The first numeric modifier, -22, increased procedural services, indicates that a procedure took a longer time than the typical service. An example of when to append this modifier would be applicable with a young child or a demented adult. If a comprehensive audiologic assessment was completed and it took longer than it typically does or with additional skill, the service would be appended as 92557-22. Documentation as to why this procedure took longer should be a part of the patient's record and may be called upon for submission if the procedure is denied and an appeal is filed.

Another common modifier for audiologists, -52, indicates reduced services. Since all diagnostic codes are binaural, this modifier is often utilized when only one ear is tested. If CPT® code 92557, comprehensive audiometry, was performed monaurally, the procedure would be appended as 92557-52. Another common application for the use of this modifier is when bone conduction was not performed but the other tests required of CPT® code 92557 were and should be appended identically.

The discontinued procedure modifier, -53, may be appended when the service is discontinued due to the patient becoming ill during the procedure and the provider chose to terminate the service. In the same example, it would be appended as 92557-53. Although this has greater applicability with surgical procedures, providers will want to consult with the payers for their guidance in using this modifier for audiologic procedures.

Finally, the -59 modifier is to be appended when indicating "distinct procedural service." In 2010, this became critical to audiologists with the creation of the new bundled CPT® code, 92540, basic vestibular evaluation. This code includes four separate and distinct tests, CPT® codes 92541, 92542, 92544, and 92545. When clinical decision-making results in one to three of the four tests being performed and not all four, the -59 modifier indicates those tests are separate and distinct and should be appended with each of these codes. Documentation in the patient's record should include why the fourth test was not performed. If all four of the tests are completed, the bundled code, 92540, is billed without any modifiers. For those providing cochlear implant services, the National Correct Coding Initiative (NCCI) has edits that also include the -59 modifier so that a cochlear implant service can be performed on the same date as CPT® code 92626. For the combination

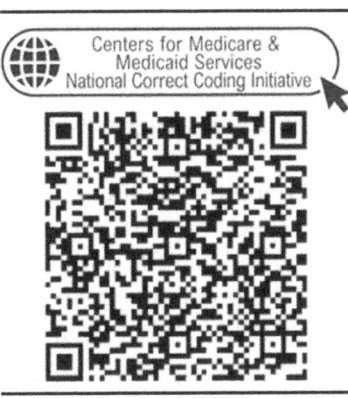

of codes that have these edits, consult the American Academy of Audiology, the American Speech-Language-Hearing Association, or the Centers for Medicare & Medicaid Services.

Medicare Modifiers

Although the numeric modifiers described above apply to all services, and some are not recognized by all payers, there are alphabetic modifiers required by Medicare that pertain to medical necessity and the use of the ABN. Those modifiers are GY, GA, GX, and GZ. The Medicare beneficiary and not the provider chooses one of three options on the ABN, directing how they want their claim to be filed (or not) to Medicare. The provider then appends the necessary modifier(s) to the claim. They are listed below.

GA Modifier

GA is the "Waiver of Liability Statement on file" and is utilized when a required (mandatory) ABN is issued for a designated covered service. This indicates that the patient has a signature on file by way of their signed ABN, but the procedure may not be a covered service due to it not being medically reasonable and/or necessary. In the event it is not reimbursed, the patient can then be billed for that service since their signature is on file and they were alerted to the possibility of their financial responsibility; if there is no patient signature, then this denial will have to be written off.

GY Modifier

GY is "Item or service statutorily excluded, does not meet the definition of a Medicare benefit," such as hearing aids, and the ABN was not given to the patient. Many third-party payers require a denial from Medicare for the patient to access the hearing aid benefit provided by that secondary payer. In this case, on line 19 of the CMS 1500, you would indicate that this is for denial by Medicare to initiate secondary payer coverage to generate that denial.

GX Modifier

The GX modifier says that "Voluntary liability notice was issued," indicating that a nonrequired or voluntary ABN would be issued for noncovered services, such as routine annual evaluations not based on medical necessity, hearing aids, tinnitus treatment, or aural rehabilitation. It is encouraged that patients be given the voluntary ABN when in doubt, so their signature attests to their understanding of their fiscal responsibility in case it is contested later.

GZ Modifier

The GZ modifier refers to "service is not covered by Medicare" and is utilized when an ABN is not on file. When claims are submitted with this modifier, billing the patient for those services is disallowed.

Multiple Modifiers

Multiple modifiers could be listed as with this example: 92557-52 GY if you performed comprehensive audiometry monaurally and you need Medicare to deny this service for the patient's secondary to reimburse for a hearing aid.

Copays, Coinsurances, and Deductibles

Copays and coinsurances are highly likely to be a part of a patient's healthcare benefit. A copay is a specified amount, typically $25.00 to $50.00 as indicated on their health insurance card, and must be collected from the patient at the time of service. Coinsurance is a percentage of the visit that needs to be paid by the patient at the time of service, usually those who are insured by PPOs, fee for service, and Medicare. Medicare Part B participating providers are required to collect the coinsurance and any unmet deductible. As an example of coinsurance, if the total of the procedures performed was $250.00 for that date of service and the patient is to pay a 20% coinsurance, they would pay $50.00 to the provider. If the patient sees a non-network provider, they can expect to pay a higher coinsurance, for example 40%, if that payer requires a coinsurance.

Deductibles are another financial responsibility the patient needs to meet before their benefits "kick in." These amounts are paid annually and typically range from $500.00 to $5,000 or higher per year for an individual. Family deductibles will be different if it is a family plan. If a patient goes to a provider in the early part of the year, barring any healthcare issues or visits, it is likely they have not met their deductible and will need to pay the entire amount, which is then applied to their deductible until it is paid.

Balance Billing

"Balance billing" allows a patient to be billed for services that their insurance did not cover, for what was allowed, per that payer's specific fee schedule and often advanced notice that noncovered services are the patient's responsibility. For PPOs that often discount the patient's fees, balance billing is disallowed as the provider has agreed to accept the discounted rate per the contract with the payer. If this is not specified in the contract, a verification of benefits is advised prior to the procedures being performed. An example of balance billing would be if $425.00 was billed to the insurance company, which paid $399.00, then the patient can be billed the remaining $26.00, as long as it is not contractually disallowed (Chapter 16).

Explanation of Benefits (EOBs)

Providers will want to trend and monitor the payments when the Explanation of Benefits (EOB) arrives in the office. This is a formal description between the payer and the provider of the covered and noncovered services for that date of service, the payment received, and the patient's responsibility for payment. The patient is also likely to be the recipient of an EOB so they will also be notified as to what was paid and what is their responsibility, if any. The payer's legend should be available to check what the abbreviations and their codes indicate as they may be specific for that payer. Especially if a private practice is just beginning, it would be beneficial to set up a spreadsheet with each payer to be billed, what the fee schedule reimbursement is for each code, and if it is permitted to bill the patient for noncovered services. This way, trends can be discovered more quickly and if there's been a unilateral change to the reimbursements, the payer may be contacted to determine a course of action. Write-offs will likely be a component illustrated on the EOB and indicates the amount that is not billable to the patient and therefore must be written "off the books," especially for those payers with whom there is a contract. For example, if services were billed to a PPO, the write-off amount would be what is contractually agreed upon by both parties and not billable to the patient.

It is necessary to establish a fee schedule for the practice of usual and customary fees, based on the hourly rate and contact hours. Chapters 11, 13, and 14 in this text will be resourceful in how to devise appropriate fees.

Evaluation and Management Codes (E&M)

Evaluation and management codes are not recognized by Medicare when performed by an audiologist. While that does not eliminate other third-party payers from reimbursing for these codes, there are several requirements to consider when billing E&M codes. The CPT® codebook is very specific in the evaluation and management code requirements for new and established patients, including the complexity of medical decision-making and other requirements. It is imperative that prior to using these codes, the section of the CPT® code book be read and fully understood. It is also necessary to consult with individual payers about their specific guidance for E&M codes prior to filing claims for those services, to ensure that audiologists are recognized for payment for E&M codes by that payer as well as if state licensure laws have any special regulations or rules. If considered a noncovered service, the patient should expect to be responsible for payment as long as it is not contractually excluded. Again, as a cautionary note, only the lower-level E&M codes may be used when providing greater than typical services such as with tinnitus and vestibular patients and not with the typical diagnostic evaluations often seen by audiologists. Further, for audiologists employed by an otolaryngology practice, if an audiologist files an E&M code on the same date of service as the ENT's E&M code, the audiology E&M will likely be denied.

Tracking all procedures and to whom they are being billed to see trends in payments, denials, and the lengths of time between billing and payment will be beneficial. Changes may occur and can then be addressed quickly. The state may have mandated prompt payment regulations and the practice's third-party payer contracts may also address timely claims filing as well as their policies regarding payment or updating claim status.

Waivers

Insurance or financial waivers are a mainstay in the practice and should be offered at the time of service for procedures that will not be covered by the patient's insurance. By having the patient sign this document with the date of service and the procedures performed, they then become responsible for any payments not paid by a third party, if allowed by that party. This will allow billing them for that difference if not contractually excluded. An example is cost sharing and upgrading to more sophisticated technology if the patient chooses to do so. The decision to upgrade is then considered beyond their covered benefit and is now a noncovered benefit, and the patient is responsible. Providers need to check with their specific payers on whether or how to proceed with these upgrades.

Although the consideration that a patient may not pay the bill for services is not pleasant, unfortunately, it does occur. Many practices send three notices to the nonpaying patient requesting payment. If nothing is received, the option of utilizing the services of a collection agency or an attorney to capture this lost balance is urged. Generally, if these mechanisms are utilized and if payment is then procured, usually only 50% or so of the full amount collected is realized. Therefore, it is incumbent to collect at the time services are provided, if allowed by the third-party payer, and should include the required copays, coinsurances, and/or deductibles, especially for larger expense items such as hearing aids or extensive testing or treatment. Know the third-party payer contract requirements as many do disallow the patient to pay for services, especially hearing aids, prior to insurance being billed, occurring after dispensing (Chapter 16).

Bundling Versus Unbundling/Itemization of Hearing Aid Fees

For the last several years, the dilemma of whether to bundle or itemize hearing aid fees, which includes separating professional fees and other related fees from the device in the delivery of hearing aids, has been a major point of discussion. Bundling fees means charging one fee for all hearing aid–related services, including professional services and the costs for the device(s). If an unbundled or itemized hearing aid–related system for fees is used, each of the incurred services for the hearing aids, such as professional fees for dispensing, orientation, verification, earmolds, earmold impressions, batteries, assistive listening devices, extended warranty packages, and follow-up visits, in addition to the actual device costs, is specified. The Healthcare Common Procedure Coding System (HCPCS) codes provide the vehicle to itemize fees in the provision of amplification devices and services. The hearing aid codes are listed as monaural versus binaural, by style (CIC, ITE, ITC, BTE, and body), and by technology (analog, programmable, and digital).

By considering the itemization model, it is obvious to the patient which of the fees are for the "hardware" of hearing aids/amplification systems and which of the fees are charged for the provision of services or the "software" of the procedure. Patients should understand and appreciate the value of the services they receive from their provider. Itemization sets the stage for patients to understand the breadth of audiologic services provided and is the suggested methodology when filing claims to third-party payers if not prohibited by state licensure laws.

From a bottom-line viewpoint, itemization should increase cash flow so that clinic days are not spent seeing no charge hearing aid rechecks all day. The American Academy of Audiology has created a step-by-step document to assist you in the itemization process.

American Academy of Audiology
Guide to Itemizing
Professional Services

Collections

One of the potential problems of maintaining a practice is having the patients pay their bills in a timely fashion. Ideally, no device should leave your office without it being paid for by the patient or knowing what the reimbursement from the third-party payer will be forthcoming. Many offices avert this problem with a verification of benefits as well as with credit card payments that are confirmed in real time and there is no issue of nonpayment with checks. There are several healthcare credit cards available so that the credit card company pays, and the patient in turn pays them if they qualify for this service. This eliminates the practice of having to bill the patient monthly, something that can only add to the cost of doing business.

Procedurally, many audiologists require half of the fee at the time of the hearing aid evaluation as a deposit for patients who are paying privately, with the other half at the time the instruments are dispensed. Audiologists need to be familiar with the return policies for hearing devices within their state as regulations are quite variable and may also specify the time frame in which the funds can be returned to the patient. Further regulations also may specify how much, if any, of the funds paid for the devices may be retained by the clinic for provider services.

If private pay patients have not paid what was agreed upon in the purchase agreement for their devices and the clinic has shown a good-faith effort to collect (industry standard appears to be sending three monthly statements), then there may not be a choice other than to submit the patient's account to a collection agency or to an attorney who provides collecting on delinquent accounts as a service. but it is likely the provider will receive approximately 50% of the full amount collected and this simply reinforces how critical it is to capture the fees at the time the patient leaves the office with their new device(s).

Medicare Audits

A Medicare audit may be triggered by several factors, but it most often occurs when there is overutilization, when billed services are outliers in comparison to like providers in the same area, when processes are not followed, if there are direct patient complaints or reports from a disgruntled employee or competitor, and/or when the payer's guidelines policy may direct this to occur. It is important to consider Medicare's use of data mining for fraud and abuse as they examine provider data and compare them to their counterparts to see if someone is filing claims not in accordance with other like providers. When Medicare recovers over $2.68 billion in 2023 as they have in the last several years, it is understandable why a magnifying glass may be focused on a practice with suspect claims. Third-party payers will perform random audits to ensure compliance with billing procedures and billing practices. Also, some third-party payers have their own fraud and abuse departments and will prosecute violators to the full extent of the law.

One of the audit methodologies that Medicare utilizes is the Comprehensive Error Rate Testing (CERT) to reduce and recover payments made incorrectly. CMS calculates the Medicare fee-for-service (FFS) improper payment rate through the CERT program. Each year, CERT evaluates a statistically valid random sample of claims to determine if they were paid properly under Medicare coverage, coding, and billing rules (CMS, 2017b).

To avoid any type of an audit, practitioners need the most appropriate and complete documentation in effect as the requested specific patient chart(s) likely will be reviewed by the auditors. One of the most common audit activities is to verify the completion of correctly billed procedures for a specific date of service as reflected in the chart notes and office management systems. The diagnosis assigned to that date of service will also be verified with the report.

In most cases, if a discrepancy is found, the auditors may assess a fee with penalties and interest, to pay for any identified offenses. The practice has the right to appeal, and it is recommended to obtain legal counsel well versed in healthcare and Medicare/Medicaid/thirty-party doctrine. A utilization review will likely occur within a specific time frame post audit to ensure that specific procedures have been implemented. As noted above, payback of funds with a penalty and/or interest fees, termination of the contract with that specific provider, and/or the potential for legal action may also ensue, post audit.

Medicare Fraud and Abuse

Due to the 2010 Affordable Care Act, changes in fraud and abuse initiatives resulted in improper payments being returned to Medicare; more than $4.3 billion were recovered in 2013, rising upward from $4.02 billion in 2010 just prior to the passage of this act. Recently, in 2023, it was reported that "Medicare loses an estimated $60 billion each year due to fraud, errors, and abuse, though that number is impossible to measure" (Senior Medical Patrol, 2024). Issues related to these problems affect people across the country, often cost-

ing them time, money, and well-being. Medicare-related errors contribute to this annual loss even though errors can be honest healthcare billing mistakes. However, repeated errors by a doctor or provider could be considered a red flag of potential fraud or abuse if not corrected. When people steal from Medicare, it hurts us all and is big business for criminals. Some common examples of fraud, errors, or abuse could include:

- Charging for services or supplies that were not provided.
- Misrepresenting a diagnosis, a person's identity, the service provided, or other facts to justify payment.
- Prescribing or providing excessive or unnecessary tests and services.

Senior Medicare Patrol
Dollars Lost to Fraud

Senior Medicare Patrol
Medicare Fraud Prevention Week

Medicare Advantage plans are also under scrutiny with "improper payments" to the tune of $16.6 billion for 2022 and 2023. Fraud includes knowingly submitting false claims or misrepresentations of fact to obtain a federal healthcare payment for which no entitlement would otherwise exist; knowingly soliciting, receiving, offering, and/or paying remuneration to induce or reward referrals for items or services reimbursed by federal healthcare programs; and making prohibited referrals for certain designated health services (CMS, 2016c). Abuse may include billing for unnecessary medical services, charging excessively for services or supplies, and misusing codes on a claim, which includes upcoding and unbundling codes (CMS, 2016c).

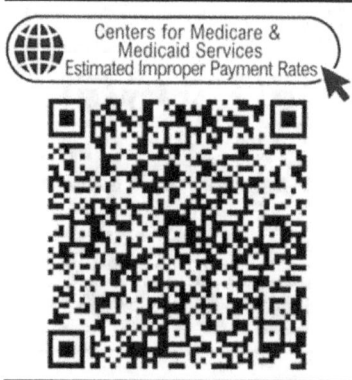

To combat fraud, Medicare has established practice patterns to predict fraud, based on overutilization in providers' offices. Licensure and background checks will be eventually investigated to ensure legitimacy, not only of the providers, but also to ensure that services are not provided to ineligible beneficiaries, such as those who are deceased, a common fraudulent and abusive practice. It is suggested that audiologists conduct internal audits of billing practices and of their documentation to ensure compliance. Providers who are aware of fraud are expected to report it and are to be protected by whistleblower laws.

Contract Negotiations

Until the last several years, many providers, including audiologists, had the stance of being grateful for any insurance company that would reimburse for services. Since the healthcare landscape has changed substantially, this has also. Although the insurance company holds the contract with the patient for the provision of healthcare services, providers are also at their mercy with the contracts they have in place with third-party payers (Chapter 16). In considering contracts, a few choice questions are in order:

■ Are patients allowed to share in the cost of an upgrade in technology beyond their covered benefit?
■ Is a waiver required? Does the payer provide one?

- If the upgrade is allowed as a noncovered service, how will that be reflected on the EOB? Is S1001, a deluxe item, patient aware and recognized?
- Is billing allowed for other noncovered services?
- What is the fee schedule and how often is it revised?
- When can payment be expected? Is there a prompt pay law in place?
- What is the denial process?
- What are the other requirements? Do I have to provide access to services 24/7 as noted in many contracts?
- How much liability do I need to carry?
- What is the length of the contract?
- How can the contract be terminated and by whom? What is the required time frame for termination?
- Can the contract be changed unilaterally by the third party, such as with a unilateral change in the fee schedule?
- Will this secure patients in a designated demographic area?
- Ease of verification of patient enrollment?
- Are prior authorizations required?

One of the most, if not the most, critical components of any contract is the reimbursement you receive for services. Many plans devise their fee schedule according to the Medicare Physician Fee Schedule. Relying on this will not keep the doors open to your practice. Practice owners need to know their hourly rate (Chapter 14), what the contracted fees are (and renegotiate with commercial payers if need dictates), and business expenses necessary to maintain a healthy practice. Other chapters in this text can assist you in determining these rates (Chapters 11 and 13).

Some commercial insurance plans continue to not include audiologists as providers. If considering the "any willing provider" clause that a state may have legislated, it is essential to contact the provider relations department of that third-party payer to educate them about audiologists and, by virtue of qualifications, the services provided. It may be helpful to stress that these services prove to be cost-effective with audiologists being the first line of contact in managing their subscriber's hearing and balance care. Assistance from state professional organizations is essential to pave new roads in enacting policy changes as well as arranging an educational meeting with the payer's provider relations department and medical director of that plan with several local colleagues. It may also be helpful to discuss with them the audiology scope of practice, the services provided, the outcomes and successes documented by patient testimonials and literature reviews, and redacted copies of several explanations of benefits (EOBs) issued by their competition, illustrating their competition's successful reimbursement of audiology services.

The example of discounting services or giving away services to acquire more hearing aid patients is illegal if offering the same service to Medicare patients since Medicare patients cannot be billed at a higher fee than another patient for the same procedure. This may be true with Medicare Advantage plans because at this writing, several third-party administrators disallowed the patient from paying for their hearing evaluation, bundling it in the cost of the device. In addition, Medicare contractors have guidance regarding the solicitation of services. The cost of goods and the cost of maintaining an office at times can be greater than what appears to be an incentive to contract with that insurance carrier. Refer to Chapter 12 in this book to learn to calculate the amount of funds needed to maintain the practice and overhead to make appropriate decisions for the financial health of a private practice. It is advised to seek legal counsel familiar with healthcare laws prior to signing any contractual agreement.

As with any third-party payer, there are many questions to be reviewed even when a contract has been in effect for years: These questions would include:

- What is the average reimbursement time frame?
- What is the denial process?
- What are the codes to be reimbursed?
- What is the fee schedule for those codes?
- Can the patient be billed for the difference between what is reimbursed by the insurance company and the fee billed?
- How often is the fee schedule updated?
- How much professional liability insurance is necessary?
- Are there administrative fees such as annual credentialing fees?
- What is the contract termination policy?
- What is the patient dismissal process?

While this certainly is not an exhaustive list, it is the beginning of the questions that should be considered of these third-party payers. For more informa-

tion on these programs and details on how to negotiate these contracts, see Chapter 16.

In the case of hearing aid reimbursement, consider if there is a covered benefit, what it is, if the patient can share in the cost of advanced technology, and if an invoice and/or prior authorization is required for payment. In addition, the following should be considered: itemizing the hearing aid acquisition fees, including batteries, earmold(s), and earmold impression(s) if applicable; the dispensing fee as well as the conformity evaluation; and other professional services as well as the policy if a hearing aid(s) is returned for credit (query about if any professional fees may be retained if allowed by state licensure laws). Again, this is not the entire list of potential questions, but those presented are designed to facilitate the best provider decisions when providing services to subscribers with audiology insurance benefits.

For those who provide vestibular rehabilitation, it is vital to know the nuances of billing and if audiologists can be reimbursed for all diagnostic and treatment codes for vestibular services by third-party payers.

Due to the changing healthcare landscape, it is rare for providers to be successful in "carving out" procedures that are more time-consuming and/or costly to avoid discounts that would apply to these services. These would include amplification, central auditory processing, aural rehabilitation, and tinnitus treatment, to name a few, but it is certainly worth an attempt.

Managed care is a different entity and is much more restrictive and dogmatic: They will "allow" providers to be on their panel or network if they require a provider in the area. The difficulty in penetrating this system is that often those panels are closed, and no new providers are accepted. This can potentially have a great financial impact for the practice if many patients or potential patients have a contract with a payer that is not accessible. Be vigilant and continue to request participation even if constantly told "no." Accessibility may be obtained by exercising the "any willing provider" law, if your state has such regulations. This means they must accept anyone as a provider if they meet their criteria. As insurance plans often limit the number of providers and if they have reached that number, new provider applications will not be accepted. These limitations are to their advantage as it allows them greater negotiating power in dealing with fewer providers within their network. The patient may have the option of going "out-of- network," but it will come at a greater out-of-pocket expense if they choose to do so. Out-of-network providers are not restricted to the in-network fee schedules, which may be advantageous.

Documentation, Documentation, Documentation

Documentation details anything related to the patient's visit, provides the continuity of care between the professionals involved in that particular patient's care, and provides a historical chronicle. It is required by third-party payers, and as a legal document, it can be subpoenaed. In hospital settings and major medical centers, the chart is likely to be reviewed for quality assurance indicators and compliance.

The patient's chart needs to include their demographics: name; date of birth; contact information; insurance information with a copy of both sides of their healthcare card; driver's license; the name of the referring professional if needed; the reason for their visit; their case history, including allergies, surgeries, hospitalizations, medications, and occupational and recreational noise exposure history; and recommendations. For the pediatric population, the prenatal, birth, and postnatal histories should be included in addition to familial history. For adults, all the above should be included as well as the age or time of onset of their hearing or balance disorder. All audiologic procedures are to be signed and dated. Given that Medicare and most commercial payers base payment on medical necessity, this must clearly be documented in the chart and should reflect the patient noting a change in hearing, balance, and or tinnitus.

In isolation, the audiogram does not constitute a report. The interpretation of the performed procedures and recommendations for patient management is required in the chart notes and placed on the audiogram and/or in the patient's record, as well as an original signature and the date of service. A case history should also be included on the audiogram if space permits.

An emergency room physician once told this author, "If it isn't in the chart, it didn't happen." Those wise words are the basis of how documentation should be considered during the course of the patient's visit for a particular date of service. Another method would be to think of the documentation as if a reviewer was reviewing a chart for an audit. It is

"SOAP" NOTES FOR DOCUMENTATION

Subjective is the description of the presenting problem as the patient relates it during discussion. This would also include the case history; referral; a review of the patient's medical history, including medications and surgeries; their occupational and recreational noise exposure history; and any other pertinent audiologic related information.

Objective should be the physical findings encountered in the examination of the patient, including otoscopic findings.

Assessment includes the procedures performed and an interpretation of their results.

Plan includes recommendations. This would include, but is not limited to, the treatment options recommended for the patient, further referrals and/or procedures, amplification options, assistive listening devices, and/or undergoing tinnitus or vestibular treatment, for example. The provider's signature should be on the audiogram as well as the chart progress notes.

imperative to include anything the patient describes during the history and physical intake, the tests performed, and the findings and recommendations.

Electronic Health Care Records (EHRs)

In 2004, President George W. Bush announced his vision of electronic health records (EHRs) being a reality by 2014 (CMS, 2007), and while it may seem this has been completed, this transition is still unfolding in healthcare, including offices where audiologists are employed. These electronic healthcare records have resulted in a paperless, computer-accessed healthcare record.

While the information listed below is a vital component of the EHR, the demographics, the progress notes, medications, history, and physical as well as outcome measures are all a part of the EHR (CMS, 2007). While not totally implemented in audiology clinics at this writing, the benefit of the EHR is that within facilities such as hospitals, any patient healthcare information will be accessible by any provider in real time who has the appropriate password to access their healthcare information. In the medical side of healthcare, these EHR programs are rapidly increasing across the United States, and the provider is the one who maintains these electronic records.

Electronic healthcare records require an encrypted signature and specific progress notes may not be able to be changed once the signature is affixed and the chart note is saved for that time/date of service. Addenda may possibly be included for information that needs to be submitted for the same date of service. At this writing in 2024, EHR is required for physicians, *not* audiologists, but is highly likely, especially with office management systems; these EHR systems will be required for audiologists in the near future. These EHR notes need to be completed in a very timely manner and not left until later in the day when there have been several patients in between, possibly blurring the facts. EHR may disallow this practice as one record may need to be completed before another record is opened and is system specific.

Letters to referral sources should be completed within 24 to 48 hours post visit and can serve as a thank you for the referral. These letters should also include the name of the patient, the date of the letter and the date of service(s), findings, and recommendations for your mutual patient to assist them in managing their patient. These communications also solidify the current physician referral requirement for Medicare patients with acute hearing loss and vestibular symptoms by addressing the medical necessity requirement. Even when not required, this letter also solidifies excellent patient care as it "closes the loop" with the physician knowing what has been provided on behalf of their particular patient.

EHR documentation has six key elements:

- Case history.
- Procedures performed.
- Findings and results.
- Recommendations.
- Signature affixing.
- Date of the evaluation and dictation.

If errors are made in the charting process, several guidelines need to be followed for a hardcopy chart:

Do not destroy what has been written. Correction fluid is *not* to be utilized; simply strike out what needs to be eliminated, initial it with three initials, and place the date of action near those initials. For EHR, addendum notes may also possibly be attached but are dependent on the software of the electronic record.

When charting in hardcopy and electronic records, a guideline to follow is that the chart may be subpoenaed in a legal action or requested for a third-party payer audit. It needs to be legible, methodical, and within the confines of the minimum standard of care for audiology. To determine what constitutes standard of care, please consult *Audiology Clinical Practice Algorithms and Statements* (AAA, 2000). There are to be no sticky notes or other papers that are affixed. Every visit, phone call, encrypted email, and any other patient contact needs to be noted, dated, and signed.

For audiology practices falling under HIPAA regulations, legal authorities do not require consent (for treatment), but authorization for a single event, such as requesting a student's educational record, is likely to be required. The Notice of Privacy Practices (NPP) directs how the patient wants their healthcare information to be treated. For those working in a hospital setting, there are guidelines to follow, courtesy of the Joint Commission in Accreditation of Healthcare Organization (JCAHO).

In addition, there are other endorsing bodies that survey and accredit specific departments of a hospital or outpatient and/or rehabilitation facilities.

Chart Composition

The following necessary components indicate what is to be included in a patient's hardcopy chart, while electronic health care records may have established modules built into their particular system, available templates, and the ability for scanned documents to be added such as audiologic tests results. These are the following requirements:

- Patient registration form (needs to include the patient's demographic information [e.g., name, address, date of birth, phone number, insurance information, and (referring) physician if applicable]).
- Copies of the healthcare card (enrollment should be verified before they are seen) and driver's license/photo identification.
- Physician order if required by payer.
- Adult or pediatric medical history form.
- Insurance waiver.
- Advance Beneficiary Notice for Medicare beneficiaries if the service provided requires an ABN or, for a noncovered service, a voluntary ABN.
- Notice of Privacy Practices for HIPAA, signed by the patient, updated annually.
- Hearing aid–related forms:
  - Medical clearance by a physician if required by state licensure regulations.

- Hearing aid waiver if required by state licensure regulations.
- Contract/purchase agreement.
- Hearing aid checklist of discussed points, signed by the patient.
- Earmold and/or cerumen waiver form, signed by the patient if either or both procedures were performed (Appendix 17–B).
- Hearing aid warranty information.
- Postwarranty hearing aid service package document, indicating the services offered and the length of time they will be offered, if applicable.

Records Retention

HIPAA forms are to be retained for 6 years after the last date of service. It is suggested that providers contact their state's insurance commission regarding record retention laws. They may be listed on that state's website. If no specific guidance is offered, records of minors typically must be retained 7 years after reaching the age of maturity, and for adults, records should typically be retained for 7 years after their last visit. Deceased patient records should be retained for 7 years past the last date of service.

Several states have differing guidance as to who owns the patient's medical record. Consulting this website will give the necessary information pertinent to the regulations regarding this topic specific for each particular state(s). As a provision of HIPAA, the patient has the right to review their chart and amend anything for which they are not in agreement. The chart, however, is to be maintained by the facility that "owns" it. If the chart is subpoenaed, the subpoena will specify if the original chart must be submitted or whether a copy will suffice; *suggested practice is to retain the original and offer a copy.* Requested chart copies by the patient, attorneys, or another third-party payer are to be issued in a timely manner and state laws may prevail. The patient may be charged for the copy of their chart and state insurance laws may dictate what that fee may be limited to on a fee-per-page basis. HIPAA regulations require that if the patient requests their record in an electronic format, it is to be provided in that format, if possible.

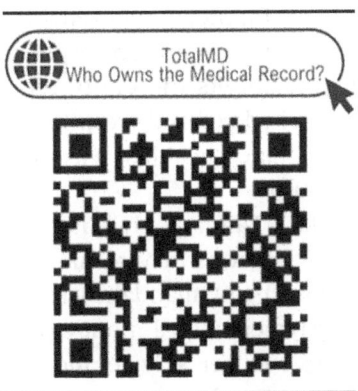

TotalMD
Who Owns the Medical Record?

Reports

The lifeline of an audiology practice's health is referrals. One way to ensure that the success of a practice continues is to inform the referral source via a well-written, succinct, and timely report as to the outcome of that patient's visit, preferably within 24 hours. This is an opportunity to have open communication regarding that patient, to demonstrate expertise, and to make recommendations that are vital to patient care. From a marketing standpoint,

it maintains the audiologist's name and the work performed on the radar of that referring professional. Reports need to be well written and concise. The SOAP format noted earlier is applicable to report writing. Many of the audiology-specific software office management systems and EHRs have report templates embedded in them. However, audiologists should consider this aspect of a patient visit as critical to patient care, the health of the practice, and fulfilling the requirements of third-party payers, if applicable.

Referrals to and From an Audiologist's Office

Referrals to other specialties such as otolaryngology, neurology, primary care, internal medicine, pediatrics, speech-language pathology, and other audiologists are a vital aspect of the standard of care. Practitioners should expect a report from a referring provider. Although audiologists are considered the experts in hearing and balance disorders, the provider may not have the expertise in certain areas of audiology practice; for example, some may not be comfortable with tinnitus or dizzy patients. If outside of the scope of an audiologist's practice or if experience with a particular treatment area is dated, it is best to refer to a colleague who is an expert in those particular diagnostics and/or treatment techniques. It is responsible patient care to conduct these referrals when necessary and is addressed by some state licensure laws and professional organizations' codes of ethics.

Conversely, referrals will be forthcoming from other providers; therefore, to maintain open lines of communication, a report and an appropriate thank you note to the referral sources are also suggested. This process closes the loop by meeting the standard of patient care and fulfilling any necessary third-party payer requirements, including those from Medicare.

The Laws That Bind: Stark Laws, Anti-Kickback Statutes, Safe Harbors, HIPAA, and State Licensure

As healthcare providers, audiologists are required to follow the federal regulations applicable to the provision of audiologic and vestibular services, which include:

- Stark Laws.
- Anti-Kickback Statutes.
- Safe Harbors.
- False Claims Act.
- Health Insurance Portability and Accountability Act (HIPAA).

Note that individual states may have more stringent counterparts of the above regulations; therefore, it is suggested this be investigated to determine whether these exist and the impact on audiologists. Each of these regulations will be examined in detail individually and their applications to audiology specified in the following sections.

Stark Laws

All audiologists should be aware of the federal antifraud laws as well as any relevant state antifraud laws. Before enter-

ing into a contractual arrangement with a physician or physician group, an audiologist should consult legal counsel familiar with healthcare fraud and abuse laws. The Stark Law and the Anti-Kickback Statute should be considered separately; activities or arrangements that are acceptable under one may violate the other (Abel & Hahn, 2006).

The Stark Law (42 U.S.C. § 1395nn) prohibits physician "self-referrals." That is, it prohibits a physician (or a physician's immediate family member) from referring patients for designated health services to an entity in which the physician (or their immediate family member) has a financial relationship, unless a specific exception applies. The law also prohibits the entity receiving the prohibited referral from billing for those designated health services (Abel & Hahn, 2006).

The Stark Law is a civil, not a criminal, law. Violations may result in denial of reimbursement, mandatory refunds of federal payments, civil money penalties up to $15,000 per service and civil assessment up to three times the amount claimed, and exclusion from federal and state healthcare programs. The Centers for Medicare & Medicaid Services (CMS) issued regulations (42 C.F.R. Part 411) implementing the Stark Law in two phases over a period of several years, with the third phase going into effect in 2007. In 2016, CMS finalized additional changes to the Stark Law in the final rule of the Medicare Physician Fee Schedule, and in 2022, there were further updates impacting physicians. Exposure to audiologists should be verified by your legal counsel, who is familiar with state and federal regulations impacting the practice of audiology in the states where audiologist is licensed.

STARK LAWS I & II

The Stark Law is sometimes referred to as "Stark II." The statute originally only prohibited physician referrals to labs in which the referring physician has a financial interest ("Stark I"). When the statute was broadened to prohibit physician referrals to any entity in which the referring physician has a financial interest, it was designated "Stark II" (Abel & Hahn, 2006).

To violate Stark, there must be a *referral* by a physician (or their immediate family member) to an *entity* in which the physician (or their immediate family member) has a *financial interest* for the furnishing of *designated health services (DHS)*.

A *referral* is any physician requesting, ordering, certifying, or recertifying the need for a DHS for which payment may be made under Medicare. An *entity* is any person (including an individual, partnership, or corporation) that furnishes DHS. If the referring physician personally performs the service, there is no referral. A person is considered to be furnishing DHS (listed below) if it is the person to which CMS makes payment or to whom the right of payment has been reassigned. Thus, an audiologist may be an entity receiving a prohibited referral if tied to Medicaid services for hearing aids if considered durable medical equipment or to devices such as cochlear implants and osseointegrated devices for Medicare beneficiaries. Audiologists should consult with legal counsel as to the implications for their specific state regulations and these Medicare and Medicaid scenarios.

A *financial interest* is broadly defined to include direct or indirect ownership or investment interest or a direct or indirect compensation arrangement. *Designated health services (DHS)* are defined as the following items and services only:

- Clinical laboratory services.
- Physical therapy, occupational therapy, and outpatient speech-language pathology services.
- Radiology and certain other imaging services.
- Radiation therapy services and supplies.
- Durable medical equipment and supplies.
- Parenteral and enteral nutrients, equipment, and supplies.
- Prosthetics, orthotics, and prosthetic devices and supplies.
- Home health services.
- Outpatient prescription drugs.
- Inpatient and outpatient hospital services.

Because of this narrow definition of DHS, the Stark Law has limited application to audiologists. The only audiology services that fall within the definition of DHS are those furnished as hospital inpatient or outpatient services; however, the hospital is the entity that receives payment from CMS for those services, not the audiologist, and is the entity that must comply with the Stark Law.

While Medicare does not consider hearing aids to be DHS, Medicaid in the state may, so seek legal counsel familiar with state and federal regulations. The Stark Law and implementing CMS regulations provide many exceptions. These include bona fide employment relationships, arm's-length agreements for the rental of office space or equipment, and "in-office ancillary services." To qualify for an exception, a transaction or arrangement must meet specific requirements. For example, to qualify for the in-office ancillary services exception, the services must meet a supervision requirement (e.g., furnished by an individual under the supervision of the referring physician), a building requirement (e.g., furnished in the same building in which the referring physician normally furnishes services to patients), and a billing requirement (e.g., billed by the supervising physician, the group practice, an entity wholly owned by the physician or group practice, or an independent third-party billing company acting as agent of the physician, group practice, or entity) (CMS, 2021) Because the Stark Law has a limited impact on audiologists, the exceptions will not be discussed in detail in this chapter.

In essence, the Stark Law prohibits a physician (or their immediate family member) from referring a patient for the furnishing of DHS to an entity in which the physician (or immediate family members) has a financial interest, unless an exception applies. Because the Stark Law only applies to referrals for the furnishing of DHS, and because the only audiology services that are DHS are inpatient and outpatient hospital services, Stark Laws have a limited impact on audiologists. In the case of hospital services, CMS makes payment to the hospital, so the hospital is the entity that must comply with Stark. Audiologists should be aware, however, that most states have their own Stark Laws, and some of these may be broader than the federal Stark Law. Whenever in doubt, audiologists are advised to consult legal counsel well versed in federal, state, and local laws (Abel & Hahn, 2006).

Anti-Kickback Statute (AKS)

The Anti-Kickback Statute [42 U.S.C. §1320a-7b(b)] was promulgated to address the soliciting and receiving of kickbacks in return for referrals of patients whose items or services are reimbursable under federal healthcare programs. It prohibits any person from "knowingly and willfully soliciting or receiving any remuneration (including any kickback, bribe, or rebate) directly or indirectly, overtly or covertly, in cash or in kind" to induce someone to refer an individual for "any item or service for which payment may be made in whole or in part under a federal health care program" (Abel & Hahn, 2006).

The AKS prohibits kickbacks because (1) they create an incentive to overutilize reimbursable services, increasing costs to Medicare and other federal healthcare programs; (2) they distort medical decision-making; and (3) they result in unfair competition by freezing out qualified providers who are unwilling to pay kickbacks (Abel & Hahn, 2006).

The AKS is a criminal statute, and violation of the AKS is a felony punishable by imprisonment (for up to 5 years), heavy fines (up to $25,000), and/or exclusion from federal healthcare program participation. "Civil Monetary Penalties may also be imposed up to $50,000 for each violation, plus the additional imposition of three times the amount of the remuneration offered, paid, solicited, or received, also known as treble damages" (Lewis, 2011; OIG, 2024). Unlike the Stark Law, in civil law, intent is a critical element that must be proved by the prosecutor. However, while intent to induce referrals or obtain money for referrals is to be proven, it is not required. The AKS is enforced by the Office of the Inspector General (OIG). Thus, the elements of an AKS violation are the following:

- Intent: acting knowingly and willfully.
- Offering, giving, soliciting, or receiving remuneration.
- Referral of patients to purchase, lease, order, or arrange for any item or service reimbursable under a federal healthcare program.

The AKS is much broader than the Stark Law. Unlike Stark, it is not limited to particular designated health services; instead, it applies to any item or service payable in whole or in part under any federal healthcare program. Many possible arrangements between audiologists and physicians may involve the AKS. Here are a few examples:

- An audiologist furnishes diagnostic tests to a physician's patients at no

or reduced charges in return for hearing aid referrals, where hearing aids are covered by the state Medicaid plan. The audiologist is giving the physician remuneration (i.e., free or reduced-price diagnostic tests) in return for referrals of hearing aid business reimbursable by Medicaid.

- An audiologist rents office space from a physician and pays the rental fee based on the number of referrals of Medicare/Medicaid patients received from the physician. The audiologist is giving the physician remuneration (i.e., above-market rent) in return for referrals of Medicare/Medicaid business. Also see the American Speech-Language-Hearing Association's website for examples applicable to audiologists.

American Speech-Language-Hearing Association Self-Referral Regulations

- An audiologist accepts remuneration (in the form of gifts, entertainment, loans, cooperative marketing funds, trips, or other benefits) from a hearing aid manufacturer in return for prescribing the manufacturer's hearing aids, where the hearing aids are covered by Medicaid or another federal program. The audiologist is receiving remuneration in return for recommending the purchase of hearing aids reimbursable by Medicaid (Abel & Hahn, 2006).

The American Academy of Audiology Ethical Practice Guideline for Relationships With Industry for Audiologists Providing Clinical Care (revised 2017) educates members about the ethics and legality of the acceptance of trips, cash, and other gifts in exchange for recommending items that may be paid for by a federal healthcare program. Abiding by these guidelines protects the audiologist from inadvertent violations of the Anti-Kickback Statute.

Safe Harbors

To avoid criminalizing innocent conduct, there are many "safe harbors" to the AKS. If a transaction meets all the requirements of a safe harbor, it is protected from prosecution. However, failure to qualify for a safe harbor does not automatically mean a transaction is not in violation of the AKS. The safe harbors include arm's-length agreements for the rental of office space or equipment, discounts, and bona fide employment relationships. While a complete discussion of the AKS safe harbors is beyond the scope of this chapter, two of the harbors are worth mentioning because of their widespread use (Abel & Hahn, 2006).

To qualify for safe harbor protection, a discount must be "a reduction in the amount a buyer (who buys either directly or through a wholesaler or a group purchasing organization) is charged for an item or service based on an arms-length transaction" (42 C.F.R. § 1001.952[h][5]). The discount must be

made at the time of sale (or, if a rebate, the terms of the rebate must be fixed and disclosed in writing to the buyer at the time of sale). The buyer receiving the discount must, upon request of the OIG or state regulators, provide certain information from the seller. In addition, the discount must be properly disclosed and reflected in the charges billed to the federal healthcare program paying for the item or service. Thus, *the discount must ensure benefit to the Medicare or Medicaid program.* The discount must be earned in the same fiscal year as the purchase of the applicable item or service. The safe harbor does not protect discounts in the form of cash payments (or cash equivalents) (Abel & Hahn, 2006).

To qualify for the office rental safe harbor, an audiologist must ensure that rental payments are not disguised kickbacks to induce referrals by the physician-landlord. Specifically:

- The rental agreement must be in writing and signed by the parties.
- The rental agreement must cover all premises rented by the parties and specify the premises.
- The term of the agreement must be at least 1 year.
- If the audiologist is renting space for periodic intervals, the agreement must specify the exact schedule of usage.
- The aggregate rental amount must be set in advance, consistent with fair market value, and may not consider the volume or value of referrals.
- The aggregate space rented may not exceed what is reasonably necessary to accomplish a commercially reasonable business purpose.

For a more detailed discussion of this safe harbor, see OIG (2000).

As previously noted, some states have their own anti-kickback and Stark laws, which may differ from the federal regulations. Whenever in doubt, consult with legal counsel well versed in both federal and state anti-kickback laws as it is beyond the purview of this chapter (Abel & Hahn, 2006).

False Claims

The False Claims Act (31 U.S.C. §3729-3733) specifies the following ill-advised actions as considered fraudulent:

- Presenting a claim that the person knows or should know is for an item or service that was not provided as claimed or is false or fraudulent.
- Presenting a claim that the person knows or should know is for an item or service for which payment may not be made.
- Violating the AKS.
- Violating Medicare assignment provisions.
- Violating the Medicare physician agreement.
- Providing false or misleading information expected to influence a decision to discharge.
- Failing to provide an adequate medical screening examination for patients who present to a hospital emergency department with an emergency medical condition or in labor.
- Making false statements or misrepresentations on applications or contracts to participate in the federal health programs.

Services that are determined to be fraudulent will result in the revocation of privileges in providing services to that insurer, potential legal action that may revoke state license(s), payback of funds with penalties and interest, and possible incarceration. There are potential criminal and civil penalties if found guilty.

Providers should bill only for services that are necessary when determining the patient's diagnosis. The Office of the Inspector General, in their pursuit of fraud and abuse, is on the lookout for false claims, especially submitting claims for services not rendered. In addition, because of the 2010 Affordable Care Act, any overpayment due to a federal payer must be paid back within 60 days of discovery, or it may be considered a false claim.

HIPAA

In 1996, the Health Insurance Portability and Accountability Act (HIPAA), Public Law 104-191, was promulgated by Congress "to improve portability and continuity of health care when there was a change of jobs, to combat waste, fraud and abuse in health insurance and health care delivery to simplify the administration of health insurance, and for other purposes". Because the deadline passed without congressional response to healthcare standards, the responsibility fell to the secretary of the Department of Health and Human Services (DHHS) and the Centers for Medicare & Medicaid Services (CMS), which has the responsibility of implementing them. According to HIPAA privacy guidelines, when treatment, payment, or operational (TPO) information is involved, a medical release is not required. However, in a litigious society, it may be prudent to obtain one for any exchange of information to protect the patients, the practice, and the audiologist. Consent according to HIPAA is optional, may be obtained once, and can be revoked. The Notice of Privacy Practices (NPP) should be updated annually with the patient's signature, attesting to how they want their Personal Health Information (PHI) handled as patients' situations change. Authorization, typically for a one-time occurrence, is required for those instances.

There are five titles that comprise HIPAA with Title II, Administrative Simplification, being the most important in most audiology practices, created to have PHI transmitted securely. Within this title are Transaction and Code Sets (effective date October 16, 2003), Privacy (April 14, 2003), and Security (April 21, 2005). The Unique Identifiers Rule, which includes the National Provider Identifier (NPI) for providers and the Tax Identification Number (TIN)/Employer Identification Number (EIN) for employers, became effective on May 23, 2007, and for small health plans, a year later to the day.

The Department of Health and Human Services (DHHS) oversees HIPAA. If any violations occur with the privacy aspect of HIPAA, the Office for Civil Rights at DHHS is responsible for the enforcement. Penalties may include criminal and civil penalties.

HIPAA has five titles, each of which addresses varied sections of this act. These are listed below.

■ TITLE I: Portability and Renewability. This title allows for the portability of healthcare for those who have changed or lost their jobs.

■ TITLE II: Administrative Simplification. This section applies to any provider or facility that transmits health information and will affect nearly all healthcare providers, as it addresses the standards of transmitting healthcare information via electronic methods. Due to concerns regarding the security of this information being processed electronically, administrative simplification was created. The following are also included with administrative simplification.

■ Transaction and Code Sets (standardization of CPT®, ICD-CM, and HCPCS codes, Unique Provider Identifiers). The transaction and code sets allow for all third-party payers to utilize uniform and standard sets of codes such as CPT®, the ICD-CMs, and the HCPCS codes. However, workers' compensation in many states (and at least one state's Medicaid agency) has additional codes they may utilize, generally for hearing aid–related procedures.

■ Privacy Rules. Protecting personal health information, Notice of Privacy Practices (NPP).

■ Security Rules. Safeguards to protect data, computers, and the information therein; disaster recovery.

■ TITLE III: Tax-Related Health Provisions

■ TITLE IV: Application and Enforcement of Group Health Plan Requirements

■ TITLE V: Revenue Offsets

Appendix 17–C presents a sample HIPPA authorization release form especially for a practice that may be designed specifically for the provider's practice. Specifically, the form must include the name and address of your practice or facility and the patient's name, address, and birth date. In addition, the information that they need released or that will be released from the provider to a third party with their identifying information should be included, as well as an expiration date for the authorization. The patient's right to revoke the authorization also needs to be addressed, as well as the notification that the information may be redisclosed by the recipient.

National Provider Identifier

Since May 23, 2007, all healthcare providers and covered entities have been required to have the 10-digit Unique Provider Identifier, the National Provider Identifier (NPI), one of the last vestiges of HIPAA's Administrative Simplification. As part of their request, healthcare facilities must have a Tax Identification Number (TIN) or Employer Identification Number (EIN). HIPAA calls for a "standard unique health identifier for each individual, employer, health plan and health care provider for use in the healthcare system" (CMS, 2004). The NPI number is managed by CMS via the NPI Enumerator. This single provider number replaced all numbers assigned to providers; it links to a provider's Medicare Provider Transaction Access Number (PTAN) and will be the only number used for a provider's entire professional career for billing purposes for all payers. If providers move to another state, they will utilize this same 10-digit number until the day of retirement but may need to obtain a new Medicare Provider Trans-

action Number (PTAN). The NPI number carries no intelligence or mechanism to identify a provider or their specialty.

The NPI application process is quite simple and can be completed online in approximately 20 minutes. Providers will need to share their NPI with entities such as an employer, clearinghouses, third-party payers, or any others who would utilize it for billing purposes. Hospital employees have their services billed by way of the hospital's NPI.

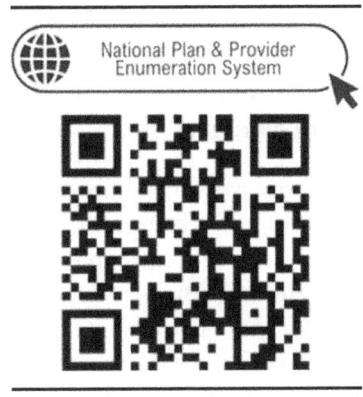

The National Employer Identifier Number (EIN) became effective in 2007, a separate and distinct number from the NPI. This nine-digit number assigned by the Internal Revenue Service to all healthcare employers is required on all healthcare plan submissions and is required on the CMS 1500 billing form, in the office management system software, or in your electronic healthcare record.

Informed Consent

Audiologists have all encountered patients that do not seek audiologic treatment under their own volition, but by that of a well-meaning relative or friend. The patient has the ultimate right to determine treatment. When that patient is incapacitated and unable to make their own decisions, a legally appointed power of attorney may act on their behalf. It is suggested that a place be included for the patient's signature on the practice's registration form, indicating the patient is granting permission to provide the necessary audiologic diagnosis and treatment options. HIPAA does not require consent for treatment. For those 18 years or younger, a note from the parent or guardian is necessary to provide audiologic services in that parent or guardian's absence (Abel & Hahn, 2006).

Minimum Necessary

HIPAA addresses the importance of disseminating the minimum information necessary for treatment, payment, and operations (TPO) in dealing with patient care and privacy issues. If recounting a very interesting clinical case in a presentation or journal article, all patient identifying information must be redacted as this is not considered TPO information. The privacy component of HIPAA addresses how personal health information is to be viewed, transmitted, and stored. Anyone who provides healthcare services is considered a Covered Entity (CE) unless they do not transmit any healthcare information electronically. A CE can include any provider who transmits PHI electronically, including health plans and clearinghouses. Electronic transmissions include Internet, dial-up, private networks, tapes, and CDs.

If a provider is a CE, as most audiologists are, the Notice of Privacy Practices (NPP) is given to the patient the first time they present to the practice. It ad-

dresses how all their PHI will be treated and what is permissible for any contact with the patient and family members and the processes if there are any complaints. This aspect of HIPAA ensures that in the cases of treatment, payment, and/or operations, consent is implied, and information may flow among any of the covered entities involved in that patient's healthcare.

As audiologists, providers may see evidence of abuse, domestic violence, and/or neglect. In cases such as this, privacy is "suspended" as the appropriate authorities are to be contacted immediately, which may include and are not restricted to law enforcement, children's services, and/or domestic violence shelters. This should be addressed in the NPP as well as in the office, clinic or facility policy, and procedures manual.

Incidental disclosures are addressed under HIPAA. This would be the inadvertent disclosure of PHI such as if a patient, lost in the office, happened to walk by as the audiologist was discussing something on the phone with another patient. Although the audiologist attempted to make it as private a conversation as possible, an unforeseen circumstance transpired.

CEs need to have a business agreement (BA) in place when PHI is exchanged, and it needs to be signed by both parties. Therefore, hearing aid manufacturers need to have BAs with the facility since there is PHI exchanged on the patient's behalf when, for example, a hearing aid is ordered. Of course, fictitious names could be substituted, but that is certainly more information to track. Other BAs that need to be in place are with anyone who processes claims, such as an insurance claims clearinghouse; those who do billing; an accountant and attorney; and, if transcription services are utilized, the transcriptionist. Due to the 2009 Health Information Technology for Economic and Clinical Health Act (HITECH), regulations were enacted so that BAs also have a contractual responsibility to the CE for providing services. HITECH also was enacted to address the processes and penalties when a data breach occurs.

HIPAA Omnibus Rule

On September 23, 2013, the HIPAA Omnibus rule went into effect, with several major additions to existing HIPAA and HITECH regulations, including the following:

"If a facility received remuneration from a third party whose product or services are marketed to patients to encourage them to purchase those products and services, that communication must be authorized prior to dispersal by the patient; the definition of BAs was expanded to include agreements with their sub-contractors to protect the PHI that is exchanged and that BAs should be updated; that if a patient refused to authorize payment submission to their insurance and privately pay for the service, the provider is obligated to comply; that patients have access to copies of their medical record in the format requested, including electronically, if they choose; if a CE chooses to raise funds for their facility, individuals have the opportunity to opt out of fundraising communications; and finally, but not limited to, the process of a data breach, should that occur in a practice, with notification to the affected patients, the local media, and for breaches of unsecured PHI affecting 500 or more individuals, the affected patients and

the local media, and the Secretary of Health and Human Services must be immediately notified when the breach is discovered."

Early in the HIPAA transition process, there were many myths about what was allowed, some of which have persisted. The patient may sign in on a sign-in sheet, but the reason for their visit *should not* be listed. Many offices that utilize the sign-in process will have a line where the patient signs their name, which can then be pulled off after their visit is noted by staff. Since "minimum necessary" is the hallmark of HIPAA, charts and computer monitors should not face the patient or be in a highly trafficked area, where they can be easily seen. Collection calls and informing patients of test results should be completed in an area where the conversation will not be overheard. Reminder postcards sent to the patient need to be in envelopes so that PHI cannot be viewed, such as the reason why the recipient will be seen, and any type of marketing requires authorization (Pessis & Williams, 2005). A newsletter that provides general information, as long as it doesn't promote a specific product and/or brand, and mass mailings that do not include PHI are permissible (Pessis, 2003).

Authorization in the form of written permission for a one-time, date-specific event or time frame is required. For example, audiologists need permission from parents to confer with school personnel regarding school-aged patients who wear amplification, such as the clinical audiologist and the educational audiologist exchanging information on a mutual patient. The Family Educational Rights and Privacy Act (FERPA), the law for those in educational settings, was promulgated to protect student education records and is the educational setting's version of HIPAA.

The security side of HIPAA addresses administrative procedures, physical safeguards, technical data security services, and technical security mechanisms (Pessis & Williams, 2005). Administrative procedures cover documentation and formal procedures for selecting and executing information and how the staff will protect that data. All information security measures are to be reviewed (Pessis & Williams, 2005). Physical safeguards are necessary to protect the information within the walls of an office such as the actual computer system and the provision for fire, theft, and disaster recovery. Hardcopy charts must be kept in locked cabinets and in locked rooms and/or offices. The technical data security services safeguard the processes used to protect, control, and monitor information access (Pessis & Williams, 2005). This includes any password application and may also include badge readers, smart cards, and biometrics (Pessis & Williams, 2005). Passwords should be changed periodically and may be required by some facilities' systems, including NOAH. Finally, technical security mechanisms address the utilization of unauthorized access to data transmitted over a communications network and may include a secure network, firewalls, and encryption (Pessis & Williams, 2005). Emails must be encrypted for any communications to patients.

Every office providing healthcare in compliance with HIPAA has specified the name of their privacy officer on their NPP. This representative is to be contacted when a patient has a complaint. The patient has the right to review their chart and request a change in their record, known as an amendment, which is then accepted or rejected by the provider and documented in the chart. A complaint may also be registered by contacting the Office of Civil Rights. Fines for HIPAA violations can be substantial and, depending on level of culpability, can range from civil monetary penalties of $100/violation to $50,000/violation for those unaware they were committing a HIPAA violation, to an annual maximum of $50,000/violation up to $1.5 million per calendar year, for those violations because of conscience neglect and no corrective action was taken to correct any violations. Exclusion from Medicare and Medicaid may also occur due to HIPAA violations. Criminal penalties range from imprisonment of 1 year for unknowingly committing a HIPAA violation or with reasonable cause, up to 10 years for malicious disregard and/or personal gain.

Security

The intent of the security component of HIPAA is to protect data integrity, confidentiality, and availability in safeguarding privacy. It was implemented on April 21, 2005 (Pessis, 2003). The security section comprises four categories: administrative procedures, physical safeguards, technical data security services, and technical security mechanisms (Pessis, 2003). The administrative procedures discuss how staff protect the data as well selecting and executing information on information security. Assessment and review of information security procedures, manuals, and records is required (Pessis, 2003).

Physical safeguards protect the actual computer system from theft, fire, intrusion, and other environmental hazards. Technical data security services safeguard the processes used to protect, control, and monitor information access (Pessis, 2003). Computer passwords are included in this component as well as biometrics, smart cards, and electronic signatures. It is recommended that passwords be changed periodically, a requirement in many facilities for many aspects of employment, including log-in computer access, payroll, email access, EHR, and NOAH. Technical security mechanisms are geared to prevent the intrusion of an unauthorized, uninvited outside source into entered data. Firewalls and encryption apply to this component.

HITECH

The HITECH (Health Information Technology for Economic and Clinical Health Act) was signed into law as part of the 2009 American Recovery and Reinvestment Act to promote the adoption of "meaningful use" of health information (not applicable to audiologists at the time of publication), to address privacy and security provisions concerning data breaches of PHI, and to define technologic specifications for secure nationwide electronic exchange of information. When a breach occurs, those affected by the breach as well as the Department of Health and Human Services must be informed within 60 days of discovery; if the breach affected 500 people or more, these entities must be informed as well as the local media outlets. Existing Business Agreements (BA) will likely need to be revised to be in compliance with HITECH, as BAs are now subject to part of HIPAA privacy and security rules and subject to HIPAA civil and criminal penalties. Civil penalties range from $100 to $50,000/violation, with an annual maximum of $1,500,000 and the criminal penalty for knowingly obtaining or disclosing PHI is up to $50,000 and imprisonment for up to 1 year. For those offenses committed under false pretenses, fines may be increased to $100,000 with up to 5 years of imprisonment.

Figure 17–1 presents the table of civil monetary penalties with the tiers based on previous history, the financial health of the facility, and the level of physical,

2024 HIPAA Penalty Structure				
Penalty Tier	**Tier 1**	**Tier 2**	**Tier 3**	**Tier 4**
Culpability	LACK OF KNOWLEDGE	REASONABLE CAUSE	WILLFUL NEGLECT	WILLFUL NEGLECT (NOT CORRECTED WITHIN 30 DAYS)
Minimim Penalty per Violation – Inflation Adjusted	$137	$1,379	$13,785	$68,928
Max Penalty per Violation – Inflation Adjusted	$68,928	$68,928	$68,928	$2,067,813
Maximum Penalty per Year – Inflation Adjusted	$2,067,813	$2,067,813	$2,067,813	$2,067,813

Figure 17–1. Civil monetary penalties. *Source:* Adapted from *What are the penalties for HIPAA violations?* (2024). The HIPAA Journal.

financial, or reputational harm incurred to the patient. A correction plan must also be created and adhered to. Criminal penalties up to $100,000 and up to 10 years imprisonment may also be imposed.

State Regulations/Licensure

At this writing, audiologists are regulated in all 50 states by state licensure. A license to practice audiology is mandated, is the only requirement to practice (for consumer protection), is what defines scope of practice, and is the only requirement for Medicare enrollment. "Minimum necessary" is the standard of care for most licensure laws, so that if services are not provided under "the standard of care," liability issues will ensue when litigated.

It is incumbent upon every audiologist to know the state licensure laws in the state(s) in which they practice and are licensed; ignorance is not a defense when dealing with federal and state laws. Scope of practice for the profession is clearly delineated in position statements and documents on professional organization websites, but it is possible that a procedure that is included in the scope of practice may not be delineated or allowed in the licensure law. If a practice wants to provide a service that is not addressed in the particular state's licensure law, an opinion from the governing board should be requested given that the liability policy covers what is in the scope of practice as noted in the state licensure law(s).

Some states have also addressed codes of ethics and have included them as part of the revised code or law, and they must be abided as such. Something

illegal may not be unethical and the reverse can also be true.

Certification

Although licensure is required to practice audiology, certification is not. Certification affirms professionalism and is a mechanism of promoting the continuing education audiologists have undertaken to hone skill sets and stay abreast of the rapid changes in the field. Currently, there are two certifications for audiologists. One is voluntary, bestowed upon meeting the requirements established by a freestanding board, whereas the other type of certification is an option for membership of that professional organization. Continuing education is a requirement for licensure in most states as well as for certification.

Other Practice Issues for Consideration

The federal regulations above create the framework in which compliance must be met. There are other issues to consider when protecting the provider and their practice, and these are listed in the following sections.

Liability

As audiologists, there are two types of liability to consider: malpractice and, for those who are in private practice, property liability. Malpractice is liability insurance that covers the provider in whole or in part if that provider errs by negligence or omission causing injury to the patient. Property liability covers the physical facility of the office for such things as fire, theft, and injuries that occur on the premises, to name a few potential catastrophes or mishaps.

An umbrella policy provides additional coverage if there is property damage or other potential calamities that exceed the limits of current coverage. The local insurance agent can be contacted for any of these insurance needs, but professional liability coverage is one of the benefits of membership of a national professional organization.

Impaired Practitioners

Rule 8b of the Code of Ethics of the American Academy of Audiology states, "Individuals shall not engage in dishonesty or illegal conduct that adversely reflects on the profession." This could certainly include the danger of being an impaired practitioner—drug or alcohol induced. If the provider suffers from the abuse of either, whether the drug is legal or not, they are placing themselves and their patients at risk; the personal and professional liability is not worth the cost. If providers know of a colleague who is impaired, there are several options for consideration and may be set forth in the policy and procedures manual of the place of employment. Intervention is often used to confront the impaired practitioner and make them aware of their problem, the impact it has had on those who participate in that intervention, and their recommendations for seeking assistance in combating that problem. Audiologists have the ethical burden to report their colleague to the ethical committee of the professional organization of which they are a member for review, and state licensure laws may compel them to report suspicions about the

licensee to that board as well (Abel & Hahn, 2006).

Incompetent Patients

A core professional rule of practice is cited as Principle 4 of the American Academy of Audiology's Code of Ethics and states, "Members shall provide only services and products that are in the best interest of those served." Rule 4a specifies that "individuals shall not exploit persons in the delivery of professional services."

As audiologists serve the elderly, confused or forgetful patients are often seen who may be unaware they are experiencing these symptoms. Dementia may be accompanied by belligerence, and these patients will require specialized care. Providers that cannot provide this care need to refer to a colleague. Working closely with the family of this challenging patient may be a guide to other avenues; for example, an assistive listening device may be recommended instead of a hearing aid (Abel & Hahn, 2006).

Dismissing a Patient

According to the American Medical Association, a physician is free to accept or decline an individual as a patient (Metz, 2006). There are many reasons as to why a patient may need to be dismissed from service. Noncompliant patients, those who do not follow your recommendations, perpetual no-shows, and those who do not pay their bills are patients whom providers may consider to be better served by another audiologist. This may also be due to personality traits or conflicts between the patient and the audiologist. Critical in making the decision to dismiss a patient is to *notify them, in writing, with 30 days' notice, providing a deadline of termination and the names of other audiologists whom they may contact for care, via certified mail with a signature request to verify their receipt of the letter, which is then placed in their chart.* Document in the patient's chart the reason they are being terminated as well as provide them with a copy of their records. As with providing any records to another healthcare professional or an attorney, the provider maintains the original chart and the patient receives the copy. Although personal thoughts may tend to color the provider's thinking, the patient's best interest must be kept tantamount (Chapter 18).

If appropriate procedures are not followed in the termination of a patient, the provider may be accused of abandonment. Abandonment generally means a unilateral severance of the professional relationship between a healthcare provider and a patient without reasonable notice at a time when there is still a need for continuing healthcare. Notification to the referring physician or healthcare provider is required (Forbes Advisor, 2024). As with many concerns discussed in this chapter, audiologists will want to consult with legal counsel familiar with healthcare issues and federal, state, and local laws.

As the groundwork is laid to realize an audiologist's professional home and ambitions, may the laws cited here offer a guide that provides the framework for practice and the coding information the mechanism for maintaining that framework.

As state and federal laws change in the healthcare arena, it behooves every practitioner to know what those changes are relative to compliance. In the next few years, there will likely be a change of core payment methodologies and less reimbursement for services. Additional bundled codes and the bundling of bundled codes may play a role in the evolution from defined moments such as the introduction of Medicare, regulations for compliance, and reduction in reimbursement paradigms, but the determination to continue to provide the utmost in care in even the most challenging situations will prevail for the benefit of those whom we serve.

References

Abel, D., & Hahn, R. (2006). Ethical issues in practice management. In T. Hamill (Ed.), *Ethics in audiology: Guidelines for ethical conduct in clinical, educational and research setting* (pp.62–74). American Academy of Audiology.

American Academy of Audiology. (2000). Audiology clinical practice algorithms and statements. *Audiology Today Special Issue,* August 2000. https://www.audiology.org/wp-content/uploads/2021/05/Clinical PracticeAlgorithms.pdf_53994824786 af8.17185566.pdf

American Academy of Audiology. (2014). *American Academy of Audiology Ethical Practice Guideline for Relationships with Industry for Audiologists Providing Clinical Care.* July 28, 2011. Revised September 2017. https://www.audiology.org/wp-content/uploads/2021/05/2017_09 -Revised Guideline_CURRENT.pdf

American Academy of Audiology. (2016a). Code of Ethics. Revised April 2023. https://www.audiology.org/wp-content/uploads/2023/05/AAA-Code-of-Ethics -and-Non-Compliance-Procedures -2023-04-1.pdf

American Academy of Audiology. (2016b). *2016 Editable superbill template.* https://www.audiology.org/academy-updates-superbill-template-2024/

American Academy of Audiology Coding and Practice Management Committee. (2006). *Capturing reimbursement: A guide for audiologists.*

American Medical Association. (2012). *HIPAA violations and enforcement.* http://www.ama-assn.org/ama/pub/physician-resources/solutions-managing-your-practice/coding-billing-insurance/hipaa health-insurance-portability-accountability-act/*hipaa*-violations-enforcement.page

American Medical Association. (2024a). *Criteria for CPT® Category I and Category III Codes.* Chicago, IL. https://www.ama-assn.org/practice-management/cpt/criteria-cpt-category-i-and-category-iii-codes

American Medical Association. (2024b). *AMA Specialty Society RVS Update Committee.* https://www.ama-assn.org/system/files/ruc-update-booklet.pdf

American Medical Association. (2024c). *Private practice checklist key considerations in providing ancillary services in your physician practice.* https://www.ama-assn.org/system/files/private-practice-checklist-ancillary-services.pdf

Centers for Medicare & Medicaid Services. (2001). *Program memorandum AB-02-080, Audiologists—payment for services furnished.* https://www.cms.gov/Regulations-and Guidance/Guidance/Transmittals/downloads/AB02080.pdf

Centers for Medicare & Medicaid Services. (2004). *CMS Announces the standard unique health identifier for health care providers for use in standard transactions under HIPAA.* https://www.cms.gov/newsroom/press-releases/cms-announces-standard-unique-health-identifier-health-care-providers-use-standard-transactions.

Centers for Medicare & Medicaid Services. (2008). *Transmittal 84.* https://www.cms.gov/transmittals/downloads/R84BP.pdf

Centers for Medicare & Medicaid Services. (2010). *Revisions and re-issuance of audiology policies-JA6447.* https://www.hhs.gov/guidance/sites/default/files/hhs-guidance-documents/JA6447.pdf

Centers for Medicare & Medicaid Services. (2011). *Medicare benefit policy manual, chapter 15.* https://www.cms.gov/Regulations-and-Guidance/Guidance/Manuals/downloads/bp102c15.pdf

Centers for Medicare & Medicaid Services. (2012). *Payment for servicesf Furnished by audiologists.* https://www.cms.gov/regulations-and-guidance/guidance/transmittals/cms-program-memoranda-items/cms024824.

Centers for Medicare & Medicaid Services. (2013). *MLN Matters® Number: SE0908.* https://www.hhs.gov/guidance/sites/default/files/hhs-guidance-documents/SE0908.pdf.

Centers for Medicare & Medicaid Services. (2016a). *MLN Matters Number SE0441. Incident to services.* https://www.cms.gov/outreach-and-education/medicare-learning-network-mln/mlnmattersarticles/downloads/se0441.pdf

Centers for Medicare & Medicaid Services. (2016b). *MLN matters number: SE0441.* https://www.cms.gov/Outreach-and-Education/Medicare-Learning-Network-MLN/MLNMattersArticles/downloads/SE0441.pdf

Centers for Medicare & Medicaid Services. (2016c). *Medicare fraud and abuse: Prevention, detection and reporting.* ICN006827. https://www.cms.gov/Outreach-and-Education/Medicare-Learning-Network-MLN/MLNProducts/Downloads/Fraud-Abuse-MLN4649244.pdf

Centers for Medicare & Medicaid Services. (2017a). First level of appeal: Redetermination by a Medicare contractor. https://www.cms.gov/medicare/appeals-and-grievances/orgmedffsappeals/redeterminationbyamedicarecontractor.html

Centers for Medicare & Medicaid Services. (2017b). Comprehensive error rate testing reports. https://www.cms.gov/data-research/monitoring-programs/improper-payment-measurement-programs/comprehensive-error-rate-testing-cert

Centers for Medicare & Medicaid Services. (2017c). Medicare learning network. Medicare Parts A and B appeals process. https://www.cms.gov/Outreach-and-Education/Medicare-Learning-Network-MLN/MLNProducts/downloads/MedicareAppealsprocess.pdf

Centers for Medicare & Medicaid Services. (2021). *Centers for Medicare and Medicaid Services physician self-referral law frequently asked questions.* https://www.cms.gov/Medicare/Fraud-and-Abuse/PhysicianSelfReferral/Downloads/FAQs-Physician-Self-Referral-Law.pdf

Centers for Medicare & Medicaid Services. (2024a). *Advanced beneficiary notice.* http://www.cms.gov/Medicare/Medicare-General-Information/BNI/ABN.html

Centers for Medicare & Medicaid Services. (2024b). *Audiology services.* https://www.cms.gov/medicare/payment/fee-schedules/physician/audiology-services

Centers for Medicare & Medicaid Services. (2024c). *What isn't covered by Part A and Part B.* https://www.medicare.gov/what-medicare-covers/what-isnt-covered-by-part-a-part-b

Centers for Medicare & Medicaid Services. (2024d). *Medicare and you: 2024.* https://www.medicare.gov/pubs/pdf/10050-Medicare-and-You.pdf

Centers for Medicare & Medicaid Services. (2024e). *Overview of electronic health care records.* https://www.cms.gov/Medicare/E-health/EHealthRecords/index.html

Centers for Medicare & Medicaid Services. (2024f). *What is a MAC and what do they do?* https://www.cms.gov/medicare/coding-billing/medicare-administrative-contractors-macs/whats-mac#WhatIsAMac

Congress.gov. (2003). *H.R.1—Medicare Prescription Drug, Improvement, and Modernization Act of 2003.* https://www.congress.gov/bill/108th-congress/house-bill/1.

Forbes Advisor. (2024). *What is patient abandonment 2024 guide.* https://www.forbes.com/advisor/legal/medical-malpractice/patient-abandonment/

Hobart, R. (2006, April). *Medicare new provider training.* American Academy of Audiology. AudiologyNOW! 2006, Learning Module, Minneapolis, MN.

Justice Department. 2023. *Justice Department recovers over $2.68 billion from false claims act cases in fiscal year 2023.* https://www.justice.gov/opa/pr/false-claims-act-settlements-and-judgments-exceed-268-billion-fiscal-year-2023

Lewis, D. (2011). Anti-kickback considerations for the audiologist. *Audiology Today, 23,* 72–74.

Metz, M. (2006). Ethics of professional communication. In T. Hamill (Ed.), *Ethics in audiology: Guide for ethical conduct in clinical, educational, and research settings* (p. 45). American Academy of Audiology.

Office of Inspector General. (2000). *Special fraud alert: Rental of space in physician offices by persons or entities to which physicians refer.* https://www.hhs.gov/guidance/document/special-fraud-alert-rental-space-physician-offices-persons-or-entities-which-physicians

Office of Inspector General. (2017). *Texas otolaryngology practice settles false and fraudulent Medicare and Medicaid claims ase.* https://oig.hhs.gov/fraud/enforcement/texas-otolaryngology-practice-settles-false-and-fraudulent-medicare-and-medicaid-claims-case/

Office of the Inspector General. (2024). *Types of civil monetary penalties and affirmative exclusions.* https://oig.hhs.gov/fraud/enforcement/types-of-civil-monetary-penalties-and-affirmative-exclusions/

Pessis, P. (2003, October). *Reimbursement: Am I playing by all of the rules?* Presentation at the Academy of Dispensing Audiologists Convention, Ft. Myers, FL.

Pessis, P., & Williams, K. (2005, March). *We're near the Capitol so let's increase YOUR capital!* American Academy of Audiology Annual Convention Pre-Convention Seminar, Washington, DC.

Senior Medical Patrol. (2024). *Preventing Medicare fraud* https://smpresource.org/.

Social Security Act. (2003). *Payment for physician's services.* Sec. 1848. [42 U.S.C. 1395w–4]. http://www.ssa.gov/OP_Home/ssact/title18/1848.htm

U.S. Federal Register. (2004). *NPI final rule.* https://www.cms.gov/Regulations-and-Guidance/Administrative-Simplification/NationalProvIdentStand/Downloads/NPIfinalrule.pdf

Appendix 17–A
Advanced Beneficiary Notice

A. Notifier:
B. Patient Name: C. Identification Number:

Advance Beneficiary Notice of Non-coverage (ABN)

<u>NOTE:</u> If Medicare doesn't pay for D._____below, you may have to pay.
Medicare does not pay for everything, even some care that you or your health care provider have good reason to think you need. We expect Medicare may not pay for the D._____below.

D.	E. Reason Medicare May Not Pay:	F. Estimated Cost

WHAT YOU NEED TO DO NOW:
- Read this notice, so you can make an informed decision about your care.
- Ask us any questions that you may have after you finish reading.
- Choose an option below about whether to receive the D._____listed above.

Note: If you choose Option 1 or 2, we may help you to use any other insurance that you might have, but Medicare cannot require us to do this.

G. OPTIONS: Check only one box. We cannot choose a box for you.

☐ **OPTION 1.** I want the D._____listed above. You may ask to be paid now, but I also want Medicare billed for an official decision on payment, which is sent to me on a Medicare Summary Notice (MSN). I understand that if Medicare doesn't pay, I am responsible for payment, but I can appeal to Medicare by following the directions on the MSN. If Medicare does pay, you will refund any payments I made to you, less co-pays or deductibles.

☐ **OPTION 2.** I want the D._____listed above, but do not bill Medicare. You may ask to be paid now as I am responsible for payment. I cannot appeal if Medicare is not billed.

☐ **OPTION 3.** I don't want the D._____listed above. I understand with this choice I am **not** responsible for payment, and I cannot appeal to see if Medicare would pay.

H. Additional Information:

This notice gives our opinion, not an official Medicare decision. If you have other questions on this notice or Medicare billing, call **1-800-MEDICARE** (1-800-633-4227/**TTY:** 1-877-486-2048).
Signing below means that you have received and understand this notice. You may ask to receive a copy.

I. Signature:	J. Date:

You have the right to get Medicare information in an accessible format, like large print, Braille, or audio. You also have the right to file a complaint if you feel you've been discriminated against. Visit Medicare.gov/about-us/accessibility-nondiscrimination-notice.

Form CMS-R-131 (Exp.01/31/2026)   Form Approved OMB No. 0938-0566

Appendix 17–B
Cerumen and Earmold Impression Waiver Forms

CERUMEN REMOVAL WAIVER

I understand that I have impacted cerumen (wax) in one or both ears. I am therefore giving <u>(name of the audiologist who will be removing the cerumen)</u> the permission to remove it by way of the method best for me. I understand in the course of the cerumen removal I may incur a canal laceration, bleeding or the worst case and highly unlikely scenario, a tympanic membrane perforation.

I give my permission to have this procedure performed (please circle) in:

Right ear   Left ear   Both ears

and understand that cerumen removal is in the scope of an audiologist's practice, for which they are licensed to perform.

_____

Patient Name

_____

Date

continues

Appendix 17–B. *continued*

EARMOLD IMPRESSION(S) WAIVER

In order to provide hearing aids, earmolds, swim plugs or custom hearing protectors, it will be necessary to obtain earmold impressions.

A block of cotton or foam with a string attached will be placed into your ear canal with an earlite. Impression material will then be injected into your ear canal. This will cure over a period of approximately 10 minutes. Your hearing may seem diminished during this time and is normal.

As with any procedure, there are rare risks. These risks can include a traumatic perforation of the eardrum, allergic reactions to the silicone impression material, cotton or foam; increased hearing loss; increased or change in tinnitus; laceration of the ear canal.

These risks have been reviewed with me, I understand them and give my permission to (name of audiologist) to have earmold impressions taken of (please circle):

Right ear   **Left ear**   **Both ears**

_____

Patient's signature

_____

Date

Appendix 17–C

Sample Authorization Form

COMPANY NAME
Address
City, State Zip

HIPAA AUTHORIZATION FORM

Phone: (xxx) xxx-xxxx   Website: www.yourwebsite.com   Fax: (xxx) xxx-xxxx

I, _____, whose date of birth is _____.
authorize _____ to disclose to and/or
obtain from _____ the
following information:

Description of Information to be Disclosed
(Patient/Client should initial each item to be disclosed.)

____	Assessment	____	Testing Information
____	Diagnosis	____	Educational Information
____	Psychosocial Evaluation	____	Presence/Participation in Treatment
____	Psychological Evaluation	____	Continuing Care Plan
____	Treatment Plan or Summary	____	Progress in Treatment
____	Current Treatment Update	____	Other _____

Purpose

The purpose of this disclosure of information is to improve assessment and treatment planning, share information relevant to treatment and when appropriate, coordinate treatment services. If other purpose, please specify: _____
_____

Revocation

I understand that I have a right to revoke this authorization, in writing, at any time by sending written notification to _____ at the above address. I further understand that a revocation of the authorization is not effective to the extent that action has been taken in reliance on the authorization.

Expiration

Unless sooner revoked, this authorization expires on _____, or as otherwise indicated: _____

Conditions

I further understand that _____ will not condition my treatment on whether I give authorization for the requested disclosure. However, it has been explained to me that failure to sign this authorization may have the following consequences: _____
_____

continues

Form of Disclosure

Unless you have specifically requested in writing that the disclosure be made in a certain format, we reserve the right to disclose information as permitted by this authorization in any manner that we deem to be appropriate and consistent with applicable law, including, but not limited to, verbally, in paper format or electronically.

Redisclosure

I understand that there is the potential that the protected health information (PHI) that is disclosed pursuant to this authorization may be redisclosed by the recipient and the protected health information will no longer be protected by the HIPAA privacy regulations, unless a State law applies that is more strict than HIPAA and provides additional privacy protections. Other types of information may be re-disclosed by the recipient of the information in the following circumstances: _____
_____

I will be given a copy of this authorization for my records.

_____
Signature of Client   Date

_____
Signature of Parent, Guardian or Personal Representative   Date

If you are signing as a personal representative of an individual, please describe your authority to act for this individual. Attach appropriate document (power of attorney, temporary orders, healthcare surrogate, etc.)
_____
_____

_____ Check here if client refuses to sign authorization.

_____
Signature of Staff Witness   Date

18 Patient Management: Creating Value to Improve Loyalty

Brian Taylor, AuD, and
Robert G. Glaser, PhD, MBA

Beyond Clinical Service Delivery—Developing Patient-Centric Practices

There was a time in healthcare when patient loyalty was not a noteworthy concern. People chose their practitioner and stayed with them throughout their lives. Commonly, the patient's children and grandchildren would be delivered and followed by the same practitioner throughout their lives. If a new associate entered the practice, the patients would rather see "Ol' Doc Jones" than the new practitioner unless there was absolutely no option beyond their perception of the urgency of their situation. Rarely did they consider leaving "Ol' Doc Jones" since he had been with the family for as long as anyone could remember: The only way out of the care and influence of the practitioner was when the patient or the practitioner died or otherwise moved elsewhere. There was little or no concern about Doc Jones's academic or clinical training. Patients generally did not care what he knew; they appreciated that he not only cared for them but about them

and their entire family. There was a reciprocal bond, a personal relationship between the caregiver and the patient that was inviolate. There was little to no risk of legal action for mismanagement or malpractice in those times. Patients appreciated whatever attempt at resolution the practitioner could come up with as an honest, forthright endeavor. A documented standard of care was nonexistent nor considered necessary at that time.

Those days are long gone. The modern era of regulated practice in healthcare was introduced when Codes of Ethics were established by the respective healthcare professions and regulatory agencies were developed to set forth statutory descriptions of academic preparation and standards of care. With this new era came a different relationship between patients and all healthcare providers. Successful patient management is now solely about assessment, therapeutic intervention, and clinical technique. There are a surprising number of patient-centric activities that can significantly affect the continuum of a patient's care. This chapter explores how these activities affect the ability to provide quality care, increase patient satisfaction, and develop patient loyalty in a practice.

Developing Patient Loyalty

Patient care begins when a member of the front office staff schedules an appointment. The person on the other end of the line moves from caller to patient in a matter of minutes if the front office professional successfully navigates the interaction. The caller, now a patient, will be arriving at the office expecting a high degree of professionalism, timely service, attentive staff, and caregivers sensitive to their specific needs. Each patient must experience seamless transitions from the waiting area to exam room, from exam room to payment window, and from departure to follow-up care as promised. Seamless transitions in any healthcare setting depend on the synchrony of the front office, professional staff members, and how well they take care of the patients at the center of their coordinated efforts.

Patient Loyalty Defined

Patient loyalty is the result of paying attention to what it takes to keep a patient and providing excellence in service on a consistent basis: Patient loyalty is critically important to a practice. Patient satisfaction is important to referral sources. Patient-centric care develops loyalty creating a partnership across patients, their families, and the provider of the professional services to ensure that decisions respect the patient's wants, needs, and preferences and that the pa-

tient receives the support and education they need to participate in their own care. Patient-centric care is, in its purest form, all about honoring the patient's perspective. In their classic study of critical business relationships, Reinartz and Kumar (2002) establish several factual statements based on customer loyalty that are directly applicable to the services provided in everyday clinical practice. Their business relationship statement is followed by an interpretational statement (in parentheses) appropriate for audiology practice:

- *Customer satisfaction is the key to customer loyalty.* (Satisfied patients will likely return for repeat services.)
- *Loyal customers expect tangible benefits for their loyalty.* (Patients expect cost breaks on batteries, special "tune ups," etc.)
- *Loyal customers become more price sensitive.* (Second or third sets of hearing instruments expected to cost "reasonably" more expensive than the last instruments.)
- *Loyal customers may not be less expensive to maintain.* (Consistent marketing efforts are necessary to retain patients—they are bombarded with opportunities to change providers.)
- *Loyal customers provide effective word-of-mouth marketing.* (Satisfied patients will recommend the clinic's services to others.)

Building patient loyalty can be expensive in both time and capital. It is, however, a task that both front office and professional staff members must continuously and consistently strive to develop. Each patient encounter is an opportunity to foster patient loyalty: Developing patient loyalty must be considered in the diagnostic phase as much as the rehabilitative segment of a patient's journey through the practice. All forms of communication with the existing database of patients must focus on developing and maintaining patient loyalty, telephone conversations, newsletters, reminder letters, special offers, and other advertising media.

Rao (2011) demonstrated that effective communication between patients and providers increases the likelihood of:

1. Positive patient outcomes.
2. Accurate diagnoses and timely treatments.
3. Patients and family members understand and adhere to recommended treatment regimens.
4. Greatly improved patient safety.
5. Patient and family satisfaction with the care they receive.

Wong et al. (2003) suggested satisfaction ratings are likely influenced more by how well patients are treated than by the sound quality and improved speech intelligibility of their hearing aids. Satisfied patients are more likely to seek provider guidance and care for the long term. If providers see most of their patient base annually, providing meaningful services delivered in a sincere and patient-centric manner, patients will likely continue with that provider's care and return to them for new hearing instruments when required. It does not, however, take much to move a loyal patient in that valuable database to one seeking an alternative location for their hearing care. The Research Institute of America reported on just how costly it is for businesses to be apathetic toward customer service. To underscore the point of importance to all in the business of providing professional services, the word "patient" has been inserted for "customer":

- The average practice will hear nothing from 96% of unhappy patients who receive rude or discourteous treatment.
- Ninety percent of patients who are dissatisfied with the services they receive will not come back or buy again from the offending practice.
- Each unhappy patient tells their story to an average of nine other people.
- Only 4% of unhappy patients bother to complain to the office— they will complain to the referral source and will do so loudly and vociferously.
- Of those patients voicing a complaint, between 54% and 70% will do business again with the organization if their complaint is resolved—that figure rises to 95% if the patient feels the complaint is resolved quickly.
- Sixty-eight percent of patients who refuse to return to a practice do so because of the perception that the practice is "indifferent."

With conventional wisdom putting the average life span of modern hearing aids at 7 to 8 years, it becomes crucial to the long-term success of the practice to have patients return consistently for their hearing care. Hopkins (2006), while highlighting the importance in developing close, clinical relationships with patients, points out another reason to maintain a loyal patient database: "Even if your product has a long lifespan and

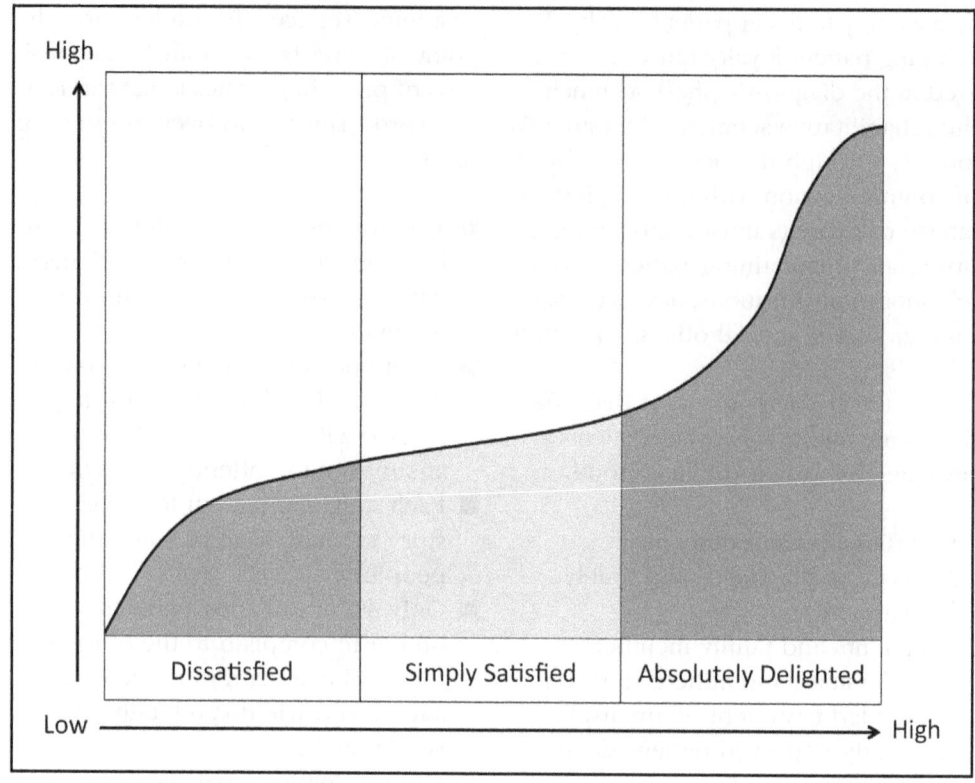

Figure 18–1. Levels of patient satisfaction and effect on loyalty to practice.

people shouldn't need to replace it for a long time, you still want to work on keeping those patients loyal to your practice. The reason: They'll tell their friends, relatives, and even strangers about what a great experience they had with you. They'll be your biggest fans and provide free advertising for your services with their testimonials and referrals."

Marketers refer to three stages of the customer/patient life cycle, each with critical points of contact with the practice: first-time customers, repeat customers, and customer advocates (Marsh, 2005). Creating a group of customer advocates who voluntarily function as true "cheerleaders" is, without doubt, the greatest form of marketing and stands as a strong tribute to any professional practice.

Patient loyalty should be considered an outcome of the practice's dedication and diligence in developing and maintaining patient satisfaction. Long-term, loyal patients will be the desired outcome if they are well satisfied and treated with respect, dignity, and technical excellence by every member of the practice team. To maintain patient loyalty, each patient must be absolutely delighted with services; *being satisfied is no longer sufficient*. Patients dissatisfied with services for whatever reason, real or imagined, are likely to be lost forever.

Figure 18–1 depicts the interrelationship and importance of patients classified in one of three, distinct categories: Dissatisfied, Simply Satisfied, and Absolutely Delighted.

Dissatisfied Patients

Dissatisfied patients are in an area of discord. They are, for whatever reason, dissatisfied with all aspects of the practice, whether the front office staff, the professional staff, or their perception of the quality of the services received. When asked about their experiences in the practice, they will quite likely issue strongly negative comments. Negative word-of-mouth comments are unequivocally damaging to the reputation of a practice.

To illustrate the impact of word-of-mouth comments, consider a recent first-time restaurant experience. Chances are high that a decision was made to try the restaurant based on a word-of-mouth recommendation by a family member, friend, or colleague. And if this person's opinion is valued because they are a good cook or an ardent gastronome that appreciates dining and knows their way around a wine list and a menu, the value of that recommendation will have added credibility and increase the likelihood of acting on their recommendation. Consider the same scenario for negative word-of-mouth comments. If the comments about the restaurant were negative from these same, credible sources, chances are strong visiting that particular restaurant would not even be considered.

The same holds true for healthcare practices. Positive word-of-mouth testimonials may not ensure a new patient appointment; however, negative word-of-mouth statements will likely derail many more potential appointments than you can imagine. Study after study in business journals and textbooks confirm that more people will be influenced by negative comments about a business or a practice than positive comments. The enduring folklore about the relative effectiveness of positive and negative word-of-mouth "reputations" suggests that a well-satisfied patient typically talks to three or five people while a disgruntled patient will replay a discordant event to as many as 10 or more individuals. Add to that the *"word-of-mouse,"* otherwise known as the World of Internet-Bolstered Communication, and the potential number of contacts a determined, dissatisfied patient can reach in a local practice area expands at an alarming rate. Improving patient satisfaction will decrease the likelihood of negative word-of-mouth comments about a practice. Nevertheless, it is best to always offer patients the opportunity to communicate their dissatisfaction with any member of the practice team. Better those patients complain to personnel within the practice who can intervene and attempt to remedy a difficult situation than to have the patient issue complaints and indications of dissatisfaction to their family and friends.

Practices with even a few patients in the dreaded Dissatisfied area depicted in Figure 18–1 are operating suboptimally. Dissatisfied patients will leave the practice to reduce their stress (real or imagined) and to avoid conflict or uncomfortable interactions in the future. Retrieving these patients requires a frank assessment of their discord and an immediate, personal response to eliminate the source of the disharmony. Once the source of the discord is identified and an affirmative plan to resolve the situation is set into motion for the individual and their family, the patient may move into the area of the Simply Satisfied. It may not take much to achieve this shift, possibly only an acknowledgment of an error, an apology, and an indication of sincere appreciation for being a patient in the practice and, perhaps, a reasonable token of appreciation for their willingness to reconsider their position.

Simply Satisfied Patients

Patients in the area of the *Simply Satisfied* may not be the best asset to the practice because they are susceptible to competitor outreach in advertising or direct solicitation offering technical advances, simplicity of operation, or compelling pricing strategies. As a group, these patients pay little attention to efforts to foster patient loyalty, and many demonstrate the attitude of *"what-have-you-done-for-me-lately?"* during each practice visit. They are less concerned about the practice and more concerned about price than most patients. They rarely recommend the practice to others or comment on their experiences when visiting their primary care physician who referred the patient to the practice. Practices dedicated to simply maintaining good, yet basic care; dwelling on avoiding mistakes; just meeting, not exceeding patient needs; and retaining staff members with limited enthusiasm will have a large section of their patient database falling in the area of the Simply Satisfied.

Absolutely Delighted Patients

Patient-centric practices that value each patient as an engaged partner in their program of hearing or balance rehabilitation will generate a substantial number of patients in the area of the *Absolutely Delighted*. These patients frequently become cheerleaders for the practice, recommending your services to family, friends, and strangers in casual conversations. They will thank the referral source for their wisdom in recommending the practice for their hearing care and will continue to sing praises of the provider and the practice at every opportunity: bridge club, church group, or social gathering. These patients are worth far more to the practice than the revenue generated by their diagnostic studies, office visits, and hearing instruments.

Several key elements, however, must be engaged in the practice from the onset of a patient's care to elevate a person to the ranks of the Absolutely Delighted. Those elements can be found in a comprehensive Patient's Bill of Rights, which sets forth what every patient should expect as a patient in the practice. There is a critically important stipulation that must be understood when a Patient's Bill of Rights is posted in the practice or written in documents the patient receives at their first visit. Everything listed in that document must be delivered on a consistent basis.

The Provider-Patient Relationship: Verbal and Nonverbal Communication

There is little doubt that negative word-of-mouth comments can destroy the reputation of a practice. Providing a patient with an avenue to express their dissatisfaction, gain resolution of their problem, and stay in the practice that cares enough to resolve issues of discord will create increased patient satisfaction. Retrieving those patients lost to internal errors gives hope to all in the practice,

PATIENT'S BILL OF RIGHTS

■ Know that quality care is our priority.

■ Expect excellent service from Audiology & Speech Associates.

■ Know that you will be respected by everyone in our practice.

■ Expect us to answer your phone call in a timely and welcoming manner.

■ You will be greeted in a friendly manner by every member of our practice.

■ Know that we recognize the importance of your time.

■ You can always expect excellent communication from us.

■ We will listen to your concerns.

■ We will deliver what we promise.

■ To optimize your success, we will use state-of-the-art assessment and treatment procedures, including the best hearing aids suited to your needs.

■ We will provide prompt attention to all your service needs.

■ Family and friends are welcomed and encouraged to accompany you to appointments—everyone will benefit from their interest and presence.

■ Questions about your hearing loss, your care plan, hearing instruments, and billing information will be answered fully at any time.

■ Expect quick and accurate resolution of questions about your account.

■ If we make an error, you will receive an apology—we will make it right.

the patients, and the staff that even the most egregious errors can be rectified to everyone's satisfaction and benefit.

The way a clinician communicates information to a patient is as important as the information being communicated (Chapter 20). Patients who understand their care providers are more likely to acknowledge their health problems, understand their treatment options, and modify their behavior accordingly (Travaline et al., 2005).

Beck et al. (2004) also reviewed an extensive body of published evidence linking specific verbal and nonverbal behaviors to short-, intermediate-, and long-term outcomes in interactions between primary care providers and their patients seen in their office practices. A total of 36 verbal and 16 nonverbal behaviors were considered from the 22 studies included in their meta-analysis. Even though these behaviors were included in controlled or descriptive studies involving primary care providers, the consistency of impact noted throughout the studies between the provider and the patient enables an appropriate

---

VERBAL BEHAVIORS LINKED TO POSITIVE PATIENT OUTCOMES

■ Empathy—intellectual appreciation of a patient's situation.
■ Provider statements of reassurance or support.
■ Encouraging patient questions.
■ Allowing the patient's point of view to guide the visit.
■ High proportion of objective statements by provider (explanation).
■ Provider's expression of approval related to positive patient actions.
■ Laughing and joking from the provider's side (tension release).
■ Provider addressing patient problems of daily living, relationships, and emotions (psychosocial issues).
■ Provider asking about and providing counseling for psychosocial issues.
■ Increased time spent on health education and sharing clinical data.
■ Provider fosters discussion of treatment parameters.
■ Friendliness and courtesy of the provider.
■ Receptivity to patient questions and statements (listening behaviors).
■ Provider talks at the patient's level.
■ Provider ready to clarify and educate patient.
■ More time spent on history taking.
■ Increased encounter length.

---

extrapolation to healthcare providers in general and audiologists specifically.

Many of the behaviors fostering positive clinical outcomes (better patient compliance, improved response to various treatments, and improved overall health status) describe a list of patient-centric behaviors needed to develop patient comfort within the practice to increase the likelihood of satisfaction with both professional staff and members of the front office staff. The list of behaviors linked to negative outcomes provides a list of behaviors to be avoided. Verbal behaviors associated with significant, positive patient outcomes are included in the box.

Behaviors associated with significantly negative patient outcomes include those listed in the box. These behaviors were found to consistently promote negative feelings and disenfranchisement to the extent that patients did not return to the providers studied. Although not reported, the literature on verbal and nonverbal behaviors suggest that it is possible to develop negative attitudes, loss of confidence, and patients exiting from practice. These issues can easily permeate the atmosphere of any practice. This is especially true of those practices that *fail to focus on the patients, their integration into the practice, and the levels of their satisfaction with each member of the practice staff.*

Beck et al. (2002) describe 16 specific nonverbal behaviors found in one or more studies that were significantly as-

---

**VERBAL BEHAVIORS LINKED TO NEGATIVE
PATIENT OUTCOMES**

- Negative social-emotional interactions.
- Passive acceptance of information provided by the patient to the provider.
- Antagonism and passive rejection of the patient by the provider.
- Formal, directive behaviors on the part of the provider.
- High rates of biomedical questioning by the provider.
- Interruptions issued by the provider.
- One-way information flow from the patient to the provider without response.
- Lack of attentiveness on the part of the provider (disengaged listening).
- Provider directives issued with apparent irritation, nervousness, or tension.
- Dominance and verbal directness on the part of the provider.
- Provider issues opinions prior to completion of the evaluation.

---

sociated with patient outcomes. Behaviors of interest to audiologists associated with positive clinical outcomes included less mutual gaze, positive head nodding of the provider, forward lean toward the patient, direct body orientation of the provider (shoulders squared to patient), and uncrossed arms and legs by the provider. Nonverbal behaviors that were associated with unfavorable clinical outcomes included more patient gaze by the provider, provider body orientation 45 to 90 degrees away from the patient, backward lean away from the patient, crossed arms by the provider, and frequent touch by the provider.

Selected Verbal Behaviors to Improve Patient Satisfaction

Professional and front office staff should be aware of both verbal and nonverbal statements and behaviors that can affect patient satisfaction and clinical outcomes. Beck et al. (2002) suggest that healthcare providers should focus on the following verbal behaviors linked statistically ($p < .05$) to patient satisfaction, compliance, comprehension, and positive perception of their provider: empathy, courtesy, friendliness, reassurance, support, encouragement of a patient's questions, explanation giving, and providing positive reinforcement regarding compliance in all aspects of their treatment.

Many of the findings reported in their analysis were commonsense; for example, empathic patient-centered verbal styles were associated with high patient satisfaction. Participatory decision-making was found to be a strong provider-patient interaction resulting in significantly better clinical outcomes. Additionally, extensive sharing of clinical information and patient education about potential effects of treatment were found to consistently improve patient comprehension and satisfaction contributing to an overall improvement in clinical outcomes.

The extensive meta-analysis by Beck et al. (2002) indicates the strong impact of verbal and nonverbal behaviors in the development of the interrelationship between clinicians and their patients. Content, method of delivery, body positioning as well as visual contact, and other physical and nonverbal postures have been shown to significantly impact clinical outcomes. The importance and impact of these findings on daily clinical practice cannot be underestimated or discounted. Practice owners and managers should include discussions and training about these opportunities for success as well as negative imagery and messaging to be avoided when interacting with patients in the practice (Chapter 20).

The Service-Profit Chain

One way to create more loyal patients is to create more loyal employees. In the 1990s, researchers at Harvard University created the service-profit chain. It outlines how the satisfaction of workers affects the satisfaction of customers. If the people who work for a company are happy, their customers are also happy; if a worker is loyal to their employer, a customer is also likely to be loyal to that same business. Workers who are happy at work may make better products or services. Buyers who get good products and services may be more likely to buy again. The service-profit chain can help companies make more money and make

their employees and customers happier. This gives the company more money, giving the workers better working conditions. The circle keeps going because the happiness and loyalty of the workers then increase.

According to Haskett et al. (1997), the service-profit chain links employee satisfaction, customer loyalty, and financial success in service-oriented businesses. It shows that focusing on employee engagement and customer satisfaction might boost a company's financial performance. The service-profit chain has several links that must be accounted for in order for it to be effective. Here are those links.

Internal Service Quality

Internal service quality is how well the company supports and helps its employees. It includes things like training, tools, funding, and the environment where the work is done. When workers get good service inside the company, they are more likely to be happy and motivated to give customers great service.

Employee Satisfaction

In the service-profit chain, employee happiness is a key link. When workers are happy, they are more likely to be engaged, committed, and motivated to do a good job. They tend to be more productive and are more likely to remain loyal to the company.

Employee Productivity and Performance

When workers are happy, they are more likely to be more productive, improving the quality of their service. Customers are more likely to be happy and stay with a company whose workers do a good job and give them a good experience.

External Service Value

External service value is how customers see the quality and worth of a company's services. It includes things like how rapid is a response, reliability, how customers are treated, and how the customer feels overall. Customers are more likely to be happy and loyal to an organization if they think the service is worth a lot.

Customer Satisfaction

Customer satisfaction is a way to measure how well a company meets or goes above and beyond what customers expect. They help the organization's long-term growth and its ability to make money. Customers who are happy with an organization are more likely to keep doing business with it, buy from it again, and tell others about it.

Customer Loyalty

Customer loyalty is how committed and willing a customer is to keep doing business with a company over time. They make a big difference in the organization's growth and profit-making ability. Loyal customers are more likely to buy from the practice again, tell their friends, and be less responsive to price changes.

Financial Performance

The by-product of the service-profit chain is how well the business does financially. Better financial success lets the company put money into employee training, better customer service, and other areas to keep the chain going. When an organization does a good job of managing the above factors, it leads to more loyal customers, which in turn leads to more sales, income, and profit.

Tips for Improving Service-Profit Chain

Improving the service-profit chain needs a strategic plan that focuses on improving the satisfaction of employees, the satisfaction of customers, and the financial performance of the business. Here are some tips to assist in improvement improve of organization's service-profit chain:

Leadership

Develop solid leadership skills that will inspire and drive all employees. Give employees a clear idea of the clinic's vision, tell them what the practice expects from them, and lead by example. Invest in leadership development programs to help managers and directors get better at their jobs. Even small businesses with fewer than five employees can benefit from leadership development.

Internal Service Quality

Make sure employees have all the tools, training, and help they need to provide great service. Streamline processes, put money into technology, and encourage them to work together as a team. Always look at and improve the quality of internal services to eliminate roadblocks and make things run more smoothly.

Employee Satisfaction

Set up a good work setting that encourages employees to be engaged and happy. Give workers competitive pay and benefits, provide chances to grow and learn, and recognize and reward their achievements. Encourage open conversation, ask for feedback, and take care of any problems or worries right away.

Customer Satisfaction

Market research, surveys, and other media can help determine what customers want and expect. Use what has been learned to make practice service more personal and improve the customer's experience. Train employees to be understanding, responsive, and proactive when it comes to meeting customer wants and needs.

Customer-Centric Culture

Create a culture in the business that puts customer happiness first. Tell employees how important it is to provide great service, encourage them to take responsibility for customer problems, and empower them to make decisions that will benefit customers. Values that focus on the customer should be part of measuring success and giving rewards.

Building Customer Loyalty

Set up plans to build strong relationships with customers that will encourage them to stay with the practice. Create customer loyalty programs, make personalized offers and suggestions, and create events that they will remember.

Providers should actively request comments and deal with customer concerns immediately to demonstrate care about their happiness.

Measure Financial Performance

Always keep a sharp eye on financial success indicators such as revenue, profit, the cost of getting a new customer, and the lifetime value of a customer. Look at trends and find places to improve or spend. Use the data to make good choices and get the most out of the available resources.

Continuous Improvement

Adopt a mindset of innovation and constant improvement. Encourage workers to talk about methods to improve customer satisfaction, service quality, and operational efficiency. Assess methods, systems, and customer feedback on a regular basis to find ways to improve.

Communication and Engagement

Encourage everyone in the company to talk to each other in a clear and open way. Keep the employees up to date on business goals, customer feedback, and success metrics. Encourage two-way communication channels and ask employees for their thoughts and comments. Involve workers in making decisions that affect the quality of service and the customer experience. During practice expansions, include employees in the business planning and ensure that they receive a copy of the business plan so that they all feel part of the business and the expansion program.

Training and Development

Invest in training and development programs to help workers improve their skills and knowledge. Offer ongoing training that highlights the best ways to serve customers, business trends, and new technologies. Give employees the tools and information they need to do their jobs well.

Generational Mindset

Today's adult society consists of five generations (ordered from oldest to youngest): The Silent Generation, Baby Boomers, Generation X, Millennials, and Generation Z. These generations were raised in different social and political atmospheres and, consequently, have different childhood upbringings and familial environments that shape their attitudes and behaviors. These differences produce different values, wants, and needs in adulthood. Early and late psychological researchers have proven this to be true: The environment in which an individual is brought up in, namely the things that they lack or are deprived of in their childhood, strongly influences their value development throughout adulthood.

According to Becton et al. (2014), generational mindset refers to thinking based on the era into which one was born. When viewing this information, care must be taken not to fall prey to developing stereotypes or biases. Table 18–1 is a richly inclusive and tremendously instructive compilation of cross-generational characteristics important to all healthcare practitioners, K–12 educators, special educators, college professors, and all who work with people in need of specialized assessment and treatment regimens (Peterson, 2011).

Fostering Patient Confidence

It is no easy task to have phones ringing, people at the payment window, and convincing a prospective patient that the office they have chosen or been referred to will be a comfortable place to receive the type of care they need. The patient must know from the initial contact with the practice that the care they will receive will be comprehensive and excellent in every way. High patient confidence at the first patient visit is the responsibility of the receptionist.

Confidence in the practice during and after the first visit is the responsibility of all members of the team, front office and professional staff alike. It takes teamwork.

The Receptionist as an Informational Source and Anxiety Reducer

The true value of the receptionist lies not solely in their abilities to organize and care for patients logistically and in a timely fashion but also in their abilities to accurately assess patient distress and respond with a solution to their problem. An invaluable asset, the best receptionists are part mechanic, part counselor, part customer service specialist, part magician. They are always dressed appropriately and, above all else, great listeners dedicated to the patient's success in the practice.

Table 18–1. Reactions of Various Generations

Workplace Characteristic	Veterans (1922–1945)	Baby Boomers (1946–1964)	Generation X (1965–1980)	Generation Y (1981–2000)
Work Ethic	Respect authority, hard work, age = seniority. Company first	Workaholics, desire quality, question authority	Eliminate the task, self-reliant, want structure and direction, skeptical	What's next, multitasking, tenacity, entrepreneurial
Work is . . .	An obligation	An exciting adventure	A difficult challenge. A contract	A means to an end
Leadership Style	Directive, command and control	Quality	Everyone is the same. Challenge others. Ask why	Remains to be seen
Communication	Formal memo	In person	Direct. Immediate	Email. Voicemail
Rewards and Feedback	No news is good news, satisfaction in a job well done	Money. Title recognition. Give me something to put on the wall	Sorry to interrupt, but how am I doing? Freedom is the best reward	Whenever I want it, at the push of a button Meaningful work
Motivated By	Being respected	Being valued and needed	Freedom and removal of rules	Working with other bright people
Work/Life Balance	Keep them separate	No balance "Live to work"	Balance "Work to live"	Balance—it's 5 p.m.— I've got another gig
Technology is . . .	Hoover dam	The microwave	What you can hold in your hand. PDA, cell	Ethereal—intangible

Source: Peterson, 2011.

They create the first and often the most lasting impression on the patient. They are responsible for explaining financial policies, obtaining insurance information, and collecting copays. Not only must they be efficient in practice operations, but they must also possess excellent interpersonal communication skills and a thorough knowledge of clinical procedures and treatment options available in the practice. Time spent instructing a receptionist to be a good listener and gatherer of information and an excellent communicator and host or hostess will contribute immensely to consistently high patient satisfaction ratings. An excellent study by Taylor (2006) indicated that the interaction with the audiologist is the most important driver of patient satisfaction, whereas the interaction with the receptionist had significant impact on overall patient satisfaction with the practice.

The receptionist must be well trained to understand not only office procedures, specifics about billing, coding, and collection, and how to successfully guide a patient to the office from across town; they must also know and understand the clinical aspects of the office. A good way to train a receptionist about what goes on in the practice is to have them become a "patient." Undergoing a comprehensive hearing evaluation, having a vestibular assessment, or watching a hearing instrument fitting provides lasting impressions and increases sensitivity to what patients experience during their visits.

The insight gained by the receptionist-as-patient will translate into valid experiential depictions of what to expect, how the patient might feel during the procedures, and what to expect on being fitted with hearing instruments for the

first time. Patients respond favorably by having prior knowledge of the clinical situation. Reduced fears and increased confidence will set the stage for a comfortable visit and a far less anxious patient.

People learn well by experience. A receptionist who has undergone a vestibular study can immediately reduce a patient's anxiety about the procedure because they have "gone through it and lived to tell about it." With firsthand experience, the receptionist will be better able to answer patient questions and resolve concerns that might otherwise result in a missed or canceled appointment.

Receptionists are critical, frontline members of the team and have as much duty to the patient on the front end of the appointment as does the professional involved in the clinical assessment, counseling, and rehabilitation on the back end of the appointment. The front line must be a strong line. Patient comfort and satisfaction is, after all, about patient outcomes, and receptionists play a large part of setting the patient up for consistent, positive outcomes. Reduced fears and increased patient confidence set the stage for a successful office visit for the patient and provider alike.

When the patient arrives for the appointment, the receptionist once again becomes the first point of contact. Their approach to each patient should vary with the patient's personal needs and anxiety level. Making the patients feel welcome and comfortable in the office should be a seamless transition from the booking conversation on the phone to the greeting at the reception room window. These interactions are crucial junctures prior to the actual patient-professional interaction. As a part of the team, the receptionist will develop observations and opinions on the patient's emotional status and perhaps a view of their expectations as well. By engaging the patient in conversation as they are about to fill out forms or as they are escorted to the examination room, the receptionist has the first opportunity to observe the patient's behaviors. Even with hearing instrument repairs, the receptionist should foster discussion about how the instrument is working, what the patient's observations have been, and when the difficulties began.

These informal discussions serve to cue the patient about questions to ask during the visit. They also provide the patient with an opportunity to vent frustrations about the difficulties that have driven them back to the office. The more inquiries the patient hears about their situation, the more the patient develops a secure sense that everyone in the practice is genuinely interested in solving their problems. When every member of the practice team demonstrates sincere empathy and interest, the probability of a positive outcome during the visit is greatly enhanced.

The Patient's Perspective

The receptionist should be viewed as an interested, caring person, fully engaged in the best interests of the patient. The patient must have confidence that the receptionist will serve, at least to some extent, as an in-office advocate, who will get them to the appropriate member of the professional staff in a timely manner. In that sense, a receptionist is as much a care provider as any member of the clinical staff. No license is needed to be involved in fostering a

patient's well-being. The goal in all patient care is to have every member of the practice working toward a positive outcome for the patient. This goal is established on behalf of the patient, their family, and the person who referred the patient to the practice.

Long-term patients value the receptionist. They expect to hear their voice on the phone when they call with questions, to order hearing aid–related items, or to schedule a visit to the office. Relationship building is as important at the front desk as it is in the exam or fitting room. The patient-receptionist relationship is important and must never be discounted in the continuum of care provided in the practice. A low turnover rate in the receptionist position is critical. Should the receptionist leave the practice, it is imperative to have the replacement spend adequate time integrating patient information and front office operations beyond their orientation.

After-Care Duties: Thank You Notes and Follow-Up Calls

The receptionist should be assigned the duty to contact patients after they have left the office. They should be responsible for sending each new patient an after-care thank you card, which encourages the patient to call if there are questions about billing, setting up another appointment, or reviewing what the next step might be after the initial appointment. Patients remember these efforts and are likely to tell their friends and families about the note and excellent service they received in the practice. Building patient loyalty is critically important to the long-term health of the practice. Every member of the team must have a strong commitment to this effort and contribute to building patient loyalty daily.

Follow-up phone calls a few days after a hearing instrument fitting or replacing a repaired device are just as important as a thank you note to a new patient. Checking on their progress with their new or repaired instruments is an effective way to show interest in their response to the treatment regimen and to provide a spot check on the adequacy of the fitting and stability of the repair. If the receptionist suspects the patient is struggling or is concerned about the effectiveness of the repair, the patient should be scheduled for a return visit at their earliest convenience. Waiting for their next scheduled visit simply prolongs the anxiety and promotes a loss of confidence in the fitting or repair.

Occasionally, a patient may have a difficult time in response to segments of the vestibular evaluation. Patients who have a prolonged refractory period in response to caloric stimulation or those who have a general weakness following the examination should be contacted by phone the same day of the test. Inquiring about their status and suggesting they return to the referring physician as scheduled will go far in assuring them that their response to the test was nothing extraordinary. Of course, if their response was beyond that which is usually anticipated, the patient should be directed to consult with their physician immediately. Additionally, the referring physician should be contacted immediately, and a course of action should be agreed upon.

Unfortunately, too few practices take the time to capitalize on easily managed opportunities like these to increase patient satisfaction and loyalty. Little time

is involved in most patient management activities. Telephone calls can be completed during lulls in activities in the office or at the end of the day. If the caller, front office or professional staff, encounters the patient's voicemail, they should leave a message that imparts interest in their progress, reassuring them that all in the practice stand ready to resolve any issues that might have developed. Additionally, the patient should be issued an invitation to call back to let the practice know how they are doing.

Handling Challenges on the Phone or at the Window

Challenging interactions with patients occur on a regular basis. A variety of factors contribute to these sometimes confrontational episodes. Beyond instrument repair issues, errors on the part of the practice staff and misinterpretation of information issued to the patient by the practitioner are two of the more common reasons for challenges by patients, their spouse, or other family members. Hearing loss, advancing cognitive deficits, multiple medications, misinformation provided to family members by the patient, and confusion about the "next steps" to be taken in their care plan also contribute to challenges.

The first responder to problem situations is usually the receptionist. They must be empowered to resolve and manage as many challenges as possible. Receptionists must be great listeners and gatherers of information. Having a sense of humor is a definitive prerequisite for the position. They must have well-developed communication skills, patience, and commitment to patient satisfaction above all else. They must

RULES OF PATIENT ENGAGEMENT FOR RECEPTIONISTS

- Patients are the priority.
- We work for them.
- Always with a smile.
- Courtesy *at all times*.
- Professional appearance is important.
- Your boss is always on the phone.
- Apologies are always appropriate.
- Solutions do not excuse.
- Excellence at the speed of light.

recognize when they are unable to satisfy the caller or person at the window and know how to deftly transfer the patient to the office manager or practice owner in a manner that appears to be part of the solution versus a means to get the patient out of their way. Receptionists must be tactful and sensitive to the patient's concerns and be readily willing to apologize for situations or circumstances over which they have neither control nor contribution to the difficulty at hand.

Every member of the practice team, however, must be able to identify patient concerns and immediately move to resolution. Prompt recovery, when mistakes or misperceptions on the part of the patient occur, will make the difference between a satisfied patient and a "former patient" in the practice. The faster a situation is resolved, the greater the likelihood the patient will be satisfied. Both professional and administrative staff must remember one of the key elements in the rules for patient engagement: "Excellence at the Speed of Light." Patients are uninterested in who

is to blame, nor should they be bothered with details of how an error or oversight occurred. If interested in an explanation, they should receive as detailed an account as seems appropriate to the situation.

The most common, clinically relatable complaints include repeat repairs (defined as a second repair within 45 to 90 days of the first repair), costs of the instruments, battery consumption, too many follow-up visits, time to adjust to the instruments is too long, instruments are too conspicuous, noise reduction features fail to meet expectations, and difficulty using instruments with the telephone. Most of these issues are outside the purview of the receptionist, but complaints must be addressed, and the patient should be encouraged to realistically assess their complaints in view of their position in the continuum of the fitting process, the extent of their hearing loss, and the goals set forth prior to and during the assessment and counseling period. Reassurance and a quick willingness to have the patient return prior to a scheduled visit are usually adequate in stemming the tide of anxiety in the early stages of adjustment to new or recently repaired instruments.

If the patient is concerned about an inordinate turnaround time for a repair or establishing their appointment time for their fitting, the receptionist should check the dates of the order or repair submission and advise the patient of the appropriateness of the time frame in question. If the repair or new order is outside the customary period from order to arrival, they should immediately call and check on the order and contact the patient the same day of their inquiry.

Patients deserve an acknowledgment of an error, an apology, and a prompt resolution of their problem with the assurance that the error will not happen again. They expect the person to whom they are talking to be empowered to resolve their situation, and they expect that person to be solution driven. Patient-centric practices embrace problem resolution without judgment and with one goal in mind: total patient satisfaction. No blame, no excuse, no fault, just resolution to maintain long-term patient loyalty.

Challenges by Prospective Patients on the Phone or at the Window

One of the most common sources of confusion and error when talking with prospective patients on the phone rests with the unknown parameters of their hearing loss. Receptionists must be able to understand the reason for their call, make sure the patient has heard and integrate the appointment date and time, and determine that the patient understands the services to be provided dur-

ing their upcoming visit. Asking the patient to repeat the appointment date and time is one way to confirm their reception of the information. If the patient is severely hampered on the telephone, the receptionist should ask to talk to another family member or friend. In some cases, having a "designated talker" for severely hearing-impaired patients or those with cognitive impairments will facilitate the process of issuing and confirming appointment dates and times.

Established Patients Who Develop Cognitive Difficulties

Long-standing patients who are developing cognitive impairments present a unique challenge. The front office staff may not be privy to their decline. Responses to questions, remembering appointment dates and times easily negotiated prior to the onset of their cognitive issues, now present distinct problems at home, on the phone, and in the exam room. Recognizing difficulties involving memory issues compared to the relatively consistent problems associated with the patient's hearing loss takes an attentive ear and a good sense of the clinical presentation of patients with memory-based difficulties. In this era of widely dispersed families, it is unwise to rely on family members to make a patient's developing cognitive issues known to the practice. By the same token, when cognitive decline is suspected, a call to the patient's attending physician will likely be appreciated by the care provider, especially if the patient has not been seen in their office for some time.

When the appointment is made, the receptionist should advise each patient about items of importance to bring to their scheduled visit. They should bring hearing instruments currently in use and information describing repair warranties and applicable healthcare coverage. New patients should be apprised of the extent of Medicare coverage. If covered by a private carrier with a hearing aid benefit, they should bring the information with them if the plan is not commonly seen in the practice. Specific policies about payment on the first visit, missed appointments, and other items of interest should be discussed on the phone or in writing prior to the first visit.

to talk so loudly as it hurts their ears. Each person has accompanied the patient for specific reasons: None should be ignored or considered less important than the patient. They deserve to be included in the information processing, the fitting process, and follow-up care. They will likely become care providers and will need guidance in proper insertion, cleaning, and battery replacement. These are the family and friends we like to see in our offices. Their involvement can only enhance the patient's experience and serve to develop realistic expectations in the circle of their family and friends.

Critical Points of Patient Contact: Difficult Patients/Families

There are several chairs in each exam or fitting room. One chair is for the patient and the other chairs are for those interested in the outcome of the professional intervention and care. These chairs are filled with family members, friends, parents, children, sons-in-law and daughters-in-law, and girlfriends or boyfriends. Each chair supports one person, and each person is present at the visit because they are inexorably intertwined with the patient. As such, they are as much a part of the diagnostic and rehabilitative process as is the patient. Each has a vested interest in the patient's success. After all, it would be nice to be able to talk to Aunt Edna without the conversation being heard above the blaring of the neighbor's television. Aunt Edna just wants everyone to stop shouting. The younger children in the family would be more likely to engage her in conversation if they did not have

Noncompliant Patient/Family/ Extended Care Facility

Individuals able to comply with a rehabilitative plan and who choose not to follow the plan must be considered noncompliant. Each takes a volitional step not to proceed as advised. Some will do so to gain a passive-aggressive advantage, others because of depression or disinterest in their living arrangements. Each will have a reason, which is, more times than not, hidden from professional care providers, family, and friends. Noncompliant patients are not unique to the practice of audiology. Physicians, dentists, and other providers see them with surprising regularity.

Consider Mrs. Filbert, who is returning to her cardiologist following a trial of a new medication for hypertension. During the office visit, the cardiologist notes that her blood pressure remains elevated and asks if she has been taking all of the five pills she is supposed to take each day. She replies that she decided it was too much trouble taking five pills, so she cut it down to three a day. Concerned about the patient's obvious noncompliance, the cardiologist stresses the need to take all five pills as prescribed. Mrs. Filbert responds by saying that she can only take three pills a day, not five. The cardiologist must now decide to either discharge the patient or increase the strength of the medication so that three pills will work or find another medicine that does not require five tablets a day.

Audiologists are faced with similar difficulties. Many practices require their new patients to begin wearing their hearing instruments with daily regularity, morning until night. Others may create a schedule for the first and second weeks. When the patient returns to the first postfitting visit and exclaims that he only needs to wear the hearing instruments when "he thinks he needs them regardless of what his wife says," the audiologist must determine the best method to convince the patient that he will be less likely to adjust to the instruments if he fails to wear them as recommended, especially during the initial fitting period. If this noncompliance continues into the second or third postfitting visit, there is an increasing chance the patient will return the instruments or keep them and become one of the dissatisfied patients who will complain how the practice and the professionals let him down and how hearing instruments simply do not work.

Much of the problem of noncompliance can be avoided by careful patient selection or at least having an idea of what a patient brings to the overall clinical mix. Traynor (2003) suggested that although formal assessment with personality inventories like the Myers-Briggs

Type Indicator would be an optimal approach to identifying difficult patients, this sort of assessment does not lend itself well to the rigors and time constraints of daily clinical practice. Informal assessment can be readily used to identify those patients in need of tailoring approaches to optimize outcomes. Observing and listening to how patients respond to questions or statements borrowed from these inventories will enable the clinician to localize each patient into one of four personality categories, each with its own characteristics to be addressed or considered during their assessment and treatment (Chapter 20).

Traynor (2003) outlined critical characteristics of noncompliant patients who fall into the category of "Intuitive-Thinking Clients." Several of their characteristics include:

- Can present as aloof, intimidating, argumentative, and arrogant.
- Often impatient with the aural rehabilitation (fitting) process.
- Complain about small problems.
- When unsuccessful, may change the recommended program on their own.
- Skeptical and often requiring references and rationale for A/R process.
- Tend to overanalyze the problem and try to fix it themselves.

Being able to identify a noncompliant patient early in the clinical process can help in determining whether the difficulties the patient will likely bring to the practice will be more strain than benefit. If too many issues arise from their treatment and a point of decision is reached—prompted by patient or professional—to consider returning the hearing instruments, it may well be in the best interests of staff and patient alike to terminate the rehabilitative effort and issue a referral to another practice. As Traynor (2003) indicated so eloquently, "Clinicians should be grateful that these patients make up only 4% to 5% of the general clinical population." (Personal style is discussed in Chapter 20.)

Despite the best efforts at identifying problem patients, some will slip through even the most vigilant audiologist's sensors. The key question is what can be done to retrieve the situation and move the patient to a satisfied or delighted hearing instrument wearer. As a matter of the usual course in dealing with patients, there may not be any conceivable adjustment or tactic available to alter the situation. There are a few measures that should always be considered: The first includes evaluating the extremes by having the patient, family, or friends assess their performance with and without the instruments. By recommending this assessment, a discussion will begin in the office and continue into their respective homes or workplaces about how much better the patient performs with the instruments in their ears than with them in a drawer or on the dresser. Another approach is to have the patient return to the office for follow-up visits until they are wearing the instruments with acceptable consistency based on the observations of their family or friends. The goal of this approach is to assist the patient in appreciating the benefits of consistent instrument use. If these patients can be moved to an acceptable schedule of consistent instrument use, they will develop increasingly greater satisfaction as the benefits of usage become apparent to both the patients and those around them.

Patients in extended care facilities (ECFs) present a different issue concerning compliant use of hearing instruments. In many of these facilities, the patient may not be able to insert the instruments and must rely on the staff of the ECF to provide the necessary and appropriate assistance to do so. If the staff fails to appropriately place the hearing instruments in or on the patient's ear or places the instruments appropriately and fails to turn them on, change the batteries, or clean the instruments, the ECF becomes the source of a noncompliance situation at the patient's expense. Finding an ECF that takes pride in the quality of care provided to their residents to the point that each patient wearing hearing instruments is functioning to their maximum hearing potential is a distinct rarity. Unfortunately, this seems to be the case no matter what the family is paying for their loved one's care. Altering the course of this catastrophe requires intervention with the nursing supervisor and staff. Recognizing that individuals with multiple morbidities— visual impairment, hearing loss, cognitive difficulties—commonly seen in ECFs will require special attention and the need for the staff to go an extra mile in planning and providing optimal care for each resident. Having the attending physician write specific orders for hearing instrument placement, care, and cleaning might help. With orders written, oversight for appropriate hearing instrument placement and assessment of use becomes part of the medical record and will likely be discussed during care conferences. The attending physician is now integrally linked to the quality of care provided under their medical management while adding a powerful ally to both the patient and the family should disputes develop over the adequacy of care regarding hearing instrument usage. However, it is more likely that these simple but time-consuming tasks will fall to the patient's family. Following the patient to the ECF and providing instructional support to the staff will help. Nothing, however, will supplant the watchful eye of demanding family members.

Angry or Disgruntled Patients

Anger fueled by declining health, frustrating encounters with insurance companies and other healthcare providers, or too many yet needed follow-up visits and out-of-pocket costs of hearing instruments can turn an otherwise kind, cooperative patient into a caustic, angry, and unsettled person bellowing at the receptionist's window.

Immediate steps must be taken to resolve the issues and assure the patient that whatever it takes to reduce frustrations or change an irritating situation will be done. Every member of the front office and professional staff of the practice is responsible for patient satisfaction and patient loyalty. Recall that 68% of patients refuse to return to a practice because they believe the practice is "indifferent" to their concerns and needs. No one wants to think they are unimportant. Recall also that if the patient's issues are delineated, discussed, and resolved quickly, the patient will likely stay with the practice and develop an odd sense of pride in generating what is perceived as positive change.

Service recovery is not just about fixing a patient's problem. It is about listening to the patient and recognizing their dissatisfaction. It should never take

two members of a practice to resolve an issue for one patient, nor should two people be required to foster patient satisfaction and loyalty. There are patients in every practice who are consistently cranky. It must be the goal of every staff person to make their visit the friendliest and most pleasant at every trip to the practice.

One patient who fit the bill for being consistently cranky had been coming to one of our offices (RGG) for many years. Every person in the office agreed to make his visits full of smiles and charm. One day, the patient exclaimed, obviously peeved, "What is it with you people? I do nothing but moan and groan and you all stay so cheerful and upbeat no matter what!" The entire office staff celebrated this minor, yet important team victory with a celebratory pizza lunch the next day. They were determined to charm his socks off and they had succeeded. In a patient-centric practice, every patient is treated in that manner every day the office is open for business.

Conflict Resolution and Staff Safety

Every member of the practice staff must be trained to resolve patient issues and calm patients down when they are agitated or overly concerned. In addition, each staff member must be able to recognize when a situation has gotten out of control and what steps to follow to resolve the issue. Patients can become highly agitated and, in some cases, combative. Just as the practice should have an exit plan in the event of a fire and a plan for calling 911 in the event of a medical emergency, so too should there be a plan in place to protect the staff from a potentially dangerous patient. Just about the time the office staff begins to think they have seen everything or that "our patients would never become physically abusive," a major eruption takes place at the payment window with the patient slamming their fist into the wall or tossing wall hangings on the floor in a frenzy.

In that event, an immediate 911 call summoning the police should be made. What about the time from the call to their arrival? What can be done to calm the situation and regain everyone's temperament and civility? Interventionists suggest that anything to defuse the situation should be done. Telling the patient not to worry about charges for the day and reassuring them that there has been no harm done will go far in lessening the tension of the situation. If the spouse or a friend is with them, ask for their intercession in the matter and have them help calm the situation. Conflict resolution needs calm more than focusing on immediate resolution in the early stages of an incident. Whatever it takes to calm the situation should be put into play. The goal is to have the patient leave the office without harming themselves or others—or for the police to arrive and secure everyone's safety. Angry patient scenarios should be considered an important topic for discussion at staff meetings, just as important as fire safety or procedures for office closure for inclement weather.

Cool-down techniques to resolve conflict should be discussed and training should be completed at least annually. A procedural description of cool-down techniques to be used in the event of significant patient conflict should be developed with the help of mental health professionals. The basic components of cool-down techniques geared to mollify patient anger include:

1. Engaging the assistance of the spouse or family member accompanying the patient to intervene.
2. If the interaction involves a member of the front office staff, immediately involve a member of the professional staff in the situation.
3. Appropriate physical distance between the patient and staff members must be maintained.
4. Immediate understanding and unequivocal agreement about the issue at the core of the disturbance should be exhibited on the part of the staff.
5. Encourage the patient to talk about the problem without being patronizing, talk, talk, talk.
6. Staff members should avoid any statement or behavioral posture that could escalate the situation—listen, listen, listen.
7. Assure the patient that resolution of the circumstance will be in their favor.
8. Resolution must be rapid, outcome(s) clear, and assurance reiterated that all will be resolved to their satisfaction.
9. If the patient remains agitated despite best efforts to cool the situation to a tolerable level, the front office staff should be prepared to dial 911 to summon the police.
10. If there is no reduction in the intensity of the situation, the professional staff member must politely yet firmly ask the patient to leave the office.

11. If the patient refuses, advise the patient that the authorities will be called.
12. If there is refusal to leave, 911 should be called—" This is Dr. ____'s office at XYZ address, we have a combative patient situation and we need help immediately—the patient's name is ____, he is a (description)."

THE BELLIGERENT PATIENT

Mr. H. came to the office on the referral of Dr. B, his primary care provider. During the history taking, Mr. H. became obviously agitated and angry in response to usual questions about the development, severity, and effects of his hearing loss in his daily activities. Mr. H's wife was in the exam room and noticed his agitation. At one point, the patient stopped the questions and demanded to know why we needed to know so much about his hearing problems. He demanded that we "just get on with the testing" and that the "rest of this stuff is none of your business." It was obvious from his breathing and the extension of his neck vessels that he was markedly angry. The wife tearfully urged him to calm down. Response to Ms. H's suggestion was to decompensate into torrid remarks and movements that suggested the patient was about to escalate the situation into a physical confrontation.

The clinician stopped the conversation with an admonishment that he needed to "cool down," that the discussion was trying to get information that would figure into a plan to help Mr. H and the family. The clinician then announced a 5-minute break to regain composure and upon the clinician's return, a decision would be made as to the next step in the clinic visit.

The patient remained agitated and angry when the clinician returned to the exam room. Mr. H announced that "you SOBs are only after the contents of my wallet so you might as well just open it up and take it now!" With that comment, the patient flung his wallet to the wall and his wife burst into tears. At that point, the clinician asked Mr. H to leave the office. Mr. H refused and told the clinician to "just go on with your damn tests and let's get this over with." At this point, the clinician informed Mr. H that the visit was finished for the day and reiterated the request to vacate the office immediately. The patient said nothing yet stayed in the exam chair. The spouse begged Mr. H to leave.

The clinician had alerted the front office to be prepared to call the police if needed and at this point informed the patient that if he did not

continued on next page

continued from previous page

leave immediately, the police would be called to forcefully remove him from the property. Mr. H muttered under his breath, told the wife to get the car, and left the exam room. This patient's insurance was billed for the visit and his primary care provider was called as soon as the property was exited. The primary care provider indicated that the patient had a recent altercation with the billing staff in their office, which the physician attributed to the patient's initial stages of dementia. Organic brain syndromes including dementia do not lessen the dangers of physical confrontation with patients. Audiologists should be aware of the possibilities of aggressive behaviors from patients known to have been mild mannered over many years of care provided in the practice.

In any event, aggressive or threatening behaviors toward professional or front office staff must not be tolerated. Staff should be well trained to identify and respond to patients with multiple morbidities as described herein. Annual reviews of emergency measures within the office should be part of a routine effort to reduce patient-related violence in the practice.

For the safety of all concerned, the practice staff must remain calm and in control of the situation. Physical contact with the patient must be avoided at all costs. Police response is usually quite rapid due to the explosive nature of these situations and the potential for physical altercations. Most municipal police departments have a community relations officer who will come to the office to discuss emergency notification and response times with specific instructions about reporting and responding to an incident involving an angry or agitated patient. Immediately following an incident, the referring physician should be contacted to explain the situation and circumstances under which the patient became agitated with a full disclosure of the resolution, no matter the outcome of the situation. A detailed, factual report of the incident from onset to outcome should be prepared by each staff member involved. The comments should be signed by each staff member, and each report should be reviewed by the attorney of record for the practice.

A follow-up letter should be sent to the referring physician to confirm the telephone conversation and the resolution of the situation. The report should be part of the patient's continuing medical record. The practice's attorney will advise how best to interact with the patient in the future such as no further contact whatsoever or possibly send a certified letter to the patient confirming the need for the patient to seek care elsewhere.

Statutory regulations governing the practice of medicine and dentistry commonly contain sections regarding patient abandonment. These sections usually stipulate the circumstances under which patients may be discharged from a practice and set forth guidelines or suggestions on how best to advise a patient that they will no longer be seen for continuing care (Chapter 17). Although required for physicians and dentists, it is not common to see these requirements in laws or other regulatory language governing the practice of audiology. A thorough reading of state licensing law and administrative rules should clarify whether there are specifically proscribed requirements or necessary means to inform a patient that they will no longer be seen as a patient in the practice. If in doubt, contact the state licensing board with a written request for clarification. When corresponding with your state licensing board or registration department, always send the correspondence, no matter the topic, via certified mail with a return receipt requested. This creates a documented record of the submission or inquiry. Should there be no response from the licensing board within a reasonable period, a phone call to the executive director of the board should be made to determine the status of your inquiry. If the executive director is unable to satisfy the request, the chairman of the board or elected state representative should be contacted on the behalf of the professional.

Baby Boomers: The Primary Population Served

Maintaining patient loyalty is becoming more difficult regardless of the profession. That may be especially true of the primary population to be served over the next 15 to 20 years. Primary care physicians, dentists, optometrists, and audiologists are becoming acutely aware of the markedly reduced tensile strength of the ties that bind Baby Boomers to their respective practitioners. As the Baby Boomer generation begins to access the healthcare system, new demands will be placed on the healthcare system in general and the hearing instrument delivery system specifically (Chapter 20).

Boomers enjoy essentially unlimited access to medical and healthcare information through the Internet. They are the best-educated generation of Americans; 33% are college graduates, and those who did not finish college attended. Boomers are generally computer literate.

Boomers approach their healthcare like no other group. They do not think of themselves as "old" but rather view their age well below their true chronologic status. When they go to their providers for assessment or routine care, they are characteristically well armed with an expansive knowledge of their healthcare issues. They commonly seek healthcare practitioners directly, scheduling visits with those with advanced degrees and specialty certification. They are abruptly critical of the quality of care provided and the surroundings in which services are delivered. They are more likely to leave a healthcare provider to seek second opinions if they do not feel they are receiving accurate and appropriate information or care.

Boomers' trust and the confidence in their healthcare providers develop from their perceptions of professionalism within the office, the efficiency and friendliness of the front office staff, and the important, yet ephemeral, doctor-to-patient relationship. They are less likely to accept mediocrity and less tolerant of problems arising from limited attention, common errors in billing, and items or issues in need of what they consider to be too much postpurchase attention.

Fortunately, Boomers are more likely to seek hearing care sooner than those in previous generations, and they readily accept well-credentialed, nonphysician practitioners as their healthcare provider for specific, well-defined healthcare needs (Traynor, 2011). As a group, they are more likely to seek alternative providers to their current providers based on price, time to schedule services, convenience of service locations, time spent in the office, and, most importantly, their perception of the quality and outcome of each encounter.

In the final report of the Clarity-Ear Foundation two-part survey, which focused on the prevalence and impact of hearing loss in Baby Boomers, several interesting and important characteristics about this generation came to light. This well-regarded and oft-quoted study began in 2004 with 437 randomly selected participants between 49 and 59 years of age. An initial online survey was completed followed by a telephone interview focusing on the prevalence of hearing loss. It focused on how Boomers felt their lives were impacted by their hearing loss. A group of 458 randomly selected participants 41 to 60 years of age completed an online survey, also followed by telephone interviews.

These findings are of special interest to audiologists since the first formal classes in audiology were begun in 1946 at Northwestern University, the same year the first group of over 75 million Boomers was born. The findings of the study confirmed many clinical observations and produced several interesting findings selected below:

- About half (53%) of Boomers have at least a "mild" hearing loss.
- Men were significantly more likely to report a hearing loss than were women (62% to 38%).
- Three-fourths of those reporting a severe hearing loss were men and 26% of those with hearing loss had their hearing loss formally diagnosed by a healthcare professional—37% had not had their hearing tested.
- Only three out of four (73%) parents whose adult children say they have a hearing loss had their hearing tested.
- One-fourth said their hearing loss affected their work; handling phone calls and conversations with coworkers were the areas most impacted.
- One-fourth said their hearing loss had an impact on their earning potential.
- Ninety-seven percent of participants stated they were aware of hearing aids.
- Seventy-eight percent indicated they were aware of amplified telephones that could help individuals with hearing loss.
- Among those with severe hearing loss, only 42% wore hearing aids.

A more contemporary view of the Baby Boomer group and how best to approach them as patients was proffered by Traynor (2012), Veto (2015), the Age Wave Group, and in an editorial by Windmill (2017). Hearing instruments have been described as "medallions of old age" rather than as exemplary technical passports to an improved, engaged life. Hearing care should be a substantial part of wellness. The message in advertising, invited lectures, and every opportunity to meet people who would likely benefit from modern hearing instrumentation should include the repositioned concept that embracing life to the fullest sets forth an image of vitality and engagement rather than retreat.

- *Rule 1:* Think life stage—not age. In the past, people were mostly doing the same things at a certain age. Boomers have very diverse lives and do not do the same things at specific ages as previous generations.
- *Rule 2:* Diverse clinical needs. Since they come from many different stages of life, Boomers have very different needs clinically. For example, Boomers prefer a one-to-one rehabilitative program. They are not inclined to accept any form of group treatment programming.
- *Rule 3:* Emotionally meaningful treatment programs. Boomers do not respond to high pressure; they respond to emotional arguments and will purchase products if the situation "feels right." Clinicians need to talk about the future and how beneficial advancements in hearing instruments will provide improved performance in real-life situations. They readily accept sophisticated technology enabling them to hear better in difficult listening situations.
- *Rule 4:* Watch out for ageism. Since they do not feel they are old, Baby Boomers do not like things that make them feel old, such as bank accounts "for seniors" or senior citizen discounts. They respond well to sophisticated, progressive treatment programs and appreci-

ate the attention counseling offers and being provided information on adaptive strategies to be used in situations of multiple talkers or noisy environments.

- *Rule 5:* More information is better. Gone are the days when a clinician selects a hearing instrument and informs the patient this is what you need—case closed. Boomers want as much information as possible about size, style, shape, adjustments, an explanation of the technology, and why the clinician has chosen the specific brand of instrument to be used. They often bring an Internet file to the clinic with varied types of products and information about care, cleaning, and postfitting follow-up. Internet files should be encouraged, and appropriate discussion should focus on their questions and concerns. The discussions enhance their perception of the clinician as a caring, professional willing to take the time they need to understand their loss and how they want to be involved in their hearing care.
- *Rule 6:* Tell a story. Boomers want to hear about other patients' success with the instruments being considered. Of equal importance, they appreciate the frankness about specific situations, which may continue to present communication difficulties.
- *Rule 7:* Understand changing values. Boomers had always focused on "becoming someone" and view themselves with their successes as "being someone." They value where they have been and what it has taken to get to this point. Even though hearing loss is more of a

threat than the hearing instrument, counseling to accept these changes can be difficult. Successful performance improvement with appropriately fitted hearing instruments will outdo objections to the use of hearing instruments every time.

■ *Rule 8:* Make it relevant to me! Boomers want to see themselves in the treatment program, and it is necessary to paint a picture of how they will fit into the process. Describe the successes various patients have experienced in their everyday lives and in their efforts in the workplace. Discuss the impact on their interactions with family and friends.

■ *Rule 9:* Pay in the gray. This generation is tired of hearing things like the "Best of the Best" or "the finest available" relative to products and treatment programs. Just as "buy one get one free" is generally unappealing to Boomers, absolute claims are equally unappealing. Better to present alternatives and give choices based on varied benefits from different circuit capabilities.

■ *Rule 10:* Learn baby learn. This is a group that will continue to make Internet files of advancing technologies, treatment techniques, implantable hearing devices, and other state-of-the-art products after they have been evaluated, fitted, and followed in the clinic. How they feel about you and your services will change over time as they view your efforts through the lens of technology and the success or limitations it brings to their lives. These patients will expect you to stay on top of advancing technologies and to let them know what, if anything, has

improved or is on the horizon when ready to consider changes in their hearing instruments.

Follow-Up Care: Critical Element of Successful Long-Term Practices

Consistent follow-up care is a requirement in any healthcare practice. Follow-up care should be highly systematized and patient centric at the office staff level and engagingly personal at the provider-patient interface. Follow-up care is an operational method to increase patient satisfaction and foster patient loyalty, and it an additional means to encourage patients to sing the praises of the practice, not just to their family and friends but to the healthcare provider responsible for their referral to your practice.

The Art of Personalization

The era of "Sign in—Sit down—Shut up" healthcare has ended.

Baby Boomers will be between 60 and 78 years old in 2024 and they will accept nothing less than active participation in their healthcare. The generation to follow them, Gen X, will be between 45 and 59 and will be no less demanding than their older cohorts. Neither practice nor practitioner can prosper long term without creating a consistent atmosphere of patient involvement. Involving patients and those interested in their well-being fosters high patient satisfaction and loyalty.

This is true for medical specialists and generalists, dentists, optometrists, and audiologists as well. It is important to personalize the patient's visit. As mentioned previously, sending a handwritten note following the initial patient encounter thanking them for choosing this practice and encouraging their active participation in subsequent visits goes a long way in building a comfortable relationship. Consider creating a brochure informing the patient what to expect at the fitting and during subsequent follow-up visits. Underscore the importance of the follow-up visits as opportunities to "dial in" the instruments for use across a variety of listening conditions. Keep in mind that even the most seasoned hearing instrument wearer will admit to at least a bit of apprehension while waiting for their new hearing instruments. These efforts provide an appreciated informational bridge between visits.

Friends, Family, and Patient Referrals

Patients referring prospective patients to the practice is the highest form of recognition for any healthcare practitioner. It sends a clear message to the incoming individual that the referring patient has had a valuable experience and that they have been well served and are confident enough to make a recommendation to a friend or member of their immediate or extended family. The referring patient should be recognized in some way: A personal thank you note or a certificate for a free pack of batteries provides important recognition and appreciation. Although it is inappropriate and breaches a variety of organizational codes of ethics, actively seeking patient-generated

---

BEFORE HEARING INSTRUMENTS: PATIENT BROCHURE

Realistic Expectations

Hearing aids are just that, devices to aid your hearing. Hearing instruments will not return your hearing function to normal, and they will not "cure" your hearing loss. If you use your hearing aids appropriately and wear them consistently, you can expect to hear better in almost all situations. There will be a few places where you may experience difficulty, such as extremely noisy restaurants. But, for the most part, you and those around you can expect improved hearing and better communication.

Adjusting Takes Time

Realistic expectations are critically important. So too is the time it takes to get used to your new hearing instruments. Although periods of adjustment

continued on next page

continued from previous page

vary, many patients report continued hearing improvement and better speech understanding over a 3- to 6-month period. Since the auditory centers in the brain have not been subjected to these sounds, processing remembered sounds gets noticeably easier day by day.

Everyday Sounds

There is also an adjustment period to everyday sounds in our environment. Many patients report they forgot how annoying certain sounds can be and would just as well do without hearing them again. Clocks ticking, noisy refrigerators, and emergency sirens are examples of noises that may not seem important, but each contributes to your environment. Modern, digital circuitry has been designed to reduce the negative effects of noise in your listening environment.

Background sounds are no longer the greatest hurdle a hearing instrument wearer needs to overcome. Better technology coupled with improved fitting techniques add up to a tremendous outlook for a successful outcome—even in areas with background noise, you will likely benefit from your hearing aids and hear those people seated at your table. It may not be perfect, but it will be far better than you can imagine with older hearing aids or by avoiding new instruments because you have heard they are so difficult to get accustomed to.

Keeping in touch with your environment is important. Enjoy all the sounds in your environment and recognize that even unwanted sounds have value. It's about taking a bit of the bad with all the good and staying in the everyday richness we call life. Welcome back to the world of all kinds of sounds!

Everyone Will Benefit From Your Hearing Instruments

Most of our patients come to us by referral from their family doctor. Others come to us by the "urgings" of their family or friends. They have a vested interest in your hearing. If you are hearing better, everyone benefits from easier and more accurate communication.

Effective communication is a two-way street. If you persevere in wearing your hearing instruments, you and your family and friends will benefit from your willingness to improve your communication situation. Although

continued on next page

continued from previous page

it may be difficult at times, the more effort you put into adjusting to and wearing your hearing instruments, the more you will benefit from them.

Ultimately, better hearing is up to you. You must wear your instruments consistently, maintain them well with regular cleaning, and have them fully charged r have an extra battery on hand at all times if your device uses replaceable batteries. Improved hearing takes but a few minutes of your time and attention daily. Our office is dedicated to your success, and we are here to assist you in any way to make your journey to better hearing the best it can be. We will be available to you as long as you need us!

referrals must not be considered a part of marketing or practice promotion. Accepting the recognition of a referral by a satisfied patient in the practice is appropriate: Actively seeking these referrals is beyond the issues of ethics and simply unprofessional.

Notes in the Margins and Photo ID

A handy way to personalize relationships with patients is to jot notes in the margins of the chart or on a separate comment sheet so that events or circumstances can be recalled that are important to the patient at the next visit. Birthdays, weddings, retirements, and funerals are items of foremost importance to patients, and when they feel comfortable sharing this information, take the time to listen and inquire about it at subsequent patient visits. Staff should consistently peruse the obituaries, and if it involves a current patient or one of their family members, a note of condolence or sympathy card should be sent. When working with a patient and their family for several years, their audiologist becomes important to them, and as such, an appropriate response will be greatly appreciated and remembered for many years. Birthdays can be programmed to come up in most Management Information Systems and patient databases. Although some patients (and clinicians as well) have stopped counting birthdays, everyone likes to be recognized on their birthday.

Going beyond what is expected should be second nature when it comes to patient care. Extra effort cannot be taught; it comes not from a book but from the heart. Patients and their families appreciate extra effort. It bolsters confidence in the care they are receiving and reinforces their perception of your interest in their success.

Loyal patients have high comfort levels within the practice—both in the interest paid to them as a patient and in the quality of the professional care they have received. Loyalty is directly related to comfort and confidence and a sense of the staff having a genuine interest in the patient as an individual, not just as a person with hearing impairment seeking and receiving professional services to improve their communication capabilities.

One of the most effective tools for front office and professional staffs to improve patient recognition is to keep a photo of the patient at the back of the chart for reference. Indeed, some third-party payers are requesting that patients be confirmed by reviewing an identifying photo on a driver's license or other form of identification bearing a photo of the patient. It is amazing how many times the practice staff will refer to a patient's photo to solidify their image with the name or to confirm they are dealing with a specific patient about a topic relevant to that patient's care or billing situation. Of course, having access to these photos can also clarify the patient's identity in a rogue's gallery sort of way. Every practice has difficult patients, and making sure who is who can serve as a means of alerting staff about problems, likes or dislikes, or patients with specific needs.

Newsletters

Practice newsletters are not only appreciated by your patients but also anticipated and a welcome update about the goings-on in the practice. Loyal patients feel a part of the practice and are interested in staff changes, training, and accomplishments. They want to know about attendance at seminars to improve technical and clinical skills. They like to read about innovative technology and will call and inquire about the need to consider "newer" technologies when discussed in the newsletter.

There are services that provide practice newsletters. The practice sends them the database, and they mail a newsletter at specified intervals. They are well written and contain a wealth of information. However, they lack the personal edge of a practice-generated newsletter. Practice newsletters are time-consuming. They should be formatted by a professional printing service, incurring both production and mailing costs. If there is not enough time, talent, or resources to develop and mail at least three newsletters per year, consider a commercial practice newsletter. Either way, a practice newsletter provides an important opportunity to stay in the patient's view and remain in the view of their significant others as well.

Net Promoter Score

Earlier sections of this chapter addressed the importance of generating loyal customers. Believe it or not, there is a way to measure it, and of course, when something can be measured, it can be improved. Measuring and improving starts with the use of patient surveys, also known as a customer comment card. Perhaps the best way to measure and improve loyalty is with just one question: How likely are you (the customer) to refer others to this business? Created by business professor Fred Reichheld in the early 2000s, the Net Promoter Score or NPS is used by many businesses today to track customer loyalty. In fact, if a business is emailing a comment card and asks, "Tell us how we are doing," chances are great that this business is using NPS to make business decisions.

According to Reichheld, only one question needs to be asked and one number (the answer to the question) that needs attention: On a scale of 1 to 10, how likely are you to recommend our "service" to a colleague or friend? Answers from 1 through 6 are "detractors," 7s and 8s are "neutrals," and 9s and 10s are "promoters." Only the enthusiastic 9s and 10s are counted as promoters. The satisfied 7s and 8s are lukewarm and don't count. The rest (1s through 6s) are customers who will likely make a negative comment if asked to recommend the service provider.

After, say, 50 or more customers are surveyed with that single question, the NPS is calculated by disregarding the neutrals (7s and 8s) and subtracting the detractors (1s to 6s) from the promoters (9s and 10s), and a net promoter percentage score of all customers surveyed is generated. So, if 1,000 customers are surveyed, and 500 of them are promoters, 100 are detractors, and the rest are neutrals or did not respond, the calculation of the NPS is:

$$\text{NPS} = \left[\frac{(500 - 100)}{1,000} \right] \times 100 = 40\%$$

Brands such as Apple, Harley Davidson, and Amazon.com have historically high net promoter scores of between 70% and 80%. As a practice manager or owner, the only number of concerns is the net promoter score, how high it is, and—more importantly—whether it is increasing. If it increases, the clinic is generating more loyal customers.

The Value Equation

Most business managers know that value is a key to driving ever-higher levels of customer loyalty. Remember, the more loyal a customer is, the more likely they are to repurchase from the clinic and not a competitor across town or online. Since value is so critical to loyalty, it makes sense to better understand the underpinnings of value and how it is created. Fortunately, the creators of the service-profit chain also devised an effective way to define value based on these four factors: Results, Process, Price, and Effort. Each of these variables requires further explanation.

Results

What is the primary need of the customer? If a person wants to go to Paris, it is just travel from Point A to Point B—nothing more, nothing less. However, if a customer wants to take a trip to celebrate their 50th wedding anniversary, then the primary result is more likely to be a memorable experience. What is a memorable experience? It can vary a great deal depending on the customer. The obvious consequence of not understanding the needs of the customer is that they might never return. For audiologists, the result is almost always better communication ability. That result varies from person to person and often is not experienced for a least a few weeks.

Process

Achieve the primary result of getting from Point A to Point B in many ways. The difference is the way it is done. In the Value Equation, there is a Process. Processes must be analyzed in terms of what creates value for the customer because it almost always increases the expenses. For audiologists, the way they help a patient move from Point A to Point B is dependent upon the quality of their clinical processes. Through the lens of the Value Equation, the way of testing and counseling patients takes on greater meaning, and thus, it is more than a simple diagnostic test; it becomes a relatable and transformative experience.

Price

The price is, of course, what the customer must pay for hearing aids and service. More precisely, it's the personal check they write, the credit card swiped, or the hard cold cash they may have taken years to earn. After all, hearing aids, after automobiles and homes, are among the most expensive purchases for many older adults.

Effort

Effort, or what is known as convenience costs, is to which degree the customer tries to receive or acquire a service. If shopping at IKEA, there is great effort by customers in picking up the furniture in stock and putting it together at home or, if they are at a cafeteria, moving through the line rather than being served. The effort used by the customer reduces the price. If room service is ordered, the service fee must be paid, as it is more convenient to have a meal in the room than going to the restaurant. Consumers are then paying for the luxury of less effort to fulfill their desires. For audiologists, effort boils down to making the patient's experience convenient and "worth the time" to make an appointment, wait in the reception area to see the clinician, and then have their problem addressed quickly.

The Monetary Value of One Loyal Customer

Audiologists often refer to embracing a "patient for life mindset." This refers to the financial value of a repeat buyer who also refers family and friends to the practice. For example, take a 65-year-old female with an expected life span of 20 years who buys a pair of hearing aids for $4,000. Given an average life span for the hearing aids of 5 years, this means this person could buy three more pairs of hearing aids, which will generate another $12,000 to $15,000 of revenue. Additionally, this person will likely buy some other services and accessories, even upgrade the next set or sets of devices from the practice. But the big number is the potential referrals. Over the lifetime of, say, four other people referred to the practice from this one loyal customer, this could be well over $50,000 in revenue for the practice. All with no marketing funds used to acquire these customers. It is easy to see why creating loyal, repeat purchasers is the name of the game and this should be the goal of every practitioner.

Summary

As the business management pioneer Peter Drucker said, "The purpose of any business is to create a customer." Of course, loyal customers who buy again and again are a natural consequence of effective leadership, sound execution, and attention to detail. Creating exceptional value leads to loyal customers. A key lesson in this chapter is that loyal customers do not happen by chance; managers and practice owners must execute a plan to create them. There is no substitute for a well-developed patient management plan. Effective patient management plans and the skills required to implement them are usually learned from the best teachers—*the patients themselves.* An ability to communicate and readily develop rapport and comfort in patients and those accompanying them to their office visit will set the practice above those merely interested in number of patients, procedures, and instruments dispensed.

Whether in an independent private practice, an ENT-audiology practice, or a nonprofit community speech and hearing center, capable patient management must be the cornerstone of excellence in the daily clinical schedule. Patients referred to or seeking the professional care of an audiologist have come to expect clinical excellence and positive outcomes in their quality of life. Anything less the whole of the profession of audiology loses important standing in the healthcare arena, one important patient at a time.

Every patient seen in the practice must know that their physician, friend, or relative issuing the referral has done so with great confidence in this practice's patient management skills. They have made the referral knowing that audiologists are the professionals uniquely qualified to provide both diagnostic studies and appropriate treatment for patients with hearing and balance difficulties. They also refer knowing that patients will, after comprehensive assessment, be appropriately referred for medical or surgical intervention when required.

Each patient coming to the practice must expect professional, dedicated service from every member of the practice staff always, every day the doors are open, and the telephones are answered.

Anything less than the items found in the Patient's Bill of Rights and the practice is not serving patients or referral sources well.

As Albert Einstein once said, "Strive not to be a success, but rather to be of value."

References

Beck, R. S., Dautridge, R., & Sloane, P. D. (2004). Physician-patient communication in the primary care office: A systematic review. *Journal of the American Board of Family Practice, 15*(1), 25–38.

Becton, J., Harvell, J., & Jones-Farmer, A. (2014). Generational differences in the workplace. *Journal of Applied Social Psychology, 44*, 175–180.

Cavitt, K. (2015). ADA and IntriCon partner to launch earVenture low-cost hearing aids; HIA expresses concerns. *Hearing Review, 22*(11), 12.

Heskett, J., Sasser, W. E., & Schlesinger, L. (1997). *The service profit chain*. Free Press.

Hopkins, T. (2006, February 6). Do your customers feel ignored? Entrepreneur.com.

Marsh, D. (2005). Turning patients into patient advocates. *The Hearing Journal, 58*(2), 48.

Peterson, D. (2011). Four generations: Can't we all get along? Arthur Maxwell 2024. https://arthur-maxwell.com/articles/2011/09-generations.php

Rao, P. R. (2011, November 17). Our role in effective patient-provider communication. *The ASHA Leader.*

Reinartz, W., & Kumar, V. (2002, July). The mismanagement of customer loyalty. *Harvard Business Review*, pp. 86–94.

Schwab, E. F. (2016, May/June). A personal journey into private practice. *Audiology Today*, pp. 14–19.

Taylor, B. (2006). How quality of service affects patient satisfaction with hearing aids. *The Hearing Journal, 59*(9), 25–34.

Travaline, J. M., Ruchinskas, R., & D'Alonzo, G. E. (2005). Patient-physician communication: Why and how. *Journal of the American Osteopathic Association, 105*(1), 13–17.

Traynor, R. M. (2003, August). Personal style and hearing aid fitting. *The Hearing Review*, pp. 16–22.

Traynor, R. (2011). Are Baby Boomer patients a world-wide phenomenon? Hearing Health and Technology Matters. http://hearinghealthmatters.org/hearinginternational/2011/are-baby-boomer-patients-a-world-wide-phenomenon/

Traynor, R. (2012). *Baby Boomers: Our new patients*. Presentation to An Interactive Workshop in The Business of Audiology, Davenport, IA.

Veto, D. (2015). Interview by B. Carroll, K. Glay, and D. Culver. *Audiology Today, 7*(4), 26–33.

Windmill, I. (2017, January/February). Where is the outrage? *Audiology Today*, pp. 10–12.

Wong, L., Hickson, L., & McPherson, B. (2003). Hearing aid satisfaction: What does research from the past 20 years say? *Trends in Amplification, 7*(4), 117–161.

19 The Hearing Industry: Navigating Vendor Relationships

Brian Taylor, AuD

Introduction

Because of their relatively large margins, the sale or dispensing of hearing aids has been a staple of most audiology practices for decades. Although these relatively large margins have eroded with the rising popularity of managed care in recent years, a rapidly aging Baby Boomer population helps to maintain a steady demand for the retail sale of hearing aids in most regions of the country. Hearing aid dispensing is a low-volume, high-margin business, which suggests many practices can remain profitable by dispensing hearing aids to 20 patients or fewer every month. Further, because hearing aids are such an integral part of many audiology clinic's revenue stream, it is imperative to have a keen understanding of the relationship between hearing instrument manufacturers, and other related vendors, and the audiologist who is making business decisions within a practice. After all, without effective business relationships with suppliers and vendors, the audiology practice's path to profitability is easily derailed. The primary aim of this chapter is to provide a deeper understanding of the

hearing care industry and the value of hearing aid vendor relationships for the owner or manager of an audiology practice.

The first lesson of this chapter is in terminology. Business-savvy audiologists tend to use three terms interchangeably: *manufacturer, supplier, and vendor*. There are some subtle differences between these terms. A manufacturer typically refers to a specific entity that produces hearing instruments. Simply stated, a manufacturer builds hearing aids. Currently, there are five major *prescriptive* hearing aid manufacturers along with the recent emergence of a few dozen *over-the-counter (OTC)* hearing aid manufacturers.

Audiologists of course buy many items, which are not hearing aids, that they often resell to consumers. This list includes assistive listening devices (ALDs), hearing protection devices, and many other components they need to operate their business. Additionally, audiologists buy all sorts of equipment that they use every day to conduct hearing assessments and fit hearing aids. Therefore, a broader term is needed to describe these entities. That brings us to the terms suppliers and vendors. Although these two terms are used interchangeably, believe it or not, there is a subtle difference between them. A supplier is a business entity that provides specific goods, services, or raw materials to another organization—typically for manufacturing purposes. Since audiologists are not making their own hearing aids these days, the term supplier is probably not accurate. That leaves the term vendor. A vendor, which is best described as a type of supplier, is an entity that sells finished goods or services directly to a business. Although three terms are commonly used interchangeably, the most accurate term is vendor. For that reason, the term vendor is used here.

"B2B" vs. "B2C"

Vendors, by definition, are engaged in what is referred to as *business-to-business* or *"B2B"* transactions. Business-to-business (B2B) is a form of transaction between businesses, such as one involving a manufacturer and wholesaler, or a wholesaler and a retailer. Business-to-business refers to transactions conducted between companies, rather than between a company and individual consumers. Prescription hearing aid companies do not sell their products directly to consumers; therefore, they are a *B2B business*. On the other hand, over-the-counter hearing aid companies do sell their devices directly to consumers. Thus, they are a good example of a "B2C" company. The term *business-to-consumer (B2C)* refers to the process of selling products and services directly between a business and consumers who are the end users of its products or services. Most companies that sell directly to consumers can be

referred to as B2C companies. For example, when you go to the mall to buy a new pair of shoes, you are buying from a B2C company. Audiologists who dispense hearing aids are engaged in *B2C* transactions.

Profession vs. Industry

Another pair of terms often used interchangeably are profession and industry. Many readers of this chapter are enrolled in an academic program that culminates in the terminal degree, doctor of audiology; other readers might be licensed hearing aid dispensers or audiology assistants. Regardless of training, credentials, or academic degree, by virtue of these qualifications, it is a *profession*. Members of a profession have common characteristics: ethical codes, specialized knowledge, skills, and training. They adhere to professional standards and follow their specific professionally mandated codes of ethics. In contrast, the term industry typically refers to a grouping of companies focused on a particular service or distinct business activities. Industries are also broader in scope than professions. Professionals may work within an industry, but there is more to an industry than just professionals. Manufacturers, suppliers, and vendors are among those entities that are part of a broader industry. This chapter focuses on the hearing care *industry* and how audiologists, members of a *profession*, interact with various vendors within that broader industry. *Stated differently, audiologists, hearing aid dispensers, and otolaryngologists are all members of separate professions, each of which resides within the larger hearing care industry.*

The objective of this chapter is two-fold: First, it outlines the current structure of the major players within the hearing care industry. Most of these players are vendors in which audiologists have an opportunity to form relationships. Second, it provides a basic approach to creating and maintaining relationships with vendors. This section will describe the nuts and bolts of nurturing a productive relationship with hearing care industry vendors as well as why those interactions are important to a practice's success.

Business Structure of Major Vendors

In Figure 19–1, Bailey (2024) illustrates the major hearing technology vendors. Think of Figure 19–1 as a roadmap of the hearing care industry. Across the top of each column in Figure 19–1, the "holding company" (also called a parent company) is listed, with the exception of column 1, which includes single-brand companies. A holding company is a parent company—usually a corporation or LLC—whose purpose is to buy and control the ownership interests of other smaller companies. The companies that are owned or controlled by a corporation holding company or an LLC holding company are called its subsidiaries. The holding companies shown across the top of Figure 19–1 from left to right, respectively, are America Hears, Amplifon, Demant, GN, Sonova, Starkey, and WS Audiology. Many of these holding companies, including Amplifon, Demant, GN, and Sonova, are public traded companies that can be found on European stock exchanges. On the

other hand, Starkey and WS Audiology are privately owned companies. Figure 19–1 provides a lot of important information about the hearing care industry that will be covered in the next few paragraphs.

For each of the holding companies shown at the top of Figure 19–1, there are several smaller companies listed directly under each of them. These smaller companies are called subsidiaries. A subsidiary is a company that belongs to another company, which is usually referred to as the *parent company or holding company*. The parent company holds a controlling interest in the subsidiary company, meaning it owns or controls more than half of its stock.

As the subsidiaries in Figure 19–1 are reviewed, note that some of these subsidiaries manufacture hearing aids, others are large retail entities that operate hearing aid centers around the country, and others still might be managed care organizations, buying groups, equipment suppliers, or consulting companies. It is interesting to point out that the only parent company that is not a hearing aid manufacturer is Amplifon. Amplifon, an Italian-based company, is the largest hearing aid retailer in the world. The brands listed under Amplifon are private-label hearing aid brands (Miracle-Ear) or smaller regional retail distributors located in all corners of the world.

It is common for a *single-parent company* to have *multiple hearing aid brands*. Some of these brands might be independently operated inside the parent company. For example, inside the WS Audiology parent company, there are two brands, *Signia* and *Widex*, which are operated independently of one another. This means that each of these brands

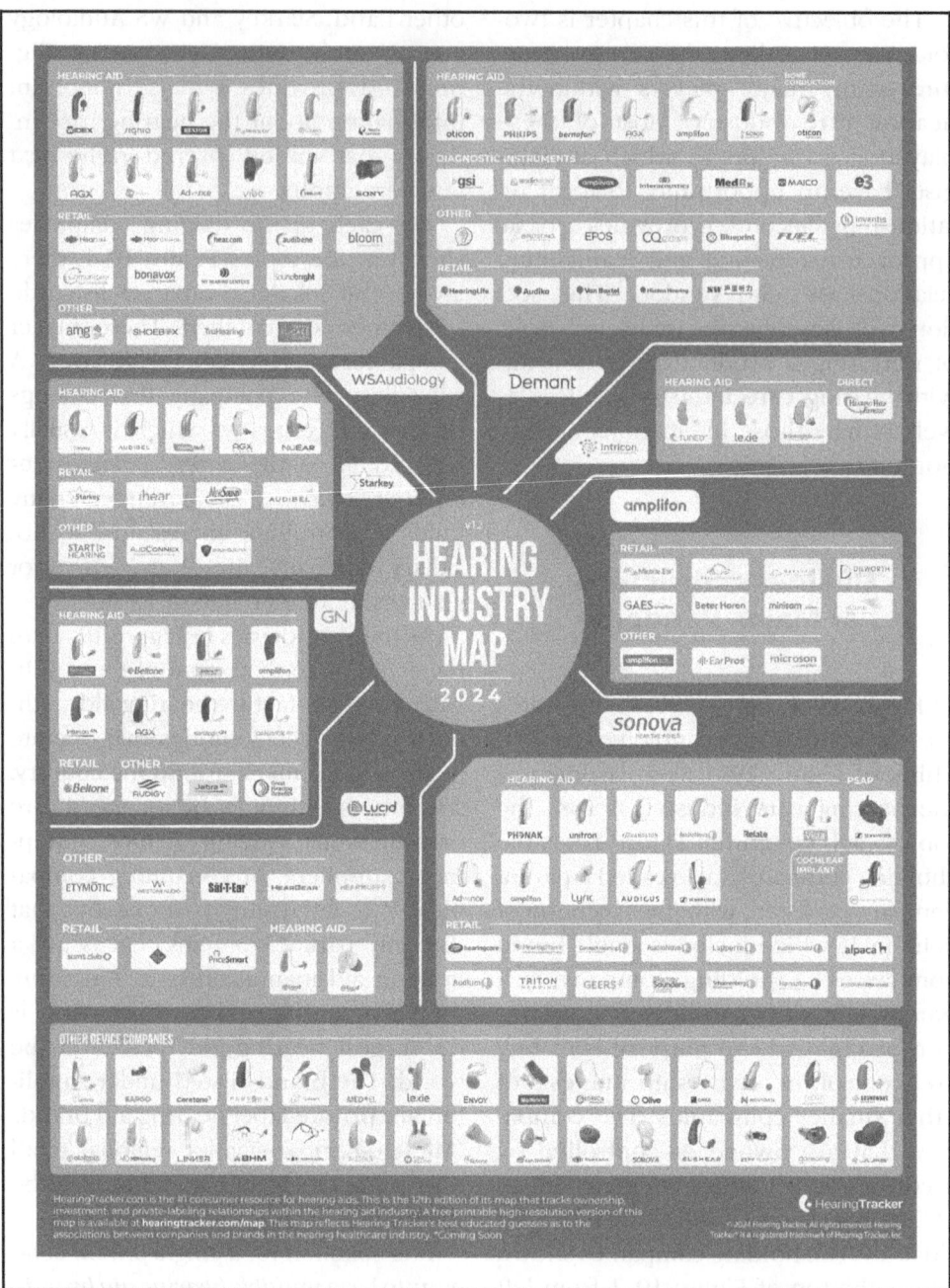

Figure 19–1. Hearing Industry Map 2024. *Source:* Reprinted with permission from Abram Bailey, Hearing Tracker (2024).

has its own signal processing platform, sales force, and fitting software even though they are part of the same parent company. Additionally, parent companies often have so-called *second brands* that have essentially the same signal processing platform as their lead brand. These second brands are often only available through managed care contracts, in a big-box store, or dispensed outside the United States. An example of a second brand is Philips or Bernafon, which are second brands of Oticon and all are within the Demant parent company.

Finally, each parent company provides *private-labeled* hearing aids that are presented to large retail chains or buying groups. Private-label hearing aids usually have the same signal processing as the lead brand, but the brand name of the hearing aid, along with the fitting software, carries a private label. The purpose, in theory, of private labels is to provide some level of exclusivity for the retail chain. Perhaps the best example of private labeling is Miracle-Ear, which has hundreds of points of sale around the United States. Currently, Signia and Starkey are two parent companies that privately label their hearing aids for the Miracle-Ear brand, which is owned by the parent company Amplifon.

One characteristic of some private-label hearing aids is "locked" fitting software. So-called locked software means that *only* the purveyor of that specific brand can program or fine-tune that particular device. If the patient of that brand goes to an independent audiologist for service, the independent audiologist cannot adjust or fine-tune the device because the software is "locked" and *can only be accessed* by purveyors or vendors of that private label. An example of "locked" software in Figure 19–1 is AGX. Note that many manufacturers produce the private label AGX for a large buying group, Audigy. The purpose of these private-label devices is to provide some level of exclusivity to Audigy members. The downside for the patient, however, is that they cannot go elsewhere for the service of that device. For example, if a patient purchased a pair of AGX hearing aids in New Jersey and went on vacation in Idaho and required service on the hearing aids, they would have to find an AGX vendor (Audigy member clinic) that had the appropriate fitting software. For this reason, there is intensive lobbying by consumer advocates for the Food and Drug Administration (FDA) to prohibit "locked" software. As of May 2024, this change in regulation *has not* gone into effect and locked devices are still available.

Buying Groups

Not all subsidiaries listed under each of the parent companies in Figure 19–1 are hearing aid manufacturers or private-label vendors. Each parent company is likely to have some type of buying group. Buying groups are a lot like Costco or Sam's Club in that the membership entitles discounts on products purchased in the store. In the case of buying groups within the hearing care industry, several audiologists from around the country agree to pool their resources and negotiate as a collective entity with vendors to receive devices at a discounted price.

The first buying group was Marcon Hearing Instruments, Inc., incorporated in 1977. The Marcon group began with a handful of retail clinic owners looking to brand themselves and their products. While this structure worked for several years, as the group changed and grew, there was interest in adding more manufacturers and using other brands. Since the mandate of most buying groups is to pool resources to create buying power with manufacturers, it works by several audiologists collectively agreeing to buy a high volume of hearing aids in exchange for a lower wholesale price. Consider, for example, that a single practice only buys 100 hearing aids per year from a certain manufacturer, but when 25 similarly sized practices around the country form a buying group, they are now buying 2,500 hearing aids. This added buying power enables smaller practices to get more favorable wholesale pricing by pooling their resources.

Group buying, also known as collective buying, offers products and services at significantly reduced prices on the condition that a minimum number of buyers would make the purchase. In the case of the hearing care industry, the buyers are audiologists in clinical practice who purchase hearing aids. There are more than a dozen buying groups in the industry. Fuel Medical, Alpaca Audiology, and Audigy are three of the largest buying groups. In addition to providing lower wholesale pricing, buying groups provide various types of business support, including marketing and human resources. Many parent companies in the hearing care industry either own outright or heavily subsidize buying groups. Because buying groups are popular, many audiologists are members of one or more buying groups; therefore, parent companies have a vested interest in supporting

buying groups. Interestingly, buying groups are one of the entities within a *vertically integrated parent company* that does not manufacture hearing aids. Instead of providing a tangible product, they provide an intangible service.

Regardless of the specific brand listed under each of the parent companies in Figure 19–1, when they are combined, they create for the parent company something called *economies of scale*. Economies of scale are cost advantages reaped by companies when production becomes efficient. Companies can achieve economies of scale by increasing production and lowering costs. This happens because costs are spread over a larger number of goods. In summary, it is these economies of scale that are achieved through the vertical integration shown in Figure 19–1.

Vertical Integration

Vertical integration is a business arrangement in which a company controls *different stages along the supply chain*. Recall that a supply chain is a network of companies and people that are involved in the production and delivery of a product or service. The components of a supply chain include producers, vendors, warehouses, transportation companies, distribution centers, and retailers. Instead of relying on external vendors, the company strives to bring processes in-house to have better control over the production or distribution process. In the case of the hearing care industry, the parent or holding company strives to control costs and increase profits by overseeing more of the supply chain. For example, when a parent or holding company owns a hearing aid manufacturer and a network of retail locations, they can control more of the distribution of the devices that they manufacture. The parent company, by owning both the manufacturer and the retail, controls the distribution of their products.

From the perspective of the audiologist, vertical integration has its pros and cons, and a detailed discussion of them is beyond the scope of this chapter, but the goal of vertical integration is to streamline processes for more efficient operations of the business. With a few exceptions shown on the far lefthand side of Figure 19–1, the hearing care industry is *highly vertically integrated*.

Vertical integration is the result of corporate roll-up mergers. A roll-up merger is when an investor, such as a private equity firm or holding company, buys up companies in the same market and merges them together. *Roll-up* mergers, also known as a "roll up" or a "rollup," combine multiple small companies into a larger entity that is better positioned to enjoy economies of scale. The fact that the oldest or often the largest subsidiary within a vertically integrated hearing care rollup is a hearing aid manufacturer is revealing. This process suggests that the hearing aid manufacturer is often the most profitable and efficient entity within the larger vertically integrated organization and that they are looking for retailers who can sell their products. By purchasing (or rolling up) these retailers into the larger parent organization, they can control the distribution of their products.

Vertically integrated companies have been a part of audiology for at least 25 years. Until the late 1990s, there were more than a dozen independently

owned hearing aid manufacturers and more than 80% of all audiology practices were independently owned and operated "mom-and-pop" shops. This all changed rather quickly around 2000, at the early stages of the so-called digital hearing aid era, when it became more costly to manufacture hearing aids. At that time, a major investment in capital was required to have the infrastructure to transition from manufacturing analog to digital devices. In the early 2000s, the market demanded digital devices and if a company was still manufacturing analog devices, that company was at great risk of going out of business because no one wanted to buy outdated analog hearing aids. Due to the added costs associated with staying competitive, many small independent analog hearing aid manufacturers could no longer keep up with market demands and were acquired by larger companies. As hearing aid manufacturers became larger, they sought more retailers who could dispense their devices to consumers. This led to hearing aid manufacturers buying retailers, which, in turn, guaranteed the distribution of their products. Over time, more hearing aid brands and other entities, such as buying groups, were also added to the vertically integrated company to remain competitive and efficient.

Although vertically integrated companies are known to be "corporate," with their own hierarchical structures and bureaucracies, and given their sheer size and the array of businesses within their "rollup," each parent company employs dozens of audiologists. These vertically integrated companies provide many employment opportunities for audiologists. For example, one large holding company can employ audiologists who are clinicians within their retail locations, sales and marketing representatives within their hearing aid manufacturers, technical support staff, research entities, and a range of management positions who oversee the various entities within the vertically integrated enterprise.

With respect to the profession of audiology, there is also a potential *downside* to vertical integration. The more vertically integrated an industry, the greater the financial and managerial resources are required to enter and compete in it. Established companies in an industry may combine their operations as a way of raising the stakes and discouraging potential new entrants (Chapter 5). This lack of competition suggests that in the future, it could be more challenging for independent audiologists to operate a private practice. Consider this from the perspective of a newly graduated audiologist who is looking for their first employment opportunity. Given the growing number of corporate-owned clinics, it might be easier (but less lucrative) to join several "big-box" retailers and forgo the chance to join a smaller, less efficiently operated private practice. Fortunately, as other chapters in this book attest, lucrative private practice opportunities still readily exist.

New OTC Entrants

Over-the-counter (OTC) hearing aids became an officially FDA-codified category of hearing devices in October 2022. Since that time, it is estimated that more than 500,000 OTC devices have been sold to consumers via either in-person or web-based channels. Currently, there are more than a dozen OTC manufacturers, including several

mainline prescription hearing aid manufacturers partnering with consumer electronic companies. For example, WS Audiology has partnered with Sony and Sonova has partnered with Sennheiser to bring OTCs to market. A detailed review of the various components of OTC regulations and types of OTCs is beyond the scope of this chapter. However, the emergence of OTC presents opportunities for clinical audiologists:

- Should I dispense OTCs?
- If I dispense them, should I sell them only on a website or in my clinic?
- Should I provide services for those who purchased their OTC devices elsewhere?
- What OTCs shall I sell?
- Will OTCs cannibalize my business?

The best business management advice that can be provided at this 2024 writing is . . . *stay tuned*. The OTC category is new, and no one knows how their availability will change the way hearing aids are sold. Early data appear to suggest that OTC buyers are about 10 years younger than buyers of traditional (or the now called "prescription") hearing aids. From a business perspective, OTCs could be a lead generator, a type of starter device for younger individuals with milder hearing loss, who eventually migrate to prescription hearing aids that are dispensed with full service through the clinical audiology channel.

Managing Vendor Relationships

The second half of this chapter deals with how audiologists can more successfully manage their relationship with vendors. The emphasis in this section focuses on all the factors associated with this relationship, including negotiating wholesale price and unit commitments. First, it points out why the audiologist-vendor relationship is so vital to the long-term success of any practice.

Consider the Following Worst-Case Scenario

It has never been more important to know how to select a manufacturing group and their line of hearing instruments. Equally important, it is critical to know when to change to another manufacturer. While selecting and departing a manufacturer-partner relationship, there are two extremely important decisions that are quite different as they both impact the quality of services provided within the practice as well as the bottom line of the operation. The story below underscores just how players are involved in the delivery of professional services throughout the patient's journey, a process that begins when an appointment is made in the clinic and continues through years of follow-up care. Any weak point along this journey, through no fault of the clinician, can derail the entire customer experience. A decade of outstanding care and service can be ruined in an instance by someone involved in the process who happens to be in an office a half a world away from the clinic where the devices were purchased. Hearing aid patients and their family members are, generally, a forgiving lot. However, this is true only up to a critical point of intolerance. When it comes to poor quality or inconsistent service, every consumer has their breaking point. Check out the situation in the boxes.

HOW MANY TIMES HAS THIS HAPPENED IN YOUR PRACTICE?

A hearing aid patient returns to pick up his repaired hearing instrument and his wife waits wearily in the room with him. The clinician enters the room with appropriate greetings, perhaps a comment on the weather and full confidence that the hearing instrument about to be replaced in the patient's ear is in full working order with the same programming, the same earmold, all ready to go when the clinician notices the serial number does not match the patient's records or the instrument fails to activate despite being fully charged. Other issues may be that it is the left instrument in your hand when a right device was sent in for repair, or the patient says the hearing aid sounds terrible in his ear and objective test box measures confirm there is a gross mismatch between actual and specified performance.

As beads of sweat develop on the audiologist's forehead, the patient and his wife look as if this situation is some sort of cruel joke since the

continued on next page

continued from previous page

responsibility rests with the clinician for all the things that make up the total picture of hearing care, including the repair, the replacement, and successful refitting of the devices. It matters not to the patient that the audiologist or case manager could not open the instrument and replace a chip or a microphone assembly if their life depended on it: It is the audiologist's responsibility, not the repair team at the manufacturing facility. Because the audiologist will bear the brunt of patient and family dissatisfaction, it is up to you as the care provider to step up to the plate and swing away as the patient's advocate. That duty is unequivocal and clearly defined, no matter the venue of your practice.

"I AM ONLY AS GOOD AS YOU WILL PERMIT ME TO BE . . ."

This aphorism should be repeated to every repair manager and inside sales representative until such time that each finally begins to see the big picture of having patients in the office appropriately disgusted by the fact that their hearing instrument needs to be sent to the manufacturing facility for its third repair in as many months. At the repair laboratory, the technician sits at their desk on the phone while the clinician faces an angry patient, convinced the hearing instrument placed in their ear will never work despite extensive diagnostic testing, counseling, and emotional preparation to the contrary.

Repair managers do not have to figure out a reasonable apology scheme for disgruntled patients and family members. It is true that the audiologist is *only as good as the repair team or manufacturer (new instruments DOA) will permit*. Virtually all clinicians have experienced a clinical problem, sometimes fantasizing about how it would feel to be able to jam our hands through the telephone and around the neck of the repair manager or inside sales representative, each of whom promised the world and delivered more problems. The key point:

The clinician, who happens to bear the brunt of responsibility because they are directly interacting with the customer, has an obligation to manage this relationship with the vendor to ensure this scenario is unlikely to occur.

Hearing Instrument Manufacturer and Audiologist: A Symbiotic Relationship

Audiologists and hearing instrument manufacturers alike have contributions to make and responsibilities to assume in a hearing aid patient's journey from diagnostic assessment to wearing hearing instruments with a high degree of satisfaction. It is the responsibility of the audiologist to blend the needs of the patient with the manufacturer who provides optimal technology for that person. It is the audiologist's significant contribution of assessment, instrument selection, and application/adjustment that forms the continuum of care for every individual seeking treatment.

The hearing instrument manufacturer has the responsibility to provide sophisticated instruments and support systems such that audiologists can readily apply these technologies within their continuum of care. A symbiotic relationship exists when reliance becomes mutually beneficial so that the patient is the direct recipient of the interdependent function of each group.

Instrument manufacturers have tremendous responsibilities in this relationship. It is their responsibility to provide audiologists with innovative solutions to hearing loss, including improved chip technology and transducers, better clarity in noise, improved reliability of operation, user-friendly fitting software, ease of modifiability, and personalized in-house service. The instrument manufacturer logically and for obvious, intrinsic reasons accepts the burden of educating audiologists about the options and instrument-specific advantages avail-

able to maximize hearing benefits in their product lines. Whether the training is delivered in the audiologist's office by a manufacturer's field representative, provided at their facility, online, or in a large Continuing Education Unit (CEU) event, the manufacturer must have a readily available and systematic training program to ensure that audiologists are maximizing the potential of their technologies. If the instruments and their technological advantages are not applied effectively in the patient's ear, the expense of extensive research and development is lost.

It is also the responsibility of instrument manufacturers to produce evidence that all claims made about their products are valid, unequivocal, and, most importantly, readily noticed by hearing aid patients. Product claims are monitored by the FDA, and manufacturers are obligated to follow their claims guidelines. The ultimate metrics of success of the relationship between manufacturers and clinicians is the level of patient satisfaction and the observations of those communicating with the patient wearing the hearing instruments.

Patient Satisfaction and Modern Hearing Aid Technology

Patient satisfaction with their hearing instruments has been steadily improving over the last several years, and it appears to be directly related to advances in newer features such as patient-controlled apps, direct Bluetooth streaming, and rechargeable devices. Recent industry reports indicate that overall patient satisfaction to be greater than 80%. MarkeTrak (MT) 2022 is the latest version of a recurring survey of hundreds of individuals with hearing loss, many of whom are owners of hearing aids. One of the most remarkable findings in MT 2022 is just how often hearing aids are reported to regularly improve the quality of life of patients. These quality-of-life improvements have steadily risen over the past three MarkeTrak reports. In 2015, 48% of respondents stated that hearing aids regularly improved their quality of life, and in 2022, this number increased to 64% (Picou, 2022).

Over the past decade, there have been a myriad of observational studies suggesting hearing aid use directly contributes to better overall quality of life. Among the many quality-of-life factors believed to be affected by hearing aid use are improved physical activity (e.g., Martinez-Amezcua et al., 2021), a slowing of cognitive decline, and increased levels of social activity (e.g., Holman et al., 2021). In one example, Campos et al. (2023) compiled survey data from 299 adult hearing aid patients. Their analysis found a 50% reduction in the odds of experiencing a fall for hearing aid users compared with nonusers. These data suggest that the use of hearing aids—especially consistent hearing aid use—is associated with lower odds of experiencing a fall.

Another example can be found in the recently published ACHIEVE study, the first randomized controlled trial to evaluate the potential for treating hearing loss stemming from cognitive decline (Lin et al., 2023). The study followed 977 participants, aged 70 to 84 with untreated hearing loss and limited cognitive decline, over 3 years. Participants were recruited from two sources: (1) existing participants in the Athero-

sclerosis Risk in Communities (ARIC) study, an ongoing study of cardiovascular health with participants initially recruited in 1987–1989, and (2) de novo community volunteers. Participants from the ARIC study had higher levels of diabetes and hypertension, and they were more likely to live alone. Each participant was assigned to a hearing loss treatment group or a health education control group. They were followed for 3 years and assessed on thinking ability and memory skills. In the higher-risk population (ARIC group), the study showed that participants in the hearing aid treatment group had a 48% reduction in cognitive decline. Those participants who did experience a significant slowing of cognitive decline had high adherence (i.e., regularly wore hearing aids every day) to the hearing intervention over the 3-year study period.

These studies, which indicate hearing aid use improves various facets of quality of life, have one commonality: The study participants who experienced significant improvements tended to wear their hearing aids several hours per day, every day. Although indisputable evidence remains elusive, it is reasonable to assume many of these quality-of-life improvements are associated with a new generation of features and app updates, most of which were not widely available in hearing aids just a few years ago. This new generation of hearing aids, for the appropriate candidate, provides additional functionality for their users. Added functionality, in turn, leads to higher levels of satisfaction, as evidenced in the MT 2022 report, which showed that patients with devices using rechargeable batteries, downloadable user-controlled apps, and wireless streamers (for the television or a companion microphone) tend to report higher levels of satisfaction compared to those who do not use these features.

products that will represent the audiologist and their practice to the consumers of products and services within their practice.

Choosing a Vendor

The choice of vendors is a major decision for any practice owner or clinic manager. There are a myriad of important factors involved in this decision. While those discussed above are very important, other components of the decision must be considered relative to the

Evolutionary Noise Suppression Technology

Audiologists should choose a hearing instrument manufacturer based on much more than price breaks and aggressive marketing campaigns. Technological and connectivity considerations, instrument costs, warranties, customer service, repair

---

EVALUATING VENDORS

In addition to the wholesale purchase of hearing aids, audiologists rely on noninstrument vendors for equipment, tools, supplies, and resale accessories used in their daily practice. Audiologists must insist vendors are transparent in all their communications. The following factors should be considered when selecting any vendor:

- *Price.* Pricing is an important factor in selecting a vendor. However, given the instability of product pricing in the hearing healthcare industry, price may not be the most critical element in choosing a vendor. Occasionally, vendors offer lower prices on a particular product as a limited, promotional effort. Vendors with greater sales volumes may pass their price breaks, and lower prices, on to their customers— but don't hold your breath waiting.
- *Breadth of product line.* Breadth of product line refers to the number and variety of products offered by a vendor. The more products offered by a vendor, the less likely a practice will have to divert staff effort engaging multiple vendors. If a good vendor is found, support them.
- *Resource capability.* Vendors committed to and effective in serving as a resource to their customers offer invaluable advantages. Those willing and able to research alternative products when items are discontinued provide an important service to busy practitioners.

continued on next page

continued from previous page

■ *Ease of doing business.* Vendors who forgo complicated credit applications and minimum purchase requirements should be considered over those with rigid requirements. Vendors should offer a variety of opportunities to order products (i.e., phone orders, fax, website, email) with varied payment methods and straightforward payment terms.

■ *Return policies.* It is important to establish a relationship with a vendor offering reasonable return policies. Vendors with limited opportunity for customers to return defective items or items that did not meet expectations may not be acting in the best interest of the audiologist or the patients served. Return policies should be unencumbered and without significant delay in issuing credits or refunds for returned products.

■ *Product availability/backorder policy.* Vendors should provide products in a timely fashion. Avoid those who are routinely out of stock or need to consistently back-order items. In the event of a back-order situation, use those vendors willing to deliver back-ordered items without additional shipping charges.

■ *Vendor independence.* Independent distributors, not owned or financially affiliated with product manufacturers, are in the best position to offer customers an unbiased, objective perspective about products.

turnaround times, and educational opportunities are but a few important items to consider when choosing a hearing instrument manufacturer for a practice.

When evaluating a manufacturer's portfolio of technologies and form factors, many characteristics should be considered. The most logical starting point in that evaluation should be the needs of the customers or patients commonly seen in the practice: What are the typical characteristics and range of hearing levels commonly seen? For example, if the practice is in a highly industrialized area, there will be a higher percentage of noise-induced hearing loss with stereotypical high-frequency "noise notch" configurations. The manufacturer's portfolio should, therefore, include high-frequency emphasis offerings with open fitting platforms. If the practice is in a pediatric hospital seeing youngsters with moderate-to-severe losses, fitting needs will differ and the manufacturer should have a well-developed series of pediatric-focused instruments with adequate power, processing capabilities, and linkability to FM systems. Fortunately, today it is possible that any of the leading vendors can provide all these features. Currently, the five major hearing aid manufacturers all offer effective noise management strategies, albeit in different ways. Additionally, all manufacturers provide a variety of form factors that appeal to a wide range of potential patients. Consequently, no single manufacturer has a competitive advantage over the others in issues related to signal processing and form factor design. Because the technology playing field is level, other factors must be considered when choosing a preferred vendor.

The first is how noise suppression technology is implemented. There are two main techniques that hearing aids use to improve speech understanding in noise:

■ Directional microphones or spatially based noise suppression.
■ Digital noise reduction or process-based noise suppression.

All modern prescription hearing aids use both types. A directional microphone will typically assume that the sound of interest for a person is the one right in front of them. The directional microphone uses beamformers to focus on the sound in the frontal hemisphere of the patient. Some manufacturers use a two-mic array beamforming system while others use a four-mic array beamforming system. Simultaneously, digital noise reduction is used to detect and reduce background noise. In this process, the devices can use clues from frequency and intensity of sound to identify the background noises. Some manufacturers rely on a fixed postfiltering system to separate noise from speech, and others rely on a deep neural network to identify noise and attenuate it. Today, four-mic arrays are most effective at improving the signal-to-noise ratio of the patient's listening environments. Presently, the manufacturers that

offer a four-mic array beamforming system are Resound, Phonak, and Signia.

Directional microphones (spatially based noise suppression) may work well in a lab setting but there are many scenarios where a person wants to hear someone who is not in their frontal hemisphere. Removing background noise with postfiltering algorithms has its own issues. The absence of all background noise makes the sound seem unnatural. People still want to hear the background sounds to maintain some sense of their listening environment, but they also want to choose to ignore them the same way as natural hearing.

Postfiltering or digital noise reduction also does not work well to identify speech if the background noise is also speech, a phenomenon known as "the cocktail party problem." Hearing aids can effectively detect that the hum of an air conditioner or the sound of a car engine is background noise. These sounds, compared to speech, are steady state and easy for modern hearing aids to detect and attenuate. In contrast, however, multiple talkers in the same room are exceedingly difficult for hearing aids to filter the sound as the talker of interest tends to shift instantaneously. In these situations, noise suppression systems of all types struggle to separate the talkers of interest from other noises, including the din of other people talking.

For the most part, improvements in the noise suppression features in hearing aids over the past 30 years have tended to be evolutionary rather than revolutionary. However, some manufacturers have already begun to incorporate them and that has demonstrated promise; therefore, artificial intelligence (AI) and machine learning could lead to extraordinary progress in hearing aids' ability to recognize the patient's listening intent. One foundation of an effective audiologist-vendor relationship is that the hearing aid manufacturer clearly and honestly communicates updates in their signal-processing platform. Given that every manufacturer of prescription hearing aids now launches new platforms and features on an annual basis, it is essential for audiologists to be kept informed about how these new platforms and features will benefit patients. Audiologists must demand they receive information about these launches from vendors in an un-varnished, evidence-based manner, devoid of marketing puffery.

Assistive Technologies and Compatibility

Hearing aid manufacturers build or distribute a range of other amplification products. There are a host of accessories to improve hearing and listening in specific conditions that are coupled to hearing instruments via direct audio input, infrared, Bluetooth integration, and electromagnetic inductance. Many

---

THE IMPORTANCE OF MANUFACTURER FIELD REPRESENTATIVES

Manufacturer field representatives provide a great service to practitioners and hearing aid patients alike. They offer quick, pragmatic information not readily available in printed bulletins or product descriptions issued by the manufacturer. Their information is gleaned from their travels within their territory interacting with their customer base. Consequently, effective sales representatives are trusted advisors who willingly share helpful information in an honest and ethical manner. Some of the valuable services they provide include:

- Training in products, software, and specific technical information.
- Establishing which patients are best suited for specific instruments.
- Offering comparisons across competitive product lines.
- Sharing tricks, gimmicks, and insights gleaned from other users of the product.
- Solving specific patient difficulties common to an instrument line.
- Assisting in developing realistic pricing for the practice's demographic.
- Advising on how others are implementing clinical best practices.
- Providing insights on pricing and positioning of bundled and unbundled packages.

of these accessories will be phased out with the advent of *Bluetooth 2.0* and *Auracast*, but that will take about a decade. Consequently, audiologists must be familiar with myriad accessories. Both assistive listening systems (ALSs) and assistive listening devices (ALDs) require specific interfacing technologies from teleloop compatibility to inductor coils specifically designed to enhance cell phone use. Compatibility with an ever-expanding group of devices developed to improve the signal-to-noise ratio and enhance speech recognition in difficult listening situations must be considered an important part of every aural rehabilitation effort. A manufacturer should have a well-developed portfolio of ALSs or ALDs or have easy access or modification routines so that their hearing instruments can interface readily with systems available elsewhere in the market. Every manufacturer now offers wireless remote microphones that significantly improve the signal-to-noise ratio of the listening situation. Additionally, rechargeable batteries have almost completely replaced conventional battery pills, something truly beneficial for those struggling with battery manipulation.

Whether it be something as simple as enjoying a sermon at church or hearing well at a meeting in a hard-walled, highly reverberant conference room, these innovative technologies are critically important to the patient and to their families as well. They not only make the products easier to use but also lend a level of patient communication/integration into difficult listening situations, reducing the numbers of environments and/or communication situations that may have been avoided altogether.

Programming Connectivity: Ease of Connecting to the Instrument

With the advent of programmable hearing instruments, a dilemma emerged for both instrument development engineers and audiologists fitting the hearing instruments: how best to connect the instrument with the programming system. This dilemma seemingly went from bad to worse in a brief period. Initially, most of the connectivity was completed with cumbersome yet "easy-to-connect" plugs to fit into capped receptacles on the instrument. Once connected, they remained connected and data transfer was relatively easily completed. Pull the connector and replace the cap to the programming port, and the commands or data were transferred and the session was done.

The ports were large and the economy of space issue inherent in the miniaturization process of hearing instruments began to win out as programming ribbons and other smaller connection systems were developed. These attempts at size reduction created, in some instances, an entirely new set of problems for the end user. The manufacturing community *could have* come together and agreed on consistent usage of size and shape of connectors, but that would have been too easy. At the time, audiologists had to have an extensive array of connecting gear and ribbons and "whatnot" to access the hearing instrument for programming or adjustment.

In this modern era (circa 2024), connectivity is no longer a problem. Bluetooth connectivity is essentially instantaneous and seamless. Nevertheless, many audiologists continue to maintain a cache of older connectors and connection boxes for those patients who continue to use older instruments.

Clinician-Friendly Software

There are many issues of equal concern to audiologists with this vendor relationship. Among the "Big 5" vendors, there are great differences in the usability, effectiveness, and simplicity of hearing instrument manufacturers' programming software systems. Some require wading through two or three screens before approaching the initial programming screen. Other programming software has little or no navigation indicators to advise the user exactly where they are in the programming sequence. Of course, an audiologist's opinion about the ease of use of a specific manufacturer's fitting software is mainly driven by familiarity with it. If a clinician seldom fits a certain brand, they are likely to believe the fitting software of that brand will be challenging to navigate. This can create a sense of being lost within the program and often results in having to restart the programming sequence. Time and confidence in the programming system are lost as the patient perceives palpable frustration. No matter the intent of the software developers, programming protocols that require disproportionate amounts of time and effort will subject the manufacturer to the financial risk of losing valuable dispensers.

Evaluating the usability of programming software systems does not require the skills or knowledge of a software developer. The audiologist working with patients every day quickly develops a sense of usability and inherent time constraints that a poorly designed program brings to the patient's visit. There are several basic aspects of software programs that can be used to evaluate hearing instrument programming software. Although not a set of absolute rules, these recommended actions, programming transformations, screen prompts, and messages provide guidelines to be used in comparing software program offerings of hearing instrument manufacturers—these recommendations remain as important in 2024 as they were when originally set forth more than 20 years ago:

1. A time-focused hearing instrument software system should permit initial programming within four keystrokes after auditory data describing the patient's hearing loss are entered in the program.
2. The software should provide an instant reading of the instruments being programmed and display the serial number and specific model details upon initial connection to the software.
3. Software users (hereinafter, audiologists will be considered the "users") must be able to accomplish their task in a naturally occurring order of events—the programming task must be in an order that makes sense to the user so that they do not have to change screens or otherwise search for solutions in other levels of the software.
4. Wording in on-screen messages should be easily understood, concise, and unambiguous.
5. All recent actions or commands completed by the user should be easily reversible by "undo" com-

mands, which would allow escape routines from specific operations in motion.

6. The programming software should be solution driven with "go to" symptom and solution selection lists to logically help the patient with their various performance complaints. The more automatic the resolution of definable problems, the faster the instruments are programmed or reprogrammed and the quicker the patient can begin to adjust to their new instruments.

7. The software must permit access to all definable parameters of the hearing instrument. Compression ratios, output by channels or frequency bands, processing speed and integration of attack and release times, and similar modifiable functions should be accessible to the audiologist programming the instrument for the patient.

8. The software must provide pulldown lists and reminders to foster recall by the clinician. With so many opportunities for optimizing the instrument fitting, it is difficult to commit to memory various routines and subroutines that may be important for the unique needs of individual patients.

9. The software must be configured to provide a printout or easily retrievable electronic record of actions by dates for each instrument programmed or adjusted after the initial programming. This record is important since it is not uncommon to have to undo programming that failed to improve a patient's particular situation. If a record is retained, the original programming configuration can be reinstated in the hearing instruments. This is an important feature since many patients will want to return to the initial settings to compare their performance in varied environments.

10. Photos of the hearing instruments in situ and patient-friendly lists of features along with audiologic findings superimposed on the effective fitting range of the instruments should be readily available to the audiologist and patients in the initial phases of counseling and preparation for the fitting.

The bottom line with respect to user-friendly fitting software is that it is much more intuitive and easier to use today than at any time in history; therefore, it is likely to become even easier to use over the next decade. The challenge is that every hearing aid manufacturer has so many models and features that it is nearly impossible for the audiologist to have intimate knowledge of every manufacturer's fitting software. Thus, it is advisable *to choose two or three manufacturers* and get to know the intricacies of their software. For audiologists employed in a large clinical setting with more than three audiologists, it is helpful for each audiologist to become intimately familiar with two or three fitting software programs. As a result, all major manufacturers are collectively known by the entire staff.

Hearing Instrument Acquisition Costs

One of the most important determinants in selecting a hearing instrument manufacturer is instrument acquisition cost. A substantial part of acquisition costs is the per-unit cost of goods or wholesale cost of each device purchased. More than just the per-unit cost should be included in the assessment. Some of these issues may not seem relatable to costs, but they will impact the practice. A good example of an important, yet nonmonetary cost factor involves the time span from placing an order to the arrival of the new or repaired hearing instrument. If Manufacturer A takes 10 days to 2 weeks to deliver a new or repaired instrument and Manufacturer B delivers in 7 days, these different schedules can be critical to patient satisfaction and, therefore, the long-term success of the practice. A few days to a week from order to arrival is often a critical time frame for a patient and family waiting for a new or repaired hearing instrument. There are other determinants involving costs and financial operations to consider in choosing a hearing instrument manufacturer. This will be covered in the following sections.

Range of Instrument Costs Across the Product Line

Most major instrument manufacturers develop a wide-ranging lineup of circuitry and instrument types within their product line. Manufacturers strive to provide a comprehensive array of offerings so that an audiologist will be able to select an instrument appropriate for a broad base of patient needs. Some of the models and features that audiologists need to ensure that their vendor of choice is carrying are:

■ Models for severe-profound hearing loss.
■ Tinnitus masking devices.

■ Custom-made earmolds for receiver-in-canal (RIC) devices.
■ Form factors in a wide range of colors.
■ Easy-to-replace receiver kits.
■ A diverse range of instant-fit ear tips.
■ Infrequently recommended features (i.e., extended bandwidth and frequency lowering).

Paying the Bills

Instrument manufacturers generally function on a 30- to 45-day payment policy. This means the practice is expected to pay the bill for the instrument completely (net) within that specified payment period. The longer the payment cycle, the greater the time the manufacturer has granted to pay the bill in full. In effect, the manufacturer is providing a loan for the period of the defined payment cycle. There might be penalties or interest charges if the bill is not paid within a specific period. Depending on the status of the practice as a customer, there may be an extended payment time period. The terms of payment should be taken into consideration when choosing a manufacturer. The longer the payment cycle, even by as little as 15 days, the longer operating funds are kept intact. Penalties for overextending the payment deadlines should be clearly stated, and if not, the Accounting Department of that respective manufacturer should be contacted to clarify the situation, preferably in writing. An additional measure of a good manufacturer is a readily available Accounting Department focused on account resolution. Most are quite pleased to review a statement and assist in resolving any confusion or incorrect entries.

The account statement should be logical and easy to read, and it should balance relative to known orders, payments, and credits for returns. If office personnel or the accountant has trouble making sense of the format of the account, request a format change. Should the Accounting Department fail to consistently provide an accurate statement, a true accounting of the orders, payments, and credits, the practice should consider another manufacturer. Resolving errors in the manufacturer's statement is time-consuming and frustrating for the audiologist and their office personnel. The clinic's part of the bargain in the business transaction is paying the bills on time. The manufacturer's part is to provide an accurate accounting of transactions in the statements.

Repair Resolution and Warranties

Hearing instrument repairs are perplexing to the patient and to the audiologist managing the person's aural rehabilitation. Despite the improvement in patient satisfaction with digital hearing instruments, there remains the ever-present issue with hearing instrument repairs. The next several sections provide insights on how to manage repairs, something that stubbornly remains an obstacle, at least to some degree, in any audiology practice. Given the added cost to the patient and the inconveniences associated with bringing the hearing aids back to the clinic because of a malfunction, having a clear strategy for managing repairs is essential. Obviously, the patient wants their hearing aid back as soon as possible; therefore, it is helpful to have a good

relationship with a manager inside the repair lab of the manufacturer, so that when questions arise about the timing of repair shipments and other issues, there is a person that can be contacted to expedite the process.

Rates of Repairs

It is difficult to determine the rates at which hearing instruments require out-of-office repairs. Although statistics on hearing instrument repairs are kept by manufacturers, neither the consuming public nor the audiology community is commonly privy to these data. Conventional wisdom (largely based on the experiences of clinicians) suggests rates of repairs on most instruments in the first year postfitting range from 10% to as much as 18% of instruments dispensed. The second- and third-year rates of repairs flatten to approximately 20% to 25%. By the fifth-year postfitting, 30% to 40% of instruments will likely undergo an out-of-office repair. Cerumen and moisture are the two leading causes of repairs.

Glaser (2017) has monitored the incidence of repairs and postfitting rates of occurrence in his practice for more than 30 years across several manufacturers, instrument styles, and various levels of circuitry. His data indicate there has been 18% fewer returns to manufacturers for repairs within the first postfitting year from 2008 to 2016. Current data have changed little; the rate of re-repairs (defined as a repaired instrument returned to the manufacturer within 45 days of the original repair date) has declined at a similar rate within the same period. The reasons for the improvements most likely include improvements in the stability of transducers and chip technology to better preventive measures to reduce repairs related to cerumen and improved manufacturing processes. There remains no substitute for training the patient and at least one other family member how to clean the hearing instruments and to do so at least three or four times per week. With the advent of electronic drying systems and better instruction in instrument care, cleaning, and maintenance, fewer returns for repairs should continue to improve. Further, given that about 80% or more of devices sold in the United States are RIC style, coupled to most ears with a noncustom, instant-fit ear tip, routine wax problems can be easily solved in the office with a quick change of the ear tip or receiver.

Establishing a Benchmark for Instrument Repairs

It is difficult to establish a benchmark for an "expected" number of hearing instrument repairs. From the patient's viewpoint, there should be zero tolerance for repairs. Audiologists agree there should be zero tolerance for repairs. The reality of the situation dictates reasonable acceptance of some repairs since electronic equipment in general and hearing instruments specifically are inherently prone to failure from time to time. It is unreasonable to assume that hearing instruments can be developed that are not subject to the need for out-of-office repairs. It is also difficult to develop a benchmark on repairs without an accurate accounting of the numbers of repairs occurring as a function of the date of the instrument being fitted. Knowing the pattern of repairs as a function of the fitting date provides an opportunity

to develop a prospective guide of what to expect of a specific model within an instrument line.

Based on well-kept anecdotal records of a single practice (Glaser, 2017) described above, the following represents an example of an anticipated repair rate that has been generated based on previous data for an approximated volume of 350 instruments per year:

■ Less than 18% of instruments fit within the first year require out-of-office repair.
■ Less than 15% of instruments in the second and third years postfitting require out-of-office repairs.
■ Less than 15% of instruments in the fourth and fifth years postfitting require out-of-office repairs.

Considering the numbers of repairs that will require a return trip to the manufacturer for repair, it becomes readily apparent that out-of-office repairs cost a great deal of time and money as well as increased levels of patient dissatisfaction and discord. However, by reducing repair rates, not only will the practice have more time to schedule new patients, but there will also be a concurrent increase in patient satisfaction. No matter how fast the return of the repaired instrument to the patient or how many warranty extensions the manufacturer is willing to issue, repairs are unacceptable to patients and family members who have come to appreciate the benefits of appropriately fitted hearing instruments.

Counseling Patients About Hearing Instrument Repairs

Beyond counseling and advising the rates of repairs, there are a few methods to assist patients in developing realistic expectations about hearing instrument repairs. As with counseling the patient and family about the importance of developing realistic expectations of improved communication performance, counseling about the incidence of hearing instrument repairs should be equally realistic. Zero percent repairs is an unrealistic expectation despite remarkable advances in contemporary hearing instrument technology. Warranty periods are made available to the patient for a reason. They stand as indicators of the possibility that instrument repairs will be needed within a 2- or 3-year period after the fitting. Why else would a manufacturer build the cost of anticipated repairs into the single unit price of their hearing instruments with additional years of coverage available with an additional cost? The fact remains that hearing instruments are subject to a variety of external and internal forces that work against developing a performance history without repairs.

Patients and family must be given appropriate training in consistent instrument care and cleaning. They must be given every opportunity to develop good maintenance habits. At the fitting and during the immediate follow-up visits, care and maintenance routines should be assessed and restated, and all involved must demonstrate competencies in care and cleaning, proper insertion and removal of the battery or proper placement of the devices in the charger, and use of dehumidifying equipment. To reduce instrument loss, advise patients and family members to place the instruments in their case or charger whenever they need to remove them. Putting their instruments in a pocket or purse is inviting loss and damage. The more the family is involved in the care and maintenance of the patient's hearing instruments, the less likely they will be lost or require an out-of-warranty repair.

Return of Repaired Instruments by the Manufacturer/Repair Facility

Repairs should be returned to the practice by the manufacturer/repair facility within 7 to 10 working days. Most repairs require a 2- or 3-day in-house period. Shipping to and from manufacturers and repair facilities is commonly facilitated by retail shippers (e.g., FedEx, UPS). Pickup and delivery at the practice door reduces critical out-of-ear time and reduces the risk of loss and damage in transit. With improvements in shipping, the onus to improve the time it takes to repair and return the repair rests with the Repair Manager and the productivity and accuracy of the staff of technicians. And then there is the extra cost of an expedited repair. Does it really warrant the extra cost? Does the repair turnaround in-house faster with the extra fee? The answer, of course, depends on the manufacturer or repair facility, but there is usually a savings of 1 or 2 days at most—perhaps worth it to the executive who has an important board meeting or to a mother who must hear her children in the middle of the night. If repair facilities can improve turnaround time to the practice for an additional charge, it seems reasonable to expect that same repair department to improve their turnaround time without an additional charge levied for expected work.

Repair turnaround time should be monitored consistently and reviewed regularly. If the data indicate turnaround time is increasing, it must be considered a critical measure in deciding whether to seek another manufacturer or repair facility. Repairs are always a rough spot for patients. The longer it takes to return the instrument to the patient's ear, the greater the probability of reduced patient satisfaction and a loss of confidence in both the hearing instrument and the practitioner.

If the patient experiences greater than three repairs in an 18- to 24-month period postfitting, manufacturers commonly replace or re-plate (replace all major components within the shell) the instrument at no charge to the patient. If they do not consider this an option, they should be urged to do so on behalf of the patient and the practice. This replacement scheme covers the patient's needs; however, it does not account for diminishing profits in the practice when greater time is spent in repeated visits, reprogramming efforts, refitting, and recounseling the patient and family to regain at least a bit of confidence lost in the instrument and the practice. Too many unplanned "re-'s" result in lost revenue and respect that will not be replaced by an instrument manufacturer or repair facility.

Beyond Improving Rates of Repair: What Can Manufacturers Do?

Since manufacturers generally do not reimburse practitioners for lost time and revenue due to multiple repairs, there are a few items or issues manufacturers could incorporate to lessen the burden of audiologists responsible for fitting their products. Repaired instru-

ments returned without the original programming is irritating, time-consuming, and an unnecessary addition to the mayhem. Granted, it may take as little as 15 minutes to reestablish patient-specific programming data to pre-repair status, but a significant number of patients perceive differences in performance with the repaired instrument, no matter the programs, the manufacturer, or whether we have informed them of the need for postrepair reprogramming. Even if the chip must be replaced, it is best for all concerned when the repair technician spends the time transferring the programming information rather than having to repeat the programming in the office with patients and family members overseeing every move the audiologist makes. Retrieving and reprogramming the instrument at the repair facility must become an institutional priority and duty of repair technicians and every instrument manufacturer or repair facility. If audiologists fitting hearing instruments are asked, each will likely report they would happily pay a bit more for repairs if those completing the repairs would at least try to replace the programming.

Warranty Extensions on Re-Repairs

Re-repairs are poison to a patient and to a practice as well. Re-repairs provide the greatest source of broken confidence in both the hearing instrument and the practice. As one irate patient said recently, "What is it with you people? You can't even get a broken instrument repaired correctly at the manufacturing plant? That damn thing hasn't worked right from day one and here

I am a year and a half later and it still doesn't work right and you can't get it right even with two tries."

Little will satisfy a frustrated patient after having had their instrument repaired only to have it fail a second time within a month or two. Re-repairs should be discussed at the initial fitting, but few practitioners dwell on the topic for obvious reasons. A realistic expectation about a repair is one thing; there is no reality to the patient when it comes to multiple repairs in a brief period. Re-repairs should not happen in this modern era of digital technology with improved transducers and manufacturing processes.

Unfortunately, re-repairs do happen and the manufacturer should provide a liberal warranty extension after the fact. Issuing an additional 6 to 12 months of warranty on a 4-year-old instrument may represent a formula for loss for a manufacturer, but it should be the minimum consideration given the patient if for no other reason than to stand as an indication of confidence by the manufacturer that another "re-repair" will not be an issue. Simply put, the repair facility should have enough confidence in their capabilities to extend warranted repairs at no charge or with attenuating costs with each successive repair.

In general, offering an extended warranty on any hearing aid that is more than 3 years old is a sensible business strategy. In addition to negotiating extended warranty terms directly with hearing aid manufacturers, there are independent companies (e.g., https:// www.ESCO.com) that offer extended warranty coverage on virtually any hearing aid. Audiologists can provide patients of out-of-warranty devices coverage with the option of an extended warranty. An extended warranty usually covers loss and damage to the hearing aids for an annual fee. Offering extended warranty coverage is commonly done during annual office visits.

Manufacturer's In-House Staff Dedicated to Rapid Resolutions

Members of the call staff in a manufacturer's repair section are the first responders in a hearing instrument repair. They must be well trained in complaint resolution, be knowledgeable about the product line in general and specific idiosyncrasies of each circuit, and know the internal tracks to resolution. They must be as efficient and accommodating as the front office associates and just as available for consultation and inquiry. They represent the human touch of a system that can quickly become impersonal and inattentive. If they cannot solve the problem over the phone or by quickly consulting with the repair section of their company, they should request the instrument be sent to their desk for personalized attention. Each member of this important team must be dedicated to complaint resolution and acknowledge the caller's problem as unique to the practice deserving an equally unique response and prompt resolution.

Incidence of Repairs

The incidence of hearing instrument repairs by manufacturers must be monitored regularly. By logging all repairs, the practice is engaged in quality control. When repaired instruments are sent or received, a few minutes spent logging information about the repair provides compelling information about the manufacturer, instrument model, and repair history of the instrument. It takes little effort to gain additional, essential information beyond counting the number of repairs. By documenting repairs by circuit class or model, the practice will get a failure rate for each class of instrument dispensed (Table 19–1). Should a spike in the incidence data occur, an analysis will be at hand and a call to the manufacturer to discuss the dilemma must be made. If the particular model of interest continues to fail, it would be appropriate to stop fitting that instrument model. It would also be appropriate to reassess the past records of repairs and determine whether it is time to consider finding another vendor for hearing instruments.

How much data should be required to contact the manufacturer? That depends on several factors. Certainly, volume should be a factor:

- If the practice is dispensing a significant number of a specific model, the data will dictate the need quite readily.
- If the data show developing evidence that one in five instruments requires a return for repair, the manufacturer should be contacted immediately.

Advise the manufacturer of the findings and ask if they have noted similar difficulties with that model. They may have a fitting or modification suggestion that will resolve the repair issue. If the Repair Manager replies they have not seen a pattern in that instrument model, advise them that in this clinic, the instrument is failing. After you have stated the case with data, make it clear that if these failures continue, there will be no more orders forthcoming from the practice for this instrument model. Confirm the telephone conversation with the Repair Manager via email and

Table 19–1. Monitoring Repair Records by Manufacturer

Records of Repairs by Manufacturer												
	Jan	Feb	Mar	Apr	May	Jun	Jul	Aug	Sep	Oct	Nov	Dec
Model #												
< 1 yr												
1–2 yrs												
2–3 yrs												
3–5 yrs												
Re-Rep												
Cost												
Turnaround												

include copies to the inside sales staff member assigned to your account and to the president of the company.

Consistent problems in the practice should become known to every level within the product side of the instrument manufacturer's hierarchy. Presidents of hearing instrument manufacturing companies are sometimes the last to know there is a flaw in a specific model or circuit class. They understand that the audiologist acts as the patient's advocate in these matters. They also understand that the clinic will cease to dispense their products if repeated failures continue.

- If the incidence of repairs exceeds established practice benchmarks.
- If turnaround time on repairs is excessive.
- If the incidence of repairs is increasing and re-repairs are on the rise.

These and other issues presented in this discussion describe the need to move to another instrument manufacturer, and in many cases, it becomes undeniably evident, a "no-brainer." The bottom line of the practice requires optimum product reliability and fast and reliable resolution of any product line difficulties.

Changing Manufacturers: When It's Time to Switch

Patient satisfaction is tied to a variety of factors. When managing the experience of hearing aid patients in any practice, audiologists must recognize and accept the fact that patient satisfaction is tied directly to the hearing instrument and to the services provided by the audiologist directing the patient's hearing care in about the same measure.

Hearing instrument manufacturers must share in the responsibility for declining patient satisfaction when data indicate the root causes of the dissatisfaction reside with a quality problem of the hearing instrument. Lack of or lethargic responses to inquiries in the face of well-documented evidence that a segment of their product line is consistently failing should be a strong factor in the decision to seek another vendor for hearing instruments. In some cases, it may be the most important or singular reason to move to another instrument manufacturer. Other concerns are:

Establishing Perspective: Continuous Monitoring of Acquisition Costs

Some practice owners and managers tend to overlook the amount of money spent on the purchase of hearing instruments. It is as if they get lulled to sleep by the fact that instrument costs never decline and always increase, so why worry about that which cannot be controlled? In today's rapidly changing economy, changes in the costs of instruments seem to be coming more frequently than ever before. As such, there is an ever-stronger need to consistently monitor acquisition costs. It takes little time to read invoices to clarify the amount of money the practice sends to each manufacturer. It will put each manufacturer into a financial perspective and appropriately embolden the practice owner or manager to become more assertive in their advocacy efforts for their patients. If a specific instrument's cost has increased a substantial

Table 19–2. Records of Instruments Ordered and Received

Records of Instruments Ordered and Received				
Patient Name	Instrument Make/Model	Acquisition Cost	Running Total Manufacturer	Dates Ordered/ Received
	/	/	/	/

amount, contact the representative and find out why the spike in cost and ask about alternative pricing or suggestions about other items in their lineup that might serve as a viable alternative. Of course, if the alternatives offer little or no benefit, it is another valid signal to seek options available from other manufacturers. The previous year's total amount spent should be in the heading of the column to further recognize the level of participation with each manufacturer. A running tabulation of acquisition costs is a simple statistic to maintain relative to the valuable perspective it provides (Table 19–2). No less than monthly reviews will deliver the timeliness necessary to monitor these important data.

Managing Returns for Credit

Industry averages suggest that about 15% of all hearing aids purchased by an audiology practice are returned to the manufacturer. Returns can take two forms; they can be exchanged for a different model, or they can be returned outright. Given the nature of age-related hearing and the many maladaptive behaviors associated with it, returns are a natural part of the audiologist-vendor relationship. It is the responsibility to track returns for credit and exchanges, as well

as find methods to keep the return rate less than a benchmark of 10% to 15%. Like repairs, it is imperative that audiologists are keenly aware of return for credit policies. Items such as the number of days postpurchasing and nonrefundable fees should be established and placed in writing by the vendor.

Hearing Aid Pricing Basics

Before delving into the topic of price, it is important to state clearly and emphatically that this section of the chapter makes absolutely no attempt to assist in any way the setting of either wholesale or retail prices within an individual clinic. Many factors go into establishing those specific prices, and to assist in setting those terms would be unethical and perhaps even a violation of price fixing statutes. It is, however, a valuable lesson to discuss at a high level the range of wholesale prices found in various audiology clinics in the United States and, more importantly, why there is such a large range in wholesale prices.

Wholesale prices refer to the cost of a product from the hearing aid manufacturer to the clinician or clinic retailer. Pricing from the manufacturer plays a vital role in determining the final retail price of the devices and ultimately plays an essential role in the profitability of a practice. Wholesale prices are generally lower than retail prices as the retailer aims to make a profit.

The wholesale per-unit price an audiology practice pays for hearing aids is largely determined by their buying power. Essentially, the more devices a business buys over a given time frame, say a month, the greater their buying power. The largest buyers of hearing aids in the United States are the Veterans Administration (VA) and the big-box retail chain, Costco. Each of these businesses buys (or procures, as behemoth companies like to say) hundreds of hearing aids each month that are shipped to a central location and then distributed to their points of sales (clinics) around the country. Their buying power is reflected in the significantly lower per-unit wholesale prices they pay.

The VA began central procurement of hearing aids in 1955 as high numbers of veterans from World War II significantly increased demand. Today, hearing aids are purchased centrally through the VA Denver Acquisition and Logistics Center on a fixed price, on what are called indefinite quantity contracts. Contracts with hearing aid manufacturers are structured as a 1-year base period with an option for the VA to renew for four additional 1-year periods. Typically, the VA will extend contracts such that they last for the full 5 years. Wholesale purchase prices are negotiated upon renewal of the 5-year period. Because these contracts involve the potential sale of thousands of hearing aids, manufacturers commit tremendous resources, often in the form of a large, dedicated sales force and technical support staff that are solely devoted to the VA system.

Centralized contracting allows the VA to pay significantly lower prices than the market average due to the program's scale, something that no ordinary practice can do. The only other entities that have the scale and buying power of the VA are Costco and managed care organizations. In the case of Costco, their procurement process is similar to the VA with a large, centralized procurement center, while managed care organizations buy hearing aids from manufacturers and ship them directly to audiologists who have contracts with these managed care organizations.

According to the Bernstein Report (2024), the average wholesale price of hearing aids (excluding remotes), based on the VA monthly data, is $440 per unit compared to the average private wholesale market price from $600 to $1,100 per device. Given their buying powers, which is similar to the VA, Costco's wholesale price per unit is estimated to be between $350 and $450, while managed care organizations' wholesale per-unit price is estimated to be about $250. You might wonder why the VA has a higher per-unit wholesale price compared to both Costco and managed care organizations. The answer is because nearly 100% of the hearing aids purchased by the VA are premium-level technology, while managed care organizations, which have an obligation to their members to hold down total costs, tend to purchase more entry-level technology.

The important lesson here for audiologists managing a small business is that the wholesale cost will always be significantly higher than what these large companies with tremendous buying power muster. Consequently, independent and other smaller practices must carve out a competitive advantage focused on professional service and personalized support. Finally, even though smaller practices do not have the buying power of the VA, Costco, or managed care organizations, there is still plenty of room to negotiate wholesale prices.

Negotiating Price

There is an old adage among experienced managers that goes something like this: "Price, quality and service, pick two because you can't have all three." When it comes to vendor relations in the hearing care industry, that maxim rings true. When looking for a reliable vendor, it is important to keep in mind that it is impossible to obtain the lowest wholesale prices, the most reliable devices, and the most personalized customer service. The practice can, however, achieve two out of three.

Negotiating wholesale pricing, a critical aspect of the vendor-audiologist relationship, is the ability to bargain wholesale pricing along with other terms. Wholesale pricing has a direct relationship to the profitability of the clinic. If the audiologist can reduce their per-unit wholesale price by say, 20%, this is added savings that goes straight to the bottom line.

There is a direct relationship between wholesale price and units purchased. That is, the more units purchased from one hearing aid vendor will usually result in a lower per-unit wholesale price. In practical terms, this means that to get a better wholesale price (or a lower cost of goods), an audiologist needs to commit most of their business to fewer manufacturers. The lesson here for the inexperienced clinician who wants to be a business manager is that a narrower number of vendors with which business is conducted will allow more favorable terms on wholesale pricing.

This is especially true in smaller practices that might dispense fewer than 30 hearing aids per month. The practice can buy those 30 hearing aids from five manufacturers or agree to buy them from two manufacturers. By agreeing to a larger unit commitment from fewer vendors, the practice gains a lower per-unit wholesale price. Manufacturers prefer to do business with practices that buy a consistent number of units each month from a practice. Consistent buyers of, for example, 30 hearing aids per month from one manufacturer tend to have a deeper knowledge of the fitting software and features. Thus, high-volume customers (practices that buy 30 or more units per month) have fewer returns, have higher satisfaction, and are less expensive to maintain.

It is also important to point out that audiologists should not commit all their business to a single manufacturer. This is a risky proposition for a few reasons:

- It is important to have a range of signal-processing and form factor choices to make available to persons with hearing loss.
- Spreading business across a few vendors mitigates risks such as a spate of poor-quality devices resulting from a transducer recall or an unforeseen delay with a new product launch.
- Independent practices differentiate themselves by offering devices from multiple vendors.

All three of these points are achieved by doing business with more than one vendor. A final point about negotiating warrants a mention. As an owner or manager, it is pivotal to negotiate favorable pricing terms with vendors. This process starts with being a trusted partner that deals honestly and fairly with each vendor. Deal earnestly and fairly with vendors and the practice will be rewarded with smooth, nearly stress-free transactions.

Stocking Hearing Aids and Buying in Bulk

Receiver in the canal (RIC) hearing aids now comprise about 80% to 85% of all hearing aids dispensed in the United States. In the clinic, there are several advantages of RIC devices; they are cosmetically appealing, they can be fitted on the same day thanks to noncustom ear tips, and, these days, they are appropriate for just about any hearing loss. There are also some big advantages of RICs for hearing aid manufacturers, too. Because no part of the device is custom made for an individual's ear, they are less expensive to manufacture. Additionally, thanks to digital chip technology, each hearing aid provides several levels of technology. With a simple click of the mouse, before the hearing aid is shipped, it can be made a premium, mid-level, or basic-level device. This also keeps the production costs down. These are all reasons as to why upward of 82% of hearing aids sold today are RICs!

Finally, considering all the customization of the acoustic parameters (gain, output, compression) and coupling to the ear is done in the office, there is a natural incentive for vendors to offer practices large stocks of hearing aids. That is, manufacturers tend to offer bulk purchases of 10 or more devices that can be purchased in advance and then sit on the shelf awaiting use. Buying in bulk can be a win-win for all concerned. Manufacturers sell a larger number of units, and the practice lowers their cost of goods, but practice managers must be cognizant of overpurchasing.

Managers must discern how many devices they need on their shelf at any given time. This can be accomplished through careful tracking and knowing appropriately how many devices of a certain model or technology level are purchased every month. One advantage of bulk purchasing of hearing aids is wholesale pricing tends to be much lower than the single-unit cost. It is the responsibility of the owner or the manager to balance "great deals" of bulk purchases and to not overstock shelves with product that sits unused for several months.

The Key to Productivity

At the end of the day, there are just three methods of unlocking productivity in hearing aid dispensing businesses. Productivity in this case is defined as generating higher sums of revenue, which is a cornerstone of profit. All three methods are predicated on the sale of hearing aids. Over the course of a business cycle—a week, a month, or a year—these three parameters must be overseen by the manager.

- *Office traffic*. Traffic within the practice is directly related to marketing. The role of the manager is to ensure that more customers who need hearing aids know that the practice exists and are willing to make an appointment. This first element of productivity is largely a function of marketing and public relations (Chapter 12).

■ *Dispense more devices over the course of the business cycle.* This requires adequate time in the schedule to see customers more likely to need hearing aids and agree to acquire them at the end of a consultation. The overall effectiveness of this second element is directly related to having methodical consultative processes that lead to more patients agreeing to purchase hearing aids at the end of the appointment.

■ *Dispense more hearing aids at a higher average selling price or with larger margins (lower cost of goods).* The third element of productivity is a function of product mix and the ability to provide patients with added value for hearing aids dispensed at a higher price point. Additionally, this third aspect of productivity, average selling price and margins, is directly related to the manager's price negotiating skills.

Managed Care and Hearing Aids

An interesting revolution in the profession of audiology began in the late 1990s when major hearing instrument manufacturers decided to solidify distribution outlets for their products. As mentioned in the first half of this chapter, this is called vertical integration. It seems fitting to end this chapter revisiting that important topic. In essence,

manufacturers determined the need to secure and manage clinical outlets that would dedicate dispensing efforts specifically within their respective product lines. These efforts paralleled ongoing activity in managed care wherein healthcare services are delivered to member-patients of health maintenance organizations (HMOs) or networks at specified locations by a panel of participating providers or employee-providers of the HMO or network. In managed care organizations, medical care, therapies, and hospitalization are controlled by corporate entities. Managers assign patients to participating providers or employee-practitioners for general or specific healthcare. Medication regimen, surgical intervention, selection of specialists, specific testing protocols, and other utilization activities are carefully controlled with strict guidelines and utilization reviews. Participating providers may suggest therapies or medications; however, these suggestions are subject to review and approval by corporate managers.

In simple terms, the rising popularity of third-party payers, including Medicare Advantage programs, that offer a hearing aid benefit is that these programs are another entity that requires the cultivation of an audiologist-vendor relationship (Chapter 16). In the case of managed care, as reviewed previously, the vendor is the managed care organization itself, which buys the hearing aids and brokers a dispensing fee with the audiologist. Careful recordkeeping of repairs, sales, and returns is an essential component to managing that relationship successfully. Audiologists should be poised to do more Medicare Advantage business, as it is estimated that 98% of all Medicare Advantage plans

THE RISE OF THE MEDICARE ADVANTAGE
HEARING AID BENEFIT

One of the biggest changes in the U.S. hearing aid market over the past 5 to 10 years has been the growth in insurance plans offering hearing aid benefits. Historically, only U.S. veterans (~6% of the adult population) had access to hearing aid reimbursement. However, today, several insurers, led primarily by Medicare Advantage ("MA") plans, offer some form of hearing aid reimbursement. Medicare Advantage (Medicare Part C) is a program for providing Medicare benefits in the United States. Under Part C, Medicare pays a sponsor a fixed payment (Chapters 16, 17). The sponsor then pays for the healthcare expenses of enrollees. Sponsors are allowed to vary the benefits from those provided by Medicare's Parts A and B if they provide the equivalent of those programs. The growth in MA hearing benefits has been driven by MA's attempt to entice eligible enrollees to become members through offering benefits such as hearing, dental, and vision, which are not included in traditional Medicare. These plans are increasingly, either directly or through a third party, administering the hearing aid purchase and delivery for their policyholders.

Currently, Humana and UnitedHealth are the two largest players in Medicare Advantage. They both work in conjunction with a hearing benefit manager to deliver hearing aid coverage to their members. These hearing aid benefit managers (e.g., TruHearing, Epic, Amplifon, Hearing Care Solutions, Nations Benefits) negotiate wholesale prices of devices directly with the manufacturers. These benefit managers have a network of clinics, which participate in their respective programs, to which they direct their policyholders (MA members) to visit to purchase hearing aids. The clinics receive a fixed fitting fee in exchange for providing audiologist service to the policyholders. Hearing aid benefit managers make money through the difference in the fees received by the insurance plan and customer (copay) versus the wholesale cost of the device, the fitting fee, and administrative costs.

The rise of MA hearing aid benefits has been a double-edged sword for audiologists in the U.S. market. The rise in MA members using their hearing aid benefit has clearly contributed to increasing penetration in the market and hence greater volumes of devices sold. On the flip side, more MA providers offering a hearing aid benefit has led to pressure on pricing. The pricing pressure has been felt most acutely in the private practice segment of the market, where clinics receive a fixed fitting fee for their services rather than the full hearing aid retail price, which

continued on next page

continued from previous page

is typically a three to four times markup on the wholesale price. An MA fitting fee can range from $250 to over $1,000 per device, depending on the specific member plan. This is generally a much lower reimbursement rate compared to the private pay market. Smaller independent practices, in particular, have felt the headwind to their business and, because of lower reimbursement rates for MA-funded fittings, regularly complain about managed care. In essence, dispensing audiologists work within two different business models: private pay and managed care (MA). Each business model has very different cost and profitability structures (Chapters 16, 17).

According to MarkeTrak surveys, in 2024, 54% of hearing aid buyers reported some form of reimbursement, up from 37% in 2004. This growth has been driven by the increase in MA plans offering hearing benefits and the overall increase in MA, which has grown to managed care for 51% of Medicare-eligible enrollees versus only 31% in 2014.

Managed care, primarily driven by these MA programs, *accounts for about 20% of total wholesale distribution* in the U.S. market in 2024, a sharp rise from around 8% in 2017. Further, managed care now comprises 30% of the retail market when the VA channel is excluded (Bernstein Report, 2024). Distribution in the retail market for managed care primarily goes through independent audiologists who are part of managed care retail networks. The rise of MA-funded hearing aid benefits presents a challenge to the audiology-vendor relationship. With the rise of MA, there are now other entities, hearing aid benefit managers (i.e., Truhearing, Epic, etc,), that require diligent management of the relationship.

have a hearing aid benefit, which enables many individuals of Medicare age to acquire hearing aids at a discounted rate with this benefit.

Since fitting fees are considerably lower with managed care contracts (the third-party payer is a middleman of sorts), this business relationship must be managed differently than the audiologist-vendor relationship. For example, managed care does offer audiologists a qualified lead, which tends to lower marketing costs and increase conversion rates, but many audiologists still struggle with the profitability in the managed care segment. Now, audiologists must cultivate a relationship with hearing aid manufacturers and these hearing aid benefit managers who work with third-party payers. Regardless of the specific entity, some general relationship building skills apply and include the following:

■ Use Excel spreadsheets to keep accurate records of all sales, repairs, and returns, as well as all billing information for each transaction. Managers should review this information, at a minimum, on a weekly basis.

- On an annual basis, review all terms and conditions with each manufacturer. Evaluate items such as per-unit wholesale price, shipping costs, and repair rates. Include an account representative from each respective manufacturer/vendor in the annual review. During these periods, schedule a review to evaluate changes in unit commitments and other terms of service.

- Request a personal visit from the outside sales representative of each company at least two times per year. Ask this individual to share market insights they have learned during their travels that can be applied to the business. Ask for personalized onboarding of new products and features as needed.

- Have a direct line of communication with each vendor. That is, have the email and direct phone number of a manager from each of the following departments for each vendor:
  - Accounting/Billing.
  - Customer Service.
  - Inside Sales.
  - Technical Support/Audiology.
  - Marketing.

A Final Note: Patient Advocacy

Patient advocacy is a time-honored tradition of all healthcare practitioners: Whatever it takes to guarantee the quality of care, dedicated healthcare practitioners work diligently on behalf of their clientele. Whether it is establishing or improving licensing and regulatory issues for audiologists or the concerted efforts of an entire profession actively advancing providers to doctoral-level training and attendant expectations, quality care must form the core of all healthcare providers' activities.

Audiologists are advocates in the relationship between hearing instrument manufacturers and the end users of their products. It is the audiologist's duty to work diligently on behalf of the patient to ensure appropriate instrumentation is placed and applied relative to the patient's particular needs. No matter the situation or circumstance, the audiologist-as-health-care-provider must first and foremost put the interests of their patients before those of the practice and the hearing instrument manufacturer. The audiologist must function as the patient's advocate in matters of conflict that may arise from time to time with vendors. The practice must insist that instrument manufacturers, suppliers, and related vendors participate as actively as any member of the practice in placing the patient at the forefront of interest in all deliberations and resolutions of conflict.

In contemporary hearing healthcare, adhering to the concept of patient-centric care is as much the responsibility of the audiologist managing the patient's aural rehabilitation as it is the responsibility of instrument manufacturers and vendors. *In the final analysis, we are all in this together with the success of those whom we serve at the core of all we do.*

References

Bailey, A. (2024). Who's Who in Audiology 2024. Hearing Tracker.com

Bernstein Report. (2024) Hearing aids: February VA data shows Sonova gaining at the expense of Demant and GN ahead of their new products in May. https://www.rbadvisors.com/insights/4-for-24-year-ahead-outlook/

Ganbo, T., Sashida, J., & Saito, M. (2023). Evaluation of the association between hearing aids and reduced cognitive decline in older adults with hearing impairment. *Otology & Neurotology, 44*(5), 425–431.

Glaser, R. G. (2017). Unpublished data on rates of return hearing aid repairs.

Holman, J. A., Drummond, A., & Naylor, G. (2021). Hearing aids reduce daily-life fatigue and increase social activity: A longitudinal study. *Trends in Hearing, 25*, 23312165211052786.

Lin, F. R., Pike, J. R., Albert, M. S., Arnold, M., Burgard, S., Chisolm, T., . . . ACHIEVE Collaborative Research Group. (2023). Hearing intervention versus health education control to reduce cognitive decline in older adults with hearing loss in the USA (ACHIEVE): A multicentre, randomised controlled trial. *The Lancet,* S0140-6736(23)01406-X. Advance online publication. https://www.nih.gov/news-events/nih-research-matters/hearing-aids-slow-cognitive-decline-people-high-risk

Martinez-Amezcua, P., Kuo, P. L., Reed, N. S., Simonsick, E. M., Agrawal, Y., Lin, F. R., . . . Schrack, J. A. (2021). Association of hearing impairment with higher-level physical functioning and walking endurance: Results from the Baltimore Longitudinal Study of Aging. *The Journals of Gerontology, Series A, Biological Sciences and Medical Sciences, 76*(10), e290–e298. https://www.ncbi.nlm.nih.gov/pmc/articles/PMC8436975/

Picou, E. M. (2022). Hearing aid benefit and satisfaction results from the MarkeTrak 2022 Survey: Importance of features and hearing care professionals. *Seminars in Hearing, 43*(4), 301–316.

20 Professional Sales Techniques

Robert M. Traynor, EdD, MBA

Introduction

Thoughts of salespeople often bring to mind used cars, vacuum cleaners, snake oil sales, or the QVC Network. While there are unprofessional and/or high-pressure salespeople for virtually all products, most professionals also sell services, procedures, and products. Consider an attorney selling time and legal skills to their client, a dentist who sells procedures and dental products, and even physicians and surgeons who sell evaluations, examinations, and operative procedures to their patients. Virtually any profession, including audiology, is a sales profession.

Selling professionally is difficult in that there are two sides to professional interaction with patients, *clinical and business*. While it is an ethical, fiduciary, and professional responsibility to clinically provide the very best in hearing care, clinicians and practice managers also need to ensure that there is enough profit in each sale to provide ongoing support for the clinic. In fact, is the utmost ethical responsibility is to stay in business so that patients are provided the proper hearing care throughout the use of the products and procedures sold to them as part of their rehabilita-

tive treatment program. Selling is an essential skill to all audiology practice specialties, but it is rarely addressed in a Doctor of Audiology (AuD) curriculum. Typically, AuD programs teach to certification standards set up by academic accreditation boards, often by those who have not seen a real patient in years. Summing up how AuD students are prepared, Wignall (2015) states that students need further education in performing hearing evaluations, relating to patients, explaining test results, *selling hearing aids*, writing a contract, asking for thousands of dollars, fitting the hearing aids, explaining the care of the aids, and conducting follow-ups. Wignall's concerns have not changed over the past 10 years as entry-level professionals still do not know much about the professional selling of products. While the winds of audiology educational programs are slowly changing to include many of these business skills, audiologists are generally not prepared to sell the products and services. Taylor (personal communication, June 27, 2024) states that so much has changed since his 2012 reminder to audiologists of their need to be salespeople. He then said, "Like it or not, most audiologists and other hearing health care professionals engage in selling everyday . . . keep in mind that all medical professions engage in selling. Surgeons often must convince their patients to undergo surgery, therapists have to persuade their clients to follow their treatment guidelines, and even dentists have to sell whiter teeth or braces. Whether you are a recent AuD graduate or a seasoned clinician, the sooner you embrace the selling process the sooner you will be successful, as the path to financial rewards and professional independence rests with your ability to sell."

Traditional Sales Techniques Do Not Work

When reading books and listening to tapes of how to sell, there are many high-pressure tactics that have been used in all professions. No matter the profession or what is being sold, traditional concepts such as "Always be closing," "Think positive and the fear of sales can be overcome," or "Your salespeople have never read any sales training books." These are the sales images that professionals, such as audiologists, when thinking of the sales process. For professionals, these outdated sales techniques fail to address the core issue of allowing the patient to arrive at their own purchase decision. The ultimate goal in professional selling is for the patients to feel they have chosen the correct course of rehabilitative treatment without feeling they have *"been sold."* Patients who have been influenced by these so-called "sales techniques" return products more often than those who have arrived at their own decision to proceed with treatment. At the basis of these professional sales techniques are some do's and don'ts in professional selling:

- *Don't:* Deliver a strong sales pitch.
- *Do:* Cease the sales pitch and begin a conversation and listen carefully.
- *Don't:* Think that the central objective is always to "close the sale."
- *Do:* Discover whether the clinician and the patient are a good fit; if not, adjust the interaction to facilitate the fit.
- *Don't:* Think that when a sale is lost it is the closing technique at the end of the sales process.
- *Do:* Realize that when a sale is lost, it usually occurs at the beginning of the sales process.
- *Don't:* Accept that rejection is a normal part of the sales process.
- *Do:* Understand that sales pressure on patients is a major cause of rejection. In a clinical situation, rejection should never occur.
- *Don't:* Keep chasing every potential patient until the answer is either yes or a no.
- *Do:* Realize that chasing patients with telephone calls and letters only leads to a perception of high sales pressure.
- *Don't:* Challenge and/or counter objections offered by the patient.
- *Do:* When a patient offers objections, uncover the truth behind them and explain the details necessary to reduce the concern as a consideration in the purchase decision.
- *Don't:* Defend and explain the value if a patient challenges the benefit of the product or service.
- *Do:* Realize that recommendations may need some explanation and rationale; getting defensive about them will only lead to perceived high sales pressure.

According to many researchers and practitioners, selling is an advanced form of communication and requires the utilization of all senses. There are hundreds of references for selling available in libraries and virtually every corner of the Internet. There are, however, some fundamental concepts that are threads woven into most of those references.

Listening Skills

In today's high-tech, high-speed, high-stress world, effective listening within the clinical situation is essential to the rehabilitative sales process. Of course, the art of listening has long been a part of audiology counseling, as well as good salespersonship (Clark, 2018; Clark & English, 2004, 2014; Crandell, personal communication, 1995; Luterman, 2001, 2020). Genuine listening builds relationships, solves problems, ensures understanding, resolves conflicts, and improves accuracy and efficiency, with less wasted clinic time. Listening is both a complex process and a learned skill; it requires conscious intellectual and emotional effort. Without intensively listening to patients, audiologists lack essential information as to their generation, personal style, lifestyle, communication needs, and other facts fundamental to the aural rehabilitative process. While there is a need for the audiologist to talk during the clinical session for informational counseling, talk should be kept at a minimum. Counselors and sales professionals suggest that 60% listening and 40% talking is a good place to begin, but that mixture can change as the relationship develops between the patient and the clinician. Most audiologists are not formally taught effective

listening skills; therefore, these skills must be developed to effectively facilitate the sale of the rehabilitative products. Ineffective listening can damage clinical relationships and deteriorate the delicate trust that has been established with the patient. Thus, a *professional sales process* is actually a *counseling process* dependent upon the specific attributes of the consumer/patient to determine their wants and needs.

Clinicians should make eye contact and relax, while not staring at the individual. While the clinician may look away now and then, it is important to be attentive to the discussion at hand. Attending to the conversation means the following:

- Be present and not distracted by other conversations or tasks.
- Offer full attention and interaction in the conversation.
- Be ready to apply or directly interact to the situation presented by the consumer (patient).
- It is necessary to mentally screen out distractions, such as background activity, noise, and speaker's accent or mannerisms.
- *Keep an open mind.* Clinicians should attempt to not be distracted by their own thoughts, feelings, or biases and listen without judging the consumer (patient) or mentally criticizing if what is said is alarming. It is OK to feel alarmed, but do not demonstrate it. As soon as judgmental bemusements are indulged, the clinical effectiveness as a listener has been compromised. It is necessary to listen without jumping to conclusions and appreciate that the consumer (patient) is using their own language to represent the thoughts and feelings inside their

brain. Clinically, the only way to learn their thoughts and feelings is by truly listening. It is essential that the clinician not be a sentence grabber by finishing sentences or put words in the mouth of the speaker. Aging and communication issues are part of our business and many consumers (patients) have difficulty expressing themselves rapidly.

■ *Listen to the words and try to picture what the speaker is saying.* The listener should allow their mind to create a mental model of the information being communicated. Whether a literal picture, or an arrangement of abstract concepts, the brain will do the necessary work if the clinician remains focused, with their senses fully alert. A listening tool for long discussions is to concentrate and remember key words and phrases, thinking only about what the other person has said, even if it is boring. If thoughts start to wander, immediately force refocusing.

■ *Don't interrupt the conversation.* Interruptions in the conversation by the clinician says the following to the consumer (patient):
  ■ "I'm more important than you are."
  ■ "What I have to say is more interesting than what you have to say."
  ■ "I don't have time for your story or opinion."
  ■ "This isn't a conversation, it's a contest, and I'm going to win."
  ■ Interruptions are a major sign that the clinician is talking too much and in need of relaxing to let the consumer (patient) tell their story or history.

■ *Wait for the speaker to pause to ask clarifying questions.* When critical points are not understood, it is necessary to have the speaker explain. Rather than interrupt, it is essential to wait until the speaker pauses. Then it might be said, "Let's back up a second. I didn't understand what you just said about . . . . "

■ *Ask questions only to ensure understanding.*

■ Questions can lead people in directions that have nothing to do with the discussion. While answering a question, the consumer (patient) will sometimes work back to their original thought but may often forget an important point fundamental to their situation. It is the clinician's responsibility to bring the conversation back to where the question was inserted to keep the discussion on track.

■ *Try to feel what the speaker is feeling.* Clinicians should attempt to feel sad as the consumer (patient) expresses sadness, joyful when joy is expressed, and fearful when describing feat; conveying those feelings through facial expressions and words ensures effectiveness as a listener. Empathy is the heart and soul of good listening. To experience empathy, it is necessary for clinicians to put themselves in the other person's place and allow the feeling of what it is like to *be them* at that moment. Empathy is not easy, as it takes energy and concentration, but it greatly facilitates communication and builds relationships.

■ *Give the speaker regular feedback.* As a listener, clinicians need to demonstrate an understanding of where the speaker is coming from by reflecting the discussion. Acknowledgments of what has been said include "You must be thrilled!"

"What a terrible ordeal for you."
"I can see that you are confused."
If the clinician feels that the speaker's feelings are hidden or unclear, then an occasional paraphrase of the content of the message may be necessary. Other interactions might simply be a nod to show understanding or through appropriate facial expressions and an occasional, well-timed "hmmm" or "uh huh."

- *Pay attention to what is not said—to nonverbal cues.* While a lot can be discussed, a significant amount of direct communication is nonverbal. Face to face with a consumer (patient), enthusiasm, boredom, or irritation can be easily detected by expressions around the eyes, the set of the mouth, or the slope of the shoulders. It is easy to determine if the consumer (patient) does not want to be there by their mannerisms.

Summarizing at the end of the listening session is extremely helpful. Summarizing will not only ensure accurate follow-through but also feel perfectly natural. Listening well improves the quality of the relationships with patients and the tips presented above can keep a good discussion on track. Actively listening to patients takes concentration, challenging work, patience, the ability to interpret other people's ideas and summarize them, and the ability to identify nonverbal communication such as body language.

As noted earlier, ineffective listening can damage clinical relationships and deteriorate the delicate trust that has been carefully built with the consumer (patient). Rosen (2024) reiterates a summary of listening errors that have been encountered by consumers (patients) in audiology clinics:

- *The clinician is doing something else when the patient is talking.*
- *The clinician is thinking about the next patient and not concentrating on the person that is talking about themselves and their situation.*
- *Waiting for pauses in the conversation so that the clinician can make specific points.*
- *Not allowing for pauses in the conversation. It is not necessary to fill pauses with speech.*
- *Clinicians need to think before they speak.*
- *Fake listening to the patient to enable getting comments into the situation.*
- *Clinicians selectively listening or only hearing what they want to hear.*
- *Not attending to body language, facial expressions, eye contact, and vocal intonation.*
- *Background noise in the room while communicating with patients.*
- *Passing judgment on people due to age, success, how they look, and so on.*

These are only some of the errors made each day in the clinic. Care must be exercised to not commit these errors as they will damage your relationship with patients.

General Patient Variables in Hearing Aid Sales

Powers and Carr (2022), in their discussion of MarkeTrak 10, presented that the majority (83%) of hearing aid users were satisfied with their devices, confirming that hearing aids are positively impacting their relationships, work performance, general ability to communicate, overall quality of life, and ability to participate in group activities. These are the successes in the use of hearing instruments that have conquered personal obstacles to the use of amplification. In a comparison of these data to that of Kochkin (1990) reporting data in MarkeTrak 1 1989, there was only 38.8% binaural hearing aid ownership; in 2022, the ownership rate was found to be 70%. While this demonstrates great success in market penetration, 30% who should use hearing aids have not obtained these devices. Chien and Lin (2012) submitted that the reasons for this lack of use were likely multifactorial and related to a general perception of hearing loss as an inconsequential portion of the aging process, the absence of adequate health insurance reimbursement for hearing rehabilitative services, and the lack of research on the impact of hearing loss treatment. Even these days, when insurance reimbursement for hearing instruments is part of many managed care programs, the multifactorial issues for the nonuse of amplification mentioned by Chien and Lin (2012) are still factors that have been known for quite some time.

There is more to the use of hearing instruments than the hearing loss itself. There is also the individual, each with their own special set of variables that cause the average person to wait 5 to 7 years after they know they have a hearing problem to seek assistance. In the 1970s, there was great confusion among rehabilitative audiologists as to why two patients with the same hearing loss would react differently to the use

of the same hearing instrument. While some of these classic patient reactions dealt with the technology of the time, many of these personal issues still prevail almost 55 years later. The variables observed by Trychin (2003), a noted hearing impairment psychologist, are still factors in the adoption of hearing instruments (Figure 20-1). The following is the classic list of reasons that patients *choose not* to use amplification:

■ *Don't realize they have a hearing loss*
Typically, hearing loss among adults is a gradual impairment that occurs over years. It is not easy sometimes to realize that there is an impairment, especially if the patient lives alone or has a limited lifestyle and those around them have good projected voices for communication.

■ *Denial 1: Do not admit they have a hearing loss*
The literature is full of examples and research that indicate the average patient who seeks rehabilitative assistance with hearing aids has known there has been a hearing deficit for about 5 to 7 years. They tend to put the burden of communication on others rather than seek treatment until it is absolutely necessary.

■ *Denial 2: Know they have a hearing loss but don't think it is a problem for them or others*
These patients know that they do not hear very well but feel that it is not a handicap. Sometimes this is perpetuated by those that always speak up to the person, or the individual does not go out much and interact with others.

■ *Denial 3: Know they have hearing loss but do not think there is anything that can be done for it*

The technology of the 21st century lends this concern a bit in the past as there is amplification for just about all but those with severe word recognition issues. Today's products truly offer significant benefit for most all hearing impairment that is tolerated well.

■ *Higher priorities*
Of course, there can be hearing impairment, but the patient and their family may have set a higher priority for something else that costs about the same as amplification. Communication may not be that important to some individuals and there is a conscious choice to spend the time, energy effort and costs somewhere else other than hearing care.

■ *Costs*
While costs are a factor and may be used as an excuse in the use of amplification, it is generally not a major concern. Further, many managed care programs now offer hearing devices as a benefit and subsidize the costs of many types and styles of hearing aids. Thus, most older people can afford the initial costs of hearing devices and their maintenance. Those that cannot afford the best products will do rather well with older technology that is readily available for a substantial reduction in cost.

■ *Lack of transportation*
Older people often have difficulty with obtaining transportation to the clinic. As eyesight fails and driving is no longer an option, patients must depend upon others to take them to their appointments. While this is usually an accommodation offered in assisted living and paid by some managed care programs, patients may not choose to use amplification due to the lack of the capability to get to the clinic for appointments.

■ *Lack of motivation to hear*
The person who lives alone may rationalize that they can hear the TV well enough by turning it up and there is no one else with whom to communicate around the house. Additionally, this issue may also be part of depression in that the person does not care to communicate with anyone and then will not choose to use amplification.

■ *Fear of being seen as failing or incompetent*
While stigma is significantly less in this century, it remains an issue. Although products are smaller and more beneficial, it is the stigma of the use of amplification that keeps some patients from considering the use of devices. Although with all the various types of hearing products in use in 2024, society tends to look at those that use hearing instruments as not as capable as those that do not use these devices.

■ *Afraid of doctors and professionals*
There is an actual phobia called iatrophobia, or the fear of doctors, that affects about 3% of the population (Esposito, 2014). Defined as the morbid and irrational fear of doctors or hospitals, this does not refer to those who simply do not like these places but rather those who are deathly afraid of them and anything associated with them, such as audiologists. Medical Economics (2021) reports that patients' general trust in doctors is also declining. Surveys have shown that nearly

40% patients in the United States believe that today's physicians do not care about patient well-being.

- **■ *Motor coordination problems***
  Fine motor skills of the hand are important in many daily activities, such as buttoning a shirt and unlocking doors. If these skills deteriorate, it will be difficult to manipulate hearing devices to put them on and off, changing batteries, and other necessary skills. Additionally, there can be cerebellar issues that cause special perception difficulties as part of the aging process that cause difficulty with the use of amplification.

- **■ *Bad prior experience with hearing aids or vendors***
  While there are many positive stories about the use of amplification, a cursory check of the Internet will glean much discussion about bad experiences with hearing devices and those that sell them. These bad experiences could be due to the purchase of the wrong device, inaccurate fitting or programming, not giving the devices the opportunities to work, or not being able to hear in noisy environments. It could be due to customer service or lack of expertise, education, or experience by the dispenser. Expensive products that do not work create a lack of wanting to repeat that terrible experience.

- **■ *Friends' or relatives' bad experiences with hearing aids or vendors***
  Hearing instruments have a terrible reputation, and it is easy to find a friend or relative that has advice for the patient who is shopping for hearing devices. Most stories are similar to those above that are not firsthand and full of bad advice.

- **■ *Overstimulation***
  While sensory overload can be a result of a disorder such as recruitment or hyperacusis, hearing devices are often fit with excessive sound or overamplification. Patients are not ready for the full recommended levels of amplification in the beginning and psycho-acoustically require a gradual introduction of sound into their lives. This is particularly true if there has been sound deprivation for an extended period of time prior to the use of hearing instruments.

- **■ *Emotional status***
  The loss of hearing causes many people to go through emotional stages similar to the loss of a loved one: denial, anger, depression, and, finally, acceptance. Adults who lose their hearing slowly without a diagnosis may undergo a slow change in personality. Isolation is common as they may be confused or fearful about their inability to communicate as clearly. The fear of losing one's income, relationships, or social standing can have a huge emotional impact, causing elevated levels of stress that then affect health in other areas. Even with diagnosis, the thought of wearing a hearing device can cause loss of self-esteem. It is not unusual for hearing loss to turn a once friendly, confident adult into an angry, isolated grump. Thus, people with hearing loss feel less comfortable and less confident in social situations, which increases psychological stress.

- **■ *Ear pain and allergies***
  Of course, if the ear hurts or there are allergies to the devices, obvious difficulty arises in the use of hearing devices.

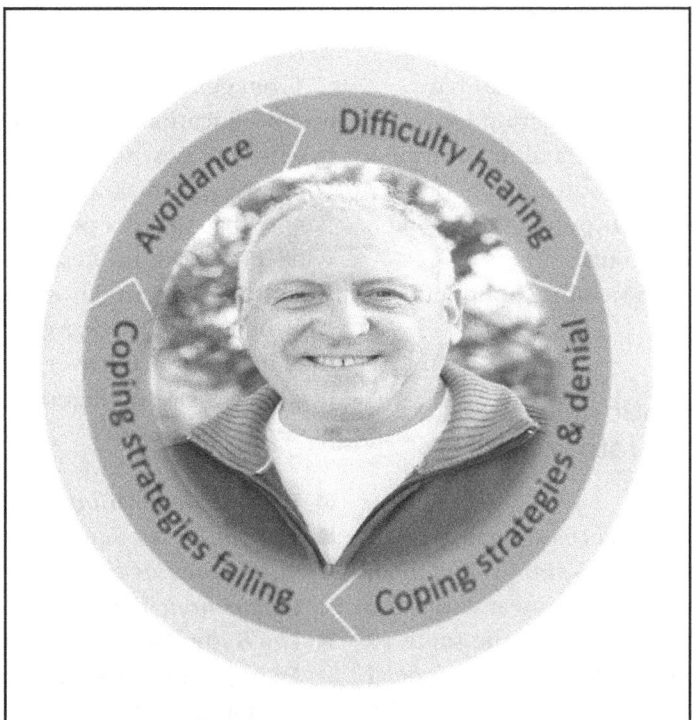

Figure 20–1. Variables of hearing loss.

■ *Vanity*
For many, the image of themselves does not fit their age and/or their hearing impairment. Many patients associate hearing problems with being old but do not *feel old*. Their self-image is that of a young, confident, robust person with successful careers and responsibilities. No matter the differences in the product, hearing instruments do not fit the self-image of the hearing-impaired person.

■ *Fear of ridicule*
Alcido and Lloyd (2024) report that there is still a pervasiveness of perceived stigma associated with hearing loss and use of hearing aids and their close association with ageism and perceptions of disability. They

also identify the potential influence of media and advertisements on maintaining hearing loss and hearing aids as stigmatizing.

■ Almost half (46%) of people diagnosed with some degree of hearing loss do not regularly wear a hearing aid.

■ Nearly half (48%) of those with hearing loss believe that there is still a stigma associated with wearing a hearing aid.

■ Over half (51%) of respondents said the main benefit of wearing a hearing aid is that it allows them to have better communications with friends and family.

■ Cost is the most common reason people do not wear hearing aids, with 56% of respondents saying they are too expensive. [Not supported by other studies.]

■ The most common social barrier people with hearing loss experience is difficulties hearing important announcements or information in public spaces like airports or train stations, as reported by 55% of respondents.

Generational Issues That Relate to Sales

Generational differences are real. By definition, the term *generation* refers to all the people born and living at about the same time and exposed to the same issues surrounding their lives. In social science, the term generation can also be described as the average period, generally considered to be about thirty years, during which children are born, grow up, become adults, and begin to have children of their own, experiencing the same momentous events within a given period.

From generation to generation, there are modifications to pop culture, world events, politics, technology, economic conditions, wars, and a myriad of other factors that shape a person's interaction with the world. In Western culture, the America's, Western Europe, and Oceania (Australia), there are several generations that have surfaced over the past hundred years or so (Figure 20–2). These generations include:

■ *The G.I. Generation:* 1901–1927
■ *The Mature or Silent Generation, also known as the Best or Greatest Generation:* 1928–1945
■ *The Baby Boomers:* 1946–1964, Two groups: Older group 1946–1954 and younger 1955–1964
■ *Generation X:* 1965–1980
■ *Generation Y/Millennials:* 1981–1996
■ *Generation Z/Boomlets/Homeland:* 1997–

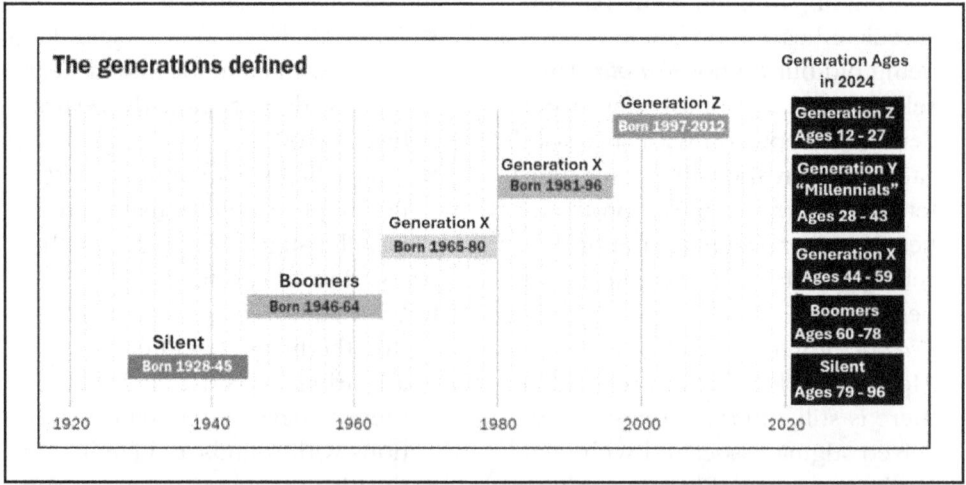

Figure 20–2. Western cultural generations. *Source*: Adapted from Pew Research Center (2019).

Baby Boomer Generation

Although generation characteristics are addressed in other chapters of this text, it is important to reiterate the attributes and traits of the generation that will most probably fill audiology clinics for many years to come.

Baby Boomers are the children of the Mature/Silent Best Generation and, thanks to their parents, had quite a different formative experience. Born between 1946 and 1964, Baby Boomers are the largest generation of children ever born in the Western world. Before World War II, there were fewer than 2 million babies born in the United States each year, and during this 18-year period, there were between 3.5 and 4 million babies born each year, generating a huge population increase (Figure 20–3 and Figure 20–4).

This was also true of the other countries that were active in World War II such as the rest of North America, Europe, and Oceania (Australia). The Baby Boomers initiated the largest population increase in the history of the world. While this increase does not include some parts of the world, it is most obvious in nations of the world that fought in World War II and in areas of the world affected by the war. Since there was such a huge increase in population at their birth, Baby Boomers will make up the bulk of hearing care patients seeking treatment until 2036 and beyond (Figure 20–5).

In the United States, this group grew up in the prosperous times of the 1950s, 1960s, and 1970s and were cuddled,

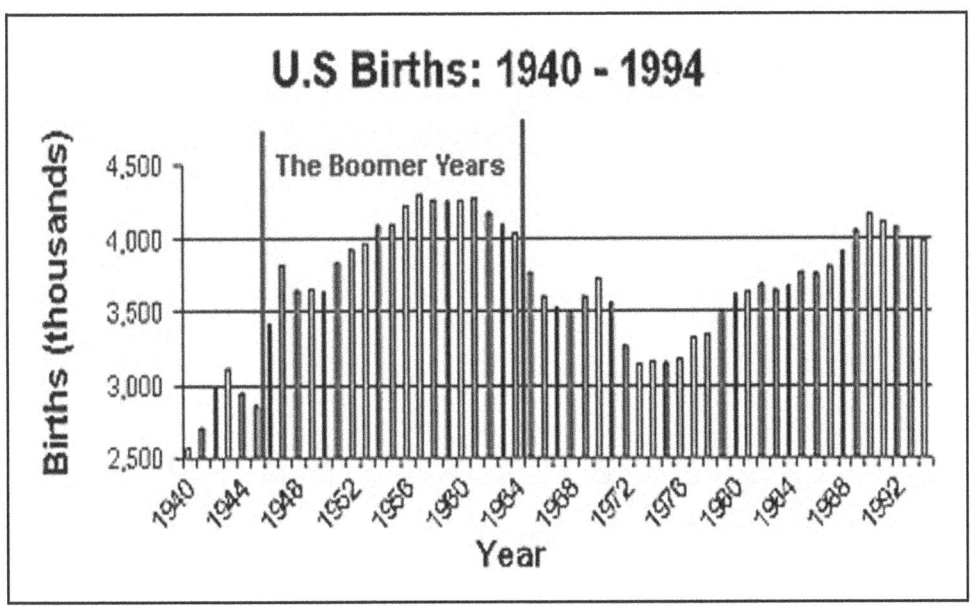

Figure 20–3. U.S. births during the Baby Boomer period (U.S. Department of Commerce, United States Bureau of the Census, 2017). *Source*: Baby Boomer Head Quarters, wwwbbhq.com.

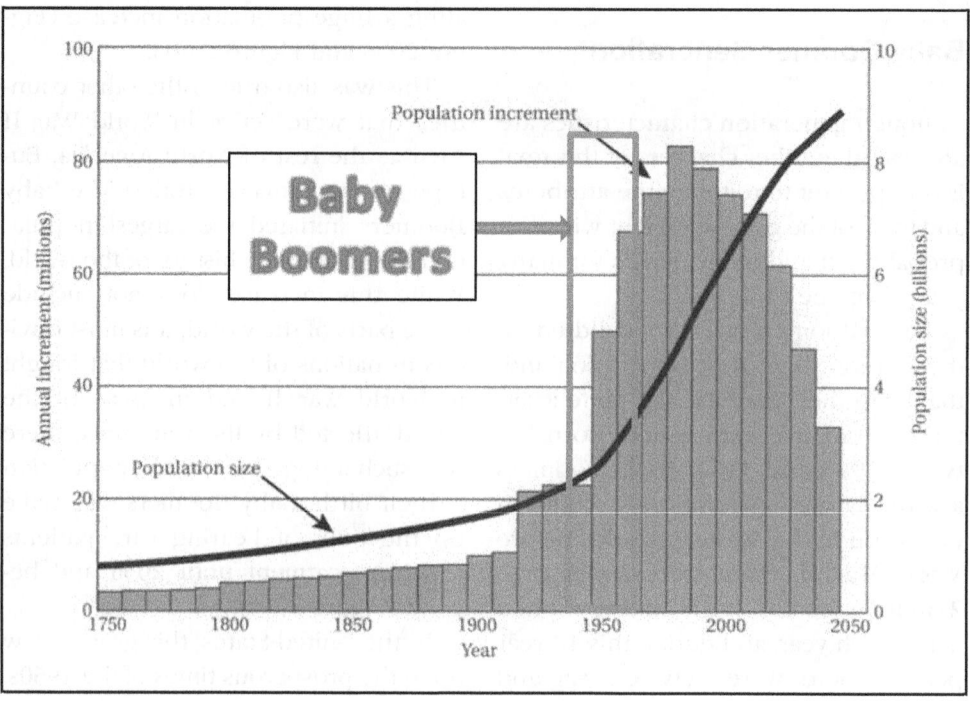

Figure 20–4. World population 1750–2050 (United Nations Population Division, 2008). *Source*: Adapted from Jeníček (2010).

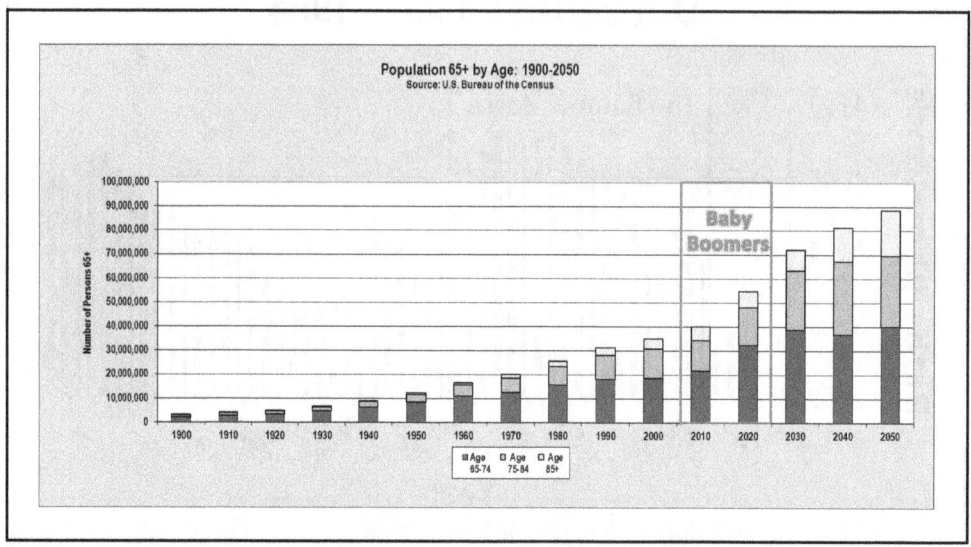

Figure 20–5. Population 65+ by age 1900–2050 (United States Bureau of the Census). *Source*: Adapted from the U.S. Bureau of Census, Administration of Aging: Department of Health and Human Services (2024).

supported, educated, and given virtually every experience that their parents could afford. Although they may have watched their favorite programs at a neighbor's house, they were the first generation to grow up in front of television. This group was greatly impacted by the Cold War with the Soviet Union and the assassinations of John Kennedy, Robert Kennedy, Martin Luther King Jr., and they grew up accepting women and minorities as equals.

The Vietnam War was a huge issue for this group as most of the young soldiers fighting the war were Baby Boomers. Many put their college or vocational education on hold for a few years as they were legally bound by the Selective Service (the draft) to spend some time in the military. The draft for the Vietnam War was an obstacle that needed to be dealt with by all males 18 years of age or older. In the initial years of the Vietnam War draft, there was a military service deferment for college students if their grade point average (GPA) was a 2.0 or higher. If the GPA went below 2.0, the Selective Service reclassified the person as 1A (ready for the draft) and they were immediately called for military service. In an attempt to make the Selective Service system fairer to all, a draft lottery was conducted to determine who went into the military and thus ended up fighting the Vietnam War. The first draft lottery drawing was held on December 1, 1969, at Selective Service National Headquarters in Washington, DC, to determine the order of the "call for induction" during calendar year 1970, that is, for registrants born between January 1, 1944, and December 31, 1950. There were 366 blue plastic capsules containing birth dates placed in a large glass container and drawn by hand to assign "order-of-call numbers" to all men within the 18 to 26 age range as specified in Selective Service law. With radio, film, and TV coverage, the capsules were drawn from the container, opened, and the dates inside posted in order. The first capsule drawn contained the date September 14, so all men born on September 14 in any year between 1944 and 1950 were assigned lottery number 1. The drawing continued until all days of the year had been paired with sequence numbers (Draft Lottery, 1969; Vietnam Extra, 2024). For young men ages 18 to 26, if their birthdate was drawn among the first 200, being drafted was very likely; if over 200, the likelihood of being drafted that year was significantly less.

Other distinctive differences between Baby Boomers and the Mature/Silent/Best Generations can be seen in three areas. The areas of marriage, jobs, and retirement offer insight into the basis for these differences.

Baby Boomer Marriage

A major difference between Baby Boomers from other generations is that of their marriage. Just as in other generations, they married in their late teens or early 20s, but the difference is the divorce rate. Matthews (2016), among others, presents that the divorce rate among Baby Boomers is about 50%. They often will remarry, divorce, marry a number of times, or never remarry, and the balance of these individuals may have never married or are among a previously unheard-of group, homosexuals who may marry as well. This lone factor creates major differences unique to this generation in that those new marriages, often to younger people, will create family situations that are quite unique from traditional situations. Thus, there are Baby Boomers with grandchildren and children at various ages, forcing a need to postpone retirement for those that are in college or still growing up at home. Coupled with these extra parenting and financial responsibilities may also be the need to assist aging parents who are living longer than ever before.

Baby Boomer Jobs

In their younger years, Baby Boomers believed that they were going to change the world and their involvement in the workforce met that goal in various areas of employment. While some Boomers went off to college to get a 4-year degree or prepare for professions, others found well-paying and stable jobs with their high school diploma. Office clerks and administrative support services were careers that provided financial stability and a convenient 9-to-5 work schedule. Those who were good with math and numbers worked in accounting and bookkeeping jobs, and many that were college graduates went to work for firms evolving in the use of computers and other technological advances. Others chose manual labor and construction jobs that were abundant in the 1960s, 1970s, and 1980s as workers could start without much formal education and learn the required skills on the job. Developments of suburbs, shopping malls, new housing, steel production, and car manufacturing were all booming during this period, creating high demand for Boomer workers.

Law enforcement is another broad field that included occupations like probation officers, customs brokers, police officers, forensic scientists, homeland se-

curity, criminal investigators, and detectives and others. Many Boomers chose this career path because they wanted to make a difference in their community. Although it was dangerous and physically demanding work with 'round-the-clock shifts, it provided generous salaries, pension plans, and health benefits. These careers typically required a high school diploma or college degree, followed by attending the police academy and on-the-job training, and it was ideal for returning veterans of the Vietnam War.

Many who went on to college worked in business as middle management, salespeople, and executives for public or private companies. This broad category included advertising executives, managers, banking, sales representatives, marketing, and so on. Boomers often worked long hours in a competitive environment, facing challenging tasks and compliance with corporate structure and strict company policies. Many of these careers involved commission-based salaries that offered additional perks and prestige, motivating people to work that much harder to earn a bigger paycheck. Elementary school teachers had the important job of preparing future leaders. They prepared students by teaching them the essential skills in subjects like math, reading, social studies, and science. Studies have shown that currently more than 50% of the country's teachers and educational administrators are Boomers. Nurses worked in the healthcare field, assessed patient health problems, implemented care plans, and maintained medical records. The clear majority of nurses currently working in the healthcare field are from the Baby Boomer era. Although salaries have increased for nurses, the day-to-day workloads, administrative tasks, long hours, and heavier patient caseloads are just some of the reasons why this field is facing a shortage of qualified workers. Many Boomers went on to become professionals, physicians, dentists, chiropractors, and even audiologists.

The huge presence of Boomers in the workforce and the marketplace has indeed caused many changes in how companies react and interact with them. The Mature/Silent/Best Generation was known for working 30 years or so and then retiring from their long-time position. Unlike their parents, the Boomers will not retire from their first real job as it is likely that the job they began in the 1960s or 1970s is no longer necessary or has been automated. While many may have retired early, others will keep on working if they are healthy and able to contribute to their chosen profession.

This unique group, no matter the profession, needed to adjust from a paper/pencil orientation to the computer world. As computers went from a hobby in the 1960s and 1970s to real work applications later, Boomers needed to learn how to use them, stay current in their use, and incorporate them within their chosen profession. Since these individuals had to learn computers for their everyday work situations, this is carried into retirement.

Distinctive Traits of the Baby Boomer Generation

For the five decades since 1946, this generation has burst into every life phase, and reactions to its wants and needs have resulted in major changes and innovations. In its early childhood, it brought success to the baby-care guidance of Dr. Spock and the geared-to-children entertainment of Howdy Doody, The Mickey Mouse Club, and early *Sesame Street*. When the first Boomers became teenagers, "Teeny Boppers" were recognized as a significant target market and, with the sixties, the world recognized the cultural impact of America's deep-thinking, soul-searching "Flower Children" (Figure 20–6). Who would have suspected then that in the seventies and eighties, the Boomers would become "Yuppies" pursuing an upscale lifestyle that contributed to both the refurbishment of urban neighborhoods and the suburban development of open farmland? This group has always thought of themselves as a young group and will not go into the aging process very gracefully. They do not consider themselves ready for "Bingo Night," "Shuffleboard," or exercises in the pool; those things are for "Old People." To better understand this group, there are some distinctive traits that define this generation (Thornhill & Martin, 2007).

■ *Entitlement.* Since the mid-1940s, they have been driving the U.S. economy in virtually every stage of life. Hospitals were built to support the births and illnesses, toys were made for them, malls were built to meet their shopping needs, schools were built to accommodate their education, and colleges and universities built classrooms and buildings to house them. As the generations grew, industry expanded to accommodate their wants and needs for the design of clothes (bell bottoms), cars (muscle cars), and other goods. Knowledge and skill in virtually every profession and discipline expanded, and as they had young families, the

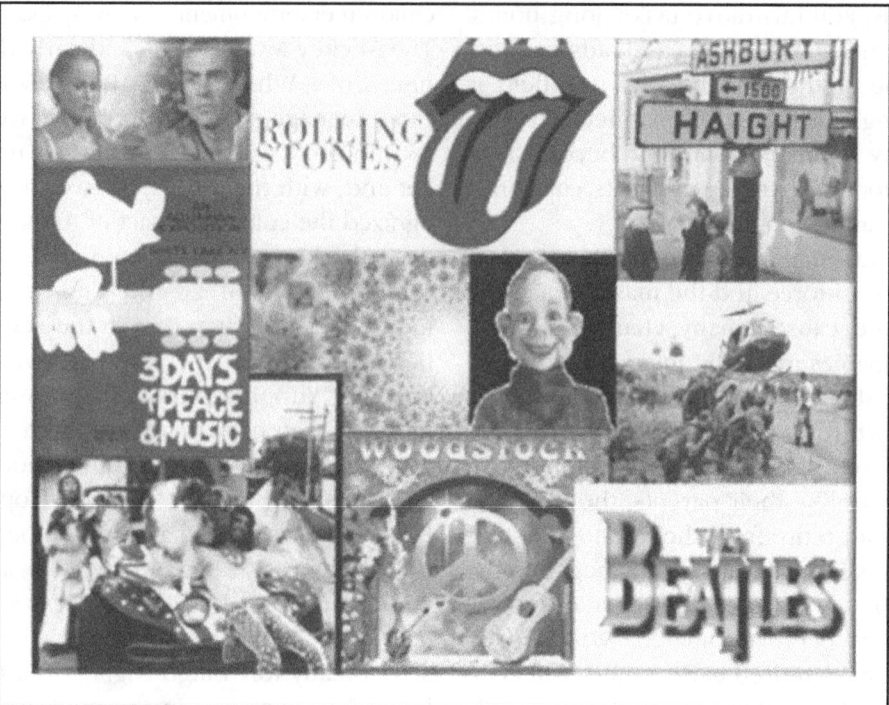

Figure 20–6. Baby Boomer generation.

housing market, cities, and their suburbs grew.

■ *Personal gratification.* Baby Boomers always had what they wanted, either from a parent's gift or assistance in obtaining their wants and needs. They have always earned more than their parents and, when married, they had two incomes to enable even a higher income due to the change in women's rights, education, and cultural changes toward women working outside the home. This change in culture provided two incomes for families and made them substantially more prosperous than the previous generation.

■ *Work ethic.* About 33% of the Boomers graduated from college and many more went to college but did not graduate. Boomers have an extremely high work ethic. They needed this as there were so many of them that it took more work and longer hours to stand out in the crowd of people seeking the same jobs or promotion to a higher level.

■ *Control.* This generation controlled and changed U.S. society and culture. They were influential in many areas such as civil rights, women's rights, fashion, foods, sports, movies, and their rock 'n' roll music.

■ *Optimism.* Sociologists feel that it was due to being reared in the 1950s and 1960s, a time of prosperity in the United States, that they often see the "glass as half full," having borne many hardships, such as the Vietnam War, the decline of the Soviet Union, Iraq/Afghanistan

Wars, the financial meltdown of 2008, ISIS, and other difficulties.

- *Will not accept "normal."* Boomers have never accepted things that were culturally supposed to be just accepted. They sought change of the rules that did not seem fair or insensitive, and they will do the same thing as they age and change how the elderly are being served and retirement programs in general.

These are traits that are part of every Baby Boomer, and they cannot be altered as they are inbred into this group. These inescapable traits are part of what make this group unique, requiring special interactions for clinical success.

Baby Boomer Retirement

Baby Boomers, their employers, and the United States are woefully unprepared to pay for the retirement of such a huge group. Since there was much downsizing and corporate reduction in pension plans in the 1980s and 1990s, many Baby Boomers are left with no guaranteed pension. Additionally, the solvency of the remaining corporate and union pension plans is very much in question (Voorhis, 2016). It is well known that without changes, Medicare will be forced to trim benefits by 2030 and Social Security by 2034.

While 55% of Boomers report having savings for retirement, nearly half of this so-called "prepared group" have less than $100,000, an amount that in today's market would generate less than $7,000 a year in retirement income. De-Vise (2023) found that nearly 50% of Boomers have no savings for retirement. Overall, one in five Boomers indicate that they will not have enough savings

to cover basic living expenses. As a group, it is not because they were foolish with their money during their earning years; it is likely the result of not earning large salaries and/or something happened, such as a health calamity, family crisis, divorce, second family expenses, a lost job, or questionable investments. Fischer (2024) offers the results of a survey relative to Baby Boomers and their retirement:

- Fifty-four percent of the respondents said they were highly confident or confident about their financial readiness for retirement and 73% reported that their financial situation was "much better" or "just as they anticipated" before they retired.
- Thirty-six percent of survey participants said Social Security is their primary source of retirement income. Sixteen percent cited traditional monthly pensions and 15% employer-sponsored retirement plans. Other responses included investments, IRAs, and outside savings.
- Regarding dependence on Social Security to defray monthly expenses, 34% of respondents said they were highly dependent (5 on a 1–5 scale). Another 37% ranked their dependence 3 or 4, indicating medium to strong reliance on their monthly Social Security checks. Only 14% said they were not at all dependent on Social Security.
- Fifty-six percent of respondents began saving in earnest for retirement between the ages of 25 and 40, while 16% either started saving for retirement after age 60 or went into retirement without any savings.

Fifty-four percent self-managed their accumulation strategies, while 27% relied on financial professionals to help them plan for retirement.

■ Fifty-seven percent of respondents said it was not at all likely that they would run out of money during their retirement years. However, 26% thought the prospect of doing so was somewhat likely, and 9% said it was either highly likely or had already happened.

■ Fifty-five percent of retirees surveyed said they had encountered no unexpected obstacles during their savings accumulation phase. Those who did face challenges reported issues such as health-related problems and expenses, market volatility, family obligations, and changes in employment status.

■ Twenty-six percent of retired Boomers blame themselves either for running out of money in their retirement or for the possibility of quickly depleting their financial resources—because they did not start saving early enough or save enough. Sixteen percent blame the government, with a Social Security payment too low to meet financial needs. Fifteen percent pointed to healthcare costs being much higher than expected.

■ Half of survey respondents said they feel financial stress and worry in retirement on par with that during their working years.

■ Adjusting to a fixed income presents significant challenges for some retirees. Twenty-nine percent of respondents cited the increasing costs of living, including healthcare expenses, while 17% noted the erosion of purchasing power due to inflation.

■ Many retirees are enjoying their free time as planned, with 58% reporting that they are doing exactly what they intended in retirement. Twenty-three percent said that they have accomplished some of their goals but regretted that their income is preventing them from doing the rest. As to their favorite retirement activities, 25% like traveling, 13% spend time with family and friends, and 13% simply enjoy their downtime.

■ Twenty-eight percent of Boomers in the survey said they plan to leave an inheritance for their heirs and have actively set aside funds. This compares with 21% of respondents who plan to use all of their financial resources during their retirement years and 34% who are undecided.

■ Twenty percent of respondents said that what surprised them most about their retirement is the joy they get from pursuing long-delayed passion and interests. Nineteen percent were surprised by the amount of free time they have available and the challenge of filling it productively. Others were caught off-guard by feeling socially disconnected, unengaged, and isolated, and still others by the effect of healthcare costs on their budgets, even with insurance.

Baby Boomers and Technology

As suggested earlier, Boomers have been involved with computers and technology as they developed during their lifetime. This is the generation most likely to have purchased some of the earliest home computers available, such as the PC Junior or the Apple II, Apple II Plus, Apple IIe, and the Apple III. As they got older, with more discretionary spending available, they were able to purchase innovative tech products as they were developed and introduced to the marketplace. As their professions and trades became computerized, they were either leading the computerizations or part of its implementation within their professions. Additionally, they often had computers at home for themselves and their children to learn how to use them, realizing a definite future need. As a result, they are a generation of computer-literate individuals and find themselves using computers and online searches almost as often as younger generations. Now that some are entering their 60s and others are approaching 80, Boomers are no less enthusiastic about modern technologies but now are as likely to learn about technologies from their children as they are from peers, who themselves are recent converts. While the use of computers was once a sign of the generational divide, Boomers have lived and worked in an era in which their use was quite common and even necessary. Thus, if they worked in occupations where computer use was essential, Boomers are often very computer literate.

A list of 10 areas of technology used by Baby Boomers routinely was compiled by Scheve (2011). While a 15-year-old list, it represented technologies that Boomers continued to use as they moved into retirement, including desktop computers and laptops, social networking, smartphones, iPads and iPods, online banking, online news sites, eReaders, flatscreen televisions and home entertainment equipment, home healthcare technology, and GPS.

James (2015) indicates that Baby Boomers are considered digital immigrants in that they did not grow up with technology but have embraced it as it developed. Eighty percent of Baby Boomers had cell phones in 2010, but by 2015, only 27% of those 65 and older who owned cell phones used smartphones. Most Baby Boomers, 68%, use more than one device: phone, tablet, and/or computer. It is the way in which they use tech that differentiates them from their younger counterparts. True to how they learned technology, Boomers have tended to use it for productivity while younger generations also use it for connectivity with friends and others. Social media is more of a Generation Y/Millennial skill, but Boomers are catching up as 56% of them use Facebook and other programs such as Twitter and Google+. Breaking up the Baby Boomer group into two age group sections, older (born 1946–1954) and younger (born 1955–1964), Rainie and Perrin (2016) compiled the following statistics regarding their use of technology☺

■ Internet use: older 76%, younger 83%
■ Broadband at home: older 60%, younger 66%
■ Cell phone: older 87%, younger 91%
■ Smartphone: older 46%, younger 59%
■ Computer tablet: older 41%, younger 35%
■ Social media: older 45%, younger 54%
  ■ Facebook: older 46%, younger 52%
  ■ Pinterest: older 17%, younger 19%
  ■ Instagram: older 8%, younger 8%
  ■ Twitter: older 8%, younger 8%

Older studies by Rainie (2012) also suggest that Boomers are familiar with

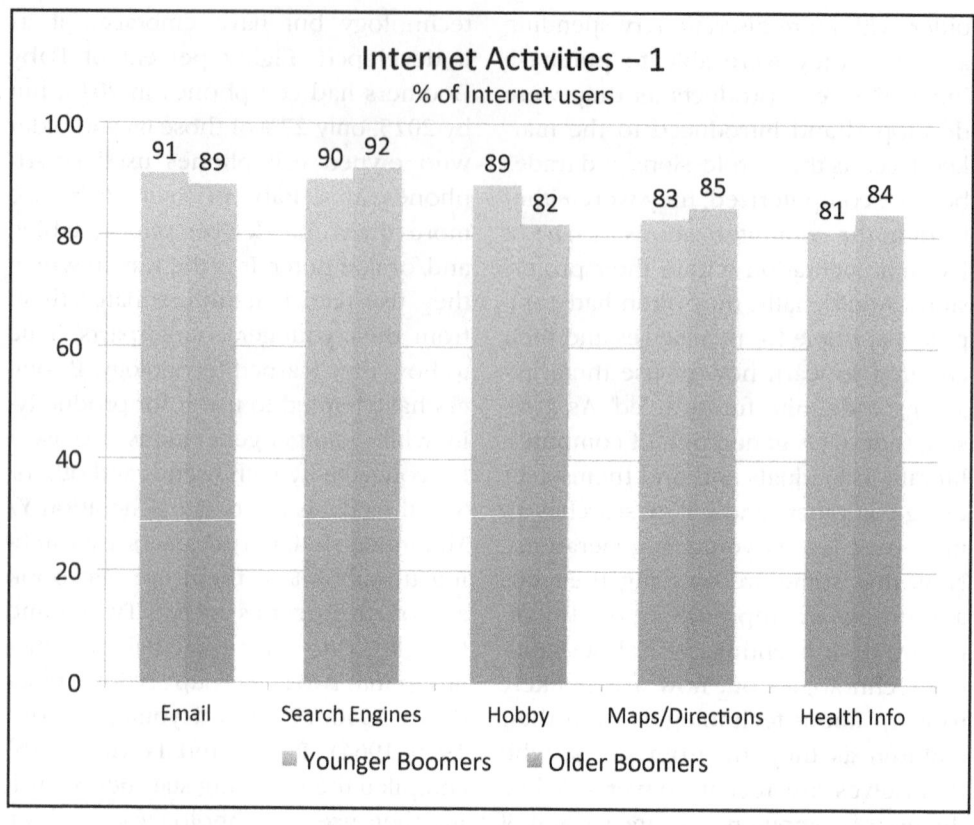

Figure 20–7. Older and younger Baby Boomer uses of technology. *Source*: Pew Research Center (2012).

technology and prepared for more. An Internet of things will not be alien or intimidating to them as they are a generation of technology adaptors and tech learners that have exploited personal networks and Internet communities to exploit life enhancement by technology. While wary of the broad societal impact of these gadgets, Boomers use computers and the Internet for a variety of activities, shown in Figure 20–7, Figure 20–8, and Figure 20–9 from Rainie (2012).

It is unique that most Baby Boomers use their computers for information that they require. Of course, most use email and search engines. Gone are the days of people thumbing through the phone book to find phone numbers or places of business when a simple entry into the computer is more convenient and gets a better result. Others use technology for hobbies, repair shops, home services, directions, and health information (Figure 20–7). Boomers also use their computers to obtain do-it-yourself information to fix things that allow them to not use a service technician, save money, and generate projects to keep themselves busy. The Internet is also their source of information about news and sports as well as government regulations for various concerns, including Social Security, Medicare, and, yes, hearing aids and audiological services.

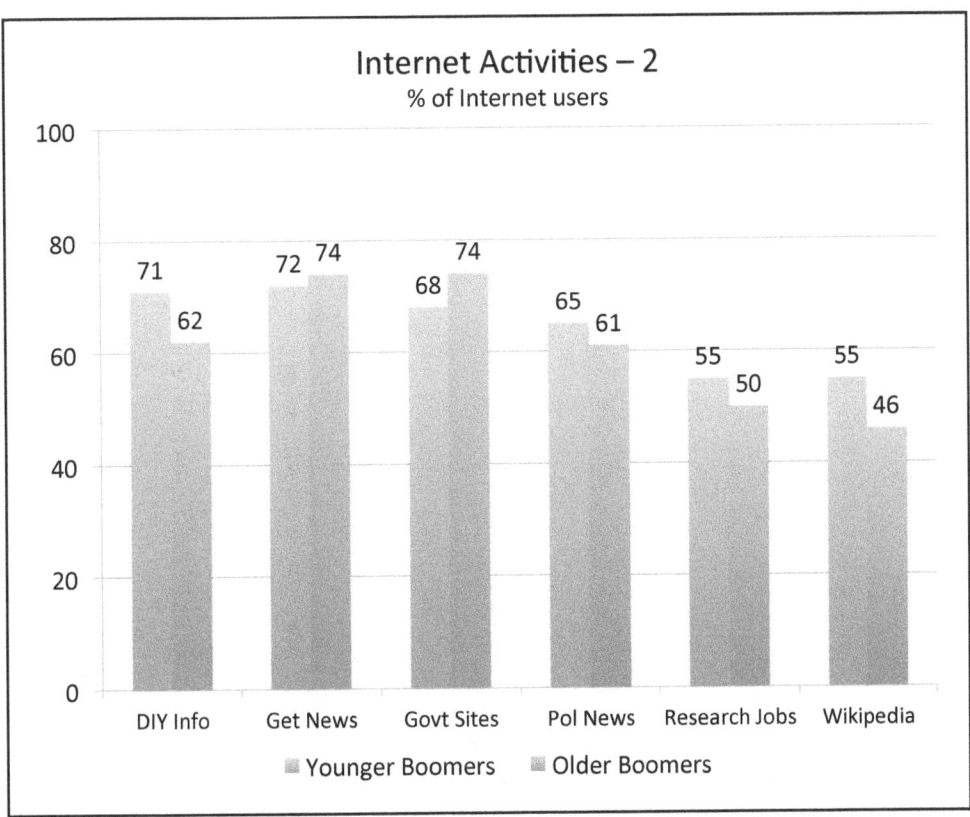

Figure 20–8. Older and younger Baby Boomer uses of technology. *Source*: Pew Research Center (2012).

They research possible jobs and other work opportunities online as well as read about interesting topics on various Wikipedia sites (Figure 20–8).

Further, Figure 20–9 indicates that they use technology to shop for the things they want and need, purchase these goods, and have them delivered to their door, allowing them to obtain what they want without walking all over town looking for those necessities. Computer hackers notwithstanding, many conduct their travel arrangements and banking online, even making online deposits when necessary. It is so much simpler than the trek downtown to the travel agent or the bank.

Some Boomers even participate in online auctions, bidding for some of the things that are treasures as well as essentials. These data are probably low in the use of technology by Baby Boomers for various purposes. Their early adoption history and use of technology suggest that their interaction with technology for everyday uses mentioned above is likely to be higher than indicated in 2012. Solutions (2024) now indicates that Boomers by 2020 were still actively embracing technology:

■ Eighty-six percent of online seniors spend at least 6 hours a day there and own, on average, five devices.

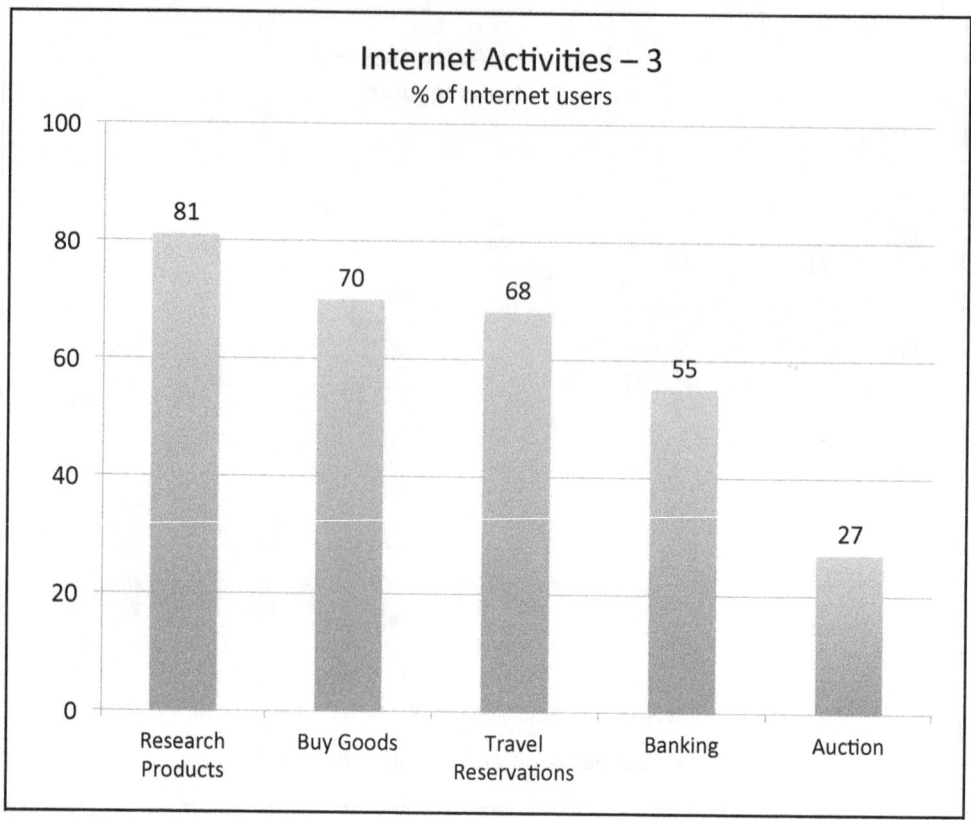

Figure 20–9. Baby Boomer uses of technology. *Source*: Pew Research Center (2012).

- Eighty-two percent of these "digital seniors" use their smartphone every day.
- Ninety-one percent go online to connect with friends and family.
- Eighty-seven percent manage their finances online.
- Seventy-three percent go online to improve their health and wellness.

The COVID-19 pandemic actually increased the use of technology for everyone, and Baby Boomers were no exception. Morris (2021) offers the data presented in Figure 20–10. During the pandemic, there was a huge increase in the use of technology by Boomers.

Boomer use of smartphones goes to 95%, smart TV use is up 10%, TV streaming devices up 20%, smart home devices such as "Alexa" and others up 36%, Smart wristbands up 64%, smart wristbands to measure health and fitness up 64%, and the use of smart watches up 57%. Obviously, Baby Boomers are using technology at a much greater rate than the previous generations and almost similar to later generations.

General and Clinical Drivers for Baby Boomers

Drivers are the motivators of people that will get them to act upon a specific

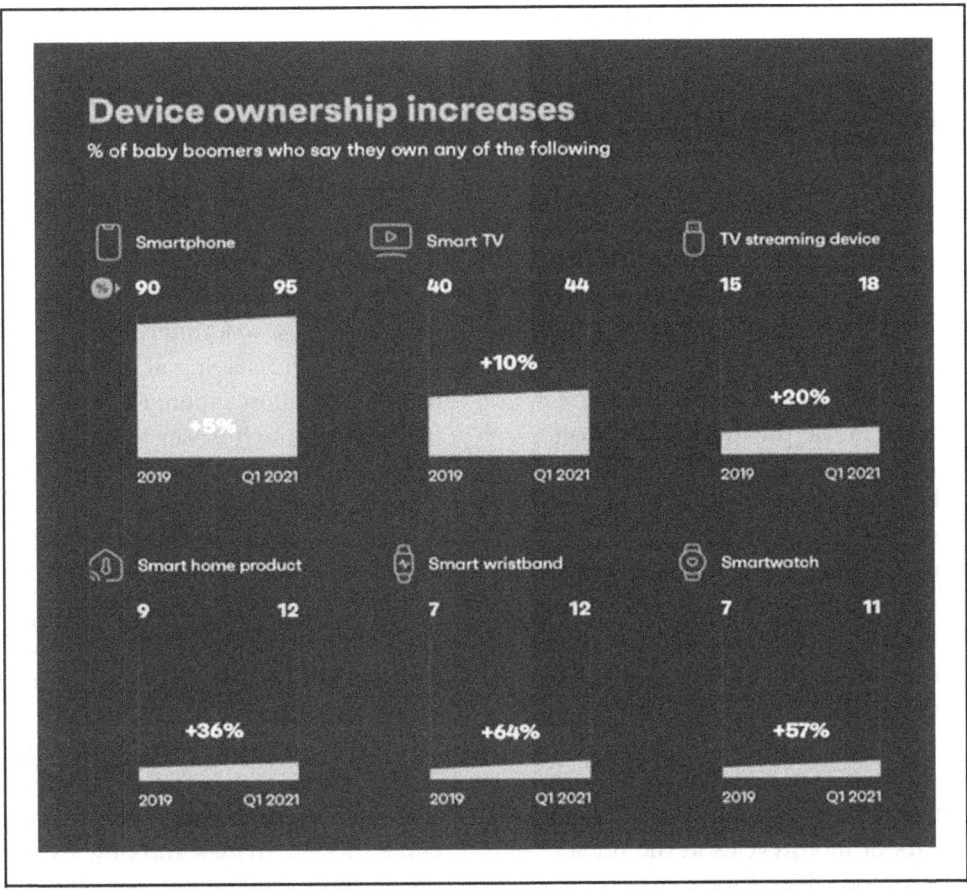

Figure 20–10. Use of technology before and after the pandemic. *Source*: Morris (2021).

issue or activity. Among Boomers, these motivators have been there all through their lives and can be used as part of a marketing program or in the clinic to facilitate action toward a rehabilitative procedure or product. These motivators or drivers include the following:

■ *Affluence.* It is well known that most of the wealth in the United States is held by Baby Boomers. While they are worried that they will outlive their retirement program, this generation can virtually afford whatever they need to con-

tinue in their lifestyle. They want to be able to do the things that they always have, and if it takes expensive hearing aids to do that, then they will buy them. Thus, they are more concerned about quality and performance, not necessarily price or the device brand.

■ *Health and wellness.* As a group, Baby Boomers are generally a healthier generation than those that have come before. While they might have started out as a sex, drugs, and rock 'n' roll culture, they have moved toward a healthy lifestyle. Most do not smoke, watch their diet, exercise often, and look for products that will keep them healthy and able to continue their lifestyle. In previous generations, age 40 is when people began to feel old, but among Boomers, this age is now 60. In fact, Thornhill and Martin (2007) state that Baby Boomers feel 14 years younger than their age. For example, a person whose age is 70 would feel like a person of 56 in the previous generation.

■ *Live for today.* Since the group has been driving the U.S. culture for such a long time, they are used to the instant gratification of their wants and needs. While they look for immediate satisfaction, high quality and special service are also expected. Since they feel younger Boomers, are seen conducting sports that are generally thought to be for the young, such as racing cars or motorcycles at the track, triathlons, marathons, mountain climbing, water sports, downhill skiing, golfing, flying, and many other activities. The "live for today" attitude is also reflected in many other areas such as travel, product purchases, education, and music, as Boomers want to get it all done while they are healthy and can participate.

■ *Working retirement.* Boomers have not saved very well for retirement but are generally healthier than those who have come before them. Where people used to retire at age 62 or age 65, there are now incentives for working longer that increase the retirement income. The difference in retiring at age 62 and age 70 is a 33% higher Social Security check each month. While some of the reasons for a working retirement are financial, another is cultural. All their life they have prepared for a career, worked in that occupation, and may have become prominent in their profession. To many, work is their identity, and giving that up totally is extremely difficult. Thus, working retirement is beneficial to staying active and technology allows them to work from home much easier than previous generations. Teaching online classes, consulting, and working from home are all possible in a high-tech society.

■ *Desire for new experiences.* They have always had new experiences, travel, education, sports, and other areas, but effective communication is essential to continue participating in new experiences. There is a need to stay competent and effective, so while these activities and new experiences will slow down somewhat, they will continue these activities well into retirement.

■ *Individualism.* Boomers have been independent and self-reliant all their life. Due to their upbringing, they feel special. Since they do feel special, they appreciate individual services and the time that is given to them by professionals. In an era when professionals take less time with everyone, the extra time taken with Boomer patients is appreciated and expected. While personal styles are able to tolerate group sessions in government clinics, such as the Veterans Administration, generally Boomers do not like the formality of a group and feel that they, in particular, need extra attention. Each

Baby Boomer is a special person with a special hearing loss, lifestyle, and situation, and the extra time is what they feel they are paying for in the rehabilitative treatment sessions.

■ *Convenience.* This group appreciates convenience and will go to the most convenient place for rehabilitative services. They appreciate easy to obtain products, close interactions, and immediate service, all on their schedule. This is the group that invented personal shoppers and dry cleaning delivered to your door; therefore, they will go to the clinic that is closest to them that offers the best personal service.

■ *Value for money.* While more concerned about performance, service, and convenience than price, Boomers do expect to obtain value for the price paid when obtaining products and services. They tend to have a "get what you pay for" attitude toward purchases, but they are not coupon cutters and expect the same deal with or without the coupon in hand.

■ *Savvy and hungry for information.* Consider how confusing the Internet is relative to hearing instruments. It is difficult for consumers (patients) to tell the real audiologists from the groups of dispensers, manufacturer clinics, ENT clinics, and other clinical operations in the area. Often patients will come in with a file that they have taken from the Internet or some other source and ask very good questions about the products, procedures, and services offered with the clinic. These files should be embraced as honestly and sincerely as pos-

sible as the clinician's answers are extremely important to prospective patients as they choose a place to obtain treatment for their hearing impairment.

■ *Ethics and environmentalism.* This group invented ethical medical interactions such as the Health Insurance Portability and Accountability Act of 1996 (HIPPA) and are concerned with how their medical records are handled. They appreciate knowing some of the specifics of office procedures and will ask about them on occasion. Additionally, they also were the first generation genuinely concerned about the environment, with "green cars," recycling, and other environmentally conscious efforts. They are concerned about battery disposal and other practical issues relative to the environment.

Previous groups of patients, patients from the Mature Best generation, have been very compliant and took recommendations at face value, but Boomers will question each and every recommendation either silently or out loud. They will ask the clinician why, look it up on the computer, or discuss it with friends and relatives to fully digest the recommendation rather than accept it at face value. Since this generation of patients will have a considerable influence on the practice of audiology for some time to come, there are six rules for clinical intervention:

■ *Rule 1: Use life stage . . . not age.* Clinicians cannot consider all Baby Boomers the same, as these patients are quite a diverse group and have many different lifestyles. Due to the divorce rate and other factors, some will be parents and grandparents at the same time, often with teenagers and/or college-age children still at home. Another group will be married or single empty nesters, and still others could be caring for aging parents. Sometimes these lifestyle situations are all happening at the same time. Clinically, it becomes necessary to consider the patient's *stage of life* rather than the *person's age* as there may be substantial diversity in lifestyle among those of the same age. Treatment techniques and product needs cannot be determined simply by their age but must be considered according to their stage of life situation. Since there is such diversity, group techniques are not very successful, and a one-to-one interaction is expected and very necessary to achieve the greatest success.

■ *Rule 2: Emotionally meaningful treatment programs.* This generation needs to be sold emotionally on treatment techniques and products as they tend to purchase on "gut-level" feelings. They have enough experience in making purchases that they will know when it is right to move forward with a purchase, but the process must be sold by stories, others that have benefited from this technique, and so on. Paint a picture of how future conversations and interactions will be conducted relating to communicative interactions with grandchildren and others. Describe how they will fit into the programs that have been designed for them, describing the type of person that benefits from the recommended device and the treatment program. Further, absolute product claims do not work with this generation. Statements like "This is the best of the best" and other similar statements do not work with this group as they have heard these things before about other products or services. Statements that suggest the type of person or lifestyle that might be successful with this program or product tend to work much better. High-pressure sales techniques do not work with Baby Boomers.

■ *Rule 3: Watch out for ageism.* Most Baby Boomers do not consider themselves old and ignore negative concepts, words, and images, such as "elderly," "senior citizen," "senior center," or "senior exercise program," as, in their opinion, these terms, issues, and programs do not apply to them and, consequently, they do not respond to senior bank accounts, senior citizen discounts, and other specials that are marketed to old people. While sensitive to these terms and programs, this group does respond to techniques and programs not specifically designed for "old people," such as Lace, Amptify, or other computer-driven rehabilitative programs.

■ *Rule 4: The more information the better.* Recall that this generation is much better educated and computer savvy, so they usually do not take a recommendation at face value. Their experience, education, and personal style motivate them to consider all the recommendations that have been presented, from friends, relatives, other professionals, readings, the Internet, and elsewhere. Embrace them when they come in with a file of computer searches as that suggests that they are considering your recommendations carefully. Often these files do not surface until after the history, evaluation, and discussion have taken place, but this is not a challenge to recommendations presented but an opportunity to answer questions that will solidify the clinical discussion, building more trust into the relationship.

■ *Rule 5: Understand their changing values.* This generation of patients worked extremely hard to stand out from the crowd of others that had aspirations as well. They worked long hours, attempting to be just that much better to get noticed by their profession or corporation. They went through the transition process of "becoming someone," and now, after much success, they are in the process of "being someone." Clinically, this can be used as an advantage in that this group is not as interested in being "cool." Thus, they accept behind-the-ear devices as they want to hear rather than insisting on a device that must not be seen. Additionally, Boomers are used to nonphysician practitioners, such as nurse practitioners, chiropractors, dentists, physical therapists, psychologists, speech pathologists, and audiologists.

■ *Rule 6: Learn baby learn.* How patients feel about their clinician and the clinic will vary from time to time. The impact of this rise and fall will be the expertise of the clinician. It is essential in this time of profound changes in technology, competition, and intervention procedures to stay ahead of the curve

in knowledge of these techniques and procedures. If the patients feel that they know more than their clinician, they will be off to seek other assistance.

In summary, an in-depth knowledge of the Baby Boomer generation is important for sales success as they are uniquely different from those that came before them. They are a very large group that will influence sales and, thus, the success of practices for several years to come. It should be remembered that the group is computer savvy and present at about 14 years younger than their chronological age and want to stay that way. They are not brand loyal to your practice or to products but simply looking for high-quality instruments, performance from the clinicians, and special treatment. For all of these reasons, Boomers will require a substantial departure from traditional sales strategies and techniques.

Personal Style

Some patients cause clinicians frustration, wonder, or worry or are just plain surprising. Sometimes those that audiologists do not expect to do well surpass their wildest expectations while others that are expected to perform in the process have difficulty in adjusting to the products and/or the treatment. It is well known that two patients with the same hearing impairment using the same hearing devices might not share the same success or failure. How could this be? Could it be lifestyle or other factors? Is it the patient's personal style that is causing the problems?

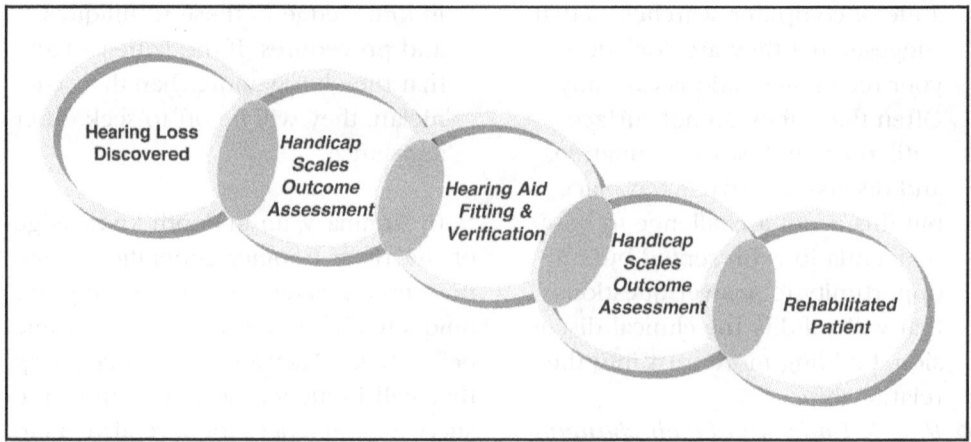

Figure 20–11. Traditional aural rehabilitation process. *Source*: Traynor (2013).

Although it may be argued that the steps in the rehabilitative process are different from those presented here, the typical aural rehabilitative chain of events includes the discovery of the hearing loss, the administration of a handicap scale, a hearing aid fitting, and another handicap scale, and then when the handicap scale is positive, we have a rehabilitated patient (Figure 20–11).

Traynor (1999, 2020) and Bray (2021) have argued for quite some time that the aural rehabilitative process is not that simple. Rehabilitative treatment is not just the hearing impairment and the fitting of amplification, but a process that occurs within the patient's personal style, their interaction with the clinician's personal style, and the hearing impairment. Personal style should be considered at the beginning of the aural rehabilitation process shortly after the discovery of the hearing impairment (Figure 20–12). It is the patient's internal process for accepting the hearing loss and adjusting to the treatment program, and the clinician must consider that those with the same hearing loss and the same hearing device will vary in their reactions

and their treatment program according to their personal style. What is personal style and how does it affect the rehabilitative and sales process? First, there must be a method of assessing this personal style, and there are many. While some use other personal style assessments, such as DSC, Colors, Tascom, and others, the concept that is the easiest and well understood to use is the Keirsey Temperament Sorter (Keirsey & Bates, 1984). The Keirsey concept is a derivative of the Myers-Briggs Type Indicator (MBTI) (Briggs & Myers, 1976), a very well researched personality assessment that is based upon the theories of Dr. Gustav Jung, a Swiss psychiatrist.

The MBTI and Audiology

The MBTI can provide audiologists with a window to view how patients react to things, situations, and other people. Moreover, the MBTI and type theory offer outstanding opportunities to provide clinical insight into patients for use in the rehabilitative treatment process. It can determine if patients are

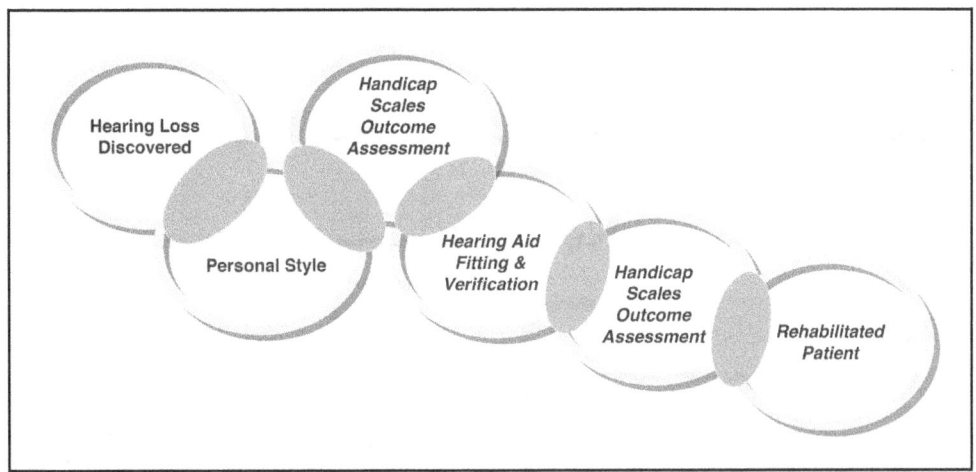

Figure 20–12. Missing link in traditional aural rehabilitation process. *Source*: Traynor (2013).

outward or inward directed, move from one project to another, give up easily, are bothered by minor details, or are generally "laid back." The use of the Myers-Briggs Type Indicator has been suggested (Traynor, 1999; Traynor & Buckles, 1996; Traynor & Holmes, 2001, 2002) for use in audiology clinics. As constructed, the MBTI identifies 16 distinctively different patterns describing how people interface with their instincts. These Jungian instincts or motivations, purposes, aims, values, drives, impulses, and urges are what create the fundamental personality differences among people. Since personal preference for a personal style characteristic reflects how that person interfaces with these instincts, these preferences can be used to categorize or type people. Based on Jung, Myers, and Briggs and portions of other psychological theories, personal situations, and reactions to word pairs, adjusted by gender, present scores on opposite scales of four continua: *Extraversion (E)/Introversion (I), Sensing (S)/ iNtuition (N), Thinking (T)/Feeling (F),* and *Judging (J)/Perceiving (P),* as shown in Figure 20–13.

In general terms, *Extraversion/Introversion* can be thought of as outgoing or shy, while *Sensing/iNtuition* may be considered as information gathering. The *Thinking/Feeling* scale can be thought of as information evaluation and *Judging/Perceiving* refers to scheduled versus flexible. Scores on these four continua make up the 16 personality types offered by the MBTI. The scores generated on the various continua are presented in Figure 20–14.

Each continuum is scored by beginning at zero in the center and progressing to a higher score, suggesting a stronger attribute toward the sides. Since the scores start at zero in the center of the continuum and become greater toward each side of the continuum, people who score in the areas that correspond to E, S, T, and J would be presented as a personal style of ESTJ (Figure 20–14), whereas those scoring in areas corresponding to I, N, F, and P would be presented as an INFP.

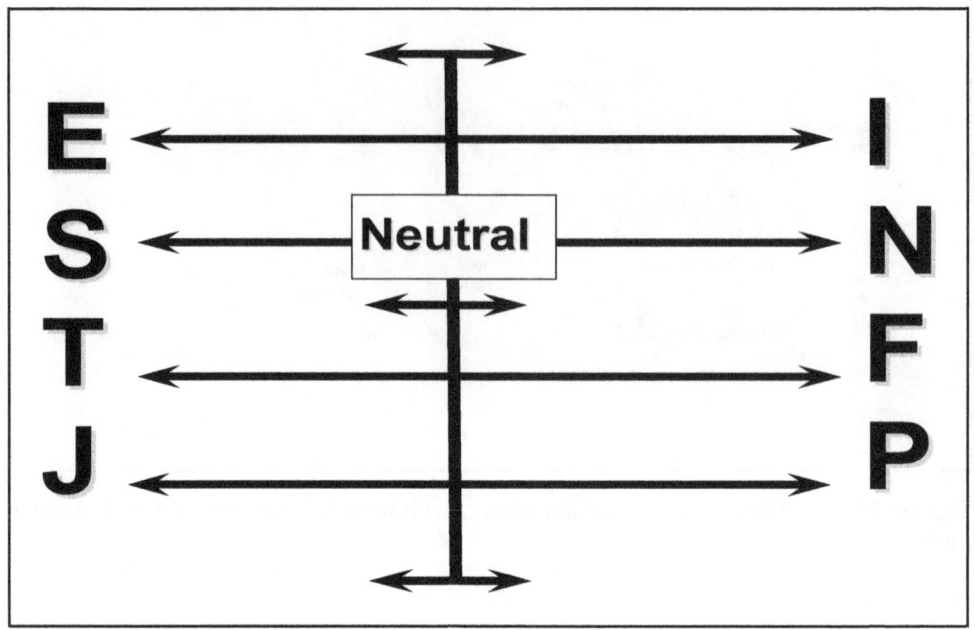

Figure 20–13. MBTI assessment continuums. *Source*: Traynor (1999).

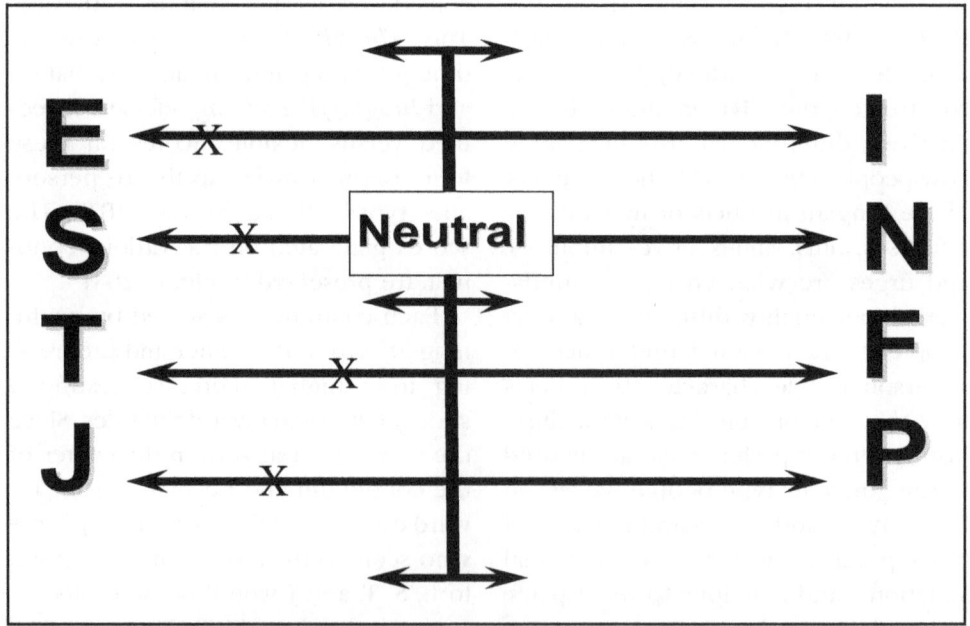

Figure 20–14. Scoring of the MBTI Personality Style Assessment. *Source*: Traynor (1999).

ISTJ	ISFJ	INFJ	INTJ
Serious, Quiet, Practical, Logical, Matter of Fact, Dependable, Realistic, Take Responsibility	Quiet, Friendly, Responsible Thorough, Painstaking Conscientious, Accurate, Concerned for Others	Succeed by Perseverance Originality, Quietly Forceful Conscientious, Principles Concerned for Others	Original Minds, Great Drive Long Range Vision, Organized Skeptical, Critical, Independent, High Standards, Determined
ISTP	**ISFP**	**INFP**	**INTP**
Quiet, Reserved, Observing, Mechanical, Cause / Effect, How and Why things work, Find Practical Solutions,	Retiring, Quietly Friendly, Sensitive, Kind, Modest, Shun Disagreements, Do not Force their Opinions	Quiet Observers, Idealistic, Loyal, Courteous, Adaptable Flexible, Little Concern for Possessions or surroundings	Quiet and Reserved, Theoretical Scientific Problem Solvers, Logical, No Small Talk Sharply defined Interests
ESTP	**ESFP**	**ENFP**	**ENTP**
On-the-Spot Problem Solvers Focus on Getting Results, Dislike long explanations,	Outgoing, Accepting, Friendly, Enjoy Everything, Sound Common Sense, Likes Facts, Not Theory	Warmly Enthusiastic, Distractible, Ingenious, Does not Plan Ahead, Rely on Ability to Improvise	Quick, Good at Many things Stimulating Company, Alert, Finds logical reasons for what they want, May Argue for Fun
ESTJ	**ESFJ**	**ENFJ**	**ENTJ**
Practical, Realistic, Decisive, Matter of Fact, Not interested in Abstract or Theories, Organizers,	Warm Hearted, Talkative, Popular, Conscientious, Need Encouragement and Praise, Need Harmony	Responsible, Responsive, Responds to Praise and Criticism, Sociable, Popular, Sympathetic,	Frank, Decisive, Leaders in activities, Good at reasoning, Enjoy adding to their knowledge, Likes to talk

Figure 20–15. Myers Briggs Personal Styles (Myers & Briggs, 1976). *Source*: Traynor, R. M., & Holmes, A. E., Personal Style and Hearing Aid Fitting. *Trends in Amplification*, 6(1), 1–31. Copyright © 2002 Sage. DOI: https://doi.org/10.1177/1084713802 00600102.

The 16 MBTI personal style types, each with its own set of characteristics, are summarized in Figure 20–15.

Extraversion (E)/ Introversion (I) Scale

Jung looked at *Extraversion* and *Introversion* as valuable opposing methods of interacting, utilized by everyone, but not in the same manner or with equal ease. Some individuals are naturally interactive, and others are not. Buetter (2012) indicates that 50% to 74% are extroverts and 16% to 50% are introverts, concurring with older studies such as Bayne (1995) that suggested there are three *Extraverts (E)* for every *Intro-* vert *(I)*. *Extraverts (E)* are more tuned into the external environment and tend to be more interested and comfortable when they are working actively with people or things. *Extroverted (E)* people prefer to communicate by conversation, often speaking first and reflecting later, and learn best by doing or discussing. People that "blurt out" answers and comments, often regretting these utterances, are *Extroverts (E)*.

To the contrary, *Introverts (I)*, make up about 16% to 50% of the population and are drawn into an inner world, preferring to communicate by writing, and reflect before acting or speaking. *Introverts (I)* learn best by reflection or mental exercise and are more comfortable when their work involves ideas. *Introverts (I)* require a good deal of their activity to take place quietly inside their heads, thinking and reanalyzing their statements and then finally responding. The word pair that differentiates an *Extravert (E)* from an *Introvert (I)* is sociability as opposed to territoriality. Where the *Extravert (E)* finds breadth appealing, the *Introvert(I)* finds the notion of depth more attractive. Other cues to preference are intensive interaction (*Extraversion*) as opposed to concentration (*Introversion*), multiplicity of relationships (*Extraversion*) as opposed to limited relationships (*Introversion*), expenditure of energy (*Extraversion*) as opposed to conservation of energy (*Introversion*), and interest in external happenings (*Extraversion*) as opposed to interest in internal reactions (*Introversion*).

Sensing (S)/iNtuition (N) Scale

As Jung's theory evolved, he was convinced that there were two strategies used for information gathering to find answers to problems or situations. These information-gathering systems were termed *Sensing (S)* or *iNtuition (N)*. *Sensing (S)* strategies use the eyes, ears, and other senses to tell what is occurring. At the other extreme, the *iNtuitor* uses meanings, relationships, and possibilities that reach beyond the senses gathering facts. These *iNtuitive (N)* skills are especially useful for seeing what might be done about a situation. It is common in type theory for one of these strategies to be preferred over the other. As the *Sensing (S)* strategy is used, the individual attains more skills, becoming an expert at noticing and rapidly assimilating all the observable facts to arrive at an analytical decision. Individuals leaning toward the *Sensing (S)* strategy

become more realistic, practical, observant, fun loving, and very adept at recalling and working with a substantial number of facts. Those that prefer *iNtuition (I)* value imagination and inspiration and are creative in projects and problem-solving. About 75% of the population utilizes the *Sensing (S)* type strategy, while 25% use *iNtuition (N)* (Priebe, 2016).

Careful listening to a person's choice of words can provide clues to how people prefer to gather information. Their choice of vocabulary, intonation, and voice quality can transmit one value over another. People who prefer *Sensing (S)*, for example, typically value experience, assess the wisdom of the past, and want to be realistic, while *iNtuititors (N)* value hunches, appraise a vision of the future, and are likely to be speculative. Words such as actual, down-to-earth, no nonsense, facts, practical, and sensible are descriptions of *Sensing (S)* people. Being risk takers and speculative, *iNtuitors (N)* prefer words such as possible, fascinating, fantasy, fiction, ingenious, and imaginative.

Thinking (T)/Feeling (F) Scale

Experience taught Jung that there were differences in how people arrived at their decisions. According to Keirsey.com (2024), the population is split about 60/40 between those that make decisions with a *Thinking (T)* strategy and those that use the *Feeling (F)* method. The *Thinking (T)* strategy (60%) predicts the logical result of any action by deciding impersonally on the basis of cause and effect, similar to the objective methods utilized by a computer. The opposite of this mechanical form of the data-based decision-making strategy is the 40% that are *Feeling (F)*. *Feeling (F)* decision-makers consider personal values as the criteria for making decisions. They give weight to anything that matters or is personally important to the individuals impacted by the decision, without considering the logical nature of the question. In decisiveness, both *Thinking (T)* and *Feeling (F)* are often utilized with equal confidence but not simultaneously. Certain personality types trust *Thinking (T)* more than *Feeling (F)* and grow skillful at dealing with the world logically without the intervention of unpredictable human reactions. Those that trust *Feeling (F)* are typically more sympathetic, appreciative, and tactful and give great weight to the personal values of themselves and others. Those that prefer impersonal choices, the *Thinkers (T)*, respond positively to words such as objective, principles, policy, laws, criteria, firmness, justice, categories, standards, critique, analysis, and allocation. Conversely, *Feelers (F)* react positively to words like subjective, values, social values, extenuating circumstances, intimacy, persuasion, humane, harmony, good or bad, appreciate, sympathy, and devotion.

Those scoring more toward the *Thinking (T)* side of the continuum give priority to objective criteria and are apt to be good at argumentation, attempting to win people over to their point of view through logic and data rather than appealing to their emotions. People scoring high on the *Feeling (F)* side of the continuum are good at persuasion based upon the personal impact of the decision on the individuals involved.

Perception (P)/ Judgment (J) Scale

Rigidness, *Judgment (J)*, or flexibility, *Perceiving (P)*, are the keys to the last of Jung's four continua. The *Judgment (J)/ Perceiving (P)* continuum describes how a person relates to the outside world. Fifty-five percent of the population are *Judgers (J)* and use a judging process to live in a planned, orderly way, to regulate and control their lives (Bayne, 1995; Statistic Brain, 2016). Individuals preferring a judging lifestyle are also scheduled, organized, systematic, and methodological. *Perceivers (P)* are the 45% of the population who typically prefer to rely on a perceptive process to deal with the outside world (Bayne, 1995). *Perceivers (P)* live in a spontaneous world, seeking to understand life and adapt to it. Individuals who prefer the *Perceiving (P)* end of the continuum tend to be spontaneous, casual, and flexible and prefer to have things loose and open-ended. *Judging(J)* people prefer words such as settled, decided, fixed, plan ahead, run one's life, closure, decision-making, planned, completed, decisive, "wrap it up," urgency, deadlines, and "get the show on the road." *Perceivers (P)*, however, prefer expressions such as pending, gather more data, flexible, adapt as you go, let life happen, keep options open, "treasure hunting," open-ended, emergent, tentative, "something will happen," "there's plenty of time," "what deadline?" and "let's wait and see."

Keirsian Temperaments: A Simpler Method

Although the MBTI may be very useful to audiologists in their rehabilitative endeavors, it can be overwhelming to clinically consider eight extraverted types (ESTP, ESFP, ENTP, ENFP, ESTJ, ESFJ, ENFJ, ENTJ) and eight introverted types (ISTJ, ISFJ, INFJ, INTJ, ISTP, ISFP,

Table 20–1. The Four Kersey Temperaments and Associated 16 MBTI Types

NF		NT		SJ		SP	
ENFJ	INFJ	ENTJ	INTJ	ESTJ	ISTJ	ESFP	ISFP
ENFP	INFP	ENTP	INTP	ESFJ	ISFJ	ESTP	ISTP

Source: Traynor, R. M., & Holmes, A. E., Personal Style and Hearing Aid Fitting. *Trends in Amplification*, 6(1), 1–31. Copyright © 2002 Sage. DOI: https://doi.org/10.1177/108471380200600102.

INFP, INTP). While there are several methods (Colors, DISC, Tascom) for considering type within a "personality shorthand" that offer clinicians specific keys to certain personal styles without having to concentrate on all the 16 MBTI traits at once, one shorthand method used quite often in personal type theory is the Keirsian Temperament (KT), originally discussed by Keirsey and Bates (1978/1984) and later clarified by Keirsey.com (2024). In this scheme, the foregoing two groups of eight types can be divided into subgroups designated by two letters, symbolizing similar characteristics. Table 20–1 presents the Keirsian Temperament categories relative to the various MBTI personal styles.

The Keirsey hypothesis suggests that the *Judging(J)/Perceiving(P)* continuum or a person's tendency toward rigidity or flexibility has the most influence on *Sensing (S)* individuals, while the *Thinking (T)/Feeling (F)* continuum or objectivity versus subjectivity has the most effect on *iNtuitive (N)* types. The first letter designation of the Keirsey Temperament reflects how the person gathers information; thus, it will always be either an *S* or an *N*. Typically, the *Sensor (S)* focuses on what is actually there, whereas *iNtuitors (N)* are optimistic and see the possibilities. Consider the concept of "Can't see the forest for the trees"; the *Sensor (S)* sees a tree, while the *iNtuitor (N)* sees a forest. Addition-

ally, *Sensors (S)* tend to be pessimistic and see the "cup as half empty," whereas the more optimistic *iNtuitor (N)* sees the "cup as half full." To *Sensors (S)*, the most important function in information gathering is not how to evaluate the data, but what to do with the data, either organize (*Judging*) it or continue to collect or seek more data (*Perceiving*). Thus, the *S* person will gather the data and evaluate what they have (*Sensing-Judging, SJ*) or they will continue to collect more data (*Sensing-Perceiving, SP*) with the expectation that more information will yield better results. *Sensors* are designated by the Keirsey Temperament as either an *SJ* or an *SP*. The *iNtuitor (N)* is more influenced how they analyze the data either objectively (*Thinking*) or subjectively (*Feeling*). The basic temperament groups for *iNtuitors (N)* are characterized by the Keirsey Temperament with the designations of *NF* and *NT*.

The Keirsey Temperament Sorter separates the 16 MBTI types into four distinct temperaments: *Sensing-Judging (SJ), Sensing-Perceiving (SP), Intuitive-Feelers (NF)*, and *Intuitive-Thinkers (NT)* (Keirsey.com, 2024; Keirsey & Bates, 1978/1984; Traynor & Holmes, 2002), facilitating easier clinical categorization. Keirsey also referred to these "letter designated styles" by names, the *SJ or the Guardian, the SP or the Artisan, the NF or the Idealist*, and *the NT or the Ratio-*

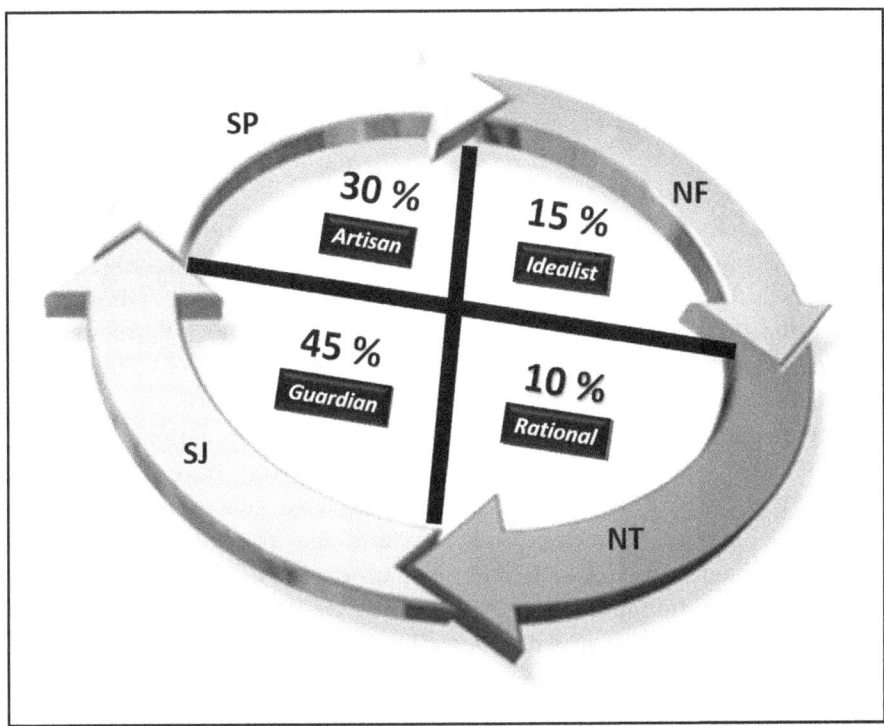

Figure 20–16. Incidence of Keirsey Personality Type in the United States population (O'Brien, 2012).

nal. Keirsey has updated their research according to the changes in personal style of the population to keep their estimates accurate. The current percentages of Keirsian Temperament types within the U.S. population in 2024 are presented in Figure 20–16.

The Keirsian *SJ or Guardian* Temperament makes up about 45% of the U.S. population. *SJs* typically observe what is going on around them and make modifications in the situation, scheduling things to keep order in their lives. Keirsian *SP or Artisan* Temperaments, approximately 30% of the population, use their observation tendencies to find favorable impulsive options. Keirsian *NF or Idealist* Temperament people, 15% of the population, are friendly people that make their decisions based upon how they will affect others, while the Keir-

sian *NT or Rational* Temperament people, only 10 % of the general population, make rational decisions based on facts.

While the online Keirsey Temperament Sorter II is designed to evaluate the four temperaments, it also provides the examinee with an MBTI type. Therefore, when considering the use of the Keirsian Temperaments, it is also prudent to consider its accuracy relative to the MBTI. Keirsey.com (2024) indicates that 62% of the time, all four of the Keirsey Temperaments will match their appropriate MBTI types. It can also be concluded that 84% of the time, the Keirsey will match three of the MBTI types, and 98% to 99% of the time, the Keirsey will match at least two of the MBTI traits. Only 1% to 2% of the time will there be no Keirsey matches with the MBTI. Thus, there is about a 98%

chance of matching at least two of the MBTI traits and an 84% chance of matching three traits. Correlations of .85, .83, .86, and .84 were found between the tests on the *Extraversion (E)/Introversion (I)*, *Sensing (S)/iNtuition (N)*, *Thinking (T)/Feeling (F)*, and *Judging (J)/Perceiving (P)* continuums, respectively, as the MBTI and the Keirsey tests are measuring the same constructs.

Obviously, it would be advantageous to be able to have a formal extensive personality profile, such as the MBTI or Keirsey, on every patient before they are seen in the clinic, but the current MBTI is time-consuming to administer (20–30 minutes), somewhat cumbersome to score, and overwhelming with the results. Therefore, the MBTI it is not as practical for general use in most clinical settings. The Keirsey Temperament Sorter II is available online in several languages at https://www.Keirsey.com and takes about 10 to 20 minutes to administer and is scored immediately. The Keirsey is not as cumbersome to score as the MBTI, is much less expensive, and allows for easy online interpretation.

Description of the Four Keirsey Temperaments

Kroeger and Thuesen (1988) summarize the Keirsey types in an analogy: *"We have a swimming pool so we can entertain a lot in the summer. Our SP guests always grab all the pool toys, head right for the water and invent a new game. The NFs sprawl on the lounge chairs and talk earnestly about life and people. The NTs dangle their feet in the water, rib each other, and critique the issues and people in their professions. Finally, the SJs always, always find some work to do like hanging up towels, husking corn,* *scrubbing the grill, or pulling weeds from the garden."*

Sensing-Judging: SJ *Individuals (Guardians)*

The *SJ* temperament consists of four MBTI types (ESTJ, ISTJ, ESFJ, and ISFJ), and they are termed "Guardians" by Keirsey (1998, 2007; Keirsey & Bates, 1984/1978; Keirsey.com, 2024). Significant proportions of the adult hearing-impaired population, the *SJs*, are individuals who have logistical intelligence, have clear objective practicality, and like to maintain control over situations. A useful summary of the overall characteristics of *SJs* with specific descriptions that can be useful in the informal identification of patients (Kroeger, 1991) is presented in Figure 20–17.

The hearing-impaired *SJ* can exhibit the following traits:

- Generally, very cooperative, active participant in A/R process.
- Value and appreciate authority but have high expectations.
- Have an intense need to maintain control of situations.
- Often take responsibility for their own rehabilitative program.
- Are impatient and frustrated if kept waiting.
- Easily follow detailed instructions and organize priorities.
- Prefer to have specified objectives.
- Have a tendency to overanalyze minor details.
- May prefer an organized group aural rehabilitation approach.
- Check out the web for a video on the *SJ* personal style at Keirsey.com.

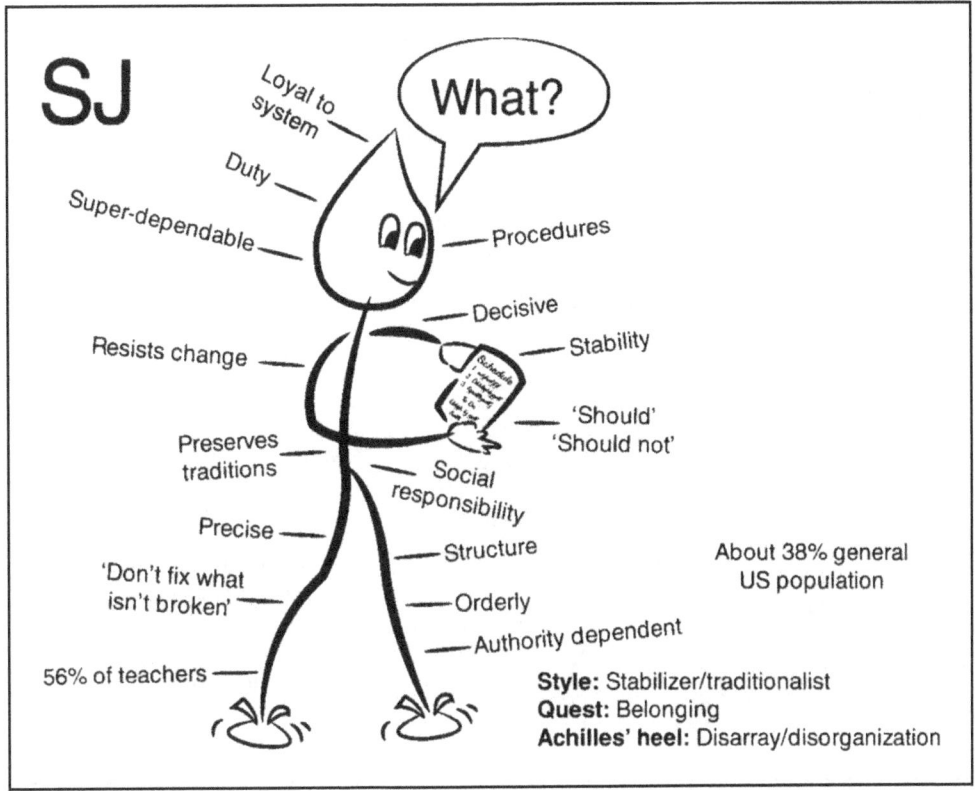

Figure 20–17. The SJ or Guardian Keirsey Personality Type (Kroeger, 1991). *Source*: Traynor, R. M., & Holmes, A. E., Personal Style and Hearing Aid Fitting. *Trends in Amplification*, *6*(1), 1–31. Copyright © 2002 Sage. DOI: https://doi.org/10.1177/108471380200600102.

Sensing-Perceiving: SP *Individuals (Artisans)*

SP individuals are tactically intellectual and are very good in crisis management. Tolerant of difficulties and their own shortcomings, the *SP* generally does not tolerate long procedures. This tolerance of imperfection is why accuracy in procedure is not of particular importance to *SP* patients. Keirsey (1998, 2007; Keirsey & Bates 1984/1978; Keirsey.com, 2024) labeled the SPs as "Artisans" and their characteristics are summarized by Kroeger (1991) and Bayne (1995). Their specific traits are presented in Figure 20–18.

The hearing-impaired *SP* can exhibit the following traits:

■ Prefer a pragmatic, concrete program—not interested in theory.
■ Prefer short explanations and have a "please fix me" attitude.
■ They have no time for the hearing impairment.
■ Have a constant drive to fix their "broken" hearing.
■ Very prone to denying the severity/impact of the hearing loss.
■ Do not prepare for their visit and prefer to just see what happens.
■ They simply jump into the process and may not follow your directions.

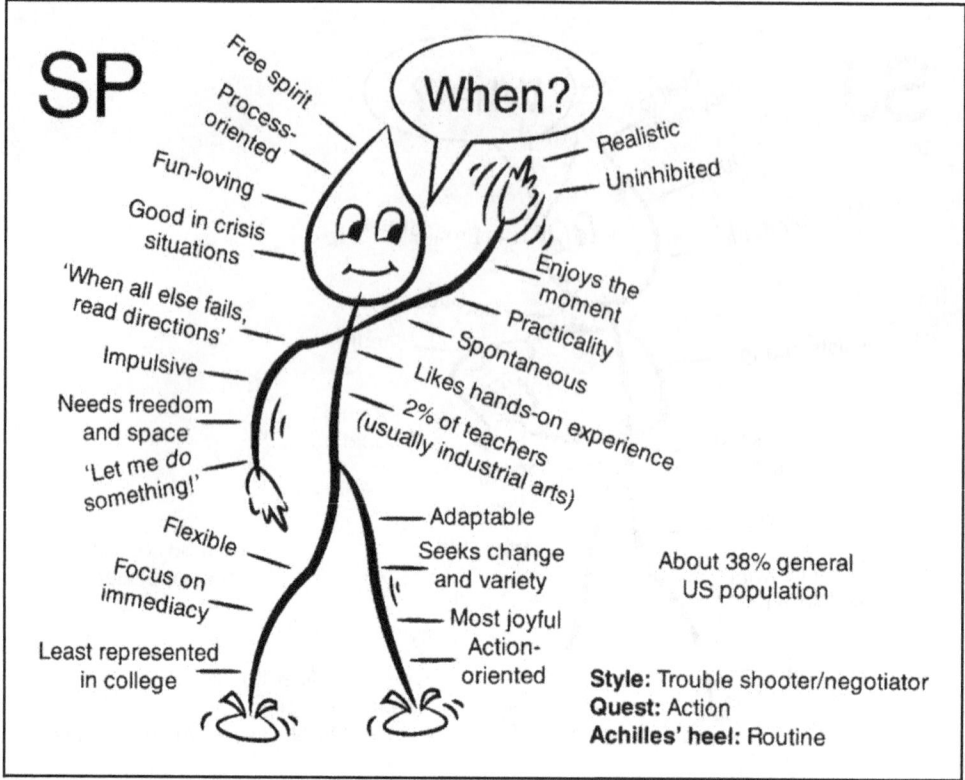

Figure 20–18. The SP or Artisan Keirsey Personality Type (Kroeger, 1991). *Source*: Traynor, R. M., & Holmes, A. E., Personal Style and Hearing Aid Fitting. *Trends in Amplification*, *6*(1), 1–31. Copyright © 2002 Sage. DOI: https://doi.org/10.1177/1084 71380200600102.

■ Have no of concept time, are distractible, and avoid discomfort and decisions.

■ They must consider the treatment program a valuable use of their time.

■ May not read any printed materials unless absolutely necessary.

■ Require immediate relevance for hearing aid fittings and aural rehabilitation program.

■ May give up if the process seems to be unsuccessful.

■ Check out the web for a video on the *SP* personal style at Keirsey.com.

iNtuitive-Feeling: NF *Individuals (Idealists)*

NFs are the abstract cooperators of the world. They have difficulty staying on task and usually have several projects going at the same time. These individuals are very diplomatic in their interactions and have an intense need for harmony in their world. Keirsey (1998, 2007; Keirsey & Bates 1984/1978; Keirsey.com, 2024) called this group "idealists" and their traits are summarized by Kroeger (1991) and Bayne (1995) as harboring a theoretically impossible need to keep everyone happy. Specific

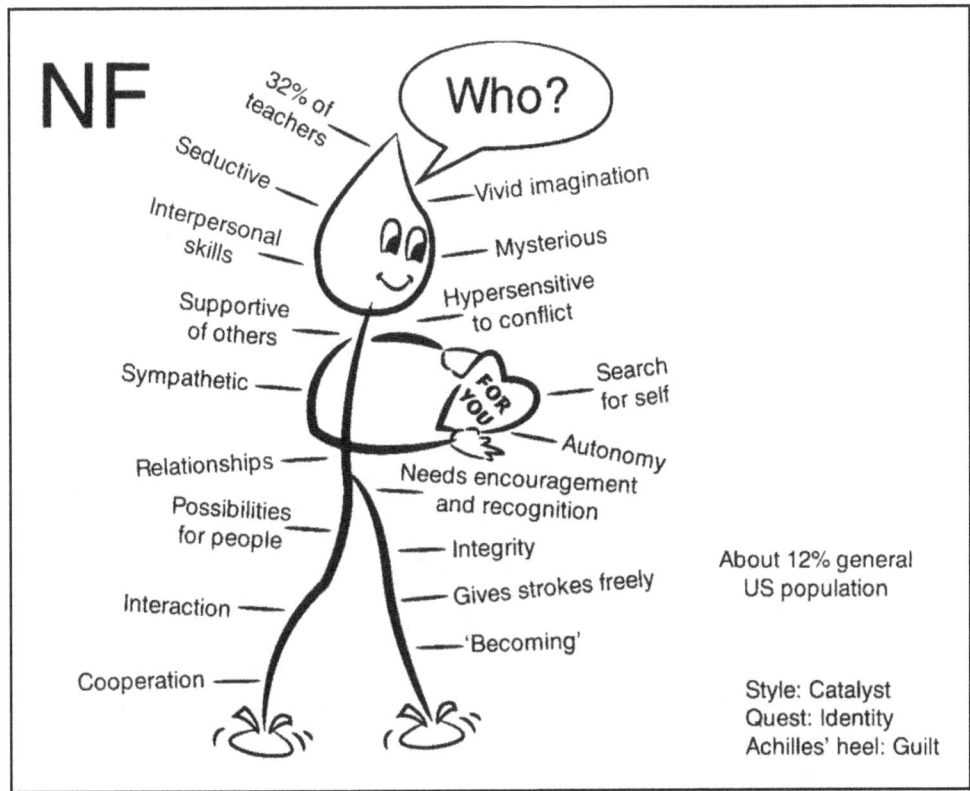

Figure 20–19. The NF or Idealist Keirsey Personality Type (Kroeger, 1991). *Source*: Traynor, R. M., & Holmes, A. E., Personal Style and Hearing Aid Fitting. *Trends in Amplification*, 6(1), 1–31. Copyright © 2002 Sage. DOI: https://doi.org/10.1177/1084 71380200600102.

traits of the NF are presented in Figure 20–19.

The hearing-impaired *NF* can exhibit the following traits:

- Have an intense need for communication with others.
- Intense need to keep harmony in their world.
- Have a feeling of obligation to others to do well in the A/R process.
- They are doing the aural rehabilitation for someone else and really want to be "good patients."
- Often have well-developed coping behaviors.
- Tend to respond best to positive reinforcement.
- Expect clear goals, objectives, and expectations.
- Can be difficult if benefits of amplification have been oversold.
- Prone to self-criticism and worry that they could have done a better job.
- Can become rigid/demanding when aural rehabilitation program is unsuccessful.
- May not offer much positive feedback.
- Generally, very cooperative in aural rehabilitation and work very hard.

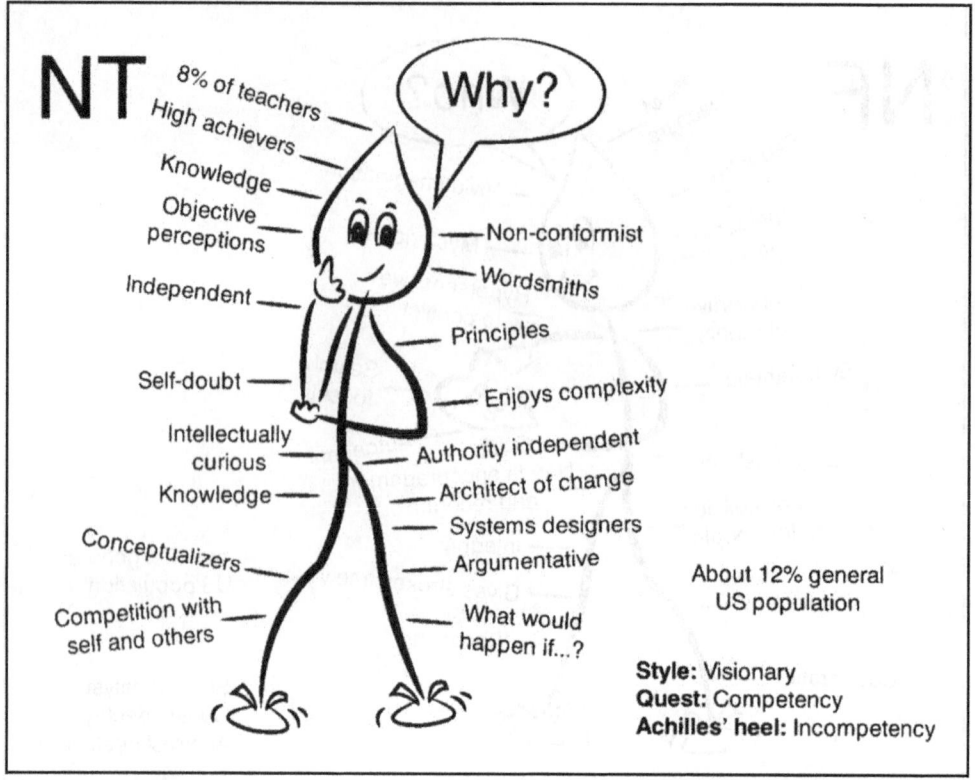

Figure 20–20. The NT or Rational Keirsey Personality Type (Kroeger, 1991). *Source*: Traynor, R. M., & Holmes, A. E., Personal Style and Hearing Aid Fitting. *Trends in Amplification*, 6(1), 1–31. Copyright © 2002 Sage. DOI: https://doi.org/10.1177/1084 71380200600102.

- Are never quite satisfied, always want a bit more hearing.
- Need to see results; to them, talk is cheap.
- Check out the web for a video on the *NF* personal style at Keirsey.com.

iNtuitive-Thinking: NT *Individuals (Rational)*

The *NTs* have very high standards and are unimpressed with authority. They prefer complexity and strategic thinking and want to be considered both logical and ingenious. The traits of the NT are discussed by Kroeger (1991)

and Bayne (1995) and summarized in Figure 20–20.

Often referred to by audiologists as the "engineer type," they are termed the "Rational" by Keirsey (1998, 2007; Keirsey & Bates 1984/1978; Keirsey .com, 2024). The hearing-impaired *NT* can exhibit the following traits:

- The most particular and independent of all types.
- Prefer to be considered logical and ingenious.
- Prefer detailed explanations.
- Are not impressed with your credentials.

- Can present as aloof, intimidating, argumentative, and arrogant.
- Often impatient with hearing aid fittings and the aural rehabilitation process.
- Complain about very small problems as they strive for perfection.
- Do not respect authority.
- Constantly pursue self-improvement.
- Tend to overanalyze problems and try to fix them themselves.
- Check out the web for a video on the *NT* personal style at Keirsey.com.

The Informal Evaluation of Keirsey Personal Style

Although many audiologists still do not consider personality type as a variable in hearing impairment, a careful, intelligent, informal estimate is certainly better than the current practice of treating all patients essentially the same. Traynor (1999) and Traynor and Holmes (2002) suggested several ways to informally estimate personality type with patients to facilitate better patient care. He indicated that experienced audiologists often do this subconsciously when comparing the current patient to those seen in the past and making adjustments in their treatment programs accordingly. While senior clinicians often modify and adjust their techniques according to various patients seen over a period of many years, the beginning and mid-career clinician cannot possibly have the experience to draw appropriate conclusions without some assessment of personal style. By conducting small-talk dialogue during the case history and discussion of the situation during a follow-up visit, the audiologist can often get a rough estimate of the patient's personality. By combining the clinical perception of the patient with the observations and information from significant others, these informal type judgments are often quite accurate. Some specific strategies for improving overall accuracy in informal assessment of personality by observation are:

1. Look for evidence of a trait and patterns of that evidence.
2. Look for evidence against the particular observed trait.
3. Look for an alternative interpretation of the evidence presented, particularly the effect of the situation.
4. Recognize the ambiguity of behavior. The same behavior can be evidence for more than one preference, and the motive for behaving in that way may matter more than the behavior itself.
5. Discover your own stereotypes and favorite terms and try to allow for them.
6. Compare your observations with those of others.
7. Have a good knowledge of theories of personality.

Looking for Extraversion or Introversion

While not a part of the general Keirsey assessment, extroversion and introversion are the easiest of all the traits to establish and can offer clues to how important communication and interaction are to the patient. Jung discovered in the early development of his theory that *Extraverts* will be inclined to speak loudly and rapidly, often make enthusiastic overstatements, use repetition and lots of gestures, and are very talkative. *Extraverts* sometimes are so talkative that they must be suppressed to finish the session in a timely manner. These patients will often present more data about themselves than needed to clinically assess the situation. Conversely, Jung found that *Introverts* are likely to express insecurity or sensitivity and speak slower in a softer voice, hesitate before speaking, are awkward in their interpersonal interactions, and sometimes appear to be aloof or reserved. *Introverts* need to be asked focused questions to get information from them that can be helpful in their treatment, both initially and during their program. *Extraverts* tend to increase their energy level and enthusiasm for the conversation as it continues, whereas *Introverts* tend to reduce their energy. In the informal assessment of *Extroversion/Introversion*, look for the following:

Extraversion
1. Patient has an expressive face, voice, and/or gestures.
2. Patient demonstrates a high level of enthusiasm and appreciates an energetic clinician with optimism.
3. Patient speaks in a loud voice.
4. Patient is talkative and appreciates a more talkative clinician.

Introversion
1. Patient expresses insecurity or sensitivity and is comfortable with silence.
2. Patient demonstrates an awkward interpersonal style.
3. Patient behaves in a fearful or timid manner.
4. Patient is reserved and unexpressive and less comfortable with action.
5. Patient keeps their partner at a distance.

6. They show a lack of interest in clinical interaction.

Informal Identification of Specific Keirsey Temperaments

Is this person an S or an N? In determining informal Keirsian cues to personality, the most difficult component to assess is the patient's use of the *Sensing (S)* or *iNtuition (N)* strategy to gather information. Generally, *Sensing* patients tend to look for specifics and examine all the components of issues, focusing more on the process than the overall outcome. Their counterparts, however, the *iNtuitors (N)*, gather information randomly while seeking its meaning. They would prefer to talk about what can happen rather than what is happening now. Those that are intuitive want to focus on possible outcomes rather than the process. Issues that can allow the clinician to determine if the patient is a Keirsian S or an N are as follows:

Sensors (S)
1. The patient may gesture very little.
2. Patient may keep hands in pockets or behind their backs.
3. Patients tend to read more realistic books and to remember specific plots and details of the story.
4. Patients relate stories, case histories, and experiences with hearing aids in great detail.
5. Patients appreciate a step-by-step, concrete, and detailed approach to situation.
6. Patients are not comfortable with novel and imaginative approaches.

iNtuitors (N)

1. Patients tend to look toward the possibilities, "what might be."
2. Patients may overemphasize the benefits.
3. Patients may jump from topic to topic.
4. Patients may see unrealistic possibilities with amplification and/or audiologic treatment.
5. Patients will often overlook facts and are not realistic about their hearing loss, the capabilities of the technology in their hearing aid, and so on.
6. Patients appreciate novel or imaginative approaches to treatment.

While not overtly observable, determining a *Thinker (T)* from a *Feeler (F)* does not take as much experience and observation skill as that required to evaluate clues for determining if the patient is an S or an N. Recall that in Keirsian type theory, the T or F traits have the most effect on the *iNtuitors (N)*. Thus, when observing for cues for Thinking or Feeling, it is assumed that there has already been a discovery that the person is an *iNtuitor (N)* and that the outcome will either be a Keirsian type of *NF* or *NT*. Specifically, *Thinkers (T)* seek clarity and want to apply the decisions uniformly while attempting to understand their feeling. They need to consider cause and effect of a particular treatment program. It is the nature of the *Thinker (T)* that they must understand the theory behind the program of treatment or the reason that a particular technology in a hearing aid is right for their impairment. *Thinkers (T)* will cooperate with the audiologic rehabilitation program or hearing aid fitting only if you explain the background and the theoretical basis is explained to them so that it "makes sense" to them. They respond well to detailed explanations of test results and logical application of rehabilitation methods and/or technology. *Feelers (F)*, however, need to experience feelings and seek harmony with other people and tend to be situational and subjective. Their reason to complete an audiologic rehabilitation program or use a hearing aid is to do it for others (i.e., wife, grandchildren, etc.). Involvement of significant others in the entire rehabilitative process is imperative, and they need the support of others to assure them that they are doing well.

To motivate *Feeling* patients, it is essential that they feel that others are affected by their hearing impairment. The decision to proceed in the rehabilitative process and/or a hearing aid fitting will be determined by how much of their life is disrupted by their hearing loss. Since they are sensitive to the needs of others, explanations should emphasize their abilities to communicate with others and how the treatment program or products will make life better or easier for those around them. Clues about whether a patient is a T or an F are as follows:

Thinkers (T)

1. Might act "irritable."
2. May express skepticism or cynicism and avoid emotions, especially in the early sessions.
3. May draw diagrams with their hands and number points on their fingers.
4. Need the rationale and logic behind the treatment approach and/or hearing aid selection.
5. May talk *at* their spouse.

Feelers (F)
1. Will probably behave in a cheerful manner.
2. May laugh frequently.
3. May gesture with open hands in flowing movements.
4. Want to be an easy, good case that is remembered and appreciated.

Judging (J) or Perceiving (P)

Is this person a J or a P? Among the easiest to informally identify is if the person is a scheduled, rigid, or inflexible Judger (J) or a flexible, easygoing Perceiver (P). In Keirsian type theory, the J or P traits have the most effect on the *Sensors (S)*. Thus, when observing for cues for Judging or Perceiving, it is assumed that there has already been a discovery that the person is a *Sensor (S)* and that the outcome would either be a Keirsian type of *SJ* or *SP*.

In the Keirsian Temperament, the patient will then be considered either an *SJ* or an *SP,* depending upon if they display a *Judging (J)* or *Perceiving (P)* behavior. *Judging (J)* types are clockwatchers and usually remain focused on a topic or task. *Judgers (J)* are patients who tend to focus on one method or product, offering decisive opinions immediately once they have obtained the necessary information. The audiologist must, therefore, be on time for appointments with these patients and provide all the information necessary to arrive at decisions in a concise and precise manner. *Judgers (J)* do not take commitment lightly and will usually carry through with a decision once it is made. Sometimes they even have their mind made up on specific products, such as the make and model of the hearing aid.

Perceiving (P) persons easily change topics and appear to have no concept of time or schedule. These patients generate and tolerate treatment alternatives, often answering questions with questions. Additionally, they have difficulty making closure and tend to need extra clinical time to answer that "one last question" that "just popped into their heads." *Perceivers (P)* cannot handle a presentation of all of the amplification options because they have too much difficulty focusing on specifics. It is usually necessary to summarize the information for them. Since decisions are difficult for these patients, it is necessary to present options and be flexible in your recommendations for the *Perceiving (P)* patient to feel comfortable.

Clues about whether a patient is a J or an P are as follows:

Judging (J)
1. The patients fear losing control.
2. The patients want to have options in difficult situations.
3. These patients find change stressful.
4. These patients work hard on projects and tolerate discomfort.
5. These patients need an organized and structured step-by-step approach.

Perceivers (P)
1. These patients will avoid decision-making.
2. These patients like to have lots of options and do not like organized group programs.
3. These patients like to have lots of flexibility in the rehabilitative program.
4. These patients do not tolerate discomfort.
5. These patients can be great time-wasters.

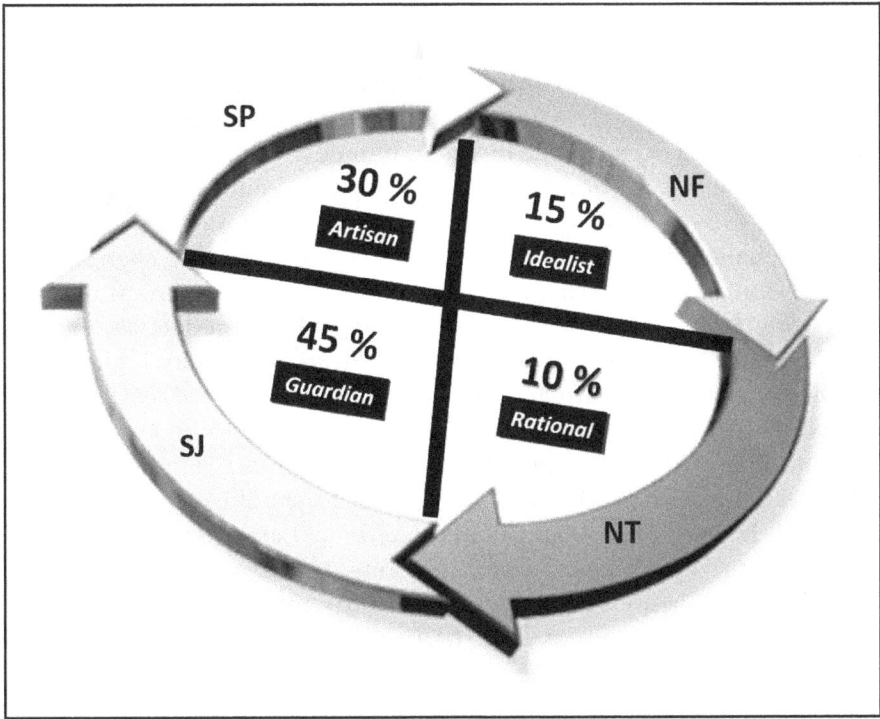

Figure 20–21. Keirsey personality type of audiologists (Traynor & Holmes, 2001).

Effect of Clinician's Personal Style

The personal style of the clinician may also make a substantial difference in successful patient interactions. Personal style may explain why certain patients do better with some clinicians than with others or why some clinicians become frustrated with certain types of patients. The job is to provide the patient with the best possible care, and the clinician must learn to work with all types. Audiologists also need to be aware that they also have their own personal style that may reflect how they perceive certain patients within the treatment process. Although a bit dated, the only study of personal style that has been conducted

is by Traynor and Holmes (2001). They evaluated 94 audiologists routinely seeing patients at the 2000 Academy of Dispensing Audiologists Convention in San Diego, California. Using an online version of the Keirsey Temperament Sorter II, it was found that 56% were *Sensing-Judging (SJ)*, 16% were *Sensing-Perceiving (SP)*, 21% were *iNtuitive-Feeling (NF)*, and 7% were *iNtuitive-Thinking (NT)*. A higher percentage of the audiologists were *NFs* (21%) than is seen in the general population of the United States (11%) (Figure 20–21).

This is not necessarily surprising since *NFs* are known to gravitate to the helping professions, but it does mean that clinicians need to be very careful not to project their own personality into treatment sessions and hearing aid selection/verification. In 2024, the Traynor and Holmes study is the only data available that offers some indication of the clinician's personal style using the Keirsey Temperament Sorter. While these data must be considered according to their age and the resultant changes in clinical personalities between 2001 and 2024, the lesson is that clinicians will be seeing mostly *SJ or Guardian* patients who are the same as their own personal style. This suggests that Guardian clinicians (about 56%) will feel comfortable with about 45% of their patients, and for those with other personal styles, the clinician will have to make changes in their interactions that might not be comfortable for them. For clinicians who possess personal styles that are not SJ or Guardian, they will need to modify their comfortable tendencies most of the time. Those clinicians new to managing patient visits need to consider some of their innate tendencies. Thus, the following insights are offered to begin an understanding of how to manage the patients of a personal style different from that of the clinician.

Generally, *Extraverted (E)* clinicians are not comfortable extracting information from *Introverted* patients, while *Introverted (I)* clinicians are not comfortable with the interactive chatter of the *Extraverted (E)* patients. *iNtuitive (N)* clinicians who have constructed positive blueprints for rehabilitative plans may need to deal with *Sensing (S)* patients who have more pessimistic, analytic attitudes toward the process, while the Sens*ing (S)* clinicians are frustrated with patients who do not follow their step-by-step aural rehabilitation program. *Feeling (F)* clinicians need to understand that they cannot make all of their patients happy, whereas *Think-*

ing (T) clinicians may need to focus less on the data and more on the patient. Finally, *Judging (J)* clinicians may find it difficult and extremely frustrating to deal with *Perceiving (P)* patients who jump from topic to topic and are never on time. Although it is impossible for audiologists to change personality totally for their clinical interactions, it is possible to reduce the adverse effects from personality interactions. For example, *Introverted (I)* clinicians must make an effort to be especially outgoing and interactive, and *Thinking (T)* clinicians should attempt to present the *Feeling (F)* arguments for various situations. Understanding one's own personality and the advantages and limitations when interacting with certain types of patients can be a major asset to clinical success. For the patients who present extremely difficult interactions for certain clinicians, it may be necessary to schedule them with another clinician to provide the best possible rehabilitative care. Based upon the literature and clinical experience using personal style as a clinical asset, the following are recommendations for clinicians of various types:

SJ Clinician
1. Do not expect every patient to be on time.
2. All patients do not want an organized step-by-step program.
3. Do not be practical for everyone, especially the NT patients.
4. Do not focus on the procedure, especially for SPs and NFs.
5. Do give clear objectives and prepare for situations.
6. Have options when one treatment program (or hearing aid) does not work.

SP Clinician

1. Tolerate long procedures when they are necessary.
2. Try to focus more on the overall outcome rather than the process.
3. Accuracy of a particular adjustment or procedure may be more accurate than thought.
4. Be tolerating of patient difficulties.

NF Clinician

1. Be aware that not all of your patients will be happy.
2. Good clinicians need to disagree with their patients sometimes.
3. Focus and concentrate on boring rehabilitative treatment tasks.
4. Do not expect everyone to care as much.

NT Clinician

1. Perfection is not always necessary.
2. Most patients need to have things simplified.
3. Most patients do not require long presentations, including the background, for each procedure.

Putting It Together: The Professional Sales Journey

Audiologists walk a fine line. On one side, there is the fiduciary responsibility to the patient to provide the best hearing care possible (aural rehabilitation), but there are also the business pressures of running and maintaining the practice (the need to make sales). Aural rehabilitative treatment and the sales process, however, are one in the same as when the rehabilitative process is conducted correctly, the sales will simply happen as a result. The process is really a journey by the patient toward a goal of bet-

ter hearing, and if conducted properly, the journey naturally leads to a "sale." By realizing that patients are on a journey toward better hearing, rather than a "sales prospect," clinicians can meet both the needs of the patients and the practice. The method involves moving the patient toward a decision to pursue treatment, building a relationship with them through first impressions, establishing trust, and offering continuous care; the "sale" comes easily and is a natural part of the aural rehabilitative process.

The Sales Journey: The Role of Patient Motivation

Before the journey can begin, however, patients must realize that there is a hearing impairment that needs attention. If the impairment has not been realized, then it will be virtually impossible to have a positive rehabilitative result. Further, if the journey begins without the patient's cooperation or with high-pressure sales tactics, it will be unsuccessful, resulting in product returns or the nonuse of the very devices that are essential to their quality of life. It is *always best to wait until the patient is ready for hearing care* rather than to "sell" them or their family on treatment when they are not invested in the process. Over time, the unaddressed issues such as avoidance, difficulty hearing, failing coping strategies, denial, and other of Trychin's classic hearing loss variables will eventually convince the patient and their family that it is time to begin treatment.

More recent studies, such as Lin et al. (2011) suggesting that dementia is reduced by obtaining treatment for hearing loss, may also make a case to the patient or their family so that they may continue activities and the interactions

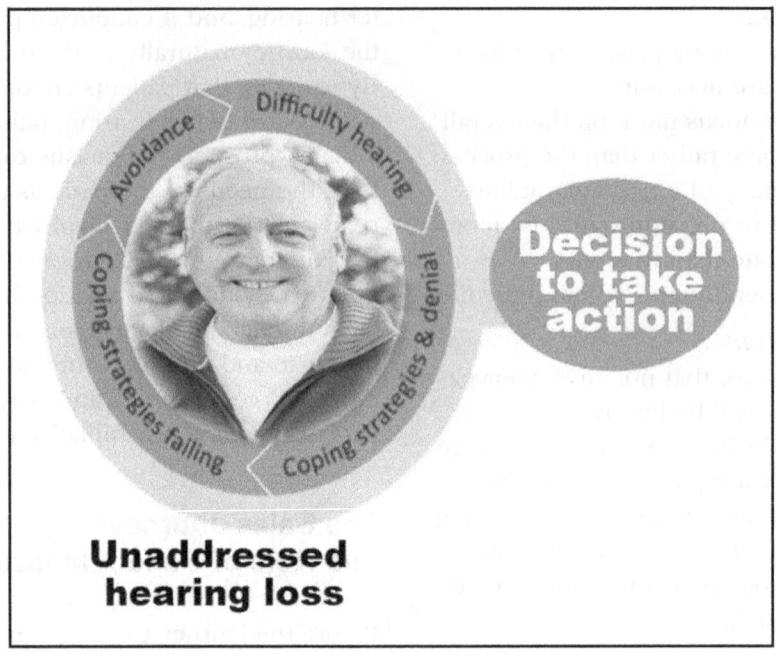

Figure 20–22. The sales journey: decision to take action (Traynor & Eagon, 2016).

that have been cherished for a lifetime. Thus, the decision to obtain treatment for hearing loss is the essential first step toward successful hearing care. Knowledge of the generations, personal style, and the use of listening skills presented earlier in this discussion are used to review the patient's readiness for treatment. Even if the patient is not quite ready for treatment, a correctly conducted hearing care discussion will usually lead the patient and their family back to the clinic when they are ready to pursue treatment (Figure 20–22).

The Sales Journey: The Relationship Phase— First Impressions

Once the patient is committed to working on their hearing impairment, the journey moves to the *relationship phase* of the clinical interaction. As presented in Figure 20–23, the relationship phase of the process consists of three components: *the first impression, building trust, and offering continuous care.*

First impressions are extremely important to the journey as it is where patients and clinicians both "feel each other out." Of course, learning for the clinician begins by meeting the patient and the initial exchange of greetings and casual conversation, as well as the informational counseling that goes with the process of getting acquainted, taking the hearing health history, audiologic evaluation, and subsequent rehabilitative discussions. While discussing their hearing health history, consider their generational issues by assessing their personal style and reviewing lifestyle. Fundamental clues to the patient's situation are

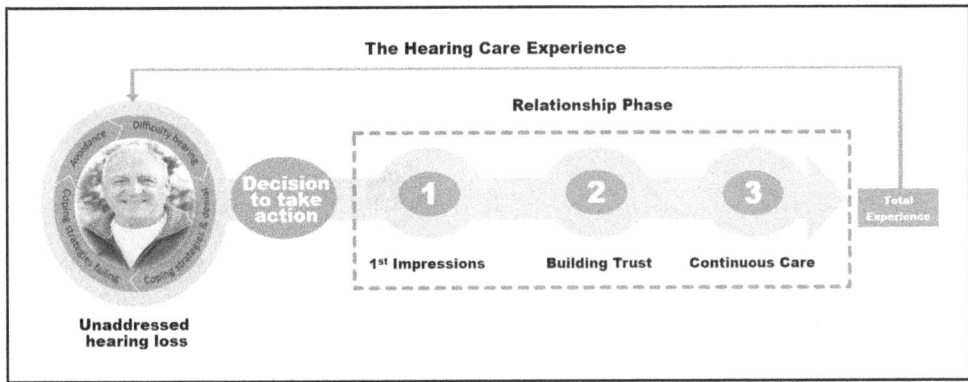

Figure 20–23. The sales journey: the relationship phase (Traynor & Eagon, 2016).

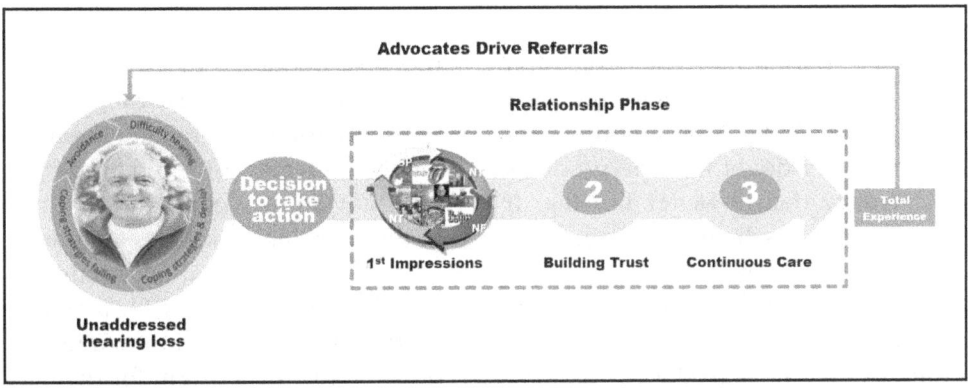

Figure 20–24. The sales journey: personality style (Traynor & Eagon, 2016).

obtained and an initial personal style can be determined from the discussion (Figure 20–24).

The first impression portion of the relationship phase of the journey is simply listening and getting to know the patient, picking up the generational and personal style issues that facilitate knowledge of how to relate on an individual and very personal level. It also involves allowing the patient to "get to know" the clinician through a relaxed interactive discussion. The first impression also is for the family to be convinced that this clinic, particularly this clinician, is the best guide for their loved one's hearing journey, allowing the building of trust.

The Sales Journey: Building Trust

Once there is an understanding of the patient's personal style, generation, and lifestyle, the process of building trust begins (Figure 20–25). Hearing aids and those who deal with them suffer from a trust problem. While the professional reputations of audiologists and the products have advanced, the lingering issue with patients is that hearing aids are not very helpful and expensive, and those who deal with them are simply *"out to get your money."* So, this is where clinicians begin with a new patient, even after developing a positive relationship

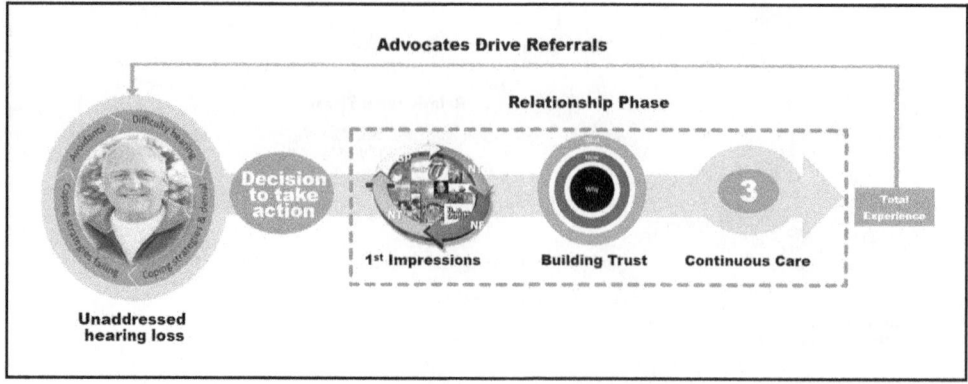

Figure 20–25. The golden circle beginning with *THE WHY* (Sinek, 2009).

with them during the first impression phase of the process. Patients often start out skeptical of the clinic and the clinician, and they doubt that the products will actually deliver better hearing. If the sales process beings with product discussions, these negative impressions taken from friends, relatives, and others are reinforced.

Sinek (2009) introduced a new method of selling that has been very successful for companies such as Apple, United Airlines, and others that is called *The Golden Circle*. The Golden Circle is essential to the understanding of the sales process and the building of trust.

Figure 20–26 presents The Golden Circle, which does not begin with product and does not even begin with the process of how to deal with the hearing loss; it begins with *Why*.

■ The *Why* is all about the patient's purpose of coming to the clinic. *Why* is the patient here today, and what do they hope to accomplish? The *Why* looks for their motivation to seek rehabilitative treatment. The conversations and discussions should center on situations that are the most important to the patient. It is communication? Hearing the birds? Hearing the grandchildren, wife, or caretaker? Keeping their job? *Why* do they get out of bed in the morning? And does anyone care? Ask open-ended questions and discover their story for action on their hearing loss. Some questions on the intake form for the *Why* should include:

■ What do your coworkers say when you . . . ?

■ How often do you and your wife go out for movies?

■ What types of activities do you like to do with friends?

■ Tell me about a recent time when communication was difficult.

■ When I talk with patients, there's frequently a key moment that caused them to schedule a hearing evaluation. What happened recently to bring you to the clinic today?

■ What impact does this have on you when _____ happens?

■ What was your reaction when . . . ?

■ How did you feel when . . . ?

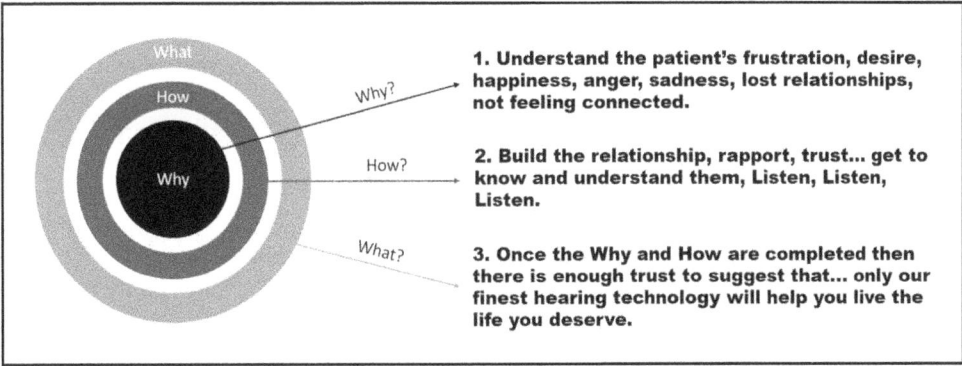

1. **Understand the patient's frustration, desire, happiness, anger, sadness, lost relationships, not feeling connected.**

2. **Build the relationship, rapport, trust... get to know and understand them, Listen, Listen, Listen.**

3. **Once the Why and How are completed then there is enough trust to suggest that... only our finest hearing technology will help you live the life you deserve.**

Figure 20–26. The sales journey: building trust (Traynor & Eagon, 2016).

- How has this affected your enjoyment of . . . ?
- Ask for the reaction/impact of friends, coworkers, and spouse as well.
- The *How* deals with the treatment process: the evaluation, the discussion, and the process of determining which products might be the best for this patient's needs. While it could be other rehabilitative techniques, most often this process involves the purchase of hearing devices. At this point in The Golden Circle process, the clinician has listened carefully to the wants and needs of the patient and knows their generational and personal style variables. Armed with this knowledge, they can present the process necessary to achieve their goals. Here, a discussion of the process is conducted, answering questions and describing the benefits and limitations of amplification and the likely outcomes of their use in their particular situation. Additionally, this is also the place where levels of technology are often discussed process. *What* can be done for the *why* issues discov-

ered earlier, and once these *"How"* issues are discussed, the patient is usually ready for the *What* products that are necessary to do something about their situation.

- *What* is the discussion of the products necessary to achieve the goals identified in the *Why* and *How* discussions. Here is where specific products, prices, and benefits of one over the other are presented. This is the easy portion of the discussion for the audiologist as they now can present products, relate their experiences with the instruments, and complete the sales process with the trust of the patient.

Now that the first impression has been made and the clinician has some idea of the patient's personal style, the trust factor has now also been solidified as the clinician did not immediately being discussing product and costs. Care has been taken to present the rationale for taking action relative to the impairment. Since the patient and their family now understand the rationale behind the recommendations, as well as the explanation of how it needs to be treated, the trust built over the relationship phase

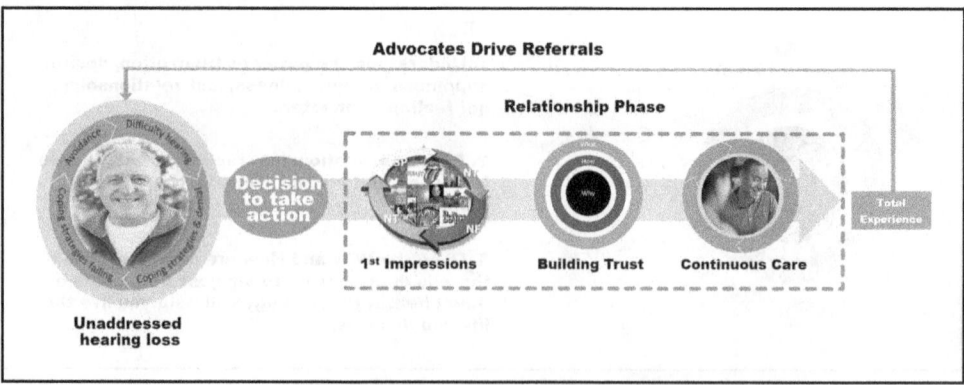

Figure 20–27. The completed sales journey (Traynor & Eagon, 2016).

moves to the continuous care phase (Figure 20–27). Seasoned clinicians know that if Phases 1 and 2 are handled well, the patient will make the decision to move forward with treatment on their own, without these "Sales Tactics" that often bring distrust. At this point, the sale has been completed as a natural progression of the aural rehabilitative process and the rest is up to total patient care ensuring that the products dispensed and services offered are consistent with the discussions held early in the process.

References

Alcido, M., & Lloyd, M. (2024). Forbes Health survey: Nearly half of people with hearing loss believe there is a hearing aid stigma. Forbes Health. https://www.forbes.com/health/hearing-aids/hearing-aids-stigma-survey/#:~:text=Nearly%20half%20(48%25)%20of,with%20wearing%20a%20hearing%20aid

Bayne, R. (1995). *The Myers-Briggs Type Indicator: A critical review and practical guide*. Chapman and Hall.

Bray, V. (2021). You tick, they tock, what's the difference in our clocks? *Audiology Now, 86,* 21–26.

Briggs, K.C., & Myers, I. B. (1976). *Myers-Briggs Type Indicator*. Consulting Psychologists Press.

Buetter, D. (2012). Are extroverts happier than introverts? *Psychology Today.* https://www.psychologytoday.com/blog/thrive/201205/are-extroverts-happier-introverts

Chien, W., & Lin, F. (2012). Prevalence of hearing aid use among older adults in the United States. *Archives of Internal Medicine, 172*(3), 292–293. https://www.ncbi.nlm.nih.gov/pmc/articles/PMC3564585/

Clark, J. (2019). Counseling considerations for patient and employee management. In R. Glaser & R. Traynor (Eds.), *Strategic practice management* (3rd ed.). Plural Publishing.

Clark, J., & English, K. (2004). *Counseling in audiologic practice: Helping patients and families adjust to hearing loss*. Pearson.

Clark, J., & English, K. (2014). *Counseling infused audiologic care*. Pearson.

DeVise. (2023). Nearly half of Baby Boomers have no retirement savings. *The Hill.* https://thehill.com/business/personal-finance/3991136-nearly-half-of-baby-boomers-have-no-retirement-savings/

Dimock, M. (2019). Where Millennials end and Generation Z begins. Pew Research

Center. https://www.pewresearch.org/short-reads/2019/01/17/where-millennials-end-and-generation-z-begins/

Draft Lottery. (1969). Selective service draft lottery for the Vietnam War. Wikipedia. https://en.wikipedia.org/wiki/Draft_lottery_(1969)

Espositio, L. (2014). How to overcome extreme fear of doctors. *U.S. News.* http://health.usnews.com/health-news/patient-advice/articles/2014/07/01/how-to-overcome-extreme-fear-of-doctors

Fischer, M. (2024). 12 Insights into Boomer's retirement realities. ALM Think Advisor. https://www.thinkadvisor.com/2024/06/27/12-insights-into-boomers-retirement-realities/#:~:text=Fifty%2Dfour%20percent%20of%20the,they%20anticipated%E2%80%9D%20before%20they%20retired

James, H. (2015). Boomers gain freedom through technology. Tech.co. http://tech.co/baby-boomers-gain-freedom-technology-2015-07

Jeníček, V. (2010). Population problem in the future—challenges, questions. *Agricultural Economics, 56*(3), 97–107.

Keirsey, D. (1998). *Please understand me II.* Prometheus Nemesis Book Co.

Keirsey, D. (2007). *Please understand me (DVD): Character and temperament types.* Prometheus Nemesis Book Company.

Keirsey, D., & Bates, M. (1984). *Please understand me.* Gnosology Books, Ltd. (Original work published 1978)

Keirsey.com. (2024). The four temperaments. https://keirsey.com/temperament/rational-overview/

Kochkin, S. (1990). Introducing MarkeTrak-1989: A consumer tracking survey of the hearing instrument market. *Hearing Review, 43*(5), 1–6. https://betterhearing.org/HIA/assets/File/public/marketrak/MR01.PDF

Kroeger, O. (1991, June). *On designing a day.* Pre-conference workshop at the IXth Annual Convention of the Association for Psychological Type. Washington, DC.

Kroeger, O., & Thusen, J. M. (1988). *Type talk.* Dell Publishing.

Lin, F., Metter, J., O'Brien, R., Resnick, S., Zenderman, A., & Ferucci, L. (2011). Hearing loss and incident dementia. *Archives of Neurology, 68*(2), 214–220. https://www.ncbi.nlm.nih.gov/pmc/articles/PMC3277836/

Luterman, D. (2001). *Counseling persons with communication disorders and their families* (4th ed.). Pro-Ed.

Luterman, D. (2020). Counseling in audiology and speech-language pathology. ASHA. https://www.asha.org/practice-portal/professional-issues/counseling-in-audiology-and-speech-language-pathology/

Matthews, C. (2016). American marriages still have a 50/50 chance of ending in divorce. *Fortune Health.* http://fortune.com/2016/06/17/baby-boomers-divorce/

Medical Economics. (2021). Top challenges of 2022, No. 5: Loss of trust in physicians, https://www.medicaleconomics.com/view/top-challenges-of-2022-no-5-loss-of-trust-in-physicians

Morris, T. (2021). The pandemic changed boomers' relationship with tech. Here's how. https://blog.gwi.com/chart-of-the-week/boomers-relationship-with-tech/

Myers, I. B., Kirby, L. K., & Myers, K. D. (1993). *Introduction to type* (5th ed.). Consulting Psychologists Press.

Novak, J. (2017). Six living generations in America. The Marketing Teacher. http://www.marketingteacher.com/the-six-living-generations-in-america/

O'Brien, C. (2012). 4 personality types according to the Keirsey personality sorter. WantInstitute. Video. https://www.youtube.com/watch?v=jrdZI3vJFPg

Pew Research Center. (2012, March 28). Baby Boomers and technology. https://www.pewresearch.org/internet/2012/03/28/baby-boomers-and-technology/

Pew Research Center. (2019, January 17). Defining generations: Where Millennials end and Generation Z begins. https://www.pewresearch.org/short-reads/2019/01/17/where-millennials-end-and-generation-z-begins/

Powers, T., & Carr, K. (2022). MarkeTrak 2022: Navigating the changing landscape of hearing healthcare. *Hearing Review*, *29*(5), 12–17. https://hearingreview.com/inside-hearing/research/marketrak-2022-navigating-the-changing-landscape-hearing-healthcare

Priebe, H. (2016). 7 reasons why the online MBTI community is dominated by intuitives. Thought Catalog. http://thoughtcatalog.com/heidi-priebe/2016/03/7-reasons-why-the-mbti-community-is-dominated-by-intuitives/

Rainie, L., & Perrin, A. (2016). Technology adoption by Baby Boomers (and everybody else). Pew Research Center. http://www.pewinternet.org/2016/03/22/technology-adoption-by-baby-boomers-and-everybody-else/

Ranie, L. (2012). Baby Boomers and technology. Pew Research Center, https://www.pewresearch.org/internet/2012/03/28/baby-boomers-and-technology/

Rosen, K. (2024). Active listening is an essential sales tool. All Business. https://www.allbusiness.com/active-listening-is-an-essential-sales-tool-34251-1.html

Scheve, T. (2011). 10 modern technologies Baby Boomers are using. How Stuff Works. https://health.howstuffworks.com/wellness/aging/baby-boomers/10-modern-technologies-baby-boomers-are-using.htm

Sinek, S. (2009). Simon Sinek—start with why—TED talk short edited. YouTube.com. https://www.youtube.com/watch?v=u4ZoJKF_VuA

Solutions. (2024). Welcome the rise of tech use by Baby Boomers. Post Solutions. https://www.postmediasolutions.com/blog/welcome-the-rise-of-tech-use-by-baby-boomers/

Statistic Brain. (2016). Myers-Briggs Statistics. https://www.man42.net/blog/2016/07/mbti-stats/

Taylor, B. (2012). *Consultative selling skills for audiologists*. Plural Publishing.

Thornhill, M., & Martin, J. (2007). *The Boomer consumer*. Linx Corporation.

Traynor, R. (1999). Relating to patients. In R. Sweetow (Ed.), *Counseling for hearing aids*. Singular Publications.

Traynor, R. (2013). *Personal style in hearing aid fitting*. Veterans Administration Workshop Series, Sonic Innovations.

Traynor, R. (2020). Competing in a new era of hearing healthcare: Differentiating your practice by relationships in the COVID-19 era and beyond. *Hearing Review*, *26*(8), 14–18.

Traynor, R., & Buckles, K. (1996). *Personal style, audiology's new crystal ball*. Hearing Review Supplement.

Traynor, R., & Eagon, S. (2016, September). *Audiology professional sales training*. A presentation to the students and faculty at Ohio State University, Columbus.

Traynor, R., & Holmes, A. (2002). Personal style and hearing aid fitting. *Trends in Amplification*, *6*(1), 1–31

Traynor, R. M., & Holmes, A. E. (2001, June). *Personal style and hearing aid fitting*. Presentation to the Annual Convention of the Academy of Dispensing Audiologists, Asheville, NC.

Trychin, S. (2003). Why don't people that need them get hearing aids. http://users.clas.ufl.edu/mcolburn/Web-links/Nursing%20Lecture/Why%20Don't%20People%20Who%20Need%20Them%20Get%20Hearing%20Aids.htm

U.S. Bureau of Census, Administration on Aging: Department of Health and Human Services. (2024). Research Gate. https://www.researchgate.net/figure/Population-of-people-65-years-older-and-over-is-projected-to-reach-72-million-in-2030_fig2_356183212

Vietnam Extra. (2024). What's your number? The Vietnam War Selective Service Lottery. *Vietnam Magazine.* http://www.historynet.com/whats-your-number.htm

Voorhis, D. (2016). Baby Boomers' retirement: The country's biggest and most predictable train wreck? *Miami Herald.* http://www.miamiherald.com/news/nation-world/national/article85981067.html

Wignall, L. (2015). Why don't universities teach students to sell hearing aids? Hearing Health and Technology Matters. https://hearinghealthmatters.org/hearing-views/2015/frustrated-private-practice-audiology/

21 Application of Teleaudiology in Practice Management

James W. Hall III, PhD

Origins of Telehealth

The term telehealth refers to the remote delivery of healthcare clinical services or the remote education of healthcare providers. The beginnings of telehealth can be traced to the late 1800s and the advent of commonplace devices for telecommunication, namely the telephone. Ready access to telephones permitted long-distance consultation among physicians, nurses, and other healthcare providers about patient care, including the accurate diagnosis and appropriate management of patient diseases and injuries. The next major advance in telehealth occurred in the 1950s and 1960s with the utilization of television and video link technology permitting transmission of audio and visual information in the remote provision of healthcare services and the education of healthcare personnel. A few decades later, in the 1980s and 1990s, the availability of facsimile or fax machines further facilitated rapid and inexpensive transmission via telephone of printed information, including text and images. In more recent years, the application of telehealth has expanded globally with increasing access to the worldwide web and the emergence of widespread Internet access. Finally, the popularity of telehealth exploded in 2020 as the COVID-19 pandemic and concerns about transmission of life-threatening infection created an unprecedented disruption in traditional face-to-face clinical healthcare. Interested readers will find multiple books and other resources describing in detail the origins and evolution of remote healthcare services via telehealth technology (e.g., Krumm & Syms, 2011; Manchaiah, Hall, Beukes, & Swanepoel, 2024; Swanepoel & Hall, 2010, 2020; Swanepoel et al., 2020; Swanepoel et al., 2024).

Overview of the Audiology Applications of Telehealth

In comparison to medicine, the profession of audiology has been slow to apply telehealth techniques and technology in the remove delivery of healthcare services. The term "teleaudiology" is used to describe the application of a telehealth approach in the provision of remote hearing healthcare and remote education and training of audiologists and support personnel.

The author and other audiologists regularly participated in simple forms of telehealth during the pre-Internet era. In the typical teleaudiology scenario, one audiologist with a challenging patient used the telephone to contact a colleague, usually someone with clinical skills and experience that would be helpful in diagnosing and/or managing the patient. The caller verbally described over the telephone relevant information from the patient's history and the patient's test findings (e.g., the audiogram). The remote expert would then offer a verbal clinical opinion.

The effectiveness of telephone audiology consultations was significantly enhanced in the late 1989s with the availability of fax machines in every clinic. Fax machines facilitated remote transmission from one clinic to another of detailed printed and graphic information, such as audiograms, tympanograms, otoacoustic emissions (OAE) findings, and printouts of auditory brainstem response (ABR) waveforms. The earliest formal studies of remote hearing healthcare service delivery, including video otoscopy, screening with otoacoustic emissions, and remote hearing aid programming, did not appear until the late 1990s (e.g., Birkmire-Peters et al., 1999; Schmiedge, 1997). The first published papers describing validation research appeared approximately a decade later. The initial studies demonstrated that test performance and findings for audiology services provided remotely via telehealth were comparable to the same services delivered in a traditional face-to-face clinical setting. The validation studies were conducted for a wide variety of audiology services, including newborn hearing with OAEs,

hearing assessment of children and adults with otoscopy, aural immittance measures, pure-tone audiometry, and even auditory brainstem response recordings (e.g., Krumm & Ferrari, 2008; Lancaster et al., 2009).

Soon after publication of the initial collection of validation studies, but well before COVID-19 pandemic, systematic reviews of teleaudiology techniques and technologies appeared in the literature (Swanepoel & Hall, 2010; Swanepoel et al., 2010). The systematic review papers included a focus on how teleaudiology could be applied to address the global burden of hearing loss and related disorders—that is, how remote provision of hearing healthcare services might meet the needs of regions of underserved patient populations throughout the world, such as developing countries with inadequate audiology resources, and specific underserved rural or urban regions of countries where audiology is well established.

The global COVID-19 pandemic dramatically highlighted major benefits of teleaudiology, namely, as an extension of universal precaution policy to minimize or eliminate the likelihood of serious illness or death secondary to infection with strains of the COVID-19 virus. The first papers describing this new clinical advantage of remote hearing healthcare via teleaudiology were published in early 2020, only a few months after COVID-19 was recognized as a global health threat (e.g., Ballachanda et al., 2020; Swanepoel & Hall, 2020). To maintain quality audiology clinical services for patients at risk for COVID-19 infections, Swanepoel and Hall (2020) suggested a three-tiered approach to patient care. "High-touch" service delivery in a traditional clinic setting was appropriate for patients who were at relatively low risk for contracting COVID-19, such as healthy young adults. Of course, typical infection control methods, such as social distancing, masking, hand hygiene, and surface decontamination, were important components of the high-touch model. A "low-touch" approach was recommended for patients with moderate risk for COVID-19 infection. This strategy did not require patients to visit a traditional clinic for hearing healthcare services. Instead, adult patients or pediatric patients and their parents would receive screening, diagnostic, or rehabilitative services from a trained hearing healthcare professional outside of a typical clinical setting, perhaps counter-side at a kiosk or in a drive-through arrangement. The infection control steps just cited are an integral part of the low-touch model. The term "no touch" was coined for the third option. Reserved for those patients at highest risk for infection (e.g., the elderly and patients with comorbidities), no-touch services are delivered in the home setting. No-touch services typically are limited to history taking, counseling, automated hearing screening, and hearing aid fitting and follow-up.

During the COVID-19 pandemic, clinical research evidence repeatedly confirmed the benefits of teleaudiology as a feasible strategy for safely providing quality hearing healthcare for children and adults at risk for hearing loss and related disorders (e.g., tinnitus, auditory processing disorders, and vestibular/balance problems). The rapidly expanding application of remote hearing healthcare and the growth in scientific literature on the topic during the

COVID-19 years was motivation for a comprehensive book on teleaudiology (Manchaiah, Hall, Beukes, & Swanepoel, 2024). The book *Teleaudiology Today: Remote Assessment and Management of Hearing Loss* is available in electronic or printed format. The topics covered in the book are directly relevant to this chapter and include:

1. A review of teleaudiology definitions, principles, and service delivery models.
2. How to develop and implement a teleaudiology practice.
3. Ethical, legal, and professional aspects of teleaudiology.
4. Remote hearing screening.
5. Remote counseling.
6. Remote hearing aid selection and fitting.
7. Rehabilitation via teleaudiology.

Readers interested in incorporating teleaudiology in the practice are encouraged to utilize the book as a supplement to this chapter.

Formal investigations of and clinical experience with teleaudiology confirm multiple benefits for patients, audiologists, and healthcare systems in general, including:

- Expanded access to clinical services.
- Enhanced quantity and quality of clinical services.
- More effective and efficient hearing healthcare.
- Reduced costs for patients seeking hearing healthcare access (e.g., costs associated with transportation, parking, etc.).
- Reduced cost to audiologists of hearing healthcare service delivery.

- Minimal patient risk of infection and injury with avoidance of busy healthcare facilities.
- More effective clinical instruction and training of audiologists and support personnel.

Teleaudiology offers a variety of practical advantages for audiologists and patients. For patients, remote provision of audiology services addresses constraints sometimes associated with traditional clinical models, including travel and transportation difficulties and expenses, mitigation of health risks for vulnerable populations, and cultural or religious factors that pose challenges to typical face-to-face services that require physical contact and touch between the audiologist and patient. Audiologists and audiology practices also derive two practical advantages, specifically: (1) reduced demand for clinical space, like waiting rooms and test areas, with services provided to more patients with less clinical space, and (2) reduced demands for clinical equipment. Services can be provided to more patients without acquisition of additional equipment for the clinical setting.

Tasks Prior to the Implementation of Teleaudiology Services

Some audiologists may be reluctant to take the steps of incorporating teleaudiology techniques and technology into their clinical practice. The task may seem daunting for a variety of reasons and perhaps because of some misconceptions. This chapter provides some practice tips and guidelines for audiologists and students enrolled in Doctor of Audiology programs who are interested in, or at least open to the idea of, integrating in their clinical practice a hybrid combination of remote offsite teleaudiology services and traditional in-clinic patient care. Readers are referred to a chapter in a new book (Kleindienst Robler et al., 2024) for a more detailed discussion of the steps in setting up and implementing teleaudiology services in an audiology practice. The practical review is based on the authors' decades of firsthand experience in planning, developing, and implementing a variety of remote hearing healthcare services in diverse clinical settings and geographical locations. Kleindienst Robler et al. (2024) identify five steps in the process of implementing teleaudiology services:

1. Defining the clinical need, such as screening, diagnostic assessment, or providing intervention.
2. Determining what equipment is needed.
3. Settling on the most effective model. Two examples are a clinic-to-clinic model and a virtual "direct-to-patient" arrangement.
4. Hiring and training support personnel.
5. Addressing billing, payment, and reimbursement issues.

Some preparation is required prior to the implementation of any remote audiology services. Audiologists should:

- Review relevant literature, including general information about telehealth, publications focusing on teleaudiology, and papers describing techniques, technology, and validation for specific components of the clinical assessment process.

- Research and verify audiology state licensure requirements for remote provision of audiology services.
- Verify third-party payment policies for remotely delivered audiology services.
- Develop a business plan that includes a description of the remote clinical services and programs, market analysis, competitive analysis, organizational framework, description of management, a marketing plan, and financial projections.
- Identify initial clinical goals for delivery of selected services via teleaudiology, such as the target populations and the specific services that will be offered first.
- Acquire necessary equipment and supplies.
- Hire or retrain audiology and support staff.
- Plan for a "soft launch" with selected services provided remotely to selected patient populations.

The intention of this chapter is to encourage and maybe even inspire audiologists and Doctor of Audiology students to incorporate and integrate teleaudiology concepts and strategies into clinical practice. Adherence to the above steps will likely contribute to the clinical and financial success of the teleaudiology effort.

Teleaudiology Terminology

Telehealth

The term telehealth refers to remote provision of healthcare services or noncli-nical services, such as education, training, and research, using telecommunications technology. Telehealth broadly encompasses a variety of healthcare services provided by any healthcare professional, not only physicians. The term telehealth also includes remote monitoring of symptoms, physiological data, and a wide range of health information, such as cardiac parameters (blood pressure, heart status), EEG, body weight, pulse oximetry, blood glucose, sleep, breathing function, and even fetal monitoring. The term telemedicine, in contrast, implies the remote delivery of medical services by a physician. The term teleaudiology was coined for audiology applications of telehealth, including identification, diagnosis, and management of hearing loss and related disorders (e.g., bothersome tinnitus), disorders of decreased sound tolerance (e.g., hyperacusis), auditory processing disorders, and vestibular/balance problems (Swanepoel & Hall, 2020; Swanepoel et al., 2020).

Asynchronous (Store-and-Forward) Versus Synchronous (Real-Time or Live) Teleaudiology

There are two general telehealth methods or models for remote delivery of hearing healthcare services: asynchronous and synchronous teleaudiology. Each method, summarized in Table 21–1, can be applied for identification, diagnosis, and rehabilitation of people with hearing loss and related disorders.

Asynchronous teleaudiology is quite straightforward. The approach involves two temporally separated components. Data are collected from a patient in a

Table 21–1. Summary of Asynchronous (Store-and-Forward) Versus Synchronous (Real-Time) Models for Remote Delivery of Hearing Healthcare Service

Asynchronous: Facilitator/ Parent Assisted	Asynchronous: Patient (Self-Service)	Synchronous: Audiologist & Facilitator
Hearing Screening	Hearing Screening	Diagnostic Assessment
Parent of pediatric patient or trained facilitator conducts hearing screening (e.g., tympanometry, DPOAEs, pure tones).	Adult patient conducts hearing screening (e.g., tympanometry, DPOAEs, pure tones).	Comprehensive diagnostic assessment of pediatric or adult patients
Reliance on automated devices	Exclusive reliance on simple user-friendly and typically automated, devices	Trained facilitator prepares the clinical setting for remote service delivery (lighting, placement of cameras and microphones).
Test findings are stored for later audiologist analysis.	Test findings are stored for later audiologist analysis.	Facilitator greets and registers patients.
		Facilitator instructs and prepares the patient for a diagnostic hearing assessment under audio-video supervision.
		Facilitator follows an audiologist-designed protocol.
		Facilitator serves as the audiologist's "hands" in placing transducers, inserting probes, attaching electrodes, etc.
		Facilitator may use automated devices for some procedures.
		Audiologist remotely controls equipment for complex clinical tests.
		Audiologist analyzes and interprets results in "real time" at the time of the assessment.

Table 21–1. *continued*

Asynchronous: Facilitator/ Parent Assisted	Asynchronous: Patient (Self-Service)	Synchronous: Audiologist & Facilitator
Rehabilitation	Rehabilitation	Rehabilitation
Parent of pediatric patient or trained facilitator assists in placing device(s).	Adult patient places and operates device(s) with adequate prior written or video instruction.	Facilitator prepares the clinical setting for remote service delivery (lighting, placement of cameras and microphones).
Reliance on self-fitting technology and objective verification of device operation	Reliance on self-fitting technology and objective verification of device operation.	Facilitator greets and registers the patient.
Data are stored for later audiologist review.	Data are stored for later audiologist review.	Facilitator prepares patient and places device(s).
		Facilitator serves as the audiologist's "hands" in performing device measurement, verification, validation, etc.
		Audiologist counsels the patient (informational or patient adjustment counseling).

remote location, that is, away from the traditional clinical setting. The data might consist of any information used to detect, diagnose, or manage a child or adult.

Typically, trained support personnel interact with and collect data from the patient in a remote location without direct audiologist involvement. The support person serving as the "hands and eyes" of the audiologist might be a hearing technician, an audiology assistant, or a Doctor of Audiology student. The term *facilitator* is most often used for the person who is in the field with a patient. The data that the facilitator collects are stored, usually electronically, for later access and analysis by an au-

diologist. The phrase *store-and-forward* rather than the term asynchronous is often used in reference to this method of teleaudiology. In the early years of teleaudiology, the facilitator would physically forward to an audiologist printed versions of data, via telephone fax, mail, or personal delivery. Now, it's more common for the facilitator to store data in an electronic location (e.g., Dropbox or a shared drive). The audiologist can then access the data at any later time.

Information contributing to detection of hearing loss or related disorders via the asynchronous teleaudiology approach might include responses on a questionnaire or inventory to identify people at risk for hearing loss, bothersome tinnitus, vestibular or balance problems, or auditory processing disorders. Alternatively, data used for identification of hearing loss might consist of findings for formal hearing screening, often conducted with objective auditory techniques like distortion product otoacoustic emissions (DPOAEs) or automated auditory brainstem response (AABR). Video otoscopy images are also an option in the identification component of teleaudiology. Diagnostic assessment of hearing loss via teleaudiology is also feasible. Findings for pure-tone audiometry, speech audiometry, and the above-noted objective auditory techniques are most often generated with automated equipment.

The *synchronous* approach for assessment and management of people at risk for hearing loss is sometimes referred to as real-time or live teleaudiology. As summarized in Table 21–1, synchronous or real-time teleaudiology services are provided with the assistance of an onsite facilitator or technician with the patient and the audiologist in another location. With the assistance of a trained facilitator, an audiologist can complete via teleaudiology with a pediatric or adult patient each step of diagnostic hearing assessment without direct face-to-face patient interaction. The comprehensive diagnostic services may include a focused history taking to rule out ear disease, remote otoscopic inspection of the ear, air and bone conduction pure-tone audiometry, measurement of aural immittance and otoacoustic emissions, and speech audiometry (e.g., word recognition in quiet and speech perception in noise).

In a relatively brief period, only a few years, the global COVID-19 pandemic contributed to widespread demand for teleaudiology services in countries with well-established audiology communities, as well as in global regions that lack adequate audiological services and access to quality hearing healthcare. In addition to the marked increase in demand, the heightened risk of infection from COVID-19 presented a new challenge for remote delivery of audiological services. In the United States, reliance on nonaudiology personnel like facilitators to directly interact with patients was not in compliance with physical distancing recommendations and with state or federal stay-at-home or self-quarantine orders. To circumvent these constraints in healthcare provision, online service delivery options and applications were introduced to permit diagnostic assessment of hearing loss and related disorders. The creative application of these technologies permitted the delivery of quality hearing health services with minimal risk of patient infection. As a result, audiologists had creative options for completing hearing assessment without face-to-face physical patient contact. With the innovative "no-touch" teleaudiology approach, patients collect their own audiological data independently with self-test systems or with the assistance of a family member (Swanepoel & Hall, 2020).

Options for the Application of Teleaudiology in Practice Management

Rationale

Audiologists provide clinical services to a remarkably small proportion of people within their referral area. Let's say an audiologist practices in one of the many moderate-size cities with a metropolitan statistical area (MSA) population of 500,000 to 600,000 people. Geographically distributed examples include cities such as Springfield (MA), Sarasota-Bradenton (FL), Akron (OH), Grand Rapids (MI), Tulsa (OK), McAllen (TX), Albuquerque (NM), and Concord (CA). Given the prevalence of hearing loss and related disorders, the potential caseload of an audiologist in the MSA in theory consists of tens of thousands of children and adults with communicatively important hearing loss, bothersome tinnitus, auditory processing disorder (APD), hyperacusis, and/or vestibular/balance problems. Among the above examples of cities, the potential patient population is presumably higher in those with greater numbers of elderly persons, such as Sarasota-Bradenton (FL). With the application of telehealth concepts and techniques, an audiologist has an opportunity to grow clinical practice by markedly expanding the number of potential patients seeking hearing healthcare. Of course, another obvious and important consequence of expanding potential patient populations with telehealth initiatives is enhanced management-related quality of life for a greater number of persons with hearing loss and related disorders.

Strategies and Approaches

A variety of strategies and approaches are available to audiologists who want to cast a wide net to reach children and adults who might require, or at least benefit from, hearing healthcare services. Implementation of the following strategies and approaches, presented in

no order, requires relatively little time, effort, equipment, or expense.

This approach is essentially an evidence-based telemarketing campaign targeting five diverse groups of people with an interest in health and education. One group consists of physicians, including pediatricians and other primary care physicians, and medical specialists who care for patients at risk for hearing loss. Another group is composed of nonphysician healthcare providers, such as speech pathologists, psychologists, occupational therapists, dieticians, and nurse practitioners representing different specialties. A third group consists of members of the community at large that includes adults, and parents of children, with risk factors for hearing loss and related disorders. The fourth group is made up of employers, or occupational health personnel, in businesses and industries with workers who are at risk for noise- or music-induced hearing loss. The fifth and rather varied group are educators or others interested in the education of children and adults, among them preschool teachers, schoolteachers, school principals, adult educators, and vocational counselors.

The above-noted groups are targets for tele-education, specifically evidence-based information about risks for and causes of hearing loss and related disorders. The information about risk factors for and causes of hearing loss and related disorders, and the targeted groups, varies somewhat for pediatric versus adult populations. Parents, and those professionals who provide healthcare or educational services to children, should be reminded of the important relation between hearing and the acquisition of speech and language, school performance, and specific academic skills, like reading. Education should include information about risk factors for pediatric hearing loss, hearing protection from high-intensity noise or music, and the feasibility of and rationale for hearing screening of infants, preschool children, and school-age children. Similarly, healthcare professionals and others who interact with adults must be educated about risk factors for hearing loss and related disorders in people across the age span (Hall, 2021), including comorbid conditions (e.g., diabetes, cardiovascular disease, kidney disease, hyperbilirubinemia, rheumatoid arthritis, and cognitive impairment or dementia), noise and music exposure, lifestyle factors (e.g., diet, exercise, smoking), and all forms of age-related hearing loss. Various techniques and technologies are readily available for this broad-based tele-education, among them:

1. Detailed patient-oriented information on audiology practice websites, YouTube videos, and email blasts.
2. The promotion of health and education stories in the traditional media (e.g., radio, newspaper, television) and information distributed via social media.
3. Publication of health and education articles in professional (health and education) magazines and journals.
4. Brief and simple live or recorded presentations for healthcare or educational personnel.

In combination, a tele-education initiative carried out by a single audiology practice or a group of audiologists in a geographical region is certain to increase awareness of the important role hearing plays in the health and welfare of children and adults, and of the availability of audiologists and audiology practices with the skills and knowledge to identify, diagnose, and manage hearing loss and related disorders in children and adults.

Identification of People at Risk for Hearing Loss and Related Disorders

Audiologists who elect to cast a wide net to generate awareness of hearing loss will undoubtedly also generate more referrals of potential patients. Depending on the focus of the tele-education effort, the potential patient population may consist mostly of children, adults, or people across the age span. The next goal is to identify the individuals within this relatively large group who are most likely to have a hearing loss, or a related disorder, that requires formal audiological assessment and management. Audiologists implementing effective and efficient hearing screening policies and programs can successfully achieve this goal. The systematic hearing screening initiative rests on several simple principles:

1. It is possible, with an evidence-based protocol, to quickly, inexpensively, and without direct audiologist participation identify children or adults who probably have a hearing loss from those who do not.
2. A substantial proportion of adults who fail a hearing screening do not require traditional face-to-face

audiology diagnostic or rehabilitation services.

3. The hearing screening process can identify adults with possible ear disease who require medical evaluation.

With an effective and efficient hearing screening process, only people who need and are likely to benefit from an audiologist's services are scheduled for a face-to-face clinic appointment. All other potential patients, particularly adults, are referred to another healthcare provider or assume responsibility for management of their hearing loss or related disorder.

The following screening options are available to audiologists for differentiating individuals who do not require referral to the audiology clinic versus those who should be scheduled for an audiology appointment. In the interest of practice efficiency and audiologist time management, responsibility for coordinating screening of prospective patients falls to support personnel, such as a front desk clerk. A trained facilitator, perhaps an audiology assistant, technician, or Doctor of Audiology student, conducts the formal hearing screening and communicates with prospective patients.

■ *General hearing questionnaires:* Many simple self-completed checklists, questionnaires, and self-tests are readily accessible for identifying adults with possible hearing loss. Identification of children with possible hearing loss is most often the responsibility of pediatricians, school personnel, speech pathologists, and audiologists.

■ *An ear disease questionnaire:* The Consumer Ear Disease Risk Assessment (CEDRA) is a paper/pencil tool for adults who are at risk for hearing loss based on a self-completed questionnaire or adults who fail formal hearing screening (Kleindienst et al., 2019; Klyn et al., 2019). Ruling out ear disease is a very important component of remote nonaudiologist identification and assessment, as well as essential before patient-directed management such as self-fitting hearing aids or self-help tinnitus programs. Physician referral is required for adults with a positive outcome on the CEDRA, before nonmedical management is considered.

■ *Bothersome tinnitus or disorders of decreased sound tolerance (e.g., hyperacusis):* Patients with the chief complaint of tinnitus complete a validated inventory designed to identify persons whose perception of tinnitus affects their quality of life (e.g., Tinnitus Handicap Inventory or Tinnitus Functional Index; see Hall, 2024).

■ *Formal hearing screening:* Formal hearing screening is appropriate for identifying children with probable hearing loss, including infants, preschool children, and school-age children. The same hearing screening approach can be applied in adult populations, particularly those at risk for hearing loss due to factors cited above. Recent research confirms the reliability and validity of an objective hearing screening strategy (Kleindienst et al., 2023). An effective and efficient hearing screening protocol is summarized in the box.

PROTOCOLS FOR EFFECTIVE AND EFFICIENT OBJECTIVE HEARING SCREENING OF PRESCHOOL CHILDREN, SCHOOL-AGE CHILDREN, AND ADULTS

Protocol 1: Children aged 6 years and younger. Also, any children who cannot complete pure-tone hearing screening. Hearing screening is performed with a combination of distortion product otoacoustic emissions and aural immittance measures (tympanometry and an acoustic reflex recording).

- Perform inspection of the right and left outer ear and (when feasible) of the external ear canal.
- Distortion-produced otoacoustic emissions (DPOAEs).
    - Test frequencies: f2 frequencies of 2000 Hz, 3000 Hz, 4000 Hz, and 5000 Hz.
    - Intensity levels: L1 = 65 dB SPL, L2 = 55 dB SPL.
    - Frequencies for pass: 4.
    - Pass criteria: (1) DPOAE – noise floor = > 6 dB *and* (2) DPOAE amplitude = > 0 dB SPL.
- Tympanometry and acoustic referral criteria (refer with one or more criterion):
    - Type B (flat) tympanogram.
    - Tympanogram peak (Pk) > –250 daPa
    - Tympanogram with abnormal gradient (Gr) > 160.
    - Absent acoustic reflex.

Protocol 2: Children aged 7 years and older. Also, children in Grades 3, 5, or higher.

- Perform inspection of outer ear and (when feasible) the external ear canal.
- Use Protocol 1 if hearing screening cannot be completed with the pure-tone technique.
- Pure-tone hearing screening:
    - Use sound-attenuating insert earphones as needed in noisy settings.
    - Instruct the child and verify that the child understands the task.
    - Screen with an intensity level of 20 dB HL at 1000, 2000, 4000 Hz, and 6000 Hz.
    - Screen the right ear and then the left ear.
    - To pass, children must respond to each frequency in each ear. Failure to respond to a single frequency in one ear is a refer outcome.

The author encourages interested readers to view a four-part series of YouTube videos describing this hearing screening approach.

These options for hearing screening are implemented remotely. Depending on the technical savvy of prospective patients, questionnaires and inventories may be completed with a hardcopy "paper-and-pencil" format or online. Formal hearing screening may be conducted in a variety of off-site locations that are convenient for prospective patients (e.g., nurseries for infants, medical clinics, or school settings for other children and workplaces, social settings, churches, skilled nursing facilities, etc., for adults). An asynchronous teleaudiology model is utilized for formal hearing screening. A trained facilitator conducts the formal hearing screening. Results are then stored electronically and "forwarded" to the audiologist for later review and analysis. Children who do not pass a formal hearing screening are usually scheduled for a diagnostic audiological assessment in a clinical setting. Some adults who do not pass the formal hearing screening may also be scheduled for a diagnostic audiological assessment in a clinical setting. However, an online self-test may be

an appropriate and the most efficient, approach for documenting hearing loss for other adults who fail the hearing screening.

Children and adults who are at risk for hearing loss or related disorder, and who appear to have a hearing loss or related disorder based on a questionnaire, inventory, or formal hearing screening test, are scheduled for a diagnostic assessment. Prospective pediatric patients may be scheduled for a clinic appointment with an audiologist. However, a diagnostic assessment in a traditional clinic setting is not necessary for many adults who appear to have a hearing loss. As reviewed next, a teleconsultation with the audiologist or a self-administered hearing test or a remote comprehensive diagnostic assessment may be a more efficient option for many prospective adult patients.

Diagnosis of Hearing Loss and Related Disorders

Multiple peer-reviewed publications, including journal articles and books, describe technology, techniques, and protocols for remote diagnosis of hearing loss and related disorders, particularly tinnitus (e.g., D'Onofrio & Zeng, 2021; Kim et al., 2021; Manchaiah, Hall, Beukes, & Swanepoel, 2024; Swanepoel & Hall, 2010). A detailed review of the topic, and even an exhaustive list of references, is far beyond the scope of this chapter. What follows are several general statements about, and practical guidelines for, remote diagnostic audiologic assessment. Extensive clinical research has produced evidence in support of the feasibility and validity of diagnostic hearing assessment outside of the confines of the traditional clinical setting.

As a result of technological advances in instrumentation, trained facilitators can perform remote comprehensive assessment of hearing in virtually any setting, including sites lacking a sound-treated booth. The evidence-based diagnostic test battery completed by an audiologist in a fully equipped clinic can be administered just as efficiently and accurately by a trained facilitator in a wide variety of off-site test environments, such as schools, places of work, generic office spaces, mobile vans, medical offices, skilled nursing facilities, and even prisons. The traditional audiology practice model requires individual patients to find their way to a "brick-and-mortar" clinical space, often from considerable distances and associated transportation expenses. In contrast, a teleaudiology model permits state-of-the art diagnostic assessment of hearing and related disorders wherever prospective patient population are located.

The expansion of remote diagnostic audiology services is directly linked to advances in equipment, particularly the development of technology and validated algorithms for automated data collection and analysis. Diagnostic hearing assessment of children and adults may be completed with the asynchronous or store-and-forward approach. That is, a facilitator using automated devices conducts the entire assessment onsite with the patient. An audiologist located in a clinic or perhaps a home office later reviews and analyzes the findings before determining whether further evaluation, referral, or management is indicated. The asynchronous model is often the most efficient for hearing assessment of healthy adults or older children. Conversely, some or all diagnostic procedures are conducted remotely by a trained facilitator under direct supervision and direction of an audiologist located elsewhere (e.g., a clinic or home office). This synchronous or live model is almost always appropriate for young children. It is also an option for assessment of prospective patients with complex medical histories, clear screening evidence of peripheral or central auditory dysfunction, or confounding listener variables such as cognitive impairment or dementia.

As already noted, the feasibility and increased popularity of remote diagnostic audiological assessment is directly due to advances in instrumentation. A short list of selected technological developments includes:

■ Asynchronous video otoscopy: Research confirms that the outcome of video otoscopy performed remotely by a facilitator and analyzed later by an audiologist or physician is equivalent to otoscopy performed in a clinic setting (e.g., Biagio et al., 2013).
■ Automated pure-tone audiometry: Audiologists have several options for instrumentation designed for automated air and bone conduction pure-tone audiometry (Eikelboom et al., 2013; Maclennan-Smith et al., 2013; Margolis et al., 2011; Margolis et al., 2010; Swanepoel et al., 2013). A facilitator situates the patient in the test setting and places the transducers. Then, the automated device instructs the patient before estimating and storing pure-tone thresholds. Valid hearing thresholds can be measured in any quiet space, without the need for a sound-treated room. Pure-tone signals are presented via circumaural or insert

earphones that effectively attenuate moderate levels of ambient noise. In addition, some automated audiometers include software for monitoring ambient noise to ensure that test conditions meet ANSI standards for permissible levels. One automated audiometer also includes features that provide information about the quality of test performance, including reaction time, reliability, and overall results (good, fair, poor). Even the presence of asymmetry in hearing thresholds and the type and degree of hearing loss are automatically reported (Margolis et al., 2010; Margolis et al., 2011).

■ Automated objective auditory measures: Multiple manufacturers offer devices for aural immittance measurements (tympanometry and acoustic reflexes) and otoacoustic emissions with automated analysis of findings. Research confirms that facilitators with minimum training are capable of consistently completing the objective auditory techniques (Hall, 2014).

■ Automated speech audiometry: Some automated audiometers include software for measurement of simple word recognition performance. There are also commercially available options for devices with software and applications for automated assessment and analysis of speech perception in noise (Hall & Swanepoel, 2024; Swanepoel & Hall, 2020).

This brief overview of diagnostic teleaudiology concludes with the reemphasis of an important practical point about patients who are candidates for remote assessment versus an assess-

ment in a traditional clinic setting. Audiologists must consider a variety of factors in deciding which approach—*remote assessment or a clinic appointment*—is most appropriate. The most important factors are patient age and audiological or medical complexity. Objective diagnostic auditory assessment of infants and very young children with techniques like aural immittance, OAEs, and ABR can be carried out via synchronous teleaudiology with the assistance of a trained facilitator. Cooperative older children and most adults are typically candidates for remote assessment. On the other hand, a clinic visit would be more fitting for children whose assessment is likely to include traditional pediatric audiology techniques, such as conditioned play audiometry or visual reinforcement audiometry. A clinic visit may also be indicated for some adults meeting certain criteria (e.g., possible false hearing loss, medical-legal concerns, cognitive decline/dementia, and/or preliminary evidence of auditory pathology).

Rehabilitation of People With Hearing Loss and Related Disorders

Patient Criteria for Implementing Telerehabilitation

Audiologists who are interested in implementing teleaudiology in their clinical practice are advised to consider several simple criteria for deciding which patients are candidates for entirely remote provision of management services versus patients who should receive traditional clinic-based services. Audiologists will also encounter some patients for whom a hybrid rehabilitation approach is appropriate, that is, an office visit preceded and/or followed by remote delivery of selected services. To some extent, criteria for patients who are candidates for remote rehabilitation resemble the guidelines already reviewed for determining which patients should undergo formal diagnostic audiologic assessment in a clinic setting versus remotely.

Provision of services face-to-face in a traditional audiology clinic or office is generally indicated when one or more of the following criteria are met:

1. Remote delivery of services might compromise patient rights, safety, and privacy. Similarly, audiologists should seriously consider a clinic visit if the delivery of remote services brings into question professional liability, including possible violation of codes of ethics, licensure laws, state or federal regulations and policy, or reduced standard of care.
2. Patients who for any reason are unable to perform tasks required for self-management, including utilizing computers, smartphones, special software, or applications; accessing the Internet; manipulating, handling, adjusting, or cleaning hearing aids; and other hearing assistive devices.
3. A clinic appointment is clearly indicated for patients if off-site delivery of standard of care cannot be ensured. This criterion would apply to a wide range of patients, including young children, requiring audiology expertise such as pediatric audiology skills, making earmold impressions, assessing

vestibular function, comprehensive assessment of auditory processing, psychoacoustic tinnitus assessment audiologic equipment (e.g., sound-treated rooms, sound-field loudspeakers with visual reinforcement audiometry (VRA), fully diagnostic audiometers, vestibular test equipment, cochlear implant programming equipment, real ear measurement systems, fully equipped hearing aid laboratory), and medical personnel like otolaryngologists, anesthesiologists, and nurses who are not available at off-site locations.

Initial Steps Following Diagnosis of Hearing Loss or Related Disorders

Remote diagnostic assessment of children or adults who do not pass hearing screening will invariably confirm hearing loss or related disorders in a subset of the patient population. An audiologist then must consider at least four options for the patient:

1. Patient referral.
2. Monitoring or long-term follow-up for selected patients who do not need to or are not ready to address their hearing loss or related disorders.
3. Audiological intervention or management in a traditional clinic setting.
4. Remote rehabilitation for patients with hearing loss or related disorders.

Patient referral to another health professional may be most appropriate for some patients based on the pattern of diagnostic test findings and/or the score on an inventory or questionnaire. The list of indications for patient referral before audiologic rehabilitation is rather lengthy. Otologic pathology is unusual in an older adult population (e.g., Zapala et al., 2010). However, patients with evidence of ear disease based on audiological findings or a questionnaire like the CEDRA must be referred to an otologist. Patients with hearing loss or related disorders and comorbid conditions that are strongly linked to hearing loss (e.g., diabetes, hyperbilirubinemia, kidney disease, cardiovascular disease, impaired vision, cognitive impairment, and dementia) are referred, usually through the patient's primary care physician, to an appropriate medical specialist (Hall, 2021). Patients with evidence or suspicion of mental health issues, such as depression, are referred to a psychologist or, again through their primary care provider (PCP), to a psychiatrist. Children with apparent speech/language delay are referred to a speech pathologist. Patients with specific types of hearing loss, such as auditory neuropathy spectrum disorder, or with certain related disorders (e.g., bothersome tinnitus, APD, vestibular/balance problems) may be referred to another audiologist with more expertise and clinical experience in their assessment and management.

The second option, monitoring or long-term follow-up, may be the most logical step for many adult patients after, for example, the diagnosis of a mild or transient hearing loss or the perception of tinnitus that is not affecting quality of life. The audiology decision to monitor a patient may be made in combination with an immediate referral of the patient for evaluation and management

of a concomitant or underlying health problem.

Option number three, audiological intervention or management in a traditional clinic setting, would almost always be the decision of choice for selected patient populations with hearing loss or related disorders, including infants and young children, any patient with moderate to severe hearing loss and/or a complex medical history, patients involved in a legal dispute, and patients at risk for loss to follow-up. The remainder of this discussion focuses on patients with hearing loss or related disorders who meet criteria for the fourth option: remote audiologic rehabilitation.

Telerehabilitation Options in Practice Management

With minimal research and Internet searching, readers will readily find a wealth of resources for and detailed reviews of various forms of audiology telerehabilitation (e.g., Bush et al., 2016; Govender & Mars, 2017), among them remote patient counseling and education, remote or self-management for patients with bothersome tinnitus (Beukes et al., 2018; Henry et al., 2020; Searchfield & Kim, 2022), computer-based auditory training for children and adults with diagnosed APD (Loo et al., 2010; Weihing et al., 2016), hearing assistive technology (e.g., personal FM systems) for patients with peripheral hearing loss or APD (Johnston et al., 2009), and remotely programmed hearing aids, or self-contained self-fitting hearing aids for patients who are likely to benefit from amplification (Brice, 2024; Euben, 2020; Keidser & Convery, 2016). The overall goal for audiologists who are ready to embrace teleaudiology in practice management is to incorporate remote services for selected patients whenever there are compelling clinical and practical advantages, with few or no disadvantages or constraints. Among the clear advantages for the patient and the audiologist are increased efficiency in delivery of quality services, with associated reduced cost and time.

Some rehabilitation services are obviously well suited for remote delivery in environments far removed from a clinic setting. One example is online or video-directed patient counseling and education (Manchaiah, Hall, & Beukes, 2024) that is a mainstay for initial hearing aid users and for management persons with bothersome tinnitus or disorders of decreased sound tolerance (Guitton, 2013; Henry et al., 2024; Searchfield & Kim, 2022). Relocating tinnitus management out of the clinic and into remote settings, such as a patient's home, almost always yields practical and clinical benefits for the patient receiving the services as well as the audiologist provider. Not only does the patient save time and money on transportation, but the benefits from tinnitus counseling may also be enhanced when delivered to the patient's comfortable home setting with family participation.

Amplification is at the heart of the most common clinical process for audiological rehabilitation with children and adults. For decades, each of the multi-steps in the hearing aid fitting process was invariably completed in a clinic or office setting with an audiologist completing each step of the process directly with the patient, including the hearing assessment to document a hearing loss, a review of hearing aid options, and a recommendation for amplifica-

tion. Sometime later, the patient would return for more steps that were each carried out by the audiologist, such as preparation of earmold impressions, patient education about hearing aid use, one or more steps for verification and validation of hearing aid benefit, and follow-up visits for adjustments, cleaning, repairs, and so on. Now this approach for audiologic management with amplification is at one end of a continuum of options available to people who are considering amplification.

An alternative near the other end of the continuum is the direct-to-consumer availability of self-contained self-fitting behind-the-ear hearing aids that offer the capability of hearing threshold estimation, an algorithm for an initial hearing aid setting, and training algorithms (e.g., Keidser & Convery, 2016). The patient is responsible for completing each component in the process of initiating amplification with no support or help from an audiologist. Within these two distinctly different models for acquiring amplification are numerous permutations that involve varying amounts of patient responsibility and participation by an audiologist or another category of hearing instrument specialist. Most of the options incorporate teleaudiology concepts, technology, and techniques.

Professional Considerations in Teleaudiology

Patient Rights and Consent

With any model or strategy for provision of audiology services, including teleaudiology, patients or parents of pediatric patients must be informed of the test procedures that will be performed and the tasks that will be expected of them during the assessment (Hall, 2019, 2020; Hall & Traynor, 2024; Keenan et al., 2021). Audiologists should maintain a written record of communications with patients or parents of pediatric patients that confirms the explanation of patient rights. Audiologists should utilize a legally acceptable form that includes a line for the patient's or parents of a pediatric patient's signature. Patients or parents of pediatric patients should provide written consent for the assessment and any subsequent management after the process is explained to them. Ensuring that patient rights are maintained may require additional effort and methods when a patient receives services in a remote location away from a traditional clinic and when the audiologist is not physically with the patient. There must be a plan and policy for verifying that patients in nontraditional clinical settings understand their rights. Options might include a written explanation delivered via email or regular mail before services are provided or a verbal explanation of rights via telephone (voice or video conversation) or a secure online chat (e.g., via Skype or Zoom).

Patient Privacy and Security

Maintaining patient privacy is an essential concern in the delivery of healthcare, including hearing healthcare. Protected health information (PHI) must remain confidential. Patient privacy and security in any healthcare setting, including the patient's home, requires physical and technical safeguards that limit and control access to PHI. Prevention of accidental or intentional disclosure of PHI to unauthorized people or entities is essential. In the United States, audiologists providing services in a nontraditional clinic environment, including a home setting, must comply with federal laws, such as the Health Insurance Portability and Accountability Act (HIPAA), as well as state laws and healthcare institution policies on patient privacy and security. Healthcare challenges during the COVID-19 crisis prompted the temporary relaxation of some regulations. Audiologists and Doctor of Audiology students in the United States should be aware of and comply with current federal and state laws and regulations regarding patient privacy and security. There are a variety of challenges associated with ensuring patient privacy and security for patients who receive remote audiology services. A major concern is the possibility of HIPAA noncompliance during the remote care delivery resulting from unsecured telephone and email patient communications or the presence of an unauthorized person in the patient's space or within earshot of the patient.

Three commonsense steps to safeguard patient privacy are likely to minimize inadvertent violations of the privacy and security of PHI:

1. When an audiologist cannot reach a patient directly via a telephone call, the safest policy is to simply leave a brief generic voice message requesting a callback, without disclosing any PHI in the message. Also, audiologists attempting telephone communication with patients or parents of a patient are

advised to use a dedicated clinical phone number or to take steps to prevent the patient from accessing a personal cell phone number.

2. Upon making telephone or online contact with a patient or parents of a patient such as a Skype or Zoom connection, audiologists are advised to ask the patient or parents of a patient to relocate to a private setting in the house, preferably a room with a door that can be closed.

3. When patient communication and services must take place within a common space in the residence, such as a living room or dining room, the audiologist should first confirm that the patient is alone or that the patient or parents of a patient formally consent to proceed with the assessment in the presence of one or more people and/ or family members. The audiologist should document in writing the patient's decisions regarding their privacy, including the names of those who are within the same space as the patient.

Patient Communication

Maintaining and documenting all professional communication with patients and family members reduces the risk of professional liability and violation of state or federal civil or criminal law. Audiologists should consistently, carefully, and completely document in writing all interactions with patients. It is a good clinic policy to supplement written notes with printouts of test findings and/or with photographic documentation, such as video-otoscopy images.

As already noted, all written communication must be safeguarded for patient privacy. Audiologists and Doctor of Audiology students must always remember that patient reports and all printed clinical data are considered legal documents. Legal advice about patient reports and records is quite straightforward: If you did not document each of your clinical services or your communications with the patient, then they never happened.

Ethical Conduct

The principles articulated in professional codes of ethics apply to the provision of clinical audiology services in all settings and with all delivery models. The most recent Code of Ethics for the American Academy of Audiology (AAA, 2023) explicitly notes in Rule 2C of Part 1. Statement Principles and Rules: "Individuals shall exercise all reasonable precautions to avoid injury to persons in the delivery of professional services or execution of research, whether in-person or via distance (e.g., telehealth) methods" (AAA, 2023, p. 1.) The following brief summary focuses mostly on ethical considerations in remote delivery of audiology services. All audiologists and Doctors of Audiology students must be well versed and up to date on the principles, concepts, and practices that underlie ethical conduct. Readers are referred to official codes of ethics, like the 2023 AAA document, and a recent review article (Hall & Traynor, 2024).

The literature on ethics and teleaudiology is not extensive; however, a recent systematic review of the literature provided some general guidance for the ethical delivery of audiology services via telehealth. Keenan et al. (2021) listed ethical principles discussed in a series of peer-reviewed articles. The five ethical principles were:

1. Autonomy.
2. The relationship between a professional and a patient.
3. Nonmaleficence.
4. Beneficence.
5. Justice.

These principles are regularly cited in ethics publications. The American Speech-Language-Hearing Association (ASHA) also published a list of general guidelines for ethical conduct in providing speech pathology or audiology services via telepractice (Euben, 2020) that highlighted the importance of appropriate training and adherence to the patient-related concerns cited herein, such as compliance with state laws, protection of patient confidentiality and privacy, and obtaining patient consent prior to the provision of services.

Patient Safety

Patient safety is always a top priority in the provision of audiology services to pediatric or adult patients. In a conventional clinic setting, maintaining patient safety includes taking universal precautions to control and prevent infection, implementing policies regarding fall prevention, and maintaining a safe environment of care. Audiologists should attempt to ensure that atypical and non-traditional clinical settings, including the home environment, meet these expectations. If there is increased concern about infection, patients should be encouraged to make use of personal protective equipment (PPE) to minimize risk, including face masks, medical gloves, disposable supplies that make bodily contact (e.g., ear tips), and efforts to disinfect equipment and surfaces.

Standard of Care

Standard of care is the degree of prudence and caution that healthcare providers, including audiologists, should exercise when providing clinical services to patients in any clinical situation. In a traditional clinical setting, standard of care implies delivery of clinical services according to published evidence-based clinical practice guidelines. Peer-reviewed and evidence-based clinical practice guidelines and recommendations are typically generated by audiology professional organizations and multidisciplinary professional groups. For audiologists in the United States who provide face-to-face or remote service in any setting, standard of care must be consistent with statements of scope of practice, codes of ethics, state licensure laws and regulations, and federal healthcare regulatory entities like the Centers for Medicare & Medicaid Services (CMS).

Summary

Audiologists who integrate teleaudiology into their practice will derive numerous clinical and financial benefits. Remote delivery of comprehensive audiology services is feasible and supported by substantial research literature. There are a variety of options for utilizing teleaudiology concepts and strategies in the identification, diagnosis, and management of hearing loss and related disorders in pediatric and adult patient populations. Audiologists incorporating teleaudiology into their practice have an opportunity to widen referral sources and increase patient volume without expanding clinic space or overhead expenses. In addition, incorporation of teleaudiology into a clinical practice offers multiple practical benefits to patients.

References

AAA. (2023). Code of ethics. American Academy of Audiology, Rev. April 2023. https://www.audiology.org/clinical-resources/code-of-ethics/

Ballachanda, B., Abrams, H., Hall, J. W., III, Manchaiah V., Minihane, D., Kleindienst Robler, S., & Swanepoel, D. (2020). Tele-audiology in a pandemic and beyond: Flexibility and suitability in audiology practice. Audiology Today. https://www.audiology.org/news-and-publications/audiology-today/articles/tele-audiology-in-a-pandemic-and-beyond-flexibility-and-suitability-in-audiology-practice/

Beukes, E. W., Andersson, G., Allen, P. M., Manchaiah, V., & Baguley, D. M. (2018). Effectiveness of guided internet-based cognitive behavioural therapy vs. face-to-face clinical care for treatment of tinnitus. A randomized clinical trial. *JAMA Otolaryngology Head and Neck Surgery*, *144*(12), 1126–1133.

Biagio, L., Swanepoel, D. W., Adeyemo, A., Hall, J. W., III, & Vinck, B. (2013). Asynchronous video-otoscopy with a telehealth facilitator. *Telemedicine and e-Health*, *19*, 1–7.

Birkmire-Peters, D. P., Peters, L. J., & Whitaker, L. A. (1999). A usability evaluation for telemedicine medical equipment: A case study. *Telemedicine Journal*, *5*, 209–212.

Brice, S. (2024). Remote hearing aid selection, fitting, and support. In V. Manchaiah, J. W. Hall III, E. W. Beukes, & D. W. Swanepoel (Eds.), *Teleaudiology today: Remote assessment and management of hearing loss*. Kindle Direct Publishing.

Bush, M. L., Thompson, R., Irungu, C., & Ayugi, J. (2016). The role of telemedicine in auditory rehabilitation: A systematic review. *Otology & Neurotology*, *37*, 1466–1474.

D'Onofrio, K. L., & Zeng, F.-G. (2021). Tele-audiology: Current state and future directions. *Frontiers in Digital Health*, *3*, 788103. https://doi.org/10.3389/fdgth.2021.788103

Eikelboom, R. H., Swanepoel, D., Motakef, S., & Upson, G.S. (2013). Clinical validation of the AMTAS automated audiometer. *International Journal of Audiology*, *52*(5), 342–349.

Euben, D. (2020). Top 10 ethical considerations in using telepractice. Leader Live. https://leader.pubs.asha.org/do/10.1044/2020-0513-ethics teleprctice/full

Govender, S. M., & Mars, M. (2017). The use of telehealth services to facilitate audiological management for children: A scoping review and content analysis. *Journal of Telemedicine and Telecare*, *23*, 392–401.

Guitton, M. J. (2013). Telemedicine in tinnitus: Feasibility, advantages, limitations. *ISRN Otolaryngology*, Article ID 218265. http://dx.doi.org/10.1155/2013/218265

Hall, J. W., III. (2014). *Introduction to audiology today*. Pearson Educational.

Hall, J. W., III. (2019). 5 steps to avoid medical errors in audiology practice. *The Hearing Journal*, *72*(3), 8–9.

Hall, J. W., III. (2020). Professional liability and teleaudiology services. *The Hearing Journal*, *72*(3), 8–9.

Hall, J. W., III. (2021). Promoting healthy hearing over the lifespan. *Auditory & Vestibular Research*, *30*, 74–94.

Hall, J. W., III. (2024). Ethical, legal, and professional aspects of teleaudiology. In V. Manchaiah, J. W. Hall III, E. W. Beukes, & D. W. Swanepoel (Eds.), *Teleaudiology today: Remote assessment and management of hearing loss*. Kindle Direct Publishing.

Hall, J. W., III, & Swanepoel, D. W. (2024). Hearing screening and assessment via teleaudiology. In V. Manchaiah, J. W. Hall III, E. W. Beukes, & D. W. Swanepoel (Eds.), *Teleaudiology today: Remote assessment and management of hearing loss*. Kindle Direct Publishing.

Hall, J. W., III, & Traynor, R. M. (2024). Ethics in audiology. *Audiology Today, 36*(2), 42–51.

Henry, J. A., Thielman, E. J., & Grush, L. D. (2022). Application of teleaudiology in the clinical management of tinnitus. In A. Deshpande & J. W. Hall III (Eds.), *Tinnitus: Advances in prevention, assessment, and management* (pp. 209–220). Plural Publishing.

Henry, J. A., Thielman, E. J., Kaelin, C., Quinn, C. M., & Goodworth, M. C. (2020). Tele-health based progressive tinnitus management. *The Hearing Journal, 73*(5), 32–35.

Johnston, K. N., John, A. B., Kreisman, N. V., Hall, J. W., III, & Crandell, C. C. (2009). Multiple benefits of personal FM system use by children with auditory processing disorder (APD). *International Journal of Audiology, 48*, 371–383.

Keenan, A. J., Tsourtos, G., & Tiernan, J. (2021). The value of applying ethical principles in telehealth practices: A systematic review. *Journal of Medical Internet Research, 23*(3), e25698. https://doi.org/10.2196/25698

Keidser, G., & Convery, E. (2016). Self-fitting hearing aids: Status quo and future predictions. *Trends in Hearing, 20*, 1–15.

Kim, J., Jeon, S., Kim, D., & Shin, Y. (2021). A review of contemporary teleaudiology: Literature review, technology, and considerations for practicing. *Journal of Audiology & Otology, 25*, 1–7.

Kleindienst Robler, S. J., Coco, L., Ballachanda, B., & Krumm, M. (2024). Set-up and implementation of teleaudiology practice. In V. Manchaiah, J. W. Hall III, E. W. Beukes, & D. W. Swanepoel (Eds.), *Teleaudiology today: Remote assessment and management of hearing loss*. Kindle Direct Publishing.

Kleindienst Robler, S., Platt, A., Jenson, C. D., Meade Inglis, S., Hofsteter, P., Ross, A. A., . . . Emmett, S. D. (2023). Changing the paradigm for school hearing screening globally: Evaluation of screening protocols from two randomized trials in rural Alaska. *Ear & Hearing*. Advance online publication. https://doi.org/10.1097/AUD.0000000000001336

Klyn, N. A. M., Kleindienst Robler, S., Bogle J., Alfakir R., Nielsen, D. W., Griffith, J. W., . . . Zapala DA (2019). CEDRA: A tool to help consumers assess risk for ear disease. *Ear & Hearing, 40*, 1261–1266.

Krumm, M., & Ferrari, D. V. (2008). Contemporary telehealth and telemedicine applications in audiology. *Audiology Today, 20*, 36–41.

Krumm, M., & Syms, M. J. (2011) Teleaudiology. *Otolaryngology Clinics of North America, 44*, 1297–1304.

Lancaster, P., Krumm, M., Ribera, J., & Klich, R. (2008). Remote hearing screenings via telehealth in a rural elementary school. *American Journal of Audiology, 17*, 114–122.

Loo, J. H., Bamiou, D.-E., Campbell, N., & Luxon, L. M. (2010). Computer-based auditory training (CBAT): Benefits for children with language- and reading-related learning difficulties. *Developmental Medicine & Child Neurology, 52*, 708–171.

Maclennan-Smith, F., Swanepoel, D., & Hall, J. W., III. (2013). Validity of diagnostic pure-tone audiometry without a sound-treated environment in older adults. *International Journal of Audiology, 52*, 66–73.

Manchaiah, V., Hall, J. W., III, & Beukes, E. (2024). Informational counseling and shared decision making. In V. Manchaiah, J. W. Hall III, E. W. Beukes, & D. W. Swanepoel (Eds.), *Teleaudiology today: Remote assessment and management of hearing loss*. Kindle Direct Publishing.

Manchaiah, V., Hall, J. W., III, Beukes, E. W., & Swanepoel, D. W. (Eds.). (2024). *Teleaudiology today: Remote assessment and management of hearing loss*. Kindle Direct Publishing.

Margolis, R. H., Frisina, R., & Walton, J. P. (2011) AMTAS: Automated method for testing auditory sensitivity: II. Air conduction audiograms in children and adults. *International Journal of Audiology, 50*, 434–439.

Margolis, R. H., Glasberg, B. R., Creeke, S., & Moore, B. C. (2010). AMTAS: Automated method for testing auditory sensitivity: Validation studies. *International Journal of Audiology, 49*, 185–194.

Schmiedge, J. (1997). *Distortion product otoacoustic emissions testing using telemedicine technology*. Unpublished master's degree thesis, Minot State University, Minot, ND.

Searchfield, G. D., & Kim, S.-J. (2022). Self-directed tinnitus therapy: A review of at-home tinnitus therapy options. In A. Deshpande & J. W. Hall III (Eds.), *Tinnitus: Advances in prevention, assessment, and management* (pp. 159–178). Plural Publishing.

Swanepoel, D. W., Clark, J. L., Koekmoer, D., Hall, J. W., III, Krumm, M., Ferrari, D. V., . . . Barajas, J. J. (2010). Telehealth in audiology: The need and potential to reach underserved communities. *International Journal of Audiology, 49*, 195–202.

Swanepoel, D. W., & Hall, J. W., III. (2010). A systematic review of telehealth applications in audiology. *Telemedicine and e-Health, 16*, 181–200.

Swanepoel, D. W., & Hall, J. W., III. (2020). Making audiology work during COVID-19 and beyond. *ENT and Audiology News, 29*(3), 22–26.

Swanepoel, D. W., & Hall, J. W., III. (2020). Making audiology work during COVID-19 and beyond. *The Hearing Journal, 73*(6). https://journals.lww.com/thehearingjournal/fulltext/2020/06000/making_audiology_work_during_covid_19_and_beyond.1.aspx

Swanepoel, D. W., Maclennan-Smith, F., & Hall, J. W., III (2013). Diagnostic pure tone audiometry in schools: Mobile testing without a sound-treated environment. *Journal of the American Academy of Audiology, 24*, 1–9.

Swanepoel, D. W., Manchaiah, V., Hall, J. W., III, & Beukes, E. (2024). Teleaudiology today: Revolutionizing hearing care practices. *The Hearing Journal, 77*(2), 6–7.

Swanepoel, D. W., Matthysen, C., Eikelboom, R. H., Clark, J. L., & Hall, J. W., III (2015). Pure tone audiometry outside a sound-booth using earphone attenuation, integrated ambient noise monitoring, and automation. *International Journal of Audiology, 54*, 777–785.

Weihing, J., Chermak, G. D., & Musiek, F. E. (2016). Auditory training for central auditory processing disorder. *Seminars in Hearing, 36*, 199–215.

Zapala, D., Stamper, G. C., Shelfer, J. S., Walker, D. A., Karatayli-Ozgursoy, S., Ozgursoy, O., & Hawkins, D. B. (2010). Safety of audiology direct access for Medicare patients complaining of impaired hearing. *Journal of the American Academy of Audiology, 21*, 385–387.

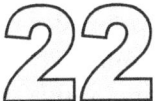 # Forensic Audiology

Dennis A. Colucci, MA, AuD, ABAC, FAAA

Introduction

As a student in audiology, a career starts with an interest in people, the desire to help others, an inquisitive mind, and an aptitude for the sciences, medicine, and rehabilitation. A calling in audiology fulfills our most human needs to find purpose and accomplishment and garner recognition. Purpose provides a direction to one's life; accomplishment supports self-esteem, and recognition from your peers maintains healthy relationships. Helping others is the best reward, as acts of kindness increase happiness, decrease stress, boost the feel-good part of the brain, and keep audiologists connected to others (Mental Health America, n.d.). Greeting patients with those famous words "How can I help you?" says it all. A career in audiology adds meaning to life, devotes kindness to others, and, for some, presents an amazing opportunity to be a forensic audiologist, which is the pinnacle of standards, professional competency, and financial stability.

The career of an audiologist lasts for decades and can take many turns. What starts as a job in a medical clinic can change over the years to working in research, evaluating veterans at the Veterans Administration (VA), opening a private practice, developing a hearing conservation program for multinational companies, operating an audiovestibular laboratory, fitting cochlear implants, teaching, and more. Each of these areas has one common denominator: advanced knowledge, skills, and abilities. Regardless of the path, each experience builds a resume of knowledge and expertise and, for some, a level of specialization capable of becoming a forensic audiologist.

The direction of any chosen path requires a high level of expertise, especially when considering the subspecialty of forensics. Building a career in forensic audiology requires extensive education, ongoing training and development, and high-quality practical experience starting at the onset. Audiology is built on the profession's doctoral-level education steeped in science, methodology, and ethics. A clinician's specific knowledge is amassed upon incontrovertible research, scientific principles, best practices, and quantifiable outcomes that improve the quality of life for those we serve (Colucci et al., 2024). Those who become forensic audiologists have the credentials to compete at every level in medical-legal cases.

Most audiologists have been unaware of the opportunity to work in the legal arena as an expert witness. This is because audiology, except for the PhD, EdD, and ScD, was not a doctoral-level profession at its inception, and the level of expertise was too limited to be recognized by legal professionals or physicians. With the advent of the AuD and advanced knowledge, forensic audiology has developed into a new and exciting subspecialty. For decades, some audiologists have worked within the legal system as experts, but few clinicians understand what it takes or how to become an expert recognized by the courts.

Audiologists as Expert Witnesses

Forensic audiology investigates and applies auditory and vestibular science and technology to criminal and civil law. The forensic audiologist is an independent expert who, by reasons of education, special training, and experience, possesses appropriate knowledge to assist the triers of fact, the jury, the judge, and counselors in understanding the evidence, information, and opinions presented to the court.

Forensic audiologists have existed for decades, but few clinicians understood how to or desired to interact with the legal system. For the most part, audiologists have lacked knowledge about expert witnessing and the role they play in the legal system. Professional witnesses are needed from every occupation, including audiology. The audiologist's advanced degrees, knowledge, skills, and abilities are sufficient credentials to ensure the efficacy of audiologists as expert witnesses. The audiologist's role as a forensic specialist is evidenced by reimbursement rates that support competency worthy of expert status equal to other professions in the legal or medical fields. Working as doctoral-level practitioners, applying the principles of research, evidence-based diagnostic assessments, and up-to-date innovation in management has widened the scope of audiology to encompass the legal arena.

The American Academy of Audiology (AAA) and American Speech-Language-Hearing Association (ASHA) include medical-legal and forensic practice within the profession's scope of practice. AAA (2023) states, "The Scope of Practice for audiology is complex, dynamic, and constantly evolving. The areas of audiology practice described in this document include screening and identification, assessment and diagnosis, treatment and management of auditory and vestibular loss, hearing conservation, neurophysiological monitoring, research and academic activities, public health, and additional expertise." This scope is appropriate for those entering forensic audiology and testifying as an expert witness within audiology. Although most audiologists are comfortable dispensing hearing aids and providing rehabilitation, many are trained and have considerable experience in audiovestibular evaluations and treatments. Forensics is a natural landing pad for those with advanced knowledge in their chosen path. Not all experts must provide a full range of diagnostics, such as auditory brainstem evoked potentials or nystagmography. However, an expert witness should understand the applications and be capable of interpreting the data when presented in reports, depositions, or trials. Several case types, such as Americans with Disabilities Act issues, educational placement disputes, and audiology or hearing aid dispensing malpractice, do not require special testing but still need experts in legal cases.

Forensic Audiology Career Building

To be an expert-level clinician capable of testifying in medical-legal cases requires training, clinical experience, and specialization. The process starts with acquiring a bachelor's degree, preferably in speech pathology, communication, or the sciences, followed by an extended graduate education and externship. The externship marks the fourth year of supervised experience in the field, where students combine their working knowledge into practice. At the end of the formal training and externship, students are granted a PhD, AuD, or AuD/PhD, depending upon their career path. The Student Academy of Audiology (SAA, n.d.) and the National Student Speech-Language-Hearing Association (NSSLHA, n.d.) have helpful resources for evaluating the options.

After receiving a doctorate, graduates take the ETS Praxis® Examination in Audiology (ETS Praxis®), which is an audiology licensure examination recognized in most states. Passing the Praxis examination is also necessary to receive the Certificate of Clinical Competence in Audiology (CCC-A) from the American Speech-Language-Hearing Association. Licensed audiologists can also obtain American Board of Audiology Certification® (ABAC), Cochlear Implant Specialty Certification® (CISC), or Pediatric Audiology Specialty Certification® (PASC) or become a Certificate Holder in Tinnitus Management (CH-TM). Some states recognize the CCC-A or ABAC with or without the Praxis scores or specified state-supervised clinical experience when applying for licensure. Licensing boards should be contacted in each state for their requirements. The National Council of State Board of Examiners (NCSB, n.d.) provides a directory of licensing boards, their contact information, degree, continuing education, state occupancy requirements, and information on support personnel, telemedicine regulations, and states in the interstate compact.

After receiving a doctoral degree, board certification, and licensure, most audiologists start their careers working in an audiology or ear, nose, and throat practice, research facilities, hospitals, public schools, the military, private practice, retail hearing aid offices, deaf education, or hearing aid manufacturing in various capacities. As audiologists gain experience, advanced training, and pursue professional interests, their path to a career in forensics starts to build. Each additional expertise supported by continuing education is among the most essential activities qualifying the clinician's integrity as a forensic expert. As the curriculum vitae expands, so does the marketability in the legal area. Examples of career-building activities include working in several areas such as rehabilitation, medicine, or industry; writing articles in journals or industry magazines, books, and other print forms; teaching at conventions; producing podcasts; or contributing to eLearning. Showing diversity in training and experience builds a better resume. However, it is not a requirement, as many experts rely on their years of experience and specialization. For example, a clinician in a university setting, veterans hospital, rehabilitation center, private practice with hearing and balance testing, or industrial hearing conservation would have a specific knowledge niche within audiovestibular disorders and treatments. Because education, clinical experience, and specialization are keys to being a good expert witness, every background in audiology has a place at the table.

Clinical Experience

The audiologist's clinical experience, as found on the curriculum vitae, will attract attorneys to accept or deny engagement based on how it meets their case needs. For example, an attorney looking for someone to be an expert witness in a gunshot accident case will be looking for someone with military, industrial, or medical audiology experience who can speak to acoustic trauma, hearing loss, tinnitus, and hyperacusis. Suppose the attorney needs someone for a head injury case involving a traumatic brain injury (TBI), migraines, tinnitus, hyperacusis, and vertigo. In that case, they will need to see some clinical or medical experience and someone who is comfortable working with and understanding neurology reports. A background in electrophysiology and balance testing can always be a plus.

Although hearing aid fitting and services are essential when discussing rehabilitation recommendations, few legal cases, other than malpractice related to state hearing aid licensing complaints, will seek an expert who provides experience in such a narrow scope of practice. Over the years, clinicians should have advanced training and several specialties that form their niche, making their information unique and desired within the legal community.

Specialization

According to legal experts, those with the greatest degree of training and experience in a specialization are more likely than not to be engaged and awarded the highest fees. For example, some expert witnesses garnish $250.00 an hour, while others with a specialization charge above $1,000.00 an hour. Audiologists have a specific niche regarding hearing loss, tinnitus, hyperacusis, and auditory processing, especially in those involving multiple injuries, including the head and neck, with or without balance disturbances. Specialization in pediatrics, cochlear implants, blast exposure, industrial noise pollution, petroleum and nuclear power plants, aircraft and community noise, and other niches are foreign to most in medicine and the general public. The audiologist is the only specialist with unique experience and knowledge in these areas. For example, an ENT specialist or neurologist would not generally be knowledgeable about industrial noise hazards, OSHA, NIOSH, fit testing, environmental and room acoustics, measuring sound transmission, competing signals, or testing auditory processing. The audiologist is a specialist who can properly educate the court, appropriately opine, and help the triers of fact to achieve a just verdict.

Principles of Forensic Audiology

The principles in forensic audiology apply across all disciplines in the medical-legal universe. The witness must demonstrate case-specific qualifications, follow the rules of the court, tell the truth, and maintain the highest ethical standards. Legal cases typically require that the expert witness perform an independent medical examination, provide a medical-legal report, be deposed, and, for a few cases, appear in court for trial. In some cases, the audiologist may not be engaged as an expert witness but as a consultant to help a firm understand the facts before them. Since attorneys and others in the legal system are unacquainted with audiovestibular issues, the audiologist is a resource who can write summary reports and rebuttals, and answer questions. As a consultant, the audiologist performs the same duties as the expert witness without testimony, and their work is privileged and not discoverable by the opposing party.

In the case of audiovestibular complaints, opining starts with determining the nexus between the accident and the injuries. As part of the discovery phase, information will be revealed requiring scrutiny, including keeping a watchful eye for malingering or bias by partisan experts. During the discovery phase, both plaintiff and defendant counsels will review all available information gathered by subpoena and other means, including the audiologist's expert witness report and their opinions. Opinions are the most essential part of the report since they assist the triers of fact in deciding a case. The first step in developing opinions is to research all the aspects of the case and evaluate all the potential causes. A forensic evaluation uses science and technology in the investigation and establishment of facts and evidence to be used in a court of law. A forensic audiologist is charged with this duty.

A nexus is formulated when a condition is qualified by the time and place, short and long outcomes, complete history, pre- and post-conditions, current findings, and the association between what research and current practices tell us. Once a nexus is determined, a differential diagnosis must be undertaken to look at all possibilities that could cause the claimed conditions. Based on the preponderance of evidence, opinions will be written, regardless of the outcome to the plaintiff or defendant.

Hearing loss, tinnitus, hyperacusis, auditory processing, and balance dysfunctions are injury outcomes oriented explicitly toward the audiologist because of training and knowledge in audiovestibular disorders, acoustics, noise, and expertise in testing, diagnosis, and rehabilitation. The methods and principles used in opining should reflect that knowledge.

When opining, the language must state they are based on a reasonable degree of audiological and scientific certainty and, more likely than not, not just a possibility. If the opinions are not qualified, they can be stricken from the record and a Daubert challenge can be filed. Opinions must be within the expert's actual field, be verified and unbiased, state the facts, and be understandable to the triers when presented.

In some cases, the report is all that is needed, and the case is settled. In other cases, a deposition is needed and, for a few, a court trial. Multiple specialties within audiology can work with legal professionals and other experts in related fields. Recommending to an attorney other specialists into a case is not uncommon. The audiologist may need the expertise of site reconstructionists, physicians, or acoustic engineers when the scope of engagement is outside their knowledge base.

Court Mechanics

Litigation and a trial can be pursued when other means of resolving a dispute between two parties, such as arbitration or mediation, are not plausible. In most cases, the best advice is not to go to court because it is expensive, time-consuming, and psychologically draining, and it can result in an undetermined and potentially undesirable outcome. However, insurance companies and defendants will challenge a complaint when injury claims have not been confirmed or appear excessive or exaggerated, harm has been misplaced, or compensation is not justified or disproportionate. For example, in a head injury case, there were multiple injuries, and the relief requested was $35,000,000, but after the trial, the jury awarded the plaintiff $1,500,000. In this case, the plaintiff, witnesses, and experts could not substantiate the claims and severity of the injuries. In fact, the experts from both sides presented similar severity findings. In an assault case, the mediated settlement was $1,750,000 because the preponderance of evidence confirmed the complaint, the burden of proof was substantiated, and expert testimony was convincing. Because experts on a case may have opposing opinions, the preponderance of evidence should be the guiding factor.

Working through the court system as an expert witness requires a reasonable understanding of how the court works. The purpose of the court is to ensure that civil procedures are followed and that justice prevails through a hierarchy of state and federal courts. Each court has different jurisdictions, and due to federalism, both state and federal governments have their own legal systems. Ultimately, the Supreme Court is the land's highest court under Article III of the U.S. Constitution. Only certain cases from the state level can request a review by the U.S. Supreme Court.

An audiologist can be an expert witness in various types of civil law cases, including contract, property, succession, and family law, depending upon the specifics, but most frequently, tort law. Tort law refers to laws that provide remedies for those who have suffered harm by unreasonable acts of another. This is based on the assumption that individuals or entities are liable for the consequences of their actions, intentional or not, if they cause harm to another individual or entity. Based on the preponderance of evidence, which must be clear and convincing, the triers of fact (judge or jury) decide if the harm that occurred was more likely than not (>50%) a result of the actions of the individual or entity. For audiology experts, the preponderance of evidence and opinions must be based on "a reasonable degree of scientific and audiological certainty."

Stages of Civil Procedure

Becoming an expert witness requires a basic understanding of the legal system, starting with the plaintiff's complaints through the appeals process. Audiologists can be engaged throughout, starting with the discovery stage. For example, the audiologist may be engaged to help draft interrogatory or deposition questions but may be deposed on their expert report. The diagram of the Stages of Civil Procedure (Traynor & Traynor, 2024) provides an overview of the process, starting with the complaint (Figure 22–1).

The Complaint

Once it is determined that a cause of action is necessary for an individual or

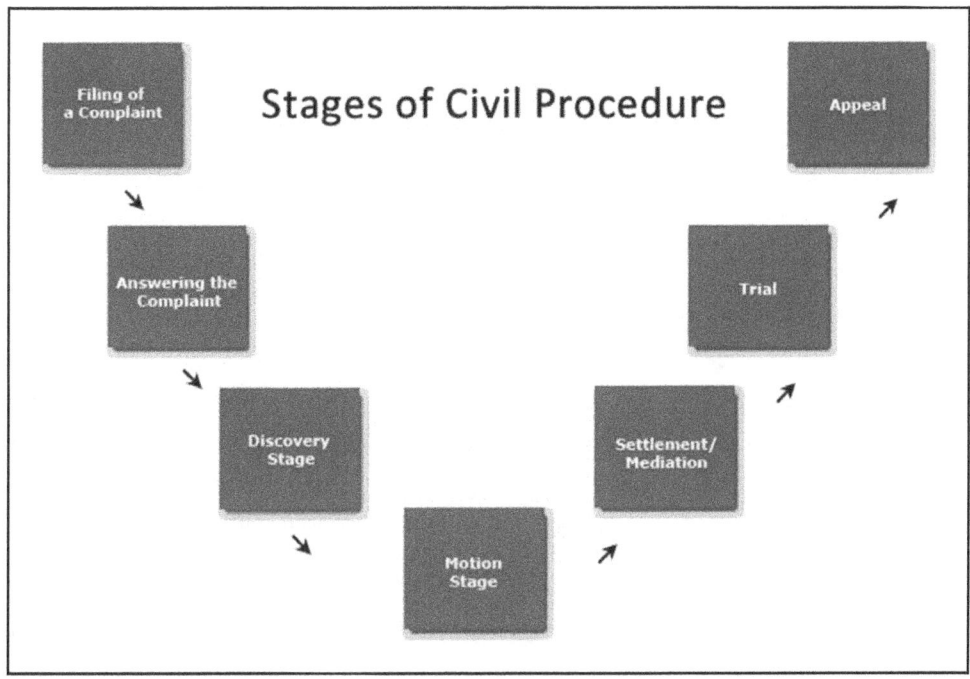

Figure 22–1. Stages of civil procedure. *Source*: From *Forensic Audiology: A Guide for the Expert Witness* (pp. 1–354) by Traynor, R. M., & Traynor, K. B. Copyright © 2024 Plural Publishing, Inc. All rights reserved.

entity (plaintiff) to obtain relief, financial or not, the process starts with the complaint. The purpose of the complaint is to present the parties involved, the plaintiff's beliefs of the case facts, the allegations and offenses, and a claim for relief. The procedure for the attorney to file a complaint can vary from state to federal, even though it is the first legal document in the lawsuit. The plaintiff's attorney is responsible for ensuring that the complaint is served to the defendant(s) and must demonstrate proof of service.

The complaint document has a caption at the top that identifies the court, such as the United States District Court Southern District of Florida or the State of California Superior Court for the County of San Diego. The caption may also include a case reference, case number, plaintiff(s) and defendant(s) names, the judge and magistrate, attorneys for the plaintiff, filing date, and more. The multidistrict litigation (MDL) number is included if the lawsuit pertains to product liability. An example of the caption and the opening statement used by an expert in a federal case is seen in Figure 22–2. Each court will have a variation of the caption depending upon the jurisdiction and type of legal case, and expert witnesses may also choose a different opening format.

Answering the Complaint

The defendants will answer the complaint in a specific period of time as

---

United States District Court
Southern District of Florida
Miami Division

IN RE: Cujoe Corporation
Replacement Prothesis Product Liability

MDL No. 4:21-md-3255

Judge X. Devin Merriott
Magistrate Judge Sandra X. Do

This document relates to:
John Doe v. Cujoe Corp., et al.
Case No. 4:30-sv-29888-XDM-SXD

REPORT OF DENNIS A. COLUCCI, M.A., Au.D., ABAC, FAAA

The following expert report is submitted on behalf of the Defendants. The independent opinions in this report are offered with a reasonable degree of audiological and scientific certainty. My curriculum vitae is labeled Exhibit A. In addition to the bibliography attached to this report, the documents I relied upon and reviewed in formulating my opinions are attached in Exhibit B. Test results can be reviewed in Exhibit C.

Figure 22–2. Lawsuit complaint caption and report header.

determined by the court, 21 days in federal court or another period as specified by jurisdiction. According to legal experts, the answer is a defense rebuttal, although the defense attorney may make preanswer motions to the court to overt or challenge the suit. The motions may include a lack of jurisdiction over the subject matter (wrong court), lack of jurisdiction over the person (wrong state), improper venue (wrong county), insufficiency of the service process, or failure to state a claim upon which relief may be granted (Mangraviti et al., 2015). Once these are finalized, an answer to the allegations is produced, and a defense posture ensues. The answer will respond to each paragraph in the complaint by admitting or denying the allegations or if there is insufficient knowledge to admit or deny the allegations. The answer will also include a list of any affirmative defenses by the defendant. The defendant can also make a counterclaim and sue the plaintiff.

The Discovery Process

Discovery provides each side of the lawsuit with a liberal means of obtaining all available evidence by requesting medical records, admissions, production of documents, evidence inspections, interrogatories, expert reports, and depositions. Under the Federal Rule of Civil Procedure 26(b)(1), the scope of discovery is defined. It clearly allows for a phishing expedition, especially during depositions. The vigorous examination of evidence helps both sides to see the entire case and qualitatively evaluate the merits and weaknesses, objectify their position, and, in most cases, settle the matter without going to trial. Over 90% of cases settle before trial, and the liberal discovery process can be credited for serving this purpose.

The discovery process is central to the audiology expert witness reporting, testimony, and credibility. Discovery includes collecting all the available information about the case, and the independent medical examinations, which provide the basis for the expert report, especially the opinions that are paramount to the case. The expert report is central to all testimony moving forward in the process. It is the guiding light of opinions to be presented at deposition or trial. Veering off statements in the report or amendments, misrepresenting findings, not telling the truth, failing to follow the science, and changing an opinion without clear justifications (i.e., new information) can ruin a case and result in a Daubert challenge, ending a forensic career.

As part of discovery, depositions are scheduled by opposing counsels of witnesses, plaintiffs, and experts. Depositions are not conducted in court but hold the same privileges of sworn testimony and perjury consequences. The purpose is to allow opposing counsels to investigate the expert's opinions and the basis for them. A direct examination or cross-examination is a unique opportunity for the audiologist to educate the attorneys and substantiate the conclusions in the report, which will be offered at trial. The deposition is the most revealing stage as opposing counsel will test the audiologist's knowledge of the subject matter, how they applied methods and scientific principles to the case,

and if they judiciously formulate their causation opinions, degree of impairment, and rehabilitation recommendations. With a calm demeanor and following the report and science, the audiology expert witness can be a valuable tool in offering educational information and opinions that are helpful to the understanding of case specifics and a basis for settlement.

Motions Stage

Once all the information has been gathered and before settlement/mediation begins, each side may present motions for the court to act upon disputed issues. Motions may be presented at any time during the litigation. However, the motions stage follows the discovery stage as new information reveals facts of the case that need adjudication for various reasons. Many motions can be filed, and the following are the most common:

- Motion to dismiss the case, typically known as getting the case "thrown out."
- Motion for a direct verdict occurs when, at trial, the plaintiff failed to prove sufficient facts such as the expert failed to prove causation.
- Motions of discovery occur when a party to the action does not provide discovery materials, and the court compels them to do so.
- Motion to compel is a request asking the court to force a party to take action on something they have refused to do, such as medical examinations.
- Motion to strike is requested when a party wants something stricken from the record because it is inappropriate or inadmissible evidence.

■ Motion for continuance occurs when the moving party requests a change in a scheduled event, such as a hearing or trial, to be moved to a later date.

■ Motion of summary judgment requests that the judge decide the case.

■ Motion to set aside judgment occurs when new information suggests the verdict should be nullified.

■ Motion for a new trial can be requested by either party when they believe a significant error has occurred, such as a motion of limine was successful, but the testimony was already presented.

■ Motion in limine, such as a Daubert motion to exclude expert testimony.

Attorneys will attempt to discredit expert witnesses for any reason, especially when they can question methodology or protocol that suggests errors, actual or not. The motion of limine is used against witnesses to remove their testimony as the jury should not hear prejudicial evidence or an expert's failure to comply with the Daubert standard. To the audiologist, a motion of limine should not occur unless there is information that has not been disclosed during discovery, administrative issues, or statements made that do not follow the science and methods. Fortunately, a Daubert hearing can be requested, and the motion can be denied upon examination by the judge.

Settlement and Mediation

After the discovery and motion stages, the next phase is determining if the opposing sides can settle the case through mediation outside the court. Mediation typically takes a half day or can last as long as 2 days. The amounts of a settlement demand and offers by the defense are confidential and will not be available during later court proceedings. A retired judge or attorney typically functions as an independent mediator paid by the opposing counsels to remain neutral during the mediation. The mediator is not financially interested in the case and is paid regardless of the outcome. The mediation starts with a case summary followed by the plaintiff's attorney stating what will be required to settle the case. The defendant then makes a counteroffer, and the negotiations commence. Should both sides come to an understanding, a settlement occurs, the trial judge is informed that the case is mediated, and the case is closed. A trial is the next stage if the mediation fails and a settlement does not occur.

The Trial

Bench and jury trials are the two types of civil trials. In a bench trial, the judge acts as the finder of facts and makes the judgment, and in a jury trial, the jury acts as the finder of fact and provides the verdict. In the jury trial, the judge will run the courtroom; make all the legal rulings, including the admissibility of the expert testimony; and instruct the jury on the applicable law. Similar to a deposition, there is a direct examination and a cross-examination. In either case, each side presents its case based on the premise that justice is served when both parties present their version of the truth. The jury has an opportunity to evaluate each case and decide if the plaintiff has met the burden of proof, demonstrating that the defendant has more likely than not harmed the plaintiff. Should a verdict not be acceptable to either side of the case, an appeal may be requested.

Court of Appeals

One of the final vestiges of legal argument at the state level falls on the appellate court. If the appeals court does not resolve the issues, the next step is to file them with the Supreme Court. An appeal can be requested in civil cases, although the court may or may not grant a hearing. The petition is explicitly asking that a new court hear the case. In court, the attorneys present the facts of their case with no new evidence or witnesses, and the panel of judges will ascertain if the trial court fairly applied the law. If it is determined that the trial was not appropriately dispensed, the appeals court may rule.

Daubert Standard

Throughout the United States, the court uses the Daubert standard or Frye rules to determine if the expert witness uses relevant and reliable methodologies in their analysis and opinions. The judge is the gatekeeper who may exclude unreliable expert testimony. The first hurdle to having testimony accepted by the court is to be deemed credible under the Federal Rules of Evidence 702, which presents guidelines for expert witness testimony (Federal Rules of Evidence, n.d.). Rule 702 asks if the following is more likely than not:

There are four primary factors bearing on the judge's decision to exclude testimony (Mangraviti et al., 2015):

1. Whether the theory or technique used by the expert can be and has been tested.

THE TESTIMONY OF EXPERT WITNESSES

Known as the Daubert standard, experts' testimony in all federal and many state courts is governed by these four criteria to be accepted by the judge in civil or criminal cases:

1. The expert's scientific, technical, or other specialized knowledge helps the trier of fact to understand the evidence or to determine a fact in issue.
2. The testimony is based on sufficient facts or data.
3. The testimony is a product of reliable principles and methods.
4. The expert's opinions reflect a reliable application of the principles and methods to the facts of the case.

Federal Rules of Evidence 2024 Edition, Quick Reference Series, Michigan Legal Publishing, Ltd.

2. Whether the theory or technique has been subjected to peer review and publication.
3. The known or potential rate of error of the method used.
4. The degree of the method's or conclusion's acceptance within the relevant scientific community.
5. In addition, numerous areas can be challenged, including the expert's qualification, reliability, misapplication of methods, false facts, invalid assumptions, or using hearsay evidence (Traynor & Traynor, 2024).

Considering that audiology is based on a doctoral-level education centered on science, methodology, and ethics and incontrovertible research, methods and principles, best practices, and quantifiable outcomes, the opportunity for a Daubert challenge should be minimal and kept to administrative complaints. Should a Daubert challenge occur, the engaging attorney should apprise the audiologist immediately, and a hearing to answer the challenge in front of the judge should ensue. The motion of limine will include specific allegations that can be addressed at the hearing. The engagement contract must include a state that requires the attorney to disclose such a motion upon receipt.

Engagement and Case Development

Civil litigation cases are based on tangible or intangible assets, such as real property versus patent rights or copyright infringement. In medical-legal cases, the claims are based on injury resulting in physical and or psychological complaints. On rare occasions, a criminal case will also need the expertise of an audiologist, such as crimes involving firearms, an accused with hearing loss, the ability of the defendant to hear in a noisy environment during the commission of a crime, or criminal offenses when in jail. For the most part, audiologists will be involved in bodily injury cases, everything from a train or car accident, airplane crash, and noise pollution to wrongful death.

From the onset, unless specifically requested, all contact with a law firm should be oral, as any written information is discoverable. Emails and texting are only for procedural materials such as timelines, court dates, scheduling, legal notices, deposition subpoenas, and discovery links.

Making a mistake by responding with a case-relevant email during the opening contact will result in the loss of engagement and admonishment.

Cases begin with a presentation by the retaining attorney. If the case's merits are within the audiologist's scope and knowledge base and are worthy of involvement, an engagement contract, curriculum vitae, W-9, and fee schedule with retainer request are sent to the attorney. The audiologist is ready to proceed after the attorney reviews the documents, agrees to the terms, and signs the engagement contract. No work should be stated until the agreement and retainer are received. Additionally, working directly with a plaintiff without an attorney is not recommended.

The expert must remember that regardless of the attorney's disposition (plaintiff or defendant), they only pay for time, not the expert's general or case-specific opinions. Although some experts are compelled to choose sides and lean in one direction or another, eventually, another expert and attorney will be able to demonstrate a lack of candor, resulting in a Daubert hearing and testimony being excluded by the court. If the court ever excludes testimony, it is generally a career-ender unless the information presented was faulty or incomplete or the parties perjured themselves. Even with this long-standing principle, some experts will take sides and damage the case outcome, hiding behind their degrees and professional status. Some do this routinely but are eventually rebuked. The best experts *take cases within their specialty*, understand the merits beforehand, and *opine based on the evidence*, even *if the outcome contradicts the case of the retaining attorney* and the plaintiff or defendant fails to win the case. Legal professionals expect experts to be impartial, upfront, and honest.

The Expert's Curriculum Vitae

The expert's curriculum vitae (CV) information is "crucially important." It is the initial document an attorney will review when considering retaining the expert, and it will be carefully scrutinized by opposing counsel, the court, and others. The CV demonstrates the expert's educational background, knowledge, skills, and capabilities in the proficiency needed to understand, present, and opine on a case. The expert must always be prepared to justify every entry,

as a poorly presented CV can discredit the witness. The CV must be current and have proper content, such as demographics, education, licenses, certifications, work history, publications, memberships, awards, CV last update, and page numbers (Mangraviti et al., 2015). Embellishing, making factual mistakes, typos, improper punctuation, or unprofessional-looking fonts is unacceptable. Red flags for cross-arguments, including gaps in employment, omission of publications or presentations, or incomplete information, intentional or not, will undoubtedly be subjects of cross-examination as opposing counsel attempts to destroy the expert's credibility. How can anyone trust the opinions presented by the expert if they cannot get the CV correct?

Engagement Contract

It goes without saying that a contract for services is always needed regardless of the profession. Without the contract, there are no guidelines for the engagement's scope, the rules outlined in the jurisdiction, fees and payments, timelines, applicable laws, disputes, notices, and more. The contract is a safety mechanism to protect the expert from undo harm, misrepresentation, and legal actions in the case of liability, motions, and arbitration. A contract is crucial to securing an engagement with the hiring attorney. In fact, attorneys appreciate a well-designed engagement agreement because it demonstrates knowledge of the legal system. An excellent example of a retention contract may be obtained at SEAK.com (2024).

Fee Schedule

A fee schedule must be presented at the onset, reflecting a reasonable fee for expertise and time spent. In the world of leading experts, qualifications in a specific topic generally command the highest fees. In wrongful death cases, the expert's fees are generally not cost-sensitive as the better qualified the expert and the quality of reporting and presentation, the more likely the outcome will be favorable. The fee schedule should include the hourly rate for all general services, including consultations with counsel, records review, report writing, research, deposition and trial preparation, and associated services. A separate level of fees should be charged for depositions (minimum 2 hours), on-site forensic evaluations, and court appearances at trial and reflect any cancellation fees, including those for the individual's independent medical examination (IME). In some instances, cases are settled at or before the deposition or trial. The fee schedule should reflect the charges and timeline for cancellation and the incurred hourly, half-day, or daily rates. Traveling out of town, requiring an overnight stay, should include a daily rate. It should also reflect out-of-pocket costs such as airplane tickets, hotel, and ground transportation.

Medical Legal Expert Report

When the retaining attorney requests a report, it must be done carefully, as a well-written report sets forth the methods and science used in formulating the opinions and prepares the expert to tes-
tify. In some cases, this may improve the case's settlement value, although when the findings support the opposing party, the opinions must seek the truth. Reports have longevity and, if not truthful and unbiased, will be used against the expert in future cases since all of the information is discoverable, and opposing counsel can use them to attack the expert's credibility. For this reason, methodology and science must guide the forensic audiologist. A poorly written report will damage the expert's reputation and make them toxic in the legal community, whereas a well-written report strongly supports the expert's credibility and standing. Using grammar software or a separate editing service can markedly improve the quality of reporting.

A medical-legal report is dramatically different from a clinical or electronic medical record (EMR). The report must be complete and detailed, and it should contain various levels of information to meet the reader's needs and help them understand, interpret, and evaluate the merits of the case, the expert's conclusions, and opinions. The judge and attorneys expect the expert report or IME to provide specific information. At a minimum, in federal court, these include complete statements of all the opinions the expert will provide and the basis, test data, and facts used for formulating the opinions, exhibits, and the witness's qualifications, including a list of all publications authored in the previous 10 years, a list of other cases in which the witness testified in the previous 4 years, and compensation and billing statements. In addition, the report should include an introduction to the case; an executive summary; appropriate referenced background information used to opine, including the science and methodology; a review of pertinent records; subject examination or interview, analysis, differential diagnosis, and opinions; and a list of materials reviewed, including all discovery, a conclusion, and bibliography. In all cases, the expert should avoid uncertainty and clearly state that the opinions in the report are based on a reasonable degree of audiological and scientific certainty.

The Law of Unintended Consequences

Actions of people, companies, and governments always have effects that can be unintended or unanticipated, but not for the expert witness. It is clear that unintentional consequences have rocked the foundation of many entities in industry and government. Making decisions without understanding the consequences has damaged societies over the ages. In the legal sense, the law of unintentional consequences takes a front seat for the expert witness because consequences from errors in analysis and testimony can damage the case. The expert witness has a duty to provide evidence-based standard-of-care opinions that use clinically acceptable principles and methods acknowledged by the scientific community. The court, counselors, and the triers of fact depend upon this standard when making their judgments and, ultimately, the verdict, which will change lives. As part of the expert's investigation, due diligence must be exhaustive, covering all potential scenarios and providing reliable and repeatable conclusions. There is no such thing as unintended consequences but excuses for not being thorough, considering all the possibilities, or being bi-

ased without regard for the truth. *For the audiology expert witness, sticking to the facts and applying the science, best practices, professional ethics, and clinical standards will prevail.*

The Universe

After India and China, the United States is the most populous country, with over 332,000,000 people (World Population Review, n.d.). There are 14 cities with over a million people, 27 with over 500,000 people, and 317 with populations of over 100,000. New York City, Los Angeles, Chicago, and Houston have the largest populations, with Phoenix, Philadelphia, San Antonio, San Diego, Dallas, and San Jose having over a million. Looking at the population density in Figure 22–3, currently, 83% live in urban areas. Since the density of the population is urban, the opportunity to provide forensic services is optimal.

When considering the incidence of nonfatal head injuries, whiplash injuries, and acoustic trauma that may result in hearing loss, synaptopathy, tinnitus, hyperacusis, and central auditory processing disorders, expert witness services in audiology are needed throughout the country. Because these injuries are frequently also seen by neurology and otology, the expert in audiology supports or denies the credibility of the claims, assesses the severity, and provides accuracy to the rehabilitation.

A broader look at the numbers puts motor vehicle accidents at the top of the list. The National Highway Traffic Safety Administration ((2022) reported that 42,795 people died in motor vehicle crashes in 2022. Statista (n.d.) states there were 9.1 million traffic crashes

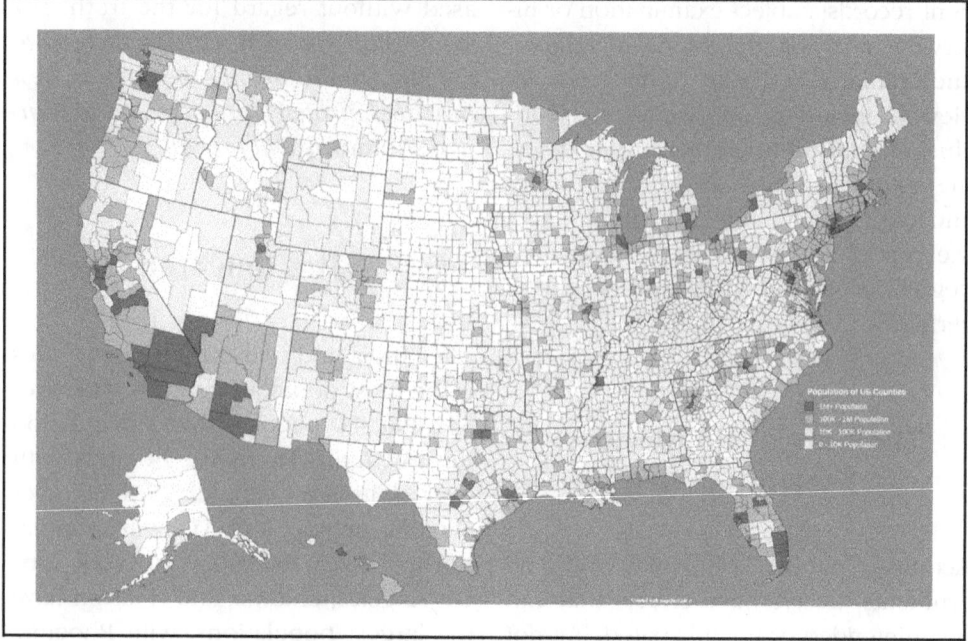

Figure 22–3. U.S. counties by population. *Source*: U.S. Department of Commerce Economic and Statistics Administration U.S. Census Bureau Complaint Caption and Report Header.

in 2021, most from passenger cars and light trucks. The Forbes Advisor (Bieber, 2023) reports that in 2022, 1,593,390 crashes resulted in injuries. Looking to data from 2020, as the COVID-19 pandemic was starting to take hold in the United States, the National Highway Traffic Safety Administration (2022) estimated nonfatal crashes on U.S. roads to be 5,215,071, with 2,282,015 people injured. These were down from the 2019 data of 2,740,140. However, the types of injuries are not reported; the occurrence of whiplash and head injury is implied and the most commonly seen by audiology expert witnesses.

A traumatic brain injury (TBI) can be devastating and cause issues with learning, memory, concentration, and problem-solving. The effects of a concussion or TBI are well known to in-clude auditory and vestibular disorders, either peripheral or central. The relationship between TBI-related hearing impairment and cognition is well known (Hwang et al., 2022). Figure 22–4 provides data collected between 2001 and 2010. Assaults, falls, environmental accidents, automobile accidents, industrial injuries, blast exposures, and sport-related concussions, for example, have a high prevalence of auditory and balance consequences, which result in litigation. According to data from the National Academies of Sciences, Engineering, and Medicine (2022), the occurrence of head trauma in the United States is approximately 2,000,000 a year with an economic cost of $4.2 Trillion.

In most bodily injury cases, the attorneys find specialists to consult and hire as experts. They present the qual-

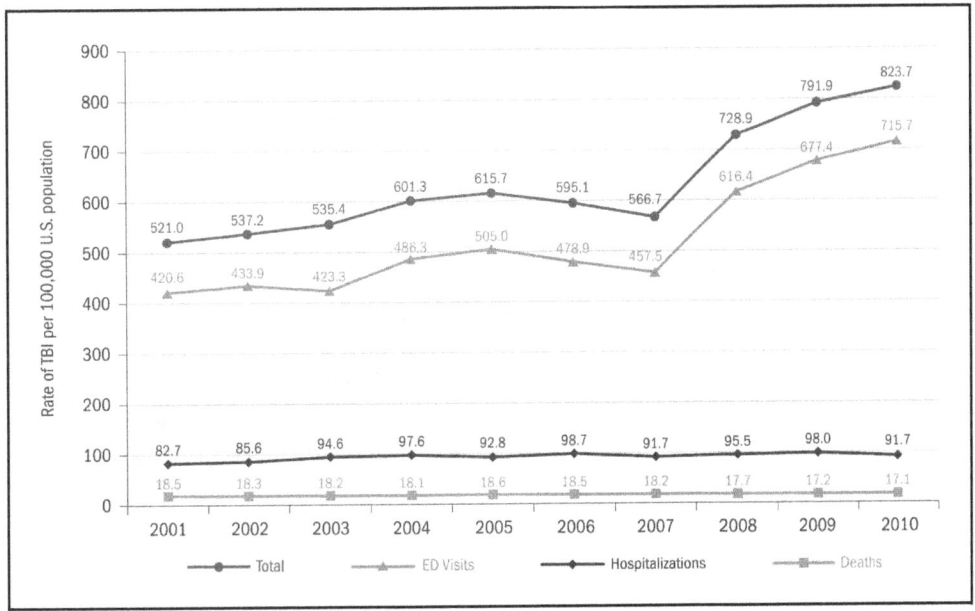

Figure 22–4. Annual age-adjusted rates of TBI-related emergency department (ED) visits, hospitalizations, and deaths—United States, 2001–2010. *Source*: Centers for Disease Control and Prevention (2015).

ifications to the opposing counsel and court. Most specialists are medical and other doctors with case-specific credentials, such as audiologists. With the number of causes related to hearing loss, tinnitus, hyperacusis, balance, and central auditory processing, the audiologist is testifying on not only causation but also severity of audiological injuries, rehabilitation needs, and outcomes of the injured party.

Case Study in Forensic Audiology

The range of medical-legal cases in which an audiologist is needed to educate the court and triers of fact concerning the nexus, claimed audiovestibular conditions, mechanisms, severity of each,

quality-of-life impingements, and rehabilitation needs is numerous. Some of these cases present consistent findings and recommendations that are repeatable across different cases, especially treatment and rehabilitation.

Audiologists interested in forensics should start with uncomplicated cases, such as acoustic trauma, and learn the proper protocol for investigation, reporting, and testifying before taking on complex cases, such as wrongful death, airplane crashes, or bellwethers. Below is the case of the vape pen explosion, which is a good example of a typical case most beginners can consider. It is similar to other cases of acoustic trauma, such as airbag deployments and explosive trauma from firearms. In the report, essential background information is important to help educate the audience and to demonstrate competency in the sub-

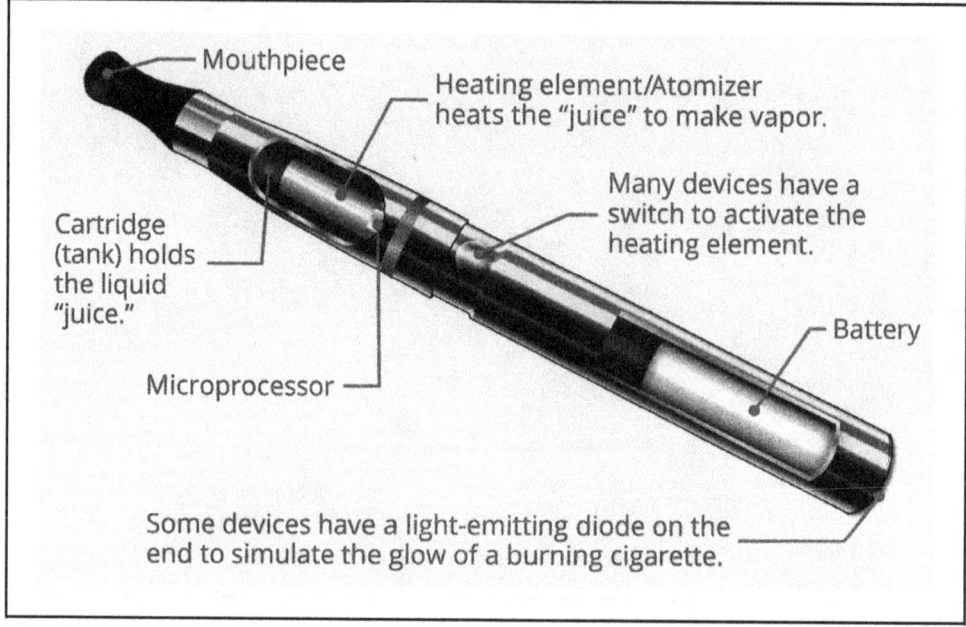

Figure 22–5. Vape pen construction. *Source*: McKenna (2017).

ject matter. Part of this background information in the following case included reviewing the mechanical mechanism of the vape pen, as seen in Figure 22–5.

The Case of the Vape Pen Explosion

The plaintiff is a 31-year-old female with a negative medical history before the accident, working full-time and living with her husband and 2-year-old infant. She had no hearing loss or tinnitus and the medical records support the claims. The plaintiff claimed hearing loss, tinnitus, and hyperacusis as a result of the lithium battery exploding without warning upon her pushing the activation button. Video recorded at the time of the accident clearly demonstrated the explosion. Although very rare, lithium batteries, mishandled or not, can ignite (McKenna,

2017). For this reason, the TSA does not allow lithium batteries in luggage and requires them to be carried onboard the plane. For this case, the defense counsel engaged the audiologist to determine the facts of the claims and provide opinions concerning the causation, severity of the injuries, and rehabilitation recommendations.

On the day of the accident, the plaintiff was using her vape pen, which she held in her right hand. After the explosion, the plaintiff claimed she could not hear from her right ear. In the emergency room, the record showed the right ear and eye required medical attention. In fact, the right eye vision was permanently damaged and, even with surgery, remained severely impaired. At medical examinations, the plaintiff claimed facial injuries, right eye damage, photophobia, hyperacusis, hearing loss, tinnitus, dizziness, headaches, anxiety, panic

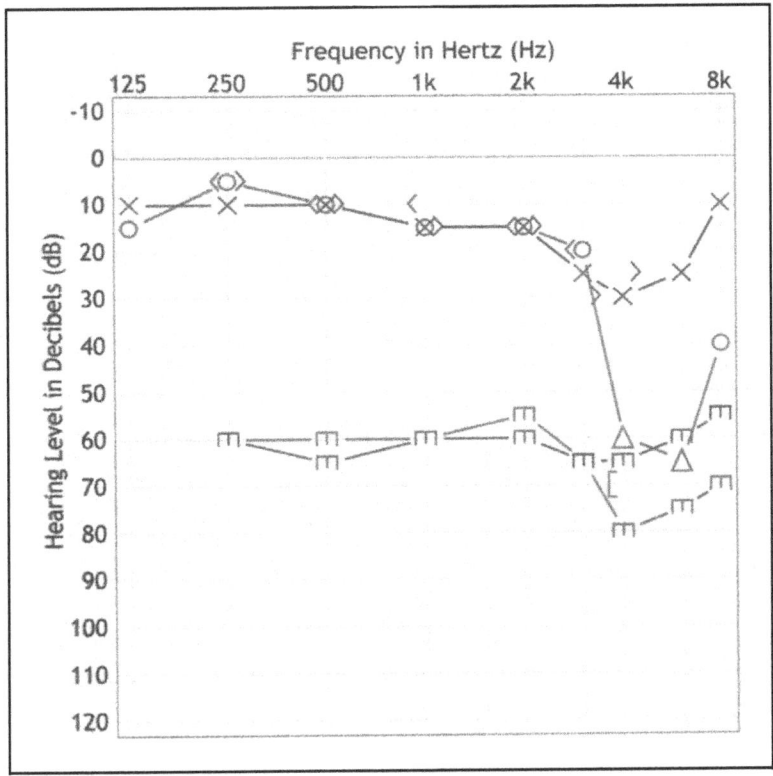

Figure 22–6. Vape pen explosion audiogram and loudness discomfort levels.

attacks, and difficulty sleeping. She did not report pain associated with her sound sensitivity.

The first action was to review all the records and video evidence accumulated as part of the discovery process. After assessing the records, an independent medical examination was conducted. During this session, an interview and audiological testing were conducted, which revealed the following findings (Figure 22–6).

Audiological Test Results

Otoscopic examination revealed normal-appearing ear canals, free of debris and tympanic membranes with robust light reflexes and appropriate translucency, position, and color bilaterally. Due to the hyperacusis, the test battery was limited to a hearing evaluation, Loudness discomfort level (LDL) testing, Quick-SIN, a limited tinnitus evaluation, and standard questionnaires. However, when possible, all cases should include cross-checking the subjective data using objective tests.

Pure-tone air and bone conduction thresholds reveal a mild to moderate, dramatically sloping, high-frequency sensorineural hearing loss in the right ear with a distinctive noise notch centered at 4000 Hz and 6000 Hz, followed by recovery at 8000 Hz. Threshold testing for the left ear revealed a mild high-frequency sensorineural hearing loss with a distinct noise notch dipping at 3000 Hz, 4000 Hz, and 6000 Hz, with recovery at 8000 Hz. Speech reception thresholds were 15 dB for the right ear and 10 dB for the left ear. Speech discrimination scores obtained at the patient's most comfortable level in quiet, using a recorded 50-word CNC word list, were 100% bilaterally. The Stenger test for the right ear revealed negative findings at 4000 Hz and 6000 Hz.

Sound sensitivity testing was measured using repeat trials for pure tones between 250 Hz and 8000 Hz in either ear. The loudness contour curves were consistent with a moderate to severe degree of sound sensitivity ranging from 55 dB to 80 dB in the right ear and 50 dB to 65 dB in the left ear. The dynamic range (difference between thresholds at 4000 Hz, 6000 Hz, and 8000 Hz and loudness discomfort measures) is significantly reduced in the right ear but consistent with the degree of hearing loss.

QuickSIN testing was conducted in each ear. Due to the patient's sound sensitivity, the test level was 50 dB in either ear, judged as loud but okay by the patient. The results were 10.5 dB SNR loss for the right ear and 5 dB SNR loss for the left ear.

Tinnitus matching revealed repeat matches to a 4000 Hz signal at 75 dB in the right ear, at a 15 dB sensation level, which is a typical finding in the tinnitus population. Tinnitus masking and inhibition were not tested due to the loudness of the required stimuli. Furthermore, the patient reports the tinnitus from the right ear was obtrusive during the evaluation, interfering with left ear testing, which, therefore, was not conducted.

The results of the Tinnitus Handicapped Inventory was 62 points or severe. The Functional score was 22, Catastrophic 16, and Emotional 24. She reports tinnitus present approximately 100% of the time, although it fluctuates in loudness. She reports tinnitus as the primary complaint, sound tolerance secondary, and then hearing loss. Her perception of tinnitus difficulty for severity is (8/10), annoyance (10/10), and effect (10/10), indicating she feels a severe impact on her quality of life.

Modified Khalfa Hyperacusis Questionnaire scores severe sound sensitivity (79 points). Scores for functional were 29, social 27, and emotional 23. The scores and loudness testing confirm the degree of reaction to sound. She did not report pain. The configuration is consistent with loudness hyperacusis, although her fear of sound was also noted in the report.

Evaluating the patient's hearing performance using the unaided APHAB (Abbreviated Profile of Hearing Aid Benefit) response tool reveals a slight to moderate loss of communication without hearing aids. For ease of communication (EC), she reported 25% difficulty; communication in reverberant rooms (RV), 37.7%; hearing in background noise (BN), 47.8%; and difficulty for aversiveness such as noise, 64%. The least amount of difficulty was in quiet listening situations, which increased in large reverberant rooms and listening in background noise. The patient's scores revealed the most unpleasantness when listening to environmental sounds. The unpleasant aversion (AV) score coincides with the patient's complaint of decreased sound sensitivity.

Reporting

As part of the background information, the audience needs to understand the differences between acoustic trauma and noise-induced hearing loss, vape pen construction, device mechanisms, and explosion history. The background information reviewed human hearing, hearing loss, tinnitus, hyperacusis, impairment, and rehabilitation. The report included an independent medical examination, complete history, records review, test data, questionnaires, differential diagnosis, opinions, and case-specific rehabilitation needs. Briefly, the opinions were as follows:

1. The plaintiff suffered asymmetrical hearing loss, tinnitus, and hyperacusis as a result of the vape pen explosion of April 5, 2019. The conclusion was based on video evidence, medical records, audiological findings, and the testimony of the plaintiff and witnesses. The report continued to describe the issues in detail.

2. The plaintiff requires rehabilitation, including tinnitus retraining therapy, cognitive behavioral therapy, and amplification. The report continued to describe each of the plaintiff's needs in detail, the standard of care, the expected outcome, and costs over a lifetime such as annual care, replacement costs, and so on.

Before the case went to trial, a settlement was reached.

Unfortunately, in this case, every physician and audiologist the patient saw failed to recommend any treatment or rehabilitation. After 4 years, the patient remained without help until the defense audiologist provided the standard-of-care recommendations in the report. Inappropriately, the patient suffered alone in isolation and in silence.

Final Word

As a career develops over the years, interests may change, and an audiologist might find the subspecialty of forensic audiology to be the most professionally stimulating and rewarding of all. Expert witnesses in every field represent the best a profession can offer because every day is a test of the integrity of one's knowledge, professionalism, and ethics. Not all doctoral-level professionals are capable of meeting this challenge. Still, most are capable of working toward that goal, especially the students who have a lifetime of experience and career-building yet to come.

As an effective expert witness, the opportunity to help the court achieve justice starts with providing technical information that is concise, accurate, and understandable to all and giving evidence-based opinions, not hearsay or assumptions. The expert witness is as much a teacher as a forensic professional. Teaching is important because the court, jury, lawyers, physicians, scientists, engineers, and others have little or no knowledge about the causes and effects of hearing loss, tinnitus, hyperacusis, or auditory processing disorders. Helping both sides of an argument understand the parameters of audiovestibular disorders improves the process.

To the experienced audiologist, the ability to work in the legal profession can become second nature. The complexity and type of cases accepted should depend upon each individual's specialties, keeping in mind that other professionals are available to consult. Those in the legal professions are well versed in what an expert witness has to offer the triers of fact, and audiologists are no exception. Although some situations can become contentious, a calm demeanor and preparation always result in a rewarding experience.

Audiologists come from many different backgrounds. Some prefer to work in rehabilitation and fit hearing aids, others like working with children in schools, and some enjoy the medical route involving complex diagnostics. Still, all have a few things in common: advanced degrees, training, and an opportunity to continue to learn and lean into their chosen profession. As a career builds over the years, a closer look at becoming an expert witness and engaging in one's areas of acquired expertise can be fulfilling, professionally rewarding, and financially beneficial. Regardless of the direction a career takes, without controversy, audiologists are the most qualified to discuss many aspects of audiovestibular disorders as expert witnesses in the legal arena.

References

American Academy of Audiology. (2023). American Academy of Audiology Scope of Practice. https://www.audiology.org/wp-content/uploads/2023/04/Scope-of-Practice_2023.pdf

American Board of Audiology. (2023). Certification 101. https://audiology.org/certification-101/

Bieber, C. (2023). Car statistics for 2023. Forbes Advisor. https://www.forbes.com/advisor/legal/car-accident-statistics/

Brainline, WETA-TV. (n.d.). Get the stats on traumatic brain injury in the United States. https://www.brainline.org/article/get-stats-traumatic-brain-injury-united-states

Centers for Disease Control and Prevention. (2015). *Report to Congress on Traumatic Brain Injury in the United States: Epidemiology and rehabilitation.* National Center for Injury Prevention and Control; Division of Unintentional Injury Prevention.

Colucci, D. A., Hall, J., Powers, T., Speankovich, C., & Traynor, R. (2024). ASHA recognizes changemakers in forensic audiology. *Hearing Journal, 77*(3), 7–11. http://DOI:10.1097/01.HJ.0001007704.80181.2e

ETS Praxis®. (n.d.). Praxis Examination in Audiology. https://www.ets.org/praxis/site/test-takers/register/how-to-register.html

Federal Rules of Evidence, Rule 702. (n.d.). Testimony by expert witnesses. Legal Information Institute, Cornell Law School. https://www.law.cornell.edu/rules/fre/rule_702

Hwang, P. H., Nelson, L. D., Sharon, J. D., McCrea, M. A., Dikman, S. S., Markowitz, A. J., . . . Temkin, N. R. (2022). Association between TBI-related hearing impairment and cognition: A TRACK-TBI study. *The Journal of Head Trauma Rehabilitation, 37*(5), E327–E335. https://doi.org/10.1097/HTR.0000000000000735

Mangraviti, J. J., Babitsky, S., & Nasser Donovan, N. (2015). *How to be a successful expert witness: SEAK'S A-Z guide to expert witnessing.* SEAK.

McKenna, L. A. (2017). *Electronic cigarette fires and explosions in the United States 2009-2016.* National Fire Data Center, U.S. Fire Administration, FEMA.

Mental Health America. (n.d.). Help others. https://mhanational.org/help-others

National Academies of Sciences, Engineering, and Medicine. 2022. *Traumatic Brain*

Injury: A Roadmap for Accelerating Progress. Washington, DC: The National Academies Press. https://www.ncbi.nlm.nih.gov/books/NBK580076/

National Council of State Boards of Examiners (NCSB). (n.d.). Directory of State Licensing Boards. https://ncsb.info/board-directory

National Highway Association. (2022). NHTSA estimates for 2022 show roadway fatalities remain flat after two years of dramatic increases. https://www.nhtsa.gov/press-releases/traffic-crash-death-estimates-2022

National Students Speech-Language-Hearing Association (NSSLHA). (n.d.). Success starts here. https://www.nsslha.org/

SEAK.com. (2024). Expert witness contract. https://store.seak.com/expert-witness-retention-contract-download/

Statista. (n.d.). Number of vehicles involved in traffic crashes in the United States in 2020. https://www.statista.com/statistics/192097/number-of-vehicles-involved-in-traffic-crashes-in-the-us/

Student Academy of Audiology. (n.d.). https://ssa.audiology.org

Traynor, R. M., & Traynor, K. B. (2024). *Forensic audiology*. Plural Publishing.

U.S. Census. (2024). US counties by population. U.S. Department of Commerce Economic and Statistics Administration. U.S. Census Bureau. https://www.census.gov/library/visualizations/2013/demo/2012-state-county-maps.html

World Population Review. (n.d.). United States—ranked by population. https://world populationreview.com

23 Ethics: The Risks We May Not See

Michael D. Page, AuD

The Risks We May Not See

"The study and practice of ethics is the complicated and convoluted navigation of vital relationships for the protection and goodwill of all."

—Michael D. Page

Thought Questions

1. What are the origins of ethics?
2. What is the etymology of the word "ethic"?
3. What stories do codes of ethics tell?
4. What stories of ethics could you tell?
5. What is the value of patients receiving unbiased healthcare?

Introduction

Healthcare providers navigate an abundance of vital relationships, including those with employers, managers, colleagues, insurance companies, communities, professional organizations, members of industry (product manufacturers), licensing boards, regulatory agencies, and even themselves! Among those important relationships is the most important connection of all: the clinician/patient relationship.

Two important aspects of ethics will be described in this chapter and utilized to explain the various categories of professional relationships and their respective ethics: *codes* of ethics and *principles* of ethics.

Codes of Ethics (COE)

Codes of ethics are usually specific living documents produced by professional entities or organizations and will naturally undergo revisions, modifications, and additions as technologies, treatments, and circumstances evolve. Codes of ethics remain dynamic to reflect the evolution of clinical circumstances and environments. While codes of ethics sometimes experience criticism and judgment, it is important to recognize that each code originates from a compelling event, experience, or story with a (potentially) unfavorable outcome. Understanding that experience or story helps connect with and embrace the code. As codes of ethics are considered and studied, one should always contemplate the following questions:

1. How did the code begin, and why?
2. What are the story origins behind each code?
3. Why have these codes risen to this level of importance?
4. How will these codes help guide my professional behavior in navigating any unseen risks?
5. How will patients benefit from our codes of ethics?

Principles of Ethics

Principles of ethics are broader and considered more general to be relevant in helping connect with all scenarios and circumstances, regardless of time, culture, nationality, or profession. The best *principles* of ethics are universal and, if designed effectively, will withstand the winds of change, decades of time, the rigors of scenarios, and every professional application.

Sometimes, clinicians default to *codes* of ethics as the "end all," the only metric to which they are accountable. One must ponder the question, "Were codes of ethics to be removed, how would they govern themselves?" The answer to that question is the very heart of the place where we should operate our ethical conduct.

The *WHY* of Ethics

For the purpose of this chapter, the *principles* of ethics to which we refer are *respect for autonomy, nonmaleficence, beneficence,* and *justice,* first introduced by Beauchamp and Childress (1979). Subsequent updates and publications have evolved into a universally recognized and accepted idea set for consid-ering aspects of ethics (Beauchamp & Childress, 2019).

Ethics Allegory

Before the days of laser measuring tools, my father used mechanical tools to ensure accuracy in building and construction projects. "True, plumb, and level!" he often said as we completed a critical section of any work project, whether building a fence, a home, or a cabin during my childhood.

A "plumb" is a tool used since ancient Egyptian times to find and ensure vertical level primarily in building construction. It is fashioned using a pointed weighted element at the bottom of a string or flexible element. A "level" is a construction tool used to achieve precision in horizontal or vertical alignments in construction efforts. A level usually contains a liquid (usually alcohol or water) inside a small container with an air bubble inside.

Good carpenters or stone masons use tools to build structures aligned with what is functionally right and true. It was true not in the "true or false" sense but rather in the sense of "accurate or exact." Even though this metaphor hails from a past generation, analogous tools (or principles) are used today to affirm stable, consistent, and trusted relationships within healthcare.

Trueness is a construct that shows alignment with a predetermined set of evidence-based research principles, standards, or codes determined by peers and/or authorities in the profession. Although *codes* and standards are often modified, honed, and refined, the truest *principles* remain universal and time-less. Their universality remains stable across professions, cultures, nationalities, and citizenships.

Ethical Practice

Ethical practice is critical at the most basic level, even pre-foundationally. Foundations are crucial for the sustainability of the code's purpose. For instance, most homeowners are unaware that soil below their homes is usually studied long before a foundation is laid and walls are erected. When I watched our home being built, the contractors were incorporating large and thick steel straps all around the top of the concrete foundation attaching to the stud walls to ensure the safety of the building in the event of hurricane-force winds known to the area only about every five years. I don't see those straps anymore and rarely even think about them. Yet, they remain in place to ensure our safety.

Foundations in homes or other buildings are rarely seen or even thought about once the structure is inhabited. Yet, given earthquakes or high winds, the foundation and the steel straps may be the only parts of the structure ensuring safety. The tools become crucial by increasing stability and sustainability for the preservation and duration of the structure. The right tools create longevity, strength, safety, and protection against unanticipated intrusions such as storms, winds, and other destructive forces, as well as other risks we cannot see.

So it is with ethics in clinical practice. Practice requires protection, especially against the winds and weather we may never anticipate (even five years later). Principles of ethics remain such an integral part of us, much like a life insurance policy, which may not be ex-

ercised for decades. *Principles* of ethics provide stability and safety not only for those who practice but also for those who receive services. Ethics increase the likelihood of independent, autonomous thinking, and clinical judgment, ensuring the best possible patient outcome free of outside influences. Ethics principles ensure a stable atmosphere that supports good clinical judgment, unencumbered by the breeze through a broken window or the storm at the doorstep of an unsecured door.

A commitment to ethical practice is a willingness to proactively seek clarity for risks we may not see, thereby creating a realm of safety for patients who trust it. It is similar to the intrusion and impact of small pests entering a home, constructing hidden nests in our moments of unawares. As it is with ethics, the smallest intrusions, left unchecked, avail the theft of the sacred geography of the clinician/patient relationship. Those intrusions become a risk we cannot see.

Ethics clarity is enhanced by the recognition that even the codes of ethics written by professional organizations may be inadequate. One can easily examine the history and evolution of codes of ethics and their impact on professional practice. Additionally, the potential for a power differential within patient relationships in ethics must drive our mindset, intentions, and actions to develop an internal compass that might far exceed the minimal requirements of a simple code of ethics. In other words, our mindset will suit us best when our actions are driven by a deep-seated commitment to ethical *principles from within*, not just because a code of ethics requires it.

While some believe that ethics provide a "sliding scale" or continuum, that there are "minimal ethics," "moderate ethics," or "excessive ethics," the author contends that there are *only ethics* that are neither minimal nor excessive. The mindset of a *continuum of ethics* is simply a *"continuum of justification,"* allowing some a level of permission to engage in marginal activities or actions while referencing a convenient tool for justification.

Ethics provides a lens through which we might evaluate the unseen risks. The key is keeping the lens clean and polished, free of smudges and smears marred by outside influences or the breezes of the day. It is a lens that must remain undistorted, thereby preserving integrity.

While ethics are primarily concerned with the impact of our intentions, actions, and relationships, ethics demand a necessary focus on oneself. Paradoxically, while ethics may protect ourselves, they are essentially focused on the safekeeping of others within our charge, exercised through our professional integrity and independent clinical judgment.

Test of Ethics

A test of the truest ethics is not only the universality of their *principles* but also the enduring and timelessness of their application. While *codes* of ethics have certainly transformed with time, the best *principles* of ethics will not. One of the most enduring principles of ethics was attributed to the ancient physician Hippocrates over two millennia ago when he demanded, "First, do no harm" (or *"primum non nocere,"* the Latin translation from the original Greek), which is not part of the Hippocratic Oath but

rather gleaned from one of Hippocrates' other works, *Of the Epidemics.*

Hippocrates' demand for doing no harm (first and foremost) indicated an acute awareness of the potential to do so (Schmerling, 2020). Therefore, before all else and before any aspect of treatment was considered or recommended, there was a strong admonition to avoid anything devious or deleterious.

In his writing, Hippocrates did not speak of standards of treatment, protocols for procedures, or methods of diagnostics, but rather only, "Do no harm." Such is a commanding signal to all professionals in every possible healthcare role, even those non-patient-facing. With Hippocrates' demand, one must ask, "How do we harm patients?"

While we often consider physical injury, the greatest potential harm may lie in aspects of objectivity, impartiality, and absence of bias prejudice. As professionals, we are blinded by the light of acclaim, the regalia of recognition, the glitz of remuneration, and the fleeting boost to self-esteem.

One of the greatest barriers to understanding and embracing ethics falls on false assumptions, lack of experience, and even one's arrogance. Professionals sometimes express, "Of course I am ethical," "I attend ethics courses because my licensure requires it," "Ethics seem to be overthinking," or "We are not ethics extremists. We are middle of the road!" A seemingly confident or overconfident stance against undiscovered or unacknowledged truth (in the form of risk) can be the greatest gamble.

The author asserts that those most at risk for unethical behavior are those who minimize, mock, or take less seriously ethics' hidden nuances. Indeed, it is one thing to acknowledge that we may not see hidden risks but quite another to deny their existence.

Ultimately, one must dismantle current perceptions of ethics and remain open to new ideas, notions, and principles designed to protect and honor relationships. Indeed, principles of ethics are merely a flashlight illuminating corners, closets, and spaces we did not know existed. Ethics provide a thought structure and template that allows us to discover unseen pitfalls, protecting not only our professional reputations but the sacred patient relationship we have worked diligently to foster and preserve.

Ethics of Self

"Self-ethics examines the relationship that exists between one's actual self and the vision one has of one's ideal self."
—Nel Noddings (Haegert, 2004)

Thought Questions

1. How do I know if I'm true to myself?
2. Of what importance is one's own ethics?
3. How do self-ethics support other professional relationships?
4. How do personal ethics impact professional ethics?
5. What might a personal code of ethics look like?
6. How should one consider principles of ethics while developing personal ethics?

Exploring Ethics of Self

Every professional must self-assess often to consider their position, role, intention, and deepest internal motivation. In Shakespeare's famed play *Hamlet*, Polonius says:

This above all:
to thine own self be true,
And it must follow,
as the night the day,
Thou canst not then
be false to any man.
Farewell, my blessing season
this in thee!
—William Shakespeare, n.d.

The "ethics of self" is our initial discussion in this chapter because, without the basis of self-awareness, self-alignment, or even self-vetting, other elements of and commitments to ethics remain moot. That is to say, it is unlikely to be intuitively ethical in our relationships with patients, colleagues, members of industry, and the profession as a whole when we are unable to find clarity about the ethical relationship with ourselves.

Without self-ethics, we will easily find ourselves bound only to *codes* of ethics (the bare minimum of ethical conduct) and find it more easily a "check-the-box" process rather than a deeply intrinsic commitment to conduct and behavior centered from within. This centering of personal principles far exceeds the routine numbered lists of *dos* and *don'ts* often contained in codes of ethics. Ethics of self include commitments to deeply rooted principles in the context of self-awareness, self-care, self-improvement, and mutual respect for all relationships. Codes of ethics are a mere symbol of the greater realm of ethics. When we understand ethics principles, codes become almost tertiary in their application.

Self-Awareness

Eurich (2018) conducted a series of surveys and reports that "95% of people believe they are self-aware, while only 10-15% are. True self-awareness is a rare quality." The disparity between those who believe they are self-aware (who are not) and those who are self-aware reinforces the likelihood of unseen compromise. With compromised ethics, should danger, weakness, bias, or peril come before us, we may be less likely able to see its potential for impact and outcome before it is too late. Therefore, the most critical acknowledgment for a clinician is recognizing a general lack of self-awareness and the risk it may pose.

Several exercises are available to increase self-awareness, and one should proactively seek opportunities to gain personal clarity. Often, clinicians are unaware of how others see them in the context of how they see themselves. One such exercise is the Johari Window (Accipio, n.d.). Increasing self-awareness may increase the propensity for healthier ethical behavior. Using the list of positive and negative adjectives, the Johari Window provides a method of evaluating how one sees themselves compared with how others perceive them.

On the list of positive adjectives, the subject (the person desiring greater self-awareness) will select positive adjectives they believe describe themselves.

Through an anonymous process, self-selected friends will use the same list of positive adjectives to choose which adjectives *they* believe describe the subject. The result produces a report where positive adjectives are sorted into four categories:

1. *Open/authentic:* Positive adjectives selected by the subject and at least one friend. These adjectives suggest that since the subject and friends select the same adjectives, these positive traits are in the open and seen by all.
2. *Hidden:* Positive adjectives selected by the subject but not by friends. These adjectives suggest that since the subject is the only one observing these traits, they may be obscure to others.
3. *Blind:* Positive adjectives selected by at least one friend but not by the subject. These adjectives suggest that others see positive traits in the subject that the subject may not see.
4. *Unknown:* Positive adjectives not selected by the subject or by any friend. These adjectives suggest that neither the subject nor their friends observe these traits in the subject; therefore, they remain unknown to all.

The same exercise is conducted with negative adjectives and processed similarly. The resulting discussion and associated coaching can be extremely valuable and insightful, although sometimes unpleasant. However, within a group, the resulting dynamics of the Johari Window can have a leveling impact on group dynamics and relationships, potentially enhancing one's view of self. Self-awareness, then, is the beginning of self-ethics.

Self-Care

Personal care is essential in supporting professional presence and engagement. Professional burnout can lead to professional compromise, with weakened character and increased vulnerability. Burnout has been linked to poorer physical and mental health among our psychotherapy counterparts, showing interference with clinical performance and possibly leading to misconduct (Simionato et al., 2019). Misconduct certainly falls into the realm of questionable ethics. Some even characterize burnout as the precursor to professional impairment. In any realm, impairment could easily cause compromised perspective and degraded performance (Abramson, 2021).

Professional burnout may be inversely proportional to the degree of engagement in self-improvement. Thus, ethics may be strengthened by honoring our responsibility to enhance our skills, honing our perceptions, and becoming more aware of unseen risks in order to improve our care for patients, as well as our responsibilities to employers. Thus, self-care is part of a holistic approach to ensuring a personal mental, emotional, and physical health regimen, which adds to the overall goal of ethical health. Baratta (2018) suggests 10 aspects of self-care, including:

1. Knowing who you are and your limits.
2. Getting the sleep you need and knowing how to rest.
3. Making sure that you're well fed.
4. Finding a way to decompress *throughout* your day, not just when you leave work.
5. Giving some thought to changing a difficult work situation.
6. Taking time to get to know *you* better, recognizing your own temperament and trying to prepare for your personal limits.
7. Identifying what you enjoy doing and what's fun for you and make a serious effort to integrate it into your day or, at the very least, your week.
8. Knowing how to decompress after a day's work.
9. Feeding your spiritual self.
10. Take time to love yourself and appreciate that there's only one you, and you're the expert on that.

Therefore, self-care contributes to the health and welfare of our commitment to professional ethics.

Self-Improvement

Our degree of self-awareness increases our self-ethics, and self-improvement may play a crucial role in its development. A personal code of ethics must exceed that of any organizational or professional code of ethics since such codes are usually broad in nature and less specific as they often provide a list of "shall" and "shall not." Ethics are mostly about our relationships with others, while self-ethics is rooted from within and strengthened through self-improvement. In consideration of our personal commitment to patients, *Psychology Today* author Thomas G. Plante (2010) suggested we ask ourselves three personal ethical questions daily:

1. How do I want to be in the world?
2. Why do I want to be this way in the world?
3. What strategies must I use to remain true to my values and principles when I'm challenged or tested?

Indeed, it is quite easy to be well behaved without tests or challenges. The true test of ethics is seen in our thoughts and actions when our circumstances are challenged or compromised. Self-improvement also includes continued education not only in professional skills but in surrounding elements of ethics, laws, and morality within the profession. Self-improvement in this context ensures that understanding and perspectives remain current and within a contemporary context.

Mutual Respect for All Relationships

Mutual respect is an often overlooked characteristic in professional relationships (Nemko, 2022) yet is the very foundation for all professional relationships (Zenger & Folkman, 2023). Some describe mutual respect as "the respect I will pay another contingent upon their respect for me." While that definition may be common, the most effective mutual respect includes an appreciation of others' opinions and their differences, with a response of politeness and the acknowledgment of unique values and perspectives *regardless of their reciprocation.* Mutual respect is a vital component of any healthy relationship.

While professionals may argue and disagree, they should maintain respect for one another. The relationship will suffer when someone disregards or belittles another's feelings, interests, opinions, or beliefs. In professional relationships, the lack of mutual respect results in a loss of unity, camaraderie, and ultimate strength required for successful business relationships. Zenger and Folkman (2023) describe seven ways to increase mutual respect in the workplace:

1. *Valuing diversity:* To establish a groundwork of respect, leaders must be aware that they may not be doing everything they can to show that they value diversity and make clear that differences are valued.
2. *Staying in touch with issues and concerns with individuals:* Staying in touch with people conveys respect. Those periodic phone calls where the boss conveyed concern only about [someone's] welfare [makes] all the difference.
3. *Being trusted:* In our research on trust, we discovered that if one person on your team distrusts you, it will significantly lower the level of trust from the rest of the team. This is a contagious emotion.
4. *Resolving conflicts:* Leaders need to resolve conflicts quickly when they occur. A respectful leader does not step back, but willingly engages in mending conflicts.
5. *Balancing "getting results" with a concern for others:* When results become more important than the people who deliver them, people feel disrespected. In most situations, this only requires making small exceptions for people (when kids get sick, accidents happen,

or someone needs a mental health break), but the impact on satisfaction and engagement will be significant. The best leaders balance getting results with the realities facing the people who produce them. Organizations and leaders must listen to the pleas to establish a culture that supports better work-life balance.

6. *Encouraging open discussion of problems and differences of opinions:* The simple act of asking another person for their opinion is a powerful way to communicate respect. But you can't just ask; you must also listen and engage. When a leader is willing to hear different perspectives and dig into problems that concern others, they show they value those team members.

7. *Giving honest feedback in a helpful way:* Direct and honest feedback can make people feel respected, as long as it's delivered in the right way. It ought to fairly reflect the person's performance. If an employee does 90% of their work correctly and 10% incorrectly, honest feedback would be 90% positive and only 10% corrective.

Respect builds trust, and trust increases the likelihood of ethical considerations and behavior. The bottom line is that self-awareness, self-care, self-improvement, and mutual respect for all relationships are the foundation for a healthy and strong self-ethic, which is the crux of all subsequent categories of ethics discussed in this chapter.

Ethics With Patients

"The sacred patient relationship acknowledges the principal connection between clinicians and their patients.
It highlights the role of clinician control, demanding the prioritization of ethical patient care above all other relationships and influences."

—Michael D. Page

Thought Questions

1. Compare and contrast the difference between a friendship and a professional relationship.
2. Why is the clinician/patient relationship often described as *sacred*?
3. How does a provider protect against patients wanting more than just a professional relationship while maintaining propriety?
4. What are the warning signs of impropriety?
5. What would you recommend to a colleague you observe as in a compromised clinician/patient relationship?

The Professional Clinician/Patient Relationship

Ethics play a crucial role in preserving the patient's dignity by providing a framework and structure that helps ensure independent and unbiased patient care. The clinician/patient relationship is the most crucial healthcare relationship. Not only is it most critical, but it is indeed the only *sacred* relationship among all professional connections. Recognizing this is recognizing an unspoken power imbalance (and potential vulnerability) between a healthcare provider and a patient.

The vulnerability confirms that the healthcare provider is in a position of power and authority over the patient and is therefore in a position demanding a level of trust unlike with other relationships. The nature of the relationship's "sacredness" suggests the need for a bond of confidentiality, trust, transparency, and independent clinical judgment, unencumbered by outside incentivizing influences. Adhering to ethical guidelines helps maintain trust and professionalism in preserving this critical relationship.

Ethics is about cultivating and maintaining trust. It is believed that this relationship has eroded over the years because of the influx and influence of outside agencies and organizations wanting some ownership within patient care models by incentivizing product and service purchasing. This includes sales representatives from any entity selling medical devices, pharmaceuticals, supplies, insurance policies, and so on.

Considering a definition of sacred as "regarded with great respect and reverence, or connected with the gods, deserving veneration" (Knowles, n.d.), healthcare providers should consider their patients' relationships as the most sacred of all professional relationships. That relationship requires the utmost respect, professionalism, and protection. Protection lies squarely and solely at the feet of the clinician provider.

Providers and a few stakeholders exist in professional realms interested in the patient relationship and "consumer protection." State licensure is specifically interested in protecting the consumer of any healthcare services. Ensuring ethical practice increases the likelihood of protecting patient rights and outcomes.

Regarding the clinician/patient relationship, it is critical to acknowledge the power differential. It is not that patients are powerless, but rather that the provider is in a more dominant role and should lead the relationship by establishing rules, structure, and boundaries around that relationship. Rules, structure, and boundaries create safety and ensure healthy engagements. While patients may often test the limits of those boundaries, some clinicians have been noted to test them, as well.

One of the primary purposes of codes of ethics is to protect the relationship between providers and consumers in the context of mitigating risks that clinicians (and consumers alike) may not see since the provider is the primary power holder of the clinician/patient relationship. Therefore, providers are in charge of engagement and should often refer to their "scope of practice," its implications, and focus.

The story is told of a neonatal intensive care unit (NICU) nurse who cared for a premature infant for many weeks. During that time, the nurse had become connected with the infant's mother, father, siblings, and grandparents. When the infant graduated from the NICU and went home, the father contacted the nurse and acknowledged her role in their child's NICU stay. The father invited her to attend a celebration dinner with the family. The nurse later acknowledged the internal discomfort but couldn't rationalize a reason not to support the celebration with the family. On the designated evening of the event, the nurse arrived at the restaurant to find only the father present . . . a clear risk the nurse did not see. It behooves all providers to anticipate such encounters, discover ways to avoid them, and maintain and support the propriety of the relationship. Often trusting a principle or code of ethics without completely understanding why may prevent impropriety.

Unlike friendships, professional relationships are not reciprocal. Friendships usually involve a mutual exchange of caring, regard, time, and obligation. Usually, no money is exchanged for friendship and good friends usually check in with each other and reciprocally grace each other with time, assistance, fun, and service. It is an equal two-way relationship.

In professional relationships, there exists only a one-way relationship that usually includes the exchange of fees for services. While it sounds callous and uncaring, it is *not* without the crucial provision of service in the context of empathy, mutual respect, integrity, and compassion while acknowledging the gratification received in providing the services.

As professional relationships become more reciprocal, boundaries become less well defined and ultimately eroded. In a conversation with an unnamed clinician and the author (personal communication, 2022), the clinician stated, "But my elderly patient is lonely and loves to take me to dinner. He's just a generous, friendly person." The question persists: "What's the unseen risk?"

While friendliness is important, it is not a friendship. Caution should be exercised whenever tempted to call patients "friends" or to engage with patients in a friend-type relationship. The professional relationship dynamics obscure independent clinical judgment by blurring the roles of bias and empathy.

Independent clinical judgment is one of the most crucial duties of a clinician.

Another story is told of a physical therapist (PT) who was an avid bicyclist. A physical therapist's patient (knowing he was an avid bicyclist) asked the PT if he would consider helping him and his family by recommending bicycles they could purchase as a family. While the PT considered the implications of this extracurricular service, he thought of the following questions:

1. Is what the patient is requesting within my scope of practice?
2. Would I be willing to chart this request and my actions?
3. What precedent would I set by engaging with this one patient in this way?
4. What if other patients heard about this through social media or otherwise?
5. What if I make recommendations and my patient is unhappy with their bicycle purchase?
6. What if one of my patient's family members is injured due to a faulty part on the bicycle I recommended?
7. What are the other risks I might not see?

After careful consideration, the PT acknowledged that the engagement might be outside of his scope of practice and politely declined the request.

Professional Guidelines for Clinician/Patient Relationship

Professional organizations provide guidelines for these relationships as follows:

American Medical Association (AMA)

The practice of medicine and its embodiment in the clinical encounter between a patient "and a physician is fundamentally a moral activity that arises from the imperative to care for patients and to alleviate suffering. *The relationship between a patient and a physician is based on trust, which gives rise to physicians' ethical responsibility to place patients' welfare above the physician's own self-interest or obligations to others, to use sound medical judgment on patients' behalf, and to advocate for their patients' welfare. A patient-physician relationship exists when a physician serves a patient's medical needs. Generally, the relationship is entered into by mutual consent between physician and patient (or surrogate)*" (AMA, n.d.-a).

American Academy of Audiology (AAA)

Nearly all sections of the AAA COE refer to and acknowledge patients. A few highlights of the code include:

- *PRINCIPLE 1: Members shall provide professional services and conduct research with honesty and compassion, and shall respect the dignity, worth, and rights of those served.*
- *Rule 1a: Individuals shall not limit the delivery of professional services on any basis that is unjustifiable or irrelevant to the need for the potential benefit from such services.*
- *Rule 1b: Individuals shall not provide services except in a professional relationship and shall not discriminate in the provision of services to individuals on the basis of culture, race, religion, sex/gender, sexual*

orientation, or general health and/or disability.
- *PRINCIPLE 3: Members shall comply with jurisdictional privacy guidelines (e.g., HIPAA, FERPA) to maintain the confidentiality of the information and records of those receiving services or involved in research. Compliance is also required in non-formal settings, including, but not limited to, social media accounts and social media groups.*
- *Rule 3a: Individuals shall not reveal to unauthorized persons any professional or personal information obtained from the person served professionally, unless authorized by law.*
- *Rule 7a: Individuals shall not use professional or commercial affiliations in any way that would limit services to or mislead patients or colleagues.* (American Academy of Audiology, 2023)

As part of protecting our consumers, clinicians are obligated under many codes of ethics to maintain their ranks by some degree of intraprofessional monitoring and policing. Most organizations require that professional impropriety be reported to the governing organization.

American Speech-Language-Hearing Association (ASHA)

Principles of Ethics I and III are devoted to acknowledging patient relationships. Principle I states, "*Individuals shall honor their responsibility to hold paramount the welfare of persons they serve professionally or who are participants in research and scholarly activities.*" Principle III states, "*In their professional role, individuals shall act with honesty and integrity when engaging with the public and shall provide accurate information involving any aspect of the professions"* (ASHA, 2023).

Academy of Doctors of Audiology (ADA)

PRINCIPLE I: To protect the welfare of persons served professionally.

- *Academy members shall use all resources, including those of other professionals, to provide the best possible service.*
- *Members shall fully inform patients of the nature and possible results of services rendered and products sold.*
  - *Members shall not misrepresent benefits of any therapeutic procedure of professional services.*
  - *Members shall not misrepresent benefits from use of hearing instruments or other assistive listening products.*
  - *Members may make reasonable statements of prognosis for both products and services, but particular care must be taken not to mislead patients to expect results that cannot be predicted or expected.*
  - *Members shall not prescribe, fit or recommend products or services which are known or suspected to be harmful to the patient's hearing or well-being without full disclosure to the patient.*
- *Members shall inform patients of the recommended services or products and any reasonable alternatives in a manner which allows the patient to become involved in, and make informed, treatment decisions.*
- *Members shall evaluate services and products rendered to determine effectiveness.*
- *Members shall not release professional and personal information obtained from the patient without the written permission of the patient in accordance with applicable state and federal law.*
- *Members shall not discriminate in the delivery of professional services on the basis of sex, marital status, age, religious preferences, nationality or race, or handicapping condition.* (Academy of Doctors of Audiology, n.d.)

All professional organizations maintain the importance of this clinician/patient relationship and its role in the patient care model. Indeed, this is the most crucial of all professional relationships.

Ultimately, clinicians should consider the following:

1. The clinician/patient relationship is sacred and must be held in the highest regard.
2. Clinicians are in complete charge of the clinician/patient relationship.
3. While clinicians are subject to the codes of ethics of the organizations to which they belong, their greater responsibility lies in the adherence to *principles* of ethics, which are the higher road of professional relationships and decision-making.

Ethics With Colleagues

"Collegial ethics must be characterized by mutual respect,

*integrity, excellence, trust,
and accountability, fostering
professional relationships and an
environment of the highest regard."*

—Michael D. Page

Thought Questions

1. Who said I have ethical obligations to my colleagues?
2. How will ethical collegial relationships influence workplace culture?
3. How do my ethical obligations to colleagues influence my team's dynamics and our service to our patients?
4. How might mutual collegial respect strengthen an entire program?
5. Why have codes of ethics included collegial relationships?

Workplace Ethics

The American Speech-Language-Hearing Association (ASHA) states, "Individuals shall not discriminate in their relationships with colleagues, members of other professions, or individuals under their supervision on the basis of age; citizenship; disability; ethnicity; gender; gender expression; gender identity; genetic information; national origin, including culture, language, dialect, and accent; race; religion; sex; sexual orientation; socioeconomic status; or veteran status" (ASHA, 2023). We often consider these requirements *for our patients*, but ASHA's COE includes the same requirements *for our colleagues*.

Because healthcare professionals belong to an exclusive tribe, they are responsible for the rules and guidelines of the tribe and for one another. Relationships with colleagues can be part of a "professional culture," one that should foster the strength of the profession, as well as the strength of the relationships within it.

Often in the profession, we characterize someone's competence by rating their skill, knowledge, and experience—the technical skills. Rarely, however, do we prioritize what some characterize as the "soft skills" or nontechnical skills such as communication, leadership, teamwork, creativity, time management, adaptability, problem-solving, work ethic, critical thinking, conflict management, and emotional intelligence (Danao, 2024). However, is it possible that the "soft skills" are actually the "hard skills"? To substantiate that, one might review each soft skill listed above by asking themselves, "To what extent would I be willing to forgo this soft skill?"

Simon Sinek argues that trust is the cornerstone upon which high-performing teams and companies are built ("Building High Performance Through Trust," 2023). Without trust (a perceived soft skill), it is challenging to achieve meaningful results or maintain healthy, long-lasting relationships. Sinek later claims that it is better to sacrifice some level of performance over any sacrifice of trust. He states, "Trust, although mostly intangible and often hard to quantify, is the more critical factor in the success of a team." In a survey of high-performing teams, Sinek found a unanimous preference for trustworthiness over sheer performance in leaders and teammates. Relationships based and built on trust then foster stronger intercollegial relationships, strengthening interactions and building foundations—the very bedrock of ethical practice (Pederson, 2023).

Workplace Behavior and Codes of Ethics

Workplace behavior and interprofessional relationships reflect the respect (or disrespect) of professional ethics. Since most professionals spend more hours with colleagues than with their own family members, the ethics of workplace environments matter. Codes of ethics speak to these relationships. The AAA's Code of Ethics (COE) states, "Members shall honor their responsibilities to the public and to professional colleagues" (American Academy of Audiology, 2023). While the COE does not define "responsibilities to the public and to the professional colleagues," one must infer the vital characteristics of mutual respect, integrity, empathy, and trust. In addition, Rule 8b states, "Individuals shall not engage in dishonesty or illegal conduct that adversely reflects on the profession" (American Academy of Audiology, 2023).

While skill, knowledge, and experience are critical in clinical care, it is possible that many of the violations of ethical practice may also include the "soft skills" highlighted above, especially in aspects of trust and communication. We are rarely adept at self-governance, simply because it is sometimes difficult to see ourselves and our behavior objectively. Therefore, it often requires the perspective of another. This perspective may include that of a supervisor, colleague, outside agency, or even a patient. Codes of ethics are overseen by a governing body, either a committee specific to ethics or a board of directors overseeing ethical practices.

This model provides some level of internal watch-care or self-governing of professionals by their peers. And while most professional behavior is exemplary, at times, some is less than stellar. Most professional organizations address this within their respective codes of ethics, which require reporting of colleagues who may exhibit compromised ethical behavior. Consider a sampling of codes regarding relationships with colleagues from the following professional organizations:

American Medical Association

"A physician shall uphold the standards of professionalism, be honest in all professional interactions, and strive to report physicians deficient in character or competence or engaging in fraud or deception to appropriate entities."

—(AMA n.d.-a)

American Speech-Language-Hearing Association

- *PRINCIPLE IV, Rule S: Individuals who have knowledge that a colleague is unable to provide professional services with reasonable skill and safety shall report this information to the appropriate authority, internally if such a mechanism exists and, when appropriate, externally to the applicable professional licensing authority or board, other professional regulatory body, or professional association.*

- *PRINCIPLE IV, Rule A: Individuals shall work collaboratively with members of their own profession and/or members of other professions, when appropriate, to deliver the highest quality of care. (ASHA, 2023)*

American Academy of Audiology

■ *PRINCIPLE 7: Members shall honor their responsibilities to the public and to professional colleagues.*
  ■ *Rule 7a: Individuals shall not use professional or commercial affiliations in any way that would limit services to or mislead patients or colleagues.*
  ■ *Rule 7b: Individuals shall inform colleagues and the public in an objective manner consistent with professional standards about products and services they have developed or research they have conducted.* (American Academy of Audiology, 2023)

Academy of Doctors of Audiology

■ *PRINCIPLE VI: To maintain ethical standards and practices of the Academy of Doctors of Audiology.*
  ■ *Members agree to govern their professional activities by this Code of Ethics.*
  ■ *Members agree to report to the Board of Directors for the Academy of Doctors of Audiology (or to its designees) any violations of the Code of Ethics, and to cooperate with any authorized inquiry or action the Board may undertake.* (Academy of Doctors of Audiology, n.d.).

Moreover, the AAA COE mandates that audiologists report to the Ethical Practices Committee "when there are reasons to believe that a member of the Academy may have been in noncompliance with the Code of Ethics" (American Academy of Audiology, 2023). These obligations include both proactive mea-sures of interprofessional support as well as policing. The tribal mindset includes mutual support and mutual accountability. Indeed, one must not only be held accountable but also hold the other tribe members accountable for their actions as outlined in the respective codes of ethics.

Workplace Behavior and Laws and Statues

One must not overlook laws and statutes dedicated to professional conduct. Virtually every state will have descriptions of what might be considered unprofessional conduct. Utah is one state that has a fairly exhaustive description of unprofessional and egregious conduct, which may be used as an example for study (Utah Code, Title 58, 2024). Ultimately, collegial relationships should be regarded with great mutual respect and regard within the context of ethical conduct and behavior.

Ethics With Members of Industry

"Recognizing when a relationship with industry is crossing the line of propriety is more important than any perceived act of impropriety."

—Michael D. Page

Thought Questions

1. How can members of industry influence the clinician/patient relationship?

2. What role do members of industry play in the clinician/patient relationship?
3. What are the risks and benefits of the triad of the clinician/patient/industry relationship?
4. While we often use the term "partnership" to describe clinical and industry relationships, how should we use the four principles of ethics to more accurately characterize this relationship to protect the sacred clinician/patient relationship?
5. While the Open Payments site is relevant to physicians only, what learning and application could be voluntarily taken by every healthcare provider?

Clinical Care and Relationships With Industry

Industry serves a critical role in healthcare and in audiology specifically. Industry provides a significant resource for devices, products, and services. Industry members include (but are not limited to) any of the following:

- Hearing aid manufacturers
- Equipment manufacturers
- Cochlear implant manufacturers
- Earmold labs
- Hearing aid repair labs
- Buying groups
- Business management groups
- Third-party administrators
- Assistive device manufacturers
- Supplies companies
- Battery companies

It is easy to see and appreciate the enormous contributions of industry in the realms of hearing aid technology, implantable devices, assistive devices, and many more products and services. Industry has spent untold millions on product development and sales. Indeed, volumes could be written about the nature, evolution, and outcomes of all products and services provided by industry. Great acknowledgment accompanies that awareness. Without industry, most healthcare clinicians would be severely limited in the degree to which they could successfully treat patients.

It is the design and purpose of clinical work versus industry work that may create conflict within the clinician role, potentially resulting in a compromised clinician/patient relationship. It is critical to note that the responsibilities of clinicians and the responsibilities of members of industry (even clinicians hired for that role) are vastly different. Clinicians who are hired by industry for sales, research, or support roles are still accountable to the codes of ethics of the organizations to which they belong. While clinicians in clinical roles may be penalized for receiving incentives, their clinician counterparts employed by industry may not be penalized for offering them. In other words, clinician sales representatives working for industry are employed by industry to support and incentivize their clinically based customer counterparts. When a licensed clinician functions in a sales role for the industry, one must ask, "Is that professional functioning as a healthcare provider or as a sales representative?"

Certainly, the topic deserves additional exploration about the potential for conflict of interest and how titles and credentials are utilized and positioned

Table 23–1. Clinicians' and Industry's Separate Responsibilities

Clinician Responsibility	Industry Role
Subject to direct patient contact.	Typically, not engaging in direct patient contact, lacking credentials and licensure to do so.
Subject to state professional practice licensing laws.	Subject to business licensing laws for industry.
Aim is to protect the clinician/patient relationship.	Aim is to protect the company viability and profit.
Primary purpose is patient treatment.	Primary purpose is product development, sales, and support.
Subject to *Consent to Treat*.	Since industry is not considered a health care provider, it has no *Consent to Treat*.
Has access to a patient's protected health information.	May not have access to a patient's protected health information unless engaged in approved patient support, intervention, or research.
Subject to professional codes of ethics (AAA, ADA, ASHA, etc.) to which they belong.	Industry generally is not subject to a clinician's code of ethics, but may have accountability to AvaMed code of ethics (AvaMed, n.d.)
Under the Anti-Kickback Statute (AKS), may not receive incentives for anything that is reimbursed under a state or federal program.	May be penalized for offering incentives under AKS.
Dispenser of healthcare devices and products directly to patients as part of their treatment plan.	Sells medical devices and products to clinicians who dispense them and may sell directly to patients with whom they have an established relationship through the patient's clinician.

by industry to incentivize professional relationships with clinical providers. So much of this complex relationship is yet to be understood. Unique aspects of clinicians' and industry's separate responsibilities are outlined in Table 23–1.

At the center of that relationship is an (often) unspoken expectation of trust, transparency, and clinical judgment free from outside influences and incentives. While clinicians want to serve patients using best practices, members of industry desire to often find themselves in a conundrum managing sales quotas with their foundational clinical commitments.

Many members of industry are paid a base salary plus commissions for sales obtained within their sales territory. Therefore, while some industry representatives may be audiologists themselves, they have an additional motive to sell devices to fellow clinicians. Too often, industry decision-makers frequently overlook issues akin to the sacred clinician/patient relationship, prioritizing corporate goals, gains, and market share over maintaining ethical integrity. The compelling reality is that even the most admired companies with ethical desires may sometimes feel pressure to make ethically compromised decisions to maintain viability and market positioning. In the context of that acknowledgment, clinicians must also align clinical best practices with the codes and principles of ethics to protect the clinician/patient relationship. It is rarely easy and often encumbered.

Open Payments and Industry Gift-Giving

Industry gifts are one of the most common methods to influence a clinician's buying behavior. The power of gift-giving is not to be overlooked or understated. Gift-giving, in general, needs to be acknowledged and accounted for in each relationship. The nature of gift-giving is significant enough that the Centers for Medicare & Medicaid Services (also known as CMS) developed the Open Payments website to account for gifts given to physicians by members of the

industry. This federally mandated program collects and publishes information about payments made by drug and medical device companies to healthcare providers and teaching hospitals. The Open Payments database is publicly accessible on the Open Payments Data website.

Open Payments requirements pertain only to physicians at this time, but the principles can easily translate into any healthcare provider subject to the sales efforts of the industry members mentioned above. The database is searchable by physician name or by the industry organization that pays physicians. While one can see what payments have been made to any physician in the United States, one can also search by any industry that makes payments (in the form of gifts, meals, grants, travel, and more) to physicians. One might find a direct correlation between the monetary value of gifts to any physician and their prescriptive or device purchase practice.

The intention of the Open Payments site is to provide full transparency to consumers and other colleagues about the financial relationships between industry and physicians. While only physicians are implicated in this federal disclosure law, it may be foreseeable that other healthcare providers could be implicated as well. Could any clinician evaluate the intention of the Open Payments efforts and modify professional behavior accordingly, even without the requirement? Yes.

The Open Payments site reinforces the ethical principles of *respect for autonomy* and *nonmaleficence*. This verifies that any outside incentive influences deserve to be seen and published. It is critical to understand that simple transparency does not mitigate the influence of the gift. The influence is still prevalent and should be considered by all entities in terms of the strength of their influence and the potential for the adulteration of the sacred clinician/patient relationship.

Researcher Barry Schwartz published an essay discussing the relevance of gift-giving to developing and maintaining professional identity. He stated, "In direct response to our findings, the authors suggest a move to include virtues-based practice, an explicit curriculum for learning ethical industry relations, theoretically-aligned ethics education approaches, and systemic and structural change" (Ng et al., 2019).

Some research suggests a link between the gifts from pharmaceutical representatives to physicians (consulting fees, free meals, trips, etc.) and opioid deaths (Hadland et al., 2019). Even "academic centers and industry partners have had love-hate relationships for more than a century. Despite many examples of socially beneficial collaborations between academia and industry, it has become increasingly difficult to find an arrangement where neither clinicians/researchers working with industry nor industry itself is demonized" (Reddy & Chao, 2020).

Numerous studies have shown the unseen risk (even increased mortality rates in some cases) of gift-giving and receiving within healthcare (Institute of Business Ethics, 2012; Murphy, 2019; Palmisano & Edelstein, 1980; Sierles, 2006). Hadland et al. (2019) stated, "Our findings suggest that direct-to-physician opioid marketing may run counter to national efforts to reduce overdose deaths and that policymakers should consider limits on marketing as part of a robust, evidence-based response to the U.S. overdose crisis." While audiologists do not prescribe medications, the crux of this article implies the unseen risk of gift-giving within healthcare. It behooves all professionals to seek deeper reasons for the practice of ethics rather than just asking what the limits are.

What's the risk of the ethical dilemma healthcare professionals face when engaging salespeople to offer tempting gifts? The article outlines cultural responses to gift-giving and ethical issues surrounding healthcare professionals' responses to pharmaceutical marketing strategies. While audiologists rarely receive gifts from pharmaceutical companies, the principles around gift-giving by any industry member remain substantially parallel.

Codes of ethics often address gifts, but sometimes with limited perspective. AAA's *Ethical Practice Guideline for Relationships With Industry for Audiologists Providing Clinical Care* (2017) states that "acceptance of in excess of $50 by a member of the American Academy of Audiology from any company that manufactures or supplies products that he or she professionally uses or recommends, may compromise, or give the appearance of compromising, the audiologist's ability to make ethical decisions, and should be avoided." Yet, Bloom and Bloom (2015) and Soo-Jin Lee (2021) claim that the value of the gift has little bearing on the influence of the recipient.

The social psychology of gift-giving is replete. "The acceptance of a gift, it is suggested, is, in fact, an acceptance of the giver's ideas as to what one's desires and needs are. Gift-giving as a mode of social control and expression of unfriendliness is considered. The relationship between gift exchange and social structure is analyzed from the standpoint of the 'gratitude imperative.' The essay concludes with a treatment of benefit exchange as a technique for the regulation of shared guilt" (Schwartz, 2021). Ultimately, a clinician recognizing when a relationship with industry is crossing the line of propriety is more important than any industry act of impropriety.

Clinical Research Relationship With Industry

Research partnerships have existed between clinical sites and industry. Given the varying motivations and operational models of both entities, it remains critical that certain principles of ethics be recognized and honored. With clinical/industry research, it becomes crucial that both parties protect human subjects and personal health information, distribute research credit appropriately, provide for adequate research design and data protection, and mitigate conflict of interest in product-oriented outcomes research (Siniger et al., 2011).

AAA (Siniger et al., 2011) makes the following noteworthy recommendations:

1. It is considered unethical for a member to conduct research in a manner that does not provide an honest, fair, accurate, and complete evaluation of the product, device, or procedure.
2. Members should disclose financial relationships between the researcher and the sponsor in all written and verbal research reports.
3. Members should avoid agreements with industry sponsors that limit the dissemination of research results.
4. Members should only enter into explicit research contracts with specific deliverables restricted to scientific issues and should not accept "no strings attached" grants and gifts.
5. Members should disclose any financial relationships between the researcher and the sponsor in any public written or verbal reports of product evaluation activities.
6. Members who conduct industry-sponsored research and who also utilize that company's products clinically should disclose that relationship to their patients in writing.

As one reviews these recommendations, each can be tied back to the *principles* of ethics: autonomy, nonmaleficence, beneficence, and justice. Each reflects on the necessity of protecting the sacred patient relationship through transparency, integrity, and trust.

Ethics Within the Profession

"...one individual has the power and strength to impact the entire tribe for good or otherwise."

— Stichler, 1998

Thought Questions

1. What ethics-related obligations do clinicians have to their profession?
2. How does one clinician's unethical or ethical behavior impact the profession as a whole?
3. How do professional standards and codes of ethics protect consumers?
4. What obligations do healthcare professionals have to the consumers of their services?

Professional Ethics

Ethics have a long history of evolution, and one should assume they will continue to evolve as circumstances change. As is already established, ethics *should* change as circumstances dictate, while the *principles* of ethics remain stable. Ultimately, ethics in a profession are regulated by the respective professional organizations. These organizations are the "tribe" to which a professional belongs. Clinicians may not always love the tribe or even all of its members. Clinicians belong to a tribe nonetheless and are subject to its requirements if they hold membership within a respective professional organization.

Professional Tribes and Tribalism

Even if clinicians don't belong to a professional organization, they remain members of the tribe simply by shared credentials. Once one becomes a part of a tribe, their actions and behavior impact the entire tribal community. Indeed, one individual has the power and strength to impact the entire tribe for good or otherwise (Stichler, 1998).

Within a professional tribe, workplace culture becomes a foundation for ethics within the environment and is defined by *Forbes* as "the shared values, belief systems, attitudes and the set of assumptions that people in a workplace share" (Agarwal, 2018). The elements of that definition integrate with the principles of ethics prolifically. Stanford University Professor Jeffry Pfeffer's research (Pfeffer, 2018) makes compelling claims, stating, "The workplace is the 5th leading cause of death in the U.S., higher than Alzheimer's or kidney disease."

Pfeffer's research shows that the mismanagement of workforces causes more than 120,000 deaths a year and accounts for 5% to 8% of annual healthcare costs. The odious cultures of many workplaces (especially within healthcare) can impact personal health, even to the point of death. Those experiencing the impacts of bad workplace cultures find themselves in the crosshairs in direct conflict with the ethics principle of nonmaleficence.

In addition to belonging to a tribe and our ethical responsibility to the tribe, let us differentiate "belonging to a tribe" from "tribalism." Dictionary.com (n.d.) defines a *tribe* as "a group or class of people with strong common traits, values, or interests," confirming the fact that audiologists and other healthcare professionals divide themselves from other professions into a unique and distinct group.

Tribalism, however, is different. Cottone (2022) speaks of tribalism, "Beyond physical survival, our various tribal memberships bestow other important benefits, like being able to buy ridiculous quantities of Lucky Charms at discount prices, for those of us who are members of the Costco tribe." As we have witnessed, a few clinicians choose fraudulent behavior over behavior of integrity, which should not detract from the overall and exemplary behavior of most professionals, but it can. The critical component is that the integrity of one impacts the integrity of the profession. After all, belonging to a tribe is about agreeing to be accountable and holding other members of the tribe accountable. Codes of ethics are replete with descriptions of ethics within the profession. While tribalism keeps others out, being a productive and contributing member of a professional tribe enhances clinical care and protects consumers by establishing minimum standards for behavior and practice, enhancing inclusivity.

Culture and Ethics

An effective and strong culture builds a substantial organization. Culture is a primary ethical obligation each clinician has with their colleagues and with their organization. Additional requirements regarding ethics within the profession include the following:

American Academy of Audiology

■ *PRINCIPLE 8: Members shall uphold the dignity of the profession and freely accept the Academy's self-imposed standards.*
  ■ *Rule 8a: Individuals shall not violate these Principles and Rules nor attempt to circumvent them.*
  ■ *Rule 8b: Individuals shall not engage in dishonesty or illegal conduct that adversely reflects on the profession.*
  ■ *Rule 8c: Individuals shall inform the Ethical Practices Committee when there are reasons to believe that a member of the Academy may have been in noncompliance with the Code of Ethics.*
  ■ *Rule 8d: Individuals shall inform the Ethical Practices Committee when their state licensure and/or other professional memberships have been revoked or suspended due to a disciplinary action.*
  ■ *Rule 8e: Individuals shall fully cooperate with reviews being conducted by the Ethical Practices Committee in any matter related to the Code of Ethics.* (American Academy of Audiology, 2023)

American Speech-Language-Hearing Association Code of Ethics

From the Preamble: *The ASHA Code of Ethics reflects professional values and expectations for scientific and clinical practice. It is based on principles of duty, accountability, fairness, and responsibility and is intended to ensure the consumer's welfare and to protect the rep-*

utation and integrity of the profession. (ASHA, 2023)

It is important to see where we might find alignment with other professional organizations. The American Medical Association (AMA n.d.-a) claims to have been founded in part to establish the world's first national code of medical ethics and claims to be the most widely recognized and the most comprehensive ethics guide for physicians.

Academy of Doctors of Audiology

- *PRINCIPLE V: To engage in conduct which shall enhance the status of the profession.*

  Members must honor their responsibility to the public, their profession, and their colleagues. (Academy of Doctors of Audiology, n.d.)

Laws and Statutes

Within professions, distinct laws, statutes, and regulations govern professional behavior and practice. Some of those are described below:

- *Stark Law.* The Stark Law (42 U.S.C. § 1395nn), is a part of U.S. federal laws that prohibit physician self-referral, specifically a referral by a physician of a Medicare or Medicaid patient to an entity for the provision of designated health services if the physician (or an immediate family member) has a financial relationship with that entity. The law aims to protect Medicare patients from receiving unnecessary medical services. The Stark Law is a strict liability statute, which means proof

of specific intent to violate the law is not required. Penalties for violating this law are severe, even when the practitioner did so unknowingly or unintentionally. While the Stark Law may not pertain to audiologists, there may be some association under some circumstances and in some professional environments. Therefore, it always behooves a clinician to "act as if" the statute applies since it certainly applies on a broader umbrella in the principle of nonmaleficence (American Medical Association, 2020).

- *The Anti-Kickback Statute 42 U.S. Code § 1320a–7b(b), and the Safe Harbors Law.* The Anti-Kickback Statute's (1972) main purpose is to protect against fraud and abuse against patients and the federal health care programs. The statute helps reduce the devious influence of money on healthcare decisions. The law states that anyone who knowingly receives or pays anything of value to influence the referral of federal health care program business, including Medicare and Medicaid, could be charged with a felony. Violations of the statute are punishable by up to 5 years in prison, criminal fines up to $25,000, administrative civil money penalties up to $50,000, and exclusion from participation in federal health care programs (Office of Inspector General, Office of Public Affairs, 1999). Responding to these concerns about the potential benefit from what appears to be "kickbacks," Congress (1987) authorized the regulations designating specific "safe harbors" for various payment and business practices that, while potentially prohibited by the law, would not be prosecuted. This would allow industry to secure contracted discount models for healthcare entities without fearing prosecution.

■ *False Claims Act.* False Claims Act 31 U.S.C. §§ 3729 - 3733 (Lincoln Law, 1863) is sometimes referred to as the Lincoln Act (referring to then U.S. President Abraham Lincoln). During Civil War times, widespread abuses were reported regarding contractors and suppliers of goods to the Union Army. Following the Civil War, the law lay somewhat dormant until 1986, when amendments were added, strengthening its authority to combat fraud and introduce allowances, rewards, and protections for whistleblowers. Today, the False Claims Act is the basis for virtually every insurance fraud claim against audiology providers billing government third-party payers (Medicare and Medicaid). Clinicians filing false claims against any government entity is deceitful constitutes maleficence and is contrary to principles of ethics, including the principles of nonmaleficence and justice (a contractor fraudulently taking more remuneration than due) (U.S. Department of Justice, 2024).

■ *Physician Payment Sunshine Act.* The Physician Payment Sunshine Act (Sunshine Act), which is part of the Affordable Care Act (ACA), requires manufacturers of drugs, medical devices, and biologicals that participate in U.S. federal health care programs to report certain payments and items of value given to physicians and teaching hospitals. While this act does not include most audiologists directly, it will include audiologists indirectly and critically if they are associated with or employed by a teaching hospital. Under this act, any type or value of gift provided to physicians (and audiologists at teaching hospitals) must be reported to a public database, creating transparency in the incentive-based relationship between providers and companies that sell to them. Reportable gifts include (but are not limited to) meals, excursions, lodging, gifts of products, travel, research grants, and more. Gifts (of any value) received by providers from any medical device (hearing aid, implantable device, or supplies company) or pharmaceutical company encourage an unseen obligatory relationship between the provider and the giver. Thus, the receiver establishes a level of loyalty (often unseen or unacknowledged). Accepting gifts of any value breaches a commitment to independent and unbiased clinical judgment and treatment. The risk of bias increases the likelihood of compromised clinical judgment. Those who fail to acknowledge the potential for compromise will likely be most susceptible to its impact (CMS.gov, 2024). While some physicians express ambivalence about whether gifts create an ethical dilemma, surveying the recipient of sometimes lavish gifts about their influence is *akin to asking the fox if he should guard the henhouse* (Brett et al., 2003).

■ *FTC Policy on Deception.* The Federal Trade Commission (FTC) publishes a policy statement regarding deception, which states that practice is deceptive either by representation or omission if it is likely to mislead consumers (patients). Section 5 of the FTC Act declares unfair or deceptive acts or practices unlawful, and Section 12 specifically prohibits false ads likely to induce the purchase of devices. The FTC considers an advertisement's overall "net impression" to determine whether it misleads consumers (U.S. Federal Trade Commission, n.d.). Audiologists may be guilty of deception if they misrepresent their treatment, services, or outcomes. The AAA Code of Ethics states that an audiologist may not guarantee outcomes or results from any form of treatment or intervention (American Academy of Audiology, 2023). The author recalls several audiology advertisements using the statement "better hearing guaranteed," which would, in fact, violate the code of ethics. Deception weakens a patient's autonomy by creating inaccurate perceptions or promises. Deception falls contrary to the principle of nonmaleficence (causing harm) and also compromises the principle of justice by the potential for failing to deliver on promises made.

Ethics in Sources of Knowledge: Artificial Intelligence (AI)

"The ethics of knowledge encompasses a range of ethical considerations related to the acquisition, creation, sharing, and use of knowledge, with the overarching goal of promoting truth, integrity, responsibility, and respect in our interactions with knowledge."

—OpenAI (2024)

Thought Questions

1. Why is it important to protect the integrity of our knowledge base?
2. What unseen risks may exist with the application of AI?
3. How can the four principles of ethics help guide our use and application of AI?
4. What proactive measures can be taken to ensure integrity in AI's clinical or research application?
5. What might be the important elements of an AI code of ethics?

Vital History

The dawn of artificial intelligence (AI) is not as recent as one might think! Its presence and influence continue to pervade all aspects of life with both "pace and scale" and aspects of its development that span decades (Hindocha & Badea, 2022). The need for ethics in AI has been long considered a primary concern. Nonetheless, its history (including its ethics) is reminiscent of the public fear of and ultimate embrace of the Internet in the 1990s. The explosion of cognitive technologies detonated a plethora of emotions, including doubt, suspicion, fear, and reticence about the credibility and trustworthiness of such knowledge whose source may not be verified or trusted. It is one thing to have access to knowledge, but dynamic knowledge or knowledge with its own decision power is quite another.

What would eventually emerge as the World Wide Web in the 1990s was a complex and arduous evolution. History reports, "The internet got its start in the United States more than 50 years ago as a government weapon in the Cold War. For years, scientists and researchers used it to communicate and share data with one another" (History.com Editors, 2019). The evolution and explosion were unpredictably prolific, so most might not imagine life without the Internet. And yet, it continues to evolve and expand.

Early on, it was the author's experience that some universities and publishing agencies failed to accept most information obtained from the Internet because credibility could not be established or vetted. It was thought that because one did not visit the library and touch the pages of the journal quoted, the information could not be reliable. Eventually, however, the Internet evolved into a very credible resource, and it was eventually embraced as a reputable source of knowledge to the extent that it could be verified, vetted, and cited.

While employed by a prominent healthcare organization in Salt Lake City, Utah (USA), the author recalls not only being assigned his first email address but eventually receiving a thick catalog-like book publishing all known Internet sites available at the time (the 1990s). They were organized alphabetically and categorically. Due to the rapid explosion of Internet sites, no other such catalog had been published to the author's knowledge. Such was the unanticipated growth of the Internet.

In 2018, *Harvard Business Review*, in a survey of 250 executives who were familiar with their companies' use of cognitive technology, reported that approximately three-quarters of them believed that AI would substantially transform their companies within 3 years. They report that "the hype surrounding artificial intelligence has been especially powerful, and some organizations have been seduced by it" (Davenport, 2018). Such seductions are common in newer technologies and solidify the thought that AI is here to stay, along with the increasing demands for ethics to guide its utility. One author describes AI as "the power to harm, pav[ing] the way to unethical behavior" (Blackman, 2020). Like most other platforms, it is the author's opinion that AI may have the potential to reveal unintended consequences by the risks not readily seen. Companies are quickly learning that AI doesn't just scale solutions. It also scales risk.

Ethical practice in using artificial intelligence is critical to maintain safety, preserve one's professional integrity, and increase trust while avoiding plagiarism, dishonesty, or the perpetuation of distorted, adulterated, or even false information. Some report that AI has the potential to enable compromises in the confidentiality of patients' sensitive data and begs for the development of AI ethics in "concordance with human values and ethics" (Solanki et al., 2022). Hindocha and Badea (2022) propose that in the process, we consider the different moral theories that may serve as a basis of thought that should build around "virtue ethics," which is focused more on character traits and less on task or duty track. There are many parallels between the onset of Internet use and the viability and credibility of AI. "While AI experts don't agree on many things, they all agree on one thing: AI technology is going to have huge effects on society and business" (Kaput, 2022).

AI's Potential for Impact

The potential impact for AI is likely immeasurable at this point in time. Once we think we understand its potential, it is the point where its potential becomes exponential. Google CEO Sundar Pichai stated, "Artificial intelligence is going to have a bigger impact on the world than some of the most ubiquitous innovations in history. AI is one of the most important things humanity is working on. It is more profound than . . . electricity or fire" (Clifford, 2018).

Clifford also states positive considerations, and thoughts about AI within our professional settings have produced some of the following ideas:

1. AI may automate repetitive, data-driven, and mundane tasks.
2. AI may reduce human error and minimize errors.
3. AI could conduct tasks that are too dangerous for us.
4. AI could help us make better, smarter, and faster decisions.
5. AI may solve problems in ways that we can't.
6. AI may make us richer.
7. AI could make us more productive.
8. AI works 24 hours per day.

Cost of Risk

Some believe that AI creates a potential risk for patient autonomy, bias, and transparency. This certainly provides op-portunities for the template proposed by Beauchamp and Childress (2019), which proposes the previously noted filters of autonomy, beneficence, non-maleficence, and justice. Risks of AI may include patient safety concerns such as providing inaccurate screening, diagnosis, treatment, and patient education.

Unfortunately, there may be room for incorrect prescriptive algorithms for hearing aids, implantable devices, or other treatments. In severe cases, risk may include compromise and even the loss of life. Ahmad et al. (2023) suggest from their research that AI significantly impacts the loss of human decision-making and makes humans lazy. It also impacts security and privacy. If in management, one must consider an actual line item that would be budgeted for risk management. Greater risk yields greater cost. The greater the cost yields, the greater the potential for loss of trust, credibility, and reputation.

Much like the development of the Internet, the ethical use of artificial intelligence in healthcare demands the consideration of the cost of risk. While metrics exist for calculating the cost of risk (Calculator Academy, 2023), suffice it to say that the cost of risk is the expense of risk management and any losses incurred (in the utility of AI), or the total cost of the components required for taking on risk (Ventiv Technology, n.d.).

Harvard Business Review (PWC, 2021) suggests that responsible AI should govern systems in accordance with the environment in which we would like to operate and should be implemented using technical and procedural capabilities to address bias, explainability, robustness, safety, security concerns, and more. The intent of responsible AI, which is sometimes referred to as or conflated with trusted AI, AI ethics, or beneficial AI, is to develop AI and analytics systems methodically, enabling high-quality and documented systems that are reflective of an organization's beliefs and values and minimizing *unintended harms*" (italics added) (Gratch & Fast, 2022). Gratch also describes AI as "the power to harm, pav[ing] the way to unethical behavior." Indeed, AI, like most other platforms, has the potential to reveal unintended consequences by the risks not readily seen.

AI Ethics Justification

The cost of risk alone is the reason why companies insure themselves against unforeseen events or occurrences (i.e., the risk they may not see). One method of reducing risk will include the development and implementation of ethical codes relevant to artificial intelligence and its use within each environment. Morley et al. (2020) find that ethical issues can be (1) epistemic, (related to misguided, inconclusive, or inscrutable evidence), (2) normative (related to unfair outcomes and transformative effectiveness), and (3) related to traceability (the origin of data). These observations respectively coincide with the principles of nonmaleficence and justice.

In an exhaustive literature search on the topic of AI ethics, Weidener and Fischer (2023) report recent findings suggesting a need to include AI ethics as part of medical curricula due to the potential implications of AI in medicine. Bias was highlighted as a challenge to be addressed in teaching content in addition to basic principles of medical ethics, which could easily be addressed with the four principles outlined by Beauchamp and Childress (2019).

Lessons learned from establishing "Internet use ethics" may also help anticipate the role of ethics in AI. Furthermore, at least one author reports "a number of pros and cons in the field of AI us[e] in healthcare (Weidener & Fischer, 2023). Undoubtedly, this is a promising area with many gaps and gray zones to fill. Morley et al. (2020) describe, "We further find that these ethical issues arise at six levels of abstraction: individual, interpersonal, group, institutional, and societal or sectoral." Ellis (2023) claims, "Among its many uses, AI (like ChatGPT) can be a valuable research tool for papers and other academic writing." Audiologists have reported the utilization of AI in such aspects as research, patient educational materials, marketing, or even candidate assessment. While such utility might sound appealing, others add, "AI is . . . going to be the most important tool in solving the biggest challenges we face" (Sharma, 2024). Could it be true? What are the biggest challenges facing healthcare? What should drive its code of ethics?

Academic Writing

Categorically, AI presents several challenges for risk within academic writing. The American Psychological Association (APA) (2023) policy states that authors are responsible for the accuracy of any information in their writing. "Failure to disclose AI use may compromise diagnostic and treatment science. Transparency and professional integrity must lead the implementation of AI technology within the healthcare realm." The APA further states authors must verify any information and citations provided to them by an AI tool. Authors may use, but must disclose, AI tools for specific purposes such as editing. This APA policy may also be translated into clinical and academic use of AI. Essentially, all users of AI are responsible for its data origins, use, and implementation, ensuring the principles of transparency, honesty, and integrity. The use of AI data in publications is no exception.

These and other writing policies are subject to rapid evolution, modification, and change. An attempt to provide current guidelines here would be impru-

dent due to the nature and speed of their evolution. Therefore, one should consult the APA Style website for the most current guidelines on how to cite AI, such as ChatGPT.

While AI emerges from its infantile stages, one of the most significant and ultimate challenges to the ethical use of AI is to "bridge [the] trust gap" (Baxter & Schlesinger, 2023). The ultimate trust in AI will hinge directly upon its transparency, integrity, and trustworthiness. Confidence in AI will be built upon its ethical use and implementation over time.

While it is difficult to find agreement on who might hold the rights of AI ethics development (its use, execution, and consequences), agencies, entities, professional associations, and government bureaus will (and have begun to) step forward to claim some aspect of AI ethics management, and every organization must assert its codes of ethics for the fruitful, rightful, and appropriate use of AI within their realm. Ultimately, however, the greatest responsibility falls on each individual user. The most deeply rooted principles of ethics must stem from within. Indeed, ethics in the use of AI requires personal commitment to principles of transparency, credibility, and integrity.

Preserving integrity and mitigating risk in the clinical and professional application of AI should include the following considerations as presented in *Harvard Business Review* (PWC, 2021), which may be considered instrumental in the development of industry-specific AI codes of ethics:

■ *Establish principles to guide:* A set of ethical principles adopted and supported by leadership provides a north star to the organization.

Principles on their own, however, are not sufficient to embed responsible AI practices. Stakeholders need to consider principles in the context of their day-to-day work to design policies and practices that the whole company can get behind.

- *Consider governance ownership:* Fortunately, many leaders within organizations are interested in establishing governance practices for AI and data. However, without specifying an owner for this governance, an organization is likely to find itself with a different problem—discrete practices that may be in conflict with one another. Identify which teams should design governance approaches and agree on an owner and a process to identify updates to existing policies.
- *Develop a well-defined and integrated process for data, model, and software life cycle:* Implement standardized processes for development and monitoring, with specific stage gates to indicate where approvals and reviews are needed to proceed. This process should connect to existing data and privacy governance mechanisms as well as the software development life cycle.
- *Break down silos:* Align across necessary stakeholder groups to connect teams for the purposes of sharing ideas and leading practices. Create common inventories for AI and data for the governance process and use this exercise as an opportunity to consider structural changes or realignments that could enable the business to run better.
- *Keep tabs on the rapidly changing regulatory climate:* It's not just

customers, investors, and employees who are demanding responsible practices. Regulators are taking notice and proposing legislation at the state, regulator, national, and supranational levels. Some regulations stem from expanded data protection and privacy efforts, some from specific regulators on narrow use case areas (such as banking) and some from a more general desire to improve accountability (such as the European Union's Artificial Intelligence Act). Keeping pace with these regulations is key to identifying future compliance activities.

In point of consideration, each entity must proactively maintain its prevalence, reliance, and dominance within ethics for AI supported by these most universal of ethics principles. Blackman (2020) explained that companies demand a plan with clarity, dealing with ethical dilemmas introduced by AI. He recommended that considerations for ethics implementation include (1) identifying existing infrastructure that a data and AI ethics program can leverage, (2) creating a data and AI ethical risk framework that is tailored to your industry, (3) changing how you think about ethics by taking cues from the successes in healthcare, (4) optimizing guidance and tools for product managers, (5) building organizational awareness, (6) formally and informally incentivizing employees to play a role in identifying AI ethical risks, and finally, (7) monitoring impacts and engaging stakeholders.

Accountability ultimately rests upon not only companies creating technology, including ethics experts, professional organizations, scientists, and those who license and regulate, but also those of us who use it for the benefit of those we serve. This accountability pays the much-needed respect to the most critical aspects of honoring the sacred patient relationship. As a colleague and friend Bill Kirst (2023) once said, "Let us not forget our humanity in all of this technology."

While any significant resource like fire is good and essential, most good resources can be responsible for destruction and death. After all, the same fire that keeps us warm, heats our food, provides light, and tempers steel is the same fire that became known as the Great Chicago fire in 1871, killing approximately 300 people and nearly 17,000 structures (History.com Editors, 2018). Thus, should we regard AI's potential as a resource capable of the full unimaginable spectrum of outcomes? It deserves measured fear, our greatest respect, and our intentional and focused efforts to create the most cautious and deliberate efforts to protect ourselves, our professions, our ethics, and our patients.

In conclusion, taking control of individual, organizational, professional, and academic ethics in AI remains crucial to its success. Morley et al. (2020) argue that if action is not swiftly taken in this regard, a new "AI Winter" could occur due to the chilling effects related to a loss of public trust in the benefits of AI for healthcare. Ultimately, the ethics of artificial intelligence must adhere to transparency, credibility, and integrity. Additionally, the universal principles of ethics (autonomy, beneficence, nonmaleficence, and justice) by Beauchamp and Childress (2019) should be considered in the design, development, and implementation of codes related to AI.

Final Pledge and Commitment

The author invites the reader to consider the following pledges and commitments, which may be formalized by sharing the pledge with a colleague or with an accountability partner who can help remind, align, and support the audiologist in the obligation to professional ethics.

1. *I have an ethics obligation to myself.* I pledge to align myself with critical principles and codes of ethics.
2. *I have an ethics obligation to my patients.* I pledge to nurture the sacred patient relationship as the paramount focus. I pledge to keep my relationships with industry not only within applicable laws and codes, but within the higher order of the *principles* of ethics, thereby sustaining and respecting the sacred patient relationship.
3. *I have an ethics obligation to my colleagues and my profession.* I pledge to maintain relationships of mutual respect and honor in all encounters with all people and in all cases.
4. *I have an ethics obligation to the source of knowledge.* I pledge to be transparent in my learning, teaching, publishing, and treatments based on credible evidence and accepted clinical practice standards.
5. *I pledge to live my professional life* not just to avoid real or perceived regrets but to live and practice with a strengthened intention to perpetuate goodness.

References

Abramson, A. (2021, April 1). *The ethical imperative of self-care.* American Psychological Association. http://www.apa.org/monitor/2021/04/feature-imperative-self-care

Academy of Doctors of Audiology. (n.d.). *Code of ethics.* http://www.audiologist.org/about-us/academy-documents/code-of-ethics

Accipio. (n.d.). *The Johari window.* Accipio. http://www.accipio.com/eleadership/building-teams/the-johari-window/

Agarwal, P. (2018, August 29). How to create a positive workplace culture. *Forbes.* http://www.forbes.com/sites/pragyaagarwaleurope/2018/08/29/how-to-create-a-positive-work-place-culture/?sh=6c8545844272

Ahmad, S. F., Heesup, H., Alam, M. M., Irshad, M., Arrano-Munoz, M., & Ariza-Montes, A. (2023). Impact of artificial intelligence on human loss in decision making, laziness and safety in education. *Nature,* Article 311. http://www.nature.com/articles/s41599-023-01787-8

AMA. (n.d.-a). *AMA principles of medical ethics.* American Medical Association. http://code-medical-ethics.ama-assn.org/principles

AMA. (n.d.-b). *Code of medical ethics.* American Medical Association Code of Medical Ethics. http://code-medical-ethics.ama-assn.org

American Academy of Audiology. (2017). *Ethical practice guideline for relationships with industry for audiologists providing clinical care.* http://www.audiology.org/practice-guideline/ethical-practice-guideline-for-relationships-with-industry-for-audiologists-providing-clinical-care/

American Academy of Audiology. (2023, April 23). *Code of ethics.* American Academy of Audiology. http://www.audiology.org/clinical-resources/code-of-ethics/

American Medical Association. (2020). *A brief summary of the Stark Law and anti-kickback statute reforms (final rules)* [White paper]. http://www.ama-assn.org/system/files/2020-12/stark-law-aks-summary-final-rules.pdf

American Psychological Association. (2023, November). *APA Journals policy on generative AI: Additional guidance.* http://www.apa.org/pubs/journals/resources/publishing-tips/policy-generative-ai

Arizona Speech-Language-Hearing Association. (2023). *Arizona Speech-Language-Hearing Association's 2023 Convention.* ArSHA. http://www.arsha.org/arsha-2023-convention/

ASHA. (2023, March 1). *Code of Ethics.* American Speech-Language-Hearing Association. http://www.asha.org/policy/ET2016-00342/

AvaMed. (n.d.). *Compliance and ethics.* http://www.advamed.org/our-work/policy-areas/compliance-ethics/

Baratta, M. (2018, May 27). Self-care 101. *Psychology Today.* http://www.psychologytoday.com/us/blog/skinny-revisited/201805/self-care-101

Baxter, K., & Schlesinger, Y. (2023, June 6). Managing the risks of generative AI. *Harvard Business Review.* http://hbr.org/2023/06/managing-the-risks-of-generative-ai

Beauchamp, T. L., & Childress, J. F. (1979). *Principles of biomedical ethics.* Oxford University Press. http://global.oup.com/ushe/product/principles-of-biomedical-ethics-9780190640873?cc=us&lang=en&

Beauchamp, T. L., & Childress, J. F. (2019). *Principles of biomedical ethics* (8th ed.). Oxford University Press. http://global.oup.com/ushe/product/principles-of-biomedical-ethics-9780190640873?cc=us&lang=en&

Blackman, R. (2020, October 15). A practical guide to building ethical AI. *Harvard Business Review.* http://hbr.org/2020/10/a-practical-guide-to-building-ethical-ai

Bloom, L., & Bloom, C. (2015, October 10). Honoring the rule of reciprocation. *Psychology Today*. http://www.psychology today.com/intl/blog/stronger-the-bro ken-places/201510/honoring-the-rule -reciprocation

Brett, A. S., Burr, A. S., & Moolo, J. (2003). Are gifts from pharmaceutical companies ethically problematic? A survey of physicians. *Archives of Internal Medicine, 18*(163), 2213–2218. https://doi.org/10.10 01/archinte.163.18.2213

Building high performance through trust: Lessons from Simon Sinek. (2023, September 24). *BPD*. http://www.thebdp.org /post/building-high-performance-through -trust-lessons-from-simon-sinek

Calculator Academy. (2023). *Total cost of risk calculator*. Total Cost of Risk Calculator. http://calculator.academy/total-cost-of -risk-calculator/

Clifford, C. (2018, February 1). *Google CEO: A.I. Is more important than fire or electricity*. CNBC. https://www.cnbc.com/2018 /02/01/google-ceo-sundar-pichai-ai-is -more-important-than-fire-electricity.html

CMS.gov. (2024, January). *Open payments data advanced search*. https://www.cnbc .com/2018/02/01/google-ceo-sundar-pi chai-ai-is-more-important-than-fire-elec tricity.html, http://openpaymentsdata.cms .gov/search

Cottone, J. G. (2022, July 31). Tribalism: How to be part of the solution, not the problem. *Psychology Today*. http://www .psychologytoday.com/us/blog/the -cube/202207/tribalism-how-be-part-the -solution-not-the-problem

Danao, M. (2024, April 28). Eleven essential soft skills in 2024 (with examples). *Forbes*. http://www.forbes.com/advisor /business/soft-skills-examples/

Davenport, T. H. (2018, January 30). Artificial intelligence for the real world. *Harvard Business Review*. http://hbr.org/webinar /2018/02/artificial-intelligence-for-the-real -world

Dictionary.com. (n.d.). *Tribe*. http://www .dictionary.com/browse/tribe

Ellis, M. (2023, July 6). *How to cite ChatGPT and AI in APA format*. Grammarly. http:// www.grammarly.com/blog/ai-citations-apa/

Eurich, T. (2018, January 4). What self-awareness is (and how to cultivate it). *Harvard Business Review*. http://hbr.org /2018/01/what-self-awareness-really-is -and-how-to-cultivate-it

General Dynamics. (n.d.). *Commitment to ethics*. http://www.gd.com/responsibility /commitment-to-ethics

Gratch, J., & Fast, N. J. (2022). The power to harm: AI assistants pave the way to unethical behavior. *Current Opinion in Psychology, 47*. https://doi.org/10.1016/j.cop sy.2022.101382

Hadland, S. E., Rivera-Aguirre, A., Marshall, B. D. L., & Cerda, M. (2019). Association of pharmaceutical industry marketing of opioid products with mortality from opioid-related overdoses. *JAMA Network Open, 2*(1). https://doi.org/10.1001/jama networkopen.2018.6007

Haegert, S. (2004). The ethics of self. *Nursing Ethics, 11*(5), 434–443. https://doi.org/10 .1191/0969733004ne722

Hindocha, S., & Badea, C. (2022). Moral exemplars for the virtuous machine: The clinician's role in ethical artificial intelligence for healthcare. *AI Ethics, 2*, 167–175. https://doi.org/doi.org/10.1007/s43681 -021-00089-6

History.com Editors. (2018, August 21). *Chicago fire of 1871*. History. http://www .history.com/topics/natural-disasters-and -environment/great-chicago-fire

History.com Editors. (2019, October 28). *The invention of the Internet*. History. https:// www.history.com/topics/inventions/in vention-of-the-internet

Holm, S. (2016). Principles of biomedical ethics. *Journal of Medical Ethics, 28*(5), 332. http://jme.bmj.com/content/28/5/332.2.info

Institute of Business Ethics. (2012, November 10). *The ethics of gifts and hospital-*

ity. http://www.ibe.org.uk/resource/the-ethics-of-gifts-hospitality.html

Kaput, M. (2022, March 14). Fifteen pros and cons of artificial intelligence you should know. *Marketing Artificial Intelligence Institute.* http://www.marketingaiinstitute.com/blog/pros-and-cons-of-artificial-intelligence

Kirst, B. (2023, March 23). *AI as copilot* [Online forum post]. LinkedIn. Retrieved May 22, 2024, from http://www.linkedin.com/pulse/leading-change-era-ai-bill-kirst/

Knowles, E. (n.d.). *ELIZABETH KNOWLES "sacred." The Oxford dictionary of phrase and fable.* Encyclopedia.com. http://encyclopedia.com/social-sciences-and-law/sociology-and-social-reform/sociology-general-terms-and-concepts/sacred

Lee, S.-J. (2021). Obligations of the "gift": Reciprocity and responsibility in precision medicine. *American Journal of Bioethics, 21*(4), 57–66. https://doi.org/10.1080/15265161.2020.1851813

Morley, J., Mac, C. C., Bur, C., Cowls, J., Taddeo, M., & Floridi, L. (2020). The ethics of AI in health care: A mapping review. *Social Science & Medicine, 260,* Article 113172. http://www.sciencedirect.com/science/article/pii/S0277953620303919?via%3Dihub

Murphy, B. (2019, October 17). *A medical resident's guide to gifts from industry.* American Medical Association. http://www.ama-assn.org/delivering-care/ethics/medical-resident-s-guide-gifts-industry#:~:text=For%20that%20reason%2C%20the%20AMA%20Code%20of%20Medical,including%20patient%20education%2C%20and%20is%20of%20minimal%20value

Nemko, M. (2022, February 28). The need for mutual respect in a relationship. *Psychology Today.* http://www.psychologytoday.com/us/blog/how-do-life/202201/the-need-mutual-respect-in-relationship

Ng, S. L., Crukley, J., Kangasjarvi, E., Poost-Foroosh, L., Aiken, S., & Phelan, S. K.

(2019). Clinician, student and faculty perspectives on the audiology-industry interface: Implications for ethics education. *International Journal of Audiology, 58,* 576–586.

Office of Inspector General, Office of Public Affairs. (1999). *Federal Anti-kickback Law and Regulatory Safe Harbors Act* [White paper]. http://www.oig.hhs.gov/fraud/docs/safeharborregulations/safefs.htm

OpenAI. (2024). *ChatGPT* [Large language model]. Retrieved May 22, 2024, from http://chat.openai.com/chat

Palmisano, P., & Edelstein, J. (1980). Teaching drug promotion abuses to health profession. students. *Journal of Medical Education, 55*(5). https://doi.org/10.1097/00001888-198005000-00013

Pashkov, V. M., Harkusha, A. O., & Harkusha, Y. O. (2020). Artificial intelligence in medical practice: regulative issues and perspectives. *Wiadomosci Lekarskie, 73,* 2722–2727. http://pubmed.ncbi.nlm.nih.gov/33611272/

Pederson, C. (2023, November 22). *Trust vs. performance: The bedrock of leadership and team success* [Online forum post]. LinkedIn. http://www.linkedin.com/pulse/trust-vs-performance-bedrock-leadership-team-success-chris-pederson-4auzc/

Pfeffer, J. (2018). *Dying for a paycheck.* HarperBusiness. https://jeffreypfeffer.com/books/dying-for-a-paycheck/

Plante, T. G. (2010, September 19). Three ethical questions that we should ask of ourselves every day. *Psychology Today.* http://www.psychologytoday.com/us/blog/do-the-right-thing/201009/three-ethical-questions-we-should-ask-ourselves-every-day

PWC. (2021, December 20). How organizations can mitigate the risks of AI. *Harvard Business Review.* http://hbr.org/sponsored/2021/12/how-organizations-can-mitigate-the-risks-of-ai

Reddy, S. S., & Chao, S. (2020). Academic collaborations with industry: Lessons for the future. *Journal of Investigative Medicine, 68*, 1305–1308. https://doi.org/10.1136/jim-2020-001636

Schmerling, R. H. (2020, June 22). First, do no harm. *Harvard Health Blog*. http://www.health.harvard.edu/blog/first-do-no-harm-201510138421#How%20Practical%20Is%20"First,%20Do%20No%20Harm

Schwartz, B. (2021). The social psychology of the gift. *American Journal of Sociology, 73*(1). http://www.audiology.org/wpcontent/uploads/2021/05/2011_Research_Ethics_Guidelines.pdf_539978b57f7708.62116006.pdf

Sharma, A. K. (2024, January 1). *Twelve risks and dangers of artificial intelligence (AI)*. Caclubindia. http://www.caclubindia.com/articles/12-risks-and-dangers-of-artificial-intelligence-ai-50844.asp

Sierles, F. S. (2006). The gift-giving influence. *AMA Journal of Ethics, 8*(6), 372–376. https://doi.org/10.1001/virtualmentor.2006.8.6.ccas3-0606

Simionato, G., Simpson, S., & Reid, C. (2019). Burnout as an ethical issue in psychotherapy. *Psychotherapy, 56*, 470–482. https://doi.org/10.1007/s43681-022-00195-z

Siniger, Y., Wilber, L. A., Fabry, D., & Jacobsen, G. (2011). *Guidelines for ethical practice in research for audiologists*. American Academy of Audiology. http://www.audiology.org/wpcontent/uploads/2021/05/2011_Research_Ethics_Guidelines.pdf_539978b57f7708.62116006.pdf

Solanki, G., Grundy, J., & Hussain, W. (2022). Operationalizing ethics in artificial intelligence for healthcare: A framework for AI developers. *AI and Ethics*. https://doi.org/10.1007/s43681-022-00195-z

Stichler, J. F. (1998). Developing collaborative relationships. *AWHONN Lifelines, 2*(3), 53–54.

U.S. Department of Justice. (2024, February 23). *The False Claims Act*. http://www.justice.gov/civil/false-claims-act

U.S. Federal Trade Commission. (n.d.). *Enforcement policy statement on deceptively formatted advertisements* [Policy brief]. http://www.ftc.gov/system/files/documents/public_statements/896923/151222deceptiveenforcement.pdf#:~:text=As%20the%20Commission%20set%20forth%20in%20its%201983,and%20unambiguously%20to%20overcome%20any%20misleading%20impression%20created

Utah Code, 58 Occupations and Professions § 501. (2024). http://le.utah.gov/xcode/Title58/Chapter1/58-1-S501.html

Ventiv Technology. (n.d.). *Five things every risk manager should know about total cost of risk*. http://www.ventivtech.com/blog/5-things-every-risk-manager-should-know-about-total-cost-of-risk

Weidener, L., & Fischer, M. (2023). Teaching AI ethics in medical education: A scoping review of current literature and practices. *Perspectives on Medical Education, 12*, 399–410. https://doi.org/10.5334/pme.954

William Shakespeare. (n.d.). Literary Devices. https://literarydevices.net/william-shakespeare/

Zenger, J., & Folkman, J. (2023). Seven ways to make employees feel respected, according to research. *Harvard Business Review*. http://hbr.org/2023/06/7-ways-to-make-employees-feel-respected-according-to-research

24 Administering a Medical School Audiology Practice: A Career Retrospective

Michael Valente, PhD

Editors' note: This chapter is a departure from all others in this book. It reflects many of the accomplishments of one of the most renowned audiologists of the past 50 years, Dr. Michael Valente. Unlike the other chapters, it is written in the first person. This is done deliberately, as it puts the reader inside the author's head. This allows for an intimate portrayal of his thoughts during critical junctures throughout his career as a clinician, researcher, and Business Manager. Readers who find themselves in a similar situation—academically trained as a clinical audiologist and then suddenly thrust into the role of managing a large not-for-profit department within an esteemed medical center—are sure to benefit from his firsthand account of his 30-plus years at Washington University School of Medicine. In this chapter, he shares many of the personal and engaging experiences that made him a legendary figure within the profession.

Introduction

The author's journey and experience with clinic administration administering an Audiology practice within a Medical School can present significant opportunities as well as significant challenges that may not be present when administering Audiology practices in other environments discussed in this textbook. This is especially true if the Medical School is rated within the top three and the Department of Otolaryngology-Head and Neck Surgery is rated within the top 10 in the country. In such an environment, the expectation for scholarly activity and research is very high for the Director and any staff members wishing to engage in such activities. Those expectations may not be part of the expectations in other environments. Also, the services provided to patients are expected to be "state of the art." Again, this expectation may not be present in other environments. In fact, the faculty and staff within the adult Audiology division are expected to contribute to developing these new "state-of-the-art" services. In addition, the Director is expected to administer the clinic so the clinic demonstrates profitability in spite of the fact that many services and policies required to support the clinic (i.e., billing and collection, scheduling, information technology [IT], Business Manager, etc.) may not provide a level of service one might hire if working in another environment. It is an environment where the Director is responsible for their staff but also responsible to meet the needs of a large, ever-changing number of Audiology interns and externs, physicians and residents within and outside of the immediate department. Finally, there can be a significant degree of "politics" present within the department and across the Medical School, in addition to interaction with professionals having egos that can be quite challenging. Some or all of these challenges may be unique in a Medical School environment that may not be present at all or perhaps to a smaller degree in other environments.

For 34 years (1986 to 2020), I directed the Adult Audiology Division within the Department of Otolaryngology-Head and Neck Surgery at Washington University in St. Louis School of Medicine (WUSM). Prior to this position, upon completing my graduate studies, I spent 6 years as a faculty member at a regional state university in the Department of Speech Pathology and Audiology. In that position, I taught undergraduate and graduate Audiology courses and supervised in the Audiology clinic 2 days a week. This was at a time when audiologists were not allowed to dispense hearing aids but rather referred patients to hearing aid dispensers. My next position was as a staff member at Veterans Administration hospitals in Omaha for

3 years and Atlanta for 1 year. This was followed by returning for a faculty appointment in the Department of Speech Pathology and Audiology at a large state university, performing essentially the same duties I had in my initial position described above at the regional state university.

At the time, I was at a large state university and felt a need to grow and challenge my comfort level. I enjoyed the teaching and patient care that were parts of my previous positions, but I found that my position felt comfortable and lacking challenges. I could have continued in this latter position for the remainder of my career and I probably would have been successful. I felt I was good at what I was doing (teaching, supervising, and patient care), but I felt an urge to take on a position that would be challenging and stimulating. I felt this need, despite the fact of it possibly resulting in being less than successful. I felt I needed to look for something that was out of my comfort zone to see if I had the physical and mental skills to be successful.

In late 1986, a position matching such a desire became available at WUSM. When I interviewed for the position to direct the Adult Audiology Division within the Department of Otolaryngology-Head and Neck Surgery at WUSM, it was made clear by the Chairperson that renewal of my faculty appointment was contingent upon demonstrating that the division was profitable. Further, I was required to demonstrate scholarly productivity by publishing in peer-reviewed journals having high impact factors.

An intriguing aspect of accepting this position was that I had no prior administrative experience at that point in my career. I had no prior business experience. I did not even know the difference between the terms "being in the red" or "being in the black." Also, at that point, I had had only one manuscript published in a peer-reviewed journal and research was not at the top of my list in what I wanted to accomplish as an audiologist. The only job responsibilities I had experienced at that point that interested me were teaching and providing high-quality patient care.

By accepting this position, I had accomplished my goal of seeking an environment that was challenging and stimulating and would test my abilities to succeed in a domain where I had no prior experience. As I started this new position, I had no idea if I would succeed. In fact, I thought the odds were that I would not succeed.

I retell this story about my career journey not to brag, but rather to encourage readers who might be experiencing self-doubt about their skills. I would suggest that you challenge yourself. Do not assume you cannot be successful. If you fail, which you will not, you will always have your prior skills to fall back on. I cannot begin to tell you how many times I repeated this advice to students and staff over my 45 years of teaching at the universities and while providing service at the Veterans Administration hospitals and WUSM.

Through information imparted within this chapter, my hopes are to relate to readers how I approached my new position managing the Adult Audiology Division within a Medical School environment, so the Division was profitable and concurrently becoming heavily engaged in academic activities. My goal in this chapter is to provide great detail in some sections to give the reader a sense of what it was like to be "in my shoes" at the moment decisions needed to be made.

Organization of the Division of Adult Audiology

Within every professional environment (e.g., Medical School, university, hospital, Veterans Administration hospital, not-for-profit, industry, big box, etc.), there will be differences in the organization and operation of an Audiology program. No two clinic operations within the same type of professional environment operate in the same way. No two directors have the same personality, life experiences, professional experience, and vision. For example, at WUSM, patient services for cochlear implants, vestibular services, and services for the pediatric population were independent divisions headed by other colleagues. In other Medical School environments, all of these services might be under the leadership of one individual.

Figure 24–1 illustrates the organization chart for the Adult Audiology Division at WUSM. It should be noted that I have been retired for 3 years and now carry the title of Professor Emeritus. Information imparted here is from my perspective, based upon work I accomplished during my years of service. As with any clinic, this information may not reflect the current state or status quo. In addition, this author recognizes there are and would have been myriad ways to structure the directorship duties. In my position, I directed the operation of three clinical sites. The largest clinic

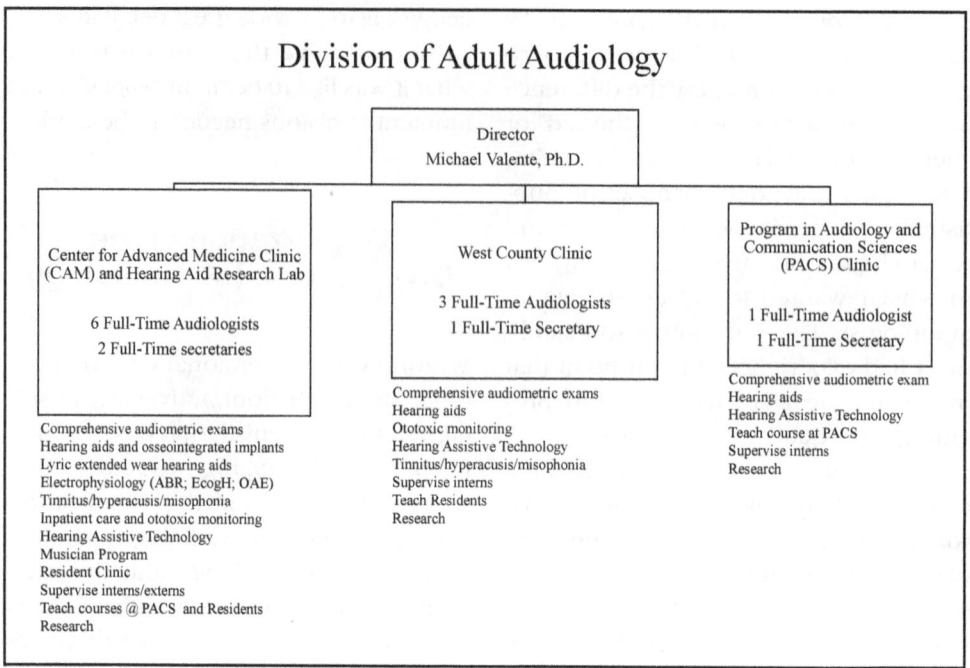

Figure 24–1. Organizational chart of the Division of Adult Audiology.

was housed in the Center for Advanced Medicine (CAM), which also housed the primary Otolaryngology physician outpatient clinic, the resident clinic, and provision of inpatient services to patients at Barnes-Jewish Hospital, which was directly affiliated with Washington University School of Medicine. The West County Clinic (WC) was a large clinic housed in the Washington University Patient Services Building and Barnes-Jewish West County Hospital, located approximately 15 miles west of CAM. This clinic served Audiology patients as well as patients referred from Otolaryngology physicians who scheduled some of their patients at WC as well as CAM. The last clinic was the Audiology clinic situated in the Central Institute for the Deaf (CID) building that was the home for the AuD program within the Program of Audiology and Communication Sciences

(PACS). In this arrangement, the "in-house" Audiology clinic was operated by the Department of Otolaryngology and the AuD program paid the department a fee to manage the clinic. This clinic saw private patients and was the primary training site for students within the AuD program. At the CAM, there were six full-time equivalent (FTE) audiologists and two FTE secretaries. At our West County Clinic, there were three FTE audiologists and one FTE secretary. At PACS, there was one FTE audiologist and one FTE secretary. Figure 24–1 lists the variety of clinical services provided at each site. What is not illustrated in Figure 24–1 is the organization of the division within the Medical School. I was directly responsible to the Chairperson of the department. The Chairperson was directly responsible to the Dean of the Medical School. The Dean was directly responsible to the chancellor of the university. Fortunately, in my 34 years, I never had to schedule a meeting with the Dean or chancellor to explain my decisions. I did, however, on many occasions explain my decisions to the Chairperson during our monthly meetings or in the hallways.

The Four Responsibilities as Director of Adult Audiology Within a Medical School

As the Director of Adult Audiology, there were four major responsibilities with many specific duties under each of these four areas, which will be described in great detail in the pages that follow. These responsibilities were clinical care, teaching, academic activities/research, and administration. One advantage of the position was how time was scheduled. While patient care appointments were scheduled on specific days and times (other than the occasional add-on or walk-in), the other three responsibilities had no definitive time within a day that the responsibility was addressed. The schedule was eventually modified to reduce patient care responsibilities to 2 full days a week, and the other three responsibilities were handled with flexibility.

A special note is required here. Although patient care was provided 2 days a week, other responsibilities tended to spill over. For example, it was not uncommon while treating patients to receive emails, text messages, and/or phone calls to address some administrative issues. There were times while walking a patient to see a physician that it would be necessary to stop in the hallway to address an issue requiring "immediate care." At other times, while in the office preparing patient notes, someone would walk into my office seeking an answer to some administrative issue. These interruptions to address administrative issues also occurred very often when while conducting "teaching moments," interacting with students in the Hearing Aid Research Laboratory.

The other aspects of this position that were enjoyable were the autonomy and lack of micromanaging by two of three Chairpersons. This autonomy was earned over time because many decisions and actions led to profitability and an active research laboratory that led to increased national and international recognition for WUSM. Also, there was little or no staff discord. Although administration comprised the majority of my time, I will discuss this responsibility later because that responsibility was the most complex.

At this point, it might be helpful to digress a bit to address the concept of the *workweek*, as it was part of my responsibility to define and implement this. That is, what were the expectations of the professional staff? On paper, the Director position was one FTE, which meant a 40-hour workweek. As Director, however, and as any director and other professionals can relate, the actual workweek far exceeded 40 hours. Sometimes it was as many as 60 to 80 hours per week. There was always the need to take unfinished work home to complete and respond to emails and phone calls in the evening and on weekends. There were weekend and evening faculty meetings and retreats. When one elects to take a position requiring scholarly work, that requirement requires

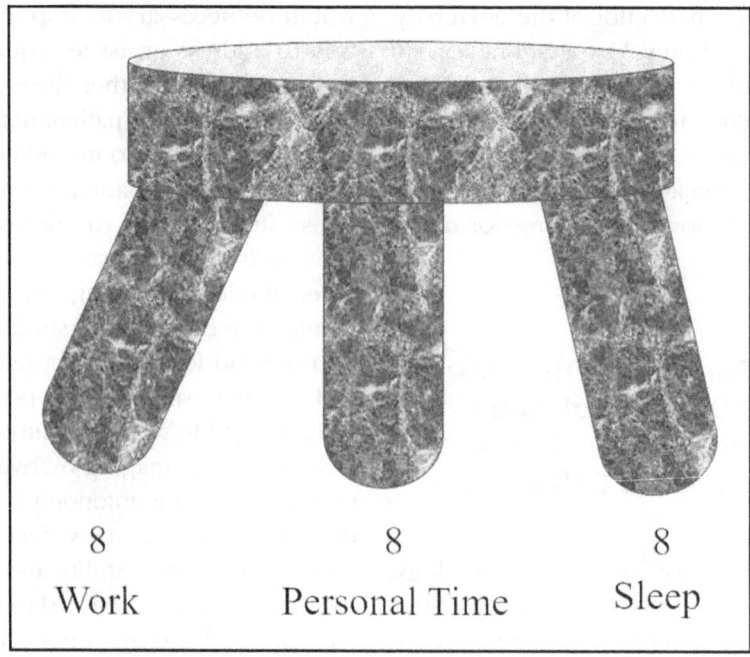

Figure 24–2. Analogy of life as a three-legged stool when life-work is balanced.

presenting the findings from the clinic or research laboratory at state, national, and international professional meetings. In my career at WUSM, I gave 344 national and international presentations, with most being invited and typically presented on weekends. In addition, while electing to take a position requiring scholarly productivity, this requirement resulted in preparing 16 textbooks, 29 chapters, 44 manuscripts in peer-reviewed journals, and 48 manuscripts in non-peer-reviewed journals. When one has a research laboratory, the responsibility includes deadlines for manuscripts and budget planning that typically creep into the evening and weekends. There was also the opportunity to chair three Best Practice Guidelines for the American Academy of Audiology (AAA) and the American Speech-Language-Hearing Association (ASHA). Again, the time to

complete those tasks was typically in the evenings and on weekends. Do not mistake this as bragging, complaining, or whining as all of these challenges and opportunities are enjoyed as career highlights.

Although a strong work ethic is essential to success, these figures should have been created much earlier. In Figure 24–2, the analogy of a three-legged stool illustrates the importance of achieving a *work-life balance*. In Figure 24–2, the length of the three legs supporting the stool is equal: 8 hours each for work, personal time, and sleep. In Figure 24–3, the stool is *imbalanced* because the leg for work has now expanded to 12 hours at the expense of personal time that is now reduced to 4 hours. Professionals should not automatically be expected to shift from a balanced to an unbalanced lifestyle as a by-product of their positions. While there are times this responsibility shift might temporarily occur due to deadlines, it should not extend for long periods of time. If it continues too long, *burnout* soon follows along with increased tension within the workplace and/or at home. This may lead to seeking a new position, leaving the profession, or worse. As discussed later, no matter the cause, the process to replace a staff member is incredibly expensive in time and money and should avoided at all costs, no matter if it is a major Medical School or a small private practice.

It should be an additional responsibility of the Director or practice owner to recognize this work-life balance and take the necessary steps to address any imbalance. Many personal issues arose with staff (e.g., maternity leave, jury duty, sick child or significant other, death of a family member, car or home repair, etc.). In all my 34 years, I was proud that I ALWAYS responded, *"Do what is necessary because family comes first. We'll find a way to make sure the clinic operates. That is not your problem."*

I was fortunate in my 34 years that no audiologist within my purview was ever dismissed. Those who did resign left to take positions closer to home, moved because a spouse took another position away from St. Louis, or transferred to another division within the department

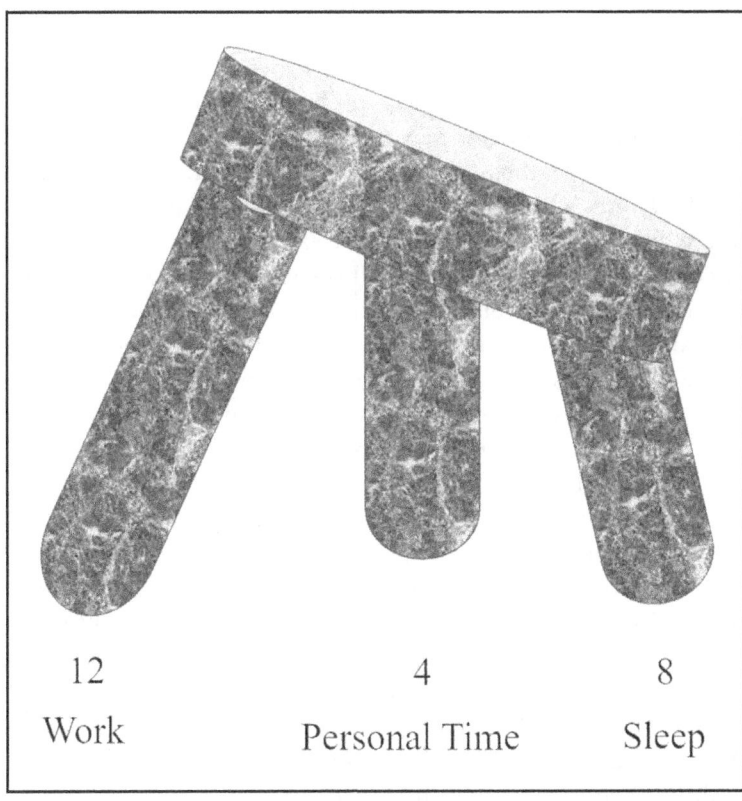

Figure 24–3. Analogy of life as a three-legged stool when life-work is unbalanced.

because they felt it was new and more challenging. In fact, three staff transferred to the Cochlear Implant Program and one transferred to the vestibular team. Six others left to pursue a PhD as a direct outcome of being involved with collaborating with the Hearing Research Laboratory within our division. A few resigned to seek part-time employment at other facilities because I required full-time employment. In a bit of humor, although it was not funny at the time, I hired an audiologist and within 2 weeks he came to my office to announce he was leaving because he decided he no longer wanted to be an audiologist. I never saw that one coming, nor could I have prevented the professional change of heart.

The remainder of this chapter will delve in great detail into how I approached each of these four areas of responsibility as Director. The reader must keep in mind that another Director may have approached each of these areas quite differently. There is no "right answer," and there are many admirable directorship styles, although these worked well for me at the time. As I mentioned above, within any similar organization (e.g., Medical School, hospital, private practice, etc.), there may be significant differences in the manner of the operation of the clinic. That is one of the wonders of human behavior: the ability and freedom to shape your daily activity in whatever vision you may have. Our critical thinking skills allow us to realize that the manner in which we make decisions today may be different tomorrow, as new information and ideas are received. We keep up with the ever-changing healthcare landscape, with no two days ever being the same.

Audiology 1986 Compared to 2020

The provision of patient care in 2020 was not the same as it was in the beginning. In 1986, computers, the World Wide Web, digital technology, Electronic Medical Records (EMRs), cell phones, email, Noah interface, telemedicine, digital signal processing and noise reduction, remote fine-tuning, rechargeable batteries, digital audio files available on audiometers, Microsoft Office, digital scanned ear impressions, video otoscopy, and so much more were not available.

In spite of these advances over time, in some respects, clinical patient care remained the same, but it was provided using newer equipment and technology. The procedures used to perform comprehensive audiometric examinations, speech audiometry, and immittance audiometry remained the same as it was in 1986. Although the equipment changed, WUSM always assessed pure-tone thresholds at 3000 Hz and any mid-frequency where there was a difference of ≥ 20 dB HL between octaves. We still always used full lists when assessing word recognition scores and always used recorded speech and not monitored live voice (MLV).

The newer audiometers and immittance units, among other things, allowed the staff to deliver speech materials via audio files downloaded to the audiometer instead of recordings on discs or CDs. This equipment also allowed staff to immediately download audiometric and immittance results completed through a commercial software package (e.g., AudBase) to the patient's EPIC EMR. This is in comparison to the previous procedure of completing the audiometric examination with red and blue pens and then copying the audiometric results manually for placement in the patient's paper medical record. Additionally, there was the manual writing of progress notes in a patient chart and, finally, placement in a *medical records room*. As technology became more advanced, audiometric and immittance results became immediately available to the Otologist, resident, or Otolaryngologist in the clinic, providing clinical care via the EPIC EMR used by the Medical School. This was quite different because previously, the audiologist was required to copy the audiometric results and escort the patient and results to the physician or nurse. Additionally, the staff member could complete the patient report via EPIC and immediately forward it to the patient's EMR. One additional advantage was the ability of patients to access their results if they were enrolled in the Medical School "MyChart" patient portal.

New Technologies and Procedures Adopted for Use at WUSM

An important component of any clinic in improving patient care is the addition of new technologies and procedures as they emerge. As Director of the clinic, the policy was to meet with the staff member to discuss their idea while assessing if the new procedure or technology added value to existing provided by the clinic.

A small sample of some of these new procedures and technologies that WUSM adopted over time is presented below:

- Tinnitus retaining therapy (TRT).
- Real ear measures (REMs).
- Misophonia and hyperacusis therapy.
- Dispensing Lyric hearing devices.
- Bone-anchored devices.
- Telehealth.

THE BLESSING AND CURSE OF NEW EQUIPMENT AND PROCEDURES

The adoption of most of these new procedures or technologies required *downtime* for one or more staff to learn the equipment or procedure, then train other staff members on its implementation into the clinical use. This downtime obviously impacts *billable hours*. The other consideration is that some of these new technologies or procedures are expected by staff, patients, and faculty to be part of a program housed in a Medical School that might not ordinarily be expected in other environments. This expectation is both a blessing and a curse. The blessing was that the WUSM clinic was always on the cutting edge of new technological advances. The curse was the substantial time and effort required to effectively introduce these procedures and technologies into the clinic.

- Over-the-counter (OTC) hearing aids.
- Musician hearing program.
- Hearing assistive technology.
- Bedside audiometry-ototoxicity.
- Hidden hearing loss.

Discussion for New Technology and Procedures

A procedure used by the WUSM to initiate use of a new technology or procedure was to request that the clinicians address:

- What would be the benefit to patients by obtaining this technology or offering this new procedure to patients?
- What would be the benefit to the clinic, interns and externs, the department, and the Medical School?
- What would be the costs affiliated with training (i.e., airline, hotel, ground transportation, registration).
- What would be the proposed number of patients who might desire or benefit from this new service?
- Is the new procedure or technology covered by Medicare, Medicaid, or other third-party reimbursement?
- What would be the time required to be away from clinic responsibilities to attend and implement training, as well as to create policy/procedures for our policy/procedure manual?

The Clinical Culture

Part of administering the clinic was the responsibility of ensuring that the Audiology staff members were never viewed as "technicians" but rather as an integral part of the success of the department in its missions of patient care, research, and teaching. The Audiology staff were fortunate at WUSM to interact with medical faculty and resident physicians that respected audiologists as vital members of the Otolaryngology team. Very few physicians over the years dictated patient care. Typically, the audiologist obtained a case history, administered whatever diagnostic procedures the audiologist deemed necessary, and counseled the patient on the results. The audiologist also scheduled whatever follow-up visits or procedures might be necessary (e.g., hearing aid evaluation, auditory brainstem response, vestibular evaluation, etc.). Patients were often directly scheduled with the audiologist upon appropriate referral from the patient's primary care physician. Patients were also referred by the audiologist to department physicians and physicians in other departments within the Medical School. Equally important were the referrals of physicians in numerous specialties who referred patients to the Audiology clinic for diagnostics and treatment. In addition, the Audiology staff members were directly involved in education and research projects with the physicians and residents. This "equal" interchange was not a "given," and it was earned over the years by the excellent care provided by the Audiology staff as well as research productivity.

Although the relationships between the audiologists and physicians at WUSM were excellent, there were two clinic issues that were particularly frustrating, in my opinion. One issue was handling physician *add-ons*. "Add-ons" often required immediate clinical care when the audiologists already had full patient schedules. It often required administrative diplomacy to provide this service without frustrating Audiology staff. This was often at the expense of the care provided by the audiologist to their patients.

The other frustration was cerumen removal. Although cerumen removal is within the scope of practice for audiologists, all the Chairpersons (otolaryngologists) during this 34-year tenure felt that cerumen removal *should not be provided* by audiologists for a variety of legal and medical reasons.

The clinic always received a very large percentage of patients arriving with excessive cerumen. Using this model presented by these chairs, the Audiology staff had two options:

- Reschedule the patient after the cerumen was removed by their physician.
- Call the Otolaryngology clinic to see if an Otologist, a resident, or other physician would agree to remove the cerumen.

The problem with this option was that it was often difficult to find a physician willing to perform this task. Second, if a physician or resident could be found, it often required a long delay before the cerumen was removed. This delay would create significant problems in evaluating that patient later in the day while concurrently caring for other patients already scheduled.

Three other frustrations in operating an efficient clinic were the large number of *no-shows*, patients arriving late for a scheduled appointment, and *walk-ins* for hearing aid care. These three issues resulted in clinical disruptions, and eventually policies were developed that reduced these issues.

Forms to Clarify Policy and Improve Communication Between Staff and Patients

As there was a need to clarify policy and communication among staff and their patients, numerous forms were required to facilitate this communication at WUSM, which may or may not be the same forms that could be used in other clinics. These forms may, however, be guidelines for other clinics and modified as necessary to facilitate their needs. At WUSM, it was found that these forms not only increased communication but also improved the efficiency of the clinical operation.

Figure 24–4 through Figure 24–13 illustrate examples of several clinical forms that were implemented. Since fees change over time, the reader should note that all forms discussed below, where charges were applied, simply will show only the $ symbol. All of these forms were reviewed and approved by legal counsel of the Washington University School of Medicine and the administrator of the department responsible for negotiating hearing aid contracts. Thus, they are proprietary and may not be reproduced. In an ever-changing clinical world, it is probable that many of these forms have been deleted, modified, or newly created within the WUSM clinic.

The Drop-Off Form

The Drop-Off Form (Figure 24–4) was designed because a fair number of patients simply arrived at the clinic and requested to see their audiologist to address a problem with their hearing aid(s) or earmold(s). The staff recognized the importance of patients having access to

Center for Advanced Medicine (CAM)-Adult Audiology
4921 Parkview Place, Suite 11A
St. Louis, MO 63110, 800-437-5430

Patient Name: _____   Date of Birth: _____

Phone Number: _____   Audiologist _____

Reported Problem: _____
_____

MAKE:_____ MODEL:_____   SERIAL NUMBER:_____

Additional Items Included: _____
....

ACTION TAKEN: _____
_____

Charge for Repair: $ _____   **Charges** (Bold indicates out-of-warranty service):

Date Patient Called: _____   **Drop Off Fee:** $

☐ **Tubing Change:** $, **Repair:** ☐ 6 mo:$ ☐ 12 mo:$

☐ **Replacement Receiver:** $

Additional Notes: _____
....

Repair Picked Up By: _____   Date of Pick-Up: _____

Figure 24–4. Form to provide care for hearing aids that were dropped off. *Source*: Washington University School of Medicine in St. Louis.

their hearing aids, but at the same time, it was difficult to address the concern due to the heavy clinic schedule. The staff's inability to immediately address their patients' needs was a source of concern, but at the same time, they had other patients to care for. Due to no-shows, cancellations, or late arrivals it was often possible to quickly resolve the problem, but this only reinforced the behavior.

To address this problem, a "drop-off" form was developed and used in all clinics. Typically, the patient arrived at the clinic and was instructed to give the hearing aid(s) to our secretary. Our secretary told the patient they would hear from their audiologist within 1 to 2 work-

ing days. The patient was also informed, when appropriate, that a loaner hearing aid would be available at no charge if they wanted to schedule an appointment. The secretary would fill out the form including the patient's name, date of birth, phone number, make/model/serial numbers of the devices, and any items left with the aids (carrying case, earmolds, etc.) and, finally, identify the patient's audiologist. Further, the secretary would document the problem(s) as described by the patient and they were informed of any potential charges depending upon if the aids were in or out of warranty. If out of warranty, the fees were highlighted, and the patient was counseled to consider purchasing an extended warranty to avoid charges in the future. Charges were made for the replacement of receivers for all devices that were not under warranty. If the aid was repaired in the clinic, an electroacoustic analysis and dehumidification was completed as part of the repair. In all cases, patients were charged a fee for dropping off the hearing aid(s). The new policies included in this form (i.e., drop-

off fee) were sufficient in many cases to stop the previous habit of dropping off hearing aids without an appointment.

Loaner Hearing Aid Form

It often became necessary for a hearing aid or hearing aids to be sent back to the manufacturer for repair because the problem could not be resolved in the

LOANER HEARING AID CONTRACT

_____

I, _____, acknowledge receipt of

Make:_____ Model:_____ Serial #:_____

hearing aid/earmold.

I assume responsibility for the condition of this aid and any repair costs

excluding those of normal maintenance and wear. Should this aid be lost or

stolen, I understand that I am fully responsible for the replacement cost and

authorize Washington University to charge the credit card listed below.

Credit Card Type:_____ CC#:_____

Expiration Date:_____ Cardholders Name:_____

I have read and understand the above.

_____
Patient's Signature (or Guardian)   Date

Figure 24–5. Loaner hearing aid form. _Source_: Washington University School of Medicine in St. Louis.

clinic. At WUSM, the patient was provided a loaner hearing aid at no charge while the aid was being repaired (Figure 24–5). Often, the loaner aid had to be programmed as closely as possible to those parameters that were in the hearing aid sent for repair. The patient was required to provide credit card information in order to receive loaner aid, although all patients returned the loaners and there was never a need for a credit card charge.

Dispensing of Hearing Aids to Patients Whose Coverage Is Not Provided by WUSM

Many of our patients had insurance coverage where third-party payers covered the cost of hearing aids completely or partially. Often, patients were informed by their insurers that WUSM was a provider for hearing aids. Unfortunately, in many cases, WUSM was not a provider for their program, and it was uncomfortable to inform the patient that they had received misinformation from their insurers. As will be reported later, our division provided hearing aids for only one or two third-party insurers who allowed the division to balance bill. (Balance billing allows the provider to bill for the balance not covered by the insurance program.) This form was used to document the patient's understanding that hearing aids through their insurance were not covered by the division. If the patient still elected to receive hearing aids through the division, then the patient and witness signed the form

---

DEPARTMENT OF OTOLARYNGOLOGY
HEAD AND NECK SURGERY

DIVISION OF AUDIOLOGY

Patient name _____
Date_____ Date of Birth_____

I understand that the Division of Adult Audiology does not contract with any insurance plans (except United Healthcare) for hearing aids and related services and full payment is expected at the time the hearing aids are dispensed. If I file for reimbursement to my insurance company, I understand that Washington Unive. "t Dept. of Otolaryngology will not apply any contractual adjustment that my i. sur. ce might apply to my hearing aid charges. Should my insurance company remit payment for the hearing aids to Washington University I will only be refunded the actual payment received from my insurance.

Patient Signature _____

Date_____

Witness Signature _____

Date _____

Figure 24–6. Form signed by patients stating the division does not dispense hearing aids to their third-party payer. *Source:* Washington University School of Medicine in St. Louis.

presented in Figure 24–6, which was then placed in their EMR. At this point, the patient understood that they would be responsible for payment at the time service was rendered. The patient was advised to submit our invoice to their insurance plan. In the rare case of insurance payment, the department would refund some or all of the actual payment received from the insurance company to the patient.

Extended Warranty

Hearing aid repairs can be expensive, and this form was used to counsel the patient on the advantages of extending their hearing aid warranty. In the patient file, staff documented the expira-

tion of the warranty for the hearing aids. At a visit prior to the expiration of the manufacturer's warranty, the staff provided patients with this form to help them understand out-of-warranty repair costs (Figure 24–7). This information was shared with the patient at the hearing aid evaluation, hearing aid fitting, and the hearing aid assessment. This form also counseled the patient on how many times the warranty can be extended regarding the specific manufacturer and the advantages of extending the warranty. The charges on this form were reviewed annually to assess any necessary fee changes. As a note, the abbreviation MRN on this form and several others stands for medical record number. This number was one of several methods of

Patient Name: _____ Date: _____ DOB_____ MRN_____

Your hearing aid(s) warranty expires on _____.

If Warranty Extended		If Warranty Not Extended	
Drop-Off Service	$0	Drop-Off Service	$
HA Check/Clean	$0	HA Check/Clean	$/$
Repair	$0	Repair	$ to $ (6 to 12 mo. warr.)
Receivers	$0	Receivers	$ to
Loss and Damage	$0 deductible/aid	Loss and Damage	New hearing aid purchase

Maximum Warranty Length by Manufacturer:

☐ **Phonak:** Four Years of Total Warranty (e.g. one-year additional warranty for Level 1, two for Level 2-3)
☐ **Resound:** Five Years of Total Warranty (e.g. two-year additional warranty for Level 1, three for Level 2-3)
☐ **Starkey:** Unlimited as Long as Device is Functioning.
☐ **Widex:** Four Years of Total Warranty (e.g. one-year additional warranty for Level 1, two for Level 2-3)

The cost of extending the warranty through _____ (one-year after expiration) is as follows:

Hearing Aid check/clean, repair, and loss/damage warranty is $ per hearing aid, per year.

This warranty covers drop-off service, hearing clean and check, receivers, and repairs at **no cost**. Also includes a loss and damage policy with a $360 deductible per aid. Loss and damage policy can only be used one-time.

Total Cost: ☐ (one hearing aid). ☐ $ (two hearing aids)

Please call us at 314-362-7509 by _____ to let us know if you wish to extend the warranty.

Figure 24–7. Form counseling patients on extending hearing aid warranty. *Source*: Washington University School of Medicine in St. Louis.

```
                    DIVISION OF AUDIOLOGY PRICES

Common Hearing Aid Supplies
Hearing Aid Batteries (Power-One, 1.45 V)...................................... $ for 8-pack
Dri-Briks (Each)..................................................... $/3; $/6 (1 yr. supply)
Phonak BR Desiccants............................................................$/2; $/8
Zephyr Dry-N-Store............................................................. $
Dri-Aid Kit/ Dri-Aid Desiccant "Pillow ................................... $/$
Hearing Aid Cleaning Spray.................................................. $
Earmold Air Blower.......................................................... $
Otoease.................................................................... $
All Other Hearing Aid Supplies (Oaktree)................................. MSRP

Earpieces
Earmold Impression for Monitors........................................... $ (includes both ears)
Custom Earmolds for Hearing Aids or Custom Hearing Protection.........$ per ear
Musicians' Earplug (includes appointment to verify).......................$ each, $ set

Loss and Damage Deductibles
ESCO L and D.............................................................$ per device
Adult Audiology L/D deductible............................................$

Out of Warranty Services:
Appointments:
Drop-Off Fee.............................................................. $
Hearing Aid Service....................................................... $ (15 min.) $ (30 min.)
Extended Comprehensive Repair  oss &  Dai. ge........................ $ per device, per year

Prices Do Not Include S rvice Fee:

Out of war anty replace nt  t re eivers (3 month warranty)
Phonak and  esound........................................................ $ per receiver
Widex..................................................................... $ per receiver
Starkey .................................................................. $ per receiver

Hearing Aid Repairs: Out of Warranty                          (Warranty)
Repair (6 month warranty)................................................ $ (6 mo.)/ (12 mo.)
All-Make Repair > 5 years old............................................ $ (6 mo.)/$ (12 mo.)
Manufacturer Repair for Hearing Aids > 5 years ........................ $ per device (6 month)

Hearing Aid Remakes + Repairs
Remake (still in repair warranty)......................................... $ per device
Remake + Repair (6 month warranty) ...................................... $ per device
Remake + Repair for Hearing Aids > 5 years (6 month warranty)........... $ per device
Remake + Repair (1 year warranty) ....................................... $ per device
```

Figure 24–8. Menu of costs for hearing aid supplies. *Source*: Washington University School of Medicine in St. Louis.

quick retrieval of a patient's record from the EMR system.

Charges for Hearing Aid Supplies

This form provided patients with the various charges for hearing aid supplies, earmolds, loss and damage, out-of-warranty repair, replacement of receivers, remakes, and repairs (Figure 24–8).

The changes in this form were reviewed annually to assess any necessary changes.

Hearing Aid Charge Invoice

This is a form provided to patients at the time hearing aids were dispensed and adhered to state licensure requirements (Figure 24–9). For patients with insurance allowing balanced billing, the insurance company was contacted by our secretary to document eligibility, authorize dispensing, and inform the patient the amount paid by the insurance company and the remainder by the patient. All communication about this conversation was documented and placed in the patient's EMR. This information was used by the audiologist to obtain approval from the patient to order the aids, earmolds, and accessories. This invoice documents the total cost of the hearing aids, earmolds, and accessories; the amount the patient will pay; and the amount that will be paid by their insurance. The patient was also informed that they would be required to pay any

HEARING AID SERVICES

MRN_____

DATE_____

PATIENT NAME_____   DIAGNOSIS

CODE_____

DATE OF BIRTH_____   BILLING

PROVIDER_____

CPT CODE_____

Hearing aid for the right ear...$_____

MAKE _____   MODEL _____   SERIAL # _____

WARRANTY _____   BATTERY SIZE _____

CPT CODE_____

Hearing aid for the left ear..$_____

MAKE _____   MODEL _____   SERIAL # _____

WARRANTY _____   BATTERY SIZE _____

ACCESSORIES

CPT CODE_____ DESCRIPTION_____
                     SERIAL#_____ $_____

CPT CODE_____ DESCRIPTION_____
                     SERIAL#_____ $_____

TOTAL CHARGES FOR THE DAY..$_____

AMOUNT PAID TODAY...$_____

<u>RIGHT TO CANCEL</u>

You may return an undamaged hearing aid for refund within 30 days after the date of your fitting. The refund will consist of the cost of the hearing aid minus a _____ service/rental fee per hearing aid.

Please note, refunds on cash or check payment may take 4-6 weeks to process.

PATIENT SIGNATURE_____ **DATE**_____

AUDIOLOGIST SIGNATURE_____

LICENSE NUMBER_____

Figure 24–9. Invoice for new hearing aids. *Source*: Washington University School of Medicine in St. Louis.

LYRIC HEARING AID SERVICES

PAT. ACCT. NO.:_____ DATE:_____

PATIENT'S NAME:_____ INSURANCE:_____

ADDRESS:_____ DX CODE:_____

_____ PROVIDER CODE:_____

PHONE:_____

The following are your charges for a Lyric device through Washington University School of Medicine:

☐ CPT CODE _____

Device for the right ear .... $ _____

_____   _____   _____
MAKE   MODEL   LYRIC ID

_____   _____   _____
CONDITION   SUBSCRIPTION EXP.   DEVICE SIZE

☐ CPT CODE _____

Device for the left ear .... $ _____

_____   _____   _____
MAKE   MODEL   LYRIC ID

_____   _____   _____
CONDITION   SUBSCRIPTION EXP.   DEVICE SIZE

Total Charges .... $ _____
Amount Paid .... $ _____
Balance .... $ _____

PATIENT: _____   DATE: _____

_____ AUDIOLOGIST

Figure 24–10. Invoice to dispense Lyric hearing device. *Source*: Washington University School of Medicine in St. Louis.

difference if the division did not receive payment. Fortunately, our division did not experience this problem for reasons described later.

Patient Invoice for Dispensing Lyric Devices

This reflected adherence to state licensure requirements as Lyric devices are leased on an annual basis, not purchased (Figure 24–10).

Form for Providing Services for Hearing Aids Purchased Elsewhere

Staff members often provided services to patients whose hearing aids were purchased elsewhere but were not sat-

---

DIVISION OF ADULT AUDIOLOGY

Service Options for Hearing Aids Purchased Outside of School of Medicine

Patient name: _____

Date: _____

_____$0 minutes or $0/hour: Unbundled hearing aid service option. The charge for hearing aid services is based on the time taken to complete the services and charges must be paid at the time of the service. Services can include: hearing aid programming and completion of real-ear measures to appropriately verify the hearing aid fitting, counseling on use, care, and maintenance of hearing aid, hearing aid cleaning, hearing aid troubleshooting, and verifying hearing aid performance. Out of warranty repairs, earmolds, and changing earmold tubing are charged separately.

_____$0/hearing aid: Bundled hearing aid service option. This one-time fee includes services for the lifetime of the hearing aid. Services include: hearing aid programming and completion of real-ear measures to appropriately verify the hearing aid fitting, counseling on use, care, and maintenance of the hearing aid, hearing aid cleaning, hearing aid troubleshooting, and verifying hearing aid performance. Out of warranty repairs, earmolds, and changing earmold tubing are not included and are charged separately.

Patient Signature: _____

Figure 24–11. Counseling patients on policy for division to provide care for hearing aids not purchased in the division. *Source*: Washington University School of Medicine in St. Louis.

isfied with their performance. Once the patient learned the division dispensed hearing aids, they would often request that one of our audiologists service the hearing aids. The patient was informed that the division can accommodate the request but that the division must charge for this service. The service agreement in Figure 24–11 provides two options. One option is simply reprogramming the aids and the other option is to provide complete care for a year. The charge for the first option was unbundled and charged in 15-minute increments. The second option was a single bundled fee providing coverage for a year. The form in Figure 24–12 required the signature of the patient.

Form Explaining Our Bundled Approach

Figure 24–12 was presented to patients at the time of their hearing aid fitting to inform them that care for aids pur-

chased using the bundled model would be provided at no charge for the duration of warranty. They were further informed that charges would begin upon the termination of the warranty. The patient was also counseled that they could pay for an extended warranty upon the expiration of the original warranty. The patient and a witness signed and dated the form. The bottom half of this form applied to patients with a third-party payer where balanced billing was applied.

Advanced Beneficiary Notice (ABN)

This notice informed the patient that the audiologist, upon obtaining the patient's signature, would provide services for the hearing aid evaluation, hearing aid fitting, and hearing aid assessment related to bone-anchored hearing devices (Cochlear and Oticon) (Figure 24–13).

DIVISION OF ADULT AUDIOLOGY

Patient Name: _____

Date: _____ Date of Birth:_____ MRN: _____

I understand all care for my hearing aids will be provided at no charge from the Division of Adult Audiology at Washington University School of Medicine to the expiration of my hearing aid warranty on _____. At the expiration on the warranty of my hearing aid(s), I understand I will be responsible for payment to the Division of Adult Audiology for all visits at the prevailing hourly rate.

Patient Signature: _____ Date: _____

Witness Signature: _____ Date: _____

☐ UHC Hearing Aid Benefit (Do Not Need to Sign)

I understand that the Division of Adult Audiology does not contract with any insurance plans (except United Healthcare) for hearing aids and related services and full payment is expected at the time the hearing aids are dispensed. If I file for reimbursement to my insurance company, I understand that Washington University Dept. of Otolaryngology will not apply any contractual adjustment that my insurance might apply to my hearing aid charges. Should my insurance company remit payment for the hearing aids to Washington University I will only be refunded the actual payment received from my insurance.

Figure 24–12. Form counseling patients purchasing hearing aids as self-pay and others using insurance with balanced billings. *Source*: Washington University School of Medicine in St. Louis.

As with other services not covered by Medicare (Chapter 17), the signed ABN form is required so that the patient understands that this service will not be covered under their insurance program.

Scholarly Academic Activity and Teaching

The most significant difference between being employed as a Medical School audiologist and a typical Audiology private practice is the opportunity to be involved in academic scholarly activities. These include, but are not limited to, supervision of interns and externs, lectures, teaching, and research. Virtually all the staff, including interns and residents, took part in these activities. Examples of these opportunities are described below.

■ *Teaching assignments within the Washington University School of*

Medicine Program in Audiology and Communication Sciences. Teaching routine courses to residents in Otolaryngology and to the community on various issues within Audiology.

■ *Audiology grand rounds.* Each month for 10 months of the year, all the audiologists and researchers investigating issues related to hearing in the Medical School (>35 audiologists) had the opportunity to plan sessions and topics for these grand rounds meetings.

■ *Research grand rounds.* Every month throughout the year, all the department research faculty and staff members met for "research grand rounds." Audiology staff presented data from the Hearing Aid Research Laboratory.

■ *Faculty grand rounds.* Every month throughout the year, all faculty, residents, and researchers involved with hearing presented data from the Hearing Aid Research Laboratory.

■ *Resident training program.* Audiologists taught courses in comprehensive audiometric examinations, electrophysiological measures, and amplification.

---

ient Name:_____Date of Birth_____MRN:_____

Insurance does NOT pay for the services required by your audiologist to properly fit your Baha. This cost will be $. I will be responsible for this cost at the time of the fitting of the Baha. This fee includes the programming and verification of the performance. It also includes all follow-up care and future appointments with the audiologist related to the processor for the duration of the warranty of the device. Which is typically two year.

WHAT YOU NEED TO DO NOW:

- Read this notice, so you can make an informed decision about your care.
- Ask any questions of your audiologist that you may have after you finish reading this.

Signing below means that you have received and understand this notice. You will also receive a copy.

Signature:_____   Date_____

I have selected _____ as the color for my sound processors. I understand that that if I wish to exchange the processor for a different color I will be charged a restocking fee by Cochlear Corporation.

Baha System: _____ Baha Attract   _____ Baha Connect

Baha Processor: _____ Baha 5   _____ Baha 5 Power   _____ Baha Super Power

Please circle your choice of accessorie (2 for first-time Baha orders, 1 for upgrades)

Remote Control – Allows for easier control of volume and program settings

Phone Clip – Uses Bluetooth to stream phone calls and music from a cell phone

Mini Microphone – Allows for easier conversation in a noisy environment

TV Streamer – Streams sound from the connected TV directly into the Baha processor

Oticon processor: _____ Ponto 3   _____ Ponto 3 Power   _____Ponto 3 Super Power

Included Accessory:

Oticon Medical Streamer: direct access to mobile phone calls, music and much more. It has a built-in telecoil and can also act as a remote control for the sound processor. No additional accessories are needed.

Figure 24–13. ABN for bone-anchored devices. *Source*: Washington University School of Medicine in St. Louis.

■ *Resident Audiology rotations.* Aside from the "formal" resident training described above, all staff members were actively involved in training of the residents as they rotated through the Audiology clinic.

■ *Clinical grand rounds.* One staff member taught a weekly 1-hour "clinical grand rounds" course that all the students in the first 3 years of the WUSM PACS AuD program were required to attend.

■ *Audiology INTERNS AND EXTERNS.* All staff members in the three clinics were involved with internship and externship training. Interns arrived at the clinics 2 full days a week for the semester and (fourth-year) externs arrived at the clinics 5 days a week for 9 to 10 months.

■ *Capstone Projects.* As part of the requirements for graduation from PACS, students were required to complete a yearlong Capstone Project. Staff members were directly involved in these Capstone Projects as either the primary advisor or a second reader.

■ *Publications and presentations.* A Medical School requires scholarly work and the staff members collaborated on books, book chapters, national meeting posters and presentations, articles for peer-reviewed and non-peer-reviewed journals, and writing grants to bring funds into the program.

■ *WUSM–PACS AuD Program.* There were many opportunities to teach courses within the AuD program.

Thus, the main difference within a Medical School program, as with some other university programs, is that scholarly activities are expected simultaneous with the maintenance of an ongoing profitable clinical operation. While this was often a monumental task at WUSM, it offered tremendous opportunities for staff to be both an academic and a clinical audiologist.

Administration Responsibilities

Introduction

The position of Director of the Adult Audiology Division constantly changes. Over time, the Director position required more administrative responsibilities. In a large Medical School program, these administrative responsibilities are continuously changing, with changes in the Chairperson and physicians who were added or departed. These changes required modification of adaptation to their preferences within the Audiology clinics as well as clinic schedule modification to provide adequate coverage. Other issues such as Medical School policy changes, new state and federal regulations that involved the opening and closing of clinics, and designing and overseeing the building of new Audiology clinics all contributed to the increased administration time relative to clinical service and research time.

Assigning Staff Administrative Responsibilities

Across the three WUSM adult Audiology clinics, there were 12,000 patient visits annually, and this number kept growing. These three clinics dispensed

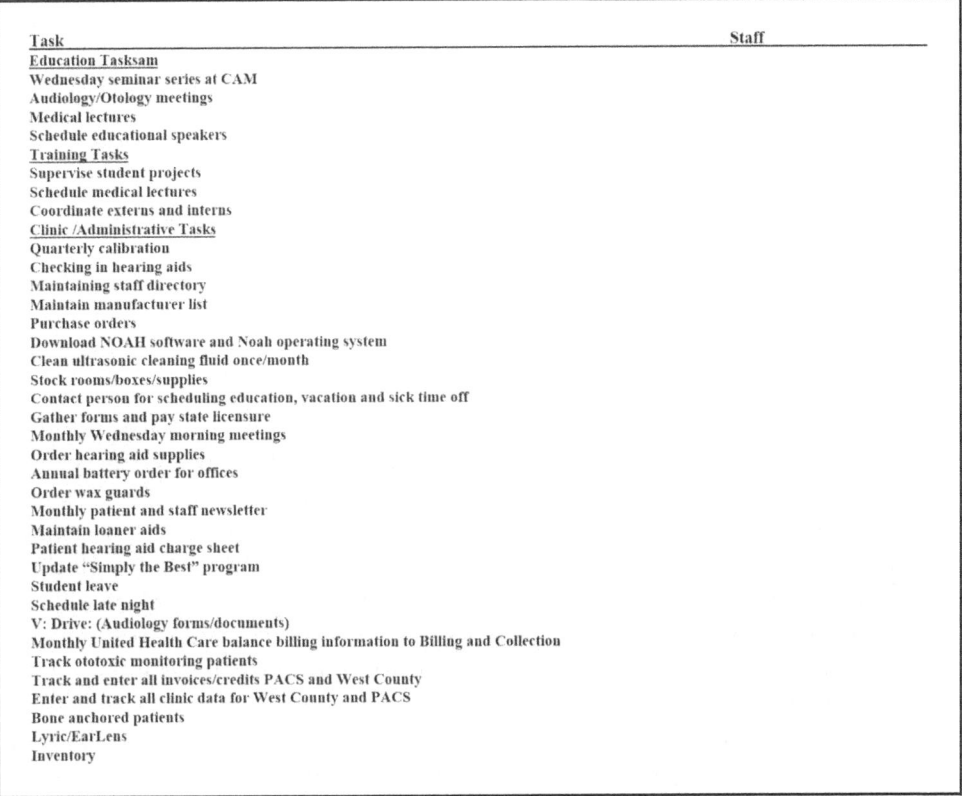

Figure 24–14. List of tasks assigned to staff.

850 hearing aids every year. These clinics all had the same type of mundane routine responsibilities related to calibration of equipment and specific issues that were relative to these individual clinics along with all the other expected scholarly activities (Figure 24–14). To handle all of the responsibilities, it was necessary to delegate many of these responsibilities to other staff members.

Figure 24–14 lists 36 tasks assigned to various staff members, and with their input, this list continued to grow. It is difficult to appreciate the degree to which these mundane tasks occupied the time of the staff and the Director, so that requires some explanation. A review of the tasks listed in Figure 24–14 provides the reader with some insight into the complexity, diversity, and time required to maintain the three clinics. Specifically, these tasks were:

Quarterly Calibration of Equipment

A staff member checked the calibration of the audiometers, sound field, and immittance units quarterly to ensure they adhered to current ANSI standards. They also checked the calibration of the hearing aid test boxes and real ear systems (reference and probe microphones and loudspeakers) at the three clinic sites. Due to the large volume of equipment pieces, this task often took the better part of a day. To facilitate these tasks, a schedule was created within each booth and with rotating audiologists, performing daily listening checks prior to patient contact for the day. In addition to these listening checks and quarterly calibrations, a local company with two or three employees came annually to complete exhaustive calibrations of all the equipment at the three clinical sites.

Download Updated Manufacturer Software and Noah Operating System

Three audiologists (one at each site) were assigned to download new versions of the hearing aid manufacturers' Noah software as well as software updates for our Frye, Aurical, and Audioscan real ear analyzers. When a new version of the Noah operating system was released, it was necessary to contact the Medical School IT department as the Noah database for all three clinical sites were on a secure network.

Scheduling of Vacations and Sick and Educational Time Off

One staff member was assigned as the "point person" for all staff members. To request vacation or time off, each staff member was instructed to call this person when the staff member or member of the family was sick requiring the staff to be out. Other reasons for calling might include the inability to work due to weather or perhaps a problem with an automobile. Still other reasons were jury duty, bereavement, and so on.

This designated staff member tracked the requests by means of a spreadsheet and these data were sent to the Director monthly so all time off could be tracked.

This method proved to be quite effective to ensure that no staff took more time away than allowed WUSM policy. I also had a policy to limit vacation requests to no more than 1 week unless international travel was involved or if there were special circumstances.

Ordering of Batteries

A large portion of the patient population still is using conventional hearing aid batteries. To reduce cost, the division purchased the various battery models in bulk twice a year. This task was assigned to one staff member to handle the purchase and delivery for all three clinics. This audiologist worked with the Director to negotiate the lowest possible price, as well as the distribution of the stock to the three clinics. These semiyearly orders were based on clinic statistics showing the battery types (e.g., 13, 10, and 312 batteries) of hearing aids dispensed.

Order Hearing Aid Supplies

As with batteries, our division ordered hearing aid supplies in bulk in order to receive a significant discount. For example, each patient was provided an electronic dehumidifier when new hearing aids were dispensed. This task was assigned to one staff member at each site.

Consignment (Loaner) Aids

All three sites had a large supply of loaner hearing aids that would be provided at no charge while a patient's hearing aid was repaired or being replaced due to loss. Each loaner aid was measured in a 2cc coupler to be sure it was in good working order. The aid and

2cc printout were placed in a cabinet at each site and an inventory was created with make/model/serial number, along with a printout from the measurement (gain, output, frequency response, equivalent input noise level, distortion, etc.). When the aid was loaned, the audiologist documented the name of the patient, date of birth, and the date it was loaned on the loaner hearing aid form (Figure 24–5).

Monthly Patient and Staff Newsletter

One staff member prepared a monthly newsletter that was emailed to patients who provided their email addresses as well as all faculty and staff members. This newsletter was placed in the waiting and counseling room at the three clinics. These newsletters imparted updated information about division activities, research studies, presentations, publications, and helpful tips about care of hearing aids, earmolds, and accessories. The newsletter also highlighted a story about a staff member and their accomplishments each month. Some newsletters also included stories about a physician, a resident, or front office, billing, and/or scheduling personnel.

Update "Simply the Best" Program

Each clinic had a large display case containing various working hearing assistive devices. These displays included personal listening devices, TV listening devices, alerting systems, amplified telephones, amplified stethoscopes, and so on. These displays were provided at no cost to the clinic by Oaktree Prod-

ucts and contributed greatly to sales of these items.

V Drive (Audiology Forms and Documents)

The V drive was a computer location where all the forms used in the clinic were available. This location offered a separate, secure drive within the computer system where all forms, brochures, and other division documents were stored.

Enter and Track All Clinic Performance Data

An audiologist at the WUSM–PACS clinic and one at the West County clinic were recruited to enter data and present the Director a monthly spreadsheet on a variety of measures related to clinic performance and costs of goods. Each audiologist at these two clinics used the same spreadsheet as the third clinic. The Director merged these data into performance spreadsheets to track the financial status of the clinics.

Monthly United Health Care (UHC) Balanced Billing Information for Billing Office

The division had an agreement to dispense hearing aids to patients who enrolled with a specific United Health Care policy, which allowed the clinic to dispense hearing aids using balanced billing. In this scenario, the patient was charged the same amount as a self-pay patient. When the devices were dispensed, part of the cost was paid by the patient and the balance billed to UHC. One audiologist was assigned to gather the information from all the audiologists

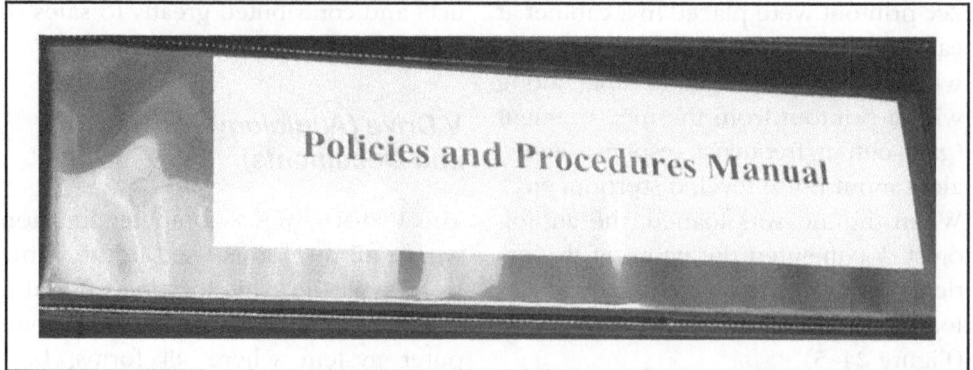

Figure 24–15. Three-ring binder containing division policy and procedure manual.

about these patients. Data were collected regarding the UHC hearing aids dispensed from the three clinics and forwarded to our billing and collection office to track payments from UHC. These data allowed a staff member from billing and collection to send this audiologist a report to document the accuracy of the UHC payments. The WUSM Adult Division arbitrarily allowed 3 months for payment to be received before we notified billing and collection to contact UHC to determine the status of the delayed payment.

Inventory

The department Business Manager required an inventory twice a year of all audiometric equipment, computers, copiers, monitors, printers, and fax machines at the three clinic sites. This task was assigned to the Director.

Education and Meetings

As can be seen in Figure 24–14, there were several educational seminars, lectures, meetings, retreats, conferences, and other professional development opportunities that the staff regularly attended. These were scheduled and forwarded to all staff members and secretaries of the department to ensure patients were not scheduled during these times (Figure 24–14).

Assigning Interns and Externs With Certain Clinical Tasks

Division philosophy was to include student interns and externs in some assignments of certain clinical tasks. This was to assist in the mentorship related to clinical operations and promote teamwork. For example, one year, an extern completely updated and revised our Clinic Policy and Procedure Manual (see Figure 24–15).

Marketing

Promotion of the division's services and clinical staff to the community is of paramount importance. As a not-for-profit facility, the WUSM had a policy that all clinical services, including the Division of Adult Audiology, could not market commercially (i.e., newspaper, radio, television). Thus, marketing was limited to internal promotional activities via brochures, patient hand-outs, and lectures within and outside the Medical School. The rules were clear that Audiology was able to market services but not products. The Medical School felt marketing would leave an impression on the public that the Medical School was promoting one product over another. These marketing activities were disallowed by the rules of the Medical School:

■ Hearing aid manufacturer marketing programs.
■ Meet-and-greet promotional events.
■ Mailers to patients.
■ Open houses hosted by hearing aid manufacturers.

While the division did allow for a 15% discount to current patients on new hearing aids, they subscribed to a *word-of-mouth* marketing concept believing that if a patient has a positive experience, that positivity would be conveyed to one or two friends or family members. If the experience was negative, however, then that experience would be extended to any number of the patient's circle of friends or family. Thus, the key was to always try and provide the best possible patient experience.

Presentations

Several methods to market that were allowed by the Medical School are discussed below. Most of these events were free and were provided by all staff members.

■ *Consumer presentations* at minimed school meetings described above and lectures to consum-

ers on tinnitus, misophonia, and hyperacusis.
■ *Lectures at senior living communities* in the St. Louis area.
■ *Social media* using Facebook, Instagram, Twitter (X), and the division website.
■ *Department grand rounds* presentation to other departments such as Aging, Internal Medicine, Neurology, Psychology, Psychiatry, Endocrinology, Pharmacy, Cardiovascular, and others.
■ *Various support group* presentations in the St. Louis area such as Hearing Loss Association of America, Meniere's Disease Support Group, Acoustic Neuroma Support Group, and Tinnitus Support Group.

In these presentations, it was important to convey to patients why the care provided in the WUSM Adult Audiology Division may be better than that in other facilities within the community. This was accomplished by sharing information on what services were part of our care provided and perhaps not provided by other clinics. This included the use of real ear measures to fit hearing aids to individual hearing losses using a validated prescriptive target. Our standard of care also included measures of performance in noise with and without hearing aids to determine benefit and if greater benefit might be achieved via accessories, such as remote microphones or a TV listening device. It was important in these marketing sessions to emphasize that staff members did not receive a commission based upon the dispensing of hearing aids. Further, we emphasized that the practices utilized in the clinic to dispense hearing aids were the same as advocated by the Best Practice

Guidelines of the American Academy of Audiology and American Speech-Language-Hearing Association.

The division did not accept invitations to participate in community hearing screenings as it was found that the number of referrals for follow-up care was very small. In addition, Medicare prohibited offering free services to generate other services such as diagnostics.

Brochures

The division was fortunate to have the services of a world-class marketing department at the Medical School. Over the years, members of the division worked with that department to create professional quality brochures that were placed in a variety of places throughout the Medical School and hospital clinics. The staff also brought these brochures along to the presentations provided within and outside the Medical School.

For example, as part of the hiring process for new employees at the Medical School and hospital, the division arranged for *Human Resources (HR)* to place a brochure that promoted the division within the *new employee* file and collection of resources. The number of employees at the Washington University Medical School and hospitals was over 46,000 and quite a pool to attract to the clinics help of a brochure. The division clinics also offered a 15% discount in the brochure for hearing aid services, which was also made available to faculty, staff, and family members of WUSM. This benefit was also extended to the large number of clinics in the St. Louis area operated by the Medical School. The same brochure was provided to Human Resources at Barnes-Jewish Hospital as part

of the WUSM complex. Other division brochures included:

- *Musicians' Hearing Program.* Brochures for this program were placed in the patient waiting room and clinic counseling rooms at all three clinics. This brochure highlighted the impact of loud sounds on hearing and the resulting tinnitus. The brochure also promoted hearing protection and the dispensing of musician custom earpieces.
- *Summary of services provided by the Division of Adult Audiology.* These summaries were placed in clinic rooms and waiting rooms at all three clinics.
- *Programs providing services for patients experiencing tinnitus, misophonia, or hyperacusis.* Information about these specialized programs was disseminated as deemed necessary.
- *Ototoxic monitoring program.* Brochures related to this program were placed in the pharmacy department and all the floors of the hospital. One brochure was for patients, and another was geared toward providers.
- *Connection between hearing loss and cognitive decline.* Brochures related to this important issue were developed, based on the evidence available at that time.
- *Offering of free hearing aid classes for the community.* Information about these classes was placed in patient counseling rooms and in the waiting room area.
- *Hearing assistive technology.* A display of these devices and their dispensing was described earlier with our "Simply the Best" program.

■ *Differences between conventional, OTC, PSAP, and basic hearing aids.* A brochure outlining the differences among conventional hearing aids, over-the-counter (OTC) aids, Personal Sound Amplifier Products (PSAPs), and basic hearing aids was devised. This included an explanation of using an unbundled service approach to compete with the advent of OTC devices. This brochure also described the advantages and disadvantages of each option.

Division Website

The division was fortunate to have the services of a faculty member responsible for assisting each colleague and the numerous programs in building the department website. Various members of the division worked very closely with this faculty member and his staff to develop and update the division website. Figure 24–16 illustrates the opening page of the division website. Figure 24–17 illustrates the opening page of the website for our Hearing Aid Research Laboratory. Both of these websites were available to patients by way of staff members and pointing out its availability during patient visits. For example, our research laboratory was well known within the Medical School and often patients would ask if they qualified for any of the current studies.

Division Intranet Website

Several years ago, a staff member felt our clinic was inefficient because forms for the provision of patient care were

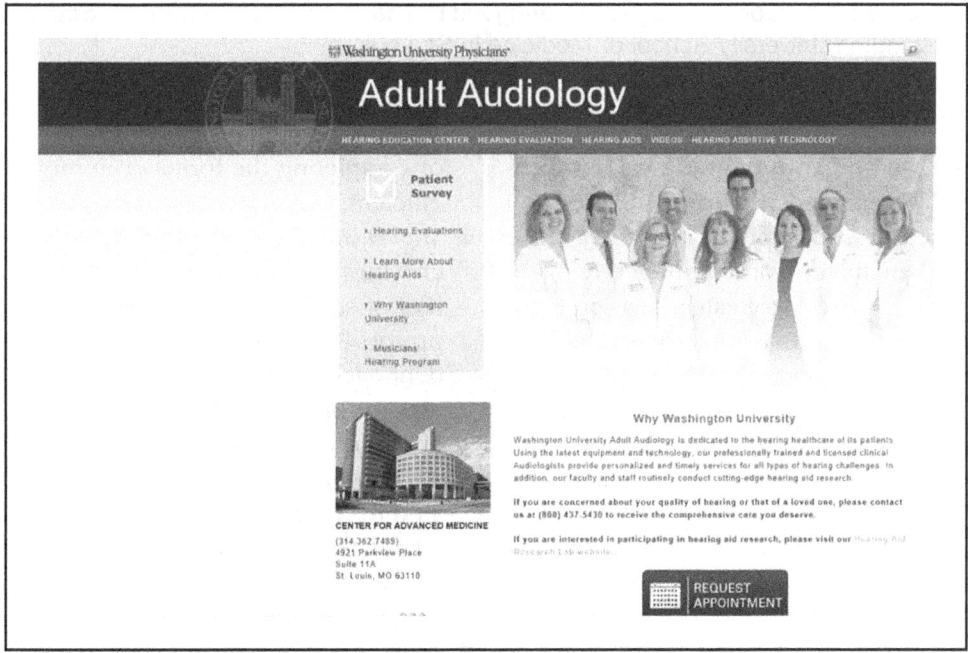

Figure 24–16. Opening page of division website. *Source*: Washington University Physicians.

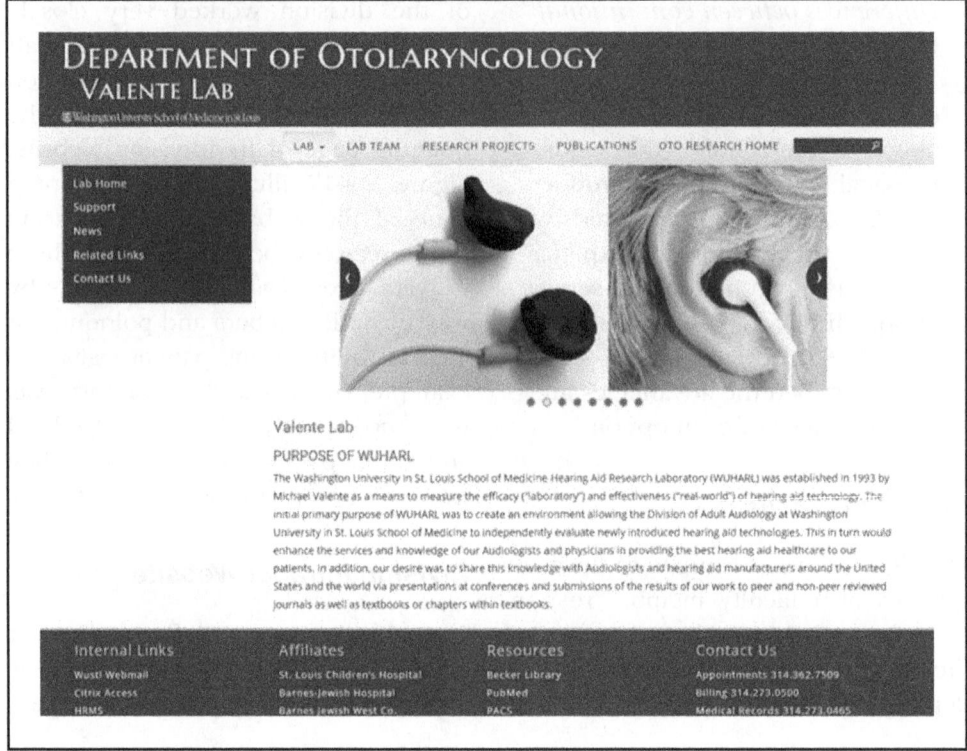

Figure 24–17. Opening page of Hearing Aid Research Laboratory website. *Source*: Washington University School of Medicine in St. Louis.

not well organized. There was no central site related to all the policies and procedures for the staff or students. The staff member worked diligently on a massive project to create a division intranet that was divided into several sections. It is important to bear in mind that the information placed in this intranet website was constantly updated with new information added or modified and older information deleted. The intranet website was divided into the following major sections:

- *Manufacturer forms for hearing aid order, repair, extended warranty, and earmold.* These forms were prepopulated to make the process of completing the forms even more efficient.

- *Supervision.* This section included checklists, instructions for testing, lists of student tasks, externship protocols, internship protocols, student evaluation information, checklists for hearing aids, and information about other supplies.

- *Personal folders.* These were created for each staff member to place whatever personal information they felt necessary to maintain within a single organized site.

- *Clinic resources.* Examples of materials housed here included the Hearing in Noise Test (HINT; Nilsson et al., 1994) test forms and

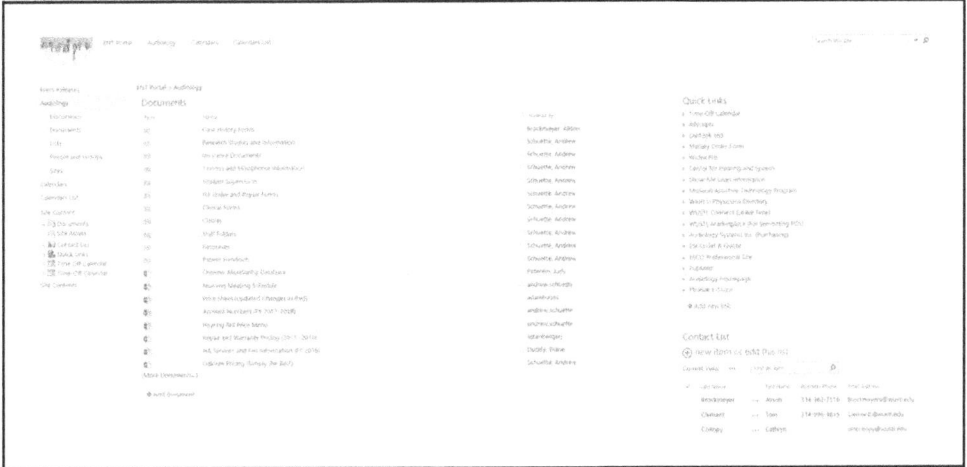

Figure 24–18. Opening page of division intranet website.

normative data, a vast quantity of PowerPoint presentations created by the staff, real measure procedures, calibration records, WUSM policies and procedures, patient information and forms on bone-anchored devices, word recognition confidence intervals, our ototoxic monitoring protocol, loaner hearing aid program information and forms, hearing aid dispensing materials and discount information, "Simply the Best" program information for assistive technology, division newsletters, Aurical Guide, Frye 7000 Guide, Audioscan Guide, AudBase Guide, EPIC EMR guide, copies of all brochures, and patient counseling handouts.

■ *Patient resources.* Links were maintained to numerous websites for a wide variety of support groups and financial assistance programs provided by the state of Missouri.

■ *Other resources.* This section included the time-off calendar, Show-Me Loan program of Missouri information, Missouri Assistive Technology Program materials, WUSM physician directory, records reflecting leave time, "Marketplace" to complete purchase orders for equipment, PubMed access information, Audiology website information, and resources relevant to our Hearing Aid Research Laboratory website.

■ *Division website.* We stored crucial information here, including that related to mechanisms for patients to request an appointment with the division (Figure 24–18).

Hiring and Maintenance Audiology Staff

Although these Human Resources procedures are generally similar to those presented within Chapter 6 relative to small businesses, universities, and major Medical Schools such as WUSM, HR procedures for major public institutions

WASHINGTON UNIVERSITY SCHOOL OF MEDICINE
JOB DESCRIPTION

DATE: 08/26/13

JOB TITLE: Clinical Audiologist
JOB CODE: H1520 **GRADE**: **FLSA**: Exempt

POSITION REPORTS TO: Director of Adult Audiology
DEPARTMENT: Otolaryngology

POSITION SUMMARY: As a clinical audiologist in the Division of Adult Audiology at Washington University School of Medicine, the candidate will divide his/her time between providing services for our Adult Audiology Clinic at the **Central Institute for the Deaf (CID) (80%)** and also serve as an integral part of student clinical education by working with the **Program in Audiology and Communication Sciences (PACS) (20%).**

For PACS:

a. Coordinate clinical placement of all 2nd and 3rd year students for the Fall, Spring and Summer semesters.

b. Supervise 1st year students who typically observe patient care in the Adult Clinic at CID.

c. Teach a one-hour course/week for the combined 3rd year students for the Fall and Spring semesters.

PRINCIPAL DUTIES & RESPONSIBILITIES OF A CLINCIAL AUDIOLOGIST:

Essential Functions:

1. Performs/interprets standard/advanced audiometric tests, selects/fits/counseling patients about hearing aids and hearing assistive technology on adult patients.
2. Evaluates central auditory dysfunction, determining level of patient condition and optional treatment methods at our Center for Advanced Medicine (CAM) Clinic.
3. Counsels on aural rehabilitation and hearing assistive technology.
4. Can conduct regular resident teaching sessions, present monthly physician briefings on research progress, and develop graphic presentations using a variety of computer based programs.
5. Supervises audiology interns and externs

Other Functions:

6. Calibrates/maintains audiologic equipment.
7. Assists with related administrative and teaching duties.

JOB LOCATION/WORKING CONDITIONS: Works in the Central Institute for the Deaf building. Normal audiology clinic environment and attendance at national/regional seminars.

CRITICAL SKILLS/EXPERTISE: Equivalent of Certificate of Clinical Competence (C-AAA) from ASHA or eligibility for clinical fellowship, with Missouri license in audiology.

MINIMUM EDUCATION & EXPERIENCE: AuD in Audiology with Missouri Audiology license.

RELATIONSHIP: Regular contact with patients, faculty and staff.

SUPERVISION: Supervises interns and externs.

The above statements are intended to describe the general nature and level of work performed by people assigned to this classification. They are not to be construed as an exhaustive list of all job duties performed by the personnel so classified.

Figure 24–19. Request to hire an audiologist. *Source*: Washington University School of Medicine.

must follow strict government regulations as to their hiring procedures. Thus, the steps to hiring a new faculty or clinical member for staff are more complicated than in a small business. Indeed, the procedures used in public institutions have a detailed process that must be followed within the Department as well as Human Resources.

The Hiring Process

At WUSM, the process begins with a meeting with the department Chairperson to discuss the need for the new position and to gain approval at the department level. After the Chairperson's approval, it was necessary to complete and submit a Job Description Form, Figure 24–19, to the department Business Manager who approved and submitted it to WUSM HR.

After the approval within the department, the WUSM Office of Human Resources assigns the position search to a staff member who reviews the job description (Figure 24–20). This description is prepared into a position announcement sent electronically to a variety of websites (American Academy of Audiology, Audiology Online) and to a distribution list of colleagues. This job description included information on responsibilities and duties, delineating that the new hire would enjoy full-time exempt employee status. Requirements of the applicant were stated, including doctoral degree, preferred years of experience, cover letter, undergraduate and graduate transcripts, vitae, three letters of recommendation on official letterhead, GRE and Praxis scores, documentation of an Audiology license if available, and the National Provider Identification (NPI) number. Applicants were also informed that if an offer was made, drug screening and a background check were required prior to hiring.

As the applications are received, there is a specific process for their reception, and processing through the search process follows Medical School and government regulations. The following outlines that process within WUSM:

■ Applicants forwarded their documents to HR, who then forwarded them to the division Director for review. The documents of all applicants were forwarded to the staff to obtain their input on which three of the applicants should be invited for an all-day interview. These interviews were held with the Director and the entire staff.

■ After interviews were completed, the staff independently ranked the three applicants. They were to express a preference as to whom should be offered the position and to express their reasons for these preferences.

■ At the interview, it was important that the Director obtained a sense

of the applicant's interest in scholarly activities such as teaching and research, honesty, sincerity, and sensitivity to the feelings of others. Each applicant was asked what they could bring to the clinic to improve clinical operations. This information offered a sense of what new procedures the applicant could bring to the program, ability to work under pressure, level of self-motivation, initiative, work ethic, being a "team player," and reliability.

■ Discussing salary can be awkward for an applicant. In presenting the offer, the Director took the initiative by immediately informing the applicant that the salary is based on years of experience and is set by the department. It was emphasized that the salary offer could not be negotiated but that salary was not the only aspect to consider about the position. The candidate should also weigh the importance of the generous fringe benefit package offered by the Medical School, department, and division. For comparison,

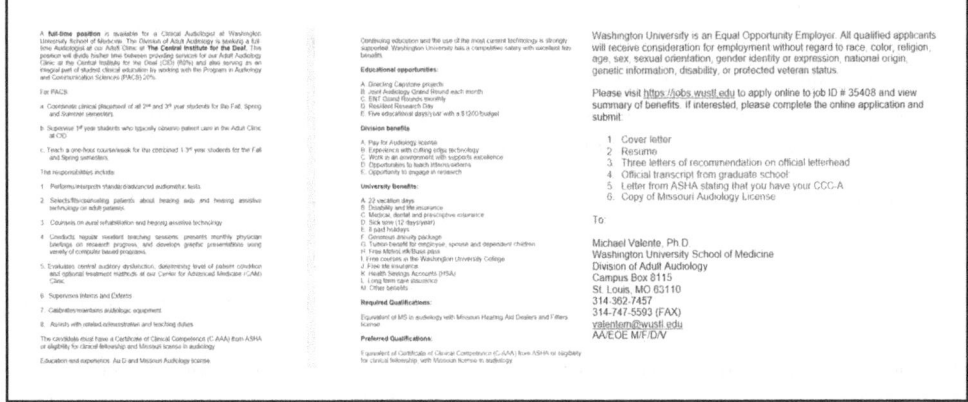

Figure 24–20. Job description for an audiologist. *Source*: Washington University School of Medicine in St. Louis.

SAMPLE MEDICAL SCHOOL AUDIOLOGY CLINIC BENEFITS PACKAGE

The following benefits package was offered to employees within the Division of Adult Audiology, Department of Otolaryngology at Washington University School of Medicine in St. Louis.

■ Excellent health, drug, dental, and vision insurance.
■ Twenty-two paid vacation days.
■ Twelve paid sick days.
■ Ten paid holidays.
■ Medical school retirement package.

To emphasize that this was an unusually generous major benefit, it was explained that the university contributes 7% to 11.5% to their retirement fund based on age, as long as the employee contributes 5% to the retirement fund. At the time, the university paid 50% of tuition for children of faculty and staff at virtually any accredited university in the United States.

■ Basic and enhanced life insurance.
■ Disability insurance.
■ Long-term care insurance.
■ Malpractice insurance.
■ Eligibility to receive a range of discounts to a wide variety of services/products because of being an employee at the Medical School.
■ Free use of mass transportation (bus and light rail) in the St. Louis area.
■ Payment for state Audiology license.
■ As previously described, there was coverage of some or all costs to attend professional meetings. Each audiologist had a $1,500 budget for educational conferences if the division was profitable.
■ Two additional days off were provided if the audiologist did not use sick days during the previous year.
■ Each staff member was allowed 5 days/year to attend educational events outside of the Medical School.

the WUSM package is quite generous, presented in the box.
■ The Director then called the selected applicant to determine if they would accept the WUSM offer and agree to a start date.

■ The department Business Manager and our contact in HR were then informed of the selected candidate and HR created an official WUSM offer for the division, and it was emailed to the applicant.

■ Upon acceptance of the offer, the unsuccessful applicants were phoned to inform them that they were not offered the position and specific reasons that they were not chosen for an offer.

■ Once the person begins their position at WUSM, the onboarding tasks for the new audiologist listed in Figure 24–21 begin. In a large medical center, the onboarding is quite detailed as there a many specific issues that must be considered.

Annual Staff Evaluation and Recommendation for Salary Increases

Each spring, the department Business Manager would present the recommended salary increases for the next fiscal year. These were mandated by the Dean of the Medical School and, typically, were between 3% and 5%. The Director of the adult division then reviews the current year budget to retrieve the

New Employee Checklist

- Start date
- Date to start scheduling patients
- Key
- ID card
- Lab coats
- Business cards
- Credentialed
- Name plate for office
- Audiology license
- Parking
- Metro pass for bus and light rail
- Orientation
- Long distance access
- OtoSecure access
- E-mail
- HIPPA training
- Username/Password (EPIC, NOAH, AUDBASE)
- Voice mail setup
- Picture for website
- Training: Frye, AudioScan, Auricle and AUDBASE
- Bio for website
- The director will audit all charts for one month or longer
- Biweekly meetings with Director
- Otology/Audiology conference
- Contact information for division directory

Figure 24–21. Form of tasks to complete when hiring a new audiologist.

total expense for salaries during the current fiscal year. For example, if the recommendation was 5%, the Director multiplied that current year budget for salaries by 0.05 to estimate the total amount of funds available to divide among the nine audiologists and four secretaries for next fiscal year. Directors' salary was recommended by the Chairperson and may differ somewhat from those recommended for staff. Additionally, this initial email regarding annual raises triggered the division's annual review process and recommendation for salary increase that was submitted to the Business Manager and Chairperson for approval.

The Annual Review Process

While this process may resemble that outlined for small business in Chapter 6, large medical centers, university positions, and other large organizations must have a significantly more detailed process.

To begin the annual review process at WUSM, the Director informed all staff members by email that it was time for their annual review. Since staff members had a copy of their review from the previous year, this was used as a reference to measure change in performance, using a number of KPIs (key performance indicators). Figure 24–22 shows the annual review form used for the nine audiologists. Figure 24–23 demonstrates the annual review form used for our four secretaries. I reminded staff members to complete the form for the current fiscal year. The secretarial staff scheduled a half-hour one-on-one meeting between each employee and Director. This was to review each staff member's performance. At the end of the review, they

were informed of the recommendation for their salary increase, but the Director emphasized that was the salary recommendation from the division, but the final decision would be made by the department Chairperson. As part of the meeting, each staff member was reminded to maintain records of all of their accomplishments throughout the current year to prepare for their next annual review. They were advised to place those accomplishments on their versions of the annual evaluation form for the next annual review meeting. The KPIs and other data points covered at the annual review were to provide their personal achievements in the following areas:

- The number of patients seen per day during the current year, as compared with the previous year. These data were collected from the current year and the previous year to access growth or retraction.
- The amount of the gross charges from the current year, as compared with those of the previous year. These data were collected from the current year and the previous year to access growth or retraction.
- Highlight any new programs or procedures they developed over the past year.
- List the presentations at local (e.g., support groups), state, or national meetings.
- Describe their research endeavors and publications in peer- and/or non-peer-reviewed journals, chapters in textbooks, or books.
- Supervision activities for externs and interns.
- Professional activities related to teaching.

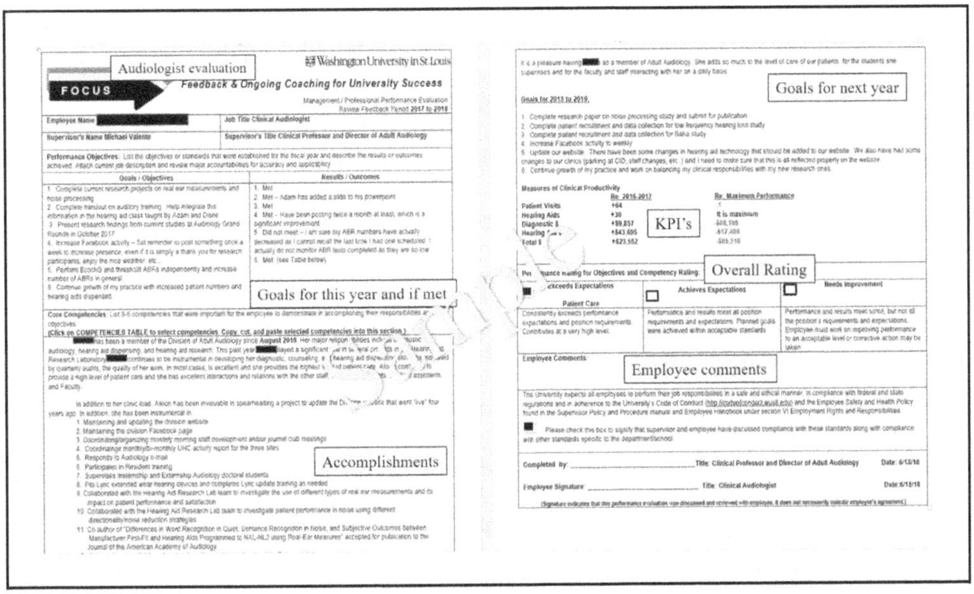

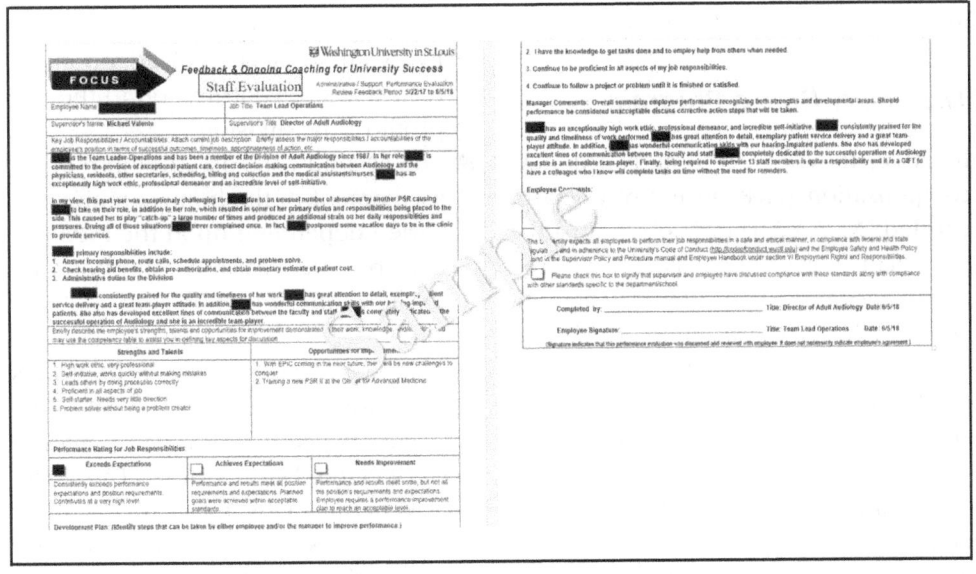

Figure 24–22. Annual evaluation form for audiologists. *Source*: Washington University in St. Louis.

Figure 24–23. Annual evaluation form for secretaries. *Source*: Washington University in St. Louis.

■ List suggestions/actions to reduce costs that they may have
implemented.

■ List suggestions/actions to enhance income that they may have
implemented.

■ List suggestions/actions to increase
efficiency that they may have
implemented.

■ List development activities of patient brochures and other instruc-
tional/counseling materials.

Audiologists were reminded that they
were not expected to evaluate patients
all day as it was reasonable to expect
that direct patient care (i.e., billable
hours) should comprise ~70% of total
work hours. This accommodation was
to provide time for the staff to accomplish the expected scholarly requirements, which was part of employment
in a Medical School environment.

The Salary Bonus Program

In 2010, the Dean announced a new
compensation package for physicians,
entitled "X, Y, Z." The X referred to the
physician's base salary. The Y referred
to the recommended annual salary increase. The Z represented a "bonus"
based on a variety of factors. Initially,
this bonus program was only for physicians, but after the Director had numerous meetings with the Chairperson and
the Dean, as well as the Office of General Counsel, the "X, Y, Z" bonus program was secured for audiologists. The
bonus program was established based
upon the Audiology division receiving
25% of the net cash profit at the end of
the fiscal year. The Director of the Division of Adult Audiology was to recommend the bonuses for the nine au-

diologists. Prior to implementing this
incentive, I met with the Chairperson and
Business Manager to create a spreadsheet identifying measures to be used to
determine the individual's contribution
to the net profit. These markers would
then be utilized to assist in the distribution of the distribution of the bonuses.
This also had to be approved by the
General Counsel's Office.

The assignment of bonuses to a very
productive clinical faculty is a difficult
process and requires some specific criteria. While the bonus amount for the
Director was determined by the Chairperson, the amounts recommended
for the nine audiologists in 2017–2018
ranged from $5,000 to $14,000. After
careful consideration of the task assigning bonuses, two rules were ultimately
part of the Director's decision for the
bonus distribution:

■ Every audiologist received a bonus
regardless of contribution to the
profit of the division.

■ The second consideration in the
assignment of the bonus amount
varied depending upon the individual's productivity and contribution
to the profit of the division.

To assist in calculation of the bonus
amount for each audiologist, the specific factors listed below were entered
into a weighted spreadsheet. These factors were similar to those reported for
the audiologist's annual evaluation reported earlier for the salary increases:

■ *Gross charges for hearing aids.* In
our division, gross charges and net
income for hearing aids were equal
because all hearing aids were "self-
pay" except for patients from the

two insurance policies where we used balanced billing. That is, the patient paid the difference between what was charged and what their insurance paid the division. This was a complicated calculation as it involved insurance companies and their payment procedures.

■ *Gross charges for diagnostics.* The net income from diagnostic services was considerably lower than the gross charge documented on the fee ticket or billing sheet and contributed less to the net profit but obviously a crucial component of the services provided by the division.

■ *Number of patients seen annually.* While an important component of clinical performance for bonus assignments, it was recognized that this was not the most accurate measure of productivity. The concern was the differences in time allocated per type of patient visit. For example, an ABR was assigned 1 hour, a hearing aid fitting was assigned 1.5 hours, and a hearing aid check was assigned a half hour.

■ *Presentations.* These were numerous and presented to a wide variety of community support groups.

■ *Growth.* This metric targeted growth in productivity, as compared with the previous year.

■ *Efforts to reduce costs.*

■ *Creation of new procedures and/or programs.*

■ *Mentoring of student research.*

■ *Supervision of interns and externs.*

■ *Teaching or presenting: resident/ physician lectures.*

■ *Publication in peer-reviewed journals.*

■ *Publication in non-peer-reviewed journals, book chapters, or books.*

■ *Attendance and presentations at national meetings.*

Figure 24–24 reports an example of a spreadsheet created and forwarded to each audiologist every month after review of the profit/loss (P/L) reports from the department Business Office. This spreadsheet reports the cumulative profit (in black) or loss (in red) for each clinical site (A, B, and C) and the sum from the three sites ("Cash P/L") as well as the calculated amount available for a bonus based on the 25% agreement. This allowed the staff to directly know if our division was achieving and maintaining a profit. In Figure 24–24, it can be seen in the lower right corner that the final net profit for the division was $276,378 and 25% of that yielded a bonus pool of $69,095 to be divided among the Audiology staff for that fiscal year. This amount was distributed among the audiologists according to the principles outlined above.

Regularly Scheduled Meetings

As Director, it was important to meet regularly with the staff, so the operation of the division was as transparent as possible. In that regard, quarterly staff meetings were scheduled, which involved travel to the peripheral clinical sites (PACS and West County) once a month to inform the staff there (audiologists and secretaries) of issues occurring at the primary clinic site (CAM), the department, and the Medical School. Annually, there were two half-day retreats for the entire staff to meet to discuss a wide variety of issues, develop goals, and answer any specific questions. In addition, monthly 1-hour meetings were conducted with all the audiologists

Monthly P/L	USE CASH BASIS FOR PROFIT/LOSS							
July		**Aug**		**Sept**		**Oct**	
A	-$5,028	A	-$11,582	A	$1,473	A	$13,463
B	$13,513	B	$4,048	B	$15,192	B	$15,578
C	$57,484	C	$76,267	C	$85,891	C	$108,634
Cost research	-$4,512	Cost research	-$8,966	Cost research	-$14,185	Cost research	-$19,404
CASH P/L	$61,457	CASH P/L	$59,767	CASH P/L	$88,371	CASH P/L	$118,271
25%	$15,364	25%	$14,942	25%	$22,093	25%	$29,568
Nov		**Dec**		**Jan**		**Feb**	
A	$32,138	A	$33,111	A	$55,500	A	$41,747
B	$17,117	B	$14,422	B	$13,734	B	$12,973
C	$134,857	C	$126,899	C	$157,591	C	$175,631
Cost research	-$24,624	Cost research	-$29,843	Cost research	-$34,356	Cost research	-$38,868
CASH P/L	$159,488	CASH P/L	$144,589	CASH P/L	$192,469	CASH P/L	$191,483
25%	$39,872	25%	$36,147	25%	$48,117	25%	$47,871
March		**April**		**May**		**June**	FINAL
A	$31,254	A	$78,880	A	$73,200	A	$30,442
B	$15,384	B	$18,920	B	$27,782	B	$42,705
C	$181,129	C	$193,893	C	$265,476	C	$260,144
Cost research	-$43,379	Cost research	-$47,890	Cost research	-$52,401	Cost research	-$56,913
CASH P/L	$184,388	CASH P/L	$243,803	CASH P/L	$314,057	CASH P/L	$276,378
25%	$46,097	25%	$60,951	25%	$78,514	25%	$69,095

Figure 24–24. Monthly spreadsheet sent to staff reporting profit or loss.

at the main clinic on campus (CAM) to discuss similar topics.

On the department level, a monthly 1-hour meeting was conducted with the Chairperson where they were updated on the activities and needs of the division. The Director also attended the monthly faculty meeting held on a Wednesday evening as well as the monthly otology/resident educational event held on a Thursday evening. Although these meetings with the Chairperson, faculty, otologists, and residents were not required, attendance was essential to keep the news of Audiology in the forefront of the minds of physicians and residents and emphasized the important role Audiology played in the department from both clinical and scholarly standpoints.

Laws That Impact Audiology

There are numerous laws, statutes, policies, and guidelines that shape the manner in which healthcare is provided to patients (Chapter 6). Many of these help to protect the rights and safety of patients and employees. The Director of an Audiology program does not need to be a lawyer, but should be aware of these laws, statutes, policies, and guidelines. Another important point is that every large organization has an Office of Human Resources. Their well-versed staff are excellent resources to seek advice to help resolve questions related to personnel issues. In addition, every large institution has some form of available legal assistance to resolve any legal issues that may arise. Often, legal assistance was sought from the WUSM Office of the General Counsel to review forms or answer questions ensuring that there was a solid legal foundation for decisions. Also, it is important to remember to retain all communication involved with the help provided by Human Resources and the institution's legal team, documenting and reinforcing the position that was taken to resolve any problem. Some important laws, statutes, policies, and guidelines with their URLs that were used in the direction of a large Audiology organization included (Chapters 6, 17):

■ *Title VII of the Civil Rights Act (1964)* (www.eeoc.gov). Covers issues related to discrimination in hiring, dismissing, or pay based on race, religion, gender, or national origin. This law also prohibits sexual harassment.

■ *Fair Labor Standards Act (FLSA)* (www.dol.gov/dol/topic/wages). Covers issues related to setting federal minimum wage but allows facilities to pay a higher minimum wage. This law mandates overtime payment for hourly employees working more than 40 hours per week (non-exempt). As mentioned earlier, audiologists were considered exempt employees and were not eligible to be paid overtime.

■ *Family and Medical Leave Act (FMLA)* (www.dol.gov/whd/fmla). Covers employees working at least a year who can take up to 12 weeks of unpaid time off but can be paid if the employee has built sufficient vacation and/or sick time. This act covers job-protected time-off for the birth or adoption of a child, care for themselves or a sick child, and care for a spouse or parent who has a serious health condition. The employee needs to apply to determine if the situation applies under FMLA guidelines. Also, it is important to recall that this law applies to organizations with 50 or more employees. These FMLA regulations do differ from state to state and should be checked for specific provisions.

■ *Age Discrimination in Employment Act* (www.eeoc.gov/laws/types/age .cfm). States that an organization cannot discriminate against applicants or employees who are greater than 40 years of age.

■ *Americans With Disabilities Act* (www.eeoc.gov/laws/types/dis ability.cfm). Prohibits job discrimination against qualified people with disabilities who can satisfy job requirements with/without reasonable accommodations. At WUSM, this law was used as a rationale to purchase new booths during several remodeling projects as the entrance to the previous sound booths did not meet requirements for wheelchair access.

■ *Uniformed Services Employment and ReEmployment Act (USERRA)* (www.esgr.org/site/USERRA/FAQ .aspx). States it is illegal to discriminate against volunteers or employees called to military duty. When reservists return from active duty of less than 5 years, the employer must reemploy the employee to their previous position or to an equal position.

- *Equal Pay Act (EPA)* (www.eeoc.gov /laws/types/sex.cfm). States that facilities cannot pay female employees less than male employees for equal work with positions requiring equal skill, effort, responsibility, and education.
- *Occupational Safety and Health Act (OSHA)* (www.osha.gov). Requires employers to provide a business free from recognized hazards and to provide education and monitoring.
- *Pregnancy Discrimination Act (PDA)* (www.eeoc.gov/laws/types /pregnancy.cfm). Prohibits job discrimination on the basis of pregnancy, childbirth, and related medical conditions. Facilities cannot dismiss employees because of pregnancy, nor can they force employees to take leave.
- *Immigration Reform and Control Act (ICRA)* (www.uscis.gov). States it is illegal to hire illegal aliens. The facility must verify identification and workplace eligibility for all employees via the employee or applicant completing an I-9 form.
- *Harassment* (www.eeoc.gov/laws /types/harassment.cfm). There are several laws prohibiting unwelcome conduct based on race, color, religion, sex (including pregnancy), national origin, age of 40 or older, disability, or genetic information. Harassment is unlawful where enduring the offensive conduct becomes a condition of continued employment or where conduct is severe or pervasive enough to create a work environment that a reasonable person would consider intimidating, hostile, or abusive.
- *Health Insurance Portability and Accountability Act (HIPPA) Privacy Rule* (www.hhs.gov/ocr/privacy). Provides protection for the privacy of individual health information. It protects the security of electronic protected health information and the confidentiality of individual health information.
- *Employee Benefit Security Administration (EBSA)* (www.dol.gov/ebsa). Deals with requirements for continuation of healthcare provisions under the Comprehensive Omnibus Budget Reconciliation Act (COBRA) and the healthcare portability requirements on group plans under HIPPA.
- *False Claims Act (FCA)–31 USC Section 3729-3733.* This act states that no one can submit a false claim, overcharge, provide substandard goods or services, or make a fraudulent request for payment. One cannot bill for services not rendered, services not medically necessary, services with an incorrect provider number, or services known not to be covered. This act prevents falsifying a patient's diagnosis, "upcoding" or billing for a service at a higher rate, and unbundling bundled codes for a greater payment. An example of the latter might be if an audiologist billed for tympanometry, acoustic reflex threshold, and reflex decay separately as opposed to billing for immittance testing.
- *Anti-Kickback Statue (AKS)– Section 11288(b) of the Social Security Act.* States that healthcare providers cannot refer patients to another provider or facility where the provider or a family member has a business interest and can draw income. It is a criminal offense to knowingly and willingly offer, pay,

solicit, or receive remuneration to entice or reward referral for items and services reimbursed by federal healthcare. No gifts, pens, note pads, trips, or cash are allowed.

■ *Food and Drug Administration Hearing Aid Dispensing Guidelines (FDA)* (www.fda.gov). These guidelines require use of referral to a healthcare provider for the red flags of ear disease. Every hearing aid sold must be accompanied by a user brochure and statements that should be contained in a purchase agreement. Each hearing aid should also be dispensed with information about hearing aid safety, the sale, the manufacturer, and correct labeling.

■ *Federal Trade Commission (FTC)* (www.ftc.gov). This agency is involved with issues related to consumer protection against deceptive or fraudulent marketing and sales practice (refund policy and warranty coverage).

Other sources of information and assistance are professional organizations where their websites contain significant information on Code of Ethics, Scope of Practice, Best Practice Guidelines, Billing, Coding, State Licensure, and Continuing Education Units (CEUs). Some of these organizations are:

■ American Academy of Audiology (AAA): www.Audiology.org
■ American Speech-Language-Hearing Association (ASHA): www.asha.org
■ Academy of Doctors of Audiology (ADA): www.audiologist.org
■ State licensure websites: these contain policies on calibration, CEUs, and Scope of Practice.

Financial Performance of the Division of Adult Audiology at WUSM

Perhaps the most time-consuming aspect of directing a large Audiology division is the constant monitoring of financial performance. While being ill-prepared for this financial responsibility, it was necessary to take some business courses within the WUSM community to facilitate the business success of the division. These courses, taken during the day and evening, were of great assistance in becoming a better administrator and improving skills in understanding the financial component of the Director responsibility.

KEY BUSINESS AND INSURANCE TERMINOLOGY

Before diving into understanding spreadsheets and the monthly profit/loss (P/L) statement, the reader should understand some of the business terms concerning the financial side of Audiology (for further explanation

continued on next page

continued from previous page

of many of these concepts, see Chapters 6, 9, 11, 14, 16, and 17). As presented here, every effort will be made to provide, when possible, examples of how the term is used in the Audiology financial reports:

■ *Gross charge(s).* This is the charge the audiologist places on a fee ticket or billing sheet for service(s). For example, in the WUSM clinics, the charge for a comprehensive audiometric examination (CPT code 92557) that included air conduction and bone conduction thresholds, speech reception thresholds, and word recognition scores was $170. This was the amount charged to the patient's insurance. When discussing finances with students and audiologists, most believe this is the income they are generating.

■ *Net income.* This is the income received as payment from the patient's insurance (Medicare, Medicaid, and other third-party payers). The rate of payment changes from year to year as contracts are renegotiated. For example, at WUSM, for the charge of $170, the division received $38.40 from Medicare, $20 from Medicaid and between $37.40 to $157.16, depending on the other third-party insurers with which the Medical School had over 150 contracts. *It should be clear that the amount collected is significantly lower than the amount billed.* Recall that it is net income that "floats the boat" and not *gross charges.* This is a very important concept to retain and understand the implications for practicing audiologists and students.

■ *Collection rate.* This term refers to the ratio between what was charged and what was received as income. In the example above for Medicare, the collect rate was 23% (i.e., $38.40/$170). Bear in mind that for Medicare, the clinic received 80% of the $38.40 (i.e., $30.72). The remaining 20% was paid by any supplemental insurance the patient might carry. If the patient did not have supplemental insurance, then either the patient was charged the 20% or this amount was written off. Also, recall the department had a resident clinic where many patients were uninsured.

■ *Payer mix.* This term relates to the percentage of patients having no insurance, Medicare, Medicaid, or private insurance (e.g., Blue Cross/ Blue Shield, United Health Care, etc.). If a clinic is heavily loaded in a payer mix of patients with no insurance, Medicare, or Medicaid, then the net income for that clinic would be poorer than that for a clinic having fewer patients in that payer mix (and more patients with private insurance). The on-campus CAM clinic had a payer mix

continued on next page

continued from previous page

more heavily filled with no insurance or Medicaid than our two other clinics. This was because the CAM clinic was the site of the resident clinic, which typically had more patients with no insurance or Medicaid.

■ *Participating provider.* This is a provider that accepts payment from Medicare. The remaining 20% of the charge may be sent to a supplemental insurance plan. If there is none or if they reject the claim, the patient may or may not be billed the remaining 20%.

■ *Nonparticipating provider.* This is a provider that does not accept Medicare patients and expects the patient to pay for services.

■ *ICD-10 CM (International Classification of Diseases–Revision 10, Clinical Modifications).* Every disease or condition and variation of a disease or condition is assigned an ICD-10 code. For example, H90.0 is a code for bilateral conductive hearing loss. H90.3 is a code for bilateral sensorineural hearing loss. Lists of these codes are available on ASHA and AAA websites. When billing, it is required to place the correct ICD-10 value on the fee ticket or billing sheet. Fortunately, these ICD-10 codes are automatically provided by electronic medical systems that audiologists typically use. The audiologist simply clicks on the correct medical condition and the software selects the correct ICD-10 number.

■ *CPT (Current Procedural Terminology).* Every test and procedure is assigned a CPT code. For example, the code for a comprehensive audiometric examination is 92557, the code for immittance is 92567, and the code for ABR is 92585. Payment for services is based on the CPT code and not the charge placed on the fee ticket or billing sheet. As presented earlier, the WUSM fee for a comprehensive audiometric examination (CPT 92557) was $170 where the Medicare reimbursement was $38.40. If the division had placed a fee of $180 on the fee ticket or billing sheet, the reimbursement would still be $38.40 because reimbursement is based on the CPT code. On a fee ticket or billing sheet, it is critical for the ICD-10 and CPT codes to align correctly, or the claim will be denied. Lists of CPT codes are also available on the ASHA and AAA websites. In addition, CPT codes are updated annually with the potential to be added or deleted (Chapter 17). Fortunately, these CPT codes are automatically provided by electronic medical systems that audiologists typically use. The audiologist simply clicks on the correct audiometric test and the software selects the correct CPT code.

continued on next page

continued from previous page

■ *Healthcare Common Procedure Coding System (HCPCS)* or *"HIC-PICs."* These are codes that identify supplies, equipment, or devices dispensed to a patient.

■ *Health Insurance Portability and Accounting Act (HIPPA).* This act protects the privacy of patients and the security of electronic information.

■ *Profit (black).* This term means that the total net income is more than total expenses.

■ *Loss (red).* In this case, the total net income is less than total expenses.

■ *Profit/loss (P/L) statement.* This term refers to a report that reports all the expenses and income and the resulting profit or loss.

■ *Cash versus accrual accounting.* In cash accounting, the profit is based upon income received. In accrual accounting, the profit is based on cash received as well as cash expected to be received at some later date. The department profit/loss was based on using the cash method of accounting.

■ *KPIs (key performance indicators).* These are various data points to measure staff performance in relative terms (e.g., current year to previous year, this year to best previous performance). KPIs can also be absolute measures (e.g., performance of a staff member, number of hearing aids dispensed in a specific month). KPIs can differ across clinical sites (e.g., private practice, Medical School, hospital, physician office, hearing aid dispensing practice). Examples of KPIs are number of patients seen, billable hours, number of specific diagnostic procedures performed, number of patient visits that were no charge, number of patient visits that were no-show, number of hearing aids dispensed, and number of hearing aids returned for credit. KPIs in a Medical School environment can also include number of presentations, number of book chapters, and number of articles published. KPIs can be used to document reasons for raises, promotions, bonuses, and so on.

■ *Loss leader.* This refers to a procedure or service that does not provide significant income to cover expenses but is important for the mission of the department or to bring other patients to the facility who require other services for which the division is paid.

■ *Bundling.* The products and services are bundled into one charge and paid at time the original service is completed. This one charge covers care for the product and associated services for the duration of a warranty. In the division, warranties ranged from 1 to 3 years depending

continued on next page

continued from previous page

upon manufacturer and level of technology. Postfit visits are completed at no charge for the professional component, but the patient may be charged for supplies. The division exclusively used the bundled method to charge for hearing aid–related services for decades.

■ *Unbundled.* The cost of the product and some essential services are combined to create a less expensive option. The patient pays when the product is dispensed. All following services that were previously included in the bundled model are instead unbundled and the patient charged separately. These services are charged from a "Menu of Services" based on the charge per hour rate and the time required to render the service. The division adopted this model in 2019 as a method to address concerns expressed by consumers as to why they did not pursue hearing aids. This concern was one reason for the introduction of PSAPs and OTC hearing devices.

■ *Direct expenses.* Typically, these are expenses that are fixed. Examples are salary, fringe benefits, and rent.

■ *Indirect expenses.* Typically, these are expenses that vary. Examples are utilities, waiting room magazines, and janitorial services.

■ *Staff bonuses.* This refers to income added to the staff base salary, based on profit and KPI measures. It is not a commission where a person receives a percentage of the income received for a product dispensed or particular service provided.

■ *Cost per hour.* This value is calculated by combining the total expenses, subtracting the expenses for products dispensed, and dividing that product by the total number of billable hours. This value is what it costs per hour to operate the clinic without obtaining a profit. Added to this value is the percentage of desired profit to create the charge/hour. This is used to determine charges for services so that the clinic is profitable at the end of the fiscal year.

■ *Procedural cost.* This term refers to the time required to complete a patient visit and attach a charge for that service based on the calculated charge per hour. The computation of time frames of 15-minute intervals was used for each type of patient visit. For example, a hearing aid check was scheduled for 30 minutes. A hearing aid evaluation was scheduled for 1 hour. A visit to complete a comprehensive audiometric examination was scheduled for 45 minutes. A hearing aid fitting was scheduled for 1.5 hours. It was important to gather this information to generate the "Menu of Services" when using an unbundled pricing approach.

continued on next page

continued from previous page

■ *Fixed cost.* These are costs that do not change from month to month. Examples are salary, fringe benefits, and rent.

■ *Variable cost.* These are costs that change from month to month. Examples are utilities, phone, marketing, and sales tax.

■ *Accounts payable.* This is a term used to denote money that is owed by the division to suppliers and others.

■ *Accounts receivable.* This is a term used to denote income received (i.e., net income).

■ *Probationary period.* This term relates to the length of time from when a new employee is hired to the time when certain benefits may be activated. For example, at WUSM, all employees received 22 days of vacation. During the probationary period, these days are accumulating but cannot be used. If the employee takes time off during this period, it is done without pay. The probationary period also relates to length of time between hiring and time when a decision is made to dismiss or convert to a permanent position. At WUSM, the probationary period was 6 months. A probationary period can be extended instead of dismissal if it is felt the staff member met many requirements but still required some additional skills training before a permanent position could be approved.

■ *Billable hours.* This term refers to the number of hours the staff members are available to bill for services. This is used to calculate cost per hour. A greater number of billable hours results in a reduced cost per hour. Fewer billable hours relate to a greater cost per hour. This explains why services provided in a Medical School may typically be greater because of the nonpatient contact requirements of scholarly production (research, teaching, etc.).

■ *Exempt employee.* Under the Fair Labor Standards Act, these employees are *professionals*. Exempt employees are paid an annual salary and are not eligible to be paid for overtime. Audiologists are exempt employees.

■ *Nonexempt employee.* Under the Fair Labor Standards Act, by definition, nonexempt employees are not professionals. Nonexempt employees are paid an hourly salary and are eligible to be paid for overtime. Secretaries are an example of nonexempt employees.

■ *Coding.* As previously discussed, it is crucial to use the correct combined ICD-10 and CPT codes to maximize payment.

■ *Reimbursement.* This is the amount received for providing services relative to gross charges. It is the same as net income, and this amount can be 0% to 100%.

continued on next page

continued from previous page

■ *FTE (full-time equivalent).* Depending on the duration of "lunch hour," this could entail a 40-hour workweek or a 37.5-hour workweek. All staff in the division were FTE and there were no part-time employees.

■ *Balance billing.* The patient pays the difference between the charge for service and the amount paid by their insurance. Net income is the same for "services applied using a combination of insurance/self-pay for remainder" and "complete self-pay."

■ *Single-unit cost.* This is the cost of a product, usually higher if purchased one at a time or infrequently.

■ *Invoice cost.* This term refers to the cost of a product appearing on the received invoice. Invoice cost is typically lower than single-unit cost, based on the volume of product purchased and negotiating skills.

■ *Continuing education units (CEUs).* These units correspond to the number of hours assigned to a course, earned at a conference, online, or within the work environment. To maintain licensure, an audiologist must receive a required number of CEUs per year.

■ *OTC/PSAP.* These abbreviations refer to over the counter and personal sound amplification products. These products were introduced to address patients' desires for less expensive options for amplification.

■ *Telemedicine.* This important term describes provision of services via the Internet or telephone. These services became very important during the pandemic when patients could not be face-to-face with healthcare providers. These services continued once the pandemic retreated. Use of telemedicine can help address the issues of accessibility and convenience that have been raised by consumers as to why they have not pursued amplification.

■ *Remote fine-tuning.* This is a service provided to a patient by an audiologist using the patient's mobile phone and manufacturer app to reprogram hearing aids remotely. In many cases, much of what can be programmed in the clinic can be programmed using remote fine-tuning. This concept also addresses patients' desires for accessibility and convenience.

■ *Advanced Beneficiary Notice (ABN).* This is a form reviewed and approved by General Counsel that is completed by an audiologist and signed by the patient. The form informs patients that the provided service is not reimbursed by Medicare (e.g., cerumen removal, fitting and programming a bone-anchored hearing aid) and must be paid by the patient.

continued on next page

continued from previous page

- *National Provider Identification (NPI).* This is required for all audiologists in order to become credentialed to bill for services. It is provided by the Centers for Medicare & Medicaid Services on its website at no cost after submitting the required form.
- *Carve out.* During the negotiation process of third-party payer contracts, hearing aid–related services are not included (i.e., carved out) for beneficiaries because reimbursement is poor. All other services, however, are provided and reimbursement submitted to the third-party payer for payment.
- *Human resources (HR).* This is the department within an organization that addresses all issues concerning employee relations. HR handles a very wide variety of services and issues such areas as hiring, dismissal, fringe benefits, and more.
- *Billing and collection.* This term refers to a department within an organization that handles all issues relative to billing for services and tracking payment for the services. All fee ticket or billing sheets are forwarded to this office for processing. These departments are often also responsible for credentialing.
- *Electronic Medical Record (EMR).* Under HIPPA regulations, all patient records are processed electronically via a secure computer network. Interactions such as billing, patient reports, X-rays, results from diagnostic tests and procedures, surgical procedures, and so forth are handled by the institution's EMR system. In many cases, these records are available electronically to a patient via a patient portal. At WUSM, this portal is called "MyChart."
- *Policy/procedure manual.* Most institutions have an HR-generated employee handbook describing all the policies and procedures of the institution. This manual is typically provided to an employee when hired, and the employee must sign a form agreeing to follow those policies and procedures or risk discipline or dismissal. In addition, departments (i.e., Otolaryngology) and divisions (adult Audiology) had their own policy and procedures manual that was readily available. The Audiology division had its own policy and procedure manual placed in the three clinics. These manuals were routinely updated to incorporate any changes.

Being an audiologist, the Director eventually viewed profitability as a signal-to-noise ratio conundrum. Imagine expenses as the *noise* and income as the *signal*. If the goal was to be *not-for-profit*, then the budget should be monitored so that *expenses* were equal to the *net income*. Staff and students often thought *income* was equivalent to *gross charges*. In this scenario, income a staff member generated was the amount they placed on the fee ticket or billing sheet submitted for reimbursement from third-party payers. It was necessary to remind staff and students that it was *net income* that "floated the boat" and the difference between *gross charge* and *net income* was quite large for diagnostic services. The difference, however, between these two values was virtually zero for the hearing aid services (e.g., hearing aids, earmolds, assistive devices, accessories, etc.) because these were self-pay services. Therefore, *gross charge* and *net income* were equal.

The goal of the division was to be *profitable*. To achieve this goal, one strategy was that the level of the *noise* (expenses) had to be reduced so the *signal* could become more prominent (i.e., greater profit). A second strategy was to increase the level of the *signal* (income) by increasing charges or scheduling more patients. The third strategy, the one ultimately selected, was to *reduce the level of the noise* and *increase the level of the signal* concurrently. The remainder of this section details how these two goals (e.g., independent of each other or combined) were accomplished.

Early Observations of Daily Operation of the Clinic Requiring Immediate Action

Usually when taking a new position, there is a "honeymoon" period where a new leader simply observes the operation but makes few changes. The new Director gathered as much information as possible to better understand the daily operation of the clinic and the overall financial health of the division. As information was gathered through

questions from the staff and the Business Manager, it was obvious that certain areas of the clinic operation could be modified to improve efficiency and profitability. In those first few months, this new Director modified the following procedures, resulting in:

- Reducing costs.
- Increasing income.
- Decreasing cost and increasing income to achieve my signal-to-noise conundrum.

The division dispensed hearing aids through a wide variety of third-party payers, and there were several significant problems with this arrangement. First, in investigating these agreements, the amount collected (i.e., net income) was significantly lower than the amount collected from self-pay patients, although the staff provided the same level of care. Second, the staff took on the task of calling the insurance companies to determine if their patients had coverage for hearing aids. Third, the problem became even greater as the staff would be told by a third-party payer that the patient was covered and they were dispensed the hearing aids, only to find after submitting charges that the patient was not covered. In this case, the division paid for the aids but did not collect income. In other cases, the staff was told by the third-party payer that the patient was covered and given the hearing aids, but later was told the bill for payment was "lost in the mail." This resulted in a need to resubmit the bill. Eventually, changing this policy ultimately reduced expenses by no longer paying for hearing aids and then finding unexpected reduced or absent payment. Further, this change increased available billable hours by eliminating the time staff members were exerting toward billing and collection. Furthermore, working conditions were improved with this change by reducing staff frustrations in dealing with third-party payers. *Finally, this change would increase income by no longer accepting the low reimbursement for the time spent with these patients.*

After another investigation of the Medical School organization, it was learned that there was a department devoted to the negotiation of third-party contracts. After a meeting with that department discussing these concerns, the problem was elevated and reduced or no reimbursement and the time the staff spent working with representatives of these third-party payers. Eventually, the existing contracts were not renewed and all future contracts that included hearing aid benefits were negotiated so that hearing aids were "carved out" if the reimbursement was found unsatisfactory. In addition, only third-party payer contracts allowing "balanced billing" were approved for hearing aid coverage. In balanced billing, the patient paid the difference between what the third-party payer paid and our charge. Typically, there were only two or three third-party payers who approved balance billing. This change significantly reduced expenses because of the unnecessary loss of income along with increased income due to improved reimbursement. *This change improved the expense and income sides of the financial ledgers.* The final step was to move the task of determining eligibility for hearing aids, and tracking payment was shifted to the billing and collection department.

It was also noticed that several staff members were ordering several models of hearing aids for the same patient. I asked about this practice and was told that by allowing the patient to experience more than one device, the patient would be in a better position to decide which was preferred. Aside from the obvious significant expenses in ordering, fitting, counseling, and returning so many devices for credit, there was the issue of "professionalism." That is, should not an audiologist be expected to know which hearing aids were or were not appropriate? This practice was discontinued because the cost in time and money was unacceptable.

As a new Director, the first P/L report from the Business Office was received. This is a very detailed spreadsheet with many rows and columns documenting the expenses and income of the division and the resulting profit or loss. As most audiologists without a business orientation, it took quite some time to learn what was included in the P/L report. It took many meetings and questions to determine that expenses attributed to Audiology in many rows were expenses that should not have been charged against Audiology. Over time and after discussions with the Business Manager, significant expense sums were removed from Audiology and shifted to physicians or other clinics within the department.

Two important lessons were learned from this experience. First, anyone responsible for directing a program must ask to receive the monthly P/L statement and take the time to understand the data in each row and column. The second lesson was to not necessarily rely on the accuracy of the data in the P/L, as it may be necessary to question the accuracy of the entries. Simply considering an expense as incorrect is insufficient; rather, it is essential to have a deep understanding of the P/L, what it means, and the data to support an argument over incorrect entries. These experiences led to the creation of divisional spreadsheets to document all of the division's expenses on daily, weekly, monthly, and annual bases. This facilitated a position of strength to argue the inaccuracies of entries on the departmental P/L. *The decision to gather and document the division's expenses helped to significantly reduce the expense side of the ledger.*

After P/Ls, for some time, it also became clear that, in some cases, income that should have been placed in the Audiology columns was inadvertently placed in some physician or other columns. These concerns were explained to the Business Manager, who would often make a change after agreeing with my assessment. *These changes improved the income side of the ledger.* Again, these examples point to the need to be vigilant and take the necessary steps to understand what is being presented in the P/L statements as well as gather and monitor the division's own data separately.

Further Efficiency Modifications for the Division of Adult Audiology at WUSM

Experience offered some opportunities to further improve the financial operation of the clinics, and with greater experience, an understanding of a better relationship with WUSM product suppliers could be obtained. Reviewing these supplier business relationships developed an understanding of the difference between *single-unit cost* versus *invoice cost* for hearing aids, earmolds,

accessories, and other supplies. Given the large volume of hearing aids the division dispensed monthly (~75 devices) and our national reputation, it seemed that the division should negotiate a bigger discount for these devices and supplies. Through many phone calls and meetings, this was accomplished, resulting in a significant reduction on the expense side of the ledger. In turn, this resulted in increased profit since the expenses for the products were lower, but our charges remained the same. *This change simultaneously improved the expense and income sides of the ledger.*

While negotiating for lower invoice costs, I also learned about and became involved with negotiations for funds from manufacturers to build the practice. These funds were placed monthly or quarterly into an account created for the division with the assistance of the Chairperson, Business Manager, and the Dean of the Medical School. This fund was created and audited quarterly by the Business Manager to be certain the funds were used only for supporting the clinic and not for personnel gain. These funds greatly enhanced the division in that the amount available over time exceeded $100,000 and was used to purchase audiological equipment, computers, and software; pay for travel to attend professional meetings; develop brochures; secure furniture; pay for consultants; and so on. *This improved the expense side of the ledger.* Over time, the use of these funds was considered unethical by manufacturers; however, when not available for use, this volume leverage was used to negotiate even greater reductions in invoice cost.

As mentioned earlier, each staff member had 22 days of paid vacation and 12 paid sick days. Unfortunately, no system was in place to track staff time off. A few observations suggested that perhaps tracking time off might be a wise solution. Another spreadsheet was created and this task was assigned to an audiologist who received an increase in salary for taking on this responsibility. From that point going forward, any request for time off was approved by this individual, and the time-off spreadsheet was monitored monthly. *This improved income by improving available billable hours.*

When dispensing medical products, many steps are involved. Specifically, all invoices contained a cost. Knowing these negotiated costs, it became easy to determine if the cost on the invoice matched this negotiated. Usually, the invoice agreed with the negotiated cost, but on occasion, the invoice cost was higher than agreed. If a discrepancy was noted, the manufacturer was contacted and the division would receive credit for the difference. This expected credit was tracked in a spreadsheet. *This decreased the expense side of the ledger.*

Another component of dispensing medical products is the return of products for credit. Initially there was no method for tracking these credits for mismatched invoices and products returned for credit to the manufacturer. Spreadsheets were created for the three clinics to document the anticipated credits and then to monitor these specific entries until the division received the credit. *This improved the expense side of the ledger.*

The Director and the supervisor of each of the three clinics kept an inventory of medical products received, signed off, and then sent to the Business Office for payment. As the product was dispensed, it was removed from the inventory. If a product was still on the spreadsheet after 60 days, the audiologist who ordered the product was contacted to determine why the product had not been dispensed. In this scenario, the secretary was contacted to schedule an appointment for dispensing of the product, or the audiologist returned the product for credit. *This new procedure improved the expense and income sides of the ledger.*

As discussed earlier, the division had contracts with two or three third-party payers who agreed to balanced billing. At the time the aids were dispensed, the patient paid a certain amount of the overall cost, and the remainder was sent to our billing and collection office to bill the third-party payer. A spreadsheet was created and an audiologist at CAM was assigned to enter the data of all transactions where payment from third-party payers was expected. Billing and collection sent a report every 30 days to that audiologist concerning which payments were received and which were still outstanding. This was important because earlier it was learned that the billing and collection office was not tracking payment. In turn, this resulted in a significant loss of income. *This was corrected by taking the described step, which improved the income side of the ledger.*

One of the biggest headaches was that many staff members provided products and services at no charge. There were many situations where not charging was appropriate, but there were many more situations where it was inappropriate or questionable. For example: For many years, our division exclusively used the bundled approach for dispensing hearing aids. In this bundled model, future visits for professional care were included in the original charge. Thus, it was appropriate for the professional component of future visits (post-dispensing) to be provided at "no charge" for the patient. There were, however, many instances where follow-up care and services for out-of-warranty hearing aids were still being provided at no charge. Not charging for those services was inappropriate, and this negatively affected the income of the division.

After many conversations with staff, it was determined that this practice was not acceptable. It negatively impacted the patient perception of Audiology and also reduced the revenue in all three clinics. While there was a slight decrease in not charging for services, this was a difficult issue to resolve and was still a concern as I left my position.

Monthly Profit and Loss Statement (P/L)

In this author's opinion, the "heart" and "brain" of managing the financial performance of the division was the profit/loss (P/L) statement delivered monthly from the Business Office (Chapter 11). At first, this P/L report was daunting. It took quite some time to better understand the data appearing in each cell (row and column). With experience, it became known that not all the data in the P/L were equally important. The P/L is simply a very detailed spreadsheet. Also, it is important to understand that P/Ls are designed differently within various organizations. Differences in design between P/Ls across institutions are primarily related to the amount of information included. Some are simpler than others, but these statements simply report all the income generated by the entity, all the expenses charged against the entity, and the resulting profit or loss. If income is greater than expense, the P/L will report a profit as well as the magnitude of the profit. If the income is less than expense, the P/L will report a loss as well as the magnitude of the loss.

Figure 24–25 illustrates an example of the WUSM P/L statement received monthly. For ease of explanation and confidentiality, the dollar amounts were deleted in most cells and simply inserted a "$" or "($)" sign. The "S" indicates the value would have been "added." The "(S)" indicates the value would have been subtracted. In the remaining cells, I inserted theoretical monetary values.

Several of the values in the "Total Column" cells to the far right represent key data used to calculate cost per hour that will be presented in the next section. Let's review this the sample P/L:

- The four **columns** represent the three clinics (Clinics A, B, and C), a column for expenses related to the research costs for the Hearing Aid Research Laboratory ("Non-Clinical"), and the sum across the rows ("Total").
- The **rows** represent numerous sources of income ("Revenue") and expenses divided in sections on "Expenses," "Allocations," and "Business Unit Allocations." The monetary values entered in the "Expenses" section were expenses for *direct costs*. The monetary values entered for "Allocations" and "Business Unit Allocations" were expenses for *indirect costs*. The sum of these three expense categories is summed to calculate "Total Dir

	Clinic A	Clinic B	Clinic C	Non-Clinical	Total
Revenue					
Gross FFS Charges	$1,770,585	$425,095	$1,409,812		$3,605,492
Discounts	(S)	(S)	(S)		(S)
Contr Adj	($464,748)	($36,022)	($204,093)		-$704,863
Net Collection FFS	S	S	S		S
less FFS Coll ps't to A R	S	S	S		S
Net Change to A R	(S)	(S)	(S)		(S)
Sales and Service	S	S	S		S
Total Revenue	S	S	S		S
Expense Alloc Credit	S	S	S		S
Total Sources	S	S	S		S
Total Rev and Sources	$1,391,676	$439,449	$1,205,000		$3,036,125
Expenses					
Faculty Salary	S	S	S		
Staff Salary	S	S	S		
Fringes	S	S	S		
Incentives	S	S	S		
Consum Supplies	S	S	S		
Prov Doubtful Accts	S	S	S		
Rental Exp	S	S	S		
Resale	$258,518	$102,676	$302,121		$663,315
Total Direct Expenses	$953,376	$319,877	$713,235	$56,913	$2,043,401
Allocations					
ACC Allocation	S	S	S		
Overhead	S	S	S		
Clinical Space to Dept	S	S	S		
Total Other Alloc	$229,914	60,222	85,435		$375,571
Business Unit Alloc					
Adm JU O and M	S	S	S		
Front End Billing	S	S	S		
School Space	S	S	S		
Allocations	S	S	S		
Registration Svc Alloc	S	S	S		
Other Clin Prac Alloc	S	S	S		
Total	$201,621	$35,163	$150,763		$387,547
Encumbrance Adj	S	S	S		(S)
Total Bus Unit Alloc	$201,621	$35,163	$150,763		S 387,547
Total Dir Exp & Alloc	$1,384,911	$415,262	$949,433	($56,913)	$ 2,806,519
Accrued Profit/Loss	S	S	S		$222,436
Cash Profit/Loss	37,612	$42,705	$302,774	($56,913)	$326,178

Figure 24–25. Monthly spreadsheet sent to staff reporting profit or loss.

Exp and Alloc" expenses near the bottom of the P/L.

■ For the "Revenue" section, various sources of income are reported on the first 10 rows for the three clinics. The row titled "Total Revenue and Sources" is the total net revenue generated by the clinics ($3,036,125). The row "Provision of Contr Adj" (–$704,863) was revenue that was lost due to "write-offs" for the various third-party payer contracts held by the Medical School. "Provision of Contr Adj" is considered to be an expense, and it will

be explained later how this value was used to calculate cost per hour. Most importantly, the data on the top row to the right report the total charges billed by the division ($3,605,492). This value represents "gross charges." As noted earlier, the bottom line of this section ("Total Revenue and Sources") reports the net income received for the division ($3,036,125). Dividing $3,036,125/$3,605,492 reports a collection rate of 84.2%. This is extremely high and reveals that for every dollar billed, the division received 84.2 cents. Collection rates for other services in the department and other specialties in the Medical School were typically closer to 50% or lower. The high collection rate of 84.2% is directly related to the large self-pay component for hearing aids provided by the staff to offset the relatively low reimbursement for diagnostic services reported above. Other less important information in this section is the total net revenue reported by each clinic. Using the same calculation described above, the collection rate for Clinic A was 78.6%, > 100% for Clinic B due to the AuD program paying an annual fee to manage the clinic, and 85.5% for Clinic C. The collection rate for Clinics B and C was higher than Clinic A because the payer mix for Clinics B and C did not include patients who were uninsured or had Medicaid because uninsured and Medicaid patients were typically scheduled to be seen by the resident clinic at Clinic A.

■ Various sources of expenses [$] are reported in the numerous rows under the sections titled "Expenses" (eight rows), "Allocations" (next three rows), and "Business Unit Allocations" (next six rows). There is one row for "Encumbrance Adj." "Expenses" were direct costs that included salaries and fringe benefits for faculty (myself) and staff (audiologists and secretaries), incentives, consumerable supplies, provision for doubtful accounts, cost for the space rented by the clinics, and resale (expenses for hearing aid related supplies). This latter expense ($663,315) will play an important role in calculating

cost/hour as will be explained below. The sum of these expenses was identified as "Total Direct Expenses" ($2,043,401). Less important information in this section are the total direct expenses reported for each clinic.

■ The next three rows ("Allocation": $375,571) and the six rows ("Business Unit Allocations": $387,547) were costs for various indirect costs. These expenses included travel, equipment, marketing, postage, web development, building maintenance, janitorial services, coffee for the kitchen, licensure, magazines in the waiting and counseling rooms, telephone, payment for e-mail addresses, long-distance access, fax line and machine, and software and software upgrades. Further, they included office equipment, purchase and maintenance of computers, laptops, monitors, printers, Electronic Medical Records, General Counsel, printing services for forms, signs, business cards, lab coats, Medical School clothing with WUSM logo for secretaries, and overhead. Also included in these costs were additional clinic space held for various departments providing service to Audiology (billing and collection, scheduling, Business Manager, etc.) and costs associated with administering the Audiology program other than by the Director (i.e., our component of the cost for the salary of the Chairperson, Business Manager and her staff, the managers and staff for billing and collection and scheduling, etc.). Other expenses included cost for IT, Human Resources, copiers, and so forth. Other less important information in this section involves total indirect expenses reported for each clinic.

■ The final row of this section reports the sum of the direct and indirect expenses for the division ($2,806,519).

■ The last two rows at the bottom report the accrued and cash profit or loss. For financial decisions and the bonuses, the department used the cash method of accounting. In this report, the "Total Cash Profit" for the division was $326,178.

Development of an Excel Spreadsheet to Calculate Cost per Hour and Charge per Hour

For over three decades, the division used a bundled approach to dispense hearing aids as did virtually every other clinic in the United States. Using this approach, the cost of the hearing aid is bundled with the professional service for one lump-sum payment. Included in this professional charge of the bundled approach in our clinics was the cost associated with the:

■ Hearing aid evaluation.
■ Taking impressions for earmolds.
■ Coupler measures of the delivered hearing aids.
■ Hearing aid fitting that ALWAYS included real ear measures to a valid prescriptive target.
■ Counseling on use and care of hearing earmolds and manufacturer app as well as any additional accessories.
■ Unaided and aided speech in noise outcome measures.
■ Follow-up care for the duration of the warranty, which could be 1 to

3 years. The follow-up care included professional services but did not include products. For example, if an out-of-warranty receiver needed to be replaced, this was charged to the patient. At the end of the warranty, the patient had the option to purchase an extended warranty to continue the services provided at the initial fit. If the patient elected not to extend the warranty, then as discussed earlier, all future care came with a charge.

This bundled model was used successfully for decades. Every year except for 2008 due to a near economic collapse in the country and 2020 (COVID-19 pandemic requiring the closing of the Medical School clinics for several months), the division was profitable.

Several years ago, there was a strong national interest in introducing PSAPs, OTC devices, and direct-to-consumer (DTC) devices (i.e., purchase on website) to address patient concerns about access to technology due to cost, accessibility, and convenience. These devices were typically less expensive than conventional hearing aids.

To address the call for lower-cost hearing aids, the division had to consider offering similar devices using an unbundled approach where the reduced charge of the device was created by dispensing devices without including many of the services offered in the bundled approach. For example, in an unbundled approach introduced in 2019, the division dispensed a basic hearing aid from a major manufacturer. This aid was purchased in bulk (i.e., 100 hearing aids) to significantly reduce our invoice cost. In the unbundled charge to the patient, the invoice cost of the aid(s) was bundled with charges for three services felt to be essential. These services included:

■ The cost for a 1-hour hearing aid evaluation.
■ A 15-minute 2cc analysis of the aids.
■ An hour slot for the hearing aid fitting using real ear measures and counseling of use and care of aids.

Using this unbundled approach significantly reduced the initial cost to the patient as they sought to obtain a quality hearing aid or hearing aids.

One of the first steps in using the unbundled approach is to very accurately calculate the cost per hour. One must then convert cost per hour to a charge per hour based on a desired profit in percent. Finally, a time analysis of all the different types of patient visits used in the hearing aid dispensing paradigm must be completed. The time analysis resulted in converting each type of patient visit into 15-minute increments. This was combined with the calculated charge per hour to create a "Menu of Services" for patients who opted to accept the unbundled approach and for patients who elected not to extend their warranty. If the calculated charge/hour was $225, for example, then visit types scheduled for 1 hour (i.e., hearing aid evaluation) would result in the patient being charged $225. If the visit type was scheduled for a half-hour, the charge was $115.

To calculate cost per hour, the audiologist needs to know:

■ Total costs associated with the operation of the division.

■ Total cost of all goods that were purchased to dispense.
■ The calculated number of billable hours when audiologists are present in the clinic to generate income.

The product of this calculation results in the cost per hour. At this point, a desired profit margin is added to create the charge per hour. Finally, a time analysis is performed to determine the amount of time set aside in the schedule to perform every patient visit type used in the hearing aid dispensing process.

In reviewing the sample P/L in Figure 24–25, it was clear that the total expenses for the division and expenses for hearing aid–related goods were included. To make the process easier and more accurate, a spreadsheet was developed to calculate cost per hour and charge per hour using a desired profit (%). These data were used to calculate the charge for the hearing aids using the unbundled approach. This also resulted in creating a "Menu of Services" for follow-up care for patients using the unbundled approach and for those electing not to extend the hearing aid warranty.

Figure 24–26 reports the spreadsheet I developed to accurately calculate the division cost/hour and then convert to charge/hour. Data are entered into this spreadsheet from key data points in the P/L:

■ *Line 1*. There were nine FTEs, resulting in 18,720 billable hours present at the start of the fiscal year (9 audiologists * 40 hour workweek * 52 weeks = 18,720 total available hours). This was used as a "starting point" to calculate billable hours for each new fiscal year. This

	2080		18,720			
Total Direct Expense			$2,043,401			
Total Oth Allocations			$375,571			
Total Business Allocations			$387,547			
Sub-Total			$2,806,519			
Resale			$663,315			
Sub-Total			$2,143,204			
Contractual Adj			$704,863			
Total Expense			$2,848,067			
Non-Billable Hours						
	Hrs/day	# days	Per Staff	# Staff	Total	
Vacation	8	22	176	9	1,584	
Holidays	8	8	64	9	576	
Sick	8	12	96	9	864	
Unrecorded	12		0	9	108	
Meetings	8	5	40	9	360	
Personal days	8	2	16	9	144	
Total					3,636	
Sub-Total Billable					15,084	
Cost/hour Non-Corrected					$188.81	

Cost/hour based on Percent Profit										
Cost/hour	10%	20%	30%	40%	50%	60%	70%	80%	90%	100%
Non-corrected	$207.70	$226.58	$245.46	$264.34	$283.22	$302.10	$320.98	$339.86	$358.75	$377.63
Cost/hour Based on Desired Profit in Dollars										
$ Profit	$50,000	$100,000	$150,000	$200,000	$250,000	$300,000	$350,000	$400,000	$450,000	$500,000
Non-corrected	$192.13	$195.44	$198.76	$202.07	$205.39	$208.70	$212.02	$215.33	$218.65	$221.96

Figure 24–26. Excel spreadsheet to calculate cost/hour and charge/hour at bottom.

value would only be meaningful if all the audiologists scheduled patients all day and had no time off. Clearly, this is not the case and will be discussed later in this section.

■ *Line 2.* I entered $2,043,401 of Total Direct Expenses from the P/L in Figure 24–25.

■ *Line 3.* I entered $375,571 of Total Other Allocation from the P/L in Figure 24–25.

■ *Line 4.* I entered $387,547 of the Total Allocations from the P/L in Figure 24–25.

■ *Line 5.* This line sums lines 2 to 4 to calculate the total expenses ($2,806,519).

■ *Line 6.* I entered the $663,315 resale expenses (hearing aid supplies) from the P/L in Figure 24–25.

■ *Line 7.* Hearing aid expenses were subtracted from total expenses to result in $2,143,204.

■ *Line 8.* I entered contractual adjustments (i.e., income lost by writing off contractual adjustments: –$704,863) from the P/L in Figure 24–25.

■ *Line 9.* Total expenses were summed from the values above ($2,848,067).

■ *The next several lines* calculated nonbillable hours due to the 22 days of vacation, 8 paid holidays, 12 sick days, 5 days for educational meetings, and 2 personal days. The sum of these for the division was 3,636 hours where the staff was not available to bill for services, leaving a total of

15,084 remaining billable hours (18,720 – 3,636).

■ When the new fiscal year began on July 1, the Director could anticipate each staff member being away from the clinic ~20% (3,636/18,720) of the time due to vacation, paid holidays, sick time, meetings, and personal days. That is equivalent to 1 day/week away from the clinic. This did not include time away from the clinic for all the scholarly opportunities discussed above as well as the number of no-shows and late cancellations.

■ Finally, $2,848,067/15,084 resulted in a cost/hour of $188.81, which was rounded to $190/hour. The numerator here represents total expense and the denominator represents number of billable hours.

A discussion about nonbillable hours is very important. The data in Figure 24–26 reflected the primary reasons for staff to be away from the clinic (vacation, holidays, sick days, days for educational meetings, and personal days). What was *not included* in the calculation for nonbillable hours included time away from the clinic for a department-wide mandatory research day, monthly Audiology grand rounds, two half-day retreats, or no-show appointments (there were 945 one year). Also not included were time away from the clinic for bereavement, maternity leave, jury duty, department and division holiday parties, required department town hall meetings, time to write reports, answering of emails and phone calls, preparing for teaching, preparing for lectures, research endeavors, writing manuscripts, calibration three times a year, obtaining normative data for new procedures, and

more. If some or all of these activities were included to calculate cost per hour, the amount would be well over $500. This amount would not be feasible to use as a base to charge for services anywhere, especially in St. Louis. So, the calculated cost per hour reported here is *very conservative* but apparently worked because the division was profitable each year. Clearly, the division would have been more profitable if we had used the greater than $500/hour charge, but that charge would far exceed any charge in the surrounding area. Patients would have quickly refrained from scheduling appointments in our clinics to be fit with hearing aids.

■ Figure 24–26 also reports data from the bottom of the spreadsheet, which takes the calculated cost/hour ($188.81) and converts this to charge/hour based on the desired profit (10%–100%). Another choice for the Director is to pick a dollar amount desired for profit at the end of the year ($50,000, $500,000, or whatever other value one may desire). At WUSM, a 20% profit seemed reasonable and this value ($226.58/charge/hour) was rounded to $225/charge/hour.

■ The next step in this process was completing a time analysis on the average time required by the staff to complete the numerous patient visit types used in the hearing aid fitting process. This was used to create a "Menu of Services" (Figure 24–27) using 15-minute increments. This was used for patients opting to pursue hearing aids using the unbundled model or for patients deciding not to renew their hearing aid warranties.

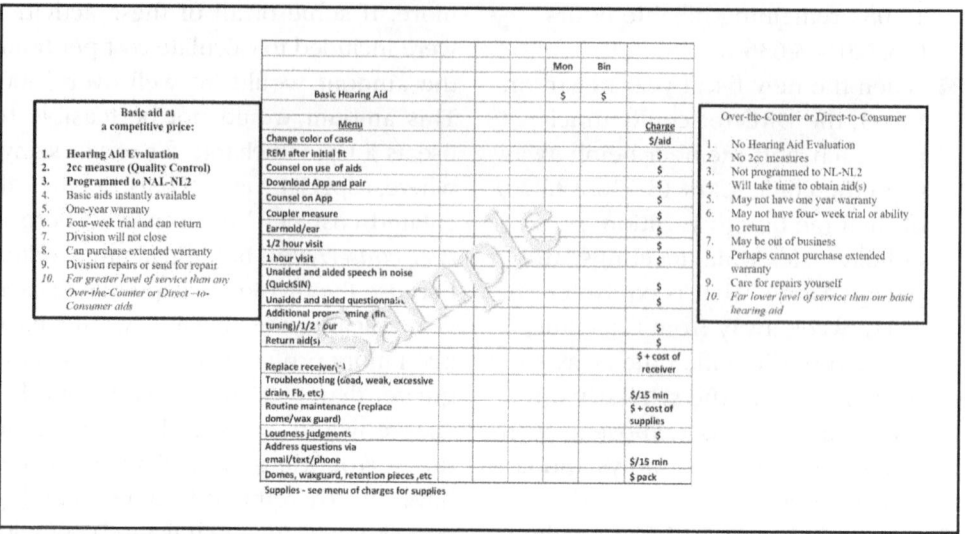

Figure 24–27. Form used to counsel on costs for unbundled purchase.

■ Also reported in Figure 24–27, the $225 charge per hour was used to calculate the charge for a monaural or binaural fit using the unbundled model by using the invoice cost of the aid(s) as the base cost. The hourly cost was then added for completing what was essential for a successful outcome. Thus, we added to the cost of the hearing aid the hourly charge per hour for a hearing aid evaluation (1 hour), 2cc analysis of aid or aids (15 minutes), and hearing aid fitting (1 hour). When the aids were dispensed via unbundling, the patient signed a form stating they understood that all future visits would be charged using the most current "Menu of Services."

■ After a significant amount of time to prepare, the division introduced this unbundled model using a basic hearing aid in 2019. Along with offering this new option, the staff created a trifold brochure inform-

ing patients of the advantages and disadvantages of the unbundled and bundled approaches. Further, the brochure delineated the advantages and disadvantages of our conventional bundled aids, the new unbundled basic hearing aid, and OTC aids purchased elsewhere. It was very interesting that in the first 8 months when patients had the choice between the more expensive bundled option and the less expensive unbundled option, only 7% of 450 fittings selected the unbundled option. Ninety-three percent preferred the bundled approach for reasons that we believed were outlined in the right and left columns of the "Menu of Services" in Figure 24–27. The left column outlines the services and advantages of our basic hearing aid at the time, using the unbundled approach. The right column outlines, in comparison to the information in the left column, what was not provided with the typical OTC/PSAP/DTC hearing aid purchased elsewhere. In many cases, the comparison outlined on this page was sufficient for patients to pursue their desire for a "less expensive alternative" within our division via the unbundled basic aid(s) rather than pursue an OT/PSAP/DTC elsewhere (such as through big-box, Costco, or direct-to-consumer websites). In most cases (93%), our patients preferred to receive the continued care of the audiologist and not, in their words, be "nickeled and dimed to death."

After these experiences, it is suggested that clinics offer unbundled *and* bundled approaches, letting the patients decide which option is a better choice for them. Retention of patients will improve and the program will grow. The finding that 93% of patients elected to purchase the more expensive hearing aids provided with professional care using the bundled approach over the significantly less expensive aids through an unbundled model bodes well for audiologists. This includes those professionals who had been feeling that the introduction of OTC aids would be the end of Audiology. At WUSM clinics, it was always viewed that OTC, PSAP, and DTC (via web) were program opportunities and not a threat.

Financial Dashboard to Manage Finances of the Division

Over the years, I developed numerous spreadsheets (see the Financial Dashboard in Figure 24–28) allowing quick monitoring of the absolute and relative (financial and other factors) productivity performance of the clinics and staff. These spreadsheets were designed to easily enter, merge, and manipulate data. Numerous decisions were made daily, monthly, or annually based on the data in these spreadsheets. In addition, decisions were based on the data tempered with "common sense" and experience. These spreadsheets served to counterbalance the accuracy of the P/L data provided by the Business Office. These spreadsheets also allowed quick communication regarding individual and site productivity and profit/loss. In gathering and analyzing the data from these spreadsheets, there was knowledge:

- Regarding reports to the Chairperson during the monthly meetings regarding adding staff, the purchase of new equipment, obtaining more space, or adding services. It is considerably easier to obtain approval for such requests if the division is profitable.
- To counterbalance the accuracy of the data generated and distributed from the Business Office via the monthly P/L statements.
- To make calculations for charges for services easier and more consistent.
- To more easily prepare the budget for the division for the next fiscal year that was due in the spring.
- To make more accurate projections of profit/loss.
- For conversations with staff members about their perceptions of how busy they were. Often some staff members thought they were busier than they actually were. A staff member would occasionally focus on the few days when they were very busy (with 10 to 12 patients) but "forget" the greater number

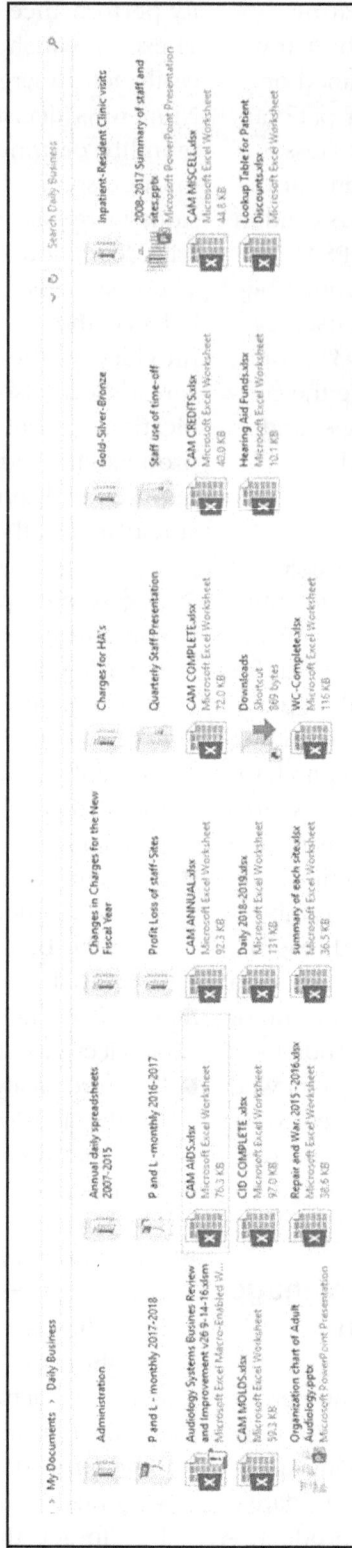

Figure 24–28. Financial dashboard.

of days when they were less busy (fewer than 6 patients) due to no-shows or late cancellations.

■ To convince the Chairperson twice to increase audiologist salaries by $10,000 each time. This was because our profit could handle this increase. This concept was also pointed out to the staff as an incentive to help with reducing costs and increasing income.

As mentioned earlier, each day I turned on my computer and saw what appears in Figure 24–28. This was my "Financial Dashboard." This dashboard contained many folders and spreadsheets that I created over time to monitor specific and general aspects of the financial activity and performance of the division. Some spreadsheets were related to specific clinical activity for all three clinics. For those spreadsheets, the data were collected by an audiologist atthe other clinic sites and sent to me. These values were merged with my spreadsheet data for CAM to create overall division data. Some spreadsheets were specific for a specific purpose.

This included data for annual evaluations and calculations for the division of the bonus. Below are some examples of what data were collected within some of these spreadsheets:

■ *Daily, weekly, and monthly performance of each site and audiologist.* Data were collected on the number of patients seen and hearing aids dispensed daily. These data were summed for each audiologist and clinic for each month. Also collected in this spreadsheet were daily "no-shows," and daily numbers were summed for the month. The spread-

sheet calculated the difference in performance for these measures for the current year versus the previous year in order to determine growth or retraction.

The data on "no-shows" were shared with the Chairperson at a monthly meeting. The large number of "no-shows" was reported to suggest implementing a policy for patients to be charged if they had not called to cancel within 24 hours of the visit. A similar policy had already been implemented by at least one specialty in the Medical School. This policy was being considered because data from other physicians and clinics within the department were reporting similar numbers of no-shows.

■ *Hearing aid invoices for each site.* These documented the patient's name and whether the invoice was for a warranty, repair, new hearing aid, accessory, or replacement for lost aid. They also documented the invoice cost and which audiologist ordered the product. The spreadsheet summed the monthly invoice cost for the aids, warranties, repairs, accessories, and assistive devices and how many aids were purchased by each audiologist for each site. This spreadsheet provided information on monthly costs for hearing aid–related invoices, and this information was merged with another spreadsheet. The clinic was able to ascertain information on the number of hearing aids ordered and then merged those data with another monthly and annual spreadsheet.

■ *Hearing aids received and pending for each site.* In this section, we listed the vendor, patient's name, audiologist, and cost information. We also documented a monthly sum of credits received. This information was merged with other monthly and annual spreadsheets in order to create running and summative tallies. There was also another spreadsheet that documented pending credits. As the credit was received, the row for that pending credit was deleted. This acted as an accurate method to track credits.

■ *Miscellaneous supplies at each site.* We were able to document supplies received (e.g., ink cartridges, response button and headset, postage, annual exhaustive calibration) and invoices. This information was summed for the month and merged with other similar monthly and annual reports.

■ *Earmolds purchased at each site.* Each row provided the name of the patient, invoice cost of earmold(s), and the patient's audiologist. This information was also summed for the month and merged with other monthly and annual reports.

■ *Annual report for each site.* Data were entered for each month and summed for the year. Entered data included fees charged for diagnostics, fees charged for hearing aids, and a sum of these two values to determine total gross monthly charges. These data were summed for the year. Also included were invoice costs for hearing aids, hearing aid credits to determine net hearing aid invoice cost, earmold costs, and miscellaneous and other hearing aid costs. All of these were also summed for the year. The final two columns calculated the total hearing aid costs (net hearing aid, earmolds, other hearing aid supplies, miscellaneous) for the month and a summation for the year. Further reported were the percentage of gross charges related to hearing aid dispensing versus performance of diagnostics.

■ *Difference in annual performance.* This spreadsheet was geared toward data described earlier for site gross charges, total number of patients seen, and hearing aids dispensed. This served to document growth or retraction for each site and for the entire division. This growth or retraction was displayed for each month and for the entire year.

■ *Summary spreadsheet.* This information was sent to the staff each month so they could view the growth or retraction of each site with respect to the previous year. This growth or retraction related to patients seen, hearing aids dispensed, and gross charges for diagnostics and hearing aids. No audiologist names were included in this report.

■ *Monthly and summed annual report.* The productivity of each staff member and site was reflected here. Included were the number of patients seen, diagnostic charges, and hearing aid charges. The monthly data were summed to yield annual results. These data were compared to the same results from the previous year to help determine growth or retraction.

■ *Calculations regarding hearing aid returns for credit (RFC).* This section summarized RFC data for each audiologist and site. Nationally, manufacturers have reported that the RFC rate has been approximately 18%. Data from the division reported a consistent RFC of ~5%. For example, if the division ordered 100 hearing aids and returned 20, the manufacturer would report a 20% RFC. Usually, the audiologist would order another hearing aid and that was dispensed. Therefore, the end result was that only 5 out of the 100 ultimately ended up in the RFC category. Thus, the total RFC was lower than the manufacturer RFC.

Documenting RFC for each staff member allowed observation of an "outlier" that a clinician that may have had a higher RFC than other staff members. When discovered, the Director would meet with that audiologist to gain a greater understanding of reasons for the RFC. In every case, the outcomes from this discussion resulted in the RFC decreasing over time. Often, the cause for these outliers was the staff member(s) providing their patients with unrealistic expectations from hearing aids. In other cases, the staff member(s) were ordering hearing aids that may not have been the best choice given the magnitude of hearing loss or preference of style desired by the patient.

In concluding this section, I often hear from colleagues and members of the audience when presenting on this topic about why I have invested so much effort in tracking financial data. This is especially the case when I received similar data from the monthly P/L. First and as mentioned earlier, there are many discrepancies reported on the P/L statement. Second, recall that the division generated $3,605,492 in charges, but at the end of the year, the division's

net profit was only $326,178. Although a profit was attained, the division generated nearly $4,000,000 in revenue and netted only slightly over $300,000. This was a bit concerning in my mind, because this allows for little "wiggle room." Thus, being vigilant in following the trail of expenses, income and productivity became essential in order to maintain profitability. Third, the P/L provides no information on absolute or relative performance of individual staff members or clinical sites. It is important to know this type of information so corrections can be made in real time and not wait until the end of the year. Fourth, the detail in documenting the performance of the division was known to the Chairperson and Business Office.

Research Responsibilities

At WUSM, research is a significant component of the institutional culture. Scholarly productivity is expected and this is part of the culture to earn promotion and job security. Over time, research would occupy a very significant part of my daily life. Meeting this research expectation at WUSM was generally achieved in two ways. One option was electing to accept a faculty position on the investigative track. The other option was electing to accept a faculty position on the clinical track. On the investigative track, faculty engaged in research full-time. These highly talented and dedicated researchers created and administered research laboratories and continually applied for grants from various federal, state, or local agencies or organizations. Some applied for grants through commercial corporations (e.g., pharmaceutical or technology companies). On the other hand, clinical track faculty engaged in research, but their primary responsibilities were patient care and/or administration.

From the beginning, I felt the clinical track was more appropriate due to my responsibilities to administer the Adult Audiology Division and provide direct patient care. Research and teaching responsibilities would come along later. Clearly, my background prior to accepting the position at WUSM did not point to the investigative track as being the appropriate option. First, my scholarly achievements prior to being recruited included only one manuscript in a low-impact peer-reviewed journal where I was the second author. I had also published five manuscripts in non-peer-reviewed journals and had 30 presentations at primarily state meetings. Second, I enjoyed patient care, the challenges of administration, and teaching. Research was not high on my list of what I wanted to accomplish.

From this meager start as a researcher outlined above, I managed in my 34 years at WUSM to present at 344 national and international conferences, author or edit 16 textbooks, and prepare 29 textbook chapters. I had 44 manuscripts accepted in peer-reviewed journals and 48 accepted in non-peer-reviewed journals. In addition, I chaired three Best Practice Guidelines for the American Academy of Audiology (AAA) and the American Speech-Language-Hearing Association (ASHA), worked on numerous national committees, and encouraged six staff members to pursue their PhD degrees through their collaboration with me in my research laboratory. As mentioned earlier, these accomplishments are not meant to be interpreted as bragging. I point these out to those readers who may be hesitant to seek a desired position, while not believing they have the skills or background to succeed. You do! In my opinion, there is more to be said for seeking and possibly failing than not seeking because of fearing failing. What follows next is how I expanded my responsibilities at WUSM to include research as a major component of my position. This process occurred gradually with the approval of the Chairperson and the understanding and assistance from the staff. For example, I started my position engaging with patients 4 days a week. As I expanded my research, these 4 days dwindled to 2 days. The patients I was scheduled to see were now scheduled with the other staff members.

My research began slowly. Initially, I was asked to collaborate with physicians who were already engaged in research and who required the need for an audiologic component. For example, physicians were engaged in research investigating the impact of several drugs on hearing or investigating the efficacy of performing ototoxic monitoring at bedside for inpatient care. I enjoyed collaborating with these physicians and learned how to develop protocols, complete the necessary forms to submit to the Institutional Review Board (IRB), create a participant Informed Consent, recruit participants, develop and enter data into spreadsheets, work with a statistician to analyze the results, develop the manuscript, and submit to a peer-reviewed journal as one of the authors. This experience improved my skills and confidence in becoming an independent researcher. These experiences whetted my appetite to become a researcher.

Over time, I now sought collaborators to join me so I could mentor them as these physicians mentored me in my early years at WUSM.

Early in my graduate education, it became apparent that the subject matter and clinical experiences that most excited me were related to hearing aid technology and the selecting and fitting of hearing aids. As described earlier, the division fit a large number of hearing aids from virtually any manufacturer. One of the manufacturers was Starkey Laboratories. At some point and for reasons I do not recall, the Director of research at Starkey Laboratories contacted me to ask if I would be interested in collaborating on researching some of their new technology. As part of the discussion, Starkey suggested helping create a Hearing Aid Research Laboratory funded by Starkey. This funding included adding a booth to our clinic dedicated to research as well as covering the salary and fringe benefits for a part-time research audiologist. I approached the Chairperson to determine the feasibility of creating such a laboratory. He, the department Business Manager, and I met with the Dean and other administrators. After many meetings, the research laboratory was approved. This began my increased role of research becoming a large part of my position.

There is an interesting sidebar concerning the booth installed by Starkey. Shortly after the booth was installed, a number of acoustical measures were completed. It was clear the internal dimensions of the booth were too small to allow for obtaining reliable sound-field measures. Our research laboratory very quickly switched to a larger booth

(1.97-m × 2.54-m × 2.73-m double-walled sound suite with volume = 14.05 m³) that was already present in our clinic and used for clinical services. This became the new home for the Hearing Aid Research Laboratory. Several years later, our division moved to the new Center for Advanced Medicine. As a result of this move, it became part of my administrative role to design new clinics. Over the course of my career, this major role in clinic design included a total of six new clinics. For this new space, a new double-walled booth was ordered and installed with the same larger internal dimensions. Soon after its installation, I contacted Mr. Larry Revit and he helped install the first R-Space sound-field system. This was a computer-controlled system allowing for a wide variety of signals and noise sources to be forwarded to an eight-loudspeaker array. This booth and the R-Space were instrumental in carrying out numerous research projects that followed.

The other part of creating the Hearing Aid Research Laboratory was the developing of the Hearing Aid Research Fund. Future funding from companies requesting our collaboration was placed in this fund. None of these funds were used for salary. Over the years, the laboratory was funded in an amount greater than $800,000. In addition, the division was allowed to keep some of the equipment used for a project after its completion. Also, the division was allowed to keep any remaining hearing aids provided for a project that participants elected not to pursue. Often, these hearing aids were provided at no charge to staff, faculty, family members of faculty, and staff. On occasion, they were provided to patients who did not have the funds to purchase hearing aids. Uniquely with this fund, there was an agreement with the Dean that the Medical School would not expect any of the income. Typically, when a faculty member receives external funding, the Medical School usually takes a significant amount to cover a wide variety of Medical School expenses to support research. I was fortunate that the Dean saw the importance of this research laboratory. I learned later that some manufacturers were hesitant or refused to fund research at several universities because of the additional cost required by universities to cover their costs for direct and indirect expenses.

Over the years, my staff and I were involved with numerous research projects with a wide variety of partners. Examples included almost all the major manufacturers of hearing aids, real ear equipment, and batteries. Some projects did not require submitting an IRB or Informed Consent because the project investigated software or other aspects of technology developed by the manufacturer. For example, our laboratory investigated differences across battery manufacturers in the buildup of rust as a result of temperature and humidity. The laboratory was often asked to investigate the ease and effectiveness of software updates or new software. Many collaborations required recruiting participants and these required submission to the Medical School Institutional Review Board along with Informed Consent. The results of many of these projects typically led to presentations at national or international conferences and publications in peer-reviewed journals.

As mentioned earlier, it is important to remind the reader that I communicated with every manufacturer-sponsored project that in order for the collaboration to move forward, the manufacturer had to understand and agree that the research staff created the protocol. Also, the manufacturer had to agree that the laboratory would submit the results for publication regardless of whether the results favored the manufacturers or did not favor the manufacturer. If the manufacturer would not agree to these requirements, then that collaboration would not move forward. For example, the laboratory engaged in a project with a manufacturer that introduced one of the first hearing aids using digital signal processing. Our results reported no significant difference in the performance between their model incorporating digital signal processing and the same model using analog signal processing. The results from this project were published.

These projects also presented opportunities for staff members and students to collaborate and participate in the entire process and to be included as authors. The reputation of the laboratory grew over time. This resulted in providing numerous opportunities for mentoring, presentations, publications in journals, and invitations to prepare textbooks and chapters. The success and positive outcomes of our laboratory also helped pave the way for my invitations to chair National Best Practice Guidelines.

Summary

My goal in preparing this chapter was to allow the reader to gain a sense of what it was like being in my shoes as I encountered some of the issues described in this chapter. I hoped to point out why administering an Audiology clinic in a Medical School was different from administering an Audiology clinic at the other clinical settings described in other chapters in this book. I wanted the reader to have a greater understanding of the challenges and opportunities that are present in a Medical School environment that may not be present in other environments.

During my tenure at Washington University, I had the honor of collaborating with two wonderful Chairpersons who supported my efforts because they saw the positive results of those efforts. There was no attempt to micromanage on their part. Of these Chairpersons, the one who stood out was Dr. Rick Chole. One day, he and I were in the clinic. I asked Rick, "How are you doing?" He responded, "I'm living the dream." I thought that was the perfect answer to describe my 34 years at Washington University directing the Adult Audiology Program. "I was living the dream."

References

American Academy of Audiology. (2006). Guidelines for the audiologic management of adult hearing impairment. http://Audiology.org/resources/documentlibrary/documents/haguidelines.pdf

ASHA Ad Hoc Committee on Hearing Aid Selection and Fitting. (1998). Guidelines for hearing aid fitting for adults. *American Journal of Audiology, 7*(1), 5–13.

Choi, J., Adams, M., Crimmins, E., Linn, F., & Ailshire, J. (2024). Association between hearing aid use and mortality in adults with hearing loss in the USA: A mortality follow-up study of a cross-sectional cohort. *Lancet Healthy Longevity, 5,* e66–e75.

Nilsson, M., Soli, S., & Sullivan, J. (1994). Development of the hearing in noise test for the measurement of speech reception thresholds in quiet and in noise. *Journal of the Acoustical Society of America, 95*(2), 1085–1099.

25 Buying and Selling Audiology Practices

Scott Myatt, MBA, MIM

Introduction: Buy, Build, or Work for Someone Else

The decision to buy a clinic, build one from scratch, or work for someone else is a very personal decision with many factors involved. Thankfully, none of these career paths are a life sentence. In fact, many audiologists change paths through their career, starting off with being an employee, then owner, then possibly back to being an employee once they sell their clinic. Most audiology clinic owners do not start or buy their clinics right after graduating. Many "fall into" ownership when the owner of the clinic decides to retire, or the ENT they worked for retired, so they decided to break off and start their own clinic.

There are many pros and cons to each of the three choices, and they vary not just between individuals but also in different stages of life. In decision-making, a "pro" to one person may be a "con" to another, and a pro in one stage of life may be a con for the same individual when they reach a different stage of life. There is a bit of overlap in pros and cons with buying and building, so an excellent place to start is with ownership versus employment.

Owning a Practice

Owning a practice has many advantages, but it is not for everyone. Particularly in the beginning stages, owning a clinic can be very stressful, as many responsibilities fall on the owner. Additionally, unless a larger practice is acquired, the amount of revenue may not allow the owner to hire the additional help they need to complement their weaknesses.

Ownership Pros

- Ability to decide location.
  - May be dictated by demographics.
  - Influenced by available opportunities.
- Operate clinic according to desires, interests.
  - Choose to do diagnostics, pediatrics, balance, etc.
- Freedom to choose teammates.
- Chart own course or destiny.
- Get to wear many hats.
  - May be the head of marketing, human resources, accounting, janitorial, etc.
- Ultimate decision-maker in the business.
- Manage people.

929

- Potential for higher earning throughout career.
- Possibility to have something to sell in the future.
- Ability to build something.
- At a certain size, the clinic can earn money without the owner being there every day.

Ownership Cons

- Be forced to wear many hats, whether or not you are good at them.
- Owning a business is not a job in that being able to go home at 5 p.m. and turn everything off is possible.
  - Many owners see patients during business hours and take care of business items like marketing after hours and on weekends.
- Managing, hiring, and firing people.
- Many audiologist owners find themselves doing less audiology than they would like to meet the demands of the business.
- Business owners feel they are not responsible only for their own home mortgages but all of their employees' mortgages as well.
- Ultimate decision-maker: The buck stops with the business owner, in both good times and bad times.
- No paid time off.

Being Employed

Employment is what most audiologists consider when entering the job market. It is the safe track where the individual can catch up on financial responsibilities such as loans and usually improve their standard of living as well as gain experience within the profession. Thus, there are also some very reasonable pros associated being employed; however, especially for seasoned veterans, there may be disenchantment with the employment situation. The following presents those positive and negatives:

Employment Pros

- Steady paycheck (possibly many compensation plans have a commission structure).
- Ability to leave work at work.
- Easier to move, relocate if needed.
- Less stress than owning the business as employees do not have the added business responsibility.
- Paid time off.

Employment Cons

- Lack of control in the direction of the clinic.
- Compensation is capped compared to an owner.
- No ability to sell the clinical operation that the employee has assisted in building.

Buying a Clinical Operation vs. Beginning a Clinic From Scratch

While there are a few uncommon routes to clinic ownership, the primary methods are buying an existing clinic or starting one from scratch. Both approaches to clinic ownership have their merits as well as their drawbacks.

Manufacturer Loan

Usually, the purchase of an audiology clinic requires the prospective owner to take out a loan. Many hearing aid manufacturers offer loans that, from a purely business and overall financial aspect, are easily the best option when compared to traditional lenders such as local banks and SBA. The interest rates and amount of down payment required by manufacturers are typically much lower than those of traditional lenders. Many manufacturers also offer the ability to pay off the loan through hearing aid purchases, so that the borrower may never make a traditional loan payment as they would to a bank. This type of loan, however, ties the borrower to that manufacturer for a specific amount of time and for a certain number of units. While manufacturers offer various specific terms, some of these loans tie the borrower to both a time commitment and a unit commitment, so even when the borrower has paid back the loan by buying the required number of units, they may still be on the hook to fulfill the time commitment. Many of these offers seem enticing, but great care must be taken to fully understand the details of what is being committed to before signing. One of the terms of many manufacturer loans is a requirement for the clinic to sell 80% or more of that manufacturer's brand of hearing aid. A typical loan period can be up to 10 years, and a lot of changes can happen in technology, market leaders, and so on in that time period. Thus, before committing to this type of a loan whether it is a hearing aid manufacturer or a buying group offering these funds, it is essential that the prospective owner have the terms interpreted by their attorney, so they fully understand their commitment. These loans also have some ethical implications and are not recommended by most audiology organizations, such as the American Speech-Language-Hearing Association or the American Academy of Audiology (Chapter 23).

Other Sources of Capital

While the majority of clinic buyers utilize loans from manufacturers, there are other options as well. Particularly for well-established clinics, SBA and other bank loans may be available. Many times, SBA loans and banks do not offer the favorable terms that manufacturers do; however, not being tied to a single manufacturer may be worth the potential added expense. Additionally, certain protected classes like minority or women-owned businesses may be able to get loans or grants with more lenient terms. Additionally, family and friend loans may work for some buyers. For lenders like this who do not need to be repaid immediately, they may be willing to accept some equity in the business as a long-term investment. Buyers considering this route should carefully consider who they want to go into business with, since a business partnership may not be as easily unwound as paying off a loan. As with other complicated legal transactions, competent legal advice should be sought. The upfront cost will certainly be worth it down the road if the partnership does not work out.

Another worthwhile avenue worth exploring is owner financing. Many audiologists do not want their clinic to "fall into" the hands of a manufacturer, and some may be adverse enough to a buyer

---

COMPARISON OF BUYING OR BUILDING A PRACTICE

■ Comparisons of buying a clinic versus building a clinic: Be advised that most manufacturers do not provide loans to new clinics as they do not have a proven track record.

■ One of the benefits of a clinic purchase rather than starting from scratch is that there is an existing database of patients who will likely continue doing business with the new owner during the first week of operations.

■ Starting a clinic and, by extension, a patient database can be daunting, potentially expensive, and time-consuming exercise.

■ The purchase of an existing clinic usually includes a group of referral sources that will typically continue to refer patients.

■ When starting a new clinic, the owner may need to spend a significant amount of time and energy in front of physicians and others who could become good referral sources.

■ By acquiring a clinic, that clinic's reputation is also being taken over, which can be good or bad. This reputation has been built through years of customer service, clinic practices, marketing, community involvement, and so on. If this reputation is good, care must be taken to ensure its continuity. If bad, careful consideration should be given prior to acquiring the practice and whether the new owner is up to the task of turning it around.

■ Starting a clinic from scratch typically costs much less than a fully functioning practice.

■ Starting a clinic from scratch allows the owner to create their own kind of reputation.

---

taking out a loan from a manufacturer that they would be willing to finance the transaction, or at least a portion of it. This can be structured as regular payments as a loan would be, or as a portion of the profits of the clinic each year. Another possibility is the buyer inserting into the clinic over time, with seat equity, cash, or a combination. Many owners are passionate about their legacy continuing, and having them as a partner can help ensure their legacy remains. In the same sense, many buyers would prefer to have the clinic, and legacy, be theirs to manage and control, so this type of structure is not for everyone.

Valuing an Audiology Practice

The value of an audiology practice is primarily determined by the amount of money or economic benefit the owner receives because they own the practice.

Part of the economic benefit owners obtain from a business is their salary, and another benefit is the reduction of their personal income by allowing the practice to pay some expenses that can be used as business expenses. Thus, the owner obtains these benefits, but the new owner may or may not use these same benefits, so before the practice can be accurately appraised, these benefits to the old owner must be accounted for and are often called *addbacks* or *normalization adjustments*.

Addback/Normalization Adjustments

The value of an audiology practice is primarily determined by the amount of money or economic benefit the owner receives because they own the practice. Many owners decide to write off certain perks to reduce their tax liabilities. Such perks should be added back to the earnings to determine the actual economic benefit a new owner may receive if they were to acquire the business. These are often referred to as *addbacks or normalization adjustments* and typically include such expenses as:

- Family cell phone plans.
- Additional retirement plan contributions that are above what is offered to employees.
- Personal automobile expenses.
- Country club dues.
- Personal travel.
- Family members who are paid above or below a market rate.
- Rents or leases that are above or below a market rate that would apply to a new owner (i.e., if the building is also owned by the business owner, but they charge themselves a nonmarket rent amount for tax purposes).
- Home office expenses.
- Other personal/business expenses.

It should be noted that not all of these increase the earnings of the business. The goal, however, is to present these addbacks to the prospective owner to enable them to determine the true economic benefit of owning the practice. As long as the owner's salary is within market range, it should not be added back. The amount above or below a market wage should be adjusted out of the earnings.

If the owner is not working in the business but is still taking a salary, this should be added back into the earnings. If the working owner of an audiology clinic makes a total of $100,000 (both salary and earnings), a reasonable wage for the owner, say $85,000, should be deducted from the earnings, bringing the business earnings down to $15,000. Assuming the owner is working in the business, their salary must be considered; otherwise, the business will likely be overvalued. In the example above, if an investor were to buy the business and they need to hire a replacement audiologist for the former owner (using the same $85,000/year salary), they would only receive $15,000 per year in earnings for that clinic. An audiologist considering buying the same clinic as an owner-operator would likely be turning down opportunities to work (as an employee) for other clinics for the same salary. Because of this, the incremental amount of money (in this case, $15,000) is what should be considered as the economic benefit of owning the clinic. There are, of course, intrinsic values to owning a clinic (being boss, controlling the future a bit more, the ability to grow, etc.); however, because they are intrinsic, only the buyer can determine their value to them personally.

A simple, real-life example may help illustrate this concept. A recently graduated AuD was considering two options: buying a small clinic where the clinic profit would be $100,000 per year or working at an established clinic as an employee making a salary of $85,000 per year. The clinic owner thought $450,000 was a fair asking price; after all, the new owner would be making $100,000 per year. The owner failed to consider the new owner/AuD would only be making $15,000 per year over what he could make as an employee elsewhere. Not considering interest, it would take 30 years of paying the difference ($15,000) to make up the $450,000 purchase price. Fortunately, the AuD realized this and did not buy the clinic.

Reviewing Financial Data

In the evaluation of the clinic's financials, there are ledger items that should not be taken into account after appropriate adjustments have been made to the earnings. Interest and taxes should be removed because they may be unique to that owner's situation and not apply to a new owner. Additionally, depreciation and amortization should be removed because they are noncash items included in the expenses for tax purposes and will most likely change when ownership changes.

The resulting number is the earnings before taxes, interest, depreciation, and amortization (EBITDA). The adjustments are applied to the EBITDA, resulting in a number that should be what a new owner could reasonably expect to earn

by owning the company and is often called "adjusted EBITDA." This is not an official tax or accounting term but is used frequently when selling, buying, or valuing a company. After determining the adjusted EBITDA, the most common method of valuing a company is to apply a multiple to it.

Assigning a Multiple

Simply stated, the multiple is a numerical reflection of the target company's attractiveness or desirability. While the adjusted EBITDA number should be objective, the multiple applied is subjective and can vary from buyer to buyer. Multiples are computed on the EBITDA and can range from 2 on the very low side to 5 on the higher side. Occasionally, very large, well-run clinics can demand a higher multiple due to both their scarcity and the fact that the buyer may want to leverage it into a platform for future growth. Such high-earning clinics may sell for a higher multiple, often reaching 7-10.

Factors That Control the Multiple

Many factors determine what multiple should be applied, some of which can be controlled by the owner while others cannot, particularly in the short term. Some of these factors include:

- Location.
  - Desirable state and city.
  - Desirable area within the city.
  - Easy to find.
  - Parking.

- If it is a medical practice, is it in a medical park or near potential referral sources?
- If it is a more retail-leaning practice, is it in an area with a lot of foot traffic?
- Competition in the area.
- Longevity.
- Employee longevity and turnover.
- Patient database.
- Look and feel of the clinic.
- Number of patients in the database.
- Number of employees.
  - Too few?
  - Too many?
- Number of providers and the amount of revenue they generate.
  - If only one or two providers bring in the majority of the revenue and one were to leave, it represents considerable risk.
- Referral sources.
  - Number of referral sources.
  - Variety of referral sources.
  - Reason they refer (do they refer to the clinic or just to the owner?).
  - Relationships with referral partners.
- Local reputation.
- Branding (is the brand built solely on the owner?).
- Consistency in revenue and earnings.
  - Sudden growth in revenue or earnings often means the owner is propping it up for a sale.
  - Steady growth.
- Number of locations.
- Revenue.
  - Clinics with higher revenues are more attractive and harder to find, so they typically command a higher multiple.
  - Greater competition among buyers for larger clinics also drives the multiple higher.

- The market for clinics in general.
  - The more buyers in a market, the more competitive it becomes, potentially driving the multiple up (seller's market).
  - Fewer buyers equal less competition, so buyers can pay lower multiples (buyer's market).

One of the most critical factors in determining an appropriate multiple is the risk associated with acquiring and owning the clinic. Risk and multiples have an inverse relationship: The higher the perceived risk, the lower the multiple, and vice versa.

Owner Risk

Creating a highly valued clinic means alleviating as much risk as possible. Much of the risk in a clinic is seen when too much of the revenue is generated by one individual, often the owner. In preparing for an eventual exit, the owner should do what they can to spread the revenue generation between multiple providers, lessening the risk of a substantial drop in revenue if one were to leave. Particularly with smaller clinics, this is often easier said than done. By the time they go to sell, wise business owners have minimized their contributions to revenue, making their practices truly turnkey.

There are a couple of methods used by buyers to hedge against risk: lowering the price and/or requiring the owner to stay on, typically with an earnout. An earnout is when a sizable part of the purchase price is earned over time. With growth goals established, the former owner has to "earn" the remaining payout. Neither a price decrease nor an earnout are the best scenarios for the seller, so owners should do all they can to address these concerns before selling.

Customer Concentration Risk

While not as common among audiology practices as many other businesses, there is some concentration risk with some clinics. This is typically seen when a clinic relies heavily on relatively few referral sources or gets a high percentage of its revenue from one source, like the VA. As much as possible, referrals should come to the clinic and not necessarily to the owner or an individual audiologist. In one extreme case, a buyer walked away from buying a clinic when they learned that 90% of the referrals and 60% of the revenue came from one ENT, who happened to be retiring within a few months and was the spouse of the office manager.

Third-Party Sales

The rise of third-party providers, or reverse networks, has been somewhat of a puzzle in the audiology industry. These companies send patients to audiology or hearing aid clinics to be fitted with aids that the patient already purchased. Utilizing these companies too much has a detrimental effect on valuations. Because manufacturers cannot dictate what hearing aids are used by these companies, they discount that amount from the revenue when valuing clinics. This holds true not only when they are considering acquiring a clinic but also when they are looking at loaning money to a buyer for a clinic. Many manufacturers will loan against the number of units that are available to convert to their brand. Historically, manufacturers have been some of the most aggressive and highest-paying buyers of audiology and hearing aid clinics. Many assume this is because they simply have deeper pockets and, while true, does not consider the whole picture. An individual buying a clinic can expect to make the adjusted EBITDA once they own the clinic. A manufacturer makes the same adjusted EBITDA, but they also make money by selling the clinic hearing aids, making a wholesale margin as well. Even if their pockets were not deeper, they make more money from owning a clinic than individuals. Applying a multiple to the adjusted EBITDA results in a clinic's price or valuation; however, terms must also be considered when evaluating offers.

Valuation Reports

There are many different reasons for obtaining a valuation of an audiology clinic; however, a written valuation report is rarely needed if the purpose is buying or selling a clinic. Detailed valuation reports can be expensive and can take a significant amount of time and work on the owner's part to prepare. For the purposes of selling or buying a clinic, a fair market value is used. The IRS (2024) defines *fair market value* as "the price that property would sell for on the open market. It is the price that would be agreed on between a willing buyer and a willing seller, with neither being required to act, and both having a reasonable knowledge of the relevant facts."

A good valuation report by someone with knowledge of the industry may be able to approximate a clinic's market value; however, a valuation report is somewhat of an educated guess, as the buyer and seller are hypothetical. The true test of a valuation is whether the owner would sell for the amount in the valuation report and if there were a buyer who would buy for that amount. Additionally, a valuation can be a single number or range but does not consider the terms of the transaction. In reality, a buyer may accept the value of a clinic, but only at a particular set of terms, which may not be acceptable to the seller, even though the owner accepted the value in the report. For example, both sides could agree upon a value of $1 million; however, the buyer would like to pay this over 5 years in a deferred or earnout structure, whereas the seller would like to receive 100% at close.

When Is a Valuation Report Required

Despite the shortcomings of a valuation report for the purposes of selling or buying, valuations have an essential role in many cases. The following are examples of when a valuation report is needed:

- A partnership dispute, particularly when one is buying out the other, and a value needs to be established.
- A divorce, when marital asset values are being determined in order to divide them.
- Creating an employee stock ownership plan, or ESOP.
- Bringing on a new partner or associate who will be buying into the clinic.
- Creating buy-sell agreements.
- Bankruptcy proceedings.
- Litigation for economic damages.
- Certain financing situations.

Particularly when there is a possibility of the need to defend a valuation report (i.e., in court or to the IRS), it is essential to find a highly qualified (and credentialed) valuation expert, preferably with experience valuing audiology practices. A valuation expert may have performed hundreds of valuations in other industries, but there are specific nuances to valuations in every industry, and audiology certainly has many nuances that are not present in other sectors and even within other healthcare businesses. One such nuance is the role that manufacturers play, both as a buyer of clinics and as a financier for private buyers. Valuation experts often rely on published market data to help establish a valuation. Other valuation experts and business brokers frequently provide these data points in exchange for access to the data provided by others. Historically, most transactions in audiology have not used brokers but have been negotiated directly between the seller and the buyer, whether that buyer be a manufacturer, consolidator, employee, owner operator, or private equity firm. Neither the buyer or the seller have an incentive to report these details of the transaction, so there is not a lot of information on past deals that is publicly available.

Buying or Selling a Clinic

One of the biggest questions when considering selling a clinic is when the best time is to sell. The best time to sell a clinic is *"when there is NO NEED to sell."* Being forced to sell a clinic for health concerns, relocating, death, or other reasons may be necessary at times, but it should be avoided when possible.

Sellers who are being forced to sell do not typically have adequate time to prepare both themselves and the business for the best buyer. They are often forced to take the first offer, which may not be the best terms, price, or buyer for their clinic, or to continue their legacy. Being forced to sell often leads to a sale of desperation.

Having established the best time not to sell (when there is a *NEED* to sell), the question remains about the best time to sell. This is a highly personal decision involving personal, career, and family goals. Sometimes offers or opportunities appear out of the blue, such as an unsolicited offer. These offers notwithstanding, careful planning for a sale or exit can be very beneficial. For a clinic owner who is still actively involved in the clinic, particularly with patient care, the ideal time to start the process of selling is 3 to 5 years before they would like to retire or exit from the practice fully. This allows for adequate time to prepare the clinic, put it on the market, find an ideal buyer, go through the selling process, and then provide adequate transition time for the new owner. Depending on the terms of the deal, the buyer may ask the owner to stay on for several months or years to assist in the transition process. Usually, this much lead time is not possible, and a successful transition can certainly happen in a much shorter time frame; however, a long time frame will result in a more successful transition to the new owner.

Preparing

The best planning for an exit starts before opening the clinic; however, as the Chinese proverb states, "The best time to plant a tree was 20 years ago. The second-best time is now." The best way to prepare for an eventual exit is by utilizing best practices throughout the clinic, from best patient care to best accounting practices. Well-run businesses are highly sought after and, therefore, much more sellable than businesses that require a lot of work to make them efficient and best in class. Best-in-class clinics sell for much higher multiples than those seen as turnaround projects.

As any business owner can testify, one of the best reasons to have a business is for the tax write-offs. This is not necessarily the case when it comes to selling the business as these write-offs typically decrease the amount of profit on paper, thereby reducing the potential tax liability for the owner. These personal perks or write-offs should be accounted for when preparing for a sale. Otherwise, the true economic value of the clinic will likely not be realized. Excessive add-backs or normalization adjustments lead to a certain amount of doubt about what is real and should be accepted by the buyer versus not considered in the final valuation.

Many buyers feel the owners received the reward of the personal write-offs while they owned the business and should not then benefit again by being able to add them back into the profits to get a higher valuation. Most buyers, however, do expect a certain number of adjustments for personal expenses, so long as they are not excessive or cross into gray areas ethically. Unscrupulous (and, in some cases, fraudulent) clinic owners have written off such things as their seasonal box seats at sporting events because they occasionally take patients, home mortgages because they have a home office, trips for board meetings when the only other board member is a spouse, and so on. When buyers see such excessive personal expenses, it causes them to doubt the integrity of the seller and if there may be other things to doubt about the business and, therefore, the transaction. In these cases, the seller is asking the buyer to trust them in how dishonest they have been.

To Whom Should the Clinic Be Sold?

There are a few options available when considering a potential buyer. Different factors, such as the size of the practice, location, type of practice, and so on, may limit the number of potential buyers, but overall, most clinics are sold to manufacturers, consolidators, or individuals, including employees.

Manufacturers

Historically, manufacturers have been the most prolific buyers; however, each seems to experience periods of aggressive acquisition and withdrawal. Many acquire under their own retail brands and try to have somewhat of a wall between their retail operations and their wholesale operations. There are pros and cons of selling to a manufacturer, with the most significant pro typically being the price offered. Not only do they have deeper pockets than other buyers, but they also make more money from each acquisition since they get both the wholesale and retail margin. One of the downsides to selling to a manufacturer is that they will often require the clinic to sell up to 90% of their brand of product. It is not a major concern if

the clinic is already selling that brand, but challenges may arise for those clinics that do not have experience selling that particular brand. Many audiologists also feel there are ethical dilemmas in selling to a manufacturer as they feel their employees and patients may not receive the same level of care under a manufacturer's ownership. Stories abound about clinics that were sold to a manufacturer that "ran it into the ground," but these stories abound in part for the same reason that negative news stories seem to be more prevalent. Stories about clinics that were acquired and then successfully run by manufacturers do not garner the same level of interest, even though there are many more of them than the failures. Manufacturers often have "well-oiled machines" running the acquisition and transition process, and they can often do it more efficiently than others due to the number of transactions they have completed. Some manufacturers rebrand the clinics and try to have a uniform look and feel to all of their clinics, while others try to keep the look and feel the previous owner established.

Consolidators

Consolidators are typically individuals or groups that buy multiple practices to put together a group of practices to sell to a manufacturer or private equity group. Because they intend to eventually "flip" these clinics to a larger buyer and because of the cost of rebranding involved, many consolidators will not rebrand the clinics into a single, unified brand. There have been some exceptions to this rule, however. Consolidators often rely on loans from manufacturers to acquire the clinics, so the clinics they acquire are often required to sell most of their hearing aids from the manufacturer who provided the funding. Because they do not intend to be providers themselves, many times their terms include some ongoing involvement by the previous owners, particularly if the owners were actively seeing patients. Like manufacturers, most consolidators have been through the process of buying an audiology clinic, so they likely have a methodology they employ for both the acquisition process as well as the transition after closing.

Individuals

Many audiologists prefer to sell to individuals, either existing employees or audiologists who will take their place in running the practice and seeing patients. While this is ideal for many, finding individuals who can acquire a practice can often be tricky. Unless the buyer is known to the owner, it can mean placing an ad online or other similar avenues to get the word out that the clinic is for sale. This can be somewhat risky in that the wrong people or groups will likely find out. This can include the employees, competition, and patients of the clinic. Individuals may not have acquired a practice before and may not know exactly the steps needed to complete the process. There is a high probability they will also need financing and will likely look to a manufacturer for this. Individuals are likely to not pay as much because their pockets are not as deep as a manufacturer, will only have the profit of the clinic, and will also likely be paying toward a loan to finance the purchase of the clinic. The upside is that they may be in a better

position to be able to carry on the legacy of the previous owner.

The Process

The first step an owner should take when considering a sale is to assemble a team of trusted advisors and let them know the plans to put the clinic on the market. This team should include an attorney and an accountant at the bare minimum. The best accountant may be the one the clinic is currently using as they will have a good understanding of the financial history of the clinic. Generally speaking, CPAs have the accounting and tax knowledge needed for the selling of a business. Lawyers, on the other hand, are much more specialized, and an attorney with experience in the buying and selling of businesses should be sought out. Deals can fall apart due to poor choices in attorneys. Too many business owners utilize attorneys because they are friends or family, thinking they will save money or that any attorney will suffice. Generally speaking, many times, attorneys who specialize in litigation, divorce, criminal defense, and bankruptcy are likely very good at what they do; however, they may not be the best choice for business transactions. Owners may also choose to utilize an experienced mergers and acquisitions advisor or business broker as well. Ideally, if the general manager or office manager can be trusted to keep everything confidential, bringing such an individual into the discussions will reduce the burden of the business owner. This is particularly true if the owner is carrying a full patient load.

Throughout the entire process, the owner's primary goal should be running the business as usual and keeping the revenues steady. The owner should continue running the business and making the same decisions as they would if they were not selling the business. Many owners get tied up in the sale process, and the revenue declines. When it comes time to finalize the purchase, the buyer may discount the price if revenues have declined significantly, or if the sale of the business does not go through for whatever reason, the owner then will be forced to revive their own business. When a close looks imminent, certain decisions with long-term potential ramifications (hiring, changes or extensions to leases, etc.) should be discussed with the buyer; however, as long as the business is owned by the seller, the decisions are to be made by them.

On paper, the process of selling a clinic is not unlike the process of selling a house. In practice, it is much more complicated. Additionally, the seller often also has full-time (or more) responsibilities of running the clinic they are trying to sell. Many chose to enlist the help of a broker or investment banker. Care should be taken to hire an advisor who has experience in selling audiology clinics because there are specific nuances to selling audiology clinics, such as the role of third parties, the role manufacturers play in financing, the current active buyers—the list goes on.

Whether or not an owner decides to use an advisor or broker, the first step is getting the necessary documents available to provide to a potential buyer. At the bare minimum, most buyers are going to request 3 years of financial statements, the types of hearing aids (and technology levels) sold, a breakdown of the manufacturers used, and the breakdown of revenue by type or category (for example, hearing aids, diagnostic

testing, services, third party, etc.). This information should not be provided to any potential buyer without both sides signing a mutual nondisclosure statement, or NDA as it is commonly referred to. While not failproof, an NDA should give a reasonable level of comfort that neither party will disclose information exchanged to other parties. Once this has been signed by both sides, the above information is commonly provided to the potential buyer. There is a fine line between too much information and not enough information prior to receiving an offer, and the seller should not provide information that could potentially be used to compete against them, like the names and salaries of their employees. Until the seller gives specific permission, the buyers should not be allowed to speak with employees. This usually does not happen until much later in the process.

Letters of Intent

Offers are typically called letters of intent (often abbreviated to LOI) and contain specific elements such as the price, payment terms, timing for the close, general expectations or requests for a transition, or post-close employment of the owner and exclusivity period. Payment terms generally contain the percentage or amount paid at close and any amounts to be paid after closing. These can be in the form of deferred payments or earnouts.

The majority of LOIs will contain an exclusivity clause, wherein the owner of the clinic cannot negotiate with other potential buyers, or entertain other offers, once signed. This is to be expected, as a potential buyer will make considerable investments in time and money in preparing to acquire the clinic and does not want to be undercut at the last moment because the owner is dealing with more than one suitor at a time. For this reason, owners should make sure the buyer is one they are comfortable with, and the LOI is one they can live with. Good letters of intent form the backbone of the purchase agreement, so the owner should get the advice of an attorney prior to signing. It is not uncommon for the letter of intent to go through a couple of versions, as both buyer and seller negotiate the details.

Asset vs. Stock

Another key element of a letter of intent will be to outline whether the transaction will be an asset deal or a stock deal. Most transactions in audiology are structured as asset deals. In an asset deal, the buyer only buys certain company assets. These assets include tangible assets like equipment and inventory but also include intangible assets such as goodwill and the company's name. It does not include any company liabilities, nor do tax ID numbers and NPI numbers transfer. In a stock deal, the buyer buys the entire company, including the liabilities (both known and unknown). One real-life example of an unknown liability was when, a few months after the transaction closed, the family of a patient sued the clinic for wrongful death. Unbeknownst to either the seller or the buyer, the patient fell on the sidewalk in front of the clinic, breaking her ankle. She later passed away from an infection she caught in the hospital. In an asset deal, the former owner would be on the hook, but in a stock deal, because the buyer bought the stock, which includes both known and unknown liabilities, they

would be on the hook, even though it happened before they purchased the clinic.

There are many tax implications to both types of transactions, and competent legal, accounting, and tax advice should be sought prior to deciding on either an asset or a stock deal. In general, sellers prefer stock deals and buyers prefer asset deals. Some flexibility is advisable though, as many buyers will refuse to do a stock deal.

Due Diligence

Once an offer is accepted by both parties, the *due diligence* period begins. Due diligence is the process of thoroughly evaluating a business before a sale or purchase. It is designed to identify any potential risks or issues that may impact the value of the business and to provide transparency to the buyer. At the outset of due diligence, the buyers will produce a list of questions and document requests to the owners. These are very in-depth, and many times, the answers (or documents) may lead to further queries. The buyers are about to spend a lot of money to purchase a business, so their goal is to make sure the business is in the expected shape. If they find anything they do not like, they can either walk away or renegotiate the offer. In this regard, it is like a home inspection—if the inspector finds a faulty water heater, they can ask to have it replaced, walk away from the deal, or ask for a price concession. Typical things an audiology practice buyer will request during due diligence include:

- Prior year tax statements.
- Bank statements.
- Copies of leases.

- Agreements with manufacturers.
- List of referring physicians.
- Advertisements.
- Human resource information.
  - List of employees, past and present.
  - Health and other benefits.
  - Salaries.
  - Tenures.
  - Handbooks.
- Copies of certificates to do business, licenses, etc.
- Manufacturer invoices.
- Pricing lists.
- Questions about lawsuits, patient complaints, etc.
- List or phone and fax numbers, emails, URLs.
- List of utility providers.
- Samples of forms or documents the clinic uses, particularly with patients.
- Business records.
- Access to patient files.
- Operating handbooks or procedure manuals.

Rather than emailing the documents back and forth, a secure online data room should be utilized, to which both buyer and seller (and their representatives) have access.

If the buyer does find out negative information during the due diligence process, they are well within their rights to either renegotiate the price and terms or walk away. Discounting the price is sometimes referred to as a "haircut." If the owners have been upfront and honest in everything prior to due diligence, the buyers should not uncover anything in due diligence that would cause them to renegotiate.

One of the most common reasons to renegotiate the purchase price is because the revenue has dropped since the conversations began. One owner decided to stop marketing as she was selling anyway and didn't want to spend the extra money. Subsequently, the revenue of the clinic dropped, and the buyer reduced the price by 25%. This haircut was more than the owner saved by not continuing her marketing efforts.

The process of selling a business can be a full-time job that can distract the owner from their other full-time job(s) as the owner of the clinic. The number one job of the owner, throughout the entire process, should be to keep the revenue at the same level as it was when it was originally presented to the buyer. Owners need to run the business as if they were not selling. Putting together an effective team can take a lot of the work from the owner to let them focus on continuing to run the business.

The Purchase Agreement

In the latter half of the due diligence period, the buyer's attorney will begin the preparation of the purchase agreement. These are typically called APA (asset purchase agreement) or SPA (stock purchase agreement) and can range in length from 30 to 60 or more pages. The document will be based on the agreed-upon letter of intent, expounding its points in detail. They typically contain references to, and perhaps place holders for, various schedules and exhibits. The seller or the seller's attorney must prepare many of these and may include such items as the leases, lists of assets, accounts receivable, bill of sale, employment agreement for the seller, and so on. Some, like the accounts receivable list, must be prepared immediately before closing; otherwise, they do not convey timely information. Much of the schedules and exhibits information will likely be contained in the due diligence information; however, because the seller guarantees the information, they should be prepared by the seller.

While their legality is currently being contested, particularly for healthcare providers, sellers should expect to receive a covenant not to compete in the purchase agreement. This makes sense in that a buyer does not want to have a seller compete with them after buying their clinic, likely taking all the clinic's former patients with them. The noncompete terms should not be overly burdensome, either in time or geography. If the owner plans to continue working in the industry, care should be taken to specify what is allowable. Performing pediatric screenings at a hospital may not compete with a hearing aid–focused clinic, but doing diagnostic testing for an ENT selling hearing aids would.

It is not uncommon for the purchase agreement to undergo multiple iterations as it is exchanged between the attorneys for each side. This is when the value of an attorney with deal-making experience makes a big difference. These types of attorneys are more focused on making the deal work while protecting their clients than those who are just out to cause the other side pain.

Once the purchase agreement is far enough along for both sides to eliminate potential dealbreakers, the buyer will likely insist on meeting with the staff.

Employees

Prior to meeting with the buyer, the owner should adequately prepare the staff by letting them know what is happening. The buyer will often meet with the staff individually and deliver offer letters and benefit packages. These meetings are typically a week or two prior to close. There needs to be enough time for the staff to ask questions and voice their concerns. The buyer usually wants these meetings sooner rather than later; however, the owners typically want to delay these meetings until close enough to the close that the deal will likely close. Both sides share in the risk—the sellers do not want to upset their employees to the point that they leave prior to close, causing the buyer to pull back, and the buyers want to be able to assess the staff with enough time to pull out or plan for changes. In no case should the buyer be allowed to speak with the staff before the seller is ready and has given permission. Sometimes employees will see the change as a time to ask for large raises or other changes. They can hold a deal hostage if they do this, threatening to leave if their demands are not met. Most buyers will continue with their current compensation and benefits packages; however, large pay increases rarely happen, as the buyer is buying the business with the existing financials. If large pay increases are added in, the business doesn't produce the same earnings and will, therefore, be worth less than what was offered.

Closing Remarks

Once all the documents are in place, including the schedules and exhibits, signature pages are signed and exchanged, and the money is wired to the seller's bank. In an asset deal, the buyer is not buying the contracts with the employees, so the seller typically terminates their employment, and they enter into new employment contracts with the buyer. The same holds true for the lease, although many landlords will allow an assignment of a lease, rather than creating a new one.

Once the documents have been signed and money wired, the transaction is considered "closed," and the business now belongs to the buyer, or new owner. As painful as it may be for the former owner, the new owner is now free to do what they choose with the business. Many times, buyers promise not to make any changes; however, changes will inevitably be made. Wise buyers hold off on making dramatic changes all at once, but many times certain changes need to be made immediately. One such example may be product choice, particularly if the buyer obtained financing from a manufacturer that the clinic did not use prior to close. Other comments on buying and selling practices are presented in Chapter 2.

Reference

IRS. (2024). IRS Publication 561 (01/2023). https://www.irs.gov/publications/p561 #en_US_202312_publink1000257933

Index